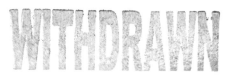

HANDBOOK OF

Medical Imaging

Volume 1. Physics and Psychophysics

Editorial Board

The cover illustration shows views of a knee obtained after trauma in which the conventional x-ray images show only minimal abnormality of the bone while the MRI shows more extensive injury to the bone and ligaments. See Chapter 12, p. 671, Effects of Anatomical Structure on Signal Detection, Ehsan Samei, William Eyler and Lisa Baron.

HANDBOOK OF
Medical Imaging

Volume 1. Physics and Psychophysics

Jacob Beutel
Harold L. Kundel
Richard L. Van Metter

Editors

SPIE PRESS

A Publication of SPIE—The International Society for Optical Engineering
Bellingham, Washington USA

Library of Congress Cataloging-in-Publication Data

Handbook of medical imaging / [edited by] Jacob Beutel, Harold L. Kundel,
    and Richard L. Van Metter.
        p. cm.
    Includes bibliographical references and index.
    Contents: v. 1. Progress in medical physics and psychophysics.
    ISBN 0-8194-3621-6 (hardcover: alk. paper)
    1. Diagnostic imaging—Handbooks, manuals, etc. 2. Imaging systems in
    medicine—Handbooks, manuals, etc. I. Beutel, Jacob. II. Kundel, Harold L.
    III. Van Metter, Richard L.
    [DNLM: 1. Diagnostic Imaging—Handbooks. 2. Health Physics—Handbooks.
    3. Image Processing, Computer-Assisted—Handbooks. 4. Psychophysics—
    Handbooks. 5. Technology, Radiologic—Handbooks. WN 39 H2363 2000]
    RC78.7.D53 H36 2000
    616.07'54—dc21   99-054487
                                                                                CIP

Published by

SPIE—The International Society for Optical Engineering
P.O. Box 10
Bellingham, Washington 98227-0010
Phone: 360/676-3290
Fax: 360/647-1445
Email: spie@spie.org
WWW: http://www.spie.org/

Printed in the United States of America.

Contents

Chapter 10. A Practical Guide to Model Observers for Visual Detection in Synthetic and Natural Noisy Images / 593

Miguel P. Eckstein, Craig K. Abbey and François O. Bochud

Chapter 11. Modeling Visual Detection Tasks in Correlated Image Noise with Linear Model Observers / 629

Craig K. Abbey, François O. Bochud

Chapter 12. Effects of Anatomical Structure on Signal Detection / 655

Ehsan Samei, William Eyler, Lisa Baron

Chapter 13. Synthesizing Anatomical Images for Image Understanding / 683

Jannick P. Rolland

x   Contents

Preface

During the last few decades of the twentieth century, partly in concert with the increasing availability of relatively inexpensive computational resources, medical imaging technology, which had for nearly 80 years been almost exclusively concerned with conventional film/screen x-ray imaging, experienced the development and commercialization of a plethora of new imaging technologies. Computed tomography, MRI imaging, digital subtraction angiography, Doppler ultrasound imaging, and various imaging techniques based on nuclear emission (PET, SPECT, etc.) have all been valuable additions to the radiologist's arsenal of imaging tools toward ever more reliable detection and diagnosis of disease. More recently, conventional x-ray imaging technology itself is being challenged by the emerging possibilities offered by flat panel x-ray detectors. In addition to the concurrent development of rapid and relatively inexpensive computational resources, this era of rapid change owes much of its success to an improved understanding of the information theoretic principles on which the development and maturation of these new technologies is based. A further important corollary of these developments in medical imaging technology has been the relatively rapid development and deployment of methods for archiving and transmitting digital images. Much of this engineering development continues to make use of the ongoing revolution in rapid communications technology offered by increasing bandwidth.

A little more than 100 years after the discovery of x rays, this three-volume *Handbook of Medical Imaging* is intended to provide a comprehensive overview of the theory and current practice of Medical Imaging as we enter the twenty-first century. Volume 1, which concerns the physics and the psychophysics of medical imaging, begins with a fundamental description of x-ray imaging physics and progresses to a review of linear systems theory and its application to an understanding of signal and noise propagation in such systems. The subsequent chapters concern the physics of the important individual imaging modalities currently in use: ultrasound, CT, MRI, the recently emerging technology of flat-panel x-ray detectors and, in particular, their application to mammography. The second half of this volume, which covers topics in psychophysics, describes the current understanding of the relationship between image quality metrics and visual perception of the diagnostic information carried by medical images. In addition, various models of perception in the presence of noise or "unwanted" signal are described. Lastly, the statistical methods used in determining the efficacy of medical imaging tasks, and ROC analysis and its variants, are discussed.

Volume 2, which concerns Medical Image Processing and Image Analysis, provides descriptions of the methods currently being used or developed for enhancing the visual perception of digital medical images obtained by a wide variety of imaging modalities and for image analysis as a possible aid to detection and diagnosis. Image analysis may be of particular significance in future developments, since, aside from the inherent efficiencies of digital imaging, the possibility of performing analytic computation on digital information offers exciting prospects for improved detection and diagnostic accuracy.

Lastly, Volume 3 describes the concurrent engineering developments that in some instances have actually enabled further developments in digital diagnostic imaging. Among the latter, the ongoing development of bright, high-resolution monitors for viewing high-resolution digital radiographs, particularly for mammography, stands out. Other efforts in this field offer exciting, previously inconceivable possibilities, e.g., the use of 3D (virtual reality) visualization for surgical planning and for image-guided surgery. Another important area of ongoing research in this field involves image compression, which in concert with increasing bandwidth enables rapid image communication and increases storage efficiency. The latter will be particularly important with the expected increase in the acceptance of digital radiography as a replacement for conventional film/screen imaging, which is expected to generate data volumes far in excess of currently available capacity. The second half of this volume describes current developments in Picture Archiving and Communications System (PACS) technology, with particular emphasis on integration of the new and emerging imaging technologies into the hospital environment and the provision of means for rapid retrieval and transmission of imaging data. Developments in rapid transmission are of particular importance since they will enable access via telemedicine to remote or underdeveloped areas.

As evidenced by the variety of the research described in these volumes, medical imaging is still undergoing very rapid change. The editors hope that this publication will provide at least some of the information required by students, researchers, and practitioners in this exciting field to make their own contributions to its ever-increasing usefulness.

Jacob Beutel
J. Michael Fitzpatrick
Steven C. Horii
Yongmin Kim
Harold L. Kundel
Milan Sonka
Richard L. Van Metter

Part I. Physics

Introduction to Part I

During the last half of the twentieth century, Medical Imaging has undergone a series of revolutionary changes. These have not only been driven by advances in the underlying science and technology, but by changes in the needs of health care providers. The diagnostic quality of images available to physicians as well as the variety and scope of available imaging technologies has expanded beyond what could have been imagined fifty years ago. The pace of this change is still accelerating. In part this revolution is attributable to advances in our fundamental understanding of the physical phenomena on which the imaging technologies are based. But the useful application of this understanding has been enabled by an increasing availability of computational power and high-speed data communications. Networked computational resources have been harnessed to support both the increasing pace of scientific research and, more importantly, to handle the vast amounts of data that digital imaging technologies require.

The best-known advances in medical imaging have applied digital imaging technology to previously unexploited physical measurables. Here the fortuitous combination of physical understanding and ever-increasing, widely available computational power have enabled the development and widespread adoption of ultrasound imaging, tomography, and magnetic resonance imaging. Further improvements and extensions of the scope of these imaging modalities are the subject of many ongoing research and development efforts. More speculative efforts are aimed toward discovering new "signals" that can be utilized for diagnostic purposes.

Even as new imaging technologies have found their place in medical diagnosis, classical x-ray projection radiography itself is undergoing a revolution. This began with the development of commercial Computed Radiography systems in the 1980s. At first large and expensive, technological advances have steadily reduced size and cost, while the usefulness of digital images has increased due to the ever-expanding information technology infrastructure in medicine. Here technological advances and the challenges of providing health care to a greater number of people more efficiently than ever before are driving revolutionary change. Research is now concentrated on the development of flat panel digital detectors whose possible applications range from digital mammography to conventional diagnostic radiography and fluoroscopy. Ultimately these detectors will lower the cost and increase

the availability of diagnostic imaging thereby completing the transition to a totally digital medical imaging environment where image information will be better
utilized to guide patient care.

Concurrent with all of these changes, our understanding of imaging science,
largely derived from information theoretic considerations developed during the
1950s, has developed to the point where it can effectively guide system optimization. This initially allowed conventional x-ray imaging systems to be optimized well beyond their prior capabilities. Now with the separation between image capture and image display enabled by digital imaging technology, we pursue
the heretofore unavailable opportunity of independently optimizing these two subsystems. This will bring image quality closer than ever before to the currently understood fundamental limits.

As we begin the new century, this volume provides a snapshot of our current
understanding of the physics of medical imaging written by authors who have contributed significantly to its development. The first three chapters describe the fundamental physics and imaging science on which x-ray projection radiography is
based. Together these provide the basis for the ongoing improvements and new
developments aimed at optimizing the performance of these imaging systems. The
unifying signal-to-noise concepts described are now accepted as the technology-
independent absolute criteria by which progress is measured for all imaging modalities. These lead naturally to a discussion of the exciting developments in detector
technology for digital radiography. Therefore, the next two chapters describe the
most recent developments in flat panel detectors for digital mammography and general projection x-ray imaging. The most exciting imaging technologies to emerge
in this information age allow us to fully visualize the three-dimensional structure
of human anatomy. They are the focus of the final three chapters in Part I. Of
these, the first two describe current practices incorporating the latest developments
in magnetic resonance imaging and computed tomography. They are followed, in
the final chapter, by a description of recent developments in volume ultrasound
imaging.

Jacob Beutel
Richard L. Van Metter

CHAPTER 1
X-ray Production, Interaction, and Detection in Diagnostic Imaging

John M. Boone
University of California, Davis

CONTENTS

1.1 X-ray production

1.1.1 Definitions and mechanisms

X rays and γ rays are forms of electromagnetic radiation that are energetic enough that when interacting with atoms, they have the potential of liberating electrons from the atoms that bind them. When an atom or molecule is stripped of an electron, an ion pair forms, consisting of the negatively charged electron (e^-) and the positive atom or molecule. X rays and γ rays, therefore, are forms of *ionizing radiation*, and this feature fundamentally distinguishes these rays from the rest of the electromagnetic spectrum.

An electromagnetic wave of frequency v has an energy proportional to v, with the constant of proportionality given by Plank's constant, h:

$$E = hv, \tag{1.1}$$

where $h = 4.135 \times 10^{-15}$ eV-s. For *diagnostic* medical x-ray imaging, the range of x-ray energies incident upon patients runs from a low of 10,000 eV (10 keV) to about 150 keV. In terms of wavelengths:

$$\lambda = \frac{c}{v}, \tag{1.2}$$

where c is the speed of light (2.997925×10^8 m/s). The range of wavelengths corresponding to diagnostic imaging span from about 0.1 nm (at 12.4 keV) to 0.01 nm (at 124 keV), compared to the visible spectrum spanning from about 400 nm (violet) to 650 nm (red). The electromagnetic spectrum is illustrated in Figure 1.1.

X rays and γ rays have different spectral characteristics, but fundamentally an x ray of energy E is exactly the same as a γ ray of energy E. By definition, γ rays originate from the nucleus of the atom, whereas x rays originate at the atomic level of the atom. Gamma rays are given off by radioactive isotopes such as technctium 99m, thallium 201, and iodine 131. A complete discussion of γ rays, which are the rays of interest in nuclear medicine imaging, is beyond the scope of this chapter.

X rays can be produced by several different methods, such as by synchrotrons, by channeling sources, by free electron lasers, etc. The most common x-ray production technology used in the vast majority of the radiology departments around the world, however, is the standard x-ray tube which emits bremsstrahlung as well as characteristic x rays. These processes are discussed below.

1.1.2 Bremsstrahlung radiation

According to classical theory, if a charged particle is accelerated it will radiate electromagnetic energy. When energetic electrons are incident upon a metal target (as in an x-ray tube), the electrons interact with the coulomb field of the nucleus of the target atoms and experience a change in their velocity, and hence undergo deceleration. *Bremsstrahlung radiation* ("braking radiation") is produced by this

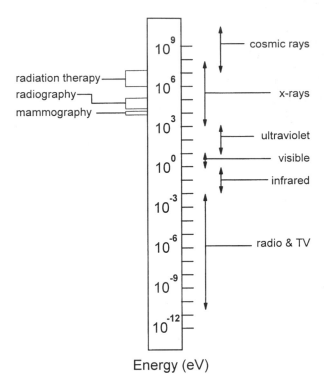

Energy (eV)

Figure 1.1: The electromagnetic spectrum is illustrated. X rays are at the high-energy, short-wavelength end of the EM spectrum. Cosmic rays of 100 GeV and higher have been observed.

process. The total intensity of bremsstrahlung radiation (integrated over all angles and all energies) resulting from a charged particle of mass m and charge ze incident onto target nuclei with charge Ze is proportional to:

$$I_{\text{bremsstrahlung}} \propto \frac{Z^2 \, z^4 \, e^6}{m^2}. \tag{1.3}$$

The bremsstrahlung efficiency is markedly reduced if a massive particle such as a proton or alpha particle is the charged particle. Relative to an electron, protons and α particles are over 3 million times less efficient (1836^{-2}) than electrons at producing bremsstrahlung x rays. Electrons therefore become the practical choice for producing bremsstrahlung. The Z^2 term in Eq. (1.3) also indicates that bremsstrahlung production increases rapidly as the atomic number of the target increases, suggesting that high-Z targets are preferred.

Bremsstrahlung production is illustrated in Figure 1.2. In Figure 1.2(a), incident electrons are shown passing near the target atom nucleus, and bremsstrahlung x rays of different energies (E_1, E_2, and E_3) are emitted. Electrons with only a grazing incidence of the atomic coulomb field (e.g., e_1^- in Figure 1.2(a)) give off

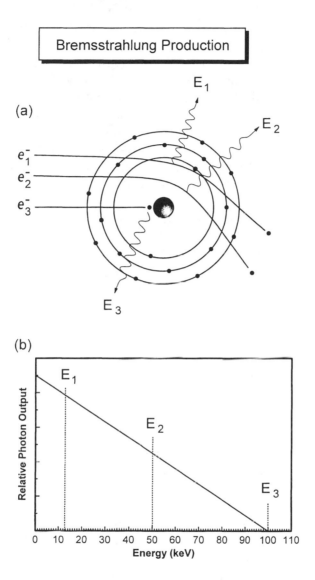

Figure 1.2: (a) Bremsstrahlung radiation is produced when energetic electrons are decelerated by the electric field of target nuclei. Electrons (e_1^-) which interact with a glancing blow emit a small fraction of their kinetic energy as an x ray (E_1), while electrons (e_3^-) which hit the nucleus directly can emit an x ray (E_3) with the total kinetic energy of the incident electron. (b) The probability of x-ray production by bremsstrahlung interaction is energy dependent. Glancing interaction between bombarding electrons and the nucleus are more probable, and therefore a larger number of low-energy x-ray photons are produced (E_1). Electrons interacting with the nucleus which give up all of their kinetic energy (100 keV in this example) occur much less frequently (E_3). Consequently, the theoretical "thick target" bremsstrahlung spectrum is the solid line shown in this figure.

only a small fraction of their incident kinetic energy. The resulting x ray has a relatively low energy, E_1, and the electron still has considerable kinetic energy and will continue to interact with other atoms in the target. On occasion, an electron (e_3^-) will interact with an atom and give up all of its kinetic energy, radiating an x ray equivalent in energy to the incident electron (see E_3 in Figures 1.2(a) and (b)). Figure 1.2(b) illustrates the theoretical energy distribution of bremsstrahlung from a thick target, produced by a monoenergetic beam of electrons (100 keV incident electrons are used as an example). The thick-target model envisions the target as layers, and due to the progressive loss of energy of more deeply penetrating electrons, the x rays produced at greater depths have a gradually decreasing maximum energy. This process is described mathematically as:

$$\Psi(E) = kZ(E_{\max} - E), \tag{1.4}$$

where $\Psi(E)$ is a histogram of the intensity (number × energy) of x rays of energy E per energy interval, k is a constant, Z is the atomic number of the target, $E_{\max}$ is the kinetic energy of the incident electron beam, and $E \leqslant E_{\max}$. The thick target spectrum is shown in Figure 1.2(b). Notice the Z dependence here is linear, unlike that seen in Eq. (1.3), because here the total bremsstrahlung emission spectrum is not considered, only that at energy E.

1.1.3 Characteristic x rays

A target used for x-ray production is usually a solid piece of metal, but when viewed from the tiny perspective of an electron it is really mostly open space filled with atomic nuclei and their bound electrons. The two constituents of the target suggests two possible types of interactions. Bremsstrahlung x rays are produced when the electrons incident upon the target interact with the nuclei, and *characteristic radiation* occurs when electrons interact with the atomic electrons in the target material.

In the classic Bohr model of the atom, electrons occupy orbitals with specific quantized energy levels. Electrons are bound to the nucleus by charge-charge interactions. A maximum of two electrons occupy the innermost electronic shell (called the K shell) and they are bound with approximately the same energy (the binding energy). The next electron shell (the L shell) is occupied with a maximum of eight electrons, each bound with approximately the same energy to the nucleus, but with substantially less binding energy than the K-shell electrons. Figure 1.3 illustrates a bombarding electron striking an atomic electron in the innermost shell, and ejecting it from its orbit. The bombarding and the ejected electrons will then go on to interact further with other target atoms, until their kinetic energy is spent.

Figure 1.4 illustrates a diagram of the energy levels of the electrons in the target atom. Compared to an unbound collection of Z electrons and a nucleus which defines the zero-energy state of the system, an atom which has electrons bound to the nucleus is *more stable* and thus the bound system has negative energy states resulting in negative binding energies. There is nothing mystical about negative

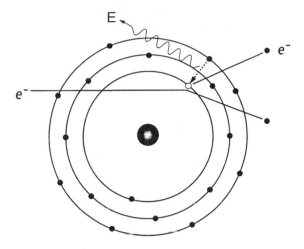

Figure 1.3: Characteristic x-ray production starts when a bombarding electron interacts with an atomic electron, ejecting it from its electronic shell. Subsequently, outer-shell electrons fill in the vacant shell, and in the process emit characteristic x rays. The energy of the characteristic x ray is the difference between the binding energies of the two shells.

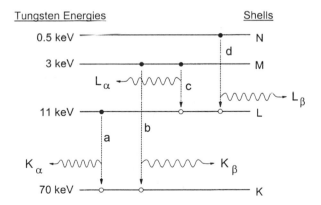

Figure 1.4: An energy diagram showing the K, L, M, and N shells is illustrated. The electron-binding energies (in keV) of each shell is illustrated for tungsten. Other elements have their own unique electron binding energies. Electrons which transition between shells emit characteristic radiation (x rays), whose energy is the difference between the binding energy of the two shells. Transitions between adjacent electron shells are called α transitions, and transitions between two or more shells are called β transitions. If the shell being filled is the K shell, then the transitions are K_α or K_β, as illustrated. L_α and L_β transitions are also shown.

energy states, they are merely a result of where the zero-energy state is defined in atomic physics. The ordering of the electron shells starts with K, and progresses alphabetically thereafter. Higher Z atoms have more orbiting electrons, and therefore have more electron shells. To give real numbers to the example, the binding energies of tungsten are indicated on the left side of Figure 1.4, where the K-shell electrons in tungsten are bound with an energy of 70 keV, the L shell with 11 keV, and the M-shell with 3 keV (using round numbers). If the kinetic energy of the bombarding electron is less than the binding energy of an orbital electron, ejection of the orbital electron is energetically unfeasible and will not occur.

When a K-shell electron is ejected by the bombarding electron, there is a vacancy left in that innermost shell of the atom, and this vacancy will be filled by an atomic electron from a different shell. This, in turn, will leave a vacancy in that shell, which will be filled by an electron from a more distant outer shell. Thus, the ejection of a K-shell electron sets up a whole cascade of electron transitions, until electrons in the outermost valence shells are filled by essentially free electrons in the environment (e.g., all those bombarding and ejected electrons, once they loose their kinetic energy, need some place to go!). Because the energy of electrons in each shell is well defined at discrete quantized values (defined by quantum numbers), the transition of an electron from one shell to another requires that energy be emitted. For example, for transition (a) shown in Figure 1.4, an electron with 11 keV moves to a shell with 70 keV, and it emits a 59 keV [(11–70 keV)] x-ray photon which is referred to as K_α emission, because the receiving shell was the K shell, and the electron was donated by the next shell up (an α transition). Transition (b) in Figure 1.4 shows an M-shell electron (3 keV) moving to the K-shell, making this a K_β emission (β means that the electron was donated from two *or more* shells away) having an energy of [(3–70)] 67 keV. Notice that the energy of a K_β x-ray photon is *higher* than that of a K_α photon. Transitions (c) and (d) illustrate the L-shell transitions, L_α and L_β. Characteristic x-rays produce discrete spectral lines.

X rays resulting from electrons transitioning between atomic shells are called characteristic x-rays; each element in the periodic table has its own unique atomic shell binding energies, and thus the energies of characteristic x rays are *characteristic* of (unique to) each atom. There is one additional nuance to the description of the last paragraph: No two electrons in the same atom actually have the *exact* same binding energy, and thus there is a slight difference in the binding energy in the electrons in each shell. For example, the two electrons in the K shell of tungsten have slightly different binding energies. Depending on which of the electrons is ejected from the K-shell, the K_α characteristic emission (for example) will be either a $K_{\alpha 1}$ (59.32 keV) or $K_{\alpha 2}$ (57.98 keV). The outer shells (L and above) have many more electrons in them, and thus transitions such as $L_{\alpha 3}$ or $L_{\beta 4}$ are possible, however these distinctions represent very small differences in energy.

Figure 1.5 illustrates the theoretical bremsstrahlung spectrum and the characteristic spectral lines for a tungsten target. The K_α emissions really are a *doublet* (the $K_{\alpha 1}$ and $K_{\alpha 2}$ lines), as is the K_β emission, but for most measured x-ray spectra, the two lines in each doublet are not resolved and they often are realized experimentally as one peak. Figure 1.5 also shows the shaded spectrum, which is

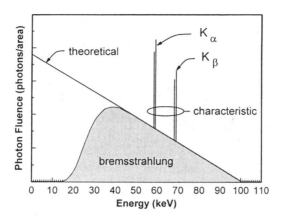

Figure 1.5: Idealized x-ray spectra are shown for 100-keV electrons striking a tungsten anode. The triangle-shaped theoretical spectrum produced inside the x-ray tube is attenuated by metallic structures in the tube, producing the shaded bremsstrahlung spectrum illustrated. Characteristic x rays appear on the spectrum as line spectra. The doublets for K_α and K_β beta characteristic x rays are illustrated.

the bremsstrahlung x-ray spectrum which is emitted from an x-ray tube. The low-energy x rays in the spectrum are preferentially absorbed by the target itself (*self absorption*) and other structures in the x-ray tube. X-ray filtration will be discussed later in this chapter.

1.1.4 General purpose x-ray tubes

1.1.4.1 Design and construction

A diagram of a general purpose x-ray tube is illustrated in Figure 1.6. A glass envelope seals the vacuum environment inside the tube. In the absence of a vacuum, energetic electrons would collide with air molecules instead of the target (anode), causing ionization of the air and a pronounced decrease in the efficiency of x-ray production of the tube. Inside the x-ray tube there are two general structures, that of the anode (left side of Figure 1.6) and the cathode (right side) assemblies.

The anode is the positively-charged pole of the high-voltage circuit inside the x-ray tube, and the anode is also the *target* of the bombarding electrons. For general diagnostic x-ray imaging applications outside of mammography, the anode is a disk made principally of tungsten. The anode is connected by a molybdenum shaft ("anode stem") to a bearing, which allows the anode and its shaft to rotate freely inside the x-ray tube. Molybdenum is a poor heat conductor, and is used as the anode stem to reduce heat transfer from the anode to the bearings. The anode shaft is surrounded inside the x-ray tube by a *rotor*. Outside the x-ray tube is the *stator*. Alternating current (AC) running through the windings of the stator produce alternating magnetic fields which cause the rotor to turn. The stator and the rotor shaft are standard components of an AC electric motor, the only difference here is that the rotor is in a vacuum environment and the magnetic field coupling the

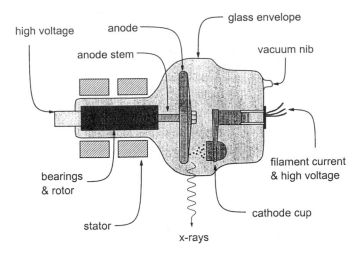

Figure 1.6: The functional components of a modern x-ray tube are illustrated.

stator and rotor therefore penetrates the glass envelope of the x-ray tube. Because the anode has to be inside the vacuum, the connected rotor and bearings need to be inside the vacuum as well, since it is not practical to pass a rotating shaft through a high-vacuum seal.

The cathode cup is the negative voltage pole of the circuit, and it is also the source of electrons that bombard the anode target. Inside the cathode cup are usually two different tungsten wire filaments, a small one and a larger one corresponding to the small and large focal spots. Only one of the filaments is used at any one time. The filaments on x-ray tubes are heavy-duty versions of the filaments inside a standard 120-V incandescent light bulb. During x-ray exposures, the filament is heated up by passing the *filament current* (e.g., 5 A at 10 V) through it. The filament heats up and electrons are emitted from the filament through a process called *thermionic emission*, similar to the operation of electron guns in TV cameras, televisions, and other electronic devices.

As electrons are boiled off of the cathode filament, the high voltage between the anode and cathode causes the electrons to be accelerated towards the tungsten target. The SI unit of energy is the joule, however in x ray practice it is more common to use the *electron volt*; an electron volt is a unit of energy equal to the kinetic energy of an electron accelerated by an applied potential of one volt. For general diagnostic x-ray imaging (outside of mammography), the applied potential across the x-ray tube ranges from about 40 kV to 150 kV. For an applied potential of (for example) 100,000 V (100 kV), an electron strikes the target with 100,000 electron-volts (100 keV) of kinetic energy. Notice that there is an important distinction here between kV (a unit of electric potential) and keV (a unit of energy).

The flow of current from the cathode to the anode inside the x-ray tube is the *x-ray tube current*, and the tube current is different (much lower) than the filament current used to heat up the filament. Typical tube currents run from around 1 mA

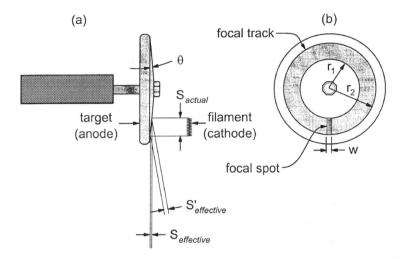

Figure 1.7: (a) A side view of the anode and cathode is shown. The angled anode design allows the use of a large actual focal spot (S_{actual}), which is beneficial for heat-loading considerations. The projection of the focal-spot towards the imaging plane is much smaller. The projected focal spot dimensions change across the field of view in the anode cathode direction ($S_{\mathrm{effective}}$ versus $S'_{\mathrm{effective}}$). (b) A front view of the anode is shown, with a rectangular focal spot and the annular focal track. The use of a rotating anode substantially increases the surface area of the target and allows higher ma studies.

in fluoroscopic mode of operation to about 1200 mA in cardiac catheterization studies. When energetic electrons strike the anode disk, they produce x rays as discussed in a previous section of this chapter. However, the efficiency of x-ray production at the energies used in diagnostic radiology is only about 0.5%, and the remainder of the kinetic energy of the electrons is deposited in the anode as heat. The choice of tungsten as the anode material is in part because of its high atomic number ($Z_W = 74$, see Eq. (1.3)), but more importantly the melting point (3300°C) of tungsten is very high compared to other metals. Nevertheless, the buildup of heat in the anode is a major engineering problem, and many advances in x-ray tube design over the past century have been aimed at increasing heat dissipation.

Figure 1.7(a) shows the side profile of the tungsten target with the filament. By incorporating a small *anode angle* (θ, where $7° \leqslant \theta \leqslant 15°$), the area of the anode bombarded by electrons (the *focal spot*) is fairly large (S_{actual}) allowing heat dissipation over a larger surface, while the dimensions of the focal spot projected downwards towards the imaging plane are small ($S_{\mathrm{effective}}$). The actual focal spot size is compressed by the tangent of the anode angle, making the effective focal spot dimensions smaller by factors from 0.12 (7°) to 0.27 (15°). This simple geometric trick is called the *line focus principle*.

In Figure 1.7(b), the front surface of the anode disk is illustrated. The disk rotates rapidly during x-ray production, and this allows the anode surface being bombarded by electrons to be constantly refreshed with cooler tungsten. Anode rotation improves the instantaneous tube loading properties, which allows higher x-ray tube currents during a shorter x ray exposure time. If the exposure time exceeds the rotation period (which at 3300 revolutions per minute is 18 ms), a region of the disk will be re-exposed to the bombarding electron beam, however because of the high heat conduction of tungsten, the heat on the surface will have had some time to diffuse from the surface into the mass of the anode. The use of a rotating anode increases the surface area for heat dissipation from a rectangle of area $(w \times [r_2 - r_1])$ to an annulus with area $(\pi (r_2^2 - r_1^2))$. Depending on the anode diameter, the increase in heat dissipation area ranges from factors of 18 to 35 for general diagnostic x-ray tubes.

The angled anode design which forms the basis of the line focus principle is not without minor problems. As shown in Figure 1.8(a), the anode angle limits the maximum dimensions of the field of view that can be exposed to x rays at a given source-to-image distance (SID). This issue of *coverage* needs to be considered when purchasing an x-ray tube for a specific application. The angled surface of the anode (Figure 1.8(b)) also causes a slight reduction in x-ray intensity on the anode side of the field of view, and this phenomenon is called the *heel effect*. X rays originate at some average depth in the target (D_{ave}), and because of the geometry

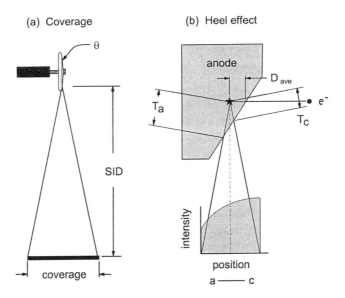

Figure 1.8: (a) Because of the line focus principle (angled anode), the field of view or *coverage* is restricted at a given source-to-image distance (SID). For instance, a 7-degree anode angle is too restrictive if 35×43 cm ($14'' \times 17''$) radiographs are to be acquired at an SID of 100 cm. (b) Another consequence of the line-focus principle is the *heel effect*. X rays are emitted at an average depth (D_{ave}) within the anode; the path length through the tungsten anode that x rays transit is different on the anode side (T_a) than on the cathode side (T_c) of the x-ray field. This difference in tungsten filtration across the field of view causes a reduction in x-ray intensity on the anode side of the x-ray field.

of the anode angle, the x ray pathlength through the anode is greater on the anode side (T_a) of the x-ray field than it is on the cathode side (T_c). The greater pathlength through the tungsten target causes more attenuation of the x-ray beam on the anode side of the field, reducing its intensity there.

The line focus principle and rotating anode design of modern x-ray tubes are used to make the effective focal spot as small as possible, and to maximize the number of x rays that can be emitted during a short period of time. Ideally, the x-ray source would be a perfect *point source* of radiation. The influence of geometry on x-ray imaging is illustrated in Figure 1.9. The x-ray shadow of an object cast onto the detector will be magnified depending upon the position of that object between the source and detector (Figure 1.9(a)). Object magnification occurs because x rays *diverge* from the small x-ray source. The magnification factor, M_{object}, of an object in the field is given by:

$$M_{\text{object}} = \frac{image\ size}{object\ size} = \frac{A + B}{A}. \tag{1.5}$$

When a thin object is in contact with the image receptor, $B = 0$, and $M_{\text{object}} = $ unity. Magnification can therefore be reduced by placing the patient as close to the detector as possible, but because the patient has appreciable thickness, anatomy that

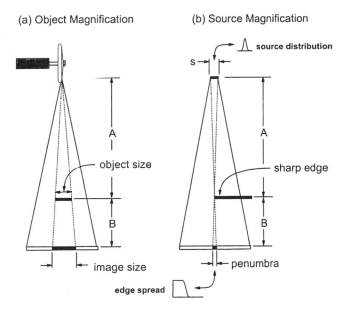

Figure 1.9: (a) An object placed between the x-ray source and the imaging plane will be magnified, with increasing magnification as the distance B increases. (b) The size of the focal spot is also magnified. For a focal spot of width S, the x-ray shadow of a sharp edge will result in a blurred edge (called the penumbra), as shown. The width of the penumbra increases with increasing magnification. Because the source distribution is usually Gaussian (or double-Gaussian) shaped, a sigmoidal edge spread is usually observed.

is closer to the x-ray tube will be magnified more than anatomy which lies closer to the detector.

The influence of a finite-size focal spot is shown in Figure 1.9(b). For objects with sharp edges which are slightly magnified, the finite dimensions of the focal spot (s) causes a geometrical broadening of the sharp edge in the imaging plane, called the *penumbra*. From similar triangles, the width of the penumbra (p) is given by:

$$p = s \times \frac{B}{A}. \tag{1.6}$$

Equation (1.6) assumes simple linear dimensions of the source and penumbra, but in reality the x-ray source has a distribution (sometimes Gaussian shaped, as illustrated in Figure 1.9(b)), and that distribution will be reflected in the penumbra as a sigmoidal *edge spread*. For anatomical structures which undergo some magnification (when $B \neq 0$), a finite-dimensioned focal spot will cause blurring of that anatomy measured at the detector plane, and hence a loss of spatial resolution will occur.

1.1.4.2 High voltage generators

The circuitry which provides the high voltage to the x-ray tube is located in the x-ray generator. The x-ray generator also provides the circuitry and control electronics for the filament current, the rotation of the anode, and the exposure timing. The basic circuit for an x-ray generator is shown in Figure 1.10. The line voltage (V_{line}) is supplied by the main power supply of the institution, and is on the order of 120 to 440 V in the United States. The line voltage can be adjusted at the control panel of the x-ray system, controlling the alternating voltage (i.e., $dV/dt \neq 0$) applied to the high voltage transformer (V_{in}). *Transformers require alternating voltage*; applying a nonchanging voltage ($dV/dt = 0$) will result in no voltage transformation or electrical exchange between the primary and secondary sides of the transformer. There are different strategies for how the line voltage is sent to the transformer, and that will be discussed below. A step-up transformer increases the voltage on the secondary side, based linearly on the ratio of windings in the generator. For example, if 100 V were fed to a step-up transformer with a ratio of windings of 1000:1 (secondary:primary), the output voltage (kV_{out}) would be 100,000 V. Of course, the electrical power (watts = volts × amperes = kV × mA) cannot be increased by the transformer, so the output current is *reduced* by the high voltage transformer by the same 1000:1 factor. In practice, since transformers are not 100% efficient, the output current will suffer greater reductions than the theoretical value.

The high voltage that is the output of the secondary side of the transformer is alternating, such that the voltage measured at one pole (i.e., at location a in the circuit) will fluctuate sinusoidally from negative to positive high voltages relative to ground. X-ray generators are usually grounded at the center tap of the transformer,

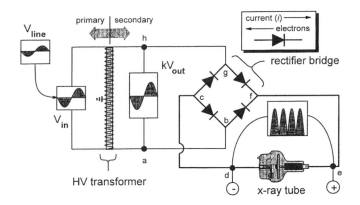

Figure 1.10: An electrical diagram of the circuit used in x-ray generators (single phase) is shown. The high-voltage transformer acts to increase the supplied voltage to the generator. The rectifier bridge serves to flip negative voltages to positive voltages so that electron flow in the x-ray tube is always from the filament to the tungsten target.

because this reduces the electrical shielding requirements of the high voltage cables running from the generator to the x-ray tube. By grounding the center tap, for example, the maximum voltages in these cables are -75 kV and $+75$ kV, instead of 0 kV and $+150$ kV, for a 150-kV generator. An alternating voltage is not wanted at the x-ray tube, because the anode should always be kept positive relative to the cathode. If the cathode voltage were to swing positive relative to the anode, electrons emitted from the hot anode (during exposure) would be accelerated towards the filament, resulting in the generation of x rays at an undesirable location and prematurely aging the filament. Therefore, a rectifier bridge is used to flip the negative voltage swings back to positive swings, producing the rectified voltage waveform as indicated (for a single phase generator) between locations d and e on Figure 1.10.

The rectifier bridge is a series of diodes (see inset), which act as one-way valves for the flow of electrons. Referring to Figure 1.10, when the voltage at location a is lower than that at location h, the path of electron flow (which is *opposite* to the flow of electrical *current*) is a-b-c-d-e-f-g-h. When the voltage at h is lower than a, the flow of electrons is h-g-c-d-e-f-b-a. In both cases, electrons transit the x-ray tube from the cathode to anode (d-e).

1.1.4.3 Generator waveforms

The circuit shown in Figure 1.10 is that of a single-phase generator (old technology). The *peak kilovoltage*, kVp, is the maximum kV value applied across the x-ray tube during the time duration of the exposure. The kV varies as a function of time, but kVp does not. For a single-phase generator, the rectified voltage waveform (kV versus time) applied across the x-ray tube theoretically swings from 0 to +kVp to 0, as shown in Figure 1.11(a). For single-phase generators, each half-sine wave occurs in 1/120th s, corresponding to the 60-Hz AC current used in the

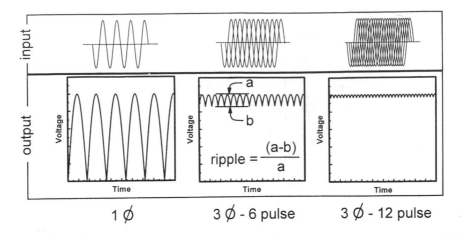

Figure 1.11: The input and output voltage wave forms are illustrated for single-phase, three-phase-6-pulse, and three-phase-12-pulse x-ray generator systems. The voltage ripple, defined in the middle pane, decreases dramatically with different generator technologies.

Table 1.1: The amount of kV ripple present in different x-ray generator technologies

Generator Type	Ripple (%)
Single phase	100%
3 phase, 6 pulse	13.4%
3 phase, 12 pulse	3.4%
Constant potential	0%
Inverter	~5%

United States. While the kV waveform produced by a single-phase generator fluctuates over time, a constant "DC" voltage applied across the x-ray tube is desired.

In an effort to come closer to the goal of a DC tube voltage, three-phase generator technology was developed and used principally during the 1960s–1980s. With a three-phase generator, three single-phase waveforms that are shifted in phase with respect to each other by $2\pi/3$ are used. The circuit diagram for three-phase generators is not shown. There are two variations in three phase generator circuits, resulting in so-called 6-pulse and 12-pulse waveforms (Figures 1.11(b) and (c)). The *ripple* in the voltage waveform is defined in Figure 1.11(b), and when ripple $\rightarrow$ 0%, the waveform reaches the desired goal of being DC. The ripple associated with different generator technologies is indicated in Table 1.1.

An extension of three-phase generator systems is the constant potential generator (CPG), which uses tetrode tanks and feedback circuits to achieve a nearly DC waveform. Representative x-ray spectra resulting from four generator technologies

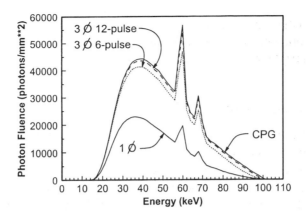

Figure 1.12: The x-ray spectra generated at 100 kVp for four generator technologies are illustrated. In going from single phase to 3-phase-6-pulse to 3-phase-12-pulse to constant-potential generators, both the *quantity* and the *quality* of the x-ray beam increases. There is a negligible difference in the x-ray spectrum between the 3-phase-12-pulse and constant potential generator systems. Modern high-frequency inverter generators produce a spectrum equivalent to 3-phase-12-pulse systems.

are shown at 100 kVp in Figure 1.12. As the ripple decreases from 100% with single-phase generators to 0% with CPG systems, the spectrum becomes slightly higher in average energy, and the output of the x-ray tube (photon fluence, or mR per mAs) increases because x-ray production becomes more efficient at higher energies. The spectra shown in Figure 1.12 were computed with a theoretical model [1] which integrates over the kV-versus-time waveforms produced by the generator technologies listed.

In the late 1980s, high frequency inverter generators were introduced to radiology. Rather than making use of the 60-Hz line frequency supplied by the local power company, high frequency inverter systems convert the primary voltage to DC, and then use a digital oscillator to chop the DC voltage to a high frequency ($\sim$2000 Hz). This voltage waveform is then input to the high voltage transformer, and the high-frequency, high-voltage waveform is rectified, smoothed, and delivered to the x-ray tube. Inverter generators are digitally controlled and by today's standards are less complicated and less expensive than three phase generators, and they produce a low-ripple ($\sim$5%) kV waveform comparable to that of a three-phase twelve-pulse generator.

1.2 X-ray interactions

1.2.1 Interaction mechanisms

X rays (and γ rays) interact with matter in several different types of interactions. Interactions, in general, can result in the local deposition of energy, and in some cases an x ray will exist after the initial interaction in the form of a scattered x ray, characteristic x rays, or annihilation radiation photons. The types of interactions are the photoelectric effect, Rayleigh scattering, Compton scattering, pair production, and triplet production. The mechanism for each of these interactions is described below.

1.2.1.1 The photoelectric effect

The photoelectric effect was discovered by Albert Einstein in 1905. In the photoelectric interaction, the incident x ray interacts with an electron in the medium. The incident x ray is completely absorbed, and all of its energy is transferred to the electron (Figure 1.13). If the electron is bound to its parent atom with binding energy E_{BE}, and the energy of the incident x ray is given by E_0, the kinetic energy T of the photoelectron is:

$$T = E_0 - E_{BE}. \tag{1.7}$$

If the energy of the incident x ray is less than the binding energy of the electron ($E_0 < E_{BE}$), photoelectric interaction with that electron is energetically unfeasible and will not occur. K-shell electrons are bound more tightly to the atom (higher $|E_{BE}|$) than outer-shell (L shell, etc.) electrons, so if photoelectric interaction is energetically not possible with K-shell electrons, interaction may still occur with an outer-shell electron. When $E_0 = E_{BE}$, then photoelectric interaction is most probable, and the interaction probability decreases with increasing E_0 thereafter. The binding energy, E_{BE}, associated with the K shell is called the K edge, and that of the L shell is called the L edge, and so on. The term *edge* refers to the abrupt jump in the probability of photoelectric interaction once the process becomes energetically possible. The photoelectric effect results in *ionization* of the atom, and a single ion pair (the e^- and the positively charged parent atom) is initially formed. The ejected photoelectron may then proceed to ionize additional atoms in the medium.

Once an electron is liberated from its parent atom, a vacancy in one of the electron shells of the atom exists. A cascade of electron transitions will occur, resulting in the production of characteristic radiation in a manner identical to that described in Section 1.1.2. In that section, atomic electrons were ejected by interaction with bombarding electrons, here the electrons are ejected by photoelectric interaction with an x ray. Either way, the sequence of subsequent events of characteristic x-ray emission is identical, and the reader is referred to Section 1.1.2 and Figure 1.4.

While the post-electron-ejection mechanism of characteristic x-ray production is the same, some practical differences should be mentioned. X rays are produced by electrons striking a high-atomic-number metal target, usually tungsten ($Z = 74$). The characteristic x-ray energies (K_α, K_β, etc.) are therefore quite high. However, x rays used for medical imaging interact first with the patient and then with the x-ray detector. The patient is composed of a medley of elements, but mostly hydrogen ($Z = 1$), carbon ($Z = 6$), nitrogen ($Z = 7$), and oxygen ($Z = 8$), that is, low-atomic-number elements. The K-shell binding energy of oxygen is 0.5 keV, and even that of calcium ($Z = 20$, a constituent of bone) is 4 keV. X rays

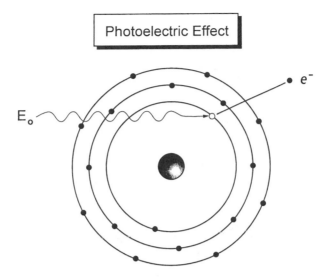

Figure 1.13: In the photoelectric effect, an x ray with energy E_0 is absorbed by an atomic electron, which is ejected from the atom causing ionization. The photoelectron will have kinetic energy equal to $E_0 - E_{BE}$, where E_{BE} is the binding energy of the electron to the nucleus.

of such low energies do not travel very far before being attenuated. For example, the mean free path of a 1-keV x ray in muscle tissue is about 2.7 μm, less than the dimensions of a typical human cell. Consequently, characteristic x rays that are produced in tissue will be re-absorbed locally in adjacent tissue.

Once the x-ray beam passes through the patient, it will strike the x-ray detector. Typical x-ray detectors are made of CsI, Gd_2O_2S, Y_2TaO_4, etc., with K-shell energies in the 30-keV to 70-keV range. The characteristic x rays produced in the detector itself can be reasonably energetic, and therefore they can propagate finite distances within the detector, or more likely escape the detector completely. This phenomenon will be discussed later.

1.2.1.2 Rayleigh scattering

The mechanism of Rayleigh scattering involves the elastic (coherent) scattering of x rays by atomic electrons (Figure 1.14). The unique feature of Rayleigh scattering is that ionization does *not* occur, and the energy of the scattered x ray is identical to that of the incident x-ray ($E' = E_0$). There is no exchange of energy from the x ray to the medium. However, the scattered x ray experiences a change in its trajectory relative to that of the incident x ray, and this has a deleterious effect in medical imaging, where the detection of scattered x rays is undesirable.

X rays scattered in a three-dimensional coordinate system (real life) require two scattering angles to describe the event. Figure 1.15 shows the geometry of scattering, where the *scattering angle* θ (which ranges from 0 to π) describes the net angular change in photon propagation (looking from the side), and the rotational

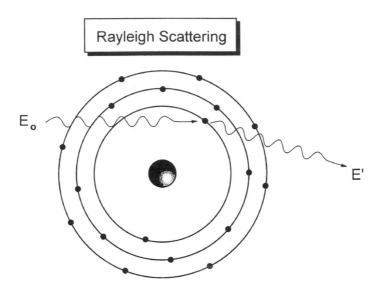

Figure 1.14: In Rayleigh scattering, the incident x ray interacts with the electric field of an orbiting electron and is scattered as a result. The energy of the scattered x ray (E') is equal to the energy of the incident x ray (E_0). No ionization occurs in Rayleigh scattering. Rayleigh scattering is most likely for low-energy x rays and for high-Z absorbers.

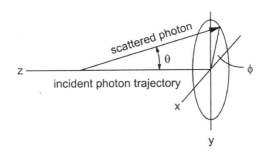

Figure 1.15: The coordinate system for x-ray scattering is illustrated. Two different angles are needed to specify the trajectory of the scattered photon. θ is the scattering angle ($0° - 180°$). The azimuthal angle (ϕ) spans between $0°$ and $360°$. The scattering angle probability density function, $p(\theta)$, depends on the x-ray energy and scattering mechanism. The probability density function $p(\phi)$ is constant over the $0°$ and $360°$.

angle ϕ (which ranges from 0 to 2π) describes the scattering angle looking down the photon's initial flight path.

Scattering angles θ for Rayleigh scattering in tissue are illustrated in Figure 1.16 for x rays of different energy. The maximum probability at each energy is normalized to 100%. Higher energy x rays (e.g., 60 keV) undergo very small angle scattering (i.e., forward peaked) compared to lower energy x rays (5 keV). This is expected, since the rules of conservation of momentum and energy hold, and the recoil imparted to the atom involved in the interaction must not result in ioniza-

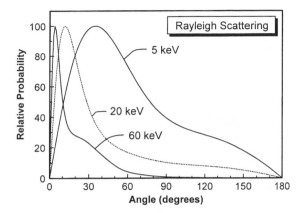

Figure 1.16: The probability density functions for Rayleigh scattering angles are illustrated for three x-ray energies in water. As the x-ray energy increases, forward scattering (small angle scattering) becomes increasingly likely. The PDF at each x-ray energy is normalized to 100%.

tion [2]. Consequently, Rayleigh scattering is more likely for low-energy x rays and high-Z materials.

1.2.1.3 Compton scattering

Compton scattering involves the inelastic (incoherent) scattering of an x-ray photon by an atomic electron (Figures 1.17). Compton scattering typically occurs at higher x-ray energies where the energy of the x-ray photon is much greater than the binding energy of the atomic electron, and therefore the Compton effect is considered to occur with outer-shell, essentially free electrons in the medium. In the Compton effect, an incident x-ray photon of energy E_0 is scattered by the medium, and the products of the interaction include a scattered x-ray photon of energy E', an electron of energy T, and an ionized atom. With Compton scattering, a relationship between the fractional energy loss and the scattering angle θ is observed:

$$\frac{E'}{E_0} = \frac{1}{1 + \alpha(1 - \cos\theta)}, \tag{1.8}$$

where

$$\alpha = \frac{E_0}{m_0 c^2} = \frac{E_0}{511\,\text{keV}},$$

and where $m_0 c^2$ is the rest mass of the electron and is equal to 511 keV. Equation (1.8) is called the Klein-Nishina equation, and qualitatively it implies that the energy of the scattered x-ray photon becomes smaller as the scattering angle increases, and this effect is amplified at higher incident photon energies.

The scattering angle distributions for Compton scattering in tissue are illustrated in Figure 1.18. Low-energy photons are preferentially backscattered,

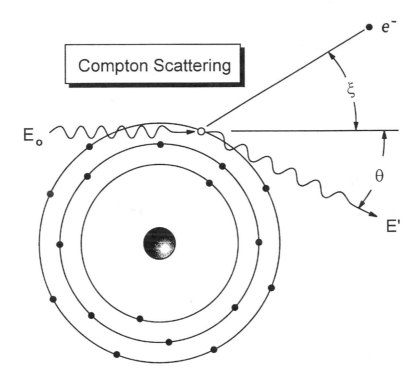

Figure 1.17: In Compton scattering, an incident x ray with energy E_0 interacts with an outer-shell electron. The electron is ejected from the atom, causing ionization. A scattered x-ray photon with energy E' emerges at an angle θ relative to the incident photon's trajectory.

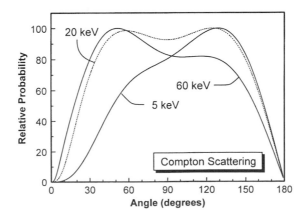

Figure 1.18: The probability density function of Compton scattering as a function of angle is illustrated for three x-ray energies in water. The height of each PDF is normalized to 100%.

whereas higher-energy x rays have a higher probability of forward scattering. At energies well above the diagnostic energy region (e.g., at 5 MeV), Compton scattering is markedly forward peaked.

1.2.1.4 Pair and triplet production

Pair production involves the interaction of an incident x ray with the electric field of the nucleus. Pair production is a classical demonstration of the interchangeability between mass and energy (Figure 1.19). After a pair production interaction, which is only feasible above 1.02 MeV, the incident x ray is completely absorbed and a positron (e^+) and an electron (e^-) are produced (hence the name *pair* production). For an incident x ray of energy E_0 (where $E_0 > 1.02$ MeV),

$$E_0 = 2m_0c^2 + T_+ + T_-, \tag{1.9}$$

where T_+ and T_- are the kinetic energies of the positron and electron, respectively, and m_0 is the rest mass of the electron (and positron). Energy of the incident x ray above 1.02 MeV ($2m_0c^2$) is realized as kinetic energy of the particle pair. It is interesting to note that the atom involved in pair production interaction is not ionized, although charged particles (e^- and e^+) are formed.

Triplet production is similar to pair production, except that the incident x-ray photon interacts with the electric field of an atomic electron instead of the nucleus (Figure 1.20). The atomic electron is ejected from the atom in the process, and it becomes the third particle. Triplet production is energetically feasible only above

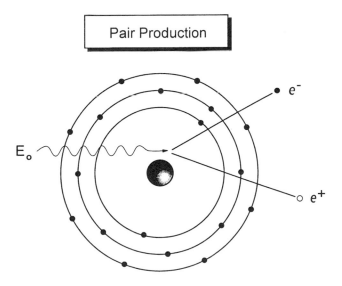

Figure 1.19: Pair production can occur when an incident x ray (with $E_0 > 1.02$ MeV) interacts with the electric field of an atom. A negatron (e^-)–positron (e^+) ion pair is formed in the interaction. Pair production does not occur at diagnostic x-ray energies.

2.04 MeV. Both pair and triplet production result in the formation of energetic electrons, which will cause subsequent ionization events. Once the positron spends its kinetic energy, it will rapidly combine with any available electron, giving rise to *annihilation radiation* as shown in Figure 1.21. The mass of the e^-/e^+ pair disappears, and two 511-keV x-ray photons are produced in nearly opposite directions. If both the e^- and the e^+ have negligible kinetic energy when they annihilate, the trajectories of the two annihilation radiation photons will be exactly opposite to each other. Annihilation radiation photons are used in positron emission tomog-

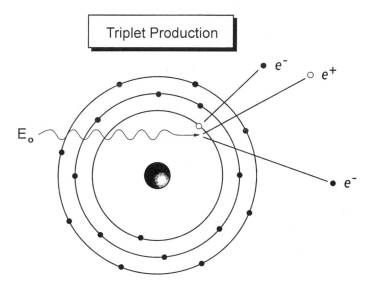

Figure 1.20:   Triplet production occurs when an incident x ray ($E_0 > 2.04$ MeV) interacts with the electric field surrounding an orbital electron. The orbital electron is ejected from the parent atom, along with a negatron/positron pair, resulting in three particles being emitted.

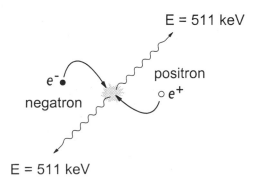

Figure 1.21:   The positrons produced in pair and triplet production will lose their kinetic energy by interaction with the medium, and then rapidly interact with any available negative electron (negatron) and *annihilate*, producing two 511-keV photons being emitted in opposite directions. The photons produced are called *annihilation radiation*.

raphy (PET) imaging, however the source of positrons is from radioactive decay, not pair or triplet production. Pair and triplet production take place at energies well above those used in diagnostic radiology, so neither of these processes occur in diagnostic medical imaging.

1.2.2 Attenuation coefficients

1.2.2.1 Linear attenuation coefficient

The interaction mechanisms discussed in the last section combine to produce *attenuation* of the incident x-ray photon beam as it passes through matter. Attenuation is the removal of x-ray photons from the x-ray beam by either absorption or scattering events. If a beam of N x-ray photons is incident upon a thin slab of material of thickness dx with a probability of interaction μ (Figure 1.22), the reduction of photons from the beam is given by dN, where:

$$dN = -\mu N \, dx. \tag{1.10}$$

Rearranging and integrating Eq. (1.10):

$$\int_{N_0}^{N} \frac{dN}{N} = -\mu \int_{0}^{t} dx. \tag{1.11}$$

Solving Eq. (1.11) with subsequent rearrangement results in the Lambert–Beers law:

$$N = N_0 e^{-\mu t}. \tag{1.12}$$

The units of thickness (t) in Eq. (1.12) are typically cm, and so the units of μ must be cm^{-1}; μ is called the *linear attenuation coefficient*. The value of μ represents the probability per centimeter thickness of matter, that an x-ray photon will be attenuated. The linear attenuation coefficient, μ, is the probability of interaction from all interaction mechanisms, and is the sum of the interaction probabilities of all the interaction types:

$$\mu = \tau + \sigma_r + \sigma + \pi + \gamma, \tag{1.13}$$

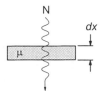

Figure 1.22: For the derivation of the Lambert–Beers Law, an x-ray beam of N photons is incident upon a slab of material with linear attenuation coefficient μ and thickness dx.

where τ is the attenuation coefficient for the photoelectric effect, σ_r is the Rayleigh scatter attenuation coefficient, σ is the Compton attenuation coefficient, π is the pair-production attenuation coefficient, and γ is the triplet attenuation coefficient.

1.2.2.2 Mass attenuation coefficient

The linear attenuation coefficient describes the attenuation properties of a specific material (take water as an example) at a specific x-ray energy. However, the value of the linear attenuation coefficient will depend linearly on the density of the material. For instance, water vapor will have a different μ than liquid water, and frozen water will have yet another value of μ. Since μ changes proportionally with the density of the material, an easy way to compensate for density is to normalize μ by the density (ρ), resulting in the mass attenuation coefficient, (μ/ρ). The mass attenuation coefficients of water vapor, liquid water, and ice are all identical (at a given energy). Since the units of μ are cm^{-1}, and the units of ρ are gm/cm^3, the units of the mass attenuation coefficient are cm^2/gm. When calculating attenuation using the mass attenuation coefficient, the units of thickness logically become the product of the known density ρ and thickness x of the material, ρx, and this product is called the *mass thickness* and has the units gm/cm^2. Thus the Lambert–Beers law becomes:

$$N = N_0 e^{-\left(\frac{\mu}{\rho}\right)\rho x}. \tag{1.14}$$

Just as the total linear attenuation coefficient μ is the sum of the linear attenuation coefficients of the individual interaction types, the total mass attenuation coefficient is the sum of its constituents as well:

$$\left(\frac{\mu}{\rho}\right) = \left(\frac{\tau}{\rho}\right) + \left(\frac{\sigma_r}{\rho}\right) + \left(\frac{\sigma}{\rho}\right) + \left(\frac{\pi}{\rho}\right) + \left(\frac{\gamma}{\rho}\right). \tag{1.15}$$

Attenuation, as calculated by the mass attenuation coefficient (Eq. (1.14)), is useful in describing the propagation of x rays through a material, but it does not tell the complete story in terms of energy deposition. Energy deposition is important both in the calculation of the radiation dose to a patient, and for the calculation of the total signal generated in an x-ray detector.

1.2.2.3 Mass energy transfer coefficient

The mass energy *transfer* coefficient is that fraction of the mass attenuation coefficient which contributes to the production of kinetic energy in charged particles. Photons which escape the interaction site do not contribute to the kinetic energy of charged particles. For the photoelectric effect, at least initially, the total energy of the incident x-ray photon, E_0, is transferred to the photoelectron. Part of this energy is used to overcome the binding energy of the atom (E_{BE}), and the remaining fraction becomes the kinetic energy T of the photoelectron:

$$\frac{T}{E_0} = \frac{E_0 - E_{\text{BE}}}{E_0}. \tag{1.16}$$

The ionized atom will either emit one or more characteristic x rays (also called *fluorescent* x rays), which will leave the interaction site, or alternatively a series of nonradiative transitions involving Auger electrons will take place, resulting in the complete local deposition of energy through charged particles. The fluorescent yield Y describes the probability of production of characteristic x rays (Y_K is the K-shell fluorescent yield and Y_L is the L-shell yield). The fluorescent yield is virtually zero for $Z < 10$, and Y_K increases with Z thereafter, reaching a value of 0.83 at $Z = 50$, and Y_L is about 0.12 at $Z = 50$. X rays with $E_0 = $ K edge can interact by the photoelectric effect with K-shell electrons, as well as by L-shell (and other shell) electrons. A function P_K describes the fraction of the photoelectric attenuation coefficient that results in K-shell interaction (τ_K / τ), for $E_0 = $ K edge. K-shell characteristic x rays have slightly different energies, depending on the transition levels which occur (e.g., $K_{\alpha 1}$, $K_{\alpha 2}$, $K_{\beta 1}$, $K_{\beta 2}$, etc.), and let the average K-shell fluorescent x-ray energy be designated as $\overline{E}_K$. Similar values (P_L and $\overline{E}_L$) can be defined for the L shell. The photoelectric mass energy transfer coefficient is given by:

$$\frac{\tau_{\text{tr}}}{\rho} = \frac{\tau}{\rho} \left[\frac{E_0 - P_K Y_K \overline{E}_K}{E_0} \right], \quad \text{for } E_0 \geqslant E_{\text{K-edge}}, \tag{1.17a}$$

and:

$$\frac{\tau_{\text{tr}}}{\rho} = \frac{\tau}{\rho} \left[\frac{E_0 - P_L Y_L \overline{E}_L}{E_0} \right], \quad \text{for } E_{\text{K-edge}} > E_0 \geqslant E_{\text{L-edge}}, \tag{1.17b}$$

since the fluorescent yield of the atoms which comprise tissue is negligible, for tissue $(\tau/\rho) = (\tau_{\text{tr}}/\rho)$. This is not the case for x-ray detector materials, however.

Rayleigh scattering does not impart energy to the media, and therefore $(\sigma_{\text{r,tr}}/\rho) = 0$, *always*. For Compton scattering, a large fraction of the incident x-ray energy leaves the site of the interaction in the form of the scattered photon (Eq. (1.8)). If the average kinetic energy imparted to electrons during Compton scattering is E_k, then the Compton mass energy transfer coefficient is given by:

$$\frac{\sigma_{\text{tr}}}{\rho} = \frac{\sigma}{\rho} \left[\frac{E_k}{E_o} \right]. \tag{1.18}$$

The mass attenuation coefficients for carbon, iodine, and lead are shown as a function of x-ray energy in Figures 1.23, 1.24, and 1.25, respectively. The mass energy transfer coefficients are also shown where appropriate. The carbon coefficients show no K-edge discontinuities in τ/ρ, because the E_{BE} is below 1 keV. For

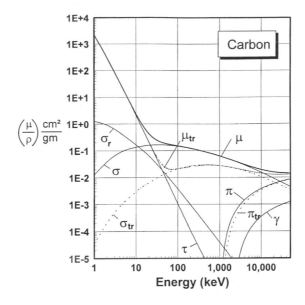

Figure 1.23: The mass attenuation coefficient for carbon is plotted as a function of x-ray energy. See text for definition of symbols.

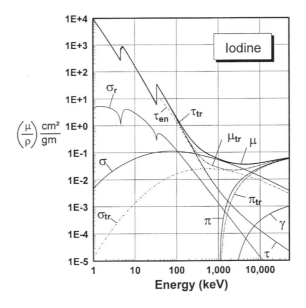

Figure 1.24: The mass attenuation coefficient for iodine is illustrated as a function of x-ray energy. The K edge of iodine (at 33 keV) and the L edge (at 5.2 keV) are apparent.

iodine (Figure 1.24) and lead (Figure 1.25), the L-edge and K-edge discontinuities are seen, and even the M edge is apparent for lead. The K-, L- and M-shell binding energies are plotted as a function of the element (Z) in Figure 1.26. The location

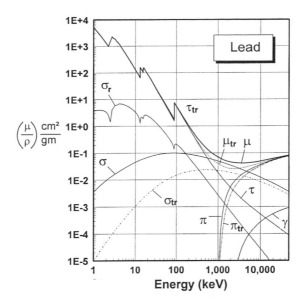

Figure 1.25: The mass attenuation coefficient of lead is shown as a function of x-ray energy. The K edge (88 keV), L edges (around 16 keV), and M edge ($\sim$3 keV) are seen.

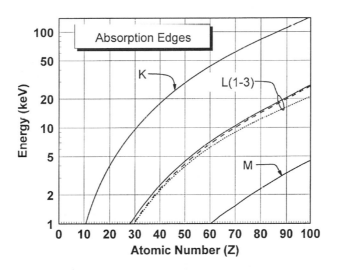

Figure 1.26: The energy of various absorption edges is illustrated as a function of the atomic number of the element. For elements below $Z = 10$ (i.e., tissue), the K edges are below 1 keV. The placement of the K edge of an x-ray detector has a relatively important role to play in the detection properties of the system.

of the K edge, and for higher Z elements the L edge, is important in the design of x-ray detectors for medical imaging, as will be discussed later in this chapter. The atomic number and energy realms in which the photoelectric, Compton, and pair interactions predominate are illustrated in Figure 1.27. The transition line be-

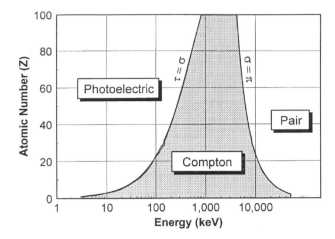

Figure 1.27: The region where each x-ray interaction process is most likely is shown as a function of atomic number and x-ray energy. The transition zones between regions correspond to the two cross sections being equal ($\tau = \sigma$ and $\sigma = \pi$).

tween the photoelectric and Compton zones is defined by $\tau/\rho = \sigma/\rho$, and the line between the Compton and pair production zones is defined by $\sigma/\rho = \pi/\rho$.

Pair and triplet production interactions do not occur at diagnostic x-ray energies, and therefore energy deposition to the patient and detector need not be discussed.

1.2.2.4 Mass energy absorption coefficient

The ratio of the mass energy transfer coefficient, (μ_{tr}/ρ), to the total attenuation coefficient, (μ/ρ), i.e., (μ_{tr}/μ), describes the fraction of the incident x-ray's energy that is transferred to charged particles in the form of kinetic energy. Let the average energy for all charged particles resulting from one interaction be represented as $\overline{E}_k$. As was discussed in Section 1.1.1, energetic electrons can interact with matter and produce bremsstrahlung radiation. The bremsstrahlung radiation that is produced, with an average energy $\overline{E}_r$, will radiate away from the site of the interaction, reducing the locally absorbed energy deposited by charged particles. The mass energy absorption coefficient, (μ_{en}/ρ), takes these radiative losses into account:

$$\left(\frac{\mu_{en}}{\rho}\right) = \left(\frac{\mu_{tr}}{\rho}\right)\left(\frac{\overline{E}_k - \overline{E}_r}{\overline{E}_k}\right). \qquad (1.19)$$

For low-Z materials such as tissue, $\overline{E}_r \approx 0$, and thus $(\mu_{en}/\rho) = (\mu_{tr}/\rho)$. Outside of the diagnostic energy range, annihilation radiation losses stemming from pair and triplet production are included in $\overline{E}_r$.

1.2.2.5 Attenuation coefficients for compounds

A compound that is a mixture of N elements will have a mass attenuation coefficient that is the weighted average (by weight) of the elemental mass attenuation coefficients. This is true for (μ_{en}/ρ) and (μ_{tr}/ρ) as well.

$$\left(\frac{\mu}{\rho}\right)_{compound} = \sum_{i=1}^{N} w_i \left(\frac{\mu}{\rho}\right)_i, \tag{1.20}$$

where w_i is the weight fraction of element i and $(\mu/\rho)_i$ is the mass attenuation coefficient (or mass energy transfer or mass energy absorption coefficients) of element i.

1.2.3 Interaction dependencies

1.2.3.1 Density

Density defines the relationship between the linear and mass attenuation coefficients. The density of each element differs depending on its state and purity, but the published values of the density of each element follow a trend of increasing density at higher Z, as shown in Figure 1.28. The noble gases and the other natural gases (H, O, N, S, Fl, etc.) are low in density, as expected. Interestingly, the rare earths ($Z = 57$ to 72) also are noticeable as a group in the context of density. Removing the gases from the calculation, the relationship between density and Z is approximately $\rho \propto Z^{0.78}$ ($r = 0.76$).

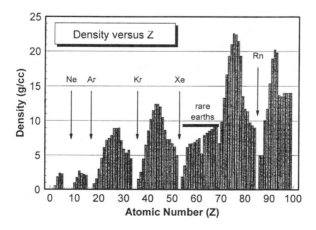

Figure 1.28: Density is shown as a function of atomic number. The low-density noble gases are indicated. The rare-earth elements are seen to disrupt an otherwise repeating pattern. Overall, the density of an element is seen to increase steadily with increasing Z.

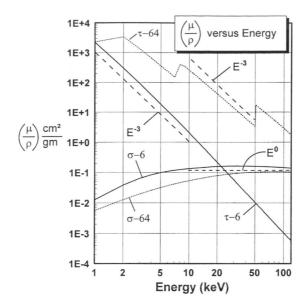

Figure 1.29: The energy dependency of the mass attenuation coefficient for two elements (carbon, $Z = 6$, and gadolinium, $Z = 64$) is illustrated. The photoelectric-effect cross sections for both elements (τ-6 and τ-64) are seen to be parallel to the dash lines indicating an E^{-3} dependency. The Compton scattering cross sections (σ-6 and σ-64) are seen to be essentially constant (proportional to E^{0}) in the diagnostic energy region from 10 keV to 200 keV.

1.2.3.2 Energy

Figure 1.29 shows the mass attenuation coefficients of carbon ($Z = 6$) and gadolinium ($Z = 64$), for the two prevalent interactions in the diagnostic energy region, the photoelectric (τ) and Compton (σ) effects. Adjacent to the photoelectric attenuation coefficients are dashed lines corresponding to an E^{-3} curve. The E^{-3} curves closely parallel the photoelectric attenuation coefficients for both carbon (τ-6) and gadolinium (τ-64). The Compton-scatter attenuation coefficients are shown, and a line corresponding to E^{0} (i.e., no energy dependency) is drawn across the diagnostic energy range from 10 to 100 keV. This E^{0} line closely parallels both the carbon (σ-6) and gadolinium (σ-64) Compton coefficients.

1.2.3.3 Atomic number

The mass attenuation coefficients as a function of atomic number (Z) are illustrated in Figure 1.30. Coefficients are shown for 20 keV and 60 keV, as indicated in the figure. Lines corresponding to a Z^{4} dependency are shown closely paralleling the photoelectric attenuation coefficients at both energies, although some bowing over occurs at higher Z. The Compton-scattering attenuation coefficients shown in Figure 1.30 are almost horizontal, indicating a Z^{0} dependency (i.e., no Z dependency).

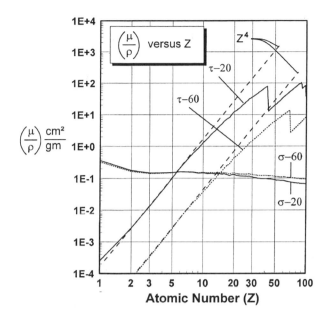

Figure 1.30: The dependency of the *mass attenuation coefficient* on atomic number is illustrated for two x-ray energies (20 keV and 60 keV). The photoelectric-effect cross sections for these two energies (τ-20 and τ-60) are seen to closely parallel dash lines corresponding to a Z^4 dependency. The Compton scattering cross sections at 20 and 60 keV (σ-20 and σ-60) are seen to be essentially constant from helium ($Z = 2$) to Fermium ($Z = 100$). Notice that this plot is for the *mass* attenuation coefficient.

Table 1.2: Attenuation coefficient dependencies

Attenuation Coefficient	Density	Atomic Number	Energy
(τ/ρ)	—	Z^4	$1/E^3$
τ	ρ	Z^3	$1/E^3$
σ	ρ	Z^0 (independent*)	E^0 (independent*)
σ_r	ρ	—	$1/E^{1.2}$

*over the diagnostic x-ray region from 10 to 100 keV.

The linear attenuation coefficient is shown versus the atomic number at 20 keV and 60 keV in Figure 1.31. Because linear attenuation coefficients are significantly effected by the density of the element, there is substantial fluctuation due to the density differences across the elements (recall Figure 1.28). The two dashed lines in Figure 1.31 represent Z^3 dependencies, and there is good agreement between these curves and the data at both x-ray energies. The gases in the periodic table were removed from Figure 1.31. The trends in x-ray attenuation coefficients relevant to diagnostic radiology are summarized below in Table 1.2.

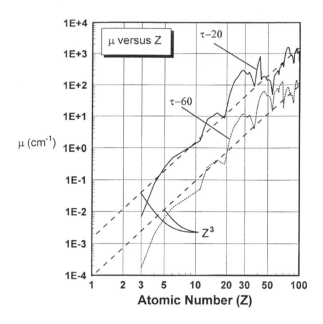

Figure 1.31:   The *linear attenuation coefficient* is shown plotted at two different x-ray energies (20 keV and 60 keV) as a function of atomic number. The linear attenuation coefficient, μ, is dependent upon the density of the element and therefore the density-dependent variations (seen in Figure 1.28) are apparent in this figure as well. Gaseous elements were removed from the graph. The linear attenuation coefficient is seen to closely parallel the dashed lines indicating a Z^3 dependency. Note that the Z^3 dependency is for the *linear* attenuation coefficient.

A $\rho \propto Z^{0.78}$ relationship was noted earlier (Figure 1.28), which is essentially the same as $\rho \propto Z^{3/4}$. Dividing the Z^3 dependency of μ by the $Z^{3/4}$ ρ dependency results in the Z^4 dependency of (μ/ρ).

1.2.4 X-ray beam attenuation

In previous sections of this chapter, the mechanisms of x-ray interaction and the energy and atomic number dependencies of the various interaction types were discussed. In this section, the discussion turns to the properties of x-ray beams that are experimentally observable in the radiology department.

1.2.4.1 Good and bad geometry

Attenuation is the removal of photons from the x-ray beam, both by absorption and scattering. To assess attenuation, the x-ray beam that is *not* removed by attenuation is what is actually measured (the primary x-ray beam). It is important that scattered photons not be included in this measurement. Because scattered x rays tend to fly about in all directions near an object being exposed to an x-ray beam, it is important to use a measurement geometry which excludes the measurement of

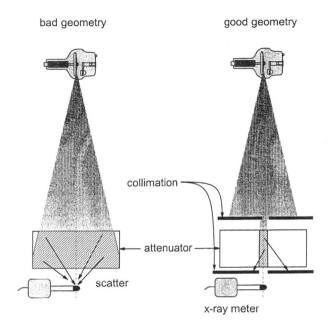

Figure 1.32: The so-called *bad geometry* and *good geometry* for making x-ray attenuation measurements are illustrated. Bad geometry exists whenever the exposure measurement includes an appreciable amount of x-ray scatter from the attenuator. The scatter contribution to the measurement can be reduced by using pre-attenuator collimation to limit the x-ray field and post-attenuator collimation to reduce the chance of scatter reaching the x-ray detector.

scattered x-ray photons, to the extent possible. Figure 1.32 demonstrates *bad* measurement geometry (Figure 1.32(a)), where the placement of the exposure meter near the exit surface of the material will result in a significant contribution of scattered photons to the measured values. *Good* geometry (Figure 1.32(b)) makes use of both pre- and post-material collimators (e.g., sheets of lead), which narrow the x-ray beam substantially. The pre-material collimator limits the area and hence the volume of the material being exposed to radiation, and this will reduce the overall number of scattered photons (specifically, the ratio of scattered to primary photons will be reduced). The post-material collimation serves to limit the scattered photons which are produced in the material so that they have a smaller chance of striking the x-ray exposure meter. Good geometry is also called *narrow-beam* geometry, and bad geometry is also called *broad-beam* geometry.

Another way to reduce the amount of scattered radiation contributing to the measurement is to move the exposure meter away from the scattering material by a reasonable distance. For example, it is a common procedure to measure the attenuation of a number of thin (e.g., 1 mm) aluminum filters (discussed below). For such a measurement, the exposure meter is placed perhaps 100 cm from the x-ray source, and the aluminum filters are placed near at the x-ray tube (typically about 20 cm from the source due to structures near the x-ray tube). Whereas the primary x-ray beam is aimed at the exposure meter and propagates in a straight line from x-ray source to exposure meter, scattered radiation produced in the filters will in general emerge from the filter with a much wider array of angles. With ample separation between the filter(s) and the exposure meter, the scattered radiation will diverge away from the primary beam and a negligible amount of scatter will be detected in this geometry.

1.2.4.2 Polyenergetic versus monoenergetic attenuation

As Figures 1.24, 1.25, and 1.26 illustrate, attenuation coefficients for a given material are energy dependent. For an x-ray beam composed of a single energy of x-ray photons (a monoenergetic beam), the attenuation of that beam will follow a perfect exponential curve according to the Lambert–Beers law (Eq. (1.12) or (1.14)). The dashed lines on Figure 1.33 shows the attenuation plot for aluminum filters (an x-ray filter is just a thin sheet of metal) at several different x-ray energies. The y axis on Figure 1.33 is logarithmic and the x axis is linear (so the plot is *semi-logarithmic*), and thus an exponential falloff will appear as a perfectly straight line, as the dashed monoenergetic lines indicate. For an x-ray spectrum consisting of many different energies (a polyenergetic spectrum), the attenuation curve (solid line on Figure 1.33) has curvature on the semi-log plot, indicating a slight deviation from exponential falloff. The attenuation, $A(x)$, of a polyenergetic x-ray spectrum,

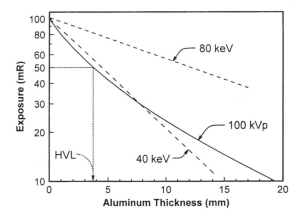

Figure 1.33: Attenuation profiles (exposure as a function of thickness) are shown for aluminum and for three different x-ray beams. The dashed lines are for monoenergetic x-ray beams at 40 keV and 80 keV. Higher-energy x rays are more *penetrating*, so the curve for 80-keV x rays is less steep than the curve for 40-keV x rays. On this semi-logarithmic plot, the attenuation curves for monoenergetic x-ray beams appear as straight lines. For a 100-kVp x-ray spectrum, the attenuation curve demonstrates curvature which is representative of *beam hardening*. The half-value layer (HVL) is the thickness of aluminum required to reduce the exposure of the x-ray beam by 50%. The HVL for the 100-kVp attenuation curve shown is approximately 3.7 mm Al.

$\Phi(E)$, from a sheet of aluminum of thickness x is given by:

$$A(x) = \frac{\int_{E=0}^{E\,max} \alpha \Phi(E)(\xi(E))^{-1} \exp\left(-\frac{\mu(E)_{al}}{\rho}\rho x\right) dE}{\int_{E=0}^{E\,max} \alpha \Phi(E)(\xi(E))^{-1} dE}, \qquad (1.21)$$

where the units of area (α) are mm^2, $\Phi(E)$ is in photons/mm^2 (at each energy E), and the function $\xi^{-1}(E)$ is in the units of mR per (photon/mm^2) (at each energy E). Attenuation is usually measured using an air ionization chamber, which reads out in units of *exposure* (roentgens). The x-ray fluence per unit exposure is given by:

$$\xi(E) = \frac{5.43 \times 10^5}{E\left(\dfrac{\mu_{en}(E)}{\rho}\right)_{air}}. \qquad (1.22a)$$

When the mass energy absorption coefficient for air, $(\mu_{en}/\rho)_{air}$, is in units of cm^2/g, and E is in keV, the units of $\xi(E)$ are photons/mm^2 per mR. $\xi(E)$ describes the photon fluence per unit of exposure, and the inverse function $\xi^{-1}(E)$ describes the exposure per unit of photon fluence. For the energy range from 1 to 150 keV, this can be calculated using:

$$\xi(E) = \left[a + b\sqrt{E}\ln(E) + \frac{c}{E^2}\right]^{-1}, \qquad (1.22b)$$

where $a = -5.023290717769674 \times 10^{-06}$, $b = 1.810595449064631 \times 10^{-07}$, $c = 0.008838658459816926$ ($r^2 = 0.9996$), E is in keV, and $\xi(E)$ is in the units of photons/mm^2 per mR. Figure 1.34 shows $\xi(E)$ over the diagnostic energy range. The $\xi^{-1}(E)$ term shows up in Eq. (1.21) because it describes the energy-dependent response of the measuring device, in this case an air-filled ionization chamber.

1.2.4.3 Half-value layer

An air-ionization exposure meter is a device capable of accurately measuring x-ray exposure. Exposure is a term which relates primarily to the x-ray beam intensity or the *beam quantity*. Measuring the x-ray energy spectrum is much more difficult, and requires sophisticated equipment that is only available in a handful of laboratories. Nevertheless, some idea of the spectral distribution (*beam quality*) of the x-ray beam is needed in the field. The x-ray attenuation coefficients are clearly energy dependent (Figure 1.29), and therefore by measuring the attenuation ($A(x)$ in Eq. (1.21)) of a known material (e.g., aluminum), a parameter relating to the x-ray beam energy distribution ($\Phi(E)$) can be assessed. The parameter used to characterize beam quality in field measurements of attenuation is called the *half-value layer* (HVL). The HVL, usually calculated using aluminum in diagnostic radiology, is the thickness of aluminum required to reduce the exposure of the x-ray beam by a factor of 2 (i.e., to 50% of its unattenuated exposure). *Exposure*

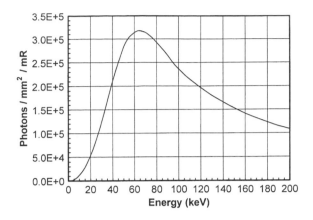

Figure 1.34:   The photon fluence (photons/mm^2) per unit exposure (mR) is shown as a function of x-ray energy across the diagnostically relevant energies. X-ray exposure measured in roentgens (or mR) demonstrates energy dependency because the mass energy absorption coefficient for air is energy dependent. This figure illustrates the function $\xi(E)$ as discussed in the text.

is defined in air (only), and therefore the HVL is properly measured only using an air ionization exposure meter; the HVL measured using a solid state x-ray detector system, for example, will be different.

Figure 1.33 illustrates three attenuation curves. For the two dashed lines corresponding to monoenergetic x-ray beams, the slope of the line (when corrected for units) is the linear attenuation coefficient. The relationship HVL = $\ln(2)/\mu$ can be easily derived. The HVL is shown graphically for the 100-kVp polychromatic x-ray beam shown in Figure 1.33, and is approximately 3.7 mm Al. For higher energy beams the HVL will increase, and for lower kVp beams the HVL will decrease.

1.2.4.4 Beam hardening

Because the polychromatic attenuation profile in Figure 1.33 shows curvature, the slope (proportional to μ) changes depending upon the amount of aluminum filtration present in the beam. This is evidence of *beam hardening*. A *hard* x-ray beam is one with higher energy, a *soft* x-ray beam is a lower-energy beam. Beam hardening is a process whereby the average energy of the x-ray beam increases as that beam passes through increasing thicknesses of an absorber. Beam hardening occurs because as a polyenergetic x-ray beam passes through an absorber, the lower-energy x-ray photons are attenuated more (per unit thickness) than are the higher-energy photons. This is a direct consequence of the energy-dependence of attenuation coefficients, which are higher at lower energies (see for example Figure 1.24).

To demonstrate beam hardening more directly, Figure 1.35 shows the same 100-kVp x-ray spectrum passed through different thicknesses of aluminum. As the thickness of the aluminum increases from 0 mm to 30 mm, two trends are observed:

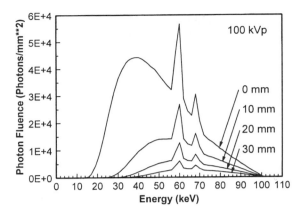

Figure 1.35: X-ray spectra corresponding to different amounts of aluminum filtration are shown. With increasing aluminum filtration thickness (indicated), the area of the x-ray spectra shown is substantially reduced (fewer x-ray photons). In addition, a gradual shift towards higher energies in the more attenuated spectra is observed. The shift in average or effective beam energy with increasing filtration thickness is called *beam hardening*.

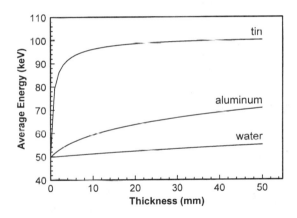

Figure 1.36: The average x-ray energy in a 100-kVp x-ray spectrum is illustrated as a function of thickness for three different attenuators. Fifty millimeters of water produces only a modest increase in average x-ray energy, whereas 50 mm of aluminum causes a more noticeable increase in average energy. Because of the high atomic number and density of tin ($Z = 50$, $\rho = 7.3$ g/cm^3), it has a profound beam-hardening effect.

(1) the number (quantity) of x rays decreases at each energy, and (2) the lower-energy photon fluence decreases proportionately more than the higher-energy fluence, that is, the beam becomes harder. The average energy of a 100-kVp x-ray beam was calculated as the beam was passed through different thicknesses of water, aluminum, and tin, as shown in Figure 1.36. The increase in the average energy of the x-ray spectrum as a function of the thickness of absorber is another direct way to illustrate beam hardening. Higher Z absorbers ($Z_{Al} = 13$, $Z_{Sn} = 50$) cause

more beam hardening per unit thickness, partially because of their higher density, and partially because of the Z^3/E^3 x-ray interaction dependency.

1.3 X-ray spectra

The physics behind the production of x rays was discussed in Section 1.1. In this section, some practical issues and applications of general radiographic and mammographic x-ray spectra are discussed. The conventional notation for *photon fluence* (e.g., photons/mm^2) at a given energy E is $\Phi(E)$. The corresponding *energy fluence* (e.g., joules/mm^2 or $\Phi(E) \times E$) is $\Psi(E)$.

1.3.1 Diagnostic x-ray spectra

1.3.1.1 X-ray filtration

X-ray spectra used for general diagnostic radiology are generally produced with tungsten target x-ray tubes at kVp's ranging between 40 kVp and 150 kVp. Even at the same kVp, each x-ray system will produce slightly different x-ray spectra. The factors which cause the variation between spectra from different x-ray systems include the calibration of the system, the generator waveform (discussed in Section 1.1.2.3), the anode angle, and the amount of filtration which is present both inside and outside the x-ray tube and its housing. The x rays produced at the x-ray tube target must pass through the glass or metal envelope of the x-ray tube, a thin layer of oil, the plastic x-ray tube port (in the housing), a mirror in some cases, in addition to aluminum or other filters which are intentionally placed in the beam (Figure 1.37). The *inherent filtration* of an x-ray tube refers to the objects in the beam path that are a part of the x-ray tube, its housing, and collimator. *Added filtration* refers to the sheets of metal (usually aluminum, but sometimes copper, erbium, or other materials) placed intentionally in the beam. The *total filtration* is the sum of the inherent and added filtration, expressed in terms of aluminum equivalence. The glass x-ray tube envelope is comprised mostly of silicon ($Z = 14$), very similar to aluminum ($Z = 13$), which makes aluminum equivalence possible.

The amount of beam filtration affects the x-ray spectra in a profound way. Because x-ray spectra at the same kVp differ, when referring to beam quality it is common to state both the kVp and the half-value layer (HVL). In the past, a term called the *homogeneity coefficient* was advocated as an additional descriptor of beam quality. The homogeneity coefficient is the ratio of the first HVL to the second HVL.

1.3.1.2 An x-ray spectral model

Many investigators have developed algorithms or models to predict the shape of an x-ray spectrum given the kVp and other parameters of the x-ray beam. A complete review of spectral models will be avoided here, but recent comparisons between various models have been made [3]. Kramer's model [4] for the bremsstrahlung spectrum was one of the first spectral models (1923), and in essence is described by Eq. (1.4). The spectral model of Tucker, Barnes, and

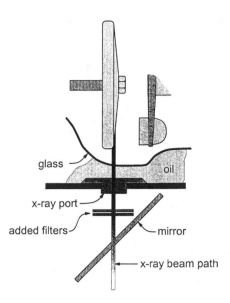

Figure 1.37: A close-up diagram of the components in an x-ray tube which an x-ray beam must pass through is shown. After production and some self filtration in the tungsten anode, x rays must pass through the glass (or sometimes metal) x-ray tube housing, a layer of oil which surrounds the x-ray tube insert for thermal and electrical insulation, the x-ray tube port, and other structures in the beam such as the mirror which is present in the collimation assembly of most clinical x-ray systems. These necessary structures in the x-ray beam constitute the *inherent* filtration. Most clinical x-ray systems have *added* filtration (usually sheets of aluminum) as well.

Chakraborty [5] is commonly used today. This model is semi-empirical, that is its derivation uses principles from basic physics coupled with phenomenological data. The Tucker, Barnes, and Chakraborty model produces high (energy) resolution x-ray spectra with excellent adherence to measured data.

Measured x-ray spectra remain the gold standard of computer-generated models. Boone and Seibert [1] recently developed a completely empirical model, based on the physically measured x-ray spectra published by Thomas Fewell [6]. Because of the accuracy and simplicity of the model (and the familiarity of this author with it), it will be briefly described. The *t*ungsten *a*node *s*pectral *m*odel using *i*nterpolating *p*olynomials (TASMIP) is based on 11 spectra measured photon-by-photon by x-ray spectroscopy. Figure 1.38 illustrates the measured spectra, where each spectrum has been normalized to a tube current of 1.0 mAs. At each energy interval, the photon fluence increases as the kVp is increased, and of course the maximum energy in each spectrum increases with increasing kVp as well. Characteristic x-ray production (the K_α and K_β lines of the tungsten anode) is not seen in spectra below 70 kVp, as described in Section 1.1.2. The vertical lines marked A, B and C in Figure 1.38(a) highlight the 40, 60 and 80 keV energy intervals. The data points where these vertical dashed lines intersect the measured spectra on Fig-

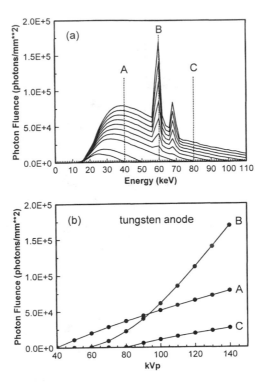

Figure 1.38: The basis of the TASMIP x-ray spectral model is shown. (a) Measured x-ray spectra reported by Fewell are shown. Where each spectra intersects a vertical line (e.g., the dotted line marked "A"), the photon fluence at that energy (e.g., 40 keV) is seen. The photon-fluence values where the dotted line "A" intersects the x-ray spectra are plotted as a function of kVp in (b). A smooth polynomial fit between the measured data points allows the calculation of the 40-keV x-ray photon fluence as a function of kVp. A similar procedure is carried out at all x-ray energies (at 1-keV intervals, the vertical lines marked "B" and "C" illustrate two other examples) to accurately compute an x-ray spectrum at any arbitrary kVp.

ure 1.38(a) are plotted as a function of the kVp as the solid circles in Figure 1.38(b). The lines interpolating the data in Figure 1.38(b) are polynomial fit results to the measured points. It is clear from the figure that an excellent fit is achieved due to the relatively smooth behavior of the data, and this fit was achieved using a maximum of 4 polynomial coefficients. The accuracy of the polynomial fit shown for 3 energies (40, 60, and 80 keV) in Figure 1.38(b) is representative of that for all other energies, and is the accuracy of the TASMIP spectral model.

The TASMIP model uses polynomial interpolation at each energy in the x-ray spectrum, from 0 keV to 140 keV in 1 keV steps. Using predetermined polynomial-fit coefficients ($a_i[E]$) derived from Fewell's measured data, an x-ray spectrum $\Phi(E)$ at any kVp can be computed:

$$\begin{aligned}\Phi(E) &= a_0[E] + a_1[E]\text{kVp} + a_2[E]\text{kVp}^2 + a_3[E]\text{kVp}^3; \quad \text{for } E \leqslant \text{kVp} \\ \Phi(E) &= 0; \qquad\qquad\qquad\qquad\qquad\qquad\qquad\qquad \text{for } E > \text{kVp}.\end{aligned} \quad (1.23)$$

A matrix of 564 coefficients (141 energies × 4 coefficients per energy) provides all the data necessary to reconstruct spectra at any kVp from 30 to 140 kVp. The TASMIP model is accurate both in terms of quality (shape of spectrum) and quantity (mR per mAs per kVp). Because the measured spectra that are the basis of the TASMIP model were from a constant potential generator, integration of the CPG spectra over a sinusoidally fluctuating kV allows the model to be adapted to produce spectra with arbitrary amounts of generator ripple (0%–100%).

The TASMIP model produces x-ray spectra for a naked tube: one with no added filtration. Several representative x-ray spectra generated with the TASMIP model are included in Table 1.3. Using published values for attenuation coefficients of the elements [7], arbitrary filtration can be applied to the naked spectra using the energy-dependent Lambert–Beers law. The coefficients and the source code for the TASMIP model can be downloaded via FTP from ftp://ftp.aip.org/epaps/medical_phys/E-MPHYA-24-1661/. All of the tungsten diagnostic x-ray spectra plotted in this chapter make use of the TASMIP model.

1.3.1.3 Effective versus average energy

It is often convenient to make estimates about the penetration capabilities or dose of an x-ray beam by assuming it is monoenergetic with some average energy. The *average energy* of an x-ray spectrum is calculated as the simple energy-weighted average:

$$\overline{E}_{\text{ave}} = \frac{\int_{E=0}^{E\max} E\Phi(E)\,\mathrm{d}E}{\int_{E=0}^{E\max} \Phi(E)\,\mathrm{d}E}. \tag{1.24}$$

The average energy is a useful measure of a spectrum that is already known (i.e., to compute the average energy, $\Phi(E)$ needs to be known). In many experimental situations, however this is not the case. Usually, only attenuation data are available. In this situation, the *effective energy* can be estimated. The effective energy is assessed as follows: The attenuation factor, N/N_0 (Eq. (1.14)) of a small thickness (t) of aluminum is measured. The monoenergetic Lambert–Beers equation (Eq. (1.14)) is then used (even though a polyenergetic beam was evaluated), and knowing N/N_0 and the aluminum thickness and density, the (μ/ρ) of aluminum is calculated. The value of (μ/ρ) is then compared to a table for aluminum of (μ/ρ) versus energy (Table 1.4 is provided below for this). Using log-log interpolation, the effective energy is calculated as that energy which matches the measured (μ/ρ). Because of beam hardening, if the effective energy of the unattenuated x-ray beam is of interest, the thickness of aluminum used for assessing attenuation should be small, e.g., 0.1 or 0.5 mm.

The average energy of various x-ray spectra is plotted in Figure 1.39. Added aluminum filtration has an appreciable effect on the average energy of the beam. For example, a 140-kVp beam with 0 mm added Al has the same average energy as a 110-kVp beam with 2 mm of added Al. The line which defines $E = 1/2$ kVp is also illustrated in Figure 1.39. For the curve corresponding to 2 mm of added

Table 1.3(a): X-ray spectra for kV 30 through 80. These spectra were generated by the TASMIP model reported in [1]. The spectra are representative of a tungsten anode x-ray tube with a 5% kV ripple (inverter generator), and with no added filtration to the x-ray tube. Each spectrum is normalized to 1.0 mR, and the tabulated numbers refer to the number of photons per mm^2 at each energy bin. Each energy bin has a width of 2 keV, and the number reported is at the center of that bin (e.g., 22.5 includes all 22 and 23 keV photons)

E (keV)	30 kV	40 kV	50 kV	60 kV	70 kV	80 kV
12.5	1.4041e + 2	9.2699e + 1	6.4350e + 1	4.8250e + 1	3.8670e + 1	3.2733e + 1
14.5	1.2540e + 3	6.9331e + 2	4.4926e + 2	3.2983e + 2	2.6301e + 2	2.2024e + 2
16.5	4.0961e + 3	2.4179e + 3	1.6510e + 3	1.2620e + 3	1.0359e + 3	8.8286e + 2
18.5	7.8961e + 3	5.0731e + 3	3.6755e + 3	2.9326e + 3	2.4833e + 3	2.1635e + 3
20.5	1.1621e + 4	7.8266e + 3	5.7929e + 3	4.6650e + 3	3.9624e + 3	3.4521e + 3
22.5	1.3420e + 4	9.9301e + 3	7.7221e + 3	6.4064e + 3	5.5474e + 3	4.8958e + 3
24.5	1.2047e + 4	1.0912e + 4	9.1883e + 3	7.9342e + 3	7.0305e + 3	6.2977e + 3
26.5	7.6392e + 3	1.0562e + 4	9.9433e + 3	9.0129e + 3	8.1916e + 3	7.4466e + 3
28.5	2.5339e + 3	9.5575e + 3	1.0162e + 4	9.6494e + 3	8.9812e + 3	8.2810e + 3
30.5	7.5966e + 2	8.7827e + 3	9.9344e + 3	9.7213e + 3	9.2436e + 3	8.6729e + 3
32.5	—	7.4717e + 3	9.4052e + 3	9.5486e + 3	9.2665e + 3	8.8181e + 3
34.5	—	5.5920e + 3	8.5233e + 3	9.1262e + 3	9.0946e + 3	8.8008e + 3
36.5	—	3.3908e + 3	7.4825e + 3	8.5701e + 3	8.7775e + 3	8.6199e + 3
38.5	—	1.2051e + 3	6.3505e + 3	7.9123e + 3	8.3658e + 3	8.3542e + 3
40.5	—	1.9783e + 2	5.4170e + 3	7.2392e + 3	7.8754e + 3	8.0009e + 3
42.5	—	—	4.3420e + 3	6.4903e + 3	7.3223e + 3	7.5807e + 3
44.5	—	—	3.0938e + 3	5.6070e + 3	6.6620e + 3	7.0749e + 3
46.5	—	—	1.8524e + 3	4.8788e + 3	6.1522e + 3	6.6695e + 3

Table 1.3(a): (Continued)

E (keV)	30 kV	40 kV	50 kV	60 kV	70 kV	80 kV
48.5	—	—	6.2079e + 2	4.0175e + 3	5.5285e + 3	6.2005e + 3
50.5	—	—	5.1687e + 1	3.3862e + 3	5.0105e + 3	5.7392e + 3
52.5	—	—	—	2.6633e + 3	4.4149e + 3	5.2400e + 3
54.5	—	—	—	1.9234e + 3	3.8361e + 3	4.7675e + 3
56.5	—	—	—	1.1592e + 3	3.2128e + 3	4.4267e + 3
58.5	—	—	—	4.3320e + 2	2.6151e + 3	4.5362e + 3
60.5	—	—	—	3.8700e + 1	2.1350e + 3	4.2471e + 3
62.5	—	—	—	—	1.6949e + 3	3.0693e + 3
64.5	—	—	—	—	1.2167e + 3	2.6052e + 3
66.5	—	—	—	—	7.1228e + 2	2.2787e + 3
68.5	—	—	—	—	2.8865e + 2	2.0599e + 3
70.5	—	—	—	—	2.3626e + 1	1.4992e + 3
72.5	—	—	—	—	—	1.0244e + 3
74.5	—	—	—	—	—	7.0927e + 2
76.5	—	—	—	—	—	4.4074e + 2
78.5	—	—	—	—	—	1.6748e + 2
80.5	—	—	—	—	—	4.9339e + 0
82.5	—	—	—	—	—	—

Table 1.3(b): X-ray spectra for kV 90 through 140

E (keV)	90 kV	100 kV	110 kV	120 kV	130 kV	140 kV
12.5	2.9408e + 1	2.8076e + 1	2.8328e + 1	2.9889e + 1	3.2580e + 1	3.6335e + 1
14.5	1.9166e + 2	1.7209e + 2	1.5847e + 2	1.4900e + 2	1.4262e + 2	1.3887e + 2
16.5	7.7304e + 2	6.9046e + 2	6.2544e + 2	5.7221e + 2	5.2747e + 2	4.8997e + 2
18.5	1.9219e + 3	1.7300e + 3	1.5695e + 3	1.4295e + 3	1.3040e + 3	1.1911e + 3
20.5	3.0627e + 3	2.7529e + 3	2.4956e + 3	2.2744e + 3	2.0798e + 3	1.9092e + 3
22.5	4.3815e + 3	3.9607e + 3	3.6027e + 3	3.2881e + 3	3.0062e + 3	2.7550e + 3
24.5	5.6985e + 3	5.2006e + 3	4.7764e + 3	4.4072e + 3	4.0826e + 3	3.8023e + 3
26.5	6.8013e + 3	6.2487e + 3	5.7712e + 3	5.3549e + 3	4.9919e + 3	4.6851e + 3
28.5	7.6354e + 3	7.0647e + 3	6.5634e + 3	6.1235e + 3	5.7408e + 3	5.4209e + 3
30.5	8.1174e + 3	7.6091e + 3	7.1486e + 3	6.7315e + 3	6.3560e + 3	6.0311e + 3
32.5	8.3462e + 3	7.8992e + 3	7.4864e + 3	7.1077e + 3	6.7645e + 3	6.4681e + 3
34.5	8.4309e + 3	8.0547e + 3	7.6927e + 3	7.3510e + 3	7.0349e + 3	6.7588e + 3
36.5	8.3363e + 3	8.0215e + 3	7.7086e + 3	7.4108e + 3	7.1370e + 3	6.9043e + 3
38.5	8.1637e + 3	7.9121e + 3	7.6449e + 3	7.3818e + 3	7.1359e + 3	6.9266e + 3
40.5	7.9135e + 3	7.7389e + 3	7.5276e + 3	7.3032e + 3	7.0807e + 3	6.8816e + 3
42.5	7.5874e + 3	7.4813e + 3	7.3205e + 3	7.1331e + 3	6.9370e + 3	6.7554e + 3
44.5	7.1936e + 3	7.1712e + 3	7.0743e + 3	6.9360e + 3	6.7774e + 3	6.6234e + 3
46.5	6.8440e + 3	6.8582e + 3	6.7936e + 3	6.6912e + 3	6.5759e + 3	6.4746e + 3
48.5	6.4790e + 3	6.5637e + 3	6.5459e + 3	6.4724e + 3	6.3722e + 3	6.2739e + 3
50.5	6.0523e + 3	6.1651e + 3	6.1769e + 3	6.1388e + 3	6.0815e + 3	6.0343e + 3
52.5	5.6269e + 3	5.7970e + 3	5.8537e + 3	5.8506e + 3	5.8201e + 3	5.7923e + 3

Table 1.3(b): (Continued)

E (keV)	90 kV	100 kV	110 kV	120 kV	130 kV	140 kV
54.5	5.2290e + 3	5.4536e + 3	5.5519e + 3	5.5814e + 3	5.5769e + 3	5.5697e + 3
56.5	5.1997e + 3	5.7213e + 3	6.0839e + 3	6.3368e + 3	6.5118e + 3	6.6416e + 3
58.5	6.1952e + 3	7.6210e + 3	8.8341e + 3	9.8486e + 3	1.0680e + 4	1.1365e + 4
60.5	6.1332e + 3	7.7888e + 3	9.2202e + 3	1.0435e + 4	1.1445e + 4	1.2287e + 4
62.5	3.8905e + 3	4.4113e + 3	4.7568e + 3	4.9939e + 3	5.1634e + 3	5.3004e + 3
64.5	3.3657e + 3	3.7955e + 3	4.0415e + 3	4.1821e + 3	4.2642e + 3	4.3243e + 3
66.5	3.2412e + 3	3.8633e + 3	4.2780e + 3	4.5575e + 3	4.7460e + 3	4.8807e + 3
68.5	3.3636e + 3	4.3512e + 3	5.1166e + 3	5.7126e + 3	6.1744e + 3	6.5377e + 3
70.5	2.4521e + 3	3.0236e + 3	3.3986e + 3	3.6756e + 3	3.9116e + 3	4.1484e + 3
72.5	1.8679e + 3	2.3428e + 3	2.6033e + 3	2.7333e + 3	2.7829e + 3	2.7882e + 3
74.5	1.6205e + 3	2.1108e + 3	2.3702e + 3	2.5011e + 3	2.5636e + 3	2.5989e + 3
76.5	1.4117e + 3	1.9449e + 3	2.2378e + 3	2.3971e + 3	2.4852e + 3	2.5449e + 3
78.5	1.1634e + 3	1.7367e + 3	2.0584e + 3	2.2396e + 3	2.3456e + 3	2.4204e + 3
80.5	9.1808e + 2	1.5344e + 3	1.8851e + 3	2.0887e + 3	2.2144e + 3	2.3084e + 3
82.5	7.1349e + 2	1.3421e + 3	1.7189e + 3	1.9496e + 3	2.0967e + 3	2.2025e + 3
84.5	4.8875e + 2	1.1681e + 3	1.5858e + 3	1.8341e + 3	1.9687e + 3	2.0285e + 3
86.5	2.8812e + 2	9.8687e + 2	1.4256e + 3	1.6952e + 3	1.8508e + 3	1.9311e + 3
88.5	1.1417e + 2	8.3759e + 2	1.3085e + 3	1.5956e + 3	1.7589e + 3	1.8399e + 3
90.5	1.6034e + 1	6.6597e + 2	1.1487e + 3	1.4526e + 3	1.6357e + 3	1.7380e + 3
92.5	—	5.1067e + 2	1.0017e − 3	1.3264e + 3	1.5381e + 3	1.6738e + 3
94.5	—	3.4443e + 2	8.5128e + 2	1.1946e + 3	1.4266e + 3	1.5831e + 3

Table 1.3(b): (Continued)

E (keV)	90 kV	100 kV	110 kV	120 kV	130 kV	140 kV
96.5	—	2.0025e + 2	7.3319e + 2	1.0897e + 3	1.3249e + 3	1.4779e + 3
98.5	—	8.1678e + 1	6.2347e + 2	9.9641e + 2	1.2337e + 3	1.3787e + 3
100.5	—	9.1437e + 0	4.9802e + 2	8.9004e + 2	1.1484e + 3	1.3156e + 3
102.5	—	—	3.9163e + 2	7.9410e + 2	1.0544e + 3	1.2176e + 3
104.5	—	—	2.5404e + 2	6.7885e + 2	9.7059e + 2	1.1707e + 3
106.5	—	—	1.4442e + 2	5.8073e + 2	8.6832e + 2	1.0500e + 3
108.5	—	—	5.7694e + 1	4.7524e + 2	7.7011e + 2	9.5777e + 2
110.5	—	—	6.7636e + 0	3.7605e + 2	6.7908e + 2	8.7644e + 2
112.5	—	—	—	2.8230e + 2	5.9396e + 2	8.0933e + 2
114.5	—	—	—	1.9598e + 2	5.3963e + 2	7.6965e + 2
116.5	—	—	—	1.0504e + 2	4.4143e + 2	6.7960e + 2
118.5	—	—	—	4.2549e + 1	3.8039e + 2	6.2953e + 2
120.5	—	—	—	5.6427e + 0	3.0589e + 2	5.5806e + 2
122.5	—	—	—	—	2.1356e + 2	4.5881e + 2
124.5	—	—	—	—	1.4691e + 2	4.1016e + 2
126.5	—	—	—	—	8.7554e + 1	3.6789e + 2
128.5	—	—	—	—	3.3858e + 1	1.6223e + 2
130.5	—	—	—	—	5.1404e + 0	1.3014e + 2
132.5	—	—	—	—	3.2930e + 0	1.5441e + 2
134.5	—	—	—	—	—	9.5672e + 1
136.5	—	—	—	—	—	6.4766e + 1
138.5	—	—	—	—	—	3.1858e + 1

Table 1.4: Mass attenuation coefficients of aluminum ($\rho = 2.699$)

E (keV)	$(\mu/\rho)_{al}$	E (keV)	$(\mu/\rho)_{al}$
10	26.048	50	0.368
11	19.678	55	0.315
12	15.330	60	0.278
13	12.264	65	0.252
14	9.731	70	0.230
15	7.980	75	0.214
16	6.576	80	0.202
17	5.500	85	0.192
18	4.647	90	0.183
19	4.034	95	0.177
20	3.423	100	0.171
25	1.830	105	0.166
30	1.131	110	0.161
35	0.769	115	0.157
40	0.567	120	0.153
45	0.446		

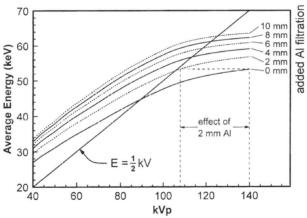

Figure 1.39: The average spectral energy as a function of kVp is shown for different amounts of added aluminum filtration. In the 80- to 100-kVp region, the average energy of the spectrum is approximately $1/2$ of the kVp. The dashed line illustrates the effect of 2 mm of added aluminum filtration.

Al, the average x-ray energy is $1/2$ of the kVp at about 105 kVp (recognizing that keV and kVp are different units); below this, the average is slightly higher than $1/2$ kVp. Federal regulations (21 CFR, Ch. I, §1020.30, 1994) require minimum HVLs at different kVps, for example HVL $= 1.2$ mm Al at 51 kVp, 1.5 mm at 70 kVp, 2.3 mm at 80 kVp, and 2.7 mm at 100 kVp. At the time of this writing, there is a move afoot (in the form of draft standards) to increase these minimum HVLs to 1.3, 1.8, 2.8, and 3.6 mm Al, respectively.

The HVL, average and effective energies for a variety of x-ray spectra are indicated in Table 1.5.

1.3.1.4 X-ray fluence

The number of x-ray quanta striking a detector per unit area (the x-ray fluence) is an important experimental parameter in determining the detective quantum efficiency of a detector system, as discussed elsewhere in this book. However, the fluence is not directly measurable in most laboratories. Knowledge of the x-ray spectrum and the exposure (mR) measured at the detector is needed to calculate the photon fluence. Previously in Eq. (1.22), the function $\xi(E)$ was defined, which is the energy-dependent (monoenergetic) photon fluence per exposure (photons/mm^2 per mR). It's inverse function, $\xi^{-1}(E)$, gives the exposure per fluence (mR per photons/mm^2). If the spectrum incident on a detector system, $\Phi(E)$, is known (for instance, it could be generated by the spectral model described in Section 1.3.1.2), and the exposure (X, in mR) measured at the detector is known, the photon fluence per exposure for the entire spectrum can be calculated using:

$$\widehat{\Phi}_{\text{spectrum}} = \frac{\int_{E=0}^{E\,\text{max}} \Phi(E)\,\mathrm{d}E}{\int_{E=0}^{E\,\text{max}} \Phi(E)\xi(E)^{-1}\,\mathrm{d}E}, \qquad (1.25)$$

where the units of $\widehat{\Phi}_{\text{spectrum}}$ are in photons/mm^2 per mR. The photon fluence, Φ (in photons/mm^2), at a specific exposure level (X) is then just:

$$\Phi = X\widehat{\Phi}_{\text{spectrum}}. \qquad (1.26)$$

For convenience, the values of $\widehat{\Phi}_{\text{spectrum}}$ for a variety of spectra were calculated using Eq. (1.25), and these values are incorporated into Table 1.5. Armed with the kVp, the HVL, and the exposure, the x-ray fluence for a wide range of spectra can be estimated.

1.3.2 Mammography x-ray spectra

Breast imaging is unique in radiography, because of the very small amount of subject contrast exhibited by the breast. In general diagnostic radiology, contrast is created by air-filled lungs, calcium-laden bones, or iodine- filled vessels. In mammography, contrast is formed by local differences in the density and composition of the breast tissue itself. In order to achieve reasonable subject contrast, therefore, the x-ray energies used are much lower than in general diagnostic radiology. At lower energies, the attenuation coefficients for tissue increase, and this contributes directly toward better subject contrast.

The x-ray tube design for mammography systems is slightly different that that shown in Figure 1.6, but the basic functionality remains the same. The biggest difference in mammography is the use of molybdenum and sometimes rhodium as

Table 1.5: Beam-quality parameters (HVL in mm Al, E_{ave} and E_{eff} in keV) and photons/cm^2 per R for beams of different kV and added filtration ($F = $ mm Al)

kV-F	HVL	E_{ave}	E_{eff}	Φ/R	kV-F	HVL	E_{ave}	E_{eff}	Φ/R
30-0	0.80	22.3	19.9	6.141e + 7	80-0	2.29	41.3	27.0	1.553e + 8
30-1	0.97	23.3	21.5	6.923e + 7	80-1	2.95	43.4	30.3	1.770e + 8
30-2	1.09	24.0	22.5	7.483e + 7	80-2	3.47	44.9	32.8	1.929e + 8
30-3	1.19	24.6	23.3	7.920e + 7	80-3	3.91	46.2	34.7	2.054e + 8
30-4	1.27	25.0	23.9	8.280e + 7	80-4	4.30	47.3	36.5	2.156e + 8
30-5	1.34	25.4	24.4	8.588e + 7	80-5	4.63	48.2	37.9	2.242e + 8
40-0	1.12	26.6	21.9	8.371e + 7	85-0	2.44	42.9	27.4	1.616e + 8
40-1	1.41	28.1	24.1	9.659e + 7	85-1	3.13	45.0	30.9	1.836e + 8
40-2	1.63	29.1	25.6	1.062e + 8	85-2	3.69	46.6	33.5	1.996e + 8
40-3	1.82	29.9	26.8	1.138e + 8	85-3	4.16	47.9	35.5	2.120e + 8
40-4	1.98	30.6	27.7	1.202e + 8	85-4	4.56	49.0	37.2	2.222e + 8
40-5	2.12	31.1	28.6	1.256e + 8	85-5	4.91	49.9	38.8	2.306e + 8
50-0	1.44	30.8	23.7	1.057e + 8	90-0	2.58	44.4	27.8	1.673e + 8
50-1	1.84	32.4	26.3	1.222e + 8	90-1	3.31	46.5	31.4	1.894e + 8
50-2	2.15	33.6	28.0	1.346e + 8	90-2	3.90	48.2	34.1	2.053e + 8
50-3	2.41	34.6	29.5	1.444e + 8	90-3	4.39	49.5	36.2	2.177e + 8
50-4	2.63	35.3	30.7	1.526e + 8	90-4	4.81	50.6	38.0	2.276e + 8
50-5	2.83	36.0	31.6	1.596e + 8	90-5	5.18	51.6	39.6	2.359e + 8
55-0	1.59	32.7	24.4	1.158e + 8	100-0	2.86	47.2	28.7	1.770e + 8
55-1	2.04	34.5	27.0	1.337e + 8	100-1	3.67	49.4	32.4	1.990e + 8
55-2	2.39	35.7	29.0	1.471e + 8	100-2	4.31	51.0	35.1	2.145e + 8
55-3	2.68	36.8	30.6	1.579e + 8	100-3	4.84	52.3	37.4	2.264e + 8
55-4	2.94	37.6	31.8	1.668e + 8	100-4	5.30	53.5	39.5	2.358e + 8
55-5	3.16	38.3	33.0	1.744e + 8	100-5	5.69	54.5	41.3	2.435e + 8
60-0	1.74	34.5	24.9	1.250e + 8	110-0	3.15	49.7	29.4	1.848e + 8
60-1	2.22	36.3	27.8	1.440e + 8	110-1	4.02	51.9	33.4	2.063e + 8
60-2	2.61	37.7	29.8	1.582e + 8	110-2	4.71	53.6	36.3	2.212e + 8
60-3	2.94	38.8	31.5	1.696e + 8	110-3	5.27	54.9	38.7	2.323e + 8
60-4	3.22	39.7	32.9	1.791e + 8	110-4	5.75	56.1	40.9	2.411e + 8
60-5	3.47	40.4	34.1	1.871e + 8	110-5	6.16	57.1	42.8	2.482e + 8
65-0	1.88	36.2	25.5	1.332e + 8	120-0	3.43	52.0	30.1	1.910e + 8
65-1	2.40	38.1	28.5	1.531e + 8	120-1	4.37	54.2	34.3	2.118e + 8
65-2	2.82	39.5	30.6	1.679e + 8	120-2	5.09	55.9	37.3	2.259e + 8
65-3	3.18	40.6	32.3	1.797e + 8	120-3	5.68	57.3	39.8	2.363e + 8
65-4	3.49	41.5	33.9	1.895e + 8	120-4	6.17	58.5	42.3	2.443e + 8
65-5	3.75	42.4	35.0	1.979e + 8	120-5	6.60	59.6	44.1	2.508e + 8
70-0	2.01	37.9	26.1	1.410e + 8	130-1	4.71	56.4	35.0	2.158e + 8
70-1	2.58	39.9	29.1	1.616e + 8	130-2	5.46	58.1	38.3	2.291e + 8
70-2	3.04	41.3	31.4	1.770e + 8	130-3	6.06	59.5	41.1	2.387e + 8
70-3	3.42	42.5	33.3	1.892e + 8	130-4	6.57	60.7	43.4	2.460e + 8
70-4	3.75	43.5	34.7	1.992e + 8	130-5	7.00	61.8	45.2	2.518e + 8
70-5	4.05	44.3	36.0	2.077e + 8	140-0	4.00	56.1	31.4	1.998e + 8

Table 1.5: (Continued)

kV-F	HVL	E_{ave}	E_{eff}	Φ/R	kV-F	HVL	E_{ave}	E_{eff}	Φ/R
75-0	2.15	39.7	26.6	1.484e + 8	140-1	5.03	58.3	35.9	2.189e + 8
75-1	2.76	41.7	29.7	1.697e + 8	140-2	5.79	60.0	39.3	2.312e + 8
75-2	3.26	43.2	32.0	1.854e + 8	140-3	6.41	61.4	42.2	2.401e + 8
75-3	3.67	44.4	34.0	1.978e + 8	140-4	6.92	62.7	44.4	2.468e + 8
75-4	4.03	45.4	35.6	2.080e + 8	140-5	7.36	63.8	46.5	2.520e + 8
75-5	4.34	46.3	37.0	2.166e + 8					

the anode (target) material, instead of tungsten. In mammography, the characteristic x-ray component of the entrance spectrum plays a more important role (it is a higher fraction of the fluence). The use of Mo and Rh is advantageous in mammography because the energies of their characteristic x-ray lines are near ideal for imaging the breast.

1.3.2.1 K-edge filtration

X-ray spectra produced in mammography are shaped by K-edge filtration. The most commonly used x-ray spectrum for screen-film mammography is produced by a Mo anode with a 30-μm Mo filter. The pre- and post-filtered spectra are illustrated in Figure 1.40. The K edge of Mo is 20.0 keV, while the characteristic x-ray emissions are at 17.4 keV (K_α) and 19.6 keV (K_β). The Mo filter acts to significantly reduce energies in the exit x-ray spectrum above 20.0 keV, because the attenuation coefficient increases abruptly at that energy. The K_α and K_β emissions from the Mo anode, therefore, pass through the filter just below the K edge, escaping the massive attenuation of the filter. The filter, therefore, reduces the bremsstrahlung component of the x-ray spectrum above the K edge, but has significantly less effect on the characteristic x rays.

The K edge of rhodium is 23.3 keV, and the characteristic x rays are at 20.2 keV (K_α) and 22.7 keV (K_β). A Rh-Rh spectrum is illustrated in Figure 1.41. The slightly higher energies of the rhodium spectrum are better for imaging thick, dense breasts, and reduce the glandular dose relative to a Mo-Mo spectrum. One of the downsides of rhodium is its low heat conductivity, making it a less-than-optimal x-ray target material. One approach to this problem used by some mammography system manufacturers is to use a molybdenum anode with a rhodium filter, and a Mo-Rh spectrum is illustrated in Figure 1.42.

1.3.2.2 Mammography spectral models

The TASMIP model presented previously in Section 1.3.1.2 was extended to x-ray spectra at low energies ranging from 18 kV to 42 kV, for tungsten (TASMIP), molybdenum (MASMIP) and rhodium (RASMIP) anodes [8]. The modeled spectra include no added filtration, other than the beryllium window of the x-ray tube.

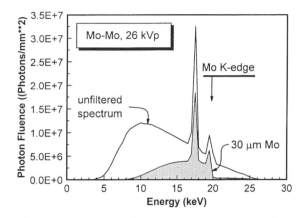

Figure 1.40: A molybdenum-anode x-ray spectrum produced at 26 kVp is illustrated. Adding 30 μm of Mo reduces much of the low-energy component of the x-ray spectrum, but also causes drastic attenuation of x-ray energies above the 20-keV K-edge of molybdenum.

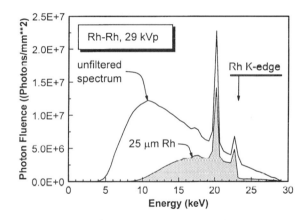

Figure 1.41: A rhodium anode spectrum produced at 29 kVp is illustrated. With the use of 25 μm of Rh, x rays in the unfiltered spectrum are significantly attenuated above the 23-keV rhodium K edge.

The influence of filtration can be added analytically with the appropriate attenuation coefficients. X-ray spectra from 20 to 40 kVp are shown in Figure 1.43(a), where the data intersecting vertical lines marked A, B and C are replotted in Figure 1.43(b) as a function of kVp. Again, the data at each energy interval (at 0.5 keV intervals) is fit with a low-order polynomial of the form given in Eq. (1.23). The ability of the spectral model to interpolate x-ray spectra at any arbitrary kVp between 18 and 42 kVp is essentially as good as the fit of the line to the data points in Figure 1.43(b). Curve B on Figure 1.43(b) rises more quickly than the other two curves because it includes both characteristic and bremsstrahlung x rays, whereas curves A and C include only bremsstrahlung production. The fit coeffi-

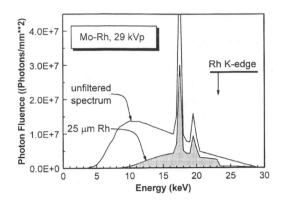

Figure 1.42: Because rhodium has poor heat loading properties, some x-ray system manufacturers make use of a molybdenum anode with rhodium filtration for patients with thicker breasts. The resulting filtered x-ray spectrum has the characteristic x rays from the molybdenum anode; however, the higher K edge of the rhodium filter allows more high-energy photons from the bremsstrahlung spectrum to be used for imaging.

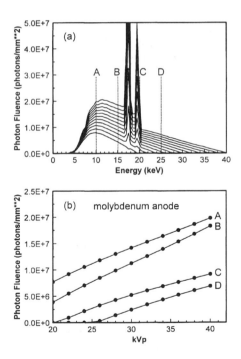

Figure 1.43: The basis of the MAMSIP spectral model is illustrated. Measured x-ray spectra from an unfiltered molybdenum x-ray tube are shown in (a). The photon fluence values where the four dotted lines (A, B, C, and D) intersect the x-ray spectra are plotted as a function of kilovoltage in (b). The smooth polynomial fit between data points allows the accurate interpolation of molybdenum anode spectra from 20 to 40 kVp.

cients and source code (in C) for producing tungsten, molybdenum, and rhodium anode spectra from 18 to 42 kVp can be downloaded at: ftp://ftp.aip.org/epaps/ medical_phys/E-MPHYA-24-1863/. In addition, selected x-ray spectra are listed in Table 1.6.

Table 1.6(a): Molybdenum anode spectra: no filtration

E (keV)	24 kVp	26 kVp	28 kVp	30 kVp
1.0	0.000000e + 0	0.000000e + 0	0.000000e + 0	0.000000e + 0
3.5	0.000000e + 0	0.000000e + 0	0.000000e + 0	0.000000e + 0
4.0	2.168454e + 5	2.469530e + 5	2.770607e + 5	3.071684e + 5
4.5	3.999241e + 5	4.350492e + 5	4.701742c + 5	5.052992c + 5
5.0	9.092965e + 5	9.657390e + 5	1.014266e + 6	1.056758e + 6
5.5	1.852189e + 6	1.960539e + 6	2.049339e + 6	2.124331e + 6
6.0	3.119855e + 6	3.309601e + 6	3.469491e + 6	3.608953e + 6
6.5	4.650150e + 6	4.996463e + 6	5.303326e + 6	5.582671e + 6
7.0	6.127157e + 6	6.591696e + 6	6.995506e + 6	7.352480e + 6
7.5	7.323179e + 6	7.861959e + 6	8.311591e + 6	8.688195e + 6
8.0	8.816939e + 6	9.648488e + 6	1.040242e + 7	1.109829e + 7
8.5	9.744869c + 6	1.073298c + 7	1.164722c + 7	1.250294c + 7
9.0	1.017125e + 7	1.121718e + 7	1.218125e + 7	1.308617e + 7
9.5	1.052994e + 7	1.168005e + 7	1.274322e + 7	1.373953e + 7
10.0	1.078209e + 7	1.203422e + 7	1.321004e + 7	1.433114e + 7
10.5	1.055093e + 7	1.182458e + 7	1.302850e + 7	1.418089e + 7
11.0	1.050428e + 7	1.180559e + 7	1.303235e + 7	1.421311e + 7
11.5	1.027428e + 7	1.163264e + 7	1.293052e + 7	1.418889e + 7
12.0	9.852025c + 6	1.121500c + 7	1.251509c + 7	1.377545e + 7
12.5	9.514555e + 6	1.092186e + 7	1.227247e + 7	1.358532e + 7
13.0	9.146336e + 6	1.053346e + 7	1.185158e + 7	1.312835e + 7
13.5	8.693804e + 6	1.008299e + 7	1.140956e + 7	1.269948e + 7
14.0	8.319038e + 6	9.725328e + 6	1.106972e + 7	1.237810e + 7
14.5	7.903160e + 6	9.325130e + 6	1.068597e + 7	1.200848e + 7
15.0	7.474432e + 6	8.910901e + 6	1.029220e + 7	1.163842e + 7
15.5	7.029001e + 6	8.480355e + 6	9.879208e + 6	1.124576e + 7
16.0	6.599079e + 6	8.062833e + 6	9.475738e + 6	1.085751e + 7
16.5	6.177217e + 6	7.666756e + 6	9.107388e + 6	1.052083e + 7
17.0	7.145661e + 6	1.007846e + 7	1.339359e + 7	1.708380e + 7
17.5	1.813264e + 7	3.255515e + 7	5.073442e + 7	7.239240e + 7
18.0	5.144513e + 6	6.901680e + 6	8.703759e + 6	1.056293e + 7
18.5	4.343736e + 6	5.771161e + 6	7.127452e + 6	8.436007e + 6
19.0	4.002346e + 6	5.471549e + 6	6.855257e + 6	8.185104e + 6
19.5	5.776796e + 6	9.425190e + 6	1.360870e + 7	1.832734e + 7
20.0	3.634076e + 6	5.697850e + 6	7.932522e + 6	1.033809e + 7
20.5	2.160767e + 6	3.277868e + 6	4.290026e + 6	5.215497e + 6
21.0	1.877515e + 6	3.018487e + 6	4.027336e + 6	4.932174e + 6

Table 1.6(a): (Continued)

E (keV)	24 kVp	26 kVp	28 kVp	30 kVp
21.5	1.566618e + 6	2.714635e + 6	3.748660e + 6	4.689933e + 6
22.0	1.305165e + 6	2.430054e + 6	3.451361e + 6	4.389296e + 6
22.5	9.111148e + 5	2.098340e + 6	3.165018e + 6	4.134167e + 6
23.0	5.580079e + 5	1.746117e + 6	2.833457e + 6	3.834781e + 6
23.5	2.062546e + 5	1.443997e + 6	2.542022e + 6	3.529125e + 6
24.0	7.354580e + 4	1.250441e + 6	2.322551e + 6	3.309835e + 6
24.5	—	9.350390e + 5	1.984457e + 6	2.993946e + 6
25.0	—	5.749190e + 5	1.688290e + 6	2.746487e + 6
25.5	—	3.106394e + 5	1.395636e + 6	2.432963e + 6
26.0	—	1.134157e + 5	1.179982e + 6	2.202884e + 6
26.5	—	—	8.765686e + 5	1.930345e + 6
27.0	—	—	4.558535e + 5	1.643381e + 6
27.5	—	—	3.223758e + 5	1.379634e + 6
28.0	—	—	1.026308e + 5	1.132229e + 6
28.5	—	—	—	8.447219e + 5
29.0	—	—	—	5.594563e + 5
29.5	—	—	—	3.093706e + 5
30.0	—	—	—	1.172057e + 5
30.5	—	—	—	—

Table 1.6(b): Rhodium anode spectra: no filtration

E (keV)	28 kVp	30 kVp	32 kVp	34 kVp
4.2	1.242933e + 5	1.310178e + 5	1.363199e + 5	1.401996e + 5
4.7	4.079981e + 5	4.268786e + 5	4.429328e + 5	4.561607e + 5
5.2	1.072115e + 6	1.113302e + 6	1.145819e + 6	1.169665e + 6
5.7	2.322837e + 6	2.412483e + 6	2.485368e + 6	2.544024e + 6
6.2	4.015591e + 6	4.217439e + 6	4.394266e + 6	4.548677e + 6
6.7	5.386873e + 6	5.656281e + 6	5.892197e + 6	6.101146e + 6
7.2	6.705502e + 6	7.087948e + 6	7.429481e + 6	7.735966e + 6
7.7	7.996216e + 6	8.512158e + 6	8.984970e + 6	9.419946e + 6
8.2	9.179753e + 6	9.808665e + 6	1.038732e + 7	1.092315e + 7
8.7	1.009174e + 7	1.083515e + 7	1.152443e + 7	1.216416e + 7
9.2	1.068639e + 7	1.153529e + 7	1.233263e + 7	1.308435e + 7
9.7	1.111798e + 7	1.206559e + 7	1.295234e + 7	1.377823e + 7
10.2	1.140856e + 7	1.238542e + 7	1.330254e + 7	1.416666e + 7
10.7	1.167703e + 7	1.278485e + 7	1.384662e + 7	1.486937e + 7
11.2	1.150456e + 7	1.262619e + 7	1.370595e + 7	1.474844e + 7
11.7	1.123614e + 7	1.237156e + 7	1.346939e + 7	1.453822e + 7
12.2	1.080819e + 7	1.196374e + 7	1.308385e + 7	1.417311e + 7
12.7	1.055307e + 7	1.173922e + 7	1.288941e + 7	1.400363e + 7

Table 1.6(b):   (Continued)

E (keV)	28 kVp	30 kVp	32 kVp	34 kVp
13.2	1.023168e + 7	1.140977e + 7	1.255328e + 7	1.366801e + 7
13.7	9.799955e + 6	1.098702e + 7	1.213848e + 7	1.325434e + 7
14.2	9.441645e + 6	1.062976e + 7	1.178654e + 7	1.291515e + 7
14.7	9.014747e + 6	1.019395e + 7	1.133610e + 7	1.244119e + 7
15.2	8.602827e + 6	9.750894e + 6	1.086698e + 7	1.195712e + 7
15.7	8.292284e + 6	9.505792e + 6	1.067377e + 7	1.178859e + 7
16.2	7.804667e + 6	8.942324e + 6	1.004904e + 7	1.113218e + 7
16.7	7.388224e + 6	8.492114e + 6	9.573392e + 6	1.064793e + 7
17.2	7.459002e + 6	8.782891e + 6	1.011712e + 7	1.147341e + 7
17.7	7.112976e + 6	8.483571e + 6	9.865162e + 6	1.126370e + 7
18.2	6.231245e + 6	7.325712e + 6	8.392394e + 6	9.442261e + 6
18.7	5.757882e + 6	6.876423e + 6	7.973396e + 6	9.048804e + 6
19.2	5.542590e + 6	6.630491e + 6	7.685562e + 6	8.722657e + 6
19.7	6.574850e + 6	8.644817e + 6	1.090517e + 7	1.335589e + 7
20.2	1.740023e + 7	2.880568e + 7	4.262994e + 7	5.853612e + 7
20.7	5.040804e + 6	6.679112e + 6	8.412025e + 6	1.021557e + 7
21.2	4.048115e + 6	5.077471e + 6	6.063153e + 6	7.020463e + 6
21.7	3.727333e + 6	4.751799e + 6	5.724808e + 6	6.661818e + 6
22.2	3.446276e + 6	4.544899e + 6	5.619037e + 6	6.668690e + 6
22.7	5.369859e + 6	8.341698e + 6	1.172659e + 7	1.547337e + 7
23.2	3.181176e + 6	4.597299e + 6	6.067501e + 6	7.591783e + 6
23.7	2.088654e + 6	2.941364e + 6	3.746706e + 6	4.504680e + 6
24.2	1.901944e + 6	2.709544e + 6	3.477765e + 6	4.206606e + 6
24.7	1.663972e + 6	2.500517e + 6	3.281741e + 6	4.007643e + 6
25.2	1.422478e + 6	2.261888e + 6	3.040427e + 6	3.765589e + 6
25.7	1.130158e + 6	1.988829e + 6	2.791033e + 6	3.536771e + 6
26.2	1.000857e + 6	1.803626e + 6	2.573315e + 6	3.309923e + 6
26.7	7.778111e + 5	1.575618e + 6	2.346923e + 6	3.091725e + 6
27.2	4.879170e + 5	1.307107e + 6	2.085432e + 6	2.822892e + 6
27.7	1.786739e + 5	1.086114e + 6	1.932466e + 6	2.717732e + 6
28.2	—	9.399850e + 5	1.701545e + 6	2.425377e + 6
28.7	—	6.489060e + 5	1.462619e + 6	2.232833e + 6
29.2	—	4.493947e + 5	1.241378e + 6	1.999084e + 6
29.7	—	1.880425e + 5	1.038327e + 6	1.824158e + 6
30.2	—	—	8.365925e + 5	1.622371e + 6
30.7	—	—	5.989440e + 5	1.371488e + 6
31.2	—	—	4.436790e + 5	1.196538e + 6
31.7	—	—	2.419280e + 5	9.390916e + 5
32.2	—	—	—	7.863929e + 5
32.7	—	—	—	6.572636e + 5
33.2	—	—	—	4.193790e + 5
33.7	—	—	—	1.907164e + 5
34.2	—	—	—	—

1.4 X-ray dosimetry

1.4.1 Exposure

X rays are silent, tasteless, and invisible. How do we measure them? X rays interact with matter by causing ionization, and this fact allows an x-ray beam to be measured using the ionization it produces. An *ionization chamber* is an air-filled chamber surrounded by electrodes (a positive and negative electrode). X rays ionize the molecules of air present in the chamber, and the electrons follow the electric field lines and are collected on the positive electrode, while the positive ions are collected on the negative electrode. The net charge is collected on the electrodes. The traditional unit of exposure is the roentgen (R), where:

$$1\,R = 2.58 \times 10^{-4}\,C/kg. \tag{1.27}$$

A typical ionization chamber for general diagnostic measurements has a volume of approximately 6 cm^3. At standard temperature and pressure, the mass of air in 6 cm^3 is about 7.8 mg. A 1-R exposure will liberate a charge of 2.0×10^{-9} coulombs inside the chamber, corresponding to 1.2×10^{10} ions. The roentgen is defined only in air, and under conditions of electron equilibrium. Electron equilibrium occurs when the number of energetic ions entering the measurement volume equal those leaving it. These conditions are met in modern exposure chambers for x-ray beams found in diagnostic radiology. For mammographic x-ray beams, special thin window chambers should be used for accurate exposure measurements.

It has been found empirically that on average, it takes 33.97 eV to produce an ion pair in air, and this is equal to 33.97 joules/C. This value is given the symbol W. Thus the energy absorbed in air by a 1-R exposure is:

$$2.58 \times 10^{-4}\,C/kg \times 33.97\,J/C = 0.00876\,J/kg = 87.6\,ergs/g. \tag{1.28}$$

Because one Rad $= 100\,erg/g$, an exposure (X) in air corresponds to a dose (also called *absorbed dose*) in air, D_{air}, of:

$$D_{air} = 0.876X. \tag{1.29}$$

Since one Gray $= J/kg$ (and thus 1 Gy $= 100$ Rads), a 1-R exposure corresponds to a dose in air of 8.76 mGy. If x rays are incident upon a medium other than air, the dose to that medium is related to that in air by:

$$D_{med} = D_{air} \frac{\left(\dfrac{\mu_{en}}{\rho}\right)_{med}}{\left(\dfrac{\mu_{en}}{\rho}\right)_{air}}. \tag{1.30}$$

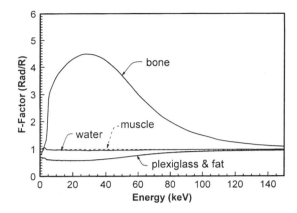

Figure 1.44: The F factor (roentgen-to-Rad conversion factor) is illustrated as a function of x-ray energy for several materials. The F factor for water and muscle are very similar, as are the F factors for plexiglas and fat. Because of the relatively high atomic number of calcium ($Z = 20$) present in bone, the F factor is substantially higher at low x-ray energies.

Combining Eqs. (1.29) and (1.30):

$$D_{med} = 0.876 \frac{\left(\dfrac{\mu_{en}}{\rho}\right)_{med}}{\left(\dfrac{\mu_{en}}{\rho}\right)_{air}} X. \tag{1.31}$$

The F factor, f, is a term defined as:

$$f = 0.876 \frac{\left(\dfrac{\mu_{en}}{\rho}\right)_{med}}{\left(\dfrac{\mu_{en}}{\rho}\right)_{air}}, \tag{1.32}$$

and so:

$$D_{med} = f X. \tag{1.33}$$

The F factor is energy-dependent for all media other than air. Figure 1.44 illustrates the F factor for various tissue types. The F factor is also called the *roentgen-to-Rad conversion factor*.

The roentgen and the Rad are traditional units, whereas C/kg (C/kg $= 3876$ R) and the Gray are proper SI units. Air Kerma is sometimes used as a substitute for exposure (especially in Europe), and is discussed below.

1.4.2 Kerma

Kerma stands for the *kinetic energy released in media*, and for a monoenergetic photon beam of N photons/cm^2 and energy E, Kerma (K) is defined as:

$$K = kNE\left(\frac{\mu_{\text{tr}}}{\rho}\right)_{\text{med}}. \qquad (1.34)$$

With E in keV, N in cm^{-2}, and $(\mu_{\text{tr}}/\rho)_{\text{med}}$ in cm^2/g, setting the constant $k = 1.6021 \times 10^{-11}$ (Rad/keV) allows K to be expressed in Rads, and with $k = 1.6021 \times 10^{-13}$ (Gray/keV), K is in the units of Gy. For a polyenergetic x-ray beam:

$$K = k \int_{E=0}^{E\max} \Phi(E)\left(\frac{\mu_{\text{tr}}(E)}{\rho}\right)_{\text{med}} E\,\mathrm{d}E. \qquad (1.35)$$

When $\Phi(E)$ is in the units of photons/cm^2 (different from previous usage) and the other units and constants are as in Eq. (1.34), the units of Kerma are the same units as for dose (Rad or Gray). Using the spectral models discussed previously, the Kerma corresponding to a 1-R exposure in air and in water was calculated for a variety of common x-ray beam energies. Only a slight energy dependence is observed. The results are provided in Table 1.7.

The primary components of air have $Z < 10$, therefore negligible fluorescence occurs and $(\mu_{\text{tr}}/\rho) = (\mu/\rho)$. Thus Kerma in air is virtually identical with absorbed dose in air. Notice that Eq. (1.35) does not contain the constant W, the value (33.97 J/C) of which was used previously in Eq. (1.28). It turns out that Eq. (1.35) can be used to compute W, and in doing so W is found to range from 33.75 J/C for a 30 kVp x-ray beam, to 34.33 J/C for a 140 kVp x-ray beam. The slight (1.7%) energy dependence in W is often considered negligible, and W is assumed to be a constant in many texts (as it was in Eq. (1.28) above).

1.4.3 Backscatter

When an x-ray beam is incident upon a low-Z solid such as a slab of water or a patient, there is an appreciable amount of *backscatter* (Figure 1.45). Backscatter refers to scatter that is generated in the solid and propagates back towards the source of x rays. Backscatter factors in diagnostic radiology can be as large as 15%, meaning that if the entrance exposure were measured with an ionization chamber placed on top of the solid (as in Figure 1.45(a)), then the exposure measurements would be about 15% higher than if they were made *free-in-air*. Free-in-air refers to making the exposure measurement with no scattering media present in the beam (Figure 1.45(b)). Roentgen-to-Rad conversion factors assume that the exposure measurements were made *without backscatter* (i.e., free-in-air). Therefore, the measurement geometry shown in Figure 1.45(a) should be avoided.

Table 1.7: Roentgen-to-Kerma factors for air and water, for a range of diagnostic x-ray spectra and HVLs. Over a wide range of spectra, the conversion factor changes by less than 2%. To change the units from mGy/R to Rad/R, multiply the conversion factors by 0.1

kVp (5% ripple)	HVL (mm Al)	KERMA in Air mGy/R	KERMA in Water mGy/R
30	1.09	8.708	9.438
40	1.63	8.726	9.420
50	2.15	8.745	9.435
60	2.61	8.767	9.460
70	3.04	8.787	9.487
80	3.47	8.806	9.514
90	3.90	8.822	9.540
100	4.31	8.834	9.561
110	4.71	8.840	9.576
120	5.09	8.845	9.590
130	5.46	8.851	9.605
140	5.79	8.857	9.618

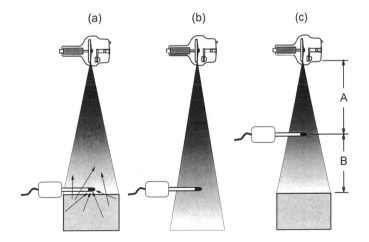

Figure 1.45: (a) Entrance exposure measurements made close to the entrance surface of a low-Z material (lucite, water, or patient) will have a large amount of backscatter contributing to the measurement. (b) Entrance exposure measurements should be made without backscatter. This figure illustrates an exposure measurement *free-in-air*, and this geometry eliminates the inclusion of backscatter in the measurement. (c) A practical compromise for measuring backscatter-free entrance-exposure values is to place the exposure meter away from the entrance surface to make the measurement. The exposure measurement is then corrected using the inverse square law to the entrance plane.

Free-in-air measurements can be made simply by moving the scattering material. For repeated experiments, however, moving and repositioning the heavy phantom is undesirable. In practice, it is common to make entrance exposure measurements using the geometry shown in Figure 1.45(c), where the exposure meter is placed a fair distance away from the surface of the phantom or patient, and the distances A and B are accurately measured. The exposure reading from the chamber, X', is then corrected by the inverse square law:

$$X = \left(\frac{A}{A + B} \right)^2 X'.$$ (1.36)

Measuring exposure with an appreciable air gap (>40 cm), with subsequent correction for the inverse square law, is equivalent to a free-in-air measurement for most practical purposes. The geometry of Figure 1.45(b or c) should also be used when measuring the entrance exposure to a detector, for example in noise power measurements (discussed elsewhere in this book). For higher-Z materials such as a detector, the majority of the backscattered secondary radiation is not Compton scatter, but rather is x-ray fluorescence.

1.4.4 Equivalent dose and effective dose

Radiation dose is a measure of the energy/mass, but different kinds of radiation have different *relative biological effectiveness (RBE)*. The RBE is a measure of relative biological harm, in essence. For example, one mGy deposited by electrons or alpha particles has a greater RBE than one mGy deposited by x rays. To compensate for this, the *equivalent dose (H)* is defined as:

$$H = w_r \text{D},$$ (1.37)

where D is the dose (in Gray) and w_r is the weighting factor for the type of radiation which delivered the dose. For x rays in diagnostic radiology, $w_r = 1$. The weighting factors w_r for other types of radiations range from 5 to 20. The unit of the equivalent dose is the Sievert (Sv, 1 Sv $=$ 100 REM).

Most risk estimates concerning radiation dose assume whole-body exposure of the individual. In diagnostic imaging, however, usually only small regions of the patient are imaged. The *effective dose, E,* is designed to essentially normalize the actual dose delivered to a small region of the body to that of a whole-body exposure. This allows an apples-to-apples comparison between two different radiation exposures at different sites in the body. To do this, tissue-specific weighting factors are used (w_t) to weight the equivalent dose H (Eq. (1.37)) to each tissue, H_t:

$$E = \sum_{t=0}^{N} w_t H_t.$$ (1.38)

Table 1.8: Tissue weighting factors for effective dose calculations (adapted from NCRP 122[9])

Tissue	w_t
Gonads	0.20
Active bone marrow	0.12
Colon	0.12
Lungs	0.12
Stomach	0.12
Bladder	0.05
Breasts	0.05
Esophagus	0.05
Liver	0.05
Thyroid	0.05
Bone surfaces	0.01
Skin	0.01
Remainder	0.05

The units of effective dose, E, are Sv, the same units as equivalent dose H. The tissue weighting factors, w_t, are given in Table 1.8.

Whereas the calculation of effective dose is beyond the needs of most scientists working on detector systems, effective dose estimates often need to be computed when applying to an investigational review board (IRB) to appraise a new detector system in clinical studies. The w_t values are given in Table 1.8, however the H_t values need to be computed from the entrance exposures to specific anatomical fields of view. How the entrance exposure at site A relates to the dose at tissue site B has been computed using Monte Carlo techniques for standard organs and typical radiographic projections. The results are compiled in tables, for instance in [10].

1.4.5 Deposition of dose in tissue

It is clear from the Lambert–Beers law (Eq. (1.14)) that the dose incident upon the surface of the patient falls off exponentially at depth within the patient. This is almost correct, but the Lambert–Beers law is valid for only the primary component of the x-ray beam and dose deposition can occur from both primary and scattered photons. To assess this, *Monte Carlo* techniques were used to estimate dose levels at various depths within a water-equivalent mathematical phantom [11]. Monte Carlo techniques are used extensively in x-ray imaging and dosimetry, e.g., [11–13]. Figure 1.46 shows the energy deposition versus depth for three different x-ray energies. The primary dose deposition (solid lines and square symbols) shows the pure exponential behavior as predicted by Eq. (1.14). The scattered dose

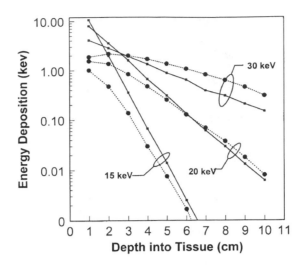

Figure 1.46: The energy deposition of x rays as a function of depth into tissue is illustrated for three different x-ray energies. The curves with solid lines and square symbols show the primary component of the x-ray beam, whereas the dotted line and circles demonstrate the scatter component of the x-ray beam. The energy deposition by primary x rays is seen to be linear on this semi-log plot, consistent with exponential behavior. The energy deposition attributable to the scatter component in the x-ray beam, however, is not linear and is seen to increase (relative to the primary component) with increasing beam energy. At 30 keV, the energy deposition coused by scatter increases in the first couple cm of tissue, indicating a dose *buildup*.

deposition (dashed lines and circle symbols) does not behave in a purely exponential manner, however. Indeed, for 30-keV x rays, the scatter dose actually increases in the first few centimeters of tissue, before falling off. This is called the *build-up* region, a very important topic in radiation oncology texts, but relevant here as well. It is also evident from Figure 1.46 that beyond the first few cm of tissue, the scatter dose is about the same magnitude as the primary dose, depending on x-ray energy. This suggests that the use of the Lambert–Beers equation (and analytical variations of it) for dose deposition is only a modest approximation, because it does not and cannot address scattered radiation. This is why Monte Carlo techniques are used so extensively in the assessment of radiation dose.

1.5 X-ray detection

1.5.1 Direct versus indirect detection

X-ray detectors can be classified as *direct* or *indirect*. A direct detector records the electrical charge (usually as a voltage or current) which results directly from ionization of the atoms in the detector. Gas detectors such as xenon detectors used in computed tomography and air ionization chambers (exposure meters) are direct detectors. Film (with no intensifying screen) is a direct detector, and it records the latent image photo-chemically. Solid-state direct detectors for x-ray imaging

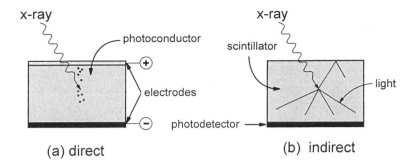

Figure 1.47: (a) The detection strategy for direct detectors is illustrated. X rays interact with a photoconductor, which is placed between two electrodes. The negative and positive ions produced during x-ray interaction migrate to the electrodes, producing charge accumulation which is then measured using sensitive electronics. (b) Indirect detection strategies make use of an x-ray *scintillator*. An x ray interacts with the scintillator, causing a burst of light photons to be emitted. The light photons then propagate by optical diffusion until they reach the photo detector (e.g., a film emulsion or Si TFT).

are made of a solid material (a photoconductor) placed between two electrodes (one electrode is pixelated). In the absence of x rays, the photoconductor acts as an insulator, and no (very little) charge flows between the two electrodes. When x rays strike the photoconductor, bound electrons are promoted to the conduction band and become conductive electrons, while mobile holes remain in the valence band of the photoconductor. These charges then migrate to the upper and lower electrodes, and the accumulated charge is measured electronically (Figure 1.47(a)). Selenium has received a great deal of attention as a direct detector for x-ray imaging, but other materials such as PbI and TlBr are being studied as solid-state direct detectors as well.

An indirect detector system, for all practical purposes, is a scintillator-based x-ray detector. X rays interact with a phosphor, causing it to emit light in or near the visible range. The visible-light photons then propagate by optical diffusion to a photodetector, such as a film emulsion or a silicon photodiode (Figure 1.47(b)). The photodetector then records the pattern of visible light given off by the phosphor as an image.

Computed radiography is the term given to a class of photostimulable phosphors, notably BaFBr:Eu. This phosphor traps excited electrons in metastable states as a result of x-ray interaction, and then when the phosphor plate is scanned with laser light, the electrons drop back to ground state and emit light. This light then propagates through the matrix of the phosphor and is detected by a photomultiplier tube. The wavelength of the emitted light is different than the laser source, and can be isolated using optical filters. This mechanism is indirect, since light photons couple the x-ray ionization event to the ultimate detection event.

Common phosphors are indicated in Table 1.9.

Table 1.9: Various x-ray detector materials used in x-ray imaging

Detector Composition	Density $(g/cm)^3$	Type
BaFBr:Eu	4.56	Indirect (CR)
$CaWO_4$	6.12	Indirect
CsI:Tl	4.51	Indirect
Gd_2O_2S:Tb	7.34	Indirect
Se	4.79	Direct
$YTaO_4$:Nb	7.57	Indirect

1.5.1.1 Activators

Some x-ray phosphors do not require activators to function as a scintillator, such as $CaWO_4$, and this phenomenon is called *host luminescence*. Many other phosphors, however, require the presence of defects in the crystal lattice structure of the phosphor for meaningful light emission to occur. To achieve defects, activators (also called dopants) are added to the phosphor at the time it is prepared. For example, Gd_2O_2S is typically doped with Tb_2O_2S, and this would be indicated as Gd_2O_2S:Tb. While Gd_2O_2S:Tb emits with a strong peak at 545 nm (green light), if Eu_2O_2S is used as the activator, the color of the principal emission shifts to 626 nm (red). Similarly, if praseodymium is used as the activator (Gd_2O_2S:Pr), the phosphor will emit 506 nm light when exposed to x rays. The wavelengths mentioned are the principal wavelengths, and other less prominent peaks in the scintillation spectra occur at other wavelengths. The activator determines not only the color of the luminescent emission, but the efficiency of the phosphor (how much light is emitted per absorbed x-ray photon) is strongly influenced as well. For a given phosphor and activator, the concentration of the activator relative to the host phosphor will also play an important role in the efficiency of the scintillator. The activators are present in only trace quantities, and their presence has negligible impact the absorption efficiency of the phosphor.

CsI is typically activated with a small concentration of thallium iodide (CsI:Tl). For use in computed radiography systems using a helium-neon laser (633 nm) as the stimulation source, BaFBr:Eu plates are used. Some CR manufacturers are now using diode-based lasers which emit around 680 nm, and this had led to imaging plates which use a combination of BaFBr:Eu ($\sim$85%) and BaFI:Eu ($\sim$15%) for improved light efficiency at this stimulation wavelength. With BaFBr, europium (as EuFBr) is in the divalent state (Eu^{+2}), and has a very fast luminescent decay (microseconds) compared to the trivalent state (Eu^{+3}, as in Eu_2O_2S), which has a slower decay (milliseconds). The rapid emission properties are very important for the fast readout times required with computed radiography—e.g., the dwell time for a 30 s readout of 2048^2 pixels is 7.1 μs/pixel.

1.5.2 Absorption efficiency

X-ray detectors need to interact with incident x-ray photons to record their presence; x rays that pass through the detector unattenuated are essentially wasted. The design goal of all x-ray detectors for medical imaging is to maximize the absorption efficiency of the detector, given the constraints of other performance parameters (such as spatial resolution) as well. The quantum detection efficiency (QDE) of a detector is given by:

$$\text{QDE} = \frac{\int_{E=0}^{E\,\text{max}} \Phi(E)(1 - e^{-\mu(E)x})\,\mathrm{d}E}{\int_{E=0}^{E\,\text{max}} \Phi(E)\,\mathrm{d}E}, \tag{1.39}$$

where x is the thickness of the detector and $\mu(E)$ is its linear attenuation coefficient, and $\Phi(E)$ is the x-ray spectrum (photon fluence per energy interval). The QDE is simply the fraction of incident x-ray *photons* which are attenuated by the detector. In both direct and indirect x-ray detectors, the signal is related to the total energy absorbed in the detector, not the number of x-ray photons. That is, x-ray detectors are not *photon counters* (like in nuclear medicine applications), but rather are *energy integrators*. The energy absorption efficiency (EAE) of an x-ray detector is given by:

$$\text{EAE} = \frac{\int_{E=0}^{E\,\text{max}} \Phi(E)E\left(\frac{\mu_{\text{en}}(E)}{\mu(E)}\right)(1 - e^{-\mu(E)x})\,\mathrm{d}E}{\int_{E=0}^{E\,\text{max}} \Phi(E)E\,\mathrm{d}E}. \tag{1.40}$$

The denominator of Eq. (1.40) is simply the amount of energy incident upon the x-ray detector (per unit area). The fraction of photons attenuated in the detector is given by the $(1 - e^{-\mu(E)x})$ term, and the amount of energy absorbed in the detector per attenuated x-ray photon is given by $E\,(\mu_{\text{en}}(E)/\mu(E))$.

1.5.2.1 X-ray energy

The QDE is shown as a function of x-ray energy in Figure 1.48 for three commonly-used x-ray phosphors: CsI, BaFBr, and Gd_2O_2S. It is widely assumed that above the K edge of the phosphor, an appreciable jump in x-ray detection is achieved. In terms of photon absorption (QDE), that is true as Figure 1.48 plainly illustrates. Figure 1.49 shows the energy absorption efficiency for the same three phosphors. It is apparent that the energy absorption efficiency above the K edge does not enjoy the large jump in magnitude as the QDE does, because the energy associated with the characteristic x-ray photons (x-ray fluorescence will be discussed later) is re-emitted by the detector.

A comparison between the QDE and the EAE is shown in Figure 1.50 for Gd_2O_2S. This figure clearly shows that the jump in photon detection at the K edge is not representative of the increase in signal detection efficiency, since it is the integrated energy that creates the signal in an x-ray detector system.

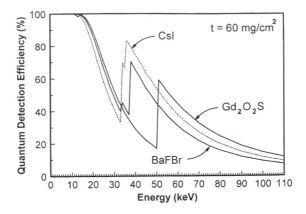

Figure 1.48: The quantum detection efficiency is illustrated as a function of x-ray energy for the three x-ray phosphors indicated. The thickness of each phosphor is 60 mg/cm^2. An abrupt jump in the QDE at the K edge of the phosphor is observed.

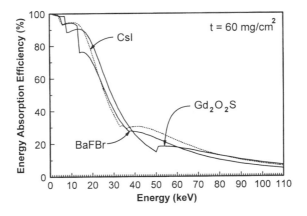

Figure 1.49: The energy-absorption efficiency is illustrated as a function of energy for three x-ray phosphors. The EAE demonstrates substantially less of a discontinuity at the K edge of the phosphor, because of the energy lost to the re-emission of characteristic x-ray photons by the detector.

1.5.2.2 Thickness

The mass thickness (mg/cm^2) required to attenuate 50% of the incident x-ray photons for four different detector systems is shown in Figure 1.51. Lower values indicate a phosphor with more stopping power. Because the mass thickness is shown, the density of the phosphor is factored out. Not surprisingly, selenium with its low Z (34) shows poor stopping power compared to the other phosphors. BaFBr, the photostimulable phosphor used in computed radiography, has stopping power comparable to CsI and Gd$_2$O$_2$S at lower x-ray energies, but a difference becomes pronounced above about ∼60 keV. Below the K edge of gadolinium, the Gd$_2$O$_2$S phosphor has poorer stopping power (based on mass thickness) than Se. However,

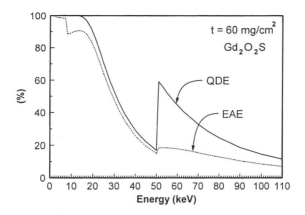

Figure 1.50: The quantum detection efficiency (QDE) and the energy absorption efficiency (EAE) are illustrated as a function of x-ray energy for a 60 mg/cm^2 Gd$_2$O$_2$S phosphor. The marked difference between the QDE and the EAE is observed.

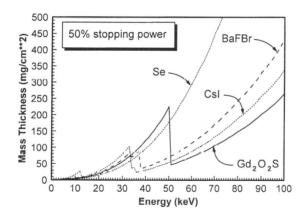

Figure 1.51: The mass thickness of the x-ray detector material required to attenuate 50% of the incident x-ray beam is illustrated as a function of x-ray energy. Selenium is seen to be a relatively poor x-ray absorber, because of its low atomic number ($Z = 34$). Gd$_2$O$_2$S is seen to have good stopping power above its K edge at 50 keV. The density of the detector material is factored out in this comparison.

the density of Gd$_2$O$_2$S is higher and thus the absolute thickness of the phosphor will therefore be less.

The fraction of energy absorbed by the detector (Eq. (1.40)) is highly dependent upon the fluorescent yield of the phosphors (which effects (μ_{en}/μ)). For example, just above the K edge of gadolinium (say at 51 keV), the ratio (μ_{en}/μ) is 0.31: This means that even if 100% of the incident 51 keV photons were attenuated by the detector, a maximum of 31% of the energy would be absorbed at the initial interaction site.

1.5.3 Conversion efficiency

Once x-ray energy is absorbed in a scintillator, it generates light either promptly for conventional phosphors or after laser-light stimulation for photostimulable phosphors (BaFBr:Eu also has a prompt emission component that is essentially wasted). Each type of phosphor has an intrinsic efficiency in which x-ray energy is converted to visible light photons. For example, $CaWO_4$ has an intrinsic conversion efficiency of about 5%, while Gd_2O_2S has an intrinsic conversion efficiency of about 15%. Depending on the quality control of the manufacturer, the conversion efficiency of a phosphor can fluctuate, for instance, depending on the precise ratio of activator that was used for a specific batch of phosphor. The efficiency is dependent on x-ray energy as well. Table 1.10 lists the number of light photons emitted at various energies for various x-ray phosphors.

Once an x-ray photon is converted into a burst of light photons at the x-ray interaction site in the screen, the light photons then propagate by optical diffusion to the surface of the screen. Optical diffusion is a process of multiple light photons each undergoing multiple scattering events. In general, a single light photon will undergo many hundreds of scattering events before emerging from a screen. At that point, light photons can interact with the film emulsion, or be imaged by an electronic photodetector. The efficiency with which light photons "get out" of the screen depend on a number of factors, including the geometry of the screen, the wavelength(s) of the emitted light, and the light transmission properties of the screen matrix.

For high-resolution screens, a light absorbing dye is sometimes added to prevent optical photons from propagating too far, improving the spatial resolution but reducing the conversion efficiency of the system. One manufacturer (Sterling "Microvision") has designed a phosphor which emits in the ultraviolet, where the optical transmission of the native screen is low. This produces an effect similar to the addition of a light-absorbing dye.

Table 1.10: Mean x ray-to-light conversion factors for various energies and phosphors (from Mickish and Beutel [14]). Based on the measurement geometry, it is estimated that the measured photon yield is about $1/2$ of the total photon yield for each phosphor

X-ray Energy (keV)	LaOBr:Tm	YTaO$_4$:Nb	Gd$_2$O$_2$S:Tb	CaWO$_4$
17.8	243	32.1	442	105
22.6	310	41.2	509	138
32.9	430	70.5	740	207
35.5	424	77.3	791	223
45.5	413	97.5	954	278
51.9	476	109.0	1016	303

1.5.3.1 Thickness

Thicker screens absorb more x-ray photons and have higher QDEs, but the light emitted in a thicker screen has a longer propagation pathlength to reach the surface of the screen. Light that diffuses through thicker layers of screen will spread out more, reducing spatial resolution (Figure 1.52). In addition to the larger blur pattern found with thicker screens (Figure 1.52(b)), light photons are absorbed more with a greater diffusion pathlength, and thus the number of photons will be reduced and the conversion efficiency may be lower.

A thick screen can be modeled as a number of layered thin screens. Each layer in the screen will contribute its own conversion efficiency and its own modulation transfer function (MTF, a spatial frequency description of resolution). Layers close to the photodetector will have higher conversion efficiencies and sharper MTFs, layers away from the photodetector will have slightly lower conversion efficiencies (due to light attenuation) and poorer MTFs.

1.5.3.2 Reflective layers

If increasing the speed of a screen is a very important design goal, a reflecting layer can be placed against the screen to reflect light initially directed away from the photodetector back toward it (Figure 1.52(c)). The addition of a reflection layer results in a broadened point-spread function and reduced spatial resolution, but a *faster* screen.

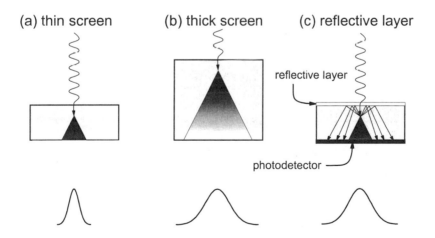

Figure 1.52: (a) A thin intensifying screen reduces the pathlength of visible-light diffusion, and thus restricts the amount of lateral spread that can occur, improving spatial resolution. (b) A thicker screen is capable of attenuating more x-ray photons; however, the pathlength of light diffusion is greater and more lateral spread of the optical signal will occur, broadening the point-spread function and reducing spatial resolution. (c) The addition of a reflective layer on the surface opposite the photodetector causes light which is emitted away from the photodetector to be reflected back and be recorded, increasing the conversion efficiency of the screen, but reducing spatial resolution.

1.5.4 Geometry

1.5.4.1 Dual screen/dual emulsion film

A dual-screen/dual-emulsion screen film system is the most commonly used type of cassette for general-purpose screen-film radiography (Figure 1.53(a)). Two screens, each containing about 60 mg/cm^2 of phosphor, are sandwiched around two film emulsions, each coated on either side of the mylar film base. This design essentially slices the intensifying screen in half, and places the photodetector (the film emulsion) in the middle. This design reduces the average pathlength that optical light photons must travel before reaching the emulsion, and is a good compromise in terms of absorption efficiency (thick screen) and spatial resolution. Notice that this design is only possible because x rays easily penetrate the film emulsion and film base to reach the more distal screen.

Dual-screen, dual-emulsion screen-film systems in which the screens are identical and the emulsion layers are identical are called *symmetrical*. *Asymmetric* screens can be matched with symmetric film-emulsion layers as well. In these systems, the film can be loaded in the cassette in either orientation with equal results. Some asymmetric screen-film systems are designed such that the top screen is matched to one emulsion layer, and the bottom screen is matched to the other emulsion layer. This type of system allows optimization for certain radiographic procedures (e.g., chest radiography), but care is necessary to assure the film is loaded into the cassette in the proper orientation.

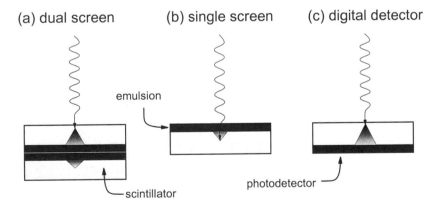

Figure 1.53: (a) The dual-screen dual-emulsion system effectively places the photodetector in the middle of the scintillator layer, reducing the average light propagation path and improving the spatial resolution of a screen-film system for a given scintillator thickness. (b) A single-screen single-emulsion detector arrangement is used in mammography and for detail cassettes. The film emulsion is placed in contact with the entrant surface of the screen, where the majority of x rays interact. This improves both spatial resolution and conversion efficiency. (c) Because digital photodetector electronics are opaque to x rays, the photodetector must be placed behind the scintillator. Consequently, the path length for optical diffusion is increased, reducing the spatial resolution and conversion efficiency in this arrangement.

1.5.4.2 Single screen/single emulsion film

Figure 1.53(b) illustrates a single screen/single-emulsion screen-film system. This design is used chiefly in mammography and for so-called *detail* cassettes in general radiography (used for extremity work—arms, hands, and feet). When x rays are incident upon the detector, they are exponentially attenuated. This means that substantially more x rays interact with the front layers of the screen than with the layers towards the back of the screen, and hence the majority of the optical photons are produced near the front surface, and fewer photons are produced near the back surface. By placing the film emulsion on top of the screen, the average light-diffusion pathlength is reduced in this orientation and the screen-film system enjoys better spatial resolution and better conversion efficiency. Here again, this geometry is only possible because x-ray photons pass through the photodetector (emulsion and film base) with little attenuation.

1.5.4.3 Digital detector systems

The geometry of a typical digital detector, for instance based on thin film transistors (TFTs, discussed elsewhere in this book), is shown in Figure 1.53(c). Because this photodetector is not transparent to x rays, the geometries of Figure 1.53(a) or Figure 1.53(b) cannot be used. Therefore, the screen orientation for solid-state digital radiographic systems (but not computed radiography) requires that the majority of light produced at the entrant surface propagate through the entire thickness of the screen to strike the photodetector. While the pixelated nature of solid-state digital detectors reduces the overall spatial-resolution potential of the imaging system, the optical blur resulting from the geometry shown in Figure 1.53(c) does contribute to a loss in spatial resolution. Perhaps more importantly, the attenuation of light photons due to the long propagation path will result in lower conversion gain (fewer light photons per absorbed x-ray photon), with negative consequences in terms of image noise (discussed in other chapters). The use of phosphors with columnar crystals such as CsI has been used in this application to reduce lateral light spread while maintaining phosphor thickness.

Direct-detection digital detectors, such as those based on selenium, do not suffer from the geometrical compromises shown in Figure 1.53(c). Unlike the unchecked spread of light photons, the spread of electrons created in direct detector systems is contained by the electric field applied across the photoconductor. Electrons follow the electric field lines, and therefore do not experience significant lateral spreading. Thus, the spatial resolution of direct detectors is virtually unaffected by lateral diffusion problems. Consequently, direct detectors can be made very thick relative to scintillator-based systems. This, in part, helps to compensate for the intrinsically poor absorption efficiency of selenium.

1.5.4.4 Other geometries

In computed radiography, the exposure of the imaging plate and the subsequent read out and image formation by a photodetector are separate events. A single imaging plate is the only detector in the cassette, and so the exposure geometry is similar to that shown in Figure 1.53(b or c), except without the photodetector. During readout, a collimated laser beam scans the imaging plate, and light is emitted. In this arrangement, two light diffusion events take place: The laser light optically diffuses into the imaging plate (with associated blur and attenuation), and then the light emitted by the imaging plate diffuses out of the screen (with associated blur and attenuation).

Most indirect imaging systems employ a design in which the photodetector is physically pressed against the intensifying screen, and screen-film systems and TFT systems are examples of this. In some systems, however, the intensifying screen and the photodetector are coupled either by fiberoptic or conventional lens systems. Examples include small-field-of-view digital biopsy systems, and some digital mammography and digital radiography systems. Intensifying screens are considered to be *Lambertian* emitters; that is, the radiance emitted from the surface of the screen will have a uniform angular distribution [15]. If the intensifying screen is coupled by a lens to the photodetector, then a reasonable fraction of the light emitted from the screen will not even strike the lens because of the physical separation between screen and lens. A fiberoptic, although physically coupled to the screen, nevertheless induces large light losses because the individual fibers accept only a small angular component of the Lambertian light emitted, because the light beyond the critical angle is absorbed in the cladding. These light losses obviously contribute to a reduction in the conversion efficiency of the imaging system.

1.5.5 X-ray fluorescence in detectors

Monte Carlo simulations were conducted with the intention of better understanding the role of x-ray fluorescence in x-ray detectors. The geometry of the Monte Carlo studies was designed [16] to measure the amount of x-ray fluorescence that is reabsorbed in the detector, and that which is emitted both in the front and towards the back of the detector. Figures 1.54(a–d) illustrate (on semilogarithmic axes) the energy deposition results of the Monte Carlo studies for Gd_2O_2S, CsI, BaFBr, and Se detectors, respectively. For brevity, only the results for the 90 mg/cm^2 thickness are shown. The term *scatter* does not technically describe x-ray fluorescence, but for the purposes here, scatter is taken to mean the combination of Compton and Rayleigh scattering, and characteristic x-ray re emission.

Figure 1.54(a) shows the situation for Gd_2O_2S. The percentages shown in this plot (and the other similar plots) refers to the percentage of the total incident x-ray energy. A small peak in Figure 1.54 is seen just above 8 keV, and this is backscattered L-shell fluorescence. There is no measurable forward-directed fluorescence, because at this energy it would be reabsorbed in the screen at a distance too close to the initial interaction to resolve, given the measurement geometry of the Monte Carlo studies. There is a small (<3%) amount of forward scatter in the 25-keV to 50-keV region, probably forward-directed (i.e., small-angle) Rayleigh scattering, which is appreciable in high-Z absorbers. At 51 keV, a huge increase in the scatter

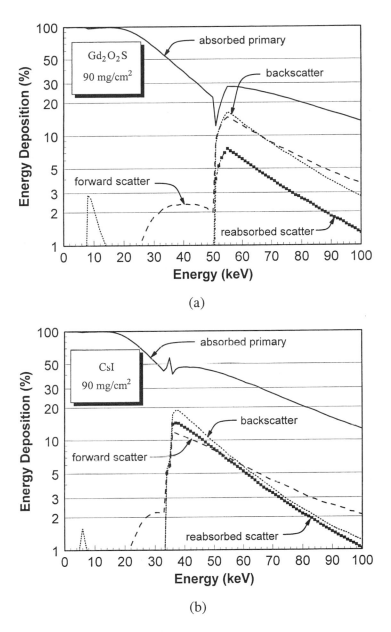

(a)

(b)

Figure 1.54: The energy deposition as a function of x-ray energy is illustrated for different components of the x-ray beam, as shown. The term *scatter* in this usage includes the
contribution of x-ray fluorescence. At the K edge of the detector material (e.g., at 50 keV
in Figure 1.54(a)), there is an enormous increase in backscatter, forward scatter, and reabsorbed scatter, and clearly x-ray fluorescence is the major contributor to these components.
This energy-deposition diagram is illustrated for (a) Gd_2O_2S, (b) CsI, (c) BaFBr, and (d) selenium. The large amount of reabsorbed scatter (fluorescence) above the K edge of the
detector may have an impact on the noise properties of the system, depending upon the
spatial distribution properties of the reabsorption.

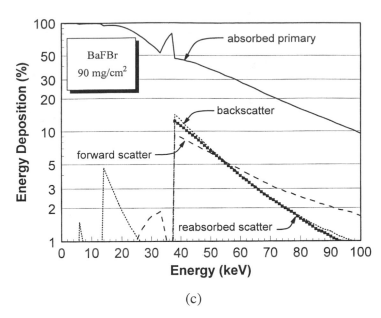

(c)

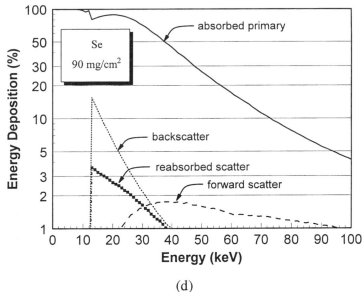

(d)

Figure 1.54: (Continued).

component occurs, but this is predominantly x-ray fluorescence as the K edge of gadolinium is 50.3 keV. The backscattered and forward-scattered components, at 55 keV (for example), are similar (backscatter: 16.5%, forward scatter: 14.8%), as would be expected because x-ray fluorescence is isotropic. As the front-to-back average position of x-ray interaction in the screen shifts towards the back with higher x-ray energy, the ratio of forward scatter to backscatter also increases.

At 55 keV, a total of 7.6% of the incident x-ray energy is reabsorbed scatter (mostly x-ray fluorescence). The vast majority of the reabsorbed x-ray fluorescence is reabsorbed within 0.5 mm of the original interaction. Depending on the pixel dimensions of the detector system and other geometric considerations, the reabsorbed x-ray fluorescence will be collected within the primary pixel and will essentially be counted as absorbed primary energy, or it will be detected in adjacent pixels and contribute toward detector blur (in a non-stochastic sense) or towards detector correlated noise (in a stochastic convolution sense, as discussed elsewhere in this book).

How large a problem is x-ray fluorescence in detectors? In the worst case, for a 55-keV monoenergetic x-ray beam incident upon the 90 mg/cm^2 Gd$_2$O$_2$S detector, 39% of the transiently-detected energy is re-emitted as x-ray fluorescence (16% backscatter +15% forward scatter +8% reabsorbed fluorescence), while 28% of the incident x-ray beam energy is absorbed as primary signal. The ratio of reabsorbed x-ray fluorescence to primary x-ray absorption (scatter/primary ratio in the detector) is 27%. The worst-case situation is mitigated in the real world by the polyenergetic x-ray spectrum. For the Gd$_2$O$_2$S detector, for three x-ray beams at 60, 80, and 100 kVp, each filtered by 20 cm of tissue, x-ray fluorescence losses are 11%, 20%, and 20%, respectively. The corresponding scatter/primary ratios are 6%, 14%, and 15%.

References

[1] Boone JM, Seibert JA. "An Accurate Method for Computer-Generating Tungsten Anode X-Ray Spectra from 30 kV to 140 kV." Medical Physics 24:1661–1670, 1997.

[2] Evans, RD. *The Atomic Nucleus.* Malabar, FL: Robert E. Krieger Publishing Company, 1982.

[3] Bissonnette JP, Schreiner LJ. "A Comparison of Semiempirical Models for Generating Tunsten Target X-Ray Spectra." Medical Physics 19:579–582, 1992.

[4] Kramers, HA. "On the Theory of X-Ray Abosrption and of the Continuous X-Ray Spectrum." Philos Mag 46:836–845, 1923.

[5] Tucker DM, Barnes GT, Chakraborty DP. "Semiempirical Model for Generating Tunsten Target X-Ray Spectra." Medical Physics 18:211–218, 1991.

[6] Fewell TR, Shuping RE, Hawkins KR. *Handbook of Computed Tomography X-ray Spectra.* Springfield, VA: HHS Pub 81-8162, 1981.

[7] Boone JM, Chavez AE. "Comparison of X-Ray Cross Sections for Diagnostic and Therapeutic Medical Physics." Medical Physics 23:1997–2005, 1996.

[8] Boone JM, Fewell TR, Jennings RJ. "Molybdenum, Rhodium, and Tungsten Anode Spectral Models Using Interpolating Polynomials with Application to Mammography." Medical Physics 24:1863–1874, 1997.

[9] NCRP 122, *Use of Personal Monitors to Estimate Effective Dose Equivalent and Effective Dose to Workers for External Exposure to Low LET Radiation.*

Bethesda, MD: National Council on Radiation Protection and Measurements, 1995.

[10] Rosenstein M. *Handbook of Selected Tissue Doses for Projections Common in Diagnostic Radiology*. Rockville, MD: HHS Publication (FDA) 89-8031, 1988.

[11] Boone JM, Seibert JA. "Monte Carlo Simulation of the Scattered Radiation Distribution in Diagnostic Radiology." Medical Physics 15:713–720, 1988.

[12] Chan H-P, Doi K. "Physical Characteristics of Scattered Radiation in Diagnostic Radiology: Monte Carlo Simulation Studies." Medical Physics 12:152–165, 1985.

[13] Morin RL (Ed.). *Monte Carlo Simulation in the Radiological Sciences*. Boca Raton, FL: CRC Press, 1988.

[14] Mickish DJ, Beutel J. "The Determination of X-Ray Phosphor Scintillation Spectra." Proc. SPIE 1231, 1990, pp. 327–336.

[15] Yu T, Sabol JM, Seibert JA, Boone JM. "Scintillating Fiber Optic Screens: A Comparison of MTF, Light Conversion Efficiency, and Emission Angle with Gd_2O_2S:Tb Screens." Medical Physics 24:279–285, 1997.

[16] Boone JM, Seibert, JA, Sabol, JM, Tecotzky M. "A Monte Carlo Study of X-Ray Fluorescence in X-Ray Detectors." Medical Physics 26:905–916, 1999.

Additional Reading:

[17] Attix Fh. *Introduction to Radiological Physics and Radiation Dosimetry*. New York, NY: John Wiley and Sons, 1986.

[18] Barrett HH, Sindell W. *Radiological Imaging: The Theory of Image Formation, Detection, and Processing, Volume 1*. New York, NY: Academic Press, 1981.

[19] Barrett HH, Sindell W. *Radiological Imaging: The Theory of Image Formation, Detection, and Processing, Volume 2*. New York, NY: Academic Press, 1981.

[20] Johns HE, Cunningham JR. *The Physics of Radiology*, 3rd Edition. Springfield, IL: Charles C. Thomas, Publisher, 1974.

[21] Dainty JC, Shaw R. *Image Science*. New York: Academic Press, 1974.

[22] Bushberg JT, Seibert JA, Leidholdt EM, Boone JM. *The Essential Physics of Medical Imaging*. Baltimore, MD: Williams and Wilkins, 1994.

CHAPTER 2
Applied Linear-Systems Theory

Ian A. Cunningham
John P. Robarts Research Institute, and London Health Sciences Centre

CONTENTS

2.1 Introduction

A wide variety of both digital and nondigital medical-imaging systems are now in clinical use and many new system designs are under development. These are all complex systems, with multiple physical processes involved in the conversion of an input signal (e.g., x rays) to the final output image viewed by the interpreting physician. For every system, a high-quality image is obtained only when all processes are properly designed so as to ensure accurate transfer of the image signal and noise from input to output.

An important aspect of imaging science is to understand the fundamental physics and engineering principles of these processes, and to predict how they influence final image quality. For instance, it has been known since the work of Rose [1–4], Shaw [5], and others that the image signal-to-noise ratio (SNR) is ultimately limited by the number of quanta used to create the image. This is illustrated in Figure 2.1, showing the improvement in image quality as the number of x-ray quanta used to produce images of a skull phantom is increased from 45 to 6720 quanta/mm^2. Negligible image noise was added by the imaging system.

The view that an imaging system must faithfully *transfer* the input image signal to the output suggested the use of foundations laid out by scientists and engineers studying communications theory, and in particular, use of the Fourier-

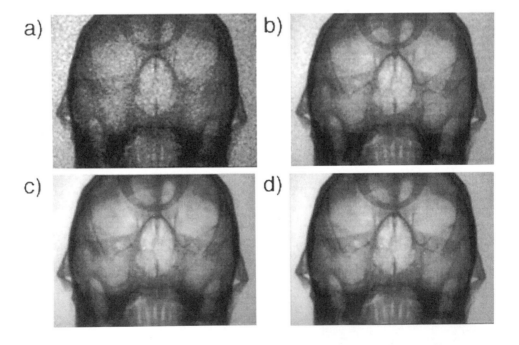

Figure 2.1: Image quality is dependent on the number of quanta used to create an image as illustrated in this example. The average detector x-ray exposure per image is approximately: a) 0.16 μR, b) 1.6 μR, c) 16 μR, and d) 24 μR.

Table 2.1: Summary of incident detector exposure and number of quanta per mm^2 used to create the images shown in Figure 2.1

	Detector Exposure	Quanta per mm^2
a)	0.16 μR	45
b)	1.6 μR	450
c)	16 μR	4500
d)	24 μR	6720

transform linear-systems approach [6]. Linear-systems theory was initially applied in the imaging sciences by Rossmann and co-workers [7, 8], including use of the modulation-transfer function (MTF) and related concepts. General works have subsequently been published by Dainty and Shaw [5], Gaskill [9], Papoulis [10], Doi, Rossmann and Haus [11], Metz and Doi [12], and others. Possibly the most extensive use of linear-systems theory in the medical-imaging field is the comprehensive text by Barrett and Swindell [13] who use this approach to describe fundamental principles and characteristics of many imaging systems in radiography, computed tomography (CT), nuclear medicine, ultrasound, and other areas.

In this chapter, principles of linear-systems theory as it pertains to the analysis of medical-imaging systems are described. The linear-systems approach is used to describe both signal and noise transfer, for both digital and nondigital systems. The link is made to metrics of image and system quality including the modulation-transfer function (MTF), noise-equivalent number of quanta (NEQ), quantum sinks, and detective quantum efficiency (DQE). For background reading, see Bracewell [14] for an excellent description of the Fourier transform, and Brigham [15] for a description of the discrete Fourier transform. General references for stochastic processes are Bendat and Piersol [16] and Papoulis [17]. The noise-power spectrum is described by Dainty and Shaw [5] and Blackman and Tukey [18].

2.2 Background concepts

2.2.1 Images and their units

The input to an x-ray imaging system is always a distribution of x-ray quanta. The output may be approximated as an analog image such as the optical density of a film transparency, or a digital image consisting of an array of digital values stored in computer memory. The term "image" may be used to represent each of these three types of quantities, giving rise to three different types of images: (1) an *analog image*, $d(r)$; (2) a *digital image*, d_n; and (3) a distribution of quanta forming a *quantum image*, $q(r)$. These particular names are the author's preference, but the distinctions are necessary as they have different units and physical meanings, and must therefore be treated differently mathematically.

Transfer theory provides a description of the relationships between these three quantities. In particular, it is used here to describe the relationship between an input quantum image (generally a distribution of x-ray quanta incident on a detector) and an output analog or digital image. In this section, these three types of images and their physical bases are described.

2.2.1.1 Analog image

The term *analog image* will be used to describe a spatially-varying sample function $d(r)$. It is expressed as a function of the continuous variable r representing position in an n-dimensional image. The units of $d(r)$ are arbitrary. Examples include the voltage from a video camera as a function of position along a trace, optical density in a radiographic film, or mean emitted intensity from a CRT monitor.

2.2.1.2 Digital image

A *digital image* generally consists of an n-dimensional array of discrete numerical values. For example, d_{n_x,n_y} represents image intensity at a particular pixel (picture element) in a two-dimensional image identified by the coordinate n_x, n_y. These values may be used as an index into a "look-up table" to produce the desired image brightness according to a specified display level and window. The values d_{n_x,n_y} are dimensionless, as are the digital values produced by an analog-to-digital converter (ADC).

2.2.1.3 Quantum image

A *quantum image* is a spatial distribution of quanta. For example, x rays transmitted through a patient and incident on an imaging detector form an x-ray quantum image. Each quantum has negligible spatial extent, and may be considered to be a point or impulse object represented as a single Dirac delta function $\delta(r - r_0)$ where r_0 is a vector describing the location of the quantum. Therefore, a quantum image may be represented as the sample function $q(r)$ consisting of the superposition of a large number of spatially-distributed δ functions.

There are two important reasons why manipulating quantum images is more complicated than manipulating analog or digital images. The first is that they must be interpreted as *distributions* in the mathematical sense, having dimension area^{-1} for a two-dimensional image. Some implications of this are described in more detail below. The second reason is that image quanta have fundamental statistical properties that cannot be ignored. It is therefore necessary to interpret $q(r)$ as a sample function of a random process. For instance, we describe the position of each quantum in an image using the random vector variable $\tilde{r}$ which has the set of values $\{r_i\}$ and where each value describes the position of one quantum. The quantum image $q(r)$ is a particular realization of these random variables, and can be expressed as the sample distribution

$$q(r) = \sum_{i=1}^{N_q} \delta(r - r_i). \tag{2.1}$$

While it is not possible to know *precisely* where the x-ray quanta are in a particular distribution because of the uncertainty principle, $q(r)$ represents a particular *possible* distribution. That is, a sample image, where the quanta may be statistically correlated—or not—in some specified way. The expected value (i.e., an ensemble average of many such realizations, see Section 2.5.2) of $q(r)$ will be written as $E\{q(r)\}$, and describes the expected distribution of quanta per unit area at position r. If the image consists only of a Poisson distribution of quanta, $\widetilde{r}$ is randomly distributed and uncorrelated over the image area, and $E\{q(r)\}$ is a constant independent of position.

Quantum images are generally two dimensional. However, it will be convenient, particularly for illustrations, to consider a one-dimensional quantum image consisting of a distribution of quanta along a line, $q(x)$, having dimension length^{-1}.

2.2.2 The Dirac δ function, sampling, and the sifting property

The Dirac δ function, or impulse function, is so important in the application of linear-systems theory, both for the representation of quantum images as described above and in the analysis of digital systems, that it is appropriate to describe its properties explicitly. The symbol $\delta(x - x_0)$ represents an impulse at position x_0 with the property that [14]

$$\delta(x - x_0) = \begin{cases} 0 & \text{for } x \neq x_0 \\ \text{undefined} & \text{for } x = x_0, \end{cases} \tag{2.2}$$

and with the constraint that

$$\int_{-\infty}^{\infty} \delta(x - x_0)\, dx = 1. \tag{2.3}$$

The δ function always has a dimension corresponding to the inverse of its argument (x^{-1} in this case). In addition, for any function $f(x)$ that is continuous at $x = x_0$,

$$\int_{a}^{b} f(x)\delta(x - x_0)\, dx = \begin{cases} f(x_0) & \text{if } a < x_0 < b \\ 0 & \text{otherwise}, \end{cases} \tag{2.4}$$

and from which comes the *sifting* property,

$$\int_{-\infty}^{\infty} f(x)\delta(x - x_0)\, dx = f(x_0) \int_{-\infty}^{\infty} \delta(x - x_0)\, dx = f(x_0) = f(x)|_{x=x_0}. \tag{2.5}$$

The sifting property provides a mechanism whereby the process of *sampling*, that is, evaluating a function at a specified position $x = x_0$, can be expressed in terms of the linear operation of multiplication with a δ function:

$$f(x)\delta(x - x_0) = f(x_0)\delta(x - x_0). \tag{2.6}$$

It is important to note that multiplication with the δ function does not result in the sample value alone—it results in a δ function *scaled* by the sample value $f(x_0)$. The sample value may be dimensionless, but the δ function is not.

The δ function is a *generalized* function in the mathematical sense as opposed to a "well-behaved" function. For this reason it is sometimes referred to as the δ symbol rather than the δ function. While it is tempting to manipulate the δ function as if it were well behaved, it is really defined only in terms of its properties, such as those given by Eqs. (2.2) to (2.5), and must be treated accordingly, and with great care.

In addition to the sifting property, other important properties of the δ function include [14]

$$\delta(ax) = \frac{1}{|a|}\delta(x), \tag{2.7}$$

$$\delta(-x) = \delta(x), \tag{2.8}$$

$$x\delta(x) = 0. \tag{2.9}$$

The Dirac δ function should not be confused with the Kronecker δ function, defined as

$$\delta_m = \begin{cases} 1 & \text{for } m = 0 \\ 0 & \text{for } m \neq 0, \end{cases} \tag{2.10}$$

often used in the description of discrete systems.

2.2.3 *Generalized functions*

While use of the δ function is often convenient, it must again be emphasized that it is a *generalized* function, and must be treated with care. The δ function was first used by physicists for the description of momentum impulses and point objects such as point charges. While the δ function is not a real function, it was often manipulated as if it were. With the subsequent development of generalized functions, it is known now that the δ function can often be manipulated as a real function but only evaluated within an integral as expressed by the sifting property in Eq. (2.5).

The class of generalized functions used here can be defined as the limit of a sequence of well-behaved functions. The one-dimensional δ function can be expressed in terms of many such limits, two being

$$\delta(x) = \lim_{\tau \to \infty} \frac{\sin(\pi\tau x)}{\pi x} = \lim_{\tau \to \infty} \tau\,\text{sinc}(\pi\tau x), \tag{2.11}$$

and

$$\delta(x) = \lim_{\tau \to \infty} \frac{\sin^2(\pi\tau x)}{\pi^2\tau x^2} = \lim_{\tau \to \infty} \tau\,\text{sinc}^2(\pi\tau x). \tag{2.12}$$

Refer to Bracewell [14] or Gaskill [9] for a description of δ functions, distributions, and generalized functions in linear-systems theory.

2.2.4 Distribution theory

Images consisting of a distribution of quanta *must* be interpreted using distribution theory. A distribution can be measured only through the use of a *sampling function*, $\phi(x)$ which describes the measurement process. The sampling function is sometimes called an *aperture function* when used to describe the sensitivity profile of a detector. Do not confuse it with the sampling operation where a waveform is multiplied with a δ function (Section 2.2.2), or a sample function of a stochastic process (Section 2.5). For example, if a measure of the one-dimensional quantum image $q(x)$ is obtained with a detector of width a, producing a signal proportional to the number of interacting quanta, the result d may be expressed as the integral

$$d = k \int_{x_0-a/2}^{x_0+a/2} q(x)\,dx = k \int_{-\infty}^{\infty} q(x) \prod\left(\frac{x-x_0}{a}\right) dx, \qquad (2.13)$$

where the detector is centered at $x = x_0$ and k is a constant relating the number of interacting quanta to the detector output signal that might be a voltage, or an analog-to-digital converter (ADC) value (assuming ADC quantization errors can be ignored). In this example, the sampling function is $\phi(x) = \prod(x/a)$ which is a rectangle of unity height and width a.

Note that while $q(x)$ is a generalized function, the expected value of $q(x)$, $E\{q(x)\}$, is a well-behaved function having the same units.

2.2.5 Transfer theory

One way of characterizing an imaging system is to describe the input-output relationships of parameters useful in the description of image signals and noise. For instance, Figure 2.2 shows input and output images, $q_{in}(r)$ and $q_{out}(r)$ respectively, of a hypothetical imaging system in which there has been a degradation of image contrast.

2.2.5.1 Signals: large-area contrast transfer

Contrast is a measure of the relative brightness difference between two locations in an image. Relative brightness is often a more important parameter than absolute brightness because the absolute brightness of a displayed image is often dependent on the display hardware (e.g., video monitor brightness setting or viewbox intensity), and may therefore have no particular significance in an absolute sense. The contrast between locations r_1 and r_2 of $q_{in}(r)$ in Figure 2.2 is C_{in}, defined as

$$C_{in} = \frac{E\{q_{in}(r_2)\} - E\{q_{in}(r_1)\}}{\frac{1}{2}[E\{q_{in}(r_2)\} + E\{q_{in}(r_1)\}]}. \qquad (2.14)$$

An alternative definition of contrast used by some omits the factor $1/2$ but is not used in this chapter. The corresponding contrast in the output image is C_{out} where

$$C_{out} = \frac{E\{q_{out}(r_2)\} - E\{q_{out}(r_1)\}}{\frac{1}{2}[E\{q_{out}(r_2)\} + E\{q_{out}(r_1)\}]}, \quad (2.15)$$

and the large-area contrast-transfer factor is therefore defined as the ratio

$$T_c = \frac{C_{out}}{C_{in}}. \quad (2.16)$$

The concepts of signal transfer are related to the spatial resolution of a system. This is illustrated in Figure 2.3 where the input-output relationship is shown for a system that transfers large-area (relative to the measurement area) contrast fairly well, but small-area contrast poorly. The result is an output image in which the contrast of fine details (small lesions and edges) is reduced, giving rise to an image that appears to be "blurred" by the system.

Transfer theory must therefore be tied somehow to concepts of both image-structure size and system spatial resolution. One way of doing this is to express

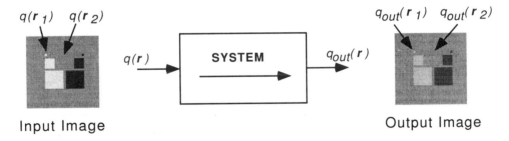

Figure 2.2: Transfer theory describes relationships between the input and output images of an imaging system. In this illustration of a deterministic system, an image is transferred accurately except for a degradation in contrast.

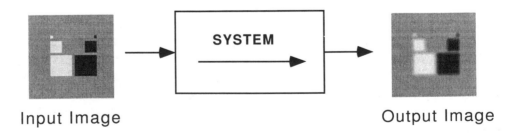

Figure 2.3: A system with poor spatial resolution transfers large-area contrast better than small-area contrast. As a result, the contrast of fine detail is reduced and the transferred image appears "blurred."

transfer relationships in the spatial-frequency domain and to make extensive use of the Fourier transform and related theorems. The uniqueness of the Fourier transform means that any problem can be solved equivalently in either the spatial (r) or the spatial-frequency (k) domains. It is often easier to find a solution in one domain than in the other, and so every imaging problem should be examined in both. In addition, important insight is often obtained when the solution to any problem is expressed in each domain. For instance, the harmful effect of signal and noise aliasing is easier to predict in the spatial-frequency domain, but it may be necessary to understand aliasing in the spatial domain to develop a physical intuition of the outcome. *The importance of being able to move fluently between the two domains cannot be overstated, and in the opinion of some, is one of the important distinguishing skills of an imaging scientist.*

2.2.5.2 Noise: variance transfer

Contrast transfer says nothing about the transfer of image noise as illustrated in Figure 2.4. Image noise is defined here as stochastic variations in image signals (see Section 2.5.2). For instance, an image of a uniform object might have a uniform intensity over a specified region of interest if not for these random variations. One way of describing noise is to calculate the variance in measurements of the image signal over a specific region of interest which has a uniform expected value. Noise variance is then given as [10]

$$\sigma_d^2 = E\{|\Delta d|^2\}, \tag{2.17}$$

where $\Delta d = d - E\{d\}$. Units of the variance σ_d^2 are the same as units of the squared signal d^2.

The variance is defined in Eq. (2.17) in terms of the expected value of $|\Delta d|^2$ which may be obtained from an average of many images (many realizations) at a particular location r. This is called an *ensemble* average. In practice, it may be necessary to use a *spatial* average of $|\Delta d|^2$ as an estimate of the ensemble average. A system for which the ensemble and spatial averages are equivalent is called *ergodic*. Ergodic systems are discussed later in Section 2.5.5.

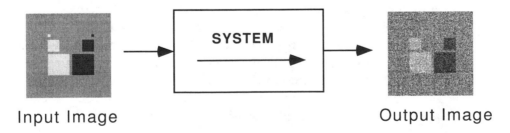

Input Image   Output Image

Figure 2.4: Noise in the output image is related to both the noise in the input image and the noise-transfer characteristics of the system. In this example, the image is transferred both with a reduction of image contrast and an increase in image-noise variance.

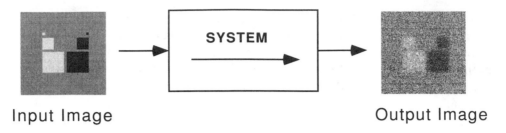

Input Image   Output Image

Figure 2.5: A system that degrades spatial resolution and also increases noise will severely compromise image quality as illustrated here, particularly for the visualization of small details.

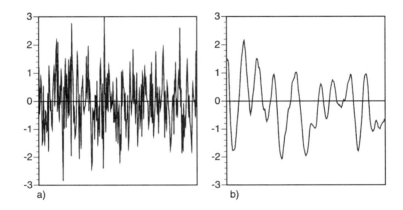

Figure 2.6: One-dimensional profiles may have the same noise variance but look very different as shown here. The noise in b) is correlated over a greater distance than the noise in a).

Figure 2.5 illustrates the input-output relationship of a system that passes contrast in a manner identical to that in Figure 2.3, but increases noise as well. The resulting image quality is severely compromised, and small structures are barely detectable, if at all.

Some insight into system performance could be obtained if a definable relationship existed between the noise variance at the input and output, and the ratio of the two would be the "noise-variance transfer" factor. However, the concept of noise-variance transfer has little meaning for the description of x-ray imaging systems for two reasons. The first is that the variance of an input x-ray quantum image is undefined as described in Section 2.6.2.3. The second is that the variance generally does not describe noise adequately in an analog or digital image. This is illustrated in Figure 2.6. Both profiles have unity noise variance; however, they look very different because the noise in a) is correlated over only a very short distance while noise in b) is correlated over a greater distance. The Fourier transform can be used to describe image noise in the presence of these correlations.

a)

b)

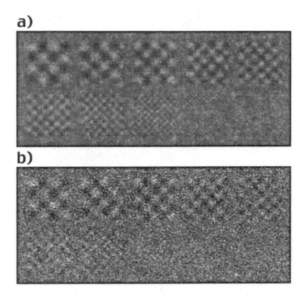

Figure 2.7: The two-dimensional images shown here have the same background noise variance but look very different as the noise in b) is correlated over a greater distance than the noise in a). The same two-dimensional sinusoidal pattern has been added to each image.

2.3 Introduction to linear-systems theory

In this section, linear-systems theory is introduced including a description of important principles and relationships required to characterize system perfor mance in the spatial-frequency domain. While most results are expressed in one-dimensional geometry in terms of the position x and spatial frequency u, similar relationships hold true using two-dimensional geometry in terms of the position vector r and spatial-frequency vector k.

2.3.1 Linear systems

A linear-system response is generally necessary before a linear-systems approach can be used to analyze or characterize system performance. Thus, the first step in any analysis is to ensure the system under study is indeed linear. Essentially, this means the output must be proportional to the input. Thus, if a system has a transfer characteristic described by S{ } such that an input $h(x)$ produces an output $S\{h(x)\}$, then for any two inputs $h_1(x)$ and $h_2(x)$, the system is linear if and only if

$$S\{h_1(x) + h_2(x)\} = S\{h_1(x)\} + S\{h_2(x)\}, \qquad (2.18)$$

and

$$S\{ah(x)\} = aS\{h(x)\}, \qquad (2.19)$$

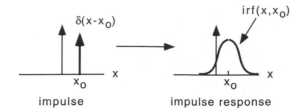

Figure 2.8: An impulse input at $x = x_0$, $\delta(x - x_0)$, produces the impulse-response output irf(x, x_0).

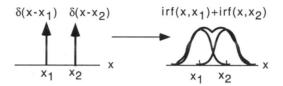

Figure 2.9: For linear systems, the output corresponding to two impulse inputs is the superposition of two impulse-response functions.

for any real constant a. Many systems that are not linear can be linearized with an appropriate calibration, or exhibit small-signal linearity. For instance, radiographic film-screen systems are not linear in their response, but can be linearized if the H&D curve (the relationship between film optical density and x-ray exposure) is known. See references [5], [9], and [20] for further discussions on using linear-systems theory for modeling radiographic systems. In general, no system is completely linear, and as such the linear-systems approach is always an approximation. The analysis of non-linear systems may be limited to their behavior with small amplitude signals [21]. In the following, we will assume a linear system except where specifically noted.

2.3.1.1 Impulse-response function, IRF

When a linear system is presented with the input $\delta(x - x_0)$, an impulse located at $x = x_0$, the corresponding output will be $S\{\delta(x - x_0)\}$ which is called the impulse-response function (IRF), i.e.,

$$\mathrm{irf}(x, x_0) = S\big\{\delta(x - x_0)\big\}. \tag{2.20}$$

The real utility of using the IRF is that for any input expressed as a superposition of many such impulse functions, the output of a linear system will consist of the superposition of one IRF for each input impulse, as shown in Figure 2.8. For instance, if the input is the two impulses shown in Figure 2.9, the output will be

$$S\big\{\delta(x - x_1) + \delta(x - x_2)\big\} = \mathrm{irf}(x, x_1) + \mathrm{irf}(x, x_2). \tag{2.21}$$

There is no requirement that the IRF be isotropic. The IRF is sometimes called the point-spread function (PSF) when used to describe a two-dimensional imaging system.

2.3.2 Linear and shift-invariant (LSI) systems

A system must also have a shift-invariant (isoplanatic) response before a Fourier-based analysis can be used. This requires that the system impulse-response function be shift invariant so that a particular structure in the image will appear the same, regardless of where in the image it is placed. In practice, analysis of systems that are not shift invariant, such as image-intensifier based systems, may be restricted to a central region where the response is approximately shift invariant. A system that is both linear *and* shift invariant in its response is sometimes referred to as an "LSI" system. Because the shape of the IRF in an LSI system is independent of position, it can be written in the form

$$\mathrm{irf}(x, x_0) = \mathrm{irf}(x - x_0). \tag{2.22}$$

2.3.2.1 The convolution integral

If a function $h(x)$ can be approximated as a large number of narrow rectangles having width Δx (see Figure 2.10), the rectangle centered at $x = j \Delta x$, where j is an index identifying the rectangle, has a height $h(j \Delta x)$ and therefore an area $h(j \Delta x) \times \Delta x$. If Δx is small relative to the width of the IRF, the shape of the rectangle is unimportant (only the area is significant) and thus each rectangle can in turn be represented as a δ function, positioned at $x = j \Delta x$, and scaled by $h(j \Delta x) \, \Delta x$. The output $S\{h(x)\}$ of a system having an IRF described by $\mathrm{irf}(x, x_0)$ can then be expressed approximately as the superposition of an IRF for each delta function:

$$S\{h(x)\} \approx \sum_{j=-\infty}^{\infty} h(j \Delta x) \, \mathrm{irf}(x, j \Delta x) \Delta x. \tag{2.23}$$

In the limit of $\Delta x \to 0$, the summation becomes the integral

$$S\{h(x)\} = \int_{-\infty}^{\infty} h(x') \, \mathrm{irf}(x, x') \, dx', \tag{2.24}$$

which is called a *superposition integral*.

When the IRF is shift invariant, the superposition integral can be simplified to

$$S\{h(x)\} = \int_{-\infty}^{\infty} h(x') \, \mathrm{irf}(x - x') \, dx', \tag{2.25}$$

which is called the *convolution integral* (see Figure 2.11). The convolution integral is of fundamental importance in the imaging sciences (and in many other areas of

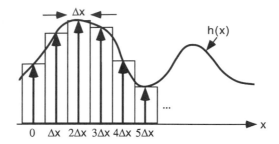

Figure 2.10:   An input signal is divided into a large number of narrow rectangles or scaled delta functions, each with area $h(j\Delta x)\Delta x$.

physics, communications theory and engineering). It describes the output signal obtained when the input $h(x)$ is passed through a linear and shift-invariant (LSI) system. The order of the integrands $h(x)$ and irf(x) can be reversed without affecting the outcome. The convolution integral is often expressed in short form as

$$S\{h(x)\} = h(x) * \text{irf}(x). \tag{2.26}$$

Selected properties of the convolution integral are listed in Table 2.2. These should be learned as one learns addition or multiplication, so that they can be used with ease.

It should be noted here that although the convolution integral (Eq. (2.25)) is a standard way of describing the response of an LSI system to an input signal, it describes a *deterministic* system only. That is, a system that has an IRF given *exactly* by irf(x). When the system has a stochastic component in its response, which includes all x-ray imaging systems, it must be viewed as a stochastic system (see Section 2.5.1) and the linear-systems approach using the convolution integral describes only the expectation value of the system response. Image noise can only be described using the linear-systems approach once stochastic theories are included as described in Section 2.5.

2.3.2.2 *System characteristic function,* T(u)

The IRF contains all the information about a system necessary to determine the expected response in any given situation. However, numerical solutions to the convolution integral are often required in practical situations, and these generally offer little physical insight toward an understanding of system performance. A useful alternative is to examine the special case of an input that varies sinusoidally with position, expressed in terms of the complex exponential

$$h(x) = e^{i2\pi u x} = \cos(2\pi u x) + i \sin(2\pi u x), \tag{2.27}$$

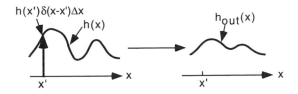

Figure 2.11: For linear and shift-invariant systems the convolution integral describes the superposition of an infinite number of IRF's weighted by the input $h(x)$.

Table 2.2: Properties of the convolution integral

Commutative:
$$f(x) * h(x) = h(x) * f(x)$$
Distributive over Addition:
$$f(x) * [h_1(x) + h_2(x)] = f(x) * h_1(x) + f(x) * h_2(x)$$
Associative:
$$f(x) * h_1(x) * h_2(x) = f(x) * [h_1(x) * h_2(x)]$$
Multiplication with a constant:
$$a[f(x) * h(x)] = af(x) * h(x) = f(x) * ah(x)$$
Addition with a constant:
$$a + [f(x) * h(x)] = [a + f(x)] * h(x) = f(x) * [a + h(x)]$$
Convolution with an impulse:
$$f(x) * \delta(x - x_0) = f(x - x_0)$$

---

where u is the "spatial" frequency (cycles/mm). The output $d(x)$ is given by the convolution integral

$$d(x) = \int_{-\infty}^{\infty} \text{irf}(x')e^{i2\pi u(x-x')}\, dx' \tag{2.28}$$

$$= e^{i2\pi ux} \int_{-\infty}^{\infty} \text{irf}(x')e^{-i2\pi ux'}\, dx', \tag{2.29}$$

where the final integral is recognized as being the Fourier transform of $\text{irf}(x)$, which we call $T(u)$. Therefore,

$$d(x) = S\{e^{i2\pi ux}\} = T(u)e^{i2\pi ux}, \tag{2.30}$$

showing that the output is identical to the input scaled by the frequency-dependent factor $T(u)$. That is, a sinusoidal input will produce a sinusoidal output at the same frequency, scaled by $T(u)$, as illustrated in Figure 2.12. Complex exponentials of the form $e^{i2\pi ux}$ are called *eigenfunctions* of the imaging system, and $T(u)$, which is complex in general, describes the *eigenvalues*. The factor $T(u)$ is called the *characteristic function* of the system. The impulse-response function and the system characteristic function are Fourier pairs:

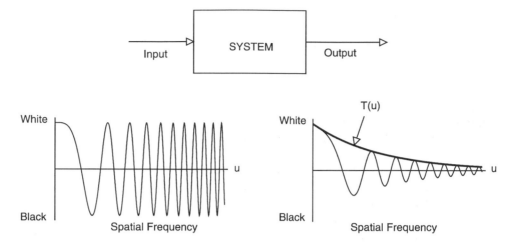

Figure 2.12: A sinusoidal signal at the input of an LSI system will produce a sinusoidal output signal with the same frequency, scaled by the frequency-dependent factor $T(u)$ which is complex in general. This illustration is approximate as the input is not a pure sine wave.

$$T(u) = F\{\mathrm{irf}(x)\}. \tag{2.31}$$

This makes it very convenient to use sinusoidal input waveforms to characterize imaging systems.

The Fourier transform expresses a function in terms of its complex sinusoidal-basis components. If a specified input $h(x)$ has the Fourier transform $H(u)$, then $h(x)$ can be expressed as the inverse Fourier transform of $H(u)$ and the corresponding output is

$$d(x) = S\{h(x)\} = S\left\{\int_{-\infty}^{\infty} H(u)e^{i2\pi ux}\, dx\right\} \tag{2.32}$$

$$= \int_{-\infty}^{\infty} H(u)T(u)e^{i2\pi ux}\, du. \tag{2.33}$$

However, because $d(x)$ can also be expressed as the inverse Fourier transform of $D(u)$ where

$$d(x) = \int_{-\infty}^{\infty} D(u)e^{i2\pi ux}\, du, \tag{2.34}$$

we get

$$D(u) = H(u)T(u). \tag{2.35}$$

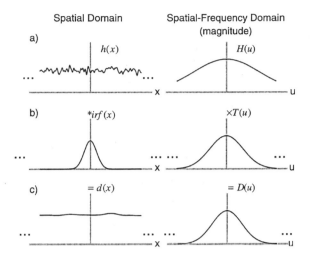

Figure 2.13: Signal-transfer characteristics can be represented either as convolution with irf(x) in the spatial domain (left column) or as multiplication with T(u) in the spatial-frequency domain (right column).

This is a very interesting result because it shows that the Fourier components $H(u)$ of the input are passed unchanged through the system other than a scaling by T(u). Thus, the signal-transfer characteristics of an LSI system can be expressed either as convolution with irf(x) in the spatial domain, or equivalently as multiplication with T(u) in the spatial-frequency domain. This relationship is illustrated graphically in Figure 2.13. In many situations it is more convenient to express imaging problems in the spatial-frequency domain than in the spatial domain, and the ability to move fluently between the two domains is critical to being able to easily solve many imaging problems.

2.3.2.3 Modulation-transfer function, MTF

As shown previously, the contrast-transfer factor, T_c, is not very useful for the description of imaging systems because it is not explicitly related to the size of image structures or to the spatial resolution characteristics of the system. However, the situation changes when we consider the transfer of sinusoidal signals. Consider the input $h(x)$ where

$$h(x) = a + be^{i2\pi ux}, \tag{2.36}$$

and where the real component of $h(x)$ corresponds to the real (measurable) input signal. Because of the sinusoidal nature of this input, it is more meaningful to characterize it in terms of its modulation than its contrast. The modulation of $h(x)$ in Figure 2.14 is given by

$$M_{in} = \frac{|h_{max}| - |h_{min}|}{|h_{max}| + |h_{min}|} = \frac{(a+b) - (a-b)}{(a+b) + (a-b)} = \frac{b}{a}. \tag{2.37}$$

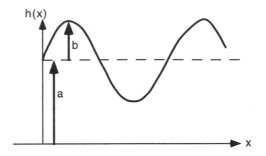

Figure 2.14: A sinusoidal signal expressed in complex exponential form as $h(x) = a + be^{i2\pi ux}$. The sinusoidal waveform is the real component of $h(x)$.

The output signal $d(x)$ is given by

$$d(x) = S\{h(x)\} = S\{a + be^{i2\pi ux}\} \tag{2.38}$$

$$= S\{a\} + S\{be^{i2\pi ux}\} \tag{2.39}$$

$$= aS\{e^{i2\pi(u=0)x}\} + bS\{e^{i2\pi ux}\} \tag{2.40}$$

$$= aT(0) + bT(u)e^{i2\pi ux}, \tag{2.41}$$

where $T(u)$ is complex in general but $T(0)$, which is equal to the area under the IRF, must be real only. The output modulation is therefore given by

$$M_{out} = \frac{|d_{max}| - |d_{min}|}{|d_{max}| + |d_{min}|} = \frac{b}{a} \frac{|T(u)|}{T(0)} = M_{in} \frac{|T(u)|}{T(0)}. \tag{2.42}$$

Similar to our definition above of the contrast-transfer factor, the ratio M_{out}/M_{in} is defined here as the *modulation* transfer function (MTF), given by

$$\text{MTF}(u) = \frac{|T(u)|}{T(0)}, \tag{2.43}$$

where $\text{MTF}(u)$ has by definition a value of unity at $u = 0$.

The MTF is not as complete a description of a system as the characteristic function $T(u)$ because phase information and a scaling constant have been discarded. However, if irf(x) is real only (i.e., has no imaginary component), which is generally true for x-ray imaging systems, both $T(u)$ and $\text{MTF}(u)$ are even functions and can be expressed in terms of positive frequencies only without loss of generalization. If irf(x) is real *and* even, $T(u)$ is also real and even, and no phase-transfer information is lost going to the MTF. The MTF is always real.

The function $\text{OTF}(u)$ given by

$$\text{OTF}(u) = \frac{T(u)}{T(0)}, \tag{2.44}$$

is sometimes called the *optical* transfer function (OTF). It is related to the MTF as $MTF(u) = |OTF(u)|$, and is similar to the MTF although it retains phase-transfer information.

In general the MTF is a two-dimensional function, expressed in terms of either a two-dimensional frequency vector k as $MTF(k)$, or orthogonal frequencies u and v as $MTF(u, v)$.

2.3.2.4 Line-spread function, LSF

The LSF describes the response of the system to a "line" delta function, normalized to unity area. This is seen if we consider a line impulse positioned at $x = x_0$ extending forever in the y direction as the line delta function $\delta(x - x_0)$. The system response along a line in the perpendicular x direction is therefore the LSF given by

$$
\begin{aligned}
lsf(x - x_0) &= \frac{\displaystyle\int_{-\infty}^{\infty}\int_{-\infty}^{\infty} \delta(x - x_0)\,psf(x, y)\,dx\,dy}{\displaystyle\int_{-\infty}^{\infty}\int_{-\infty}^{\infty} psf(x, y)\,dx\,dy} \\[2em]
&= \frac{\displaystyle\int_{-\infty}^{\infty} psf(x - x_0, y)\,dy}{\displaystyle\int_{-\infty}^{\infty}\int_{-\infty}^{\infty} psf(x, y)\,dx\,dy}.
\end{aligned}
\tag{2.45}
$$

For shift-invariant systems this relationship simplifies to

$$
lsf(x) = \frac{\displaystyle\int_{-\infty}^{\infty} psf(x, y)\,dy}{\displaystyle\int_{-\infty}^{\infty}\int_{-\infty}^{\infty} psf(x, y)\,dx\,dy},
\tag{2.46}
$$

where $lsf(x)$ is the LSF in the x direction. The LSF describes the response of a system in one direction when details of the response in the orthogonal direction have been "integrated out" as shown by Eq. (2.46).

The one-dimensional OTF in Eq. (2.44) and the line-spread function are Fourier pairs [5]:

$$
OTF(u) = F\{lsf(x)\},
\tag{2.47}
$$

where u is the spatial frequency in the x direction. Integration of $psf(x, y)$ in the y direction in Eq. (2.46) corresponds to evaluation of $MTF(u, v)$ along the $v = 0$ axis. Therefore,

$$
MTF(u) = MTF(u, v)|_{v=0}.
\tag{2.48}
$$

For systems with a rotationally symmetric IRF, MTF(u, v) is also rotationally symmetric and can be expressed in terms of a single radial spatial frequency u without loss of generality.

2.3.2.5 The correlation integral

A quantity closely related to the convolution integral that will also be used later is the correlation integral, not to be confused with the statistical correlation function described in Section 2.5. The correlation integral of two functions $f(x)$ and $h(x)$ is given as

$$d(x', x' + x) = \int_{-\infty}^{\infty} f(x')h(x' + x)\,dx'. \tag{2.49}$$

When $f(x)$ and $h(x)$ are stationary in x, then this relationship simplifies to

$$d(x) = \int_{-\infty}^{\infty} f(x')h(x' + x)\,dx', \tag{2.50}$$

which is written in short form as

$$d(x) = f(x) \star h(x). \tag{2.51}$$

The correlation integral is not commutative, and so

$$f(x) \star h(x) \neq h(x) \star f(x), \tag{2.52}$$

in general. It can also be shown that

$$f(x) \star h(x) = f(x) * h^*(-x) = h(x) * f^*(-x), \tag{2.53}$$

where $h^*(x)$ is the complex conjugate of $h(x)$.

2.4 The spatial-frequency domain

Great emphasis has been placed on being able to solve imaging-physics problems in either the spatial or spatial-frequency domain. The choice is determined by which is easier, and it is often necessary to solve parts of a problem in one domain and other parts in the conjugate domain. In this section, properties of the Fourier transform are described which are invaluable to successfully use this approach.

2.4.1 The Fourier transform

There are several excellent texts describing the Fourier transform including Bracewell [14] and Brigham [15]. See Peters and Williams [22] for a description of the Fourier transform as applied to several concepts in medical imaging.

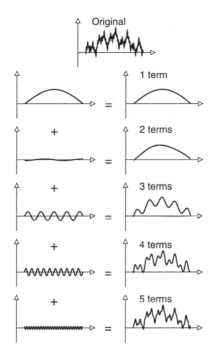

Figure 2.15: The sum of the Fourier components of a function looks more and more like the original function (shown at the top of the figure) as more and more components are added with increasing frequencies. In this figure, five such components are shown in the left-hand column, and the accumulated sum of the components are shown in the right-hand column. In this example, the imaginary terms are all zero.

The Fourier transform of $d(x)$ is $D(u)$, and the inverse Fourier transform of $D(u)$ is again $d(x)$. This reciprocal relationship is expressed by

$$D(u) = \int_{-\infty}^{\infty} d(x) e^{-i2\pi ux} \, dx, \tag{2.54}$$

$$d(x) = \int_{-\infty}^{\infty} D(u) e^{i2\pi ux} \, du, \tag{2.55}$$

where u is the spatial frequency along the x axis. It is seen that the units of $D(u)$ will always be those of $d(x) \times x$.

The Fourier transform of $d(x)$ exists for any well-behaved function $d(x)$. Thus, $D(u)$ always exists when $d(x)$ represents some sort of physical quantity, or at least a function which *could* represent a physical quantity, such as image brightness. The Fourier transform of generalized functions also exists, albeit possibly as generalized functions. Thus, the transform of a distribution of quanta exists when each quantum is represented as a δ function, which will be used a great deal later. In general, both $d(x)$ and $D(u)$ are complex, and may be expressed either as a real

Table 2.3: Summary of Fourier-transform relationships in one and two dimensions for LSI systems. $\mathrm{MTF}(u) = |\mathrm{OTF}(u)|$

Spatial Domain	Fourier Transform	Spatial-Frequency Domain
$\mathrm{irf}(x)$	1D	$T(u)$
$\mathrm{lsf}(x)$	1D	$\mathrm{OTF}(u)$
$\mathrm{psf}(x, y)$	2D	$T(u, v)$

and imaginary pair, or as a magnitude and phase pair,

$$D(u) = \mathrm{Re}\{D(u)\} + i\,\mathrm{Im}\{D(u)\} \qquad (2.56)$$

$$= |D(u)|e^{i\phi(u)}, \qquad (2.57)$$

where $\phi(u)$ is the spatial-frequency-dependent phase angle given by

$$\phi(u) = \tan^{-1}\left(\frac{\mathrm{Im}\{D(u)\}}{\mathrm{Re}\{D(u)\}}\right), \qquad (2.58)$$

through the Euler-angle relation $e^{i\phi} = \cos\phi + i\sin\phi$.

The Fourier transform expresses the fact that $d(x)$ can be written as the sum of a distribution of sinusoidal components (Figure 2.15). As more components are included, the sum looks more and more like the original function. If all non-zero components are included, the sum is identical to the original.

2.4.1.1 The two-dimensional fourier transform

The two-dimensional Fourier transform of $d(x, y)$, $D(u, v)$, is given by

$$D(u, v) = \int_{-\infty}^{\infty}\int_{-\infty}^{\infty} d(x, y)e^{-i2\pi(ux+vy)}\,\mathrm{d}x\,\mathrm{d}y, \qquad (2.59)$$

and the inverse Fourier transform by

$$d(x, y) = \int_{-\infty}^{\infty}\int_{-\infty}^{\infty} D(u, v)e^{i2\pi(ux+vy)}\,\mathrm{d}u\,\mathrm{d}v. \qquad (2.60)$$

These integrals can also be written as vector integrals in terms of the position and frequency vectors $\boldsymbol{r}$ and $\boldsymbol{k}$ as

$$D(\boldsymbol{k}) = \int_{-\infty}^{\infty} d(\boldsymbol{r})e^{-i2\pi\boldsymbol{k}\cdot\boldsymbol{r}}\,\mathrm{d}^2\boldsymbol{r}, \qquad (2.61)$$

and

$$d(\boldsymbol{r}) = \int_{-\infty}^{\infty} D(\boldsymbol{k})e^{i2\pi \boldsymbol{k}\cdot\boldsymbol{r}}\,\mathrm{d}^2\boldsymbol{k}. \tag{2.62}$$

The product $\boldsymbol{k}\cdot\boldsymbol{r}$ is a vector dot product such that $\boldsymbol{k}\cdot\boldsymbol{r}=ux+vy$.

2.4.2 The discrete fourier transform

Manipulation of digital image data in the Fourier domain requires the use of a numerical implementation of the Fourier transform, called a discrete Fourier transform (DFT), which differs from the Fourier transform in subtle ways. The fast Fourier transform (FFT) refers to a number of implementations of the DFT which make use of clever programming to increase computational efficiency. Several implementations of the FFT are available which differ in sophistication, the allowable size and form (real or complex) of the input data sequence, speed of execution, and sometimes a scaler constant.

One commonly used form for the DFT of a sequence of N values d_n for $0 \leqslant n \leqslant N-1$ is given by

$$D_m = \mathrm{DFT}\{d_n\} = \sum_{n=0}^{N-1} d_n e^{-i2\pi nm/N}, \tag{2.63}$$

which consists of a sequence of the N complex values D_m for $0 \leqslant m \leqslant N-1$. The inverse DFT is given by

$$d_n = \mathrm{DFT}^{-1}\{D_m\} = \frac{1}{N}\sum_{m=0}^{N-1} D_m e^{i2\pi nm/N}. \tag{2.64}$$

Other forms of the DFT exist, differing primarily by a scaler constant of N or $\sqrt{N}$. The user of any DFT should be aware of what DFT algorithm is being used before attempting any quantitative work. We shall use Eqs. (2.63) and (2.64) as definitions of the DFT.

The dimensions of d_n and D_m must necessarily be the same, and they are often dimensionless. This is one way in which the Fourier transform and the discrete Fourier transform differ. Another important consideration when using any DFT is to know which index value (which value of n or m) corresponds to the zero positions $x = 0$ and $u = 0$. In many DFT implementations, the central position $x = 0$ corresponds to $n = N/2 - 1$, while the central frequency $u = 0$ corresponds to $m = 0$. Erroneous placement of the zero position in one domain results in errors in the phase angle of the complex value in the conjugate domain as known from the shift theorem.

When the sequence d_n represents the function $d(x)$ evaluated at uniform spacings x_0, it is sometimes written as $d(nx_0)$ to retain this spatial relevance. However, this relationship is not as simple in the spatial-frequency domain, as the sequence D_m is *not* equivalent to samples of $D(u)$ at uniform spatial-frequency spacings of $1/Nx_0$, $D(m/Nx_0)$. While it may be tempting to view the DFT as a numerical implementation of the Fourier integral in Eq. (2.55) and write

$$D\left(\frac{m}{Nx_0}\right) = D(u)|_{u=\frac{m}{Nx_0}} \approx x_0 D_m, \tag{2.65}$$

or

$$D_m \approx \frac{1}{x_0} D\left(\frac{m}{Nx_0}\right), \tag{2.66}$$

extreme care must be used as the DFT is really a separate transform in its own right. The practical problems associated with this interpretation become clear when the DFT is viewed as a special case of the Fourier transform and is understood in the two domains (Brigham [15]). The problems include:

(a) aliasing;

(b) spectral leakage and side lobes;

(c) truncation and windowing;

(d) zero-position and phase errors (mentioned above);

(e) frequency wrap-around; and,

(f) scaling factors and units (particularly in the frequency domain).

They have been described by various authors. Excellent general works are given by Brigham [15], Bracewell [14], and Peters and Williams [22].

2.4.3 *Sampling and aliasing*

Many imaging systems of practical importance produce digital images in which image brightness is represented as a sequence of numerical values. In this section, the relationship between a function and its "sampled" (discrete) representation is described in a way that is still amenable to the analytic graphical techniques used previously.

When the function $d(x)$ is represented numerically with the N discrete values d_n for $0 \leqslant n \leqslant N - 1$, each value corresponds to $d(nx_0) = d(x)|_{x=nx_0}$, an evaluation of $d(x)$ at $x = nx_0$. The process of evaluating a function is called "sampling". One way of describing the sampling process is by making use of the sifting property of the δ function, which says that if $d(x)$ is continuous at $x = x_0$, it has a value

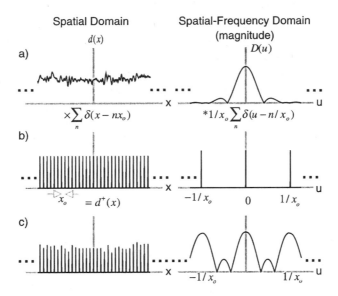

Figure 2.16: Sampling the function $d(x)$ is represented as $d^\dagger(x) = d(x) \sum_{n=-\infty}^{\infty} \delta(x - nx_0)$ and consists of a sequence of δ functions scaled by the discrete values d_n where n is an integer over $-\infty \leqslant n \leqslant \infty$. Spectral aliasing occurs when the aliases overlap in the spatial-frequency domain. Only the magnitude is shown in the frequency domain.

at x_0 given by

$$d(x)|_{x=x_0} = \int_{-\infty}^{\infty} d(x)\delta(x - x_0)\, dx = d(x_0) \int_{-\infty}^{\infty} \delta(x - x_0)\, dx = d(x_0). \quad (2.67)$$

Following Brigham [15], we adopt a graphical representation of this sampling process as shown in Figure 2.16, where each horizontal pair of figures represents a Fourier-transform pair. Sampling $d(x)$ at $x = x_0$ is represented as multiplication with $\delta(x - x_0)$ with the result being an impulse at $x = x_0$ having an undefined amplitude and area equal to $d(x_0)$:

$$d(x)\delta(x - x_0) = d(x_0)\delta(x - x_0). \quad (2.68)$$

This use of the δ function is important because it provides a mechanism whereby sampling can be represented as the linear process of multiplication. This makes it relatively straightforward to interpret the effects of sampling in the conjugate domain.

Note that multiplication with the δ function is not *equivalent* to sampling the function. Rather, multiplication with $\delta(x - x_0)$ results in a δ function positioned at $x = x_0$ that is *scaled* by the sample value of the function. The distinction is important and the δ function cannot be omitted. In addition, the δ function carries the positional information associated with the numerical value.

If a function of infinite extent is sampled at points with uniform spacing x_0, this gives an (infinite) sequence of sample values, $d(nx_0)$ or equivalently d_n, corresponding to values of $d(x)$ at positions $x = nx_0$ where n is an integer. The sampling of a function is therefore represented as multiplication of $d(x)$ with an infinite array of δ functions (Figure 2.16) resulting in $d^\dagger(x)$ where

$$d^\dagger(x) = d(x) \sum_{n=-\infty}^{\infty} \delta(x - nx_0) = \sum_{n=-\infty}^{\infty} d(nx_0)\delta(x - nx_0) \qquad (2.69)$$

$$= \sum_{n=-\infty}^{\infty} d_n \delta(x - nx_0). \qquad (2.70)$$

We use Eqs. (2.69) and (2.70) as our definition of sampling, where $d(x)$ is called the "presampling" signal and $d^\dagger(x)$ is a sequence of scaled δ functions. Note that this definition of sampling does not represent a physical measurement process, only the evaluation of a function. A physical measurement would require the use of a sampling function having finite spatial extent that would reflect the spatial sensitivity of the detector as used in Section 2.2.4 in the description of distribution theory. The δ function can be interpreted as an "ideal" sampling function having infinitesimal width.

The function $d^\dagger(x)$ is also referred to as a pulse-amplitude modulated (PAM) signal, consisting of a sum of modulated pulses at uniform spacings x_0. Many important concepts used to describe digital images come from the electronic communication field, where signals are sampled at uniform time intervals rather than uniform space intervals.

A comment on units is warranted here. A δ function has units equal to the inverse of its argument—see Eq. (2.11). In Eq. (2.69), $\delta(x - nx_0)$ therefore has dimensions of length^{-1} and hence $d^\dagger(x)$ has dimensions equal to those of $d(x) \times x^{-1}$ which are different from those of $d(x)$.

The effect of spatial sampling in both the spatial and spatial-frequency domains is shown in Figure 2.16, where each graph in the right column is the Fourier transform of the corresponding graph in the left. Multiplication in the x domain corresponds to convolution in the u domain. Thus, the Fourier transform of $d^\dagger(x)$, as shown in the lower right of Figure 2.16, is given by

$$F\{d^\dagger(x)\} = D(u) * \frac{1}{x_0} \sum_{n=-\infty}^{\infty} \delta\left(u - \frac{n}{x_0}\right), \qquad (2.71)$$

where $D(u)$ is the Fourier transform of $d(x)$. The Fourier transform of $d^\dagger(x)$ therefore consists of $D(u)$ scaled by $1/x_0$ and superimposed with an infinite number of similarly scaled aliases of $D(u)$ centered at frequencies $u = n/x_0$. As shown in Figure 2.16, the aliases may overlap if $D(u)$ extends beyond $u = \pm 1/2x_0$ where $1/x_0$ is the "sampling frequency," and $1/2x_0$ is called the sampling "cutoff frequency." If aliasing occurs, the true Fourier transform $D(u)$ cannot be determined from the aliased Fourier transform alone. This is equivalent to saying that the original function $d(x)$ cannot be determined from the sample values $d(nx_0)$ alone once aliasing has occurred.

2.4.3.1 The sampling theorem

The above considerations lead directly to a statement of the sampling theorem, adapted from Bracewell [14]:

Any band-limited function having infinite extent and no component frequencies at frequencies greater than $u = u_{max}$ can be fully determined from an infinite set of discrete samples if sampled at a frequency greater than $u_{Ny} = 2u_{max}$ where u_{Ny} is called the Nyquist sampling frequency.

This is just the condition to prevent overlap of the aliases in Figure 2.16. An even function (e.g., a cosine wave relative to the sampling grid) can be fully determined when sampled right at the Nyquist frequency, but an odd function (e.g., a sine wave relative to the sampling grid) must be sampled slightly above the Nyquist frequency. As a rule of thumb, it is wise to sample at a frequency greater than the Nyquist sampling frequency, such as u_s given by

$$u_s = f_k \times u_{Ny} = f_k \times 2u_{max}, \qquad (2.72)$$

where $f_k \approx 1.2$ is an empirically determined constant called the "Kell" factor.

2.4.3.2 Recovering a continuous function from sample values

The question should be asked whether the original presampling function $d(x)$ can be recovered exactly from the sample values d_n. In the conjugate domain this question is equivalent to asking whether $D(u)$ can be recovered exactly from the aliased spectrum $\Gamma\{d^\dagger(x)\}$ in the lower right of Figure 2.16. In the absence of aliasing such that there is no overlap of the aliases, the original primary spectral component can indeed be isolated from its aliases by multiplication with the rectangular function $x_0\Pi(x_0u)$ having a value x_0 over $-1/2x_0 \leqslant u \leqslant 1/2x_0$ and zero elsewhere where x_0 is the sample spacing. This rectangular function has an inverse Fourier transform $\mathrm{sinc}(\pi x/x_0)$, and hence the recovered signal $\hat{d}(x)$ is obtained as a convolution of $d^\dagger(x)$ with the sinc-function

$$\hat{d}(x) = d^\dagger(x) * \mathrm{sinc}(\pi x/x_0) \qquad (2.73)$$

$$= \int_{-\infty}^{\infty} \sum_{n=-\infty}^{\infty} d_n\delta(x' - nx_0)\,\mathrm{sinc}\left(\pi\frac{x - x'}{x_0}\right)\,dx' \qquad (2.74)$$

$$= \sum_{n=-\infty}^{\infty} d_n \int_{-\infty}^{\infty} \delta(x' - nx_0)\,\mathrm{sinc}\left(\pi\frac{x - x'}{x_0}\right)\,dx' \qquad (2.75)$$

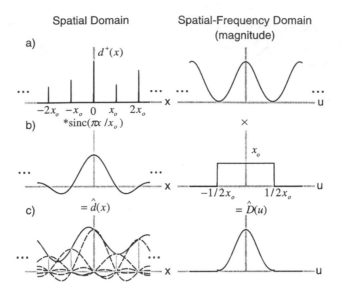

Figure 2.17: The recovered function $\hat{d}(x)$ is obtained by convolving $d^\dagger(x)$ with $\text{sinc}(\pi x/x_0)$, resulting in the superposition of a scaled sinc function for each sampled point as indicated by the dashed lines in c). Only the magnitude is shown in the frequency domain.

$$= \sum_{n=-\infty}^{\infty} d_n \, \text{sinc}\left(\pi \, \frac{x - nx_0}{x_0}\right), \tag{2.76}$$

again using the sifting theorem. Convolution of the sample values with the sinc function is sometimes referred to as sinc interpolation.

Thus, as illustrated in Figure 2.17, recovering the continuous function is achieved by the superposition of a series of scaled sinc functions corresponding to each sampled valued. Each sinc function has a value of zero at positions corresponding to all other sample locations, and hence the value of $\hat{d}(x)$ is still equal to $d(x)$ for $x = nx_0$. Use of the sampled function $d^\dagger(x)$ with δ functions is key to enabling this elegant representation.

The recovered continuous function $\hat{d}(x)$ is exactly equal to the original presampling function $d(x)$ *only* if there is no aliasing resulting from the sampling process. Aliasing would correspond to an overlap of the central component with the shifted spectral aliases (as illustrated in Figure 2.16) which could therefore not normally be isolated from the aliases.

2.5 Stochastic processes in linear systems

A random (stochastic) process can be viewed here as any mechanism giving rise to random fluctuations in a signal, generally represented as a random variable. It is not possible to precisely predict the future values of a random variable, but it may be possible to determine its statistical properties. Excellent general references for a description of stochastic processes are Papoulis [17] or Bendat and Piersol [16].

In this section, the mathematical tools required to characterize noise in medical imaging systems are summarized.

2.5.1 Deterministic versus stochastic systems

A distinction can be made between deterministic systems and stochastic systems [17]. A deterministic system, when presented with two identical inputs, will produce *exactly* the same output both times. There will be absolutely no difference, even under close examination. On the other hand, a stochastic system, when presented with two identical inputs, may produce similar outputs but they will not be exactly the same. There are many reasons why the two sample outputs may differ. For instance, some systems may use secondary image quanta (e.g., light generated in a screen, electron-hole pairs in a detector, etc.) to transfer the image from input to output, and the statistical properties of these quanta may introduce a random component in the output image. These systems are therefore fundamentally stochastic systems, independent of the statistical properties of the incident x-ray quanta.

2.5.2 Expected value and variance

The simplest way of characterizing a random variable is in terms of its expected value and variance. The expected value of the random variable a is $E\{a\}$ given by [17]

$$E\{a\} = \int_{-\infty}^{\infty} \alpha \lambda_a(\alpha)\, d\alpha, \tag{2.77}$$

where $\lambda_a(\alpha)$ is the probability of a having the value α. The variance expresses the expected value of the squared deviation from the expected value, given by [17]

$$\sigma_a^2 = E\{|\Delta a|^2\} = E\{|a - E\{a\}|^2\} = E\{a^2\} - |E\{a\}|^2, \tag{2.78}$$

where $\Delta a = a - E\{a\}$.

2.5.3 Autocorrelation and autocovariance

If $a(x)$ is a complex random variable expressed as a function of x, the autocorrelation of $a(x)$ is $R_a(x', x' + x)$ given by [17]

$$R_a(x', x' + x) = E\{a(x')a^*(x' + x)\}, \tag{2.79}$$

where $*$ indicates a complex conjugate. When $a(x)$ is a real-only value, $a^*(x) = a(x)$. The autocorrelation describes the correlation of $a(x')$ with itself at a location displaced by x.

The autocovariance describes the correlation of $a(x')$ with itself at a location displaced by x about the expected values. Thus, the autocovariance of the random variable $a(x)$ is [17]

$$K_a(x', x' + x) = E\{\Delta a(x')\Delta a^*(x' + x)\} \tag{2.80}$$

$$= R_a(x', x' + x) - E\{a(x')\}E\{a^*(x' + x)\}. \tag{2.81}$$

2.5.4 Wide-sense stationary (WSS) random processes

If a is a real-valued random variable for which the expected value and variance are stationary, that is, have fixed values, the expected value $E\{a\}$ is given by the sample mean in the limit of $N \to \infty$,

$$E\{a\} = \lim_{N \to \infty} \frac{1}{N} \sum_{n=1}^{N} a_n, \tag{2.82}$$

where a_n is the nth value of a, and the variance by

$$\sigma_a^2 = \lim_{N \to \infty} \frac{1}{N} \sum_{n=1}^{N} (a_n - E\{a\})^2 \tag{2.83}$$

$$= \lim_{N \to \infty} \frac{1}{N-1} \left[\sum_{n=1}^{N} a_n^2 - \frac{1}{N} \left(\sum_{n=1}^{N} a_n \right)^2 \right]. \tag{2.84}$$

A random process in x having all statistical properties stationary with x is called *strict-sense stationary* (SSS). A process having at least the expected value and autocorrelation stationary in x is called *wide-sense stationary* (WSS). For instance, if $a(x)$ is a WSS random process, the autocorrelation in Eq. (2.79) depends on the separation x, but not on the position x'. This simplification means that [17]

$$R_a(x', x' + x) = R_a(x), \tag{2.85}$$

and

$$K_a(x', x' + x) = K_a(x). \tag{2.86}$$

If $a(x)$ is a real process, $R_a(x)$ and $K_a(x)$ are real and even.

2.5.4.1 Noise power spectrum of a WSS random process

The autocovariance of a WSS random process, $K_a(x)$, provides a complete description of the second-order second-moment statistics in the spatial domain. In the spatial-frequency domain, the same statistics are described by the Wiener spectrum, equal to the Fourier transform of the autocovariance function. The Wiener spectrum describes the spectral decomposition of the noise variance of a WSS random process. That is, it describes the contribution to the variance from spatial frequencies between u and $(u + du)$.

For historical reasons, the Wiener spectrum is also called the noise-power spectrum (NPS). This resulted from the fact that if $a(t)$ represents a random (in time) voltage fluctuation across a pure resistance of one ohm, the expected average power dissipated by the resistance is given by the variance of $a(t)$. Thus, the spectral decomposition of the variance is called the power spectrum, or noise power spectrum, or sometimes the covariance spectrum [17].

In an imaging context, the NPS of a random process $a(x)$, $\text{NPS}_a(u)$, is expressed as a function of spatial frequencies (u) rather than temporal frequencies (t), and can be written in terms of the autocovariance as

$$\text{NPS}_a(u) = \text{F}\{\text{K}_a(x)\}. \tag{2.87}$$

Thus, the NPS and the autocovariance of a WSS random process are Fourier-transform pairs. If $a(x)$ is a real function, $\text{NPS}_a(u)$ is real and even.

2.5.5 Ergodic WSS random processes

Use of Eqs. (2.80) to characterize image noise requires the expected values $\text{E}\{a(x)\}$ and $\text{E}\{a(x')a^*(x' + x)\}$ for each x value, which may be difficult or impossible to obtain in practice. Fortunately, many random processes responsible for noise in medical imaging systems are ergodic or can be approximated as being ergodic. Being ergodic means that expected values can be determined equivalently from *ensemble* averages or *spatial* averages [17]. Thus, while the autocovariance is given by Eq. (2.80) based on true expectation values, an estimate of the autocovariance for a WSS mean ergodic random process is given by the *sample autocovariance*, $\text{K}_{a,X}(x)$, which is a spatial average,

$$\text{K}_{a,X}(x) = \frac{1}{X} \int_X \Delta a(x') \Delta . a^*(x' + x) \, dx' \tag{2.88}$$

In the limit of $X \to \infty$, the sample covariance gives the autocovariance:

$$\text{K}_a(x) = \lim_{X \to \infty} \text{K}_{a,X}(x) \tag{2.89}$$

$$= \lim_{X \to \infty} \left[\frac{1}{X} \int_X a(x')a^*(x' + x) \, dx' \right.$$
$$\left. - \frac{1}{X} \int_X a(x') \, dx' \frac{1}{X} \int_X a^*(x' + x) \, dx' \right] \tag{2.90}$$

$$= \lim_{X \to \infty} \frac{1}{X} \int_X \Delta a(x') \Delta a^*(x' + x) \, dx' \tag{2.91}$$

$$= \Delta a(x) \star \Delta a^*(x), \tag{2.92}$$

where $\star$ represents the correlation operation.

2.5.5.1 Noise power spectrum of an ergodic WSS random process

The NPS of a WSS random process is given by Eq. (2.87), and $K_a(x)$ for a WSS ergodic random process is given by Eq. (2.91). From this it can be shown that the NPS of a WSS ergodic random process is given by

$$\text{NPS}_a(u) = \lim_{X \to \infty} \frac{1}{X} \text{E}\left\{ \left| \int_X \Delta a(x) e^{-i2\pi ux} \, dx \right|^2 \right\} \qquad (2.93)$$

$$= \lim_{X \to \infty} \frac{1}{X} \text{E}\left\{ \left| F_X\{\Delta a(x)\} \right|^2 \right\}, \qquad (2.94)$$

where $F_X\{\Delta a(x)\}$ is the Fourier transform of the zero-mean function $\Delta a(x)$ truncated to the region $-X/2 \leqslant x \leqslant X/2$. Equations (2.87) and (2.94) can each be used to determine the NPS of a WSS ergodic random process. The units of $\text{NPS}_a(u)$ are equal to those of $a^2(x) \times x$.

The variance of an ergodic WSS random process $a(x)$ is given by

$$\sigma_a^2 = \text{E}\{a(x)a^*(x)\} - \text{E}\{a(x)\}\text{E}\{a^*(x)\} \qquad (2.95)$$

$$= \text{E}\{\Delta a(x)\Delta a^*(x)\} \qquad (2.96)$$

$$= K_a(x)|_{x=0}, \qquad (2.97)$$

and therefore the Fourier DC theorem shows that the variance of $a(x)$ can also be written in terms of the NPS as

$$\sigma_a^2 = \int_{-\infty}^{\infty} \text{NPS}_a(u) \, du. \qquad (2.98)$$

In summary, use of Fourier-based descriptions of image noise requires two important assumptions. The first is that processes responsible for noise both in the input signal and within the imaging chain be wide-sense stationary (WSS). This means that the mean and autocovariance of the noise processes, and the second-order noise-transfer characteristics of the imaging system, are stationary in x. This condition is often satisfied for the analysis of noise in low-contrast imaging tasks. The second assumption is that the system be ergodic. While it can be difficult to prove ergodicity, many systems of practical importance can be considered ergodic if practical approximations are made. For instance, the expectation values of image-intensifier-based video systems can be determined from multiple sequential video frames and the system can be considered ergodic if the analysis is restricted to central regions of the image. Stimulable phosphor or film-screen-based systems have grain noise that is not ergodic, and which may have to be addressed as a separate noise source.

2.5.6 Ergodic wide-sense cyclostationary (WSCS) random processes

Another important category of stochastic processes are those that exhibit some periodic behavior but which have statistical properties that are still invariant to a shift of any multiple of that period (Papoulis [17], Gardner and Franks [23]). A process is called *strict-sense cyclostationary* (SSCS) with period x_0 if all its statistical properties are invariant to a shift of nx_0 for any integer n, and *wide-sense cyclostationary* (WSCS) if only the mean and correlation are invariant. Thus, $a(x)$ is WSCS with period x_0 if

$$E\{a(x + nx_0)\} = E\{a(x)\},\qquad(2.99)$$

and

$$R_a(x' + nx_0, x' + x + nx_0) = R_a(x', x' + x),\qquad(2.100)$$

for any integer n. In imaging, an important type of cyclostationary process is that which can be written in the form

$$a(x) = \sum_{n=-\infty}^{\infty} a_n s(x - nx_0),\qquad(2.101)$$

where $s(x)$ is called the *sensing* function of the WSCS process. The expected value of $a(x)$ is given by

$$E\{a(x)\} = E\{a_n\} \sum_{n=-\infty}^{\infty} s(x - nx_0),\qquad(2.102)$$

where $E\{a_n\}$ is the expected value of a_n. For WSCS ergodic random processes, the autocorrelation is given by

$$R_a(x) = \frac{1}{x_0} \sum_{n=-\infty}^{\infty} R_a(nx_0)\tau(x),\qquad(2.103)$$

where

$$\tau(x) = \int_{-\infty}^{\infty} s(x')s(x' + x)\,dx' = s(x) \star s(x).\qquad(2.104)$$

Wide-sense cyclostationary ergodic random processes are important in the description of digital-imaging systems. For instance, if $a(x)$ is a WSS ergodic stochastic process that is represented with the digital samples $a_n = a(nx_0)$ obtained using impulse sensing functions at uniform spacing x_0, $s(x) = \sum_{n=-\infty}^{\infty} \delta(x - nx_0)$, then $a^{\dagger}(x)$, given by

$$a^{\dagger}(x) = \sum_{n=-\infty}^{\infty} a_n \delta(x - nx_0), \qquad (2.105)$$

is an infinite train of amplitude-modulated δ functions and is a WSCS ergodic random process with period x_0. The expected value of $a^{\dagger}(x)$ is given by [17, 23]

$$\mathrm{E}\{a^{\dagger}(x)\} = \mathrm{E}\{a_n\} \sum_{n=-\infty}^{\infty} \delta(x - nx_0). \qquad (2.106)$$

The autocorrelation of $a^{\dagger}(x)$, $\mathrm{R}_{a^{\dagger}}(x)$, is given by

$$\mathrm{R}_{a^{\dagger}}(x) = \frac{1}{x_0} \sum_{n=-\infty}^{\infty} R_a(nx_0)\delta(x - nx_0) = \frac{1}{x_0} R_a(x) \sum_{n=-\infty}^{\infty} \delta(x - nx_0), \quad (2.107)$$

where $R_a(x)$ is the autocorrelation of $a(x)$. Similarly, the autocovariance, $\mathrm{K}_{a^{\dagger}}(x)$, is given by

$$\mathrm{K}_{a^{\dagger}}(x) = \frac{1}{x_0} \sum_{n=-\infty}^{\infty} K_a(nx_0)\delta(x - nx_0) = \frac{1}{x_0} K_a(x) \sum_{n=-\infty}^{\infty} \delta(x - nx_0), \quad (2.108)$$

where $K_a(x)$ is the autocovariance of $a(x)$. The units of $\mathrm{K}_{a^{\dagger}}(x)$ are equal to those of $a^2(x) \times x^{-2}$.

2.5.6.1 Noise-power spectrum of an ergodic WSCS random process

In the previous section, $\mathrm{NPS}_a(u)$ was introduced as the NPS of a WSS random process, given by the Fourier transform of the autocovariance of that random process. Following Gardner and Franks [23], we introduce $\mathrm{NPS}_{a^{\dagger}}(u)$ as the Fourier transform of $\mathrm{K}_{a^{\dagger}}(x)$, the autocovariance of the WSCS random process $a(x)$ is given by

$$\mathrm{NPS}_{a^{\dagger}}(u) = \mathrm{F}\{\mathrm{K}_{a^{\dagger}}(x)\} \qquad (2.109)$$

$$= \frac{1}{x_0^2} \mathrm{NPS}_a(u) * \sum_{n=-\infty}^{\infty} \delta\left(u - \frac{n}{x_0}\right), \qquad (2.110)$$

with units of $a^2(x) \times x^{-1}$. It is important to note that these units are different from those of $\mathrm{NPS}_a(u)$, which are $a^2(x) \times x$.

This result shows that the NPS of a random-process periodic in the spatial domain with period x_0 is periodic also in the spatial-frequency domain with period $1/x_0$. This has important implications when used to describe noise in digital-imaging systems which may suffer from noise aliasing (Section 2.9.3).

2.6 Metrics of system performance

The stochastic nature of image quanta imposes a fundamental limitation on the performance of imaging systems, and gives rise to stochastic fluctuations in the image signals contributing to image formation. In this section, metrics developed to describe image quality in terms of signal and noise are described within a linear-systems framework.

2.6.1 Rose model signal-to-noise ratio

The importance of the statistical nature of image quanta to imaging was first recognized in 1948 by Rose [2, 3] and his contemporaries [24–26], and their work forms the basis of many introductory texts on the nature of signal and noise in radiography. The relationship between the number of image quanta and perception of detail is embodied in the "Rose Model," as it has come to be known, describing the signal-to-noise ratio (SNR) for the detection of a uniform object in a uniform background having a mean $\overline{q}_b$ quanta per unit area. If $\overline{q}_0$ is the mean number of quanta per unit area in the region of the object, the resulting contrast C can be written as

$$C = (\overline{q}_b - \overline{q}_0)/\overline{q}_b. \tag{2.111}$$

Rose defined "signal" to be the *incremental change* in the number of image quanta caused by to the object integrated over the area of that object. This is different from the definition of signal used elsewhere in this chapter, and hence we will call his signal the "Rose signal," ΔS_{Rose}, or difference signal, where

$$\Delta S_{Rose} = (\overline{q}_b - \overline{q}_0)A, \tag{2.112}$$

for a uniform object of area A. The noise in Rose's signal is the standard deviation in the number of quanta in an equal area of uniform background, σ_b. For the special case of uncorrelated background quanta, noise is described by Poisson statistics and $\sigma_b = \sqrt{A\overline{q}_b}$ so that the Rose SNR, ΔSNR_{Rose}, is given by

$$\Delta SNR_{Rose} = \frac{A(\overline{q}_b - \overline{q}_0)}{\sqrt{A\overline{q}_b}} = C\sqrt{A\overline{q}_b}. \tag{2.113}$$

Rose showed that ΔSNR_{Rose} must have a value of approximately five or greater for reliable detection of a uniform object under these conditions.

This result led to the general expectation that lesion detectibility should be proportional to object contrast and to the square root of object area and radiation dose (at a single x-ray energy). Under the Rose conditions (uniform object, uniform background, and uncorrelated Poisson-distributed noise), this relationship is found to be approximately correct. For instance, Figure 2.18 shows an image of a contrast-detail phantom obtained using a prototype digital x-ray mammography detector. Examination of this image shows that detectibility of these low-contrast lesions increases with lesion diameter (square root of area) and contrast, consistent with the Rose model.

Some implications and limitations of the Rose model are described in terms of modern detection theory by Burgess [27]. He shows that the Rose model corresponds to the very specific detection task called "signal known exactly" (SKE) and "background known exactly" (BKE) detection task [27, 28].

The Rose model played an essential role in establishing the fact that image quality is ultimately limited by the statistical nature of image quanta. However, its limitations quickly become apparent when used to assess image quality in many practical situations. The primary restriction is the definition of noise used by Rose in Eq. (2.113), which is valid only for uncorrelated Poisson-distributed noise. In general, noise in a recorded image is neither uncorrelated nor Poisson distributed. This may be because of the presence of additive system noise (e.g., electronic or film noise), quantum amplification stages in a cascaded system (described later), or statistical correlations introduced into the image signals by the scatter of x rays or secondary image quanta in the detector system (e.g., light in a radiographic screen). For all of these reasons, the original Rose model needs appropriate extension and elaboration to be of practical value in the analysis of most modern medical-imaging systems. The use of Fourier-based metrics of image signal and noise facilitates this extension.

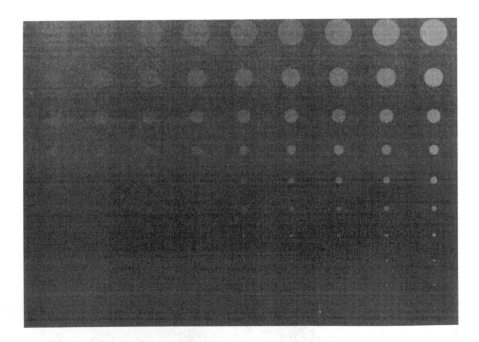

Figure 2.18: Image of a contrast-detail test phantom obtained with a prototype digital x-ray mammography detector. Lesion contrast increases in the horizontal direction and lesion diameter increases in the vertical direction (courtesy M. Yaffe).

2.6.2 Noise-power spectrum (NPS) and variance

The NPS of a one-dimensional random process $d(x)$, $\mathrm{NPS}_d(u)$, is given by Eq. (2.87) for a WSS random process, and by Eqs. (2.87) or (2.93) for an ergodic WSS random process. Thus, $\mathrm{NPS}_d(u)$ has units of $d^2(x) \times x$.

The NPS of a two-dimensional ergodic WSS random process $d(x, y)$, $\mathrm{NPS}_d(u, v)$, is given by

$$
\begin{aligned}
\mathrm{NPS}_d(u, v) & \\
&= \lim_{X,Y \to \infty, \infty} \frac{1}{XY} \mathrm{E}\left\{ \left| \int_X \int_Y \Delta d(x, y) e^{-i2\pi(ux+vy)} \, dx \, dy \right|^2 \right\} \quad (2.114) \\
&= \lim_{X,Y \to \infty, \infty} \frac{1}{XY} \mathrm{E}\left\{ \left| \mathrm{F}_{X,Y}\{\Delta d(x, y)\} \right|^2 \right\} \quad (2.115) \\
&= \lim_{X,Y \to \infty, \infty} \mathrm{E}\left\{ S_{\Delta d, X, Y}(u, v) \right\}, \quad (2.116)
\end{aligned}
$$

where $\mathrm{F}_{X,Y}\{d(x, y)\}$ is the Fourier transform of $d(x, y)$ truncated to the region $-X/2 \leqslant x \leqslant X/2$, $-Y/2 \leqslant y \leqslant Y/2$, and $S_{\Delta d, X, Y}(u, v)$ is the two-dimensional sample spectrum of $\Delta d(x, y)$ over the same range. The units of $\mathrm{NPS}_d(u, v)$ are equal to those of $d^2(x, y) \times x^2$.

2.6.2.1 NPS in one and two dimensions

While a two-dimensional analysis of the NPS is sometimes necessary [29], visualization in two dimensions can be problematic. In many situations it is adequate to examine the two-dimensional NPS in only one specified direction at a time (which we will call the x direction with corresponding spatial frequency u), where the dependence in the perpendicular direction has been removed by integration. For instance, if we define $d_Y(x)$ as the integral of $d(x, y)$ over a distance Y in the y direction, then

$$
d_Y(x) = \int_Y d(x, y) \, dy, \quad (2.117)
$$

and the NPS of $d_Y(x)$, $\mathrm{NPS}_{d_Y}(u)$, is given by

$$
\begin{aligned}
\mathrm{NPS}_{d_Y}(u) & \\
&= \lim_{X,Y \to \infty, \infty} \mathrm{E}\left\{ \frac{1}{XY} \left| \int_X \Delta d_Y(x) e^{-i2\pi ux} \, dx \right|^2 \right\} \quad (2.118) \\
&= \lim_{X,Y \to \infty, \infty} \mathrm{E}\left\{ \frac{1}{XY} \left| \int_X \left[\int_Y \Delta d(x, y) e^{-i2\pi(ux+vy)} \, dy \right]_{v=0} dx \right|^2 \right\}, \quad (2.119)
\end{aligned}
$$

which is the two-dimensional NPS of $d(x, y)$ evaluated along the $v = 0$ axis. Therefore,

$$\text{NPS}_{d_Y}(u) = \text{NPS}_d(u, v)|_{v=0}. \tag{2.120}$$

Thus, the NPS of a two-dimensional random process, $d(x, y)$, whether expressed as a one-dimensional or two-dimensional NPS, will have the units of $|d(x, y)|^2 \times x^2$. The NPS of both analog and digital images is generally expressed in units of mm^2.

The NPS and the autocovariance are Fourier pairs. The autocovariance of $d_Y(x)$ is therefore related to that of $d(x, y)$ by

$$K_{d_Y}(x) = \lim_{Y \to \infty} \frac{1}{Y} \int_Y K_d(x, y) \, dy, \tag{2.121}$$

as a direct consequence of the central-slice theorem.

2.6.2.2 The zero-frequency value of the NPS

The value of $\text{NPS}_a(u)$ for $u = 0$ is called the zero-frequency, or scale, value of the NPS. Using the Fourier DC theorem and Eq. (2.87), the zero-frequency value can be written as the autocovariance integrated over all x:

$$\text{NPS}_a(u)|_{u=0} = \int_{-\infty}^{\infty} K_a(x) \, dx \tag{2.122}$$

$$= \int_{-\infty}^{\infty} E\{\Delta a(x')\Delta a(x' + x)\} \, dx. \tag{2.123}$$

The zero-frequency value of $\text{NPS}_a(u)$ therefore depends on the extent to which $\Delta a(x)$ may be correlated.

To facilitate further analysis, it is useful to define an average correlation length of the random process $a(x)$, X_{cor}. It is defined such that if $a(x)$ has the autocovariance $K_a(x)$, the area of the rectangle formed by X_{cor} and $K_a(0)$ is the same as that

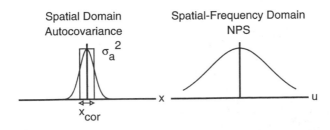

Figure 2.19: The average correlation length of $a(x)$ is defined as X_{cor}, the effective width of the autocovariance function $K_a(x)$ forming a rectangle with the same area as $K_a(x)$.

of $K_a(x)$, as illustrated in Figure 2.19. That is,

$$\int_{-\infty}^{\infty} K_a(x)\,dx = X_{cor}K_a(0).$$ (2.124)

The value $K_a(0)$ is equal to the variance σ_a^2, and hence combining this result with Eq. (2.122) gives

$$NPS_a(u)|_{u=0} = X_{cor}\sigma_a^2.$$ (2.125)

In an analogous way, the zero-frequency value of a two-dimensional NPS is given as

$$NPS_a(u,v)|_{u,v=0,0} = \iint_{A_{cor}} \sigma_a^2\,dx\,dy = A_{cor}\sigma_a^2,$$ (2.126)

where A_{cor} is the two-dimensional average correlation area.

An important special case occurs when measurements are made of a random process, such as variations in optical density of an exposed film. For instance, if $OD(x, y)$ describes the "true" optical density at position (x, y), measurements of film density obtained using a rectangular aperture (sampling function) with dimensions X by Y and area $A = XY$ can be written as $d(x, y)$ where

$$d(x,y) = \frac{1}{A}\int_{x-X/2}^{x+X/2}\int_{y-Y/2}^{y+Y/2} OD(x,y)\,dx'\,dy'$$

$$= \frac{1}{A}OD(x,y) * \prod\left(\frac{x}{X},\frac{y}{Y}\right).$$ (2.127)

As will be shown in Section 2.7.2, the NPS of $d(x, y)$ is therefore given by

$$NPS_d(u,v) = NPS_{OD}(u,v)\left|\text{sinc}(\pi Xu)\text{sinc}(\pi Yv)\right|^2,$$ (2.128)

where $NPS_{OD}(u, v)$ is the NPS of $OD(x, y)$, and therefore,

$$NPS_d(0,0) = NPS_{OD}(0,0).$$ (2.129)

If both dimensions of the measurement area X and Y are large with respect to any correlation distance in $OD(x, y)$, $NPS_{OD}(u, v)$ can be approximated as a constant value for all frequencies at which the sinc functions have a non-negligible value. The variance in $d(x, y)$ can then be written as

$$\sigma_d^2 = \int_{-\infty}^{\infty} NPS_d(u,v)\,du\,dv$$ (2.130)

$$\approx NPS_{OD}(0,0)\int_{-\infty}^{\infty}\left|\text{sinc}(\pi Xu)\text{sinc}(\pi Yv)\right|^2\,du\,dv$$ (2.131)

$$= NPS_d(0,0)\frac{1}{XY},$$ (2.132)

and therefore

$$\mathrm{NPS}_d(0, 0) \approx A\sigma_d^2, \tag{2.133}$$

where $A = XY$ is the measurement area. Equation (2.133) is in the form expressed on page 222 of Dainty and Shaw [5]. It shows that for this special case where measurements are made with an aperture (the sampling function) that is large relative to any correlation distance in the quantity being measured, the zero-frequency value is approximately equal to the measured variance multiplied by the measurement area.

This result may be useful when an accurate measure of the zero-frequency value is required. In practice, if Eq. (2.114) is used to calculate the NPS, a zero-frequency value of zero (or some other erroneous value) may be obtained when the sample mean is used as an estimate of the expectation value. It is important to note that the zero-frequency value is generally non-zero, and that its value can be affected by the measurement process. See the next section and Eq. (2.252) for additional specific implications of the zero-frequency value.

2.6.2.3 NPS, autocovariance and variance of a distribution of uncorrelated quanta

An uncorrelated two-dimensional distribution of image quanta $q(x, y)$, such as a uniform distribution of x rays, has an NPS given by [5]

$$\mathrm{NPS}_q(u, v) = \mathrm{E}\{q(x, y)\} = \mathrm{E}\{q\}, \tag{2.134}$$

which is equal to $\mathrm{E}\{q\}$, the expected number of quanta per mm^2, and is independent of spatial frequency. Note that the units of the NPS of a quantum image are different from that of an analog or digital image (which are mm^2, see Section 2.2.1). This is because quantum images are distributions, requiring distribution theory for interpretation, while analog images and digital images are not.

The corresponding autocovariance is given by

$$K_q(x, y) = \mathrm{E}\{\Delta q(x', y')\Delta q(x' + x, y' + y)\} \tag{2.135}$$

$$= \begin{cases} \mathrm{E}\{|\Delta q(x, y)|^2\} & \text{for } x = 0, \ y = 0 \\ 0 & \text{for } x \neq 0, \ y \neq 0 \end{cases} \tag{2.136}$$

$$= \mathrm{E}\{q\}\delta(x, y), \tag{2.137}$$

which is a δ function scaled by $\mathrm{E}\{q\}$. The fact that the autocovariance is proportional to a δ function is equivalent to stating that the image quanta are uncorrelated. That is, there is no statistical correlation of quanta at any position x, y with any other position x', y'.

For this special case of a distribution of uncorrelated quanta, the zero-frequency value of the NPS is obtained by combining Eqs. (2.122) and (2.137), giving

$$\text{NPS}_q(u, v)|_{u,v=0,0} = \int_{-\infty}^{\infty} \int_{-\infty}^{\infty} K_q(u, v) \, du \, dv \tag{2.138}$$

$$= \int_{-\infty}^{\infty} \int_{-\infty}^{\infty} E\{q\}\delta(x, y) \, du \, dv \tag{2.139}$$

$$= E\{q\}. \tag{2.140}$$

The variance of this distribution of image quanta, given by

$$\sigma_q^2 = \int_{-\infty}^{\infty} \int_{-\infty}^{\infty} \text{NPS}_q(u, v) \, du \, dv = \int_{-\infty}^{\infty} \int_{-\infty}^{\infty} E\{q\} \, du \, dv, \tag{2.141}$$

is undefined.

In practice, a uniform distribution of x rays coming from a medical x-ray tube will be uncorrelated and as a result have a flat NPS as given by Eq. (2.134) [5]. However, it should be noted that while a distribution of secondary quanta (such as light from a radiographic screen) will always have an uncorrelated component, they may also be partially correlated. Thus, the NPS of a distribution of secondary quanta may not be flat but will always have a non-zero component extending to essentially infinite frequencies.

2.6.3 Noise-equivalent number of quanta (NEQ)

As indicated above, units of the NPS depend on the physical basis of the image signal $d(x)$ and may be arbitrary or specific to a particular imaging system. Thus, use of the NPS for quantifying image noise brought the practical problem of absolute scaling of signal and noise-power spectra. By expressing image noise in terms of the number of Poisson-distributed input photons per unit area at each spatial frequency, Shaw obtained a common *absolute* scale of noise—the noise-equivalent number of quanta (NEQ) [5, 30]. The NEQ of a linear system can be defined as

$$\text{NEQ}(\bar{q}, u) = \frac{|\bar{q}\,T(u)|^2}{\text{NPS}(u)}, \tag{2.142}$$

for an average input of $\bar{q}$ quanta per unit area where $T(u)$ is the system characteristic function describing signal transfer from input to output of an imaging system (Section 2.3.2.2). The numerator describes the (squared) expected output signal in terms of the spatial-frequency response of the system, $|\bar{q}\,T(u)|^2$. The denominator describes the corresponding output noise power. In general, if the average output signal from a linear system is $\bar{d}$, corresponding to an average uniform input of $\bar{q}$ quanta per unit area, the system large-area gain factor is $G = \bar{d}/\bar{q}$ and

$|T(u)| = G\text{MTF}(u)$. Therefore,

$$\text{NEQ}(\overline{q}, u) = \frac{\overline{q}^2 \overline{G}^2 \text{MTF}^2(u)}{\text{NPS}_d(u)} \qquad (2.143)$$

$$= \frac{\text{MTF}^2(u)}{\text{NPS}_d(u)/\overline{d}^2}, \qquad (2.144)$$

where $\text{NPS}_d(u)$ is the output image NPS. The units of NEQ are equal to those of $\overline{q}$.

Equation (2.144) is particularly convenient to use in many practical situations as it only requires $\text{MTF}^2(u)$ and the NPS normalized by the mean signal squared, $\text{NPS}_d(u)/\overline{d}^2$, both of which are readily determined experimentally from measured image data.

Some systems have a nonlinear response and exhibit only small-signal linearity. A more general form of the NEQ that is still valid for these systems can be written as [28]

$$\text{NEQ}(\overline{q}, u) = \frac{\overline{q}^2 \left|\dfrac{\partial \overline{d}}{\partial \overline{q}}\right|^2 \text{MTF}^2(u)}{\text{NPS}_d(u)}, \qquad (2.145)$$

where $\partial \overline{d}/\partial \overline{q}$ is the incremental change in average output signal $\overline{d}$ attributable to an incremental change in the average input signal $\overline{q}$ at an average input level $\overline{q}$. For example, film-screen systems have a nonlinear response to x-ray exposure. Using Eq. (2.145), the NEQ for these systems can be written as [5]

$$\text{NEQ}(\overline{q}, u) = \frac{\overline{q}^2 |\gamma \log_{10}(e)(1/\overline{q})|^2 \text{MTF}^2(u)}{\text{NPS}_{OD}(u)} \qquad (2.146)$$

$$= \frac{(\gamma \log_{10} e)^2 \text{MTF}^2(u)}{\text{NPS}_{OD}(u)}, \qquad (2.147)$$

where γ is the slope of the characteristic optical density versus log-exposure curve (and therefore the system gain factor is $\overline{G} = \gamma \log_{10}(e)(1/\overline{q})$) corresponding to the same exposure level (and therefore mean optical density, $\overline{OD}$) as the optical-density NPS measurement, and the MTF corresponds to a small-signal MTF.

The NEQ concept expresses image quality on an absolute scale, independent of specific system parameters. It gives the number of Poisson-distributed quanta that would produce the same SNR given an ideal detector. It can be measured for specific systems at specified exposure levels in various laboratories, and the results can be directly compared. An image with a greater NEQ corresponds to lower image noise. An ideal system that transfers both signal and noise with only a scaler gain factor G results in an NEQ given by

$$\mathrm{NEQ}(\overline{q}, u) = \frac{|\overline{q}G|^2}{G^2\overline{q}} = \overline{q}, \tag{2.148}$$

which has no frequency dependence and is the best possible NEQ for an input $\overline{q}$.

Interpretation of the NEQ often requires considerable thought, but provides a great deal of insight regarding the information content of an image. It is a measure of the density of quanta the image is "worth" [31]. Wagner and co-workers [31–34] have shown that the NEQ concept can be generalized to other imaging modalities including computed tomography (CT), magnetic resonance imaging (MRI), and ultrasound imaging. They introduced the concept of a "system aperture," a_{ap}, and showed that it is related to the NEQ through the equation

$$a_{ap}^{-1} = \int_{-\infty}^{\infty} \frac{\mathrm{NEQ}(k)}{\mathrm{NEQ}(0)} \mathrm{d}^2k. \tag{2.149}$$

The system aperture is the fundamental measure of resolution in a noise-limited imaging system [31]. They also showed that for the detection of an object $\Delta s(x)$ having frequency components $\Delta S(u)$, the NEQ is directly related to the "ideal observer SNR," SNR_i, according to

$$\mathrm{SNR}_i^2 = \int_{-\infty}^{\infty} |\Delta S(u)|^2 \mathrm{NEQ}(u) \, \mathrm{d}u. \tag{2.150}$$

The ideal observer detects all of the information in the image for the required task, and SNR_i determines the performance of the observer in detection tasks.

Decision-making theory is a complex subject. A summary of important aspects of image quality, observer performance and detection theory, including the NEQ, is available as an ICRU report [28] "Medical imaging—the assessment of image quality" written by some of the most important figures in this field, including Barber, Brown, Burgess, Metz, Myers, Taylor, and Wagner.

2.6.4 Detective quantum efficiency (DQE)

The NEQ describes the effective number of Poisson-distributed x-ray quanta contributing to image SNR. Using a similar approach, the detective quantum efficiency (DQE) is a measure of the effective *fraction* of incident Poisson-distributed quanta contributing to image SNR. Thus, the NEQ is a measure of image quality while the DQE is a similar measure of system performance. The spatial-frequency-dependent DQE was first used during the mid-seventies in an attempt to develop measures of system performance common to a variety of imaging technologies by Shaw, Wagner, and co-workers [35, 36], with Wagner and co-workers [28, 36] deserving much of the credit for championing the widespread application of the noise-equivalent approach and providing some of the first absolute sets of DQE measurements. The DQE is defined as [30]

$$\mathrm{DQE}(\overline{q}, u) = \frac{\mathrm{NEQ}(\overline{q}, u)}{\overline{q}} \tag{2.151}$$

$$= \frac{\overline{q}\left|\frac{\partial \overline{d}}{\partial \overline{q}}\right|^2 \mathrm{MTF}^2(u)}{\mathrm{NPS}_d(u)}. \tag{2.152}$$

A practical expression for use when measuring the DQE of a linear system is given by

$$\mathrm{DQE}(\overline{q}, u) = \frac{\overline{q}\,\overline{G}^2\mathrm{MTF}^2(u)}{\mathrm{NPS}_d(u)} \tag{2.153}$$

$$= \frac{\overline{d}^2\mathrm{MTF}^2(u)}{\overline{q}\,\mathrm{NPS}_d(u)}. \tag{2.154}$$

In the absence of additive system noise or multiplicative noise such as fixed-pattern noise, the DQE is independent of $\overline{q}$ and $\mathrm{DQE}(\overline{q}, u) = \mathrm{DQE}(u)$ for a linear imaging system. The DQE also depends on $\overline{q}$ for nonlinear systems such as film-screen systems. The DQE is always dimensionless, and can have a value no greater than unity.

The term $\overline{q}$ in Eq. (2.154) is normally interpreted as the total number of incident quanta per unit area, independent of energy of the quanta. It can be estimated from a measurement of the actual exposure X at the detector input (excluding backscatter) with the expression

$$\overline{q} = X\left(\frac{\Phi}{X}\right), \tag{2.155}$$

where X is the measured exposure (in roentgens), and (Φ/X) is the x ray fluence per R for the particular spectrum used. X-ray tube manufacturers may provide this factor for particular test conditions. Alternatively, if the incident spectrum $\Phi(E)$ (quanta mm^{-2} keV^{-1}) can be either measured or calculated, (Φ/X) can be estimated for that spectrum as

$$\left(\frac{\Phi}{X}\right) = \int_0^{kVp} \Phi_{rel}(E)\left[\frac{\Phi}{X}(E)\right] dE, \tag{2.156}$$

where $\Phi_{rel}(E)$ is the normalized incident x-ray spectrum, and $(\Phi/X)(E)$ is the fluence per unit exposure for a mono-energetic beam with energy E and is given by [37]

$$\frac{\Phi}{X}(E) = \frac{WQ}{\left(\frac{\mu_{en}(E)}{\rho}\right)_{air} E e 10^8}, \tag{2.157}$$

where $(\mu_{en}/\rho)_{air}$ is the mass energy absorption coefficient (cm^2/g) for air, E is the x-ray energy (keV), e is the electronic charge (1.6022×10^{-19} Coul), W is

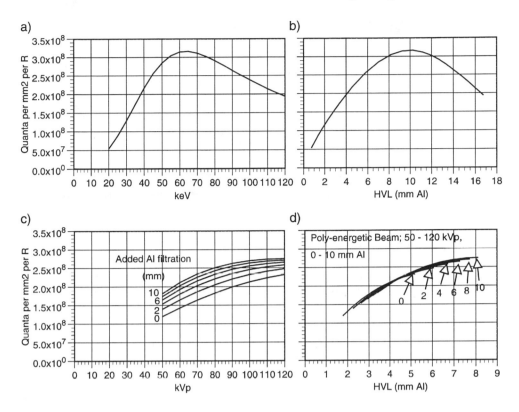

Figure 2.20: The conversion factor Φ/X (quanta mm^{-2} R^{-1}) is shown: a) as a function of mono-energetic keV; b) as a function of beam HVL for a mono-energetic beam; c) as a function of kVp for a poly-energetic beam with various thicknesses of added aluminum; and d) as a function of HVL for the same poly-energetic beams with added aluminum.

the work function of air (33.97 eV), and Q is the charge liberated in air by one Roentgen (exactly 2.580×10^{-4} Coul kg^{-1}R^{-1}). Values of (Φ/X) obtained with Eq. (2.157) are shown in Figure 2.20(a) for mono-energetic beams with energies between 20 and 120 keV, and in Figure 2.20(b) as a function of half-value layer (HVL) in mm of Al for the same beams.

Knowing an actual spectrum accurately is difficult or impractical in most situations. However, spectra can be calculated theoretically for specific situations and used to estimate (Φ/X) as a function of kVp. Figure 2.20(c) shows values of (Φ/X) calculated using Eq. (2.157) for various thicknesses of added aluminum and spectra generated using the method of Tucker [38]. It is clear that the actual value of (Φ/X) is specific to details of the spectrum used, but *insensitive* to both kVp and thickness of added aluminum when expressed as a function of the beam HVL as shown in Figure 2.20(d). Thus, an estimate of (Φ/X) with sufficient accuracy can often be obtained using Figure 2.20(d) if the HVL can be measured for the particular test conditions.

The DQE is sometimes written as

$$DQE(u) = \frac{SNR_{out}^2(u)}{SNR_{in}^2(u)},\tag{2.158}$$

although this form must be used with caution. It is only correct if the squared output SNR is given by $SNR_{out}^2(u) = \bar{d}^2 MTF^2(u)/NPS_d(u)$ and the squared input SNR by $SNR_{in}^2(u) = SNR_{ideal}^2(u) = \bar{q}$ where $SNR_{ideal}^2(u)$ corresponds to a photon-counting detector rather than any other type of detector such as an energy-integrating detector. Equation (2.152) should be taken as the general definition of the DQE.

2.7 Noise transfer in cascaded imaging systems

As discussed in the previous section, image quality is directly tied to the number of image quanta interacting with the imaging system. However, there may be additional factors degrading image quality if the imaging system is not optimally designed. For instance, when input quanta are converted to secondary quanta, such as the conversion of interacting x rays into optical quanta in a scintillating phosphor, image quality may also be influenced by the number of secondary quanta. One way of understanding the effect of these conversions is to represent the system as a "cascade" of multiple processes, and use *transfer theory* to describe the transfer of signals and noise through the system.

In addition to understanding the different approaches available for specifying system performance as described in the previous section, it is often necessary to determine whether a particular imaging system is performing at a level close to what can be expected for a particular design. In this section, methods are described which can be used to predict system performance based on design parameters. The approach is based on *transfer theory*, in which a system is modeled as a serial cascade of many stages. Transfer of signal and noise through the entire system is predicted from an understanding of the transfer properties of each stage.

In many systems, input x-ray quanta are converted to other forms of energy before producing a final image. For instance, x rays may be converted to light quanta in a radiographic screen, which may subsequently be converted to electron-hole carrier pairs in a detector. In an image intensifier, x rays are converted to light and then to photo-electrons which are accelerated before being converted to light again in the output phosphor. In some cases, the number of quanta transferred through each stage, as well as statistical correlations introduced into the distributions of these quanta, play critical roles in determining the final image quality. For instance, an inadequate number of quanta may result in a secondary "quantum sink" (see below) which will degrade image quality. In this section, methods of representing a complex system as a cascade of elementary stages are described. Transfer relationships are given for the transfer of signal and noise through these stages, and can be combined to predict the overall system DQE.

There are three elementary processes that play an important role in under-standing noise transfer: (a) quantum amplification; (b) deterministic blurring; and, (c) quantum scattering. They can be cascaded in appropriate serial combinations where the output of one stage forms a virtual input to the next. Many systems of practical importance can be modeled, and overall system signal-and-noise trans-fer determined to a good approximation. In most cases, the input and output of each stage is a distribution of quanta. These quanta may be of any form, including x rays, light, and other forms, as long as they can be considered to be independent of each other. The input and output may even represent the spatial distribution of some type of event, such as interacting quanta or just photo-electric interactions. In the following section, noise-transfer characteristics through each elementary pro-cess and methods of cascading multiple stages to predict system performance are described.

2.7.1 Quantum amplification

The first elementary process represents a conversion of quanta from one form to another, such as the conversion of x-ray quanta to optical quanta in a radio-graphic screen. Both the input and output of this stage are quantum images (Sec-tion 2.2.1.3). Each input quantum is converted to $\widetilde{g}$ output quanta where $\widetilde{g}$ is a random variable characterized in terms of a mean gain factor, $\overline{g}$, and variance, σ_g^2. Thus, if $q_{in}(r)$ is a sample function describing a sample distribution of input quanta,

$$q_{out}(r) = \widetilde{g} q_{in}(r). \qquad (2.159)$$

Rabbani, Shaw and Van Metter [39] showed that the mean number of quanta in a quantum image passing through this amplification stage is transferred according to

$$\overline{q}_{out} = \overline{g}\,\overline{q}_{in}, \qquad (2.160)$$

where $\overline{q}_{in}$ is the expected number of quanta per unit area in the input and $\overline{q}_{out}$ is the expected number in the output. They also showed that the NPS is transferred according to

$$\text{NPS}_{out}(k) = \overline{g}^2 \text{NPS}_{in}(k) + \overline{q}_{in}\sigma_g^2. \qquad (2.161)$$

These expressions can be used to describe the transfer of a uniform distribution of image quanta through an amplification process as represented graphically in Figure 2.21, and can be combined with signal-and-noise transfer expressions for other elementary processes described below to predict the performance of complex systems.

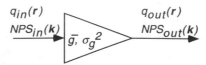

Quantum Amplification or Selection

Figure 2.21: The process of quantum amplification (and binomial selection) is represented as shown here, characterized by a mean gain $\overline{g}$ and variance σ_g^2.

2.7.1.1 Binomial selection

The amplification stage described above can also be used to represent a binomial selection process, such as the quantum efficiency of a detector. This is a special case of the amplification process in which $\widetilde{g}$ is a random variable that can have a value of 1 or 0 only. That is, each quantum incident on this selection stage is either transferred (probability $\overline{g}$), or not (probability $1 - \overline{g}$), to the output where the average value $\overline{g}$ is the quantum efficiency of the process. As a consequence of the binomial theorem, the variance σ_g^2 becomes [17]

$$\sigma_g^2 = \overline{g}(1 - \overline{g}). \tag{2.162}$$

Noise transfer through a quantum selection process is therefore given by

$$\text{NPS}_{out}(k) = \overline{g}^2 \text{NPS}_{in}(k) + \overline{q}_{in}\overline{g}(1 - \overline{g}) \tag{2.163}$$
$$= \overline{g}^2 \left[\text{NPS}_{in}(k) - \overline{q}_{in} \right] + \overline{q}_{in}\overline{g}. \tag{2.164}$$

The component $\text{NPS}_{in}(k) - \overline{q}_{in}$ is called the *correlated noise* component, and $\overline{q}_{in}$ is called the *uncorrelated noise* component. As shown by Eq. (2.164), it is sometimes said that the correlated component is "passed through" the squared conversion gain $\overline{g}^2$ in keeping with the ideal of a transfer model, while the uncorrelated component is passed though $\overline{g}$. A significant correlated component occurs when $\text{NPS}_{in}(k) \ll \overline{q}_{in}$. When the input quanta are uncorrelated, in other words, randomly distributed, then $\text{NPS}_{in}(k) = \overline{q}_{in}$. This corresponds to the smallest value that $\text{NPS}_{in}(k)$ can have, and results in an output NPS given by

$$\text{NPS}_{out}(k) = \overline{q}_{in}\overline{g}, \tag{2.165}$$

which is the expected result.

2.7.2 Deterministic blur

The second elementary process is called deterministic blurring (Figure 3.22), describing situations where image blur is accurately expressed as a convolution of

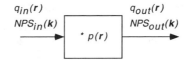

Deterministic Blur (Convolution)

Figure 2.22: Deterministic blur is represented as a convolution (linear filter). It occurs when the input signal is redistributed with a *weighting* given by the PSF.

the input with a point-spread function. The input can be either a quantum image $q(r)$ or an analog signal, but the output can only be an analog signal $d(x)$ where

$$d(r) = q(r) * \mathrm{psf}(r),\qquad(2.166)$$

and $\mathrm{psf}(r)$ is the blur PSF. When the PSF is normalized to unity area,

$$\overline{d}_{out} = \overline{q}_{in},\qquad(2.167)$$

and

$$\mathrm{NPS}_{out}(k) = \mathrm{NPS}_{in}(k)\mathrm{MTF}^2(k),\qquad(2.168)$$

where $\mathrm{psf}(r)$ and $\mathrm{MTF}(k)$ are the PSF and MTF describing the weighting of the blur. Thus, the NPS is passed through the squared MTF. An example of deterministic blur is given later in the description of the integration of image quanta in a digital detector element (Section 2.9.1).

2.7.3 Quantum scatter

Most image-blurring mechanisms, including blur caused by the scattering of optical quanta in a radiographic screen, are fundamentally scattering processes. That is, each quantum is randomly relocated to a new location with a probability described by the normalized PSF of the blur (Figure 2.23). This differs from deterministic blur which can be viewed as a redistribution of signal by weights (as described by the convolution integral), while scatter must be viewed as a redistribution by probabilities. This distinction has been recognized for some time (e.g., Dainty and Shaw [5], Wagner [32], Metz [12], Sandrik and Wagner [34], Metz and Vyborny [40], and Barrett and Swindell [13]). It was first expressed by Shaw and Van Metter [19], derived theoretically by Rabbani, Shaw and Van Metter [39], and derived again more recently using point-process theory by Barrett [41].

The output of a scatter stage must necessarily be a sample quantum image and can be written as

$$q_{out}(r) = q_{in}(r) *_s \mathrm{psf}(r),\qquad(2.169)$$

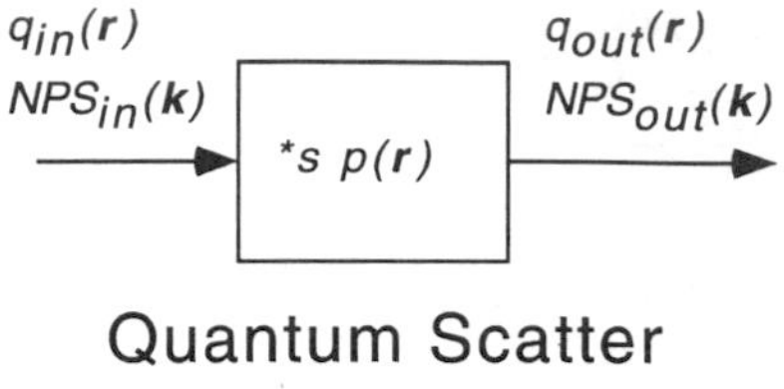

$$q_{in}(r)$$
$$NPS_{in}(k)$$
$$*_s \ p(r)$$
$$q_{out}(r)$$
$$NPS_{out}(k)$$

Quantum Scatter

Figure 2.23: Scatter was described by Rabbani *et al.* [39] and occurs when individual quanta are redistributed with a *probability* given by the normalized PSF. It is represented as a scatter operator in this transfer-theory formalism.

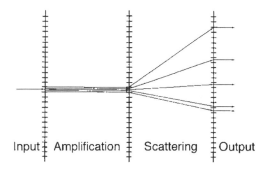

Input   Amplification   Scattering   Output

Figure 2.24: Quantum amplification and scatter operators are cascaded to describe processes involving image quanta. An amplification stage followed by a scattering stage as illustrated here is used to represent the conversion of x rays to light in a radiographic screen.

where psf(r) is the scatter PSF normalized to unity area and $*_s$ represents a scatter operator [42]. Rabbani *et al.* [39] showed that $\overline{q}$ and NPS(k) are transferred through a scatter process according to

$$\overline{q}_{out} = \overline{q}_{in}, \tag{2.170}$$

and

$$\mathrm{NPS}_{out}(k) = \left[\mathrm{NPS}_{in}(k) - \overline{q}_{in} \right] \mathrm{MTF}^2(k) + \overline{q}_{in}, \tag{2.171}$$

where psf(x) and MTF(k) are the PSF and MTF describing the scattering probabilities normalized to unity area.

It is worth noting other differences (and similarities) between deterministic blur (Eq. (2.168)) and quantum scatter (Eq. (2.171)). For instance, deterministic blur will always pass the NPS through the squared MTF. This blur corresponds to the linear filter described in many standard texts on linear systems and Fourier transforms. Scatter is a stochastic translated point process and will pass the correlated component of the NPS through the squared MTF, resulting in a frequency-dependent noise term. The frequency-independent term corresponds to the uncorrelated noise component, and is not passed through the MTF [39]. Other properties of this scatter operator, which has also been called a "stochastic convolution," are described elsewhere [42].

The three elementary processes, amplification, convolution, and scatter, can be cascaded to represent a wide variety of physical process. Of particular importance is the simple cascade of an amplification stage followed by a scattering stage as illustrated in Figure 2.24. This combination can be used to represent the conversion of x rays into light in a radiographic screen, including the scatter of light within the screen.

2.8 Cascaded DQE and quantum sinks

2.8.1 Particle-based approach

Noise transfer through a cascaded system was first examined for the analysis of cascaded multi-stage photo-multiplier detectors by Shockley and Pierce [43]. In particular, Zwieg [25] showed that the DQE of a system consisting of M Poisson gain stages is given by

$$\text{DQE}(u) = \frac{1}{1 + \dfrac{1}{\overline{g}_1} + \dfrac{1}{\overline{g}_1\overline{g}_2} + \cdots + \dfrac{1}{\overline{g}_1 \cdots \overline{g}_M}} \tag{2.172}$$

$$= \frac{1}{1 + \dfrac{1}{P_1} + \dfrac{1}{P_2} + \cdots + \dfrac{1}{P_M}}, \tag{2.173}$$

where P_j is the product of the gains for all stages preceding and including the jth stage:

$$P_j = \prod_{i=1}^{j} \overline{g}_i. \tag{2.174}$$

Equation (2.173) is particularly useful. It shows that the system DQE is degraded if the value of P_j for any stage is less than approximately one. P_j gives the number of quanta at the jth stage normalized to the number of input quanta and, if this number is less than one, the system is said to have a "quantum sink" at that stage. In this type of analysis, the first factor P_1 is generally the quantum efficiency of the detector, which is always less than unity. This is sometimes called the primary quantum sink. It is particularly important during the design of any system to ensure that an adequate number of quanta will exist at each subsequent stage to avoid any secondary quantum sinks. In general, Eq. (2.173) suggests that a secondary quantum sink would be avoided so long as the condition

$$P_j > 10, \tag{2.175}$$

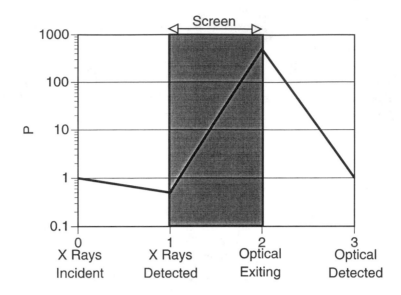

Figure 2.25: Particle-based QAD analysis showing P_j as a function of stage number j.

is satisfied. However, as shown in the next section, this condition is not restrictive enough to be useful in practice.

This simple quantum-sink analysis can be performed for an imaging system based on design parameters by representing the system as a simple cascade of amplification stages. The factors P_j can be illustrated graphically as a function of the stage number j as illustrated in Figure 2.25, clearly showing the existence of a quantum sink if any of the factors is less than, or close to, unity. It is often the first step in assessing the potential of any system design for producing high-quality images [44–48].

This type of analysis in imaging can be traced directly to Albert Rose in the nineteen-forties. He published what is thought to be the first analysis of this type in which he assessed a video chain using a model that included the television pickup tube and lenses, video amplifiers and CRT display, and the retina in an observer. He plotted the number of image quanta at each stage and showed that two quantum sinks were predicted: one at the photo cathode of the pickup tube and the other at the photo surface of the retina [3].

This approach is useful for "back-of-the-envelope"-type calculations of the DQE. However, it is now known to be overly simplistic and responsible for much wasted effort in the development of some new designs because of its failure to predict quantum sinks at non-zero spatial frequencies. Even today, Eq. (2.173) is sometimes used to predict a high DQE for system designs that have no chance of success. For this reason, it is labeled as a "particle approach," and must be interpreted with caution.

2.8.2 Fourier-based Approach

The particle-based Zwieg-type model was generalized to include second-order statistics by Cunningham *et al.* [49] using the noise-transfer relationships of Rabbani *et al.* [39]. They showed that the frequency-dependent DQE of a cascaded system consisting of M amplification and scattering stages is described by

$$\text{DQE}(u)$$
$$= \frac{1}{1 + \dfrac{1 + \varepsilon_{g_1} \text{MTF}_1^2(u)}{\overline{g}_1 \text{MTF}_1^2(u)} + \cdots + \dfrac{1 + \varepsilon_{g_M} \text{MTF}_M^2(u)}{\overline{g}_1 \ldots \overline{g}_M \text{MTF}_1^2(u) \ldots \text{MTF}_M^2(u)}}, \quad (2.176)$$

where ε_{g_j} is called the amplification Poisson excess of the jth stage given by

$$\varepsilon_{g_j} = \frac{\sigma_{g_j}^2}{\overline{g}_j} - 1. \quad (2.177)$$

The amplification Poisson excess is the relative amount by which the variance exceeds that of Poisson amplification. Poisson amplification corresponds to a variance $\sigma_{g_j}^2 = \overline{g}_j$ and excess $\varepsilon_{g_j} = 0$. Deterministic gain (a gain with no random variability) corresponds to a variance $\sigma_{g_j}^2 = 0$ and excess $\varepsilon_{g_j} = -1$. $\text{MTF}_j(u)$ is the MTF resulting from the scattering process at the jth stage. Each stage can represent only an amplification or scattering process, but not both. For amplification at the jth stage, $\text{MTF}_j(u) = 1$. For a scattering jth stage, $\overline{g}_j = 1$ and $\varepsilon_{g_j} = -1$.

In practice, the excess terms are often small enough to be neglected and Eq. (2.176) then simplifies to

$$\text{DQE}(u) \approx \frac{1}{1 + \dfrac{1}{\overline{g}_1 \text{MTF}_1^2(u)} + \cdots + \dfrac{1}{\overline{g}_1 \ldots \overline{g}_M \text{MTF}_1^2(u) \ldots \text{MTF}_M^2(u)}} \quad (2.178)$$

$$= \frac{1}{1 + \dfrac{1}{P_1(u)} + \cdots + \dfrac{1}{P_M(u)}}, \quad (2.179)$$

where $P_j(u)$ is the product of all gains and squared MTF's for all stages preceding and including the jth stage:

$$P_j(u) = \prod_{i=1}^{j} \overline{g}_i \text{MTF}_i^2(u). \quad (2.180)$$

The Fourier-based Eq. (2.179) has a pleasing symmetry with the particle-based Eq. (2.173), although it differs in an important respect. It shows that scattering stages degrade the DQE dramatically when the MTF value drops with increasing spatial frequency. The simpler particle-based analysis may not predict a secondary quantum sink when in fact image quality is being degraded for that reason at non-zero spatial frequencies.

Additive noise may, in principle, be added to the image by components in the imaging chain. This source of noise is ignored here for simplicity, but can be incorporated into an estimate of the DQE if necessary [49]. In addition, it should be noted that for systems that may incorporate geometric magnification or demagnification of the image (such as with an image-intensifier based system), $\bar{q}$ and NPS(u) must be expressed relative to a fixed plane of reference. For convenience, that plane of reference is often the input surface of the detector.

2.8.3 General criteria to avoid a secondary quantum sink

A general criteria can be developed to ensure that a secondary quantum sink does not degrade the DQE for any frequency of interest. If the maximum frequency of interest u_{max} is taken as the maximum frequency passed corresponding to MTF(u_{max}) ≈ 0.33, then MTF$^2(u_{max}) \approx 0.1$ and the following statement applies:

A secondary quantum sink can be avoided if the condition $P_j(u) > 10$ is satisfied at each stage in a cascaded system for all spatial frequencies of interest. This can generally be achieved if all quantum amplification factors subsequent to the primary selection stage are sufficiently large to ensure that

$$P_j(0) > 100. \tag{2.181}$$

Specific values will depend on system particulars, but it is clear that the frequency dependence of this type of analysis results in a much more stringent condition as given by Eq. (2.181) than that predicted by the simpler particle approach given by Eq. (2.175).

2.8.4 Quantum accounting diagrams (QAD)

The significance of $P_j(u)$ is so great in an analysis of system performance that it is informative to plot $P_j(u)$ as a function of stage number j for any spatial frequency of interest. These graphs have been called "quantum accounting diagrams" (QADs) [49]. They illustrate an "effective number of quanta" (not to be confused with the noise-equivalent number of quanta, NEQ [5, 28, 32]) at each stage of the system as a function of spatial frequency.

The QAD for the hypothetical system (assuming typical values for the various parameters) is shown in Figure 2.26. The abscissa is the stage number, j, for $j = 0 \ldots M$ (stage 0 corresponds to the x rays incident on stage 1). The ordinate is the value of $P_j(u)$. Multiple lines are drawn indicating multiple spatial frequencies of

QUANTUM ACCOUNTING DIAGRAM

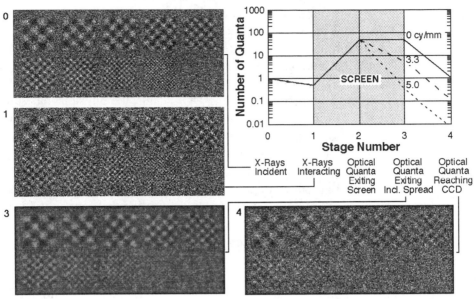

Figure 2.26: Quantum Accounting Diagram of the hypothetical system and simulated images using a Monte Carlo calculation illustrating the visual impact of the non-zero spatial-frequency quantum sink.

interest. The lines all start at $P_0(u) = 1$, corresponding to a single incident x-ray quantum.

The first step is detection of the incident x rays to select those x rays which interact assuming a quantum efficiency $\alpha = 0.5$. The QAD lines for all frequencies therefore decrease from 1.0 to 0.5.

This is followed by conversion of the interacting x rays to optical quanta, assuming a conversion factor $\bar{g} = 1000$. This value is of course x-ray energy dependent. Therefore, the value chosen is the appropriate average for the actual spectrum of *interacting* (not incident) x rays.

The third stage describes the spatial spreading of light in the screen attributable to geometric considerations and scattering. Details of what causes the spread are unimportant as long as the MTF of the blur is known, and all optical quanta are independent. The lines corresponding to each spatial frequency diverge as each line is decreased to a new value according to the square of the MTF (for that stage) at each frequency. Thus, at a frequency corresponding to $\mathrm{MTF}_r(u) = 0.1$, the QAD value is reduced by a factor of 0.01 while the QAD value at $u = 0$ is not decreased at all. This separation of the various frequency lines may cause a large decrease in the DQE at high spatial frequencies, with little or none at low spatial frequencies.

The final stage in the model is selection of those optical quanta that escape from the screen and are coupled from the screen to the detector by the lens assembly, and are detected by the imaging detector. It may be noted that this process could also be reasonably represented as several individual selection stages, corresponding to escape from the screen, collection by the lens (solid angle considerations), transmission through the lens, detection by the detector, etc. However, it has been shown [42] that multiple selection stages can be combined into a single stage and, in fact, the relative order of selection and stochastic spreading stages can be reversed without affecting the resulting DQE. Thus, the physicist has some discretion in choosing how the system is to be represented. The coupling efficiency giving the probability that an optical quantum exiting from the screen is detected by the optical detector in the hypothetical system is $\beta = 0.02$.

Examination of Eq. (2.176) shows that if a single stage has a $P_j(u)$ value much less than both unity and all other stages, that value will effectively determine the DQE of the system. That limiting stage is sometimes called the dominant "quantum sink" because it is the stage with the fewest number of quanta. Figure 2.26 shows that for this system, the dominant quantum sink is frequency dependent. For example, when $u = 0$, there is not one single dominant quantum sink, but the system DQE will be determined largely by the number of x-ray quanta interacting in the screen (stage 1) with a minor additional degradation due to the number of optical quanta at stage 4. It is said that a minor secondary quantum sink exists in the number of optical quanta coupled to the detector. At higher spatial frequencies, the picture changes. For instance, when $u \approx 6.0$ cycles/mm or more, there is a dominant secondary quantum sink at stage 4.

The visual effect of quantum sinks in images is illustrated in Figure 2.26. A Monte Carlo study was performed [50] to simulate the images produced by a system with the QAD shown. Images are shown for each step in the cascaded model to illustrate how they are degraded while transferred through the system. The images contain 10 two-dimensional sinusoidal patterns with frequencies of 1.0, 1.1, 1.25, 1.4, 1.7, 2.0, 2.5, 3.3, 5.0, and 10.0 cycles/mm. Image 0 is an image composed of the quanta incident on the system, and represents the best possible image that could be produced with any system. Image 1 is composed of the detected quanta assuming a quantum efficiency of 0.5. The noise in this image has increased by a factor of the square root of two. Image 3 is composed of the optical quanta as they exit the screen. Spatial blurring of the light degrades the MTF, and the high-frequency patterns are harder to distinguish. Noise in this image has also been smoothed by the effect of optical blur. The large number of light quanta generated for each interacting x ray causes the stochastic blur to behave much like a deterministic blur. Image 4 is composed of the optical quanta that are coupled through a lens system to an optical detector. The light collection efficiency of the lens is not enough to avoid a secondary quantum sink at this stage for spatial frequencies above approximately 2.5 cycles/mm (as shown in the QAD). As a result, image noise masks patterns above this frequency, corresponding to a degraded DQE. The quantum sink also changes the appearance of noise in the image, which becomes more uniform for all spatial frequencies because of the frequency-independent term in Eq. (2.171). This represents the component of noise resulting from the uncorrelated optical quanta.

The secondary quantum sink makes this noise component dominant. Details of the appearance of the images depends on system parameters as well as the value chosen for $\overline{q}$; however, it is clear that image quality in this example is degraded because of the secondary quantum sink. This system also clearly fails the above condition expressed by Eq. (2.181) required to avoid a secondary quantum sink.

Image quality (at high frequencies) is therefore being compromised by an inadequate number of secondary quanta, and can only be improved by increasing the value of $P_4(u)$. This could be achieved by changing the screen to increase the number of optical quanta generated per interacting x ray (if that is possible without significantly degrading the screen MTF), or by increasing the optical collection efficiency by increasing the size (and therefore cost) of the lens assembly. See reference [50] for more simulated images illustrating the effect of quantum sinks.

The QAD analysis must be considered a "first approximation" to noise analysis, and reflects only the fundamental noise limitations imposed by Poisson statistics. It does not reflect noise limitations imposed by additive noise sources such as electronic amplifier noise. In addition, it will be noted that the gain variances do not appear in a calculation of the QAD. This is another reason why the QAD is a less accurate measure of image quality than an evaluation of the DQE with Eq. (2.176) which can include additive noise [49]. The utility of the QAD approach is that it is simple, visual, physically intuitive, and clearly identifies where quantum sinks may exist and what must be done to avoid them.

2.9 Metrics of digital-system performance

An analysis of noise in digital imaging systems is more complex, and the Fourier-based approach is almost always required. In this section, concepts of the digital MTF and digital NPS are introduced. These are then used to describe one way in which the NEQ and DQE of digital systems might be expressed.

A digital-imaging detector is viewed as a two-dimensional array of discrete detector elements. (Physical detector elements are called "dels" by Dr. Martin Yaffe to make a distinction from picture elements—"pixels"—as often they are not the same thing.) The detector produces a signal that is proportional to the number of quanta interacting in each detector element (Figure 2.27). Thus, each element functions as a spatial integrator of image quanta.

2.9.1 Detector-element size and the aperture MTF

Integration of quanta in each detector element can be represented as convolution with an aperture function in the spatial domain, giving rise to a corresponding "aperture MTF" in the spatial-frequency domain. This is illustrated in Figure 2.28, where a sample distribution of x-ray quanta $q(x)$ are incident on a detector. The left column shows $q(x)$ in one dimension, and the right column shows $|Q(u)|$ where $Q(u)$ is the Fourier transform of $q(x)$.

In the following it is assumed that each detector element has unity quantum efficiency and a width of a_x. The signal from the nth element centered at $x = nx_0$,

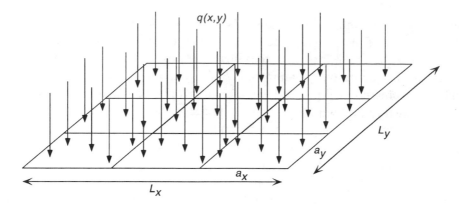

Figure 2.27: The detector array consists of an array of detector elements. Each element produces a signal proportional to the number of quanta interacting in the element.

d_n, is therefore given by the integral

$$d_n = k \int_{nx_0 - a_x/2}^{nx_0 + a_x/2} q(x)\, dx, \qquad (2.182)$$

where k is a constant relating the number of interacting quanta to the detector output as a digital value. This integral can also be written as

$$d_n = k \int_{-\infty}^{\infty} q(x) \prod\left(\frac{x - nx_0}{a_x}\right) dx, \qquad (2.183)$$

where

$$\prod\left(\frac{x}{a_x}\right) = \begin{cases} 1 & \text{for } -a_x/2 \leqslant x \leqslant a_x/2 \\ 0 & \text{otherwise.} \end{cases} \qquad (2.184)$$

Equation (2.183) is recognized as being a correlation integral evaluated at the center of the element, $x = nx_0$, and hence

$$d_n = k\, q(x) \star \prod\left(\frac{x}{a_x}\right)\bigg|_{x=nx_0}, \qquad (2.185)$$

or similarly as the convolution of $q(x)$ with $\prod(-x/a_x)$,

$$d_n = k\, q(x) * \prod\left(\frac{-x}{a_x}\right)\bigg|_{x=nx_0} = d(x)|_{x=nx_0}, \qquad (2.186)$$

where

$$d(x) = kq(x) * \prod(-x/a_x). \qquad (2.187)$$

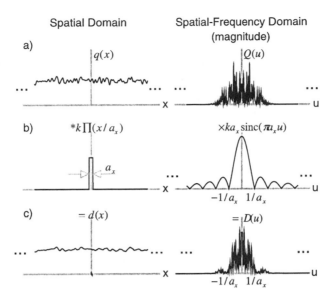

Figure 2.28: Integration of quanta in detector elements of width a_x is represented as convolution of $q(x)$ with $k\Pi(x/a_x)$ in the spatial domain, and multiplication with $ka_x\,\mathrm{sinc}(\pi a_x u)$ in the frequency domain.

The function $d(x)$ is called the *detector presampling signal*. It is a sample function that, when evaluated at positions corresponding to the center of each element, gives the detector output values for each element. Thus, $d(x)$ describes the detector signal for all possible detector-element positions, physical and non-physical.

This is a general result, showing that the effect of integrating quanta in a detector element can be represented as a convolution integral. The function $\Pi(-x/a_x)$ is the sampling function in the sense of distribution theory (Section 2.2.4), describing the measurement of $q(x)$. Convolution in the spatial domain corresponds to multiplication in the spatial-frequency domain, and Eq. (2.187) can therefore be expressed in the spatial-frequency domain as

$$D(u) = Q(u)T_{a_x}(u), \qquad (2.188)$$

where $D(u)$ is the Fourier transform of $d(x)$ and $T_{a_x}(u)$ is a characteristic function given by the Fourier transform of $\Pi(-x/a_x)$. The aperture MTF, or "del" MTF, describes how spatial frequencies are passed through the detector elements. When quanta are integrated in elements of width a_x, the aperture MTF is given by

$$\mathrm{MTF}_{a_x}(u) = \frac{|T_{a_x}(u)|}{T_{a_x}(0)} = \left|\mathrm{sinc}(\pi a_x u)\right|. \qquad (2.189)$$

As the widths of detector elements are decreased, the bandwidth of the aperture MTF is increased.

2.9.2 Digital MTF: presampling MTF and aliasing

The quantity $d(x)$ is the presampling detector signal as described in the previous section, and evaluation of $d(x)$ at the centers of each detector element gives the detector signal for each element. The process of evaluating a function is called sampling (Section 2.2.2). Evaluating $d(x)$ at positions $x = nx_0$ for all n can be represented as multiplication with the comb function $\sum \delta(x - nx_0)$ giving $d^{\dagger}(x)$, where

$$d^{\dagger}(x) = d(x) \sum_{n=-\infty}^{\infty} \delta(x - nx_0) = \sum_{n=-\infty}^{\infty} d_n \delta(x - nx_0), \qquad (2.190)$$

which consists of an infinite train of δ functions scaled by the detector values d_n. This process is illustrated in the two domains in Figure 2.29. Multiplication with $\sum_{n=-\infty}^{\infty} \delta(x - nx_0)$ in the spatial domain corresponds to convolution with $(1/x_0) \sum_{n=-\infty}^{\infty} \delta(u - 1/nx_0)$ in the spatial-frequency domain. Therefore, the Fourier transform of $d^{\dagger}(x)$ is given by

$$\mathrm{F}\{d^{\dagger}(x)\} = D(u) * \frac{1}{x_0} \sum_{n=-\infty}^{\infty} \delta\left(u - \frac{1}{nx_0}\right), \qquad (2.191)$$

as illustrated in Figure 2.29 where $D(u)$ is the Fourier transform of $d(x)$. This illustration shows that sampling $d(x)$ at uniform spacings of x_0 corresponds to

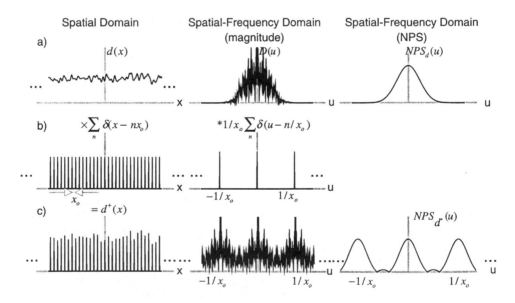

Figure 2.29: Sampling a function at uniform spacing x_0 results in spectral aliasing if the presampling signal $d(x)$ has frequency components above the sampling cut-off frequency $u_c = 1/2x_0$.

the production of aliases of $D(u)$ at spacings of $u = 1/x_0$. If the aliases over-lap, aliasing occurs, resulting in a distortion of the image signal at frequencies below the sampling cut-off frequency, $u_c = 1/(2x_0)$. Excellent descriptions of sampling and aliasing in medical-imaging systems are given elsewhere by Barrett and Swindell [13], and Metz and Doi [12] among others.

In this section, the effect of the digital detector has been described as a two-step process: (1) integration of interacting input quanta in each element to produce a presampling detector signal; and, (2) evaluation (sampling) of the presampling detector signal to generate the individual detector-element values d_n. In the spatial-frequency domain, these two processes are described in terms of: (1) the presampling MTF, $\text{MTF}_{pre}(u)$; and, (2) aliasing as determined by the sample spacing x_0. The overall effect of the detector in the Fourier domain therefore is to attenuate spatial frequencies by the presampling MTF and to introduce aliasing if frequencies remain that are greater than the sampling cut-off frequency given by $u_c = 1/(2x_0)$. Both steps are required for the description of digital detectors. The presampling MTF can be measured on real systems using techniques such as the slanted-edge method [29, 51, 52]. Dobbins *et al.* [53] describe the effects of aliasing and Fourier-domain phase errors resulting from an inadequate sampling frequency that may be encountered with digital detectors.

Of particular importance is the case of ideal dels of width x_0 with no spaces between the active regions of each del, corresponding to a unity detector fill factor. The presampling MTF is given by $\text{MTF}_{pre}(u) = |\text{sinc}(\pi x/x_0)|$ which has the first zero at $u = 1/x_0$, twice the sampling cut-off frequency, and aliasing may be hard to avoid. If the detector fill factor is less than unity, the bandwidth of the presampling MTF is increased further, resulting in more aliasing. Aliasing can sometimes be reduced with the appropriate use of a spatial "anti-aliasing" filter of some sort, such as the scattering of light in the scintillating screen of indirect flat-panel detector.

2.9.3 Digital NPS: presampling NPS and noise aliasing

The NPS has been defined in Sections 2.5.5 and 2.5.6 for only WSS and WSCS random processes. However, a digital image consists of an array of discrete values, d_n, which represent neither a WSS nor a WSCS random process. This minor dilemma is avoided with the linear-systems approach by noting that d_n are samples of the detector presampling signal $d(x)$ where $d(x)$ describes a WSS random process, and the resulting sampled signal $d^\dagger(x)$, an array of δ functions scaled by the values d_n, represents a WSCS random process. The NPS of $d^\dagger(x)$ is therefore given by Eq. (2.110) as

$$\text{NPS}_{d^\dagger}(u) = \frac{1}{x_0^2} \text{NPS}_d(u) * \sum_{n=-\infty}^{\infty} \delta\left(u - \frac{n}{x_0}\right) \qquad (2.192)$$

$$= \frac{1}{x_0^2}\left[\text{NPS}_d(u) + \sum_{n=1}^{\infty} \text{NPS}_d\left(u \pm \frac{n}{x_0}\right) \right], \qquad (2.193)$$

as illustrated in Figure 2.30(c). It is clear from Eq. (2.193) that the NPS of $d^\dagger(x)$ consists of a fundamental presampling NPS, $NPS_d(u)$, plus aliases centered at the frequencies $u = n/x_0$, scaled by the factor $1/x_0^2$. If the aliases overlap, noise aliasing takes place, potentially increasing image noise at all frequencies below the sampling cut-off frequency.

The sampling theorem states that frequencies above the cut-off frequency $u_c = 1/(2x_0)$ cannot be represented with samples obtained with a uniform sampling frequency of $u_s = 1/x_0$. We therefore introduce $NPS_{\hat{d}}(u)$ which is truncated to this frequency range, and is the NPS of $\hat{d}(x)$. Truncation in the frequency domain corresponds to convolution with a sinc function in the spatial domain, and hence $\hat{d}(x)$ is given by

$$\hat{d}(x) = \sum_{n=-\infty}^{\infty} d_n \operatorname{sinc}\left(\pi \frac{x - nx_0}{x_0}\right) \tag{2.194}$$

$$= d^\dagger(x) * \operatorname{sinc}(\pi x_0 u), \tag{2.195}$$

which is an estimate of $d(x)$, equal to a "sinc" interpolation of the digital values d_n, as illustrated in Figure 2.30(e). The NPS of $\hat{d}(x)$ is $NPS_{\hat{d}}(u)$ given by

$$NPS_{\hat{d}}(u) = NPS_{d^\dagger}(u) x_0^2 \prod(x_0 u). \tag{2.196}$$

The functions $d(x)$ and $\hat{d}(x)$ are equal only if there is no aliasing of $d(x)$.

When the DFT is defined by Eq. (2.63), the NPS estimated from one-dimensional digital data can be written as

$$NPS_{dig}(u)\Big|_{u=\frac{m}{Nx_0}} = \frac{x_0}{N} E\{|\mathrm{DFT}\{\Delta d_n\}|^2\}, \tag{2.197}$$

where $\Delta d_n = d_n - E\{d_n\}$ and is called here the *digital NPS*. It is defined only for the frequencies evaluated by the DFT, which are $u = m/Nx_0$ for $-N/2 \leqslant m \leqslant N/2 - 1$. At these frequencies it is also equal to $NPS_{\hat{d}}(u)$, and therefore $NPS_{dig}(u)$ is related to the presampling NPS, $NPS_d(u)$, by

$$NPS_{dig}(u) = NPS_{\hat{d}}(u) \tag{2.198}$$

$$= x_0^2 NPS_{d^\dagger}(u) \tag{2.199}$$

$$= NPS_d(u) + \sum_{n=1}^{\infty} NPS_d\left(u \pm \frac{n}{x_0}\right), \tag{2.200}$$

explicitly stating the undesirable effects of noise aliasing with the second term. It is satisfying to note that Eq. (2.197) can be viewed as a numerical estimate of the NPS of $d(x)$ given by Eq. (2.93). Equation (2.200) for the digital NPS was first described to the medical imaging community by Giger [54].

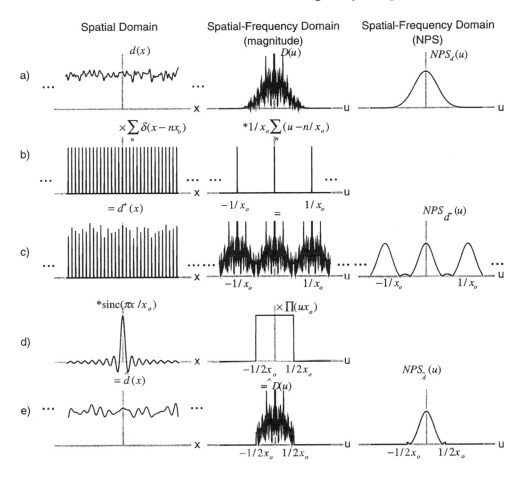

Figure 2.30: Schematic illustration describing the NPS of a digital image in terms of the Fourier transform. Left: spatial domain. Center: magnitude, spatial-frequency domain. Right: NPS.

2.9.3.1 Digital NPS in two dimensions

The digital NPS for a one-dimensional noise process is given by Eq. (2.197). However, digital images represent two-dimensional noise processes and hence it is necessary to make use of the two-dimensional digital NPS for image analyses which is given by

$$\text{NPS}_{dig}(u, v) = \frac{x_0 y_0}{N_x N_y} \text{E}\left\{\left|\text{DFT}^{2D}\{\Delta d_{n_x, n_y}\}\right|^2\right\}, \qquad (2.201)$$

for the frequencies evaluated by the two-dimensional DFT, DFT^{2D}, where x_0 and y_0 are the x and y spacings of the discrete values respectively. The one-dimensional NPS of the two-dimensional noise process represented by a digital image is given by

$$\text{NPS}_{dig}(u) = \frac{x_0 y_0}{N_x N_y} \, \text{E} \left\{ \left| \text{DFT} \left\{ \sum_{n_y=0}^{N_y-1} \Delta d_{n_x, n_y} \right\} \right|^2 \right\}. \tag{2.202}$$

Equation (2.202) should be considered a working definition of the digital NPS for systems analysis after ensuring that the DFT being used is consistent with Eq. (2.63). The expectation value of the squared DFT can be estimated by squaring and averaging the DFT of many digital noise images.

2.9.3.2 Digital-detector noise variance

The noise variance in $d(x)$ is conserved by the process of noise aliasing so that

$$\sigma_d^2 = \int_{-\infty}^{\infty} \text{NPS}_d(u) \, du \tag{2.203}$$

$$= x_0^2 \int_{-1/2x_0}^{1/2x_0} \text{NPS}_{d^{\dagger}}(u) \, du \tag{2.204}$$

$$= \int_{-1/2x_0}^{1/2x_0} \text{NPS}_d(u) + \sum_{n=1}^{\infty} \text{NPS}_d \left(u \pm \frac{n}{x_0} \right) du. \tag{2.205}$$

Noise aliasing cannot be undone once it has occurred. It can be prevented only by implementing a spatial anti-aliasing filter which would reduce the bandwidth of the presampling NPS, $\text{NPS}_d(u)$, such that negligible noise power exists at frequencies above the sampling cut-off frequency. The calculated pixel variance is given by

$$\sigma_d^2 = \frac{1}{N-1} \sum_{n=0}^{N-1} |\Delta d_n|^2. \tag{2.206}$$

2.9.4 Digital NEQ

The NEQ as given by Eq. (2.145) applies to digital systems although made more complicated by the potential presence of signal and noise aliasing. The numerator describes the system transfer of signals from the input to the output, and thus the MTF for digital systems is the presampling MTF which includes the aperture MTF. Noise in a digital image is given by Eq. (2.200) and so the digital NEQ is given by

$$\text{NEQ}_{dig}(\overline{q}, u) = \frac{\overline{q}^2 \left| \dfrac{\partial \overline{d}}{\partial \overline{q}} \right|^2 \text{MTF}_{pre}^2(u)}{\text{NPS}_{dig}(u)}, \tag{2.207}$$

for $u = m/Nx_0$ and $-N/2 \leqslant m \leqslant N/2 - 1$, where x_0 is the center-to-center spacing of detector elements. Thus, for linear digital systems, the NEQ can be calculated using

$$\text{NEQ}_{dig}(\overline{q}, u) = \frac{\text{MTF}^2_{pre}(u)}{\text{NPS}_{dig}(u)/\overline{d}^2}, \tag{2.208}$$

for $u = m/Nx_0$ and $-N/2 \leqslant m \leqslant N/2 - 1$ when using a DFT given by Eq. (2.63) and where $\text{NPS}_{dig}(u)$ is given by Eq. (2.202). Interpretation of the digital NEQ is possibly easier when expressed in the form

$$\text{NEQ}_{dig}(\overline{q}, u) = \frac{\overline{d}^2\text{MTF}^2_{pre}(u)}{\left[\text{NPS}_d(u) + \sum_{n-1}^{\infty} \text{NPS}_d\left(u \pm \frac{n}{x_0}\right)\right]}, \tag{2.209}$$

for $u = m/Nx_0$ and $-N/2 \leqslant m \leqslant N/2 - 1$. The NEQ is a measure of the noise-equivalent number of quanta, and is affected by noise aliasing. Signal aliasing adds an additional artifact that is not included in the NEQ. The digital NEQ is defined only for frequencies less than the sampling cut-off frequency, $u_c = 1/2x_0$.

2.9.5 Digital DQE

Similar to the digital NEQ, the digital DQE is defined here as

$$\text{DQE}_{dig}(\overline{q}, u) = \frac{\text{NEQ}_{dig}(\overline{q}, u)}{\overline{q}} \tag{2.210}$$

$$= \frac{\overline{d}^2\text{MTF}^2_{pre}(u)}{\overline{q}\left[\text{NPS}_d(u) + \sum_{n=1}^{\infty} \text{NPS}_d\left(u \pm \frac{n}{x_0}\right)\right]}, \tag{2.211}$$

for $u = m/Nx_0$ and $-N/2 \leqslant m \leqslant N/2 - 1$.

2.9.6 Signal aliasing

Signal aliasing can also be viewed as a form of image noise, but depends on specifics of particular images and is not WSS or WSCS. It is therefore not included in the calculations presented in this chapter. However, it is still important to remember that signal aliasing may result in additional artifacts and image degradation.

2.10 Analysis of a simple digital detector array

The DQE of a (hypothetical) simple digital detector is described here as an illustrative example of principles presented here. The detector is illustrated in Figure 2.31. It consists of a thin scintillating screen bonded to an optical detector array.

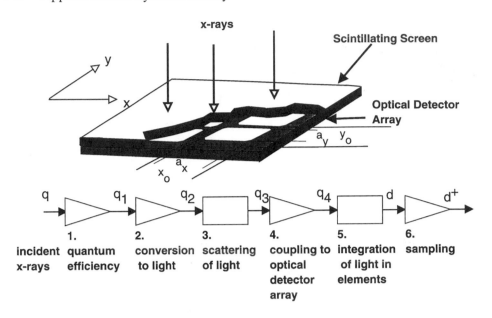

Figure 2.31: Schematic illustration of the hypothetical simple digital detector. The linear-systems model consists of 6 stages.

While this model is not intended to represent any particular imaging system, it is essentially a simple model of a hypothetical flat-panel thin-film-transistor (TFT) array detector, similar to any of several designs being developed elsewhere for radiographic and fluoroscopic applications [55, 56].

2.10.1 Cascaded model

The detector array is modeled as a cascade of six linear stages (Figure 2.31). The input is a uniform distribution of x-ray quanta represented as the quantum image $q_0(x, y)$ (Section 2.2.1.3) with an expected value of $\bar{q}_0$ quanta/mm^2. The NPS of this input quantum image is therefore $\text{NPS}_0(k) = \bar{q}_0$ (see Section 2.6.2.3). Transfer of the expected value and NPS through stage 5 and 6 is illustrated in Figure 2.32.

2.10.1.1 Stage 1: selection of x-ray quanta that interact in screen

Selection of incident x-ray quanta that interact in the screen is represented as a quantum selection stage (Section 2.7.1.1), which is a special case of quantum amplification. If the quantum efficiency is α, $\tilde{\alpha}$ is introduced as a random variable having the values 0 and 1 only with an expected value α. Therefore, using Eqs. (2.160) and (2.164), the distribution of interacting quanta can be represented as $q_1(r)$ having an expected value of $\bar{q}_1$ and NPS of $\text{NPS}_1(k)$ where

$$q_1(r) = q_0(r)\tilde{\alpha}, \qquad (2.212)$$

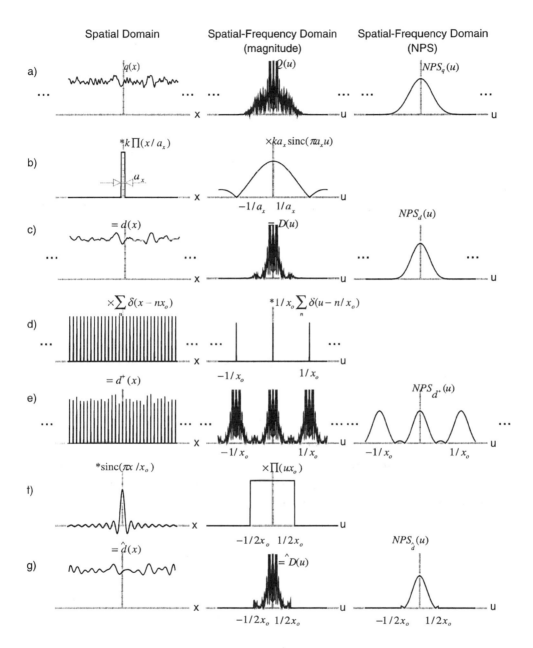

Figure 2.32: Transfer of the expected number of image quanta and corresponding NPS at each stage of the cascaded model. Left: spatial domain. Center: spatial-frequency domain (magnitude). Right: NPS.

$$\overline{q}_1 = \alpha \overline{q}_0, \tag{2.213}$$

and

$$\mathrm{NPS}_1(k) = \alpha \overline{q}_0, \tag{2.214}$$

in units of mm^{-2}.

2.10.1.2 Stage 2: conversion to optical quanta in screen

It is assumed that each interacting quantum produces an average of $\overline{m}$ optical quanta per interaction with a variance σ_m^2. This variance accounts for all variations in the conversion gain, including Swank noise and a polychromatic x-ray beam. The conversion gain (Section 2.7.1) is therefore represented as the random variable $\widetilde{m}$ and the resulting distribution of optical quanta, expected value and NPS is obtained using Eqs. (2.160) and (2.161) giving

$$q_2(\mathbf{r}) = q_0(\mathbf{r})\widetilde{m}\widetilde{\alpha}, \tag{2.215}$$

$$\overline{q}_2 = \alpha \overline{m}\,\overline{q}_0, \tag{2.216}$$

and

$$\mathrm{NPS}_2(k) = \alpha \overline{m}^2 \overline{q}_0 \left(1 + \frac{\varepsilon_m}{\overline{m}}\right) + \alpha \overline{m}\,\overline{q}_0, \tag{2.217}$$

in units of mm^{-2}.

2.10.1.3 Stage 3: scattering of optical quanta in screen

It is assumed that all light quanta scatter (Section 2.7.3) with the same point-spread function $\mathrm{psf}_s(x, y)$ normalized to unity area, neglecting variable interaction depths in the screen. The resulting quantum image, expected value and NPS are obtained using Eqs. (2.170) and (2.171) giving

$$q_3(\mathbf{r}) = q_0(\mathbf{r})\widetilde{m}\widetilde{\alpha} *_s \mathrm{psf}_s(\mathbf{r}), \tag{2.218}$$

$$\overline{q}_3 = \alpha \overline{m}\,\overline{q}_0, \tag{2.219}$$

and

$$\mathrm{NPS}_3(k) = \alpha \overline{m}^2 \overline{q}_0 \left(1 + \frac{\varepsilon_m}{\overline{m}}\right) |\mathrm{MTF}_s(k)|^2 + \alpha \overline{m}\,\overline{q}_0, \tag{2.220}$$

in units of mm^{-2} where $*_s$ represents the scattering process [42] and $\mathrm{MTF}_s(k)$ is the scatter MTF. The gain Poisson excess ε_m is related to the gain variance as given by Eq. (2.177).

2.10.1.4 Stage 4: selection of light quanta that interact

It is assumed that a fraction β of all light quanta will interact somewhere in the optical detector array. The factor β must include the coupling efficiency of light from the screen as well as the quantum efficiency of the detector array. It does not matter *where* the light quanta interact, and it does not matter if they interact in an active or inactive region. The factor β describes only the probability of interaction. The expected value and NPS of the distribution of interacting light quanta is therefore obtained using Eqs. (2.160) and (2.164), giving

$$q_4(r) = q_0(r)\widetilde{m}\widetilde{\alpha} *_s \text{psf}_s(r)\widetilde{\beta}, \qquad (2.221)$$

$$\overline{q}_4 = \alpha\overline{m}\beta\overline{q}_0, \qquad (2.222)$$

and

$$\text{NPS}_4(k) = \alpha\overline{m}^2\beta^2\overline{q}_0\left(1 + \frac{\varepsilon_m}{\overline{m}}\right)|\text{MTF}_s(k)|^2 + \alpha\overline{m}\beta\overline{q}_0, \qquad (2.223)$$

in units of mm^{-2}.

2.10.1.5 Stage 5: spatial integration of interacting light quanta in elements

The detector presampling signal is given by the integral of $q_4(r)$ over rectangles with width a_x and a_y corresponding to the width of active regions of the detector elements, corresponding to a deterministic blur stage (Section 2.7.2). If k is the scaling factor relating the number of interacting light quanta to the output signal, the detector presampling signal is given in Cartesian coordinates by

$$d(x, y) = k\left\{[q_0(x, y)\widetilde{m}\widetilde{\alpha}] *_s \text{psf}_s(x, y)\widetilde{\beta} * \prod\left(\frac{x}{a_x}, \frac{y}{a_y}\right)\right\}, \qquad (2.224)$$

where $*$ represents a two-dimensional convolution integral. The expected detector signal $\overline{d}$ is given by

$$\overline{d} = ka_x a_y \alpha\overline{m}\beta\overline{q}_0, \qquad (2.225)$$

which is unitless, and the NPS by

$$\text{NPS}_d(u, v) = k^2 a_x^2 a_y^2\left[\alpha\overline{m}^2\beta^2\overline{q}_0\left(1 + \frac{\varepsilon_m}{\overline{m}}\right)|\text{MTF}_s(u, v)|^2 + \alpha\overline{m}\beta\overline{q}_0\right]$$
$$\times |\text{sinc}(\pi a_x u)|^2|\text{sinc}(\pi a_y v)|^2, \qquad (2.226)$$

in units of mm^2. Note that it is at this stage, after integration of quanta in detector elements, one must start representing the image as an analog image rather than as a quantum image. As a consequence, units of the NPS are mm^2 rather than mm^{-2}.

2.10.1.6 Stage 6: output from discrete detector elements

The process of obtaining the discrete output signals from each detector element is represented as a sampling process. If each detector element has a center-to-center spacing of x_0 and y_0 in the x and y directions respectively, the sampled detector signal $d^\dagger(x, y)$ is given by

$$d^\dagger(x, y) = k \left\{ \left[q_0(x, y) \widetilde{m}\widetilde{\alpha} \right] *_s \text{psf}_s(x, y) \widetilde{\beta} * \prod \left(\frac{x}{a_x}, \frac{y}{a_y} \right) \right\}$$

$$\times \sum_{n_x=-\infty}^{\infty} \sum_{n_y=-\infty}^{\infty} \delta(x - n_x x_0, y - n_y y_0) \quad (2.227)$$

The expected value is given by

$$\text{E}\{d^\dagger(x, y)\} = k a_x a_y \alpha \overline{m} \beta \overline{q}_0 \sum_{n_x=-\infty}^{\infty} \sum_{n_y=-\infty}^{\infty} \delta(x - n_x x_0, y - n_y y_0), \quad (2.228)$$

consisting of two-dimensional δ functions scaled by the digital values d_{n_x,n_y} where the expected value of d_{n_x,n_y} is

$$\text{E}\{d_{n_x,n_y}\} = k a_x a_y \alpha \overline{m} \beta \overline{q}_0. \quad (2.229)$$

The NPS of $d^\dagger(x, y)$, obtained using Eq. (2.193) and generalized to two dimensions, is given by

$$\text{NPS}_d^\dagger(u, v) = \frac{1}{x_0^2 y_0^2} \left[\text{NPS}_d(u, v) + \sum_{n_x=1}^{\infty} \sum_{n_y=1}^{\infty} \text{NPS}_d \left(u \pm \frac{n_x}{x_0}, v \pm \frac{n_y}{y_0} \right) \right]. \quad (2.230)$$

Combining this result with Eqs. (2.199) and (2.226) gives the two-dimensional digital NPS as

$$\text{NPS}_{dig}(u, v) = \text{NPS}_d(u, v) + \sum_{n_x=1}^{\infty} \sum_{n_y=1}^{\infty} \text{NPS}_d \left(u \pm \frac{n_x}{x_0}, v \pm \frac{n_y}{y_0} \right), \quad (2.231)$$

for frequencies below the sampling cut-off frequencies of $u_c = 1/2x_0$ and $v_c = 1/2y_0$. The digital NPS has units of mm^2.

The one-dimensional NPS of this two-dimensional noise process is obtained by evaluating Eq. (2.231) along the appropriate axis. The NPS in the x direction is obtained by setting $v = 0$ and substituting d_n for d_{n_x}, giving

$$\text{NPS}_{dig}(u) = \text{NPS}_d(u) + \sum_{n=1}^{\infty} \text{NPS}_d\left(u \pm \frac{n}{x_0}\right), \tag{2.232}$$

which also has units mm^2 and where $\text{NPS}_d(u)$ is the presampling NPS of $d(x)$.

2.10.2 Detector DQE

The DQE of this hypothetical detector is evaluated in the x direction only to simplify the mathematical expressions by setting $v = 0$. The DQE is given by Eq. (2.211) where the presampling MTF is given by

$$\text{MTF}_{pre}(u) = \text{MTF}_s(u)\left|\text{sinc}(\pi a_x u)\right|, \tag{2.233}$$

and the presampling NPS by Eq. (2.226). In the absence of additive noise, these results can be combined, giving

$$\text{DQE}(u) = \frac{\alpha\text{MTF}_s^2(u)\text{sinc}^2(\pi a_x u)}{F(u) + \sum_{n=1}^{\infty} F\left(u \pm \frac{n}{x_0}\right)}, \tag{2.234}$$

where

$$F(u) = \left[\left(1 + \frac{\varepsilon_m}{\overline{m}}\right)\text{MTF}_s^2(u) + \frac{1}{\overline{m}\beta}\right]\text{sinc}^2(\pi a_x u). \tag{2.235}$$

This result offers little insight into important physical processes without making some simplifications. For instance, if $\overline{m}\beta > 100$ as required by the QAD condition (Section 2.8.3) to prevent secondary quantum sinks, then $(\overline{m}\beta)^{-1} \ll |\text{MTF}_{pre}(u)|^2$ for all frequencies passed by $\text{MTF}_{pre}(u)$ with any significance. If it is further assumed that the conversion gain from X rays to light is approximately Poisson so that $|\varepsilon_m/\overline{m}| \ll 1$ (a good assumption for many scintillating screens including CsI), the DQE simplifies to

$\text{DQE}(u)$

$$\approx \frac{\alpha\text{MTF}_s^2(u)\text{sinc}^2(\pi a_x u)}{\text{MTF}_s^2(u)\text{sinc}^2(\pi a_x u) + \sum_{n=1}^{\infty}\text{MTF}_s^2\left(u \pm \frac{n}{x_0}\right)\text{sinc}^2\left(\pi a_x\left[u \pm \frac{n}{x_0}\right]\right)} \tag{2.236}$$

$$= \frac{\alpha\text{MTF}_{pre}^2(u)}{\text{MTF}_{pre}^2(u) + \sum_{n=1}^{\infty}\text{MTF}_{pre}^2\left(u \pm \frac{n}{x_0}\right)}. \tag{2.237}$$

2.10.3 Noise aliasing, detector fill factor and variance

The effect of noise aliasing on the DQE is given by the second term in the denominator of Eq. (2.237). Noise aliasing can only be avoided if $MTF_{pre}^2(u) \ll 1$ for all frequencies above the sampling cut-off frequency $|u| \geqslant u_c$ where $u_c = 1/2x_0$ (Figure 2.32). Two limiting cases are considered as described below.

2.10.3.1 Low-resolution scintillator (correlated quantum noise on detector array)

A "low"-resolution scintillator implies that the system MTF in the x direction is limited by the screen and not by the detector element size a_x. The screen causes the quantum noise in the optical image incident on the optical detector array to be correlated, which reduces the noise bandwidth. Thus, $sinc^2(\pi a_x u)$ is approximately constant for all frequencies of significance passed by $MTF_s^2(u)$ and the DQE simplifies to

$$DQE(u) \approx \frac{\alpha MTF_s^2(u)}{MTF_s^2(u) + \sum\limits_{n=1}^{\infty} MTF_s^2\left(u \pm \frac{n}{x_0}\right)}. \tag{2.238}$$

If the detector elements are sufficiently small and close together that aliasing can be neglected, that is, $MTF_s^2(u)|_{u=u_c} \ll 1$ for $u_c = 1/2x_0$, the DQE reduces to

$$DQE(u) \approx \frac{\alpha MTF_s^2(u)}{MTF_s^2(u)} = \alpha. \tag{2.239}$$

Thus, for this special case of a quantum-noise-limited detector with sufficiently small detector elements and no secondary quantum sink, both image signal and noise are proportional to the MTF in the same way and the DQE is therefore flat with frequencies and determined entirely by the quantum efficiency of the screen α, not by the optical digital detector array. In particular, the DQE is not degraded by the detector fill factor $\gamma_x \gamma_y$, defined by $\gamma_x = a_x/x_0$ and $\gamma_y = a_y/y_0$, having a value less than unity. This result is only valid as long as additive detector noise can be neglected. For instance, if the detector fill factor is decreased, the signal decreases and there may be a point at which detector noise can no longer be neglected and where this result is not valid. The DQE of a two-dimensional detector array is given by the same result.

Image noise measured as the variance σ_d^2 in detector element values d_n is calculated by

$$\sigma_d^2 = \frac{1}{N-1} \sum\limits_{n=0}^{N-1} [d_n - \overline{d}]^2. \tag{2.240}$$

The variance is also equal to the presampling NPS integrated over all frequencies (in two dimensions), given by

$$\sigma_d^2 = \int_{-\infty}^{\infty} \int_{-\infty}^{\infty} \mathrm{NPS}_d(u, v) \, du \, dv \tag{2.241}$$

$$= \int_{-\infty}^{\infty} \int_{-\infty}^{\infty} k^2 a_x^2 a_y^2 \left[\alpha \overline{m}^2 \beta^2 \overline{q}_0 \left(1 + \frac{\varepsilon_m}{\overline{m}} \right) \mathrm{MTF}_s^2(u, v) + \alpha m \beta \overline{q}_0 \right]$$

$$\times \mathrm{sinc}^2(\pi a_x u) \mathrm{sinc}^2(\pi a_y v) \, du \, dv, \tag{2.242}$$

which simplifies to

$$\sigma_d^2 \approx k^2 a_x^2 a_y^2 \alpha \overline{m}^2 \beta^2 \overline{q}_0 \int_{-\infty}^{\infty} \int_{-\infty}^{\infty} \mathrm{MTF}_s^2(u, v) \, du \, dv. \tag{2.243}$$

Thus, for the low-resolution scintillator detector, noise variance is proportional to the integral of the squared MTF. If the spatial resolution of the scintillator is degraded, the width of the MTF is reduced and detector variance decreases. This means that for a specified detector-element size, less detector noise will be obtained if a lower-resolution scintillator is used and a compromise must be found between noise and resolution.

2.10.3.2 High-resolution scintillator (uncorrelated quantum noise on detector array)

A "high"-resolution scintillator implies that the system MTF in the x direction is limited by the detector-array aperture function rather than by the scintillator. This corresponds to system designs using very-high-resolution scintillators, and also to amorphous selenium "direct-detection" flat-panel detectors. Therefore, $\mathrm{MTF}_s^2(u)$ is approximately constant over frequencies passed by $\mathrm{sinc}^2(\pi a_x u)$ and the DQE simplifies to

$$\mathrm{DQE}(u) \approx \frac{\alpha \mathrm{sinc}^2(\pi a_x u)}{\mathrm{sinc}^2(\pi a_x u) + \sum_{n=1}^{\infty} \mathrm{sinc}^2\left(\pi a_x \left[u \pm \frac{n}{x_0} \right]\right)}. \tag{2.244}$$

Zhao et al. [57] have shown that the sum of $\mathrm{sinc}^2(\pi a_x u)$ and its aliases at harmonics of $u = 1/x_0$ is always equal to a constant given by

$$\mathrm{sinc}^2(\pi a_x u) + \sum_{n=1}^{\infty} \mathrm{sinc}^2\left(\pi a_x \left[u \pm \frac{n}{x_0} \right]\right) = \frac{x_0}{a_x} = \frac{1}{\gamma_x}, \tag{2.245}$$

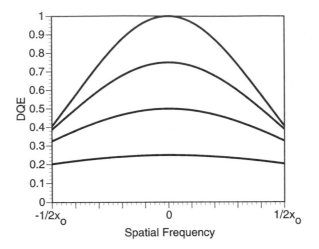

Figure 2.33: Illustration of the DQE for a two-dimensional detector with a high-resolution converter and fill-factor values $\gamma = \gamma_x\gamma_y$ (for $\gamma_x = \gamma_y$) equal to 1.0, 0.75, 0.50, and 0.25. The scintillator quantum efficiency, α, is assumed to be unity.

where $\gamma_x = a_x/x_0$ is the detector fill factor in the x direction. The DQE therefore reduces to

$$\text{DQE}(u) \approx \alpha\,\frac{a_x}{x_0}\,\text{sinc}^2(\pi a_x u) = \alpha\gamma_x\text{sinc}^2(\pi a_x u), \tag{2.246}$$

for a one-dimensional detector and to

$$\text{DQE}(u, v) \approx \alpha\gamma_x\gamma_y\text{sinc}^2(\pi a_x u)\text{sinc}^2(\pi a_y v), \tag{2.247}$$

for a two-dimensional detector. The one-dimensional DQE of this two-dimensional detector, evaluated along the $v = 0$ axis of the two-dimensional detector, is therefore given by

$$\text{DQE}(u) \approx \alpha\gamma_x\gamma_y\text{sinc}^2(\pi a_x u). \tag{2.248}$$

Thus, for this special case of a quantum-noise-limited detector with a very-high-resolution converter, the DQE is proportional to the converter quantum efficiency α, and the detector fill factor $\gamma_x\gamma_y$, and always has a shape given by $\text{sinc}^2(\pi a_x u)$, which is dependent on the x-direction fill factor. Figure 2.33 illustrates the DQE for a two-dimensional detector with a high-resolution scintillator for various fill factor values $\gamma = \gamma_x\gamma_y$ assuming $\gamma_x = \gamma_y$ based on Eq. (2.248). As the fill factor decreases, higher frequencies are passed by the detector-element apertures and noise aliasing increases. This is directly responsible for the decreasing DQE.

The detector variance is given by

$$\sigma_d^2 = \int_{-\infty}^{\infty}\int_{-\infty}^{\infty}\text{NPS}_d(u, v)\,\mathrm{d}u\,\mathrm{d}v \tag{2.249}$$

$$\approx k^2 a_x^2 a_y^2 \alpha \overline{m}^2 \beta^2 \overline{q}_0 \int_{-\infty}^{\infty} \int_{-\infty}^{\infty} \text{sinc}^2(\pi a_x u) \text{sinc}^2(\pi a_y v) \, du \, dv \quad (2.250)$$

$$= k^2 a_x a_y \alpha \overline{m}^2 \beta^2 \overline{q}_0. \qquad (2.251)$$

Thus, with the inclusion of noise aliasing, the noise variance predicted with this Fourier-based approach is equal to the variance that would be expected for a simple photon-counting detector of size $a_x \times a_y$.

It should also be noted that for this high-resolution scintillator (uncorrelated quantum noise incident on the detector array), the variance is related to the zero-frequency value of the NPS according to

$$\text{NPS}_d(0, 0) \approx a_x a_y \sigma_d^2, \qquad (2.252)$$

consistent with Eq. (2.133).

2.11 Summary

In this chapter, principles of linear-systems theory have been summarized, including the point-spread function (PSF), line-spread function (LSF), modulation-transfer function (MTF), and other simple metrics of system performance. It has been shown how images may be classified as either quantum images (distributions of quanta), analog images, or digital images. Particular attention has been paid to the issue of units for each, and an introduction given to the principles of distribution theory and generalized functions that are essential for the description of quantum images.

These simple linear-systems metrics can be used to describe the *expected*, or *noise-free*, performance of an imaging system. However, they do not describe the transfer of image noise. The stochastic-theory relationships necessary to describe noise transfer are a very recent addition to the linear-systems approach, developed primarily by Shaw, Rabbani, Van Metter, and co-workers. In addition, the introduction of a photon-scatter operator to the linear-systems repertoire has allowed this approach to be extended to include the description of quantum-based *stochastic* systems, a necessary step for the description of medical-imaging systems. As a result, the extended linear-systems approach forms the basis from which comprehensive theoretical models of noise transfer through realistic imaging systems can be developed, and the connection is made to more complex metrics of system performance including the noise-power spectrum (NPS) and noise-equivalent number of quanta (NEQ).

It has also been shown how the linear-systems approach is used to develop cascaded-systems models that can be used to *predict*, based on theoretical design considerations, metrics of system performance including the spatial-frequency-dependent detective quantum efficiency (DQE). Complex imaging systems are represented as serial cascades of multiple "elementary" processes. This approach has been very successful for the theoretical analysis of many systems, and gives a physical interpretation to the idea of a spatial-frequency-dependent quantum sink. These quantum sinks are responsible for the frequency dependence of the DQE except where limited by detector-noise sources. The cascaded approach provides a physically intuitive model that can be very helpful for understanding limitations of system performance and particular system designs, a necessary step for understanding and optimizing system performance in the design of new imaging systems.

Digital imaging systems add additional complexity to a systems analysis, requiring a description of noise aliasing. This has been accomplished using the theories of wide-sense cyclostationary (WSCS) random processes. While the description of WSCS processes has an established basis in communications theory, this author is unaware of their prior use in linear-systems theory or for the analysis or description of medical-imaging systems.

An illustrative example is given of the analysis of a hypothetical digital detector. The detector is essentially a simple model of a flat-panel active matrix detector similar to any of several designs currently under investigation and commercial production. The analysis shows how the DQE can be predicted from simple design parameters, and includes the effects of detector fill factor and noise aliasing on the DQE.

Acknowledgements

The author is grateful to The Medical Research Council of Canada and the U.S. Army Medical Research and Materiel Command, Breast Cancer Research Program, for financial support. The assistance of V. Subotic is also gratefully acknowledged for Matlab programming and creation of figures, as well as helpful suggestions and ideas from discussions with many friends and associates including H. Lai and Drs. A. Fenster, A.E. Burgess, R. Shaw, J.H. Siewerdsen, R.L. Van Metter, J. Beutel, R.F. Wagner, and G.E. Parraga.

References

[1] Rose A. "A Unified Approach to the Performance of Photographic Film, Television Pick-Up Tubes, and the Human Eye." J Soc Motion Pict Telev Eng 47:273–294, 1946.

[2] Rose A. "Sensitivity Performance of the Human Eye on an Absolute Scale." J Opt Soc Am 38:196–208, 1948.

[3] Rose A. "Television Pickup Tubes and the Problem of Vision." In Marston (Ed.) *Advances in Electronics and Electron Physics*. New York: Academic Press, 1948, pp. 131–166.

[4] Rose A. "Quantum and Noise Limitations of the Visual Process." J Opt Soc Am 43:715–716, 1953.

[5] Dainty JC, Shaw R. *Image Science*. New York: Academic Press, 1974.

[6] Cunningham IA, Shaw R. "Signal-to-Noise Optimization of Medical Imaging Systems." J Opt Soc Am A16:621–632, 1999.

[7] Rossmann K. "Measurement of the Modulation Transfer Function of Radiographic Systems Containing Fluoroscent Screens." Phys Med Biol 9:551–557, 1964.

[8] Rossmann K. "The Spatial Frequency Spectrum: A Means for Studying the Quality of Radiographic Imaging Systems." Radiology 90:1–13, 1968.

[9] Gaskill JD. *Linear Systems, Fourier Transforms, and Optics*. New York: John Wiley & Sons, 1978.

[10] Papoulis A. *Systems and Transforms with Applications in Optics*. New York: McGraw-Hill, 1968.

[11] Doi K, Rossmann K, Haus AG. "Image Quality and Patient Exposure in Diagnostic Radiology." Photographic Science and Engineering 21:269–277, 1977.

[12] Metz CE, Doi K. "Transfer Function Analysis of Radiographic Imaging Systems." Phys Med Biol 24:1079–1106, 1979.

[13] Barrett HH, Swindell W. *Radiological Imaging—The Theory of Image Formation, Detection, and Processing*. New York: Academic Press, 1981.

[14] Bracewell RN. *The Fourier Transform and its Applications*, 2 Edition. New York: McGraw-Hill Book Company, 1978.

[15] Brigham EO. *The Fast Fourier Transform*. Englewood Cliffs, NJ: Prentice-Hall, 1974.

[16] Bendat JS, Piersol AG. *Random Data—Analysis and Measurement Procedures*, 2 Edition. New York: John Wiley & Sons, 1986.

[17] Papoulis A. *Probability, Random Variables, and Stochastic Processes*, 3 Edition. New York: McGraw Hill, 1991.

[18] Blackman RB, Tukey JW. *The Measurement of Power Spectra*. New York: Dover Publications, Inc, 1958.

[19] Shaw R, Van Metter RL. "An Analysis of the Fundamental Limitations of Screen-Film Systems for X-Ray Detection I. General Theory." In Schneider RH, Dwyer SJ (Eds.) *Application of Optical Instrumentation in Medicine XII*. Proc SPIE 454, 1984, pp. 128–132.

[20] Shaw R, Van Metter RL. "An Analysis of the Fundamental Limitations of Screen-Film Systems for X-Ray Detection II. Model Calculations." In Schneider RH, Dwyer SJ (Eds.) *Application of Optical Instrumentation in Medicine XII*. Proc SPIE 454, 1984, pp. 133–141.

[21] Van Metter RL. "Describing the Signal-Transfer Characteristics of Asymmetrical Radiographic Screen-Film Systems." Med Phys 19:53–58, 1992.

[22] Peters TM, Williams JC. *The Fourier Transform in Biomedical Engineering*. Boston: Birkhauser, 1998.

[23] Gardner NA, Franks LE. "Characteristics of Cyclostationary Random Signal Processes." IEEE Transactions in Information Theory IT-21: 1975.

[24] Fellgett PB. "On the Ultimate Sensitivity and Practical Performance of Radiation Detectors." J Opt Soc Am 39:970, 1949.

[25] Zwieg HJ. "Performance Criteria for Photo-Detectors—Concepts in Evolution." Photo Sc Eng 8:305–311, 1964.

[26] Jones RC. "A New Classification System for Radiation Detectors." J Opt Soc Am 39:327, 1949.

[27] Burgess AE. "The Rose Model, Revisited." J Opt Soc Am A16:633–646, 1999.

[28] "Medical Imaging—The Assessment of Image Quality." ICRU Report 54, 1995.

[29] Dobbins JT, Ergun DL, Rutz L, Hinshaw DA, Blume H, Clark DC. "DQE(f) of Four Generations of Computed Radiography Acquisition Devices." Med Phys 22:1581–1593, 1995.

[30] Shaw R. "The Equivalent Quantum Efficiency of the Photographic Process." J Photogr Sc 11:199–204, 1963.

[31] Wagner RF, Brown DG. "Unified SNR Analysis of Medical Imaging Systems." Phys Med Biol 30:489–518, 1985.

[32] Wagner RF. "Toward a Unified View of Radiological Imaging Systems. Part II: Noise Images." Med Phys 4:279–296, 1977.

[33] Wagner RF, Brown DG, Pastel MS. "Application of Information Theory to the Assessment of Computed Tomography." Med Phys 6:83–94, 1979.

[34] Sandrik JM, Wagner RF. "Absolute Measures of Physical Image Quality: Measurement and Application to Radiographic Magnification." Med Phys 9:540–549, 1982.

[35] Shaw R. "Some Fundamental Properties of Xeroradiographic Images." In Gray JE, Hendee WR (Eds.) *Application of Optical Instrumentation in Medicine IV*. Proc SPIE 70, 1975, pp. 359–363.

[36] Wagner RF, Muntz EP. "Detective Quantum Efficiency (DQE) Analysis of Electrostatic Imaging and Screen-Film Imaging in Mammography." In Gray JE (Ed.) *Application of Optical Instrumentation in Medicine VII*. Proc SPIE 173, 1979, pp. 162–165.

[37] Johns HE, Cunningham JR. *The Physics of Radiology*. Springfield IL: Charles C Thomas, 1983.

[38] Tucker DM, Barnes GT, Chakraborty DP. "Semiempirical Model for Generating Tungsten Target X-Ray Spectra." Med Phys 18:211–218, 1991.

[39] Rabbani M, Shaw R, Van Metter RL. "Detective Quantum Efficiency of Imaging Systems with Amplifying and Scattering Mechanisms." J Opt Soc Am A4:895–901, 1987.

[40] Metz CE, Vyborny CJ. "Wiener Spectral Effects of Spatial Correlation Between the Sites of Characteristic X-Ray Emission and Reabsorption in Radiographic Screen-Film Systems." Phys Med Biol 28:547–564, 1983.

[41] Barrett HH, Wagner RF, Myers KJ. "Correlated Point Processes in Radiological Imaging." In Van Metter RL, Beutel J (Eds.) *Medical Imaging 1997: Physics of Medical Imaging*. Proc SPIE 3032, 1997, pp. 110–125.

[42] Cunningham IA, Westmore MS, Fenster A. "Unification of Image Blur and Noise in Linear-Systems Transfer Theory Using a Quantum Scattering Operator." Med Phys 27:(accepted) 2000.

[43] Shockley W, Pierce JR. "A Theory of Noise for Electron Multipliers." Proc Inst Radio Eng 26:321–332, 1938.

[44] Ter-Pogossian MM. *The Physical Aspects of Diagnostic Radiology*. New York: Harper & Row, 1967.

[45] Mistretta CA. "X-Ray Image Intensifiers." In Haus AG (Ed.) AAPM No 3, *The Physics of Medical Imaging: Recording System Measurements and Techniques*. New York: American Institute of Physics, 1979, pp. 182–205.

[46] Macovski A. *Medical Imaging Systems*. Englewood Cliffs, NJ: Prentice-Hall, Inc., 1983.

[47] Roehrig H, Nudelman S, Fu TY. "Electro-Optical Devices for Use in Photoelectronic-Digital Radiology." In Fullerton GD, Hendee WR, Lasher JC, Properzio WS, Riederer SJ (Eds.) AAPM No 11, *Electronic Imaging in Medicine*. New York: American Institute of Physics, 1984, pp. 82–129.

[48] Roehrig H, Fu TY. "Physical Properties of Photoelectronic Imaging Devices and Systems." In Doi K, Lanzl L, Lin PJP (Eds.) AAPM No 12, *Recent Developments in Digital Imaging*. New York: American Institute of Physics, 1985, pp. 82–140.

[49] Cunningham IA, Westmore MS, Fenster A. "A Spatial-Frequency Dependent Quantum Accounting Diagram and Detective Quantum Efficiency Model of Signal and Noise Propagation in Cascaded Imaging Systems." Med Phys 21:417–427, 1994.

[50] Cunningham IA, Westmore MS, Fenster A. "Visual Impact of the Non-Zero Spatial Frequency Quantum Sink." In Shaw R (Ed.) *Medical Imaging 1994: Physics of Medical Imaging*. Proc SPIE 2163, 1994, pp. 274–283.

[51] Fujita H, Doi K, Giger ML. "Investigation of Basic Imaging Properties in Digital Radiography. 6. MTFs of II-TV Digital Imaging Systems." Med Phys 12:713–720, 1985.

[52] Holdsworth DW, Gerson RK, Fenster A. "A Time-Delay Integration Charge-Coupled Device Camera for Slot-Scanned Digital Radiography." Med Phys 17:876–886, 1990.

[53] Dobbins JT. "Effects of Undersampling on the Proper Interpretation of Modulation Transfer Function, Noise Power Spectra, and Noise Equivalent Quanta of Digital Imaging Systems." Med Phys 22:171–181, 1995.

[54] Giger ML, Doi K, Metz CE. "Investigation of Basic Imaging Properties in Digital Radiography. 2. Noise Wiener Spectrum." Med Phys 11:797–805, 1984.

[55] Antonuk LE, El-Mohri Y, Siewerdsen JH, Yorkston J, Huang W, Scarpine VE, Street RA. "Empirical Investigation of the Signal Performance of a High-Resolution, Indirect Detection, Active Matrix Flat-Panel Imager (AMFPI) for Fluoroscopic and Radiographic Operation." Med Phys 24:51–70, 1997.

[56] Siewerdsen JH, Antonuk LE, El-Mohri Y, Yorkston J, Huang W, Boudry JM, Cunningham IA. "Empirical and Theoretical Investigation of the Noise Performance of Indirect Detection, Active Matrix Flat-Panel Imagers (AMFPIs) for Diagnostic Radiology." Med Phys 24:71–89, 1997.

[57] Zhao W, Ji WG, Rowlands JA. "X-Ray Imaging Using Active Matrix Readout of Amorphous Selenium: Analysis of Detective Quantum Efficiency." Med Phys 1997.

CHAPTER 3
Image Quality Metrics for Digital Systems

James T. Dobbins III
Duke University Medical Center

CONTENTS

3.1 Introduction

The last few years have seen a rapid increase in the number of digital imaging devices produced for radiographic applications. With digitized video/image intensifiers, computed radiography (CR), and more recently the advent of flat-panel imagers, an almost bewildering number of choices of digital imaging devices is available. The good news from this rapid progress in digital radiography is that devices are becoming available with image quality superior to that available just a few years ago. The challenge from this proliferation of digital devices is making the difficult decision about which device is most suitable for a particular application.

Radiologists will rightly ask, "How can I know which device I should purchase for my clinical imaging needs?" Imaging physicists, on the other hand, will be concerned with verifying the image quality specifications of the various manufacturers, developing appropriate algorithms to extend the utility of the devices, and developing appropriate clinical imaging protocols to take best advantage of the devices' imaging performance. Physicists and radiologists will need to work collaboratively to determine the appropriate applications for these devices, and the performance that may be expected from them.

In order to assess the performance of these devices, it is necessary to consider both physical image-quality parameters as well as the observer's perceptual response. Both of these areas are more difficult with digital devices than with screen film. Because the image has been sampled, quantized, and processed, there are a number of changes necessary in traditional measurements of image-quality. Furthermore, because there is an almost unlimited degree of image processing that can be done to the images, it becomes more difficult to gauge observer acceptance of the resulting images. There are a number of physical and observer-based measurements which can be used to gauge image-quality, and these will be considered in this chapter.

This chapter is divided into four sections. First, global measures of image-quality will be addressed, using measurements in Cartesian (or image-intensity) space. Second, measures in spatial frequency space will be considered. Third, methods of assessing image processing will be considered, and last, observer assessment will be addressed. Of course, the final stage in assessment of image-quality is the ability of a particular imaging device and clinical protocol to improve diagnostic accuracy. The issue of diagnostic accuracy, while very important, is an entire field of study in itself, and is therefore beyond the scope of this chapter. The interested reader is referred to other chapters in this volume on measuring diagnostic accuracy.

3.2 Global parameter assessment

Scientists and engineers customarily describe the performance of an imaging device in two domains: the $x - y$ domain of Cartesian space and the conjugate $u - v$ domain of spatial frequency space. The reason for this dual description is partly historical, but has its basis in the fact that there are certain global—that is, the same at all points of the image—responses of the system, and there are also spatially-correlated system-response characteristics. The global response characteristics are covered in this section, and generally include features that are independent of position. The spatially-correlated system-response is typically described in frequency space, and will be covered in Section 3.3.

3.2.1 Linearity

The relationship between input intensity and output signal in an imaging system influences the range over which suitable imaging performance may be obtained. This response is referred to as the characteristic curve of the device, and in the case of photographic film has the well-known sigmoid shape of the Hurter-Driffield (HD) curve. Screen-film systems have a characteristic curve that is linear (with respect to the logarithm of incident intensity) over about 1 to 2 orders of magnitude. Digital systems, on the other hand, measure their characteristic response directly with respect to exposure (rather than the log of exposure as with film), and typically have a range of linear response of 3 to 4 orders of magnitude. The range (or ratio) of highest to lowest response is often called the dynamic range of the system. Often the limit of the digital system's dynamic range is attributable to practical issues of available digitization bits rather than an inherent limitation of the x-ray detection substrate.

The linearity (or more precisely, the characteristic curve) of a system should be measured using good experimental technique and a high-quality (preferably calibrated) exposure meter. The imaging technique should be chosen to minimize confounding factors that might bias the true system response. For example, it is crucial that all image processing be turned off (except correction for bad pixels), and that "raw" data be examined. Depending on the design of the digital system, it may be difficult or even impossible to get access to true "raw" unprocessed data. It would be wise to ask the device manufacturer if it is possible to get access to unprocessed data for the linearity measurements. (Sometimes the image processing can be easily turned off by the user, but other times it will require access to special intermediate image files.)

The one exception to turning off image processing is that any pixel-by-pixel correction in the device should be used, if there is such a correction. Image intensifier/digitized video and CR systems typically may have no such correction, but most of the newer flat-panel and selenium-drum devices do. These corrections adjust for variations in the gain or offset of individual pixels, and interpolate across bad pixels. If these corrections are not used, the incorrect response of various bad pixels might bias the measurement of the desired overall system response.

Some systems have an automatic gain or sensitivity adjustment. Ideally, this should be turned off for characteristic curve measurement. However, if it may not be turned off, or if there is some question as to the linearity of response of the automatic sensitivity-adjustment itself, it may be possible to measure the response of the system in automatic sensitivity mode. To measure the linearity of the system in those conditions, one may either use the detected sensitivity value (if provided) or else one may measure the system response over a range of exposures and detect how accurately the device tracks with exposure.

Data-acquisition timing is also important in experimental measurements of absolute characteristic curve response. Most systems have some decay of detected signal over time, so it is important to measure the image response at a time following exposure that is consistent with expected clinical use. For many detectors this is not a concern, because internal device timing reads out the system at the appropriate time. However, with CR systems, the time between plate exposure and readout is entirely up to the operator. For that reason, it is recommended that a consistent delay time be used between exposure and plate readout. In some published results, a delay of 10 min was used to ensure minimal variability of response with different exposures [1, 2], based on earlier measurements of the temporal response of CR units [3].

The shape of the characteristic curve for most systems is not highly dependent on beam spectrum. However, if one wants a quantitative characteristic curve that relates image-pixel value to absolute exposure, then the beam spectrum to be employed clinically should be used, or at least a reasonable approximation to it. If the system is to be used at a range of kV_ps, for example, and one does not wish to measure the absolute response of the system at multiple kV_ps, then a compromise beam spectrum may be used. A reasonable compromise spectrum might be 70 kV_p with 0.5-mm Cu filtration under those conditions, because that is the spectrum that has been used for a number of MTF and DQE measurements [1, 2, 4].

The experimental imaging geometry is also not highly critical unless one wishes to have pixel-value response versus absolute exposure. In that case, it would make sense to minimize the impact of any scattered radiation by using a narrow pencil beam with as large a source-to-image (SID) distance as possible. The exposed area of the detector should be placed so that the region of interest (ROI) used for analysis is as close to the center of the detector as possible.

The range of exposure values to be evaluated depends somewhat on the expected range of response of the system. At the very least, measurements every tenfold variation in exposure should be used; for example, in a study of CR, exposures were made at 0.03, 0.3, 3, and 30 mR, which covered the majority of the usable range of clinical exposures to be encountered [1]. Ideally, more exposure values than these should be used, but it is often difficult to obtain the very lowest values. If at all possible, the various exposure values should be obtained by varying mA, time, and SID, keeping the same beam spectrum. However, if it is not possible to get exposure values low enough by this approach, beam filtration may be added, as long as enough additional data points are acquired to ensure adequate overlap of the response curves obtained at different beam filtration.

The increment of exposure values used should be sufficient to adequately fit a curve to the data on both a logarithmic curve and a linear curve. For example, this could be accomplished in the following way if exposures in the range 0.01–10 mR were desired: measurements at 0.01, 0.03, 0.1, 0.3, 1, 3, and 10 mR would provide relatively uniform sampling on a log curve, and additional measurements at 0.06,

0.6, and 6 mR would provide more uniform sampling on a linear curve. It is generally not necessary to make repeated measurements of the image data, because about 10 data points should be sufficient to characterize the standard error of estimate if a polynomial curve is fit to the characteristic curve. However, it is important to make multiple measurements of the exposure (but not image data) for the low-exposure range of the curve. This need for multiple measurements of exposure is because of the limited precision of most exposure meters at low exposure. One should choose a tube mAs and distance appropriate for the low-exposure conditions, then make multiple repeated measurements of recorded exposure in integration mode on the meter, in order to better determine the reading for any one individual exposure. For example, making 10 sequential shots at about 0.03 mR each might yield an integrated reading on the meter of perhaps 0.32 mR; this would indicate that any of the individual exposures would be 0.032 mR; this three-decimal-place precision exceeds that found on most meters. Of course, only one individual exposure would then be made on the actual detector for measuring the pixel value.

The analysis of mean value in the digital images is straightforward, assuming a large enough ROI is used (about 1 cm × 1 cm is recommended). The main difficulty in measuring the mean value is if there is noticeable background trending in the image. Background trending, or nonuniform shading, is usually not important in measuring the relative characteristic curve, but may bias the value of the characteristic curve versus absolute exposure. The data may be detrended, if necessary, by fitting the two-dimensional pixel-value surface with a low-order two-dimensional polynomial (typically no more than third order).

3.2.2 Artifacts

Various artifacts can occur in digital imaging systems. Often, these do not hamper clinical interpretation of the images, but it is wise to evaluate how severe the artifacts are in a particular system, and how effectively the manufacturer has corrected for them (if at all).

Digital device artifacts fall into several categories, depending on the type of device used. In the case of image-intensifier/digitized-video systems, there are artifacts associated with the image intensifier, optics, and camera. The principal artifacts from the intensifier itself include pincushion distortion, magnetic-field distortion, and vignetting. Pincushion distortion refers to the geometric distortion toward the edge of the image resulting from the curved surface of the intensifier. This type of distortion is typically measured using an array of lead beam dots. Algorithms have been developed to correct for this artifact [5]. It should be noted that because the intensifier's susceptibility to the earth's magnetic field, certain geometric distortions may change as the orientation of the tube is changed [5]. Vignetting is the drop off in intensity toward the periphery of the image attributable the optics used between the intensifier and the camera. If the optical configuration is well characterized, this distortion may be corrected by normalizing by a flat-field image. The principal artifacts associated with the camera are bad pixels (with a CCD camera) or scan distortion (with a vidicon tube).

The type of artifact most commonly encountered with laser-scanning devices (CR and film digitizers) is banding or shading in the image perpendicular to the direction of laser scan. This faint banding may be the result of dust on scanning optical mirrors, or may result from inaccurate correction for system response along the scan line (typically accomplished by some type of multiplicative correction to account for variations in light-detection efficiency across the laser-scan path). These artifacts may not easily be eliminated except by service personnel, who can sometimes clean the mirror or recalibrate the device. These artifacts are not normally noticed unless there is a large area of uniform gray level and a high-contrast digital window used. This shading artifact is one of the principal sources of low-frequency noise power in these images. In the case of CR, there may also be scratches or imperfections in the imaging plate, which of course can only be corrected by purchasing a new plate.

A scanning-drum selenium detector [6–8] has two predominant types of artifacts: ghosting and detector drop outs. The ghosting is due to deep charge trapping, and manifests itself by seeing a residual image of a previous exposure. This artifact has been described as being particularly noticeable when a postero-anterior (PA) chest image is acquired following a lateral chest image [9]. The second type of artifact, drop outs, results from regional variations in the selenium, such as may occur from crystallization. The device may be recalibrated to correct for some of the drop-out areas, but if the condition becomes too severe, the entire drum may need to be replaced. Because there may be variations in the response of the various electrometers reading out each row of the image, horizontal striping may occur in the image. This should be corrected internally by calibration of the device, but careful examination at high contrast will reveal if there is any substantial row-to-row variation.

The type of artifacts associated with self-scanned flat-panel imagers typically result from local imperfections in pixel response or to "dead" pixels, columns, or rows. These detectors consist of an x-ray absorptive layer (typically amorphous selenium or a phosphor such as CsI) coupled to an array of readout electronics (such as photodiodes and/or thin-film transistors). The response of each readout element may not be exactly the same, and furthermore, there may be local variations in the amount of deposited x-ray-sensitive layer. The result is that the gain of individual pixels may vary from location to location. Also, there may be variations in the image offset (such as from dark current) over the extent of the image. Fortunately, the self-scanned nature of the flat-panel devices makes it possible in principle to correct for the pixel-to-pixel variations in gain and offset. The gain correction is usually performed by acquiring a flat-field map of pixel response and storing that map to normalize the response of subsequent exposures. However, there may be nonuniformity in that pixel map attributable to gross variations in intensity (e.g., heel effect) or from quantum noise in the flat-field image used to form the gain correction map. The latter problem should be addressed by the manufacturer by either acquiring a very high-dose (and hence, low-noise) image for the flat field, or else by acquiring multiple moderate-dose flat-field images and averaging them.

It has been pointed out that the two approaches do not yield the same results [10], because of nonlinearity in response with increasing exposure and effects of off-set correction in the gain correction map. The offset correction is typically done automatically by measuring the image response in the dark just before or after an exposure; measuring this periodically allows the system to adjust to variations in dark current with time and temperature.

Measurement of the accuracy of the gain and offset corrections will involve taking a series of exposures (perhaps three or four) covering a range from low to high exposure. A flat-field image should be acquired, without anything in the beam except some filtration (e.g., 0.5-mm Cu placed near the tube). By exaggerating the contrast, one may visually inspect for any obvious structured patterns in the flat-field images. High-pass filtering of the image with a small kernel (e.g., 3×3) will also tend to highlight any small structured variation in detector response. This process should be repeated for high-, low-, and intermediate-exposure flat-field images to ensure that gain variations are properly handled at a variety of exposure levels.

One further concern for flat-panel devices is the distribution of completely dead pixels. In early flat-panel plates, it has been observed that there may be $>10,000$ dead pixels. While this may seem like a large number, it should be realized that this represents about 0.3% of the total number of pixels. Improvements in clean-room processing procedures are steadily reducing this number. Unless these bad pixels are somehow clustered, they usually are not noticeable in the image. Manufacturers have varying specifications for how many bad pixels are acceptable, and it usually depends on ensuring that they are not clustered in such a way that they cannot be corrected. The bad pixels are corrected by averaging adjacent pixel values. The only time the bad pixels really become a potential problem is if they occur in multiple adjacent rows or columns. One, or possibly even two, adjacent rows or columns may not be noticed after correction. However, one should be cautious in evaluating whether a given flat-panel device has an unacceptable number of bad rows, columns, or clusters.

One may ask the manufacturer for a "bad pixel map," which specifies the location of bad pixels. If that is not available, a method for finding bad rows and columns is to acquire sequential flat-field images (about 10). Then write a simple program to evaluate the standard deviation of the 10 values at each pixel location. Any corrected pixel will tend to have a smaller standard deviation over time because of local spatial averaging, and thus if an image of the pixel standard deviations is displayed, it may be possible to identify rows and columns that are probably bad. One word of caution with this approach is that there is a statistical fluctuation in measured standard deviations because of statistical sampling, so not every pixel that has a lower standard deviation will represent a truly bad pixel. But this method may be useful in looking for trends such as bad rows or columns.

3.2.3 Signal-to-noise ratio

There are many performance parameters of interest in a complete digital imaging system, including resolution, signal-response linearity, and noise properties. While signal sensitivity and image-noise properties are important by themselves, it is really the ratio of them that carries the most significance. For a given number of detected photons, N, and a stochastic signal fluctuation, σ, the maximum available signal-to-noise (SNR) is

$$\frac{S}{\sigma} = \frac{N}{\sqrt{N}} = \sqrt{N}, \tag{3.1}$$

because, for Poisson-distributed x-ray quanta, the standard deviation of measured pixel values goes as the square root of the mean number of quanta. This is the "raw" signal-to-noise ratio, because all detected quanta are included in "signal." Often of more interest is the differential signal-to-noise ratio, $\mathrm{SNR_{diff}}$, which uses the difference in signal behind the object of interest relative to its background (see Figure 3.1):

$$\mathrm{SNR_{diff}} = \frac{\Delta S}{\sigma} = \frac{CS}{\sigma} = \frac{CN}{\sqrt{N}} = C\sqrt{N}, \tag{3.2}$$

where C is the contrast, $\Delta S/S$.

If an object has area A, and there are N_a photons per unit area detected, then the measured $\mathrm{SNR_{diff}}$ of the object is

$$\mathrm{SNR_{diff}} = C\sqrt{N} = C\sqrt{N_a A}. \tag{3.3}$$

From this, one can derive the expression relating contrast and area to the number of photons per unit area required to have a given $\mathrm{SNR_{diff}}$:

$$N_a = \frac{\mathrm{SNR_{diff}^2}}{C^2 A}. \tag{3.4}$$

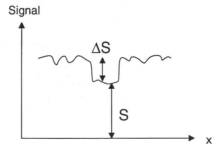

Figure 3.1: A profile of image intensity across an image containing an opacity. The differential signal, ΔS, is the difference between the raw signal S and the background signal. The differential signal is assumed to be small compared to S.

This relation is termed the Rose model after Albert Rose, an early pioneer of imaging science. Rose [11] used data from earlier experiments by Blackwell [12], which showed that the SNR needs to be about 5 for there to be reliable detection by human observers.

There are several matters of practical importance in making these measurements of SNR: (1) the assumption is made that the signal is small, so that the noise in the vicinity of the object of interest is only minimally influenced by the exposure variation across the object; (2) the ROI used to measure the standard deviation must be large enough (typically 2 cm × 2 cm) so that a reliable estimate of the mean can be determined, and so that all spatial frequencies of interest are included in the noise measurement; and (3) any background shading attributable to artifacts or nonuniformities in the detector must be eliminated as much as possible. These latter two points will be considered in more detail in the next section on DQE.

3.2.4 NEQ and DQE

If the imaging device were an ideal device, that is to say a perfect photon counter, the SNR measured in the final image would simply be proportional to the square root of the number of photons in the region of interest:

$$\text{SNR}_{\text{meas}} = \frac{N_{\text{meas}}}{\sqrt{N_{\text{meas}}}} = \sqrt{N_{\text{meas}}}. \tag{3.5}$$

Thus in a photon counting device, $N_{\text{meas}} = \text{SNR}_{\text{meas}}^2$.

However, devices used in radiography are not ideal, in that they contain sources of noise not related to the Poisson-distributed x-ray flux, and they also are usually energy-integrating devices rather than photon counters. (An integrating device is one whose signal output is related to an amount of integrated detected photon energy rather than a number of detected photons.) Thus, the SNR measured in such a non-ideal device contains noise properties worse than that due to x-ray quantum statistics alone:

$$\text{SNR}_{\text{non-ideal}} = \frac{S_{\text{non-ideal}}}{\sigma_{\text{non-ideal}}} < \sqrt{N_{\text{meas}}}. \tag{3.6}$$

If the noise in the real-world imaging device is translated back to the input stage of the device, one has a measure of noise that can be related to an effective number of incident photons had the device been an ideal photon counter. One can relate a number of quanta N' to the measured non-ideal SNR:

$$N' = \text{SNR}_{\text{non-ideal}}^2. \tag{3.7}$$

This quantity N' is called the noise-equivalent quanta (NEQ). It gives the effective number of quanta used by the device, based on the measured SNR. If the NEQ is divided by the number of quanta incident, N_{inc}, then it gives the efficiency with which the device uses the available quanta; it maps $N_{inc} \rightarrow$ *measured SNR^2*. This ratio is termed the detective quantum efficiency (DQE).

One is left with these relations:

$$NEQ = SNR^2_{non\text{-}ideal}, \tag{3.8}$$

$$DQE = \frac{NEQ}{N_{inc}} = \frac{SNR^2_{non\text{-}ideal}}{SNR^2_{inc}}. \tag{3.9}$$

As an example, consider the case with a device that has 10,000 photons incident in a given area of interest. If this device were an ideal photon counter it would have a measured SNR of sqrt(10,000) = 100. But because the device is not ideal, it may have a measured image SNR of 80, for example. In an ideal detector, an SNR of 80 would correspond to an incident number of photons of 6400. This value of 6400 is the noise-equivalent quanta (NEQ) of the device. Alternatively, one may look at the fraction of photons available that the device uses. The above device effectively uses only 64% of the number of photons available, thus having a DQE of 0.64.

A challenging part of the DQE computation is the proper determination of SNR^2_{inc} in the denominator. For a monoenergetic beam, SNR^2_{inc} is just the same as the number of incident photons. However, for a polychromatic beam, the "noise" is an energy-weighed variance, depending on the energy spectrum. Technically, the term detective quantum efficiency relates to a photon number variance (where the SNR^2_{inc} is the summed variance of photon numbers in each energy bin), but for energy-integrating detectors authors sometimes quote SNR^2_{inc} as an energy-weighted variance, because the detector signal records integrated energy rather than integrated photon number. There is some debate about which approach makes the most sense for radiographic detectors; be sure to specify whether you used a photon-number weighted variance or an energy-weighted variance in determining SNR^2_{inc} for the incident polychromatic spectrum. Fortunately, the SNR^2_{inc} computed from the two approaches does not differ by more than a few percent for most beams.

The SNR, NEQ, and DQE thus far described are local scalar quantities, and do not inform us about the resolution properties of a system. For that, one must evaluate NEQ and DQE as functions of spatial frequency. Development of the theory and methods for measuring $NEQ(f)$ and $DQE(f)$ will be given in Section 3.3. An excellent theoretical background for $NEQ(f)$ and $DQE(f)$ is given in Chapter 2 of this volume by Cunningham.

3.2.5 Inherent contrast

Inherent contrast refers to the contrast of intensity patterns in the radiographic image prior to image processing or display. It is influenced by several factors: beam spectrum, energy response of the detector, variation of anatomical thickness and composition from position to position, and scattered radiation. Some of these factors are properties of the system (kV_p, energy response of the detector, and geometry-dependence of the scattered radiation), and some are properties of the individual patient being imaged (position-dependent thickness and composition, and thickness-dependence of scattered radiation). Obviously, there is no control over the factors that are patient dependent, but it is possible to estimate the average predictable contrast from the system by considering what happens when imaging an "average" patient.

In considering the influences on inherent contrast, it is first important to describe the effect of tissue type and thickness on contrast. (This discussion is review for most readers; those interested in more detail concerning the interaction between x rays and matter may consult a suitable textbook in radiographic physics [13] or Chapter 1 of this book by Boone.) The transmission of x-ray intensity as it traverses a thickness t of material is given by the relation

$$I(t) = I_0 e^{-\mu t}, \qquad (3.10)$$

where I_0 is the incident intensity, and the attenuation coefficient μ describes the rate at which the beam is attenuated with thickness. The attenuation coefficient is the result of three physical processes at diagnostic energies: photoelectric effect, Compton scatter, and coherent scatter. Because coherent scatter accounts for less that 10% of total interactions in soft tissues above about 50 keV, it is typically ignored (coherent scatter does contribute a much larger fractional attenuation at mammographic energies). The photoelectric attenuation coefficient goes as Z^3/E^3, where Z is the effective atomic number of the material being imaged and E is the mean energy of the transmitted beam. The Compton-scatter component of attenuation changes only slowly with energy over the range 10 to 150 keV, and does not show a strong Z dependence for elements other than hydrogen.

Because both the Compton and photoelectric coefficients of tissue decrease with energy, the attenuation (and hence, the contrast) also decreases as the mean beam energy increases in most circumstances. The only circumstance in which the attenuation (and contrast) may increase rather than decrease with increasing beam energy is when the energy of the beam passes the binding energy of electron shells in the material being imaged (most commonly, only the K-shell binding energy is considered because it is the largest of the binding energies). As the beam energy passes the K-shell binding energy of the material being imaged, the photoelectric component rises sharply, giving rise to the "K-edge" effect. It is this K-edge increase in attenuation coefficient that accounts for the utility of most radiographic contrast agents (such as iodinated compounds for angiography).

The contrast of an object relative to its background is defined as

$$C = \frac{I_b - I}{I_b}, \qquad (3.11)$$

where I is the image intensity in the region of the object of interest, and I_b is the image intensity in the background surrounding the object. Consider the example

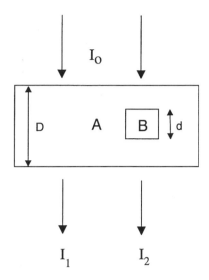

Figure 3.2: Transmission of x-ray intensity through materials. There is a section of material B inserted in the middle of another material of type A.

given in Figure 3.2. There is a large slab of material A into which a small thickness of material B has been inserted. Each of the two materials has its own attenuation coefficient, μ_A or μ_B. One may use Eqs. (3.10) and (3.11) to derive the contrast of the object B relative to its background. The intensity transmitted through the background material A is

$$I_1 = I_0 e^{-\mu_A D}, \tag{3.12}$$

and the intensity transmitted through the region containing material B is

$$\begin{aligned} I_2 &= I_0 e^{-\mu_B d} e^{-\mu_A(D-d)} \\ &= I_1 e^{-\mu_B d} e^{\mu_A d} \\ &= I_1 e^{-(\mu_B-\mu_A)d}. \end{aligned} \tag{3.13}$$

The contrast is then computed as

$$\begin{aligned} C &= \frac{I_1 - I_2}{I_1} \\ &= 1 - \frac{I_2}{I_1} \\ &= 1 - e^{-(\mu_B-\mu_A)d}. \end{aligned} \tag{3.14}$$

Thus one sees that the total thickness D of the background material cancels out of the equation, leaving just the thickness of material B and the difference in attenuation coefficients between B and its surrounding.

Equation (3.14) explains the nature of inherent contrast seen in radiographic exams. In the case of imaging the lungs, for example, the material A is air, whose linear attenuation coefficient is essentially zero when compared to tissue, yielding contrast from point-to-point in the image largely caused by local variations in traversed thickness of lung parenchyma. In the case of contrast-agent imaging, such as with angiography, the attenuation coefficient of the contrast agent is so much higher than that of blood that the contrast is largely attributable to the thickness of the contrast agent in the vessel.

Consider another example which illustrates the utility of Eq. (3.14) computing inherent contrast, namely that of a pulmonary nodule. The kilovoltage of an x-ray beam used for chest imaging is typically 120 kV$_p$, yielding a mean beam energy of about 63 keV after passing through the upper thorax. The attenuation coefficient of "average" lung tissue at this energy is approximately 0.05 cm^{-1} and the attenuation coefficient of a pulmonary nodule is about 0.20 cm^{-1}. If the nodule is 3 mm in diameter, then the contrast as given by Eq. (3.14) will be

$$C = 1 - e^{-(0.20-0.05)(0.3)} = 1 - 0.956 = 4.4\%.$$

This contrast does not include any degradation from scattered radiation (which will be considered in the next section). Thus, a 3-mm nodule of this contrast will be minimally visible in a chest radiograph.

Because the contrast of an object depends on the mean beam energy, it is important to examine those factors that affect beam energy. Of obvious note is the tube kilovoltage (kV$_p$), because it determines the highest energy in the bremsstrahlung spectrum. Likewise, the filtration in the x-ray beam also affects mean beam energy because the introduction of any material in the beam will preferentially remove low-energy photons more than high-energy photons (because the attenuation coefficient is greater at lower energies, except when considering K-edge materials).

Consider the following examples of how kV$_p$ affects image contrast in chest imaging and mammography. Table 3.1 lists the mean beam energy for two different kV$_p$s in chest imaging: 120 kV$_p$ typical of upright chest imaging and 90 kV$_p$ typical of bedside imaging. The contrast of a 3-mm nodule goes from 4.9% at 90 kV$_p$ to 4.4% at 120 kV$_p$. Based on the consideration of pulmonary nodule contrast alone, one would assume that 90 kV$_p$ is the better kV$_p$. However, the attenuation coefficient of calcium goes from 1.35 cm^{-1} to 0.90 cm^{-1} as the kV$_p$ changes from 90 to 120; hence rib contrast will be less at 120 kV$_p$. Furthermore, note that the transmission of the mediastinum increases from 0.3% to 0.7% as the kV$_p$ is raised from 90 to 120 kV$_p$. The higher penetration of the mediastinum and the reduced contrast of ribs is why the higher kV$_p$ is selected for upright chest imaging, even though the contrast of a particular soft-tissue detail (lung nodule) may not be at its optimum. In the case of mammography, Table 3.2 lists the approximate attenuation coefficients of fat, fibroglandular tissue, and calcium for a 4-cm compressed breast (50/50 mixture) at two kilovoltages, 26 and 40 kV$_p$ (molybdenum tube with 0.03-mm molybdenum filtration). At the lower kV$_p$, the difference

Table 3.1: Effects of kilovoltage on chest radiography. The assumption is made that the patient is comprised of 4 cm of soft-tissue-equivalent material and 16-cm lung-equivalent material. Scattered radiation is ignored

	90 kV$_p$	120 kV$_p$
Approx. mean beam energy	53 keV	63 keV
μ_{calcium}	1.35 cm^{-1}	0.90 cm^{-1}
Contrast of 3 mm nodule	4.9%	4.4%
Transmission through 25 cm		
mediastinum	0.3%	0.7%

Table 3.2: Effects of kilovoltage on mammography. The assumption is made that the patient is comprised of a 4-cm-compressed breast of 50/50 composition, and a molybdenum tube with 0.03-mm molybdenum filtration is used. Scattered radiation is ignored. All values are approximate

	26 kV$_p$	40 kV$_p$
Approx. mean beam energy	19 keV	24 keV
$\mu_{\text{fibroglandular}}$	0.89 cm^{-1}	0.54 cm^{-1}
μ_{fat}	0.58 cm^{-1}	0.40 cm^{-1}
μ_{calcium}	23 cm^{-1}	12 cm^{-1}

between the attenuation coefficients of fat and fibroglandular tissue, and the difference between calcium and fat, increase. In this case, the desire to have adequate contrast of microcalcifications, as well as the desire to have good contrast between fat and fibroglandular tissue, determine that a lower kV$_p$ such as 26 kV$_p$ is better.

As mentioned above, the energy response of the detector also plays a part in determining the contrast of objects. If a detector has relatively poor response at higher photon energies, then it will further reduce the contrast in addition to the reduction of tissue attenuation coefficient, and would not be a good candidate for high-kV$_p$ imaging. To precisely compute the contrast of a particular detector for a particular anatomical application at a particular beam spectrum, it is necessary to compute the following integral ratio:

$$C = 1 - \frac{\int \left(\dfrac{\mathrm{d}I_{\text{inc}}}{\mathrm{d}E}\right) e^{-\mu_A(D-d) - \mu_B d} \eta(E)\,\mathrm{d}E}{\int \left(\dfrac{\mathrm{d}I_{\text{inc}}}{\mathrm{d}E}\right) e^{-\mu_A D} \eta(E)\,\mathrm{d}E}, \tag{3.15}$$

where dI_{inc}/dE is the spectrum incident on the patient from the x-ray tube, $\eta(E)$ is the relative energy response of the detector at energy E, and the thicknesses D and d are as defined in Figure 3.2.

There are two methods for determining inherent contrast, including the energy dependence of the detector: computer simulation and experimental measurement. The computer modeling approach is customarily followed in designing an imaging device. In this approach, Eq. (3.15) is computed for various combinations of anatomical thicknesses and tissue compositions relevant to a particular application, using tabulated attenuation coefficients and beam spectra. In the simulations in this chapter, the method by Ergun *et al.* [14], and modified by the present author, will be used.

The computer-simulation approach allows the developer of a system to evaluate many combinations of detector materials and kV$_p$s for imaging specific anatomy. However, it is also important to experimentally measure the true image contrast to confirm the theoretical modeling. In an experimental measurement of inherent contrast, it is important to eliminate as much as possible the effects of scattered radiation (scattered radiation is an important factor in image contrast, but will be considered separately in the next section). To measure contrast, a narrow-beam geometry is used. This geometry includes a narrow pencil beam (with an upstream collimator), a large air gap between the sample and detector, and an aft collimator. Typically, exposed areas of the beam are no more than 1 cm × 1 cm, with an SID of several meters (the details of this depend somewhat on the image device being used; for example, with mammography tubes an SID of several meters is not possible). The sample of material to be measured is placed just downstream of the upstream collimator, to reduce unwanted scattered radiation from reaching the detector as much as possible.

3.2.6 Scattered radiation and the use of grids

Scattered radiation is a significant problem in radiography, and causes a substantial loss of contrast. Investigators have evaluated the amount of scattered radiation in chest radiography, and have found that more than 60% of transmitted intensity in the lungs and 90% in the mediastinum can be scatter [15], unless some means of controlling scatter is used. Estimates place the amount of scatter in mammography at about 30% [16]. Abdominal imaging is another clinical application where scatter is a significant problem.

As an example of the effect of scatter, consider again the case of a 3-mm pulmonary nodule. As derived in the previous section the contrast of this nodule without scatter is 4.4% at 120 kV$_p$. Using a scatter fraction of 66% for the lungs (without a grid), one can determine how much the contrast of the nodule diminishes when scatter is present. The scatter can be considered approximately as an increase in the overall background intensity. Thus, Eq. (3.11) becomes

$$C = \frac{(I_1 + I_s) - (I_2 + I_s)}{(I_1 + I_s)} = \frac{I_1 - I_2}{I_1 + I_s} = \frac{I_1 - I_2}{I_1 \left[\dfrac{1}{1 - SF} \right]} = C_{\text{no scat}} \cdot (1 - SF).$$

(3.16)

For the 3-mm nodule with 66% scatter fraction, the resulting contrast is 1.5%. Thus, in the presence of scatter, a 3-mm nodule will be minimally visible in a chest radiograph.

Scattered radiation is minimized in one of three ways: (1) by the use of a grid; (2) an airgap; or (3) a scanning slit. Each of these has been implemented with digital detectors, although grids are the most commonly used. When used in mammography units, the grid usually reciprocates, and hence the grid lines are generally not visible in the image. With stationary grids (as used in upright chest imaging), it is important to select a grid with a very high strip density so that objectionable grid-line aliasing does not occur. Grids with a strip density of 60 cm^{-1} have been used with CR without noticeable grid line artifacts, but in flat-panel detectors a slightly higher strip density of 70 cm^{-1} is currently being used. With these higher strip densities, there are no visible grid lines (or aliased grid lines which would appear as "corduroy stripes"). However, one can usually find a spike in the two-dimensional power spectrum at the aliased frequency of the grid lines. This spike of frequencies can be suppressed by spatial-frequency filtering, but doing so is usually not necessary with the high strip density grids.

As mentioned, airgaps are also used with some digital devices. A scanning-drum selenium device (Thoravision, Philips Medical) [6] was provided originally with an internal airgap of 15 cm at the center of the image. The developers of this device published results that indicate that in the imaging geometry of their device the airgap performs better than a grid when signal-to-noise ratio per patient dose is considered [17]. Nonetheless, some radiologists preferred the appearance of the images with a grid [7], and so a grid is now offered on the device.

Slits are also used for scatter reduction on selected digital devices that employ a scanning beam mechanism. These devices include some mammography devices under development, and an equalizing chest-imaging device [18, 19]. Slits can be quite effective at scatter removal if they are narrow enough [20, 21], but when a slit is much wider than about 1 cm in width, it no longer functions as an effective scatter-reduction device.

With any scatter-reducing device, it is important to consider two things. First, are there objectionable artifacts? As mentioned, with high strip density grids the grid-line artifacts are not likely to pose a problem. If grid lines are noticeable, then a different grid should be tried, or else a digital filtering method used to remove the spike of aliased grid lines. Second, is the contrast improvement satisfactory? This may be evaluated by imaging thin plastic discs in regions of high and low scatter fraction. The approximate contrast of the discs with and without the scatter-reducing mechanism should be compared to the theoretical limiting contrast (based on attenuation coefficient and disc thickness). A 10-cm thickness of Lucite may be used to simulate the scatter in the lungs of a chest radiograph; a 25-cm thickness may be used for abdominal imaging, and 4 to 6-cm-thick section of breast-equivalent plastic should be used for mammography. Better yet, imaging disks on an anthropomorphic phantom will provide a truer estimate of scatter. An easy method for using an anthropomorphic phantom is to acquire two images, one with the plastic discs, and one without, and then subtract the two images. It is then easy to measure the signal of the disc itself. It may be difficult to determine what constitutes "acceptable" contrast improvement for a digital device, but a rough estimate would be that the scatter-reducing device should provide at least equivalent performance to that obtained with conventional screen-film chest, mammographic, or abdominal imaging using standard grids.

3.3 Spatial-frequency assessment

Section 3.2 described the assessment of image parameters that were global (i.e., shift-invariant). It is also customary to describe the characteristics of imaging performance in the spatial-frequency domain. This frequency-space description is a carryover from the engineering disciplines, and is frequently referred to as classical systems analysis.

The main reason for describing system-response in frequency space is that there are spatial correlations of the response of the system. If the system response were truly the same at all points, then the global descriptions explained above would be completely satisfactory to characterize all behaviors of the system. However, the fact that both signal and noise are spatially correlated to some degree makes it useful to consider a frequency-response characterization.

3.3.1 Difficulties with linear systems analysis of digital systems

The main concepts of system response in a spatial-frequency description include modulation transfer function, noise-power spectra (NPS), and noise-equivalent quanta. These have been well described [22–25] and are very useful descriptors of resolution, noise, and signal-to-noise ratio. These concepts have been applied in a straightforward fashion to the measurement of image quality in many analog systems, such as screen-film radiography [26–33]. They have also been applied to the description of digital systems [1, 4, 34–38], but their interpretation with digital systems is not as straightforward as with analog systems when the digital system is undersampled.

Undersampling in digital systems occurs when the image is not sampled finely enough to record all spatial frequencies without aliasing. Aliasing is the masquerading of one frequency as another following digital sampling. For example, in a system with 200-μm pixels, the cutoff frequency, u_c, is 2.5 mm^{-1}, meaning that the sampled image can only contain frequencies up to 2.5 mm^{-1}. Any frequency higher than that in the presampled image will appear as a frequency lower than the cutoff frequency in the sampled image. A frequency of 3.0 mm^{-1} in the 200 μm-pixel system will appear as a 2.0-mm^{-1} frequency in the sampled image. Thus, it masquerades as, or takes the "alias" of, another frequency.

Almost all digital systems are undersampled to some degree because designers of digital imaging systems face practical constraints that must be considered in designing suitable systems. It is possible of course to sample an image finely enough that no aliasing takes place; however, such an image would contain such a large volume of data that it would strain current networking and storage technologies in a busy hospital. (For example, in chest radiography, image sampling with pixel sizes of about 100 μm or less would be required to avoid undersampling; the resulting image would require about 40 Mbytes of storage space uncompressed.) Ideally, device manufacturers would like to adjust the MTF so that there were a sharp cutoff in frequency response just at the limit of required frequency content, allowing for complete image fidelity with a relatively coarse pixel size. Unfortunately, there is usually limited ability to change the shape of the MTF curve, so that it is not possible to prevent undersampling completely without actually using very small pixels. Because the MTF has a relatively low value at higher frequencies, a compromise is usually chosen that selects a relatively coarse pixel size with modest extension of the presampled MTF beyond the cutoff of the imaging system. Such a compromise is not ideal, but allows the majority of frequency content of an image to be recorded with adequate fidelity, but also leaves a bit of aliasing at the higher frequencies. Clearly, in the future as storage and networking costs diminish, smaller pixels (which would eliminate any aliasing) may become practical; at present it is almost always the case that some aliasing is found in medical-imaging systems.

The difficulty with undersampling, and the incumbent aliasing that occurs, is that the system is no longer adequately described by a linear-systems model. An important requirement of the linear-systems approach, spatial invariance, no longer holds when the system is undersampled and there are overlapping aliased frequency components. Lack of spatial invariance means the local response of the system depends on where the sampling comb is located with respect to objects in the input image.

The practical problem then is how to compare undersampled digital-imaging systems with one another and with previous analog systems, because linear-systems analysis has been the traditional formalism. Strictly speaking, the mathematics of the sampling theorem provides understandable predictions with undersampled systems of known frequency input, but with arbitrary input frequency content the problem is not so simple. Is there some way in which the concepts of MTF, NPS, and DQE may be salvaged for use with undersampled digital systems, if only in an approximate way? The answer is yes, assuming several caveats are understood, as explained further in this section. The presampling MTF (PMTF) may be used to correctly describe a system's response to a single sinusoid input, but it does not describe the composite response of the system to an input with a broad range of frequencies (such as a delta function) at the frequencies affected by aliasing. The approximate response of the system with a broad-band input of frequencies may be described by an average, or expectation, MTF (EMTF), which takes into account the average aliasing, but doing so will not accurately describe the response of the system to a single sinusoid.

In this author's opinion, a practical compromise—though not an ideal one—is to report both the presampled MTF and expectation MTF of a digital system. Doing so should indicate the range of response anticipated between having a single sinusoid or a delta function incident on the undersampled system. The two descriptions will agree over the range of frequencies at which there is no aliasing, but will diverge at frequencies for which the system is aliased. This approach will allow a reasonable comparison to previous analog systems, but it must be understood with the caveats mentioned above.

3.3.2 MTF

Technically, the "resolution" of a system is the minimum distance that two objects can be placed and still be distinguished as distinct objects. This meaning of resolution is not very practical, because it depends to some degree on the shape of the small objects used. Of greater utility is the shape of the response of the system to a delta-function. This response is call the point spread function (PSF). It contains all of the deterministic spatial-transfer information of the system.

The engineering and scientific communities have adopted a different descriptor of system spatial-response properties, namely the modulation transfer function. The MTF is just the two-dimensional Fourier-transform amplitude, as a function of spatial frequency, of the PSF. The MTF is a handy descriptor of system spatial response because the stages of system response can be thought of as "filters," and the composite MTF of a system is the product of the MTF of all individual stages; this is contrasted to the convolution of the PSF of all stages in Cartesian space, which is a more mathematically cumbersome procedure.

The MTF traditionally has been described mathematically in one of two ways: (1) as the ratio of frequency content output vs frequency content input:

$$\text{MTF}(u, v) = \frac{|\text{FT}_{\text{out}}(u, v)|}{|\text{FT}_{\text{in}}(u, v)|}, \tag{3.17}$$

(2) as the Fourier amplitude of the response to a delta-function input to the system:

$$\text{MTF}(u, v) = |\text{OTF}(u, v)|, \tag{3.18}$$

where $\text{OTF}(u, v)$ is the optical transfer function, the Fourier transform (FT) of PSF. Both of these descriptions are equivalent for systems without aliasing. However, with aliasing, the two give different results.

3.3.2.1 Presampled MTF

The presampled MTF describes the system response up to, but not including, the stage of sampling. Typically this includes the response of the system to the blur from an x-ray detection substrate (such as the optical blur in a fluorescent screen) and an aperture function. The aperture function may include different things, depending on the design of the system. In a scanning system (such as a laser-scanned CR system or digitized-video system), the aperture function includes the beam-spot response function. In flat-panel systems, the aperture function may simply be the shape and size of the active response area of the pixel. The only part of a system's overall response function that is not included in the presampled MTF is geometric blur from the focal spot; this is excluded because it depends on the geometry of image acquisition rather than an intrinsic property of the detector itself.

In most digital imaging systems, the presampled MTF will be found to extend beyond the cutoff frequency imposed by the sampling interval. Again, this is because of the compromises of design that usually allow a slight bit of aliasing. All frequencies in the presampled MTF that extend beyond the cutoff frequency are aliased in the final sampled image; the amplitude of an aliased frequency component is also given by the presampling MTF at the frequency prior to aliasing [38].

The presampling MTF accurately describes the response of a system to a single sinusoid input (i.e., amplitude out as a fraction of amplitude in). This is consistent with definition #1 of MTF given in Eq. (3.17).

3.3.2.2 Expectation MTF

As mentioned previously, if a digital system is undersampled, the system will no longer have spatially-invariant response. The response of the system to a delta function will then depend on the phase of the sampling comb with respect to the impulse function. Under these conditions, the linear-systems approach breaks down, and there is no such thing as a true digital MTF. However, if the OTF of the digital system, OTF_d, is computed and averaged over all phases of the sampling comb, an approximate average "MTF" may be obtained that includes the effect of the aliased delta-function input.

The OTF_d is determined by taking the FT of system response when a delta function is the input. (See reference [38] for a detailed derivation of the following.) OTF_d has a phase dependence related to the position of the delta function relative to the sampling comb. If the delta function is at a distance a relative to the origin, then the amplitude of OTF_d is given as

$$\left|OTF_d(u_1;a)\right| = \left\{ \sum_{i=1}^{\infty} MTF_{pre}^2(u_i) + \sum_{i=1}^{\infty} \sum_{\substack{j=1 \\ j\neq i}}^{\infty} \left[R(u_i)R(u_j) - P_{ij}M(u_i)M(u_j) \right] \cos\left[2\pi a(u_i + P_{ij}u_j) \right] \right.$$

$$\left. + \sum_{i=1}^{\infty} \sum_{\substack{j=1 \\ j\neq i}}^{\infty} \left[M(u_i)R(u_j) + P_{ij}R(u_i)M(u_j) \right] \sin\left[2\pi a(u_i + P_{ij}u_j) \right] \right\}^{1/2}, \qquad (3.19)$$

$$0 \leqslant u_1 \leqslant u_c$$

where $P_{ij} = -1$ if i and j are both odd or both even, and $P_{ij} = 1$ if i and j have opposite parities. $R(u)$ and $M(u)$ are the real and imaginary components of OTF_{pre}.

$|\text{OTF}_d|$ is symmetric about zero frequency, so its value only need be calculated in the frequency range 0 to u_c. The frequencies in the sum are denoted u_1, u_2, u_3, etc. (all positive), and are in the ranges $0 < u_1 < u_c, u_c < u_2 < 2u_c, 2u_c < u_3 < 3u_c$, etc. (see Figure 3.3). These frequencies are defined as

$$u_i = u_1 + (i-1)u_c \qquad \text{for } i \text{ odd}, \qquad (3.20)$$

$$u_i = (2u_c - u_1) + (i-2)u_c \quad \text{for } i \text{ even}. \qquad (3.21)$$

Typically, only 2 or 3 terms of each summation will be needed because of the limited bandwidth of OTF_{pre}.

Finally, the value of MTF_d is given by

$$\text{MTF}_d(u_1; a) = \frac{|\text{OTF}_d(u_1; a)|}{|\text{OTF}_d(0; a)|} \qquad 0 \leqslant u_1 \leqslant u_c. \qquad (3.22)$$

The value of MTF_d outside the range $0 \leqslant u_1 \leqslant u_c$ may be found by reflecting $\text{MTF}_d(u_1; a)$ about zero frequency and replicating it every $2u_c$ in frequency space.

The phase dependence of MTF_d for undersampled systems is thereby demonstrated because MTF_d is explicitly a function of the phase a. If the digital system were not undersampled, then there would be no overlap of aliased frequency components, and the sum in Eq. (3.19) would have only one term, leaving $|\text{OTF}_d(u_1; a)| = \text{MTF}_{\text{pre}}(u_1)$ in the range $0 < u_1 < u_c$, which is independent of phase a.

The phase dependence of MTF_d resulting from undersampling poses a conceptual problem in that it violates the desired stationarity property of MTF. One solution to this dilemma is to consider the expectation value of MTF_d averaged over all phases (EMTF). As an approximation, the EMTF is a reasonable descriptor of digital MTF because it satisfies the requirements of being defined approximately as $|\text{OTF}_d|$ and is spatially invariant.

EMTF is calculated by averaging $\text{MTF}_d(u_1; a)$ over all possible phase values. For the image of a slit, the phase factor is just the displacement of the slit center from the origin of the image because all cosinusoids in a slit image have their origins at the slit center. The phase of a slit in a digital image may vary from $-w/2$ to $w/2$, where w is the width of the image. However, it can be shown that $\text{MTF}_d(u_1; a)$ is the same if a is shifted by multiples of one pixel (see [38]). Therefore, the average over all possible phases need only include the range 0 to b, where b is the pixel spacing. EMTF is then

$$\text{EMTF}(u_1) = \langle \text{MTF}(u_1; a) \rangle = \frac{1}{b} \int_0^b da \frac{|\text{OTF}_d(u_1; a)|}{|\text{OTF}_d(0; a)|} \qquad 0 < u_1 < u_c. \qquad (3.23)$$

As an example of this procedure, the EMTF of a CR system was measured (Philips Computed Radiography, model ACe, Type IIIN plates) [38]. The OTF_{pre} of the CR system was used to evaluate Eq. (3.23) at each sampled frequency. This

Re { OTF$_d$ }

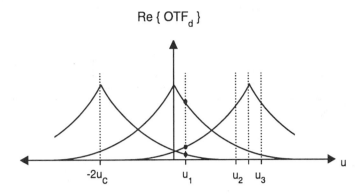

Figure 3.3: The definition of overlapping frequency components in an undersampled system. Shown are the overlapping replications of the real part of OTF$_d$ for a system. In this example, at a given primary frequency u_1, there are two positive frequencies, u_2 and u_3, that overlap it due to aliasing. The values of the overlapped frequency components at u_1 are indicated by dots. A similar graph can be drawn for the imaginary part of OTF$_d$ (from Ref. [38]).

integral is not easily evaluated analytically, so numerical integration using Simpson's rule was used (with da of $10^{-5}b$). Figure 3.4 shows EMTF as well as MTF$_{pre}$ and minimum and maximum MTF$_d$ (maximum and minimum MTF$_d$ correspond to MTF$_d$ calculated with the slit aligned approximately at the pixel center and halfway between pixels, respectively). The EMTF was found to be very close to the value of MTF$_{pre}$ up to $u \cong 2$ mm^{-1} and 4.4 mm^{-1} for the standard (ST) and high-resolution (HR) plates (with $b = 0.2$ and 0.1 mm), respectively. EMTF differed from MTF$_{pre}$ by 27% and 21% at the cutoff frequency for the standard and high-resolution plates, respectively. The maximum and minimum values of MTF$_d$ varied considerably from MTF$_{pre}$ and EMTF over a wide range of frequencies.

3.3.2.3 Errors of interpretation with digital MTF

Undersampling leads to two significant difficulties when trying to compute a digital MTF: loss of the signal-transfer property of MTF (i.e., single sinusoid response) and phase dependence of the MTF. The EMTF (or its equivalent) is sometimes used to address the phase-dependence problem, but it still leaves unresolved the problem of lack of signal transfer. If one is to make sense of the meaning of digital MTF in an undersampled system, these issues must be thoroughly understood.

Failure to properly understand these issues leads to two common misunderstandings of digital MTF. The first misunderstanding is the false notion that digital sampling *always* imposes a phase dependence on digital MTF. Such is not the case, as was shown in Eq. (3.19). When the system is not undersampled, there are no overlapping frequency components and MTF$_d$ reduces to MTF$_{pre}$. The digital MTF then has replicated segments but no phase dependence. Thus, replication of FT segments (in a sampled system) in itself does not lead to phase dependence.

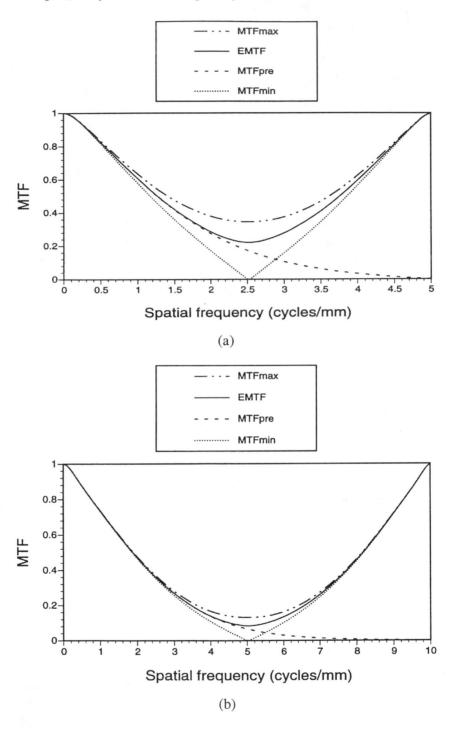

Figure 3.4: MTF values of a computed radiography system parallel to the scan direction for (a) a standard resolution imaging plate and (b) a high-resolution imaging plate. Shown are the presampling MTF (MTF_{pre}), and the maximum and minimum digital MTF (MTF_{max} and MTF_{min}), and the expectation MTF (EMTF) (from Ref. [38]).

The second common misinterpretation of digital MTF, and by far the more serious, is that digital MTF allows a reliable quantitative comparison of two digital-imaging systems. When a system is not undersampled, and therefore there is no degradation of signal-transfer information and no phase dependence, this assumption is quite valid. However, when there is undersampling, the comparison of the two systems is not at all straightforward, as illustrated in the following example.

Consider the digital MTFs of two hypothetical systems to illustrate the difficulties of comparing MTF_d (Figure 3.5). System 1 has a very typical looking MTF_{pre}, which falls off gradually to zero just beyond the cutoff frequency. There is overlap (aliasing) because the system is undersampled, which means that the digital MTF (as defined as $|OTF_d|$) contains information from both above and below u_c. System 2 is a nicely band-limited system, with an MTF_{pre} that extends just to u_c and no further. The two systems have vastly different presampling MTFs, but identical digital MTFs in this example. The two systems would respond equivalently to the image of a slit, but System 2 would be superior for imaging single sinusoids near the cutoff frequency. Thus, the nature of what was being imaged would determine whether a comparison of MTF_d or MTF_{pre} would give the more reliable conclusion about the "better" system.

As a further example, consider the two CR digital systems whose frequency responses are depicted in Figure 3.4. Both are somewhat undersampled. The frequency response at 2.5 mm^{-1} is approximately 0.36 for the HR plate, and 0.0, 0.35, or 0.22 for the ST plate (depending on whether the minimum, maximum or expectation value of MTF_d is considered). The HR plate has an EMTF value 64% higher

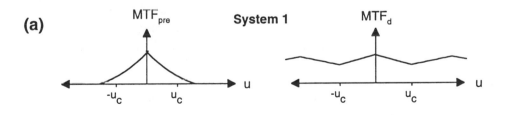

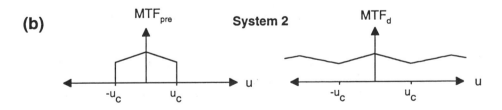

Figure 3.5: Unreliability of digital MTF for comparing systems when undersampling is present. The presampling MTF and digital MTF are shown for two hypothetical systems. Note that the presampling MTF curves are quite different, but the digital MTF_d curves are identical (from Ref. [38]).

than that of the ST plate at 2.5 mm^{-1}. However, this does not tell how much better the amplitude of a single sinusoid of frequency 2.5 mm^{-1} would be processed by the two systems. For that comparison, MTF$_{pre}$ must be used, and one finds that the HR plate is 106% better. Thus, there is a difference in the magnitude of improvement in the HR system depending on whether a broad spectrum of frequencies are imaged (e.g., a slit) or whether a narrow spectrum of frequencies are imaged (e.g., a single sinusoid). The qualitative impression of which is the better system is the same in this case regardless of whether EMTF or MTF$_{pre}$ are compared; however, the quantitative comparisons are more different.

A very important conclusion, which is often missed, is that when aliasing is present because of undersampling, MTF$_d$ is only useful for comparing the relative response of digital systems to a delta function (e.g., slit); a comparison of the systems for single sinusoids *must use the relative presampling MTFs*. When undersampled, digital signal response depends not only on the properties of the system itself, but also on the data incident on it. Although the EMTF is sometimes used as an approximate MTF for digital systems, *there is no input-independent measure of signal frequency response for an undersampled digital system over the range of frequencies affected by aliasing.*

3.3.2.4 Best way to measure MTF

Various methods of measuring the MTF have been used in the literature: the square wave method, the edge method, and the slit method.

3.3.2.4.1 Square wave method.   The square wave method uses a bar pattern with progressively narrower patterns of dark and light to determine the approximate frequency response of a system. The bar pattern is placed in the image, either parallel to the x or y axes, or along a 45° diagonal, and an image is obtained. The pixel values behind the bar pattern are then analyzed to determine the amplitude of response at each of the discrete frequencies included in the bar pattern. This amplitude reflects the square wave response of the system, not the response to a sinusoid. Thus it is not directly a measure of the MTF, although some published reports erroneously describe it as such. It may be converted to a sinusoid response by using the following approximate formula:

$$M(u) = \frac{\pi}{4}\left[M'(u) + \frac{1}{3}M'(3u) - \frac{1}{5}M'(5u) + \cdots \right], \qquad (3.24)$$

where $M(u)$ is the sinusoid response at frequency u (i.e., the MTF) and $M'(u)$ is the square wave "transfer function" derived from the bar pattern [24].

There are several difficulties with the square wave method. First, it is difficult to determine the correct amplitude from the digital image of the bar pattern. With image noise, the rounded edges of the bar pattern trace are difficult to use to determine the amplitude. Often the peak-to-peak values of several replications of the bar pattern trace are used, but again, they are limited in their precision. Second, the use of Eq. (3.24) to invert and determine the sinusoid response from the square wave response requires harmonics of the frequency being analyzed. Often there are not sufficient harmonics of each frequency in the bar pattern to reliably make such an estimate. Third, the few frequencies included in a typical commercially available bar pattern leaves an estimate of frequency response that is quite coarse.

For these reasons, the square wave response is not recommended for serious determination of the MTF of a given system, although it may be used as a quick and convenient method for following the response of a system over time to see if gross degradation has occurred.

3.3.2.4.2 Slit method.   The slit method has been very nicely described by Fujita *et al.* [39], and adopted by other users [1, 2]. The slit method measures the response of the system to an impulse function, but rather than a delta function, it uses a slit. Thus, the response of the system is given by the convolution of the PSF with the slit. The result is the line spread function (LSF). The slit method determines the MTF perpendicular to the axis of the slit by taking the Fourier amplitude of the LSF. (Technically, the MTF is a two-dimensional function, and the value of the MTF along one of the frequency axes is just the same as the Fourier amplitude of the convolution of the PSF with an infinite slit.)

The slit method uses a slit placed at a shallow angle (typically 1.5–3°) with respect to the pixel matrix to measure the LSF at a sampling interval much finer that that provided by the pixel-to-pixel distance. Pixel values in the vicinity of the angled slit represent samplings of the line spread function (LSF) at distances equal to the length from the slit center to the pixel center. The LSF is synthesized as a plot of pixel value versus distance from the slit.

The image data are first converted to be proportional to detected exposure, based on the measured characteristic curve as described in Section 3.2.1. (Note that if the digital detector is truly linear over the range of exposures used for MTF measurement, then it is unnecessary to convert pixel values to exposure.) Next, the integral of digital values across the slit (perpendicular to the direction of the slit) is computed for each point along the length of the slit (Figure 3.6). These perpendicular profile integrals are used to normalize all pixels in the vicinity of the slit. This normalization procedure, as described in more detail in Ref. [1], corrects for variations in x-ray intensity attributable to imperfections in the slit, such as from slight variations in slit width. All subsequent analyses of slit data use the normalized image values.

A plot is then made of the maximum pixel value in the perpendicular profile for each point along the length of the slit (Figure 3.7). The graph of maximum profile values is used to identify the range of the slit over which acceptable data are available for analysis. The local minima of this curve indicate the points at which the center of the slit is halfway between pixels. The distance in pixels between two of these local minima is used to determine the angle of the slit. Several of these angle determinations are averaged in order to give better precision.

The LSF is next computed by plotting the image intensity versus distance from the center of the slit for each pixel in a region of interest surrounding the slit. It is necessary to fill in any missing values and resample the LSF so that an identical

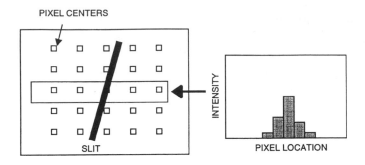

Figure 3.6: Measuring the transverse slit profile for normalization. The pixels inside the rectangular box are summed to get an integral intensity of the slit profile perpendicular to the direction of the slit. All the pixels in that row are then normalized by dividing by the profile integral. This is repeated for each row along the slit. This technique reduces problems from slit nonuniformity (from Ref. [1]).

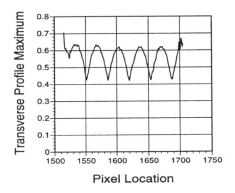

Figure 3.7: Transverse profile maximum along the length of the slit. After normalizing by the transverse profile integral (as in Figure 3.6), the maximum pixel value is found in each row along the length of the slit. The local minima of this curve indicate the points at which the center of the slit is halfway between pixels. This plot helps determine the range of reliable data along the slit (from Ref. [1]).

spacing is used between all points. The MTF is then computed by taking the Fourier transform of the LSF. The zero-frequency value of the FT is used to normalize the MTF to 1.0 at zero frequency. The MTF must be corrected for the finite width of the slit, by dividing by $\mathrm{sinc}(ua)$, where a is the estimated slit width including focal spot blurring. (In the case of the CR data cited above, for example, this correction was very small: for example, 0.8% at 5 mm^{-1} and 3.2% at 10 mm^{-1}.) MTF curves from several segments along the slit may be averaged in order to improve precision. Under these conditions, the standard error of MTF measurement was better than ± 0.005 at low frequencies and ± 0.002 at high frequencies in the CR data [1].

In order to promote consistency in measuring LSFs with very long tails, Fujita *et al.* [39] extrapolated the measured LSFs exponentially beyond the point where

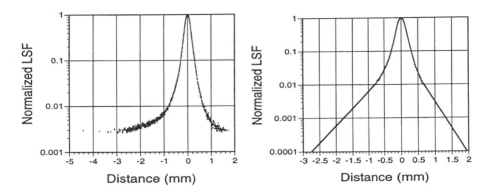

Figure 3.8: Extrapolation procedure for the line spread function. Type IIIN ST plates (200 μm pixel) with the Philips Computed Radiography Model 7000 reader are shown as (a) raw data and (b) after exponential extrapolation below the 0.01 level. LSFs have been normalized to 1.0 at their maxima (from Ref. [1]).

the LSF was at 1% of its peak value (similar to earlier work by Doi *et al.* [40]). Others have adopted the same exponential extrapolation. Figure 3.8a shows the LSF of a CR system without extrapolation; Figure 3.8b shows the same LSF after extrapolation. There is some small discrepancy between the MTFs calculated with and without extrapolation: typically about 1.5–2.5% up to the cutoff frequency. This discrepancy is caused by truncation of the very broad tails without extrapolation. Even though there is some small uncertainty introduced by extrapolation, it is recommended to use it because it tends to make the overall MTF curve better behaved by forcing a smoother transition of the LSF curve to zero.

3.3.2.4.3 Edge method. The edge method is similar to the slit method except that a sharp edge made of tungsten or lead is used [41–43]. The edge is situated at a shallow angle with respect to the pixel matrix, just as with the slit method, and the pixel values vs distance from the edge is tabulated to form a finely sampled edge response function. The derivative of the edge-response function is the LSF perpendicular to the edge; the Fourier amplitude of the LSF is the MTF.

The edge method has disadvantages and advantages relative to the slit method. An advantage of the edge method is that it produces an LSF with accurate measurement of the zero-frequency component. With the slit method, the low-frequency components will change by perhaps a few percent depending on the tail extrapolation used. A second advantage of the edge method is that it does not have the severe tube loading constraints of the slit method. There are, however, two disadvantages to the edge method. First, in this author's opinion, it is more difficult to align the edge with respect to the central beam axis than it is to align the slit. (This opinion is not shared by some who have published the edge method [43].) The difficulty with aligning the edge is that because of the tremendous image brightness, it is hard to tell from the image itself when the edge is sharply aligned. Otherwise, some type of laser device is needed to align the edge. This is in contrast to the slit, which will not produce a satisfactory slit image unless almost perfectly aligned. Thus, by rotating the slit through a narrow angle, it is easy to determine the brightest slit, and hence the optimum slit orientation. A second disadvantage of the edge method is that the derivative of the edge response function is needed to produce the LSF. Taking the derivative leaves a noisy estimate of the LSF.

In summary, the best procedure for measuring the presampling MTF would be to use both the slit and edge methods. The edge method would be used to determine the low-frequency components and the slit would be used to determine the mid- and high-frequency components. Because it is difficult and time consuming to make these measurements, if a single method is to be employed, this author recommends the slit method with exponential tail extrapolation beyond the 1% LSF level. The MTF curves determined by these methods are the presampling MTFs. The EMTF may be computed, if desired, from the PMTF using the equations in Section 3.3.2.2.

3.3.3 Noise-power spectrum

The noise-power spectrum may be understood in several ways. First, it may be thought of as the variance of image intensity (i.e., image noise) divided among the various frequency components of the image. Alternatively, the NPS may be pictured as the variance (per frequency bin) of a given spatial-frequency component in an ensemble of measurements of that spatial-frequency. These concepts are equivalent.

3.3.3.1 Theoretical background

In the case of continuous variables, Dainty and Shaw [24] give the NPS as

$$
\text{NPS}(u, v)
$$

$$
= \lim_{X,Y \to \infty} \frac{1}{2X \cdot 2Y} \left\langle \left| \int_{-X}^{X} \int_{-Y}^{Y} [I(x, y) - \overline{I}] e^{-2\pi i(ux+vy)} \, \mathrm{d}x \, \mathrm{d}y \right|^2 \right\rangle, \quad (3.25)
$$

where I is the image intensity, $\overline{I}$ is the average background intensity, and the angled brackets denote ensemble average. In the case of digital detectors, derivation of the NPS requires consideration of the discrete frequency components of the sampled image. (To simplify nomenclature, the one-dimensional case will be derived and later generalized to two dimensions.)

There are various discrete Fourier transforms available, but for the purposes of derivation the following form will be used:

$$
I(x_k) = \sum_{n=-N/2}^{N/2-1} a_n \cos(2\pi u_n x_k) + \sum_{n=-N/2}^{N/2-1} b_n \sin(2\pi u_n x_k), \quad (3.26)
$$

where $I(x_k)$ is the image intensity at the location of the kth pixel, $u_n = n/(N \Delta x)$, N = number of pixels, and Δx = pixel spacing. (Note that equivalent results are obtained if the sum over n runs from 1 to N, but to make explicit the symmetry of NPS about zero frequency, the sum from $-N/2$ to $N/2 - 1$ will be used.) The Fourier components are then given by

$$a_n = \frac{1}{N} \sum_{i=1}^{N} I(x_i) \cos(2\pi u_n x_i), \tag{3.27}$$

$$b_n = \frac{1}{N} \sum_{i=1}^{N} I(x_i) \sin(2\pi u_n x_i). \tag{3.28}$$

Using this transform it is possible to see how the variance of pixel values is related to the variance of the individual frequency components in the image. Taking the sum of squares of the Fourier amplitudes provides a useful identity:

$$\sum_{n=-N/2}^{N/2-1} |FT_n|^2$$

$$= \sum_{n=-N/2}^{N/2-1} (a_n^2 + b_n^2)$$

$$= \frac{1}{N^2} \sum_{n=-N/2}^{N/2-1} \left[\left(\sum_{i=1}^{N} I_i \cos(2\pi u_n x_i) \right)^2 + \left(\sum_{i=1}^{N} I_i \sin(2\pi u_n x_i) \right)^2 \right]$$

$$= \frac{1}{N^2} \sum_{n=-N/2}^{N/2-1} \left[I_1 \cos_{n1} I_1 \cos_{n1} + I_1 \cos_{n1} I_2 \cos_{n2} + \cdots \right. \tag{3.29}$$

$$\left. + I_1 \sin_{n1} I_1 \sin_{n1} + I_1 \sin_{n1} I_2 \sin_{n2} + \cdots \right]$$

$$= \frac{1}{N^2} \left[N I_1^2 + N I_2^2 + \cdots \right]$$

$$= \frac{1}{N} \sum_{i=1}^{N} I_i^2,$$

where $|FT_n|$ is the amplitude of the Fourier transform at frequency u_n, I_i is the intensity at the ith pixel, and $\cos_{ni}$ is $\cos(2\pi u_n x_i)$. The next to last line of Eq. (3.29) makes use of the orthogonality of sines and cosines:

$$\sum_{n=-N/2}^{N/2-1} \cos(2\pi u_n x_i) \cos(2\pi u_n x_j)$$

$$= \sum_{n=-N/2}^{N/2-1} \sin(2\pi u_n x_i) \sin(2\pi u_n x_j) = 0 \quad \text{for } i \neq j. \tag{3.30}$$

Equation (3.29) is essentially Parseval's Theorem which relates the integral of the square of a function to the integral of the square of its Fourier transform. Note that the relationship between the square of pixel values and the square of Fourier amplitudes is an exact identity; it does not depend on whether the pixel values are random. However, when the pixel values are randomly distributed with zero mean (as with Gaussian noise), it is useful to compute the ensemble average of many realizations of the noise pattern:

$$\left\langle \sum_{n=-N/2}^{N/2-1} |FT_n|^2 \right\rangle = \left\langle \frac{1}{N} \sum_{i=1}^{N} I_i^2 \right\rangle = \frac{1}{N} \sum_{i=1}^{N} \langle I_i^2 \rangle. \tag{3.31}$$

Note that for zero-mean noise, $\langle I_i^2 \rangle$ is just the variance of intensity values at the ith pixel. The variance of each pixel is the same, however, because the noise is assumed to be stationary. This equivalence of variance at all pixels is true even if there is spatial correlation of the noise, because on average over many measurements the phase will be random and each pixel will experience all possible phases of the correlation. (This is just the same as saying that with correlated photon noise from an x-ray screen, for example, any location on the screen will have the same measured intensity variance if an infinite number of measurements of the random x-ray noise are made.) Thus, Eq. (3.31) may be simplified as

$$\sum_{n=-N/2}^{N/2-1} \left\langle |FT_n|^2 \right\rangle = \sigma_{\text{pixel}}^2, \tag{3.32}$$

making use of the further relation

$$\left\langle \sum_{n=-N/2}^{N/2-1} |FT|^2 \right\rangle = \sum_{n=-N/2}^{N/2-1} \left\langle |FT|^2 \right\rangle. \tag{3.33}$$

The NPS is defined as the terms within the sum on the left-hand side of Eq. (3.32), divided by the frequency bin:

$$\begin{aligned} NPS(u_n) &= \frac{1}{(freq\ bin)} \left\langle |FT(u_n)|^2 \right\rangle \\ &= N \Delta x \left\langle |FT(u_n)|^2 \right\rangle. \end{aligned} \tag{3.34}$$

As described at the beginning, this can easily be seen to be the variance of a particular frequency component, and Eq. (3.32) shows that it is also the pixel variance spread over all frequencies, which when integrated over all frequencies yields σ_{pixel}^2.

In the case where there is not a zero mean, as would happen if there were a signal in addition to the noise, then the following modification may be made to Eq. (3.29):

$$\sum_{n=-N/2}^{N/2-1} |FT_n\{Q+S\}|^2$$

$$= \sum_{n=-N/2}^{N/2-1} \left[(a_n + A_n)^2 + (b_n + B_n)^2\right]$$

$$= \sum_{n=-N/2}^{N/2-1} (a_n^2 + b_n^2) + \sum_{n=-N/2}^{N/2-1} (A_n^2 + B_n^2) + 2\sum_{n=-N/2}^{N/2-1} (a_n A_n + b_n B_n)$$

$$= \frac{1}{N}\sum_{i=1}^{N} Q_i^2 + \sum_{n=-N/2}^{N/2-1} |FT_n\{S\}|^2 + 2\sum_{n=-N/2}^{N/2-1} (a_n A_n + b_n B_n), \qquad (3.35)$$

where Q is the zero-mean noise and S is the nonstochastic signal. A_n and B_n are the Fourier components of S at frequency u_n. When the ensemble average is taken, the first term on the right-hand side of the last line of Eq. (3.35) is just the pixel variance resulting from the zero-mean noise (as before), the second term remains unchanged because it is not random, and the last term vanishes because the linear quantities a_n and b_n represent the zero-mean noise. This leaves

$$\sum_{n=-N/2}^{N/2-1} \left[\left\langle |FT_n\{Q+S\}|^2\right\rangle - |FT_n\{S\}|^2\right] = \sigma_{\text{pixel}}^2\big|_{\text{noiseonly}}. \qquad (3.36)$$

This relation shows that there are two options for computing the NPS in the presence of a background signal. One may either subtract the background signal from the image prior to NPS analysis, or may compute the ensemble-averaged Fourier-transform square of the noise+signal and then subtract the square of the Fourier transform of the background signal. Numerical simulation reveals that both are equivalent if an infinite number of values are averaged in the ensemble. However, the certainty in measurement is better when one first subtracts off the background signal; this is because the last term in the last line of Eq. (3.35) contributes uncertainty to the measurement unless an infinite number of ensemble averages are taken (in which case it reduces to zero). Thus, the best approach is to subtract any background signal before NPS analysis.

If the signal S is subtracted out, then the NPS is given by

$$NPS(u_n) = N\Delta x \left\langle |FT_n\{I - S\}|^2\right\rangle$$

$$= \frac{N\Delta x}{N^2} \left\langle \left\{\sum_{i=1}^{N} [I(x_i) - S(x_i)]\cos(2\pi u_n x_i)\right\}^2 \right.$$

$$+ \left\{ \sum_{i=1}^{N} \left[I(x_i) - S(x_i) \right] \sin(2\pi u_n x_i) \right\}^2 \Bigg\rangle$$

$$= \frac{1}{N \Delta x} \Bigg\langle \left| \sum_{i=1}^{N} \left[I(x_i) - S(x_i) \right] e^{-2\pi i u_n x_i} \Delta x \right|^2 \Bigg\rangle. \qquad (3.37)$$

If one notes the congruence between sum and integral:

$$\lim_{\Delta x \to 0} \sum \Delta x \to \int dx,$$

then in the continuous limit one can easily see that Eq. (3.37) takes on the form in Eq. (3.25). There are two differences, however. The first difference is the limit $X, Y \to \infty$ in Eq. (3.25). This, too, will be included below in the description of the discrete NPS as a limit $N \to \infty$. The second difference is that in Eq. (3.25) there is a subtraction of only a uniform mean from the quantity $I(x)$. Subtraction of $S(x)$ would also have applied in the continuous limit had Dainty and Shaw considered the more general case of an intensity pattern with a complicated background nonstochastic signal. They considered only the more specific case of a uniform nonstochastic signal.

Before deriving the need for the limit $N \to \infty$, it is useful to note an important property of the zero-frequency component of NPS. The zero-frequency component from Eq. (3.37) is:

$$\begin{aligned}
\text{NPS}(0) &= \frac{\Delta x}{N} \Bigg\langle \left\{ \sum_{i=1}^{N} \left[I(x_i) - S(x_i) \right] \right\}^2 \Bigg\rangle \\
&= \lim_{M \to \infty} \frac{1}{M} \frac{\Delta x}{N} \sum_{m=1}^{M} \left\{ \sum_{i=1}^{N} \left[I(x_i) - S(x_i) \right] \right\}^2 \\
&= \lim_{M \to \infty} \frac{\Delta x N}{M} \sum_{m=1}^{M} \left\{ \frac{1}{N} \sum_{i=1}^{N} \left[I(x_i) - S(x_i) \right] \right\}^2 \\
&= \lim_{M \to \infty} \frac{\Delta x N}{M} \sum_{m=1}^{M} \left\{ ROImean - Truemean \right\}^2,
\end{aligned} \qquad (3.38)$$

where $ROImean$ is the mean of the actually measured N values, and $Truemean$ is the true mean of $I(x_i)$ (i.e., the mean as determined from an infinite number of measurements; also it is the mean of the known signal S). As $N \to \infty$, $ROImean \to Truemean$ and so one might assume then that $\text{NPS}(0) \to 0$. However, that is not the case. Note that

$$\sigma_{ROImean}^2 = \lim_{M \to \infty} \frac{1}{M} \sum_{m=1}^{M} [ROImean - Truemean]^2, \qquad (3.39)$$

is just the variance of the measured *ROImean* (i.e., the square of the standard error of the mean), which decreases as $1/N$ if the noise is a Gaussian random variable.

Because NPS(0) is just $N\Delta x$ times the above,

$$\text{NPS}(0) = (N\Delta x)\sigma^2_{ROImean}, \tag{3.40}$$

and the factor of N cancels the $1/N$ decrease in $\sigma^2_{ROImean}$ as $N \to \infty$, meaning that $\text{NPS}(0) \to const$ as $N \to \infty$. This is also the same result quoted in Dainty and Shaw [24] as $\text{NPS}(0) = A\sigma^2_A$, where σ^2_A is the variance of the mean signal measured with an aperture of area A.

Returning to the issue of the limit $N \to \infty$, the need for the limit may be seen by considering the consequences of having a finite extent of data. In Eq. (3.25) for continuous data, the limits of integration extend to $\pm X, Y$, which reflect the finite area over which the noise signal is measured. The integral in Eq. (3.25) may be rewritten as

$$\text{FT}\left\{[I(x, y) - \overline{I}] \cdot \text{BOX}\left(\frac{x}{2X}\right) \cdot \text{BOX}\left(\frac{y}{2Y}\right)\right\}, \tag{3.41}$$

where $\text{BOX}(x/a)$ equals 1 in the range $-a/2 \leqslant x \leqslant a/2$ and is zero elsewhere. Eq. (3.41) may be rewritten as

$$\text{FT}\left\{[I(x, y) - \overline{I}]\right\} \otimes 2X\text{sinc}(2Xu) \otimes 2Y\text{sinc}(2Yv), \tag{3.42}$$

where $\otimes$ denotes convolution. It may then be shown that

$$\text{NPS} = \text{NPS}_{\text{true}} \otimes (2X)^2\text{sinc}^2(2Xu) \otimes (2Y)^2\text{sinc}^2(2Yv). \tag{3.43}$$

In order to avoid smearing of NPS_{true} by the sinc^2 functions, it is necessary to have $X, Y \to \infty$ so that $2X\text{sinc}(2Xu) \to \delta(u)$ and $2Y\text{sinc}(2Yv) \to \delta(v)$. In the discrete case, the corresponding limit is $N \to \infty$. When sampling a limited set of noise fluctuations, one does not get a good representation of the very lowest frequencies, which can only be appreciated with a long string of data.

There is one subtlety with $N \to \infty$ in the discrete case that can cause confusion. The sinc^2 in $\text{NPS}_{\text{true}} \otimes \text{sinc}^2$ is such that its zeroes occur at spacings of the frequency bins in the optimally sampled case $[\Delta u = (N\Delta x)^{-1}]$. Thus, one may be inclined to say that the convolution by a sinc^2 function whose zeroes are at the frequency bin spacings has no blurring effect. Such is not the case, as may be seen by considering in detail how the sampling in frequency space arises.

An arbitrarily fine frequency sampling may be chosen for a given spatially sampled image by padding the edges of the image with zeroes (the frequency sampling may not be made coarser than $\Delta u = (N\Delta x)^{-1}$, which corresponds to no padding). The sampling in frequency space is therefore somewhat arbitrary, and occurs after NPS_{true} has been convolved with the sinc^2. Furthermore, even in the optimally sampled condition where the zeroes of the sinc function coincide with the frequency sampling, the amplitude of NPS is measurably diminished by the convolution of NPS_{true} with the $sinc^2$ function where NPS has a spike or a peak. The bottom line is that, to give as undistorted a rendition of the true NPS as possible, one needs to have a wide sampling of data, which in the discrete case is the same as having $N \rightarrow \infty$.

Thus, the equation for the NPS needs to be modified to include a limit as $N \rightarrow \infty$, which may be written for the full two-dimensional case as

$$
\begin{aligned}
&\text{NPS}(u_n, v_k) \\
&= \lim_{N_x, N_y \rightarrow \infty} (N_x N_y \Delta x \Delta y) \left\langle \left| \text{FT}_{nk}\{I(x, y) - S(x, y)\} \right|^2 \right\rangle \\
&= \lim_{N_x, N_y \rightarrow \infty} \lim_{M \rightarrow \infty} \frac{(N_x N_y \Delta x \Delta y)}{M} \sum_{m=1}^{M} \left| \text{FT}_{nk}\{I(x, y) - S(x, y)\} \right|^2 \qquad (3.44) \\
&= \lim_{N_x, N_y, M \rightarrow \infty} \frac{\Delta x \Delta y}{M \cdot N_x N_y} \sum_{m=1}^{M} \left| \sum_{i=1}^{N_x} \sum_{j=1}^{N_y} \left[I(x_i, y_j) - S(x_i, y_j) \right] e^{-2\pi i (u_n x_i + v_k y_j)} \right|^2 .
\end{aligned}
$$

If one has available a fast Fourier transform (FFT), then NPS is most conveniently computed from line 2 of Eq. (3.44), making sure that the normalization of the FFT is such that the forward transform includes the factor $(N_x N_y)^{-1}$ (i.e., the forward FFT need not be divided by $N_x N_y$ before inverse transforming to return the original function).

The NPS may also be computed by taking the Fourier transform of the autocovariance function (as given by the Wiener–Khintchin Theorem). Similar results will be obtained as with the method described above, as can be demonstrated to the interested reader by computer simulation using Gaussian-noise generators. However, because of the wide availability of FFT routines, it is usually most straightforward to do the so-called direct computation [as given in line 2 of Eq. (3.44)].

3.3.3.2 Noise aliasing

One of the same problems that plagues the interpretation of MTF in a digital system also applies to the interpretation of NPS. Namely, the noise components with frequency greater than u_c get aliased into the image noise at lower frequencies. The problems from undersampling the deterministic part of the signal, treated in the section on MTF, can in principal be avoided if the image is sampled finely enough. Unfortunately, the problems from undersampling the noise are not as easy to eliminate. Fortunately, the problem of phase dependence does not occur with digital NPS because the NPS is defined as an ensemble average; the ensemble average includes contributions from all possible random phases of the noise. Therefore, the digital NPS should be equally applicable at all spatial locations.

The aliasing problem arises because any noise component of a frequency higher than u_c will be replicated in frequency space and overlap other noise frequencies in a fashion identical to that described for the overlap of signal frequencies. It has been shown [37] that the measured NPS in a digital system may be described as

$$\mathrm{NPS}_d(u) = \mathrm{NPS}_{\mathrm{pre}}(u) \otimes \mathrm{III}(u; b^{-1}), \qquad (3.45)$$

where $\mathrm{NPS}_{\mathrm{pre}}$ is a "presampling" NPS arising from the noise components in the incident data before sampling, and $\mathrm{III}(u; b^{-1})$ is a sampling comb (i.e., a string of delta functions separated in frequency space by the reciprocal of the pixel spacing, b). In practice, measurement of NPS will also include an effect from the finite window used for measurement.

At first, it may be surprising that the replication and overlap of NPS_d in Eq. (3.45) appears identical in form to that for the MTF, because the NPS is related to the square of the FT components but the MTF was related to the FT components linearly. However, one may intuitively grasp the aliasing of frequency components of NPS by the following argument. The NPS is the measure of variance of a given frequency component of an image. There are frequency components above the cut-off frequency that mimic frequency components below u_c, all of whose amplitudes are given by $\mathrm{NPS}_{\mathrm{pre}}$. If one assumes that the various frequency components of image noise are uncorrelated, then the variance of one frequency component just adds to the variance of a different aliased frequency component which it overlaps, because variances add for uncorrelated random variables. Thus, overlapping frequency components of NPS_d simply add, with weightings given by $\mathrm{NPS}_{\mathrm{pre}}$. The result of this simple addition of overlapping frequencies is the standard overlapping of aliased replicated NPS components. A more rigorous derivation is given elsewhere [37].

In practice, it is not possible to measure $\mathrm{NPS}_{\mathrm{pre}}$ because the input to a system is going to contain all noise frequencies simultaneously, including those above u_c. Therefore, for any system (digital or analog) the NPS consisting of the full complement of input frequencies is the only NPS readily available to us.

3.3.3.3 Measuring NPS experimentally

The appropriate x-ray spectrum for the study must be selected. Ideally, the same x-ray spectrum should be used for NPS measurement as was used for measurement of MTF. There is unfortunately no accepted standard x-ray spectra for NPS measurements in the literature. This author believes the scientific community should pick a standard in order to promote consistency between experimental methods. Many measurements have been made at 70 kV (including screen-film and some CR measurements). Several beam filtrations have been quoted with 70 kV: 0.5 mm Cu [1, 2, 4] and 19 mm Al [44], and probably many others. These spectra are similar, and simulate the spectrum exiting an "average" patient. It is also important in the future that exposure be made at chest radiography and mammography energies. This author recommends 120 kV be selected for chest, because that is the kV used for some of the most popular asymmetric screen-film chest work. For mammography the kV depends on the tube and filtration, but 26 kV with 0.03-mm molybdenum filtration with a molybdenum tube, using filtration to simulate an average thickness of compressed breast, would seem reasonable. At this point, there is no consensus on filtration for NPS measurements, although there are some committees working on developing standards, such as the American Association of Physicists in Medicine (AAPM), which plans to publish a handbook on NPS in late 1999 or early 2000. This publication should contain some further detailed discussion about NPS measurements and spectral choices. It is recommended to check this source, as well as other standardization publications that may come out of Europe or Asia, to see if a consensus spectrum is selected. In the meantime, it is important to select kVs representative of the clinical applications of a digital detector, and to specify the filtration used in the studies.

Once the spectrum has been selected, flat-field images over a range of exposure must be acquired. Exposure values covering the usable dynamic range of the device should be used because the NPS is often exposure dependent. Exposures of 0.03, 0.3, 3, and 30 mR were used in a study of CR NPS [1], for example. Data should be acquired as the unit would be used clinically (i.e., if a grid is a standard part of the device, it should be included; however, in CR, where the plates are often used without grids, studies were done without grids [1, 2, 4]. Note, however, that if a grid is used there will be a substantial increase in low-frequency noise and one may wish to report the NPS both with and without grid for comparison). Pixel values from the detector must be converted to be linearly proportional to exposure before any data are processed by the NPS routine. The characteristic curve of the device should actually be measured, such as by the procedure in Section 3.2.1, rather than relying on a characteristic curve provided by the manufacturer.

Once the flat-field images have been acquired, the next thing to be determined for NPS measurement is the size of ROI to be used for the analysis, and the number of ROIs to be averaged. In practice, it is necessary to select the best possible values of ROI size (as given by N) and the number of ROIs in the ensemble average (as given by M), under the constraint of a finite amount of available data. The following procedure is often useful: (1) first choose N such that there is minimal distortion of the NPS; then (2) compute what certainty in the estimate of NPS is required. This latter step gives the number of ensemble averages, M, required. For limited data, there may need to be a compromise between the constraints imposed by steps (1) and (2).

Determining the best practical value of N for limited data depends on the approximate shape of the NPS function, because a greater N will be required to maintain the shape of a more sharply peaked NPS_{true}. The approximate shape may be determined by taking a single exposure with the detector, then dividing the center of the image into an array of ROIs of modest size (perhaps 64^2). This should yield 256 sample ROIs in a 1024×1024 region in the center of the image. The NPS is then computed by averaging the squared Fourier transforms in the ROIs according to line 2 of Eq. (3.44). By fitting a line through the ensemble-averaged NPS estimate in the region of its greatest slope, one may obtain an approximation to the greatest slope of the true NPS (Figure 3.9).

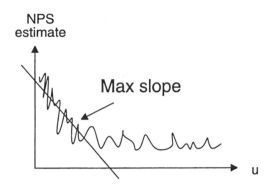

Figure 3.9: Method for determining the maximum slope of the NPS estimate. After a rough estimate of the NPS is made, a line is fit through the NPS data to determine the approximate maximum slope along the NPS curve.

A computer simulation may then be performed to estimate the most reasonable value of N. The computer simulation uses a pseudo-random Gaussian-noise generator to obtain a one-dimensional *NPS* with the same approximate maximum slope as determined above. A suitable Gaussian-noise generator may be obtained by averaging 10 values from any typical flat-distribution pseudo-random number generator (such as erand48 in C). A one-dimensional string of perhaps 4096 Gaussian noise values can be computed, the Fourier transform taken, and the FT multiplied by a filter that has the same slope as the maximum slope measured above, but with the peak of the slope at zero frequency. Then the inverse Fourier transform of the 4096 data values is taken. The result is a string of filtered noise whose NPS has a maximum slope approximating that of the actual data from the detector.

Because the maximum slope of the simulated NPS is positioned at zero-frequency, the value of NPS(0) may be examined to determine the best value of N. To do so, a one-dimensional (1-D) NPS with $N = 32, 64, 128, 256$, and 512 is computed using a subset of the string of 4096 filtered data values. The value of NPS(0) at each N is computed by averaging many trials of the procedure (perhaps 10,000), using a fresh set of initial 4096 values for each trial. The value of NPS(0) will approach an asymptote as N gets sufficiently large that the sinc^2 which convolves NPS$_{\text{true}}$ has an insignificant degradation of NPS$_{\text{true}}$. For a relatively flat NPS, almost any value of N will do, whereas for a sharply peaked NPS, an N of 256 or greater may be required. This value of N should then be used to compute the NPS of the actual data from the digital detector. The number of ensemble averages, M, may be selected by trial and error, depending on the precision desired for the NPS curve.

Over the years of noise-power analysis, considerable effort has been given to finding appropriate weighting functions for the original data to reduce the impact of the sinc^2 smearing of NPS$_{\text{true}}$. This is sometimes referred to as "window carpentry" because it attempts to build a suitable frame for the finite "window" of data available. Blackman and Tukey [25] provide a nice description of this window manipulation, which can be shown to virtually eliminate the side-lobes of the sinc^2 convolving function. However, the side lobes of sinc^2 are already small, and today when computing power is ample to handle even large data sets, there is little additional benefit to doing window weighting rather than just making N larger. Windows provide a little better result but are probably not worth the extra effort based on how easy it is to increase N by factor a of 2 in most cases. If there are cases where data is extremely limited, then windowing may be a useful option.

3.3.3.4 Fixed pattern noise

An additional point to consider is what to do when there is fixed pattern noise in the image. It is important philosophically to include this structured noise, such as would occur from phosphor granularity in a phosphor screen, in the estimate of NPS. It is included by default in all screen film NPS calculations. It is important to include structured noise because it is part of the spatially-stochastic intensity variation that affects the ability of the observer to pick out a signal from the noise. The fact that the structured noise is temporally static does not change the deleterious effect it has on the detection of an object in an image, because it can't be distinguished by the eye from spatially stochastic noise from the x-ray quanta. Even with contemporary flat-panel detectors that generally subtract out additive noise (e.g., dark current) and normalize out gain variations, it is still important to measure the entire noise including any possible residual structured noise. That is because these detectors' correction for fixed pattern noise may depend on exposure level, and the corrections may possibly vary over time and temperature. Thus the entire detector, including the corrections for fixed pattern noise, should be included in determination of NPS.

When including structured noise into the NPS, it is important to properly select the ROIs. Because the structured noise is temporally static, it would not be appropriate to use an ensemble average of $|\text{FFT}|^2$ of the same ROI measured at different times. The fixed pattern noise would be the same in each such measurement. In this case, the "noise" measured would not be ergodic; in other words, the temporal average of values would not yield the same variance as a spatial average. Ergodicity is what makes the ensemble variance (sum over m) and the spatial variance (sum over i) equivalent in Eqs. (3.29) through (3.32).

In digital detectors where there is fixed pattern noise (essentially all detectors), it is important to use a different ROI for each measurement in the ensemble of measurements. As an example, consider the case with CR [1], where a large 1024×1024 area was subdivided into 64 128×128 ROIs, and the ensemble average of $|\text{FFT}|^2$ in each of these 64 ROIs was used to calculate NPS. If more than one image is required to give as many ROIs as needed (based on the previously described optimization of N and M), then the same ROIs should not be used in the multiple images. This may require shifting the ROIs partially between subsequent exposures. The goal is to make the various ROIs in the ensemble as different as possible, to average over many realizations of the detector structured noise. For example, if 128 ROIs were needed, each being 128×128 pixels in size, one could acquire two images, use an 8×8 array of ROIs in each image, but shift the array of ROIs by 64 pixels in both x and y directions in image 2.

Once the composite NPS has been generated, it may be desirable to evaluate how much of the NPS is attributable to structured noise in the detector. In order to determine that, a second set of NPS measurements must be made. In this second set of measurements, a single ROI is selected near the center of the field of exposure. Numerous snapshots of the noise pattern in this one ROI are taken (perhaps 32), and the average of the 32 snapshots is computed. This average then represents to some reasonable precision the structured noise of the detector. [In this case the "true" structured noise may be considered a known signal, $S(x, y)$, to be subtracted as in Eq. (3.44).] This background signal is then subtracted from the ROI data in each of the 32 snapshots and the NPS computed as the average of the 32 $|\text{FFT}|^2$ according to Eq. (3.44). The resulting NPS must be multiplied by 32/31 in this example to correct for residual variance in the subtracted average. The NPS thus determined contains all noise sources except the structured noise of the detector. The precision of this method may then be improved by using multiple ROIs rather than just one ROI at the center of the image. This subtraction NPS may be compared to the composite NPS determined previously to see the relative contributions of the structured noise to the total noise.

3.3.3.5 Normalized NPS

Precision of noise-power measurements may be improved if the normalized NPS (NNPS) is computed and averaged at each ROI, rather than averaging the NPS itself. The NNPS is

$$\text{NNPS}(u, v) = \frac{\text{NPS}(u, v)}{(large\ area\ signal)^2}. \tag{3.46}$$

This quantity is readily used in the equation for NEQ, and has the benefit that if there are gross exposure variations over the measurement area (such as from the heel effect), computing the NNPS separately for each ROI and then averaging will tend to cancel some (but not all) of the variation in noise-power resulting from regional variations in x-ray exposure. If one wishes to report the NPS rather than the NNPS, then the NNPS averaged over all ROIs may simply be multiplied by the appropriate $(large\ area\ signal)^2$ corresponding to the desired exposure to yield NPS.

The "large area signal" is basically a measure of the gain of the system (i.e., the value recorded for a particular exposure incident on to the system). It is measured in the same units as the data used to determine NPS. Hence, the ratio of these two numbers leaves only units of area, typically designated as mm^2.

3.3.3.6 Low-frequency artifacts

When evaluating the NPS, it is very important to examine the full two-dimensional NPS, because there may be noise spikes in parts of frequency space that would not easily show up if only a one-dimensional curve were taken directly from the NPS data. For example, in CR systems it was found that early systems had numerous noise spikes, but subsequent systems had substantially improved and only a few noise spikes remained.

If one looks at the two-dimensional NPS (or NNPS), one will note that for many detectors the noise-power has an unusually large value along the u and v frequency axes. This is particularly true for detectors that have some strong x and y dependence to the detector structure (CR being a good example, with a different response in the scan and subscan directions). The large noise-power values along the axes are largely a result of artifacts and exposure variations (such as dust on the scanning optics or the heel effect) that are not representative of stochastic noise. Hence, when making a one-dimensional graph of NPS, it is unfair to penalize the reported performance of the device by reporting the NPS (or NNPS) along the axes themselves, because those values are not reflective of the noise-power in the great majority of frequency space.

Often investigators ignore the very lowest frequencies because it is hard to distinguish between low-frequency artifacts and low-frequency stochastic noise. However, there are several methods to address the problem of low-frequency arti-facts. The first is detrending. Detrending is subtracting some type of fit to the gross intensity variations in an ROI. For example, a plane may be fit to the exposure sur-face in an ROI, and then the plane subtracted from the ROI. Or a second-order sur-face may be fit and then subtracted. It is important when doing detrending that the mean value remain unchanged by the detrending process. Detrending is successful at minimizing the excessively large values along the u and v axes, but usually does not completely remove the large axis values.

In a report on CR devices, it was elected to avoid the u and v axes altogether [1]. Instead, a few rows of data on either side of the each axis were selected and the NNPS value plotted versus sqrt($u^2 + v^2$) in that slice of data. By doing so, the NNPS values were determined near the axis in a slice through frequency space. The data values were then binned into bins of 0.05 mm^{-1} before plotting. The procedure was performed independently for both axes. Alternatively, if one has a detector that is nicely isotropic, then a radial average of NNPS may be plotted. The u and v axes may be skipped in the radial average if adequate detrending cannot remove the sharp rise in values along the axes.

3.3.4 NEQ(f) and DQE(f)

The MTF describes the signal response of a system at a given frequency, and the NPS describes the amplitude variance at a given frequency. The ratio of these quantities, properly normalized, gives information about the maximum available signal-to-noise ratio as a function of frequency. The square of this ratio is the fre-quency dependent NEQ:

$$\mathrm{NEQ}(u, v) = \mathrm{SNR}^2_{\text{non-ideal}}(u, v) = \frac{(\textit{large area signal})^2 \mathrm{MTF}^2(u, v)}{\mathrm{NPS}(u, v)}. \quad (3.47)$$

(This definition applies to detectors whose output has been linearized with respect to incident intensity.)

One must decide whether to use the PMTF or EMTF in the above equations. Both have been reported. It gives a good estimate of the upper and lower bounds on measured NEQ(u, v) and DQE(u, v) if plots are made both ways (corresponding to understanding the MTF as the ratio of single sinusoid amplitudes out vs in, or as the FT of the response of the system to a delta function).

The NEQ(u, v) for linearized detectors may be computed from the NNPS as well:

$$\text{NEQ}(u, v) = \frac{\text{MTF}^2(u, v)}{\text{NNPS}(u, v)}. \tag{3.48}$$

Usually, a one-dimensional NEQ is plotted along the u and v orientations, unless the device is truly isotropic. A one-dimensional plot is usually used because it is almost impossible to measure a true two-dimensional MTF (usually the MTF is measured as a one-dimensional plot from the LSF along a particular orientation).

The DQE is computed as

$$\text{DQE}(u, v) = \frac{\text{NEQ}(u, v)}{\text{SNR}_{\text{inc}}^2}. \tag{3.49}$$

As with NEQ, DQE is usually plotted as a one-dimensional graph along the u or v direction (or as a one-dimensional graph in arbitrary direction if isotropic).

Once the full DQE(u, v) has been computed, it is often desired to report not only the shape of the curve, but the DQE($0, 0$) value in particular. DQE($0, 0$) is the same as the global DQE described in Section 3.2.4. It is dangerous to assume, however, that DQE($0, 0$) as given by the DQE curve is a reliable estimate of the system-response to stochastic noise. As pointed out before, it likely contains a large amount of low-frequency artifact. It is more appropriate to extrapolate the low-frequency part of the DQE(f) curve back to zero frequency when reporting the "DQE(0)" of a system.

3.4 Image-processing assessment

There are numerous combinations of image-processing algorithms that can be applied to digital radiographic images. Often these algorithms function interdependently and may involve nonlinear processing steps that prevent them from being evaluated individually. Thus, the task of evaluating image processing is quite daunting.

In this section several strategies are given. These strategies are only suggestions, and may not be applicable to every imaging situation. In addition to making physical measurements, it is also important to have radiologists evaluate actual clinical images, including a range of body habitus and disease state, before concluding that an image-processing scheme is acceptable. (Strategies for more quantitative observer evaluations are covered in Section 3.5.) Determining which processing is "optimum" is quite difficult indeed, and may involve a number of iterative cycles in which physicists and radiologists try, improve, and retry various approaches until one is found that gives good technical performance and is acceptable to the radiology community.

3.4.1 Effect of image processing on perceived image noise

There is the common experience that when a low-pass spatial filter is employed, images get less noisy, and when a high-frequency enhancement filter is applied, images get more noisy. This is sometimes true, but needs careful exploration because it depends on the distribution of frequencies in the signal and noise, and on the amount of contrast enhancement applied after filtering.

As an example, consider the case of data acquired with a CR device. A flat-field exposure was acquired at 3 mR incident on the detector. The standard deviation of pixel values in a 100×100 ROI at the center of the image was 1.7 gray level values. The data were next convolved with a square kernel 20×20 pixels in size. The standard deviation of pixel values dropped to 0.8 gray levels. The data were next high-pass filtered by subtracting the image blurred with the 20×20 kernel from the original image. The standard deviation of pixel values was then 1.5 gray levels. With both low-pass and high-pass filtering, the standard deviation of pixel values diminished because some of the noise-power spectrum had been removed.

Now consider the case of a hypothetical vessel 15 pixels wide superimposed on the same flat-field image. If the image is again high-pass filtered with a 20×20 pixel kernel, there will be some undershoot at the edges of the vessel, and the central opacity of the vessel will be reduced relative to the flat-field surrounding it. Often in a case such as this, the image is contrast adjusted to restore the central opacity of the vessel to its original contrast relative to the flat-field background. With a vessel size so close to the size of the convolving kernel, a contrast enhancement by a factor of 1.5 to 2.0 might be required. The standard deviation of pixel values would then measure approximately 2.3 to 3.0 gray levels. Thus, contrast enhancement following high-pass filtering caused almost a two-fold increase in image noise, although the high-pass filtering itself reduced the image noise. This is the effect most commonly experienced by observers: high-frequency enhancement followed by contrast enhancement increases the apparent noise compared to the anatomy contrast. The severity of this phenomenon depends on how much the signal-power spectrum of the anatomy of interest overlaps with the noise-power spectrum.

Thus, in an image-processing algorithm that modifies the frequency content, there is the potential for altering the perceived image noise. Often, digital filtering which gives rise to this effect is dependent on image intensity, so that different amounts of filtering, or different filtering kernels, may be used in different parts of the image. Coupled with the fact that the image noise texture may change from transmissive to dense patient regions because of differences in NPS in those regions, it becomes important to evaluate whether the perceived noise is acceptable or not.

Two approaches may be helpful. First, a measure of image variance may be acquired in different regions of an image, in order to see how well it tracks with exposure. The variance will be influenced of course by variations in pixel value from the overlying anatomy, so it is important to eliminate the anatomy before evaluating the variance. This may be done by two methods. A suitable phantom may be used that has flat areas for measurement of variance without background anatomy [45]. Alternatively, a subtraction of two images of an anthropomorphic phantom may be used. In the subtraction approach, the resulting variance attributable to noise will be twice that in an individual image; however, the anatomical variations will have been removed. One caveat about the subtraction method is that it also will subtract structured noise from the detector, which will artificially reduce some of the spatial noise observed in clinical images. If the measures of variance obtained by one of the above two methods tracks linearly with exposure, (as measured by the image-pixel values converted to exposure in the respective parts of the image under evaluation), then one may infer that the system is performing in a reasonably x-ray quantum-limited fashion.

It is also common to find that the noise varies not only by magnitude but by texture from region to region in an image. This is to be expected because the NPS changes shape as a function of exposure, because of the relative contribution of MTF^2-dominated x-ray noise and white-noise sources as exposure changes. This variation of noise texture from region to region can be seen in the newer asymmetric screen film combinations (such as described in [46, 47]). A change in texture from region to region only becomes a problem when the noise is judged to be unacceptable at some point in the image.

A more instructive test is to measure the NPS in dense and transmissive regions of subtraction images as described above. A relatively small ROI (perhaps 128×128) should be used, so that NPS is measured in a region of fairly uniform intensity. A number of images must be acquired and averaged to improve the NPS estimate. Again, it should be remembered that the stochastic contribution to the NPS from the structured noise in the detector will be artificially subtracted out by this method. An alternative method which maintains the structured detector noise is to measure the NPS in unsubtracted flat-field images taken at a wide range of detected exposures. However, scattering material must also be placed in the beam to get a realistic estimate of the contribution of beam-hardening and scatter to the measured NPS.

It is also useful to obtain a qualitative observer assessment from radiologists when evaluating image noise. Radiologists have become acutely sensitive to the cues they pick up from noise in an image. If they see more noise in one part of the image (the mediastinum, for example) than they are accustomed to, they may infer that the detector is not functioning reliably, or that the patient is quite obese. This inference is influenced by the years of experience reading screen-film images, with its own distribution of noise textures over the image. It is helpful in evaluating a new digital imaging detector to ask several radiologist colleagues for their assessment of the noise in the image. The goal of this strictly qualitative assessment is to determine if the noise is generally felt to be acceptable or not. If it is deemed to be not acceptable, the above study of noise texture, as measured by the NPS, may shed some light on whether high- or low-frequency noise is causing the problem. This information may help determine whether image processing is the culprit, or whether the detector itself possesses unacceptable noise properties.

3.4.2 Sufficient bit depth

Ideally, the number of bits in the initial data acquired by a detector is sufficient so there are no observed contours after image processing. Contours are where the image takes on discrete visible transitions between gray levels as in the appearance of a contour map. Contours are most noticeable in areas of low local gradient and low noise. Sometimes the contours will be observed as a "clumpiness" or "globbiness" in the image, where it appears that the noise or regional anatomy is comprised of only a few discrete gray-level values. The cause of this subtle appearance is a difficult problem to track down, as contours can sometimes be a result of image-processing quirks rather than inadequate bits.

It is generally safest to program processing algorithms so that they use floating-point math and then convert back to integer at the end of all processing, with appropriate rounding. Sometimes manufacturers code each image-processing step as integer in/integer out. Such coding is adequate in some circumstances but not all. Particularly susceptible to contouring are nonlinear grayscale transform curves and spatial filtering.

A method to check for contouring or inadequate bits is to look at the histogram of ROIs in various regions (both transmissive and dense) in actual patient images. The histogram should be well populated, without significant empty bins and relatively smooth transitions. ROIs of at least 100×100 pixels should be used to ensure an adequate sampling of local gray levels. This test should be done in both high- and low-exposure conditions. It is not always adequate to look in dark and light portions of a single radiograph, because the grayscale range may have been adjusted by the processing; rather look in images acquired in high- and low-exposure conditions. One caveat: empty or overpopulated histogram bins do not necessarily indicate a problem; it depends on whether the grey level spacing of the empty or overpopulated bins constitute a just-noticeable difference in grayscale.

It is also useful to compare the appearance of the anatomy and noise to that in a screen-film image of the same phantom (or patient, if available), bearing in mind that noise texture may be different between screen-film and digital images. If local regions appear more contoury in the digital image than in the screen-film, then there is cause for further investigation. Be sure to use anthropomorphic phantoms, not uniform phantoms, for these tests, because the image processing may function differently depending on the histogram of the image. It is also useful to obtain the assessment of a radiologist as to whether noise contouring is apparent, because the normal appearance of anatomy will be more familiar to the experienced radiologist than a physicist.

3.4.3 Grayscale fidelity

Grayscale fidelity refers to the appropriateness of the grayscale map in the image. Almost every digital imaging system modifies the grayscale map by applying a nonlinear transform curve to the output, in order to match the highest contrast to the most significant portion of the anatomical information, and to avoid clipping by appropriately handling values at the very highest and lowest exposures. The grayscale transform should contain smoothly varying monotonically changing gray levels and, if intended to mimic a particular screen-film combination, should do so with reasonable accuracy.

The first check to make on the grayscale is to check monotonicity and smoothness. If there is direct access to input digital data going into the grayscale transform, then a digital ramp covering the entire range of input values may be used to evaluate the transform. The output of the ramp should be evaluated for any noticeable breaks, plateaus, or reversal of slope.

If there is no direct access to the transform input, then an image of a plastic wedge may be tried. The wedge should be smooth, without any seams. It should be placed at a 45° angle, to avoid mistaking any artifacts associated with the detector with the ramp response from the wedge. Evaluate the image for any lines, breaks, or plateaus in the ramp. Employing a small-kernel high-pass filter may highlight small-scale abnormalities on the image of the ramp.

There is one example familiar to the author of a prototype flat-panel device that had unacceptable bends in the output transform curve provided for calibration to the laser printer. The images appeared to be blotchy, and at certain gray levels the contrast seemed to be diminished. This was a very confusing image artifact to figure out. It was discovered that the look-up table for the hardcopy printer had recently been recalibrated, using a series of discrete gray-level steps. When the look-up table (LUT) was examined, it was found to contain non-monotonic slope; in fact, there were portions of the LUT curve where the contrast (i.e., derivative) of the curve dropped by half. These gray levels corresponded to the regions with the observed loss of contrast. By forcing the LUT to be smoothed by a low-order polynomial fit, these problems were solved. The reader is encouraged to carefully examine all transform curves and LUT, even for the final-output hardcopy devices, if there are regions of anomalous contrast.

If the grayscale transform is intended to match a particular screen-film combination, as is sometimes the case, the grayscale agreement may be evaluated in several ways. First, if there is access to the digital input and output of the transform, then it may be evaluated for correspondence to an experimentally obtained characteristic curve of the desired film. Second, observers may assess qualitatively the congruence of the digital image to the screen-film being matched. Either anthropomorphic phantom images or images of patients may be used, with a panel of radiologists asked to assess the overall grayscale congruence. While not a definitive evaluation of the grayscale fidelity, this observer test can confirm if the grayscale is acceptable, which is important in clinical acceptance.

Sometimes a grayscale transform is not intended to directly match a particular film HD curve. One may still evaluate if adequate contrast exists in different regions of the image (e.g., lung and retrodiaphragm in chest imaging). This contrast test may be done experimentally by placing 5-mm-thick plastic discs in the field of view in the lung and retrodiaphragm, and taking one image with the discs and one without. A subtraction of the two images should yield an image with only the discs present, which can then be measured for differential signal. The differential signal may be compared at different locations in the image to check relative contrast in dense and transmissive regions. The image with the discs may also be hardcopy printed and the approximate optical density difference of the discs relative to their backgrounds measured with a densitometer. These optical density (OD) differences may be compared to those for a conventional screen film used in clinical practice.

One important advisory regarding the comparison of digitally processed images with conventional screen-film images: various image-processing algorithms may use nonlinear processing or combinations of algorithms (such as unsharp masking or multi-spectral analysis) so that the images will not be identical even if the same grayscale-transform curve is used. For this reason, it is important to also have a panel of radiologists evaluate the image for suitable contrast in various regions of intensity. As an example, it is important to determine whether structures in the low-OD portions of the image are adequately visualized, such as tubes and lines in the mediastinum of a chest film image. A panel of trained observers may sometimes be able to assess whether grayscale performance is satisfactory, even though physical measurements may be difficult or impossible.

3.4.4 Spatial-frequency enhancement

The most common spatial-frequency enhancements to be used are variations of high-frequency enhancement (e.g., unsharp masking) or multi-spectral analysis (where several frequency bands are processed separately). The usual goals of spatial-frequency enhancement are to improve sharpness, to suppress overall dynamic range, or to enhance regional contrast. Because there are many forms of spatial-frequency enhancement, it is not possible to describe strategies for evaluating each of them. However, several general approaches may prove useful for many of these algorithms.

First, it is important to evaluate the shape and size of the kernel used for the enhancement. In order to measure the kernel shape and size, it is necessary to input very tiny dots to the imaging system. This may be done by using metal filings or other small objects. Images of these dots should reveal the shape and size of the effective filter kernel. The morphology or appearance of the dots should be checked to ensure that they are not going to cause misinterpretation for small-scale structures, such as microcalcifications in mammography. For larger kernels, such as may be used for dynamic range suppression, it is important that the kernels not reveal an objectionable halo around a dot, which might mistakenly be identified as air, for example. The kernels should ideally be isotropic, although for some large kernels used in dynamic range suppression, square kernels may perform adequately.

The effect of the enhancement at regions of sharp intensity discontinuities should also be checked (e.g., lung/diaphragm border) to see if any ringing is present. The transition should be smooth from dark to light. Also, it should be determined if a bipolar response is noted at regions of sharp discontinuity—such a dark/light band may be misinterpreted as air around the heart for example. Imaging the edge of a uniform 1-mm thick sheet of copper is a convenient method for assessing performance at sharp discontinuities. Because some algorithms base the kernel on the surrounding image intensity, it may be helpful to place the edge of the copper sheet so that it lines up with the lung/diaphragm border, for example. A subtraction of two images, one containing the copper and one without it, will reveal the shape of any spatial filtering taking place at the lung/diaphragm boundary.

It is also important to evaluate how the enhancement affects an image where texture is important, such as in diagnosis of interstitial disease. Sometimes excessive edge-enhancement can make the image appear "busy" and give a false impression of interstitial disease where there is none. Also, with unsharp masking one should be aware of the tendency toward suppression of general opacity. In the case where diffuse disease gives a slightly less transmissive appearance to one lung, there may be a noticeable difference in overall density of the contralateral lung in a conventional film. However, with unsharp masking, this difference may be suppressed, thereby minimizing some of the difference in appearance of the two lungs [48].

It is also important to have a panel of trained radiologists evaluate overall image appearance in digital images compared to film images of actual patients. There are subtle changes in lung density that may be suspect to the radiologist but not to an imaging physicist. A panel of trained observers might be asked to rate both film and digital images for sharpness, and general anatomical appearance in various regions of anatomy. For example, if the goal of the enhancement is to sharpen the image, then it should be evaluated in both transmissive areas (lungs or fatty breast) as well as in dense regions (mediastinum or dense fibroglandular regions). It is important for the panel to evaluate the acceptability of the images over a wide range of body habitus and diseases. Again, as mentioned before, such an observer study is not intended to define how well a particular image-processing scheme will affect diagnosis, but does involve the very important element of clinical acceptability that only radiologists can give.

3.4.5 Histogram-based processing

Histogram-based processing is often performed for two reasons: to restrict the overall dynamic range displayed, and to allow histogram-based contrast optimization. Techniques for evaluating the latter are similar to evaluating spatial-frequency enhancement outlined above. For dynamic range suppression, however, it is important to determine how accurately the algorithm finds the appropriate beginning and ending grayscale values for the input data. In order to evaluate this, a range of patients from thin to medium to large must be imaged, and compared to conventional screen-film images. They should be compared for overall image darkness, and whether the brights or darks of the image appear clipped or saturated. Gross optical densities can be measured in regions of low, medium, and high optical density to compare digital hardcopy against screen-film. Input from radiologists is also crucial in this process, in order to determine if the image presentation will be judged adequate.

3.4.6 X-ray beam equalization

Most digital radiographic imaging systems do not include equalization, but there is one device manufactured that allows equalization (Oldelft, Delft, the Netherlands). Equalization is the process of modifying the spatial distribution of x-ray flux incident on the patient, in order to make the intensity transmitted through the patient more uniform. This uniformity improves the signal-to-noise ratio in dense patient regions, and although not as important with digital devices as with film, also allows more anatomy to be displayed in the linear range of hardcopy film.

The equalization is accomplished by having a beam modulator in the beam, upstream of the patient, connected through a feedback loop to a detector downstream of the patient. Based on the feedback detector signal, the modulator is opened or closed to vary the flux at a particular part of the patient. In the Oldelft device, the modulator is comprised of a scanning beam slit with about 20 modulators across the beam.

The same evaluation procedures as listed for conventional digital imaging devices should be followed with equalization devices, but two additional evaluations are also necessary. First, it is important to evaluate the image for artifacts from the modulating devices. If the individual modulators are not functioning with equivalent feedback response, then it is possible to obtain vertical stripes in the image. This may be tested by placing an edge phantom (such as a 1-mm-thick Cu sheet) in the beam. As the modulators pass over the edge, the response should be visually the same for all modulators. This image should also be evaluated for an ringing artifacts, as evidenced by alternating dark and light bands at the boundary.

Equalized images should also be evaluated for partial volume artifacts as the modulator crosses an edge which is almost vertical (such as the cardiac border). Radiologists should evaluate the films of actual patients to determine if there is any edge effect at the cardiac border which might be confused with pathology.

It is also important to be aware of patient dose with the equalization device. It may be programmed so that the same overall average dose is delivered with equalization as without, by reducing the exposure to the lungs while increasing it to the mediastinum. But it is also possible to program the device so that the dose to the lungs is maintained at conventional levels, but the dose to dense patient regions is increased. Choosing this latter approach will increase the overall patient exposure. Measurements of incident exposure on an anthropomorphic phantom may be used to determine which of these operating modes is used, and whether the mode chosen follows the exposure recommendations of a particular medical center.

3.5 Observer assessment

The last, and sometimes overlooked, stage in the imaging chain is the observer. Because it is the observer who takes the final presentation of spatial-intensity data and converts that into a diagnostic finding, it is important to include some characterization of the observer's performance in the overall scheme of assessing "image quality." Unfortunately, a rigorous observer study can be quite difficult, and the literature is full of many nonrigorous observer studies. On the other hand, as has been pointed out many times in this chapter, there is a very valuable, even essential, role for the end observer (the radiologist) in the design and evaluation of a digital device, even if the evaluation is somewhat subjective. There is tension for many imaging scientists between the extremes of conducting a "subjective" observer study (feeling that such a study is too wishy-washy to be good science) and the task of conducting a diagnostic accuracy study for every possible diagnosis (which is overly daunting, probably even impossible considering the large number of diagnostic tasks required in areas such as chest imaging). In this section, a hopefully rational plan is proposed that incorporates the need for rigorous scientific analysis with the practical constraints of limited observer time and available number of research subjects.

A four-phase approach is proposed for evaluating the performance of any digital imaging device: (1) Quantitative *physical* measurements are made of parameters that characterize device performance. This category includes such measurements as $DQE(f)$, inherent contrast and artifact assessment. (2) Quantitative *observer* measurements are made of inherent information content. These measurements include some form of contrast-detail-dose measurement. (3) Quantitative, but *subjective*, observer assessments are made of the suitability of a particular device for a particular radiographic application (e.g., chest imaging, mammography, or angiography). (4) Quantitative measurement of *diagnostic detection accuracy* for specific diagnostic tasks is performed. This type of measurement is typically an ROC study.

The above four-phase plan deserves some elaboration. First, it is important that the physical image characteristics, such as $DQE(f)$ be assessed before any other measurements are made. If one device has poorer $DQE(f)$ than another device, it is safe to assume that the poorer device will not outperform the better device, because the information content is inferior. That is not to say that some devices with excellent $DQE(f)$ are not sold with inferior image processing or display, so that they may actually be less suitable than devices with worse $DQE(f)$ but better image processing or display. Unfortunately, it is sometimes the case that poor choices of image processing and display ruin an otherwise good detector. However, if the fundamental information content of one detector is worse than another, there will be an ultimate limit to what can be achieved with that device.

Unfortunately, $DQE(f)$ alone cannot adequately predict the ultimate observer performance of a device for a specific clinical task, because the relationship between physical image-quality and observer performance is quite complex. There is some excellent work being done at various institutions to model the observer performance mathematically. This work is very important and should yield a better understanding of how physical image-quality translates into observed image-quality. A good description of this work is given in later chapters in this volume. For the present, some type of experimental observer measurement is likely to be needed. The contrast-detail-dose measurement (CDD) is a useful first study because it permits an assessment of observer-threshold detection performance for objects of known contrast and size. This study permits a determination of the minimum contrast and area of objects that are detectable with a given device at a given dose, and thus defines the hard limit of object detectability. The CDD study also permits the optimum patient dose to be estimated.

While the CDD study permits the threshold detection to be determined for signal-known-exactly targets in a uniform background, it does not predict how well a particularly pathology will be observed in a clinical film. The detection of actual anatomy or pathology depends on the conspicuity of a target object in the midst of its complex background. Conspicuity is very difficult to assess quantitatively, and ultimately only comes into play indirectly as diagnostic accuracy is measured. The gold standard measurement for diagnostic accuracy is ROC analysis for most situations. Measurement of diagnostic accuracy is a challenging field unto itself, and requires far more detail that can be provided in one chapter of this handbook. Thus the fourth phase of device evaluation will not be covered here; the reader is referred to later chapters in this volume for a treatment of this topic.

The one part of the four-part device evaluation process not described so far is the subjective observer phase (phase 3). There is debate about the role of subjective observer analyses, and some scientists do not place much stock in them. But in the opinion of this author, subjective (but quantitative) studies do serve two important purposes. First, it presents an assessment of the *likely* diagnostic performance in circumstances such as chest imaging where it would be all but impossible to do exhaustive studies of diagnostic accuracy for all possible diagnoses prior to releasing a new imaging device on the market. For this reason, the FDA 510K allowance process permits quantitative subjective analysis in comparing whether a device is considered to be "equivalent" to existing devices. It should be clear that this is not the same as actually doing diagnostic accuracy studies; for that reason the accuracy studies are also a part of the four-part evaluation presented here. It also should be clear that there are cases where subjective analyses are poorly done and thus of dubious value; an example of this would be a study where the questions were phrased in such as way as to simply highlight the features a manufacturer wished to exploit. But in this author's opinion, a well-constructed evaluation of "visibility of anatomy" in different regions of the image can be useful.

The second reason that subjective studies are useful is that they measure observer acceptance, which is far more critical to device utilization than may first be expected. For example, consider the case of equalization in chest radiography: although there is clearly superior physical image-quality in the dense mediastinum (and hence the radiographs have potentially better overall accuracy), the altered appearance of the lungs tends to accentuate the appearance of possible interstitial disease, and equalization has struggled to live up to its potential in the marketplace. In some work done in our laboratory, it was found that if the equalized appearance of a digital radiograph was altered, a highly equalized appearance was judged to be "noisier" by the radiologists even though actual measurements revealed the signal-to-noise was identical to images with lesser equalized appearance [48]. Thus, the subjective assessment of radiologists regarding a particular radiographic image will determine, for good or for bad, whether that device will be widely adopted for clinical diagnosis. A properly constructed subjective study can be useful in measuring radiologist acceptance.

The physical measures of image-quality, comprising the first stage of the four-part evaluation process, were described in Sections 3.2–3.4 of this chapter. In this last section, step 2 regarding CDD analysis and step 3 regarding quantitative subjective analysis are covered.

3.5.1 Contrast-detail analysis

Contrast-detail analysis is a well known technique for assessing observer performance of a system. There are numerous examples in the literature regarding CD analysis with CT [49, 50], mostly from the late 1970s and early 1980s, and also some recent CD evaluation of other imaging systems including digital radiographic ones [51–54]. The CD approach may be done for a particular imaging system at a given dose, and compared to another imaging system at the same dose, or else the CD response of systems may be assessed at a range of exposures. This latter approach, termed contrast-detail-dose (CDD), is the most useful because it allows the observer performance with a system to be quantified as a function of dose. Frequently, the detectability of objects changes with dose in ways not predicted by simple quantum statistics; namely, the noise texture also changes with exposure, as seen in the NPS measurements at different exposures.

The theoretical foundation for CDD is in the detection work of Rose, who incorporated the vast experimental human visual performance data of Blackwell, as mentioned earlier. The Rose model (Eq. (3.4)) predicts that, based on quantum statistics alone, there is an inverse relationship between area and the square of contrast for comparable detection. Thus, if one were presented with a two-dimensional array of dots of increasingly smaller contrast and smaller diameter, one would expect a diagonal line of detectability through this array, with every dot on one side of this diagonal line detectable, and dots on the other side of the line undetectable. This is exactly what is observed with typical contrast detail phantoms.

Real imaging systems are not ideal, and the noise properties are determined by the detector as well as by the incident quantum flux; hence the area and contrast that are just detectable with a given system will not be exactly as predicted by the Rose model for an ideal detector. Nonetheless, the array of dots of progressively smaller area and contrast still defines the threshold detection limits for the system, and hence provides very valuable information. The one thing that CDD analysis does not provide is an estimate of the required minimum-detectable contrast and area to detect an arbitrary target in the midst of complex backgrounds; that must be measured using ROC or other observer studies as described in later chapters in this volume.

3.5.1.1 Thickness-detail versus contrast-detail

The minimum-detectable contrast is measurable by CDD analysis, but the anatomical meaning of a particular contrast in terms of how thick a section of tissue is being detected is a more difficult question. For this reason, it is useful to consider the thickness-detail rather than the contrast-detail approach. In the thickness-detail method, the same phantom with an arrays of dots of decreasing area and contrast are presented to observers, but the tabulation of the data plots minimum-detectable area versus thickness of phantom material rather than minimum-detectable area versus contrast of phantom material. The significance of this difference may be illustrated by the following example.

Consider two imaging "systems," both using radiographic imaging, but one employs a 60-kV$_p$ beam with a lower Z detector and the other employs a 120-kV$_p$ beam with a higher Z detector. Both are evaluated using the same Lucite phantom, with holes drilled at varying depths and diameters. At 1-mm diameter, for example, both systems have a minimum-detectable contrast of 5% at the same incident x-ray exposure. However, the 5% contrast hole in the phantom is 1 mm deep with System A, but 2 mm deep with System B. Which system has better performance? The CDD approach would say that both systems had identical performance, because the same contrast and diameter object was observed for the same incident exposure. However, as far as the patient anatomy would be concerned, one would easily conclude that the system that could detect a 1-mm-thick vessel, for example, would be superior to a system that could only detect a minimum 2-mm-thick vessel. Thus, it is better to measure the performance based on some physical quantity such as thicknesses rather than contrast.

This point regarding thickness detail as compared to contrast detail was vigorously debated in the literature several decades ago by Hasegawa [55] and Cohen and DiBianca [49]. Hasegawa pointed out the shortcomings of using contrast as the measurement variable, as in the example above, while Cohen maintained that contrast is what the human actually observes, so it is the better quantity for observer characterization. Both sides finally pointed out in this debate that it is important to specify the physical relationship that the contrast derives from (such as detecting objects of different attenuation coefficients in CT). For that reason, this author prefers the use of thickness rather than contrast alone for radiographic applications, although it is important to note what material is compared to what other material (i.e., bone thickness in a surround of soft-tissue, or air thickness in a surround of Lucite). The relative thickness of which materials depends on the clinical application. For example, air thickness relative to soft tissue makes sense for chest imaging, but calcium thickness relative to fat makes sense in mammographic imaging. A thickness-detail phantom could be constructed of any of these material pairs, but air thickness in soft-tissue-equivalent plastic is the easiest to construct. The reader should be aware though that the measurement should ideally be made with the material of interest clinically relative to its normal anatomical surrounding tissue (or tissue equivalents).

3.5.1.2 Measurement procedure

Once the materials to be used for the detection study are selected, it is necessary to construct an appropriate phantom for the measurements. For simplicity, the example of a Lucite phantom with air-thickness contrast objects will be used, because that type of phantom only involves milling holes of different diameters in Lucite.

There are several designs described in the literature for how to present the dots of varying area and contrast (or thickness). The most common type is an array of round holes with decreasing diameter and depth. In these types of phantoms, observers are asked to specify the smallest hole visible at a given contrast, or equivalently the lowest-contrast hole visible at a given diameter. Another type of phantom uses a series of squares in the image, each containing a dot of given contrast and area in the center of each square, and another identical dot at one of the four quadrants of the square. This type of phantom requires the observer to state which quadrant a particular dot is in, for each of the sizes and contrasts. Thus, it provides a truer test of detection; if the observer mistakenly identifies that a particular dot is visible, but gets the wrong quadrant, the answer is regarded as incorrect. This procedure requires a much larger phantom (because there are two dots for each contrast/area combination), but provides a better estimate of true threshold detection.

Observers view images from the system being evaluated (or from several images if multiple systems are being simultaneously being evaluated), taken at a range of exposures. Ideally, multiple images of the same system and same exposure will be part of the data set so that analysis of variance of the results will allow an estimate of repeated measures on each observer.

The results are plotted as curves depicting either minimum-detectable thickness as a function of diameter, or minimum-detectable diameter as a function of thickness. Either is acceptable, but this author recommends thickness as a function of diameter because that is easier to compare mentally with the MTF (visible contrast vs spatial frequency). By tabulating the results from many observers, an average threshold detection curve with error bars may be obtained.

3.5.2 Subjective observer preference analysis

Following the physical measurements of image-quality, as outlined above, it is important to measure the response of observers to clinical images with the digital imaging system. A subjective but quantitative observer assessment can play a useful role at this stage of evaluation. These subjective evaluations do not in any way substitute for the ultimate clinical evaluation, which is diagnostic accuracy, but can provide three types of useful information in the design and evaluation of systems.

First, these subjective evaluations can indicate the acceptability of the presentation and appearance of these images to radiologists. The assessment of image-noise levels and image processing really cannot be judged apart from viewing clinical images. If radiologists are uncomfortable reading a particular type of image, no matter how well it scores in physical quality measures, the device is unlikely to be used with confidence.

A second benefit to this type of subjective evaluation is to provide an overall assessment of how well anatomy can be visualized in a situation where it is unlikely that trials of diagnostic accuracy are going to be accomplished for the wide range of imaging tasks possible. For example, in screening mammography there is one primary observer task: to identify opacities suspicious for breast cancer and assess appropriate clinical action. A single diagnostic-accuracy test for breast cancer detection (sensitivity and specificity) would be sufficient to evaluate the vast majority of clinical uses of a digital mammographic unit used for screening (which is not to say that a careful ROC study of this task is by any means trivial). In contrast, though, the vast array of potential diagnostic assessments in chest radiography make it difficult to find one or two diagnostic-accuracy studies that will define the majority of clinical uses for chest radiography. There are infectious diseases, malignant diseases, degenerative bone processes, inflammatory processes, interstitial diseases, airway obstructions, placement of tubes and line, and many other tasks which confront the diagnostician in chest radiography. For an imaging situation such as chest radiography, an overall assessment of how well anatomy can be visualized can be a useful assessment measure, even though final diagnostic-accuracy studies will be the definitive tests.

A third benefit to subjective observer evaluations is that they can provide context for interpreting the physical imaging measures. For example, if two imaging devices are evaluated, and one has 30% better MTF at high frequencies, the manufacturer may make a strong selling point about the product's MTF. However, if both devices are rated by trained observers as excellent for visualization of fine detail, then perhaps the strong claims by the manufacture are not as significant as they may be touted to be. On the other hand, if that 30% improvement in MTF of one device relative to the other corresponds to one device being rated as excellent and the other as merely good, then that may have clinical importance. In short, while it is always better to have a system that performs at a higher level than another, the subjective observer evaluation can provide context as to whether the improvement is important enough to warrant additional cost or to offset other potential drawbacks of the "better" system.

There are a number of these tests in the literature which can be included in this category of subjective but *quantitative* evaluations. From the outset, studies which are subjective and *qualitative* are not of interest, because they often provide only anecdotal evidence at best. However, the tests that are well designed and quantitative can be of use. These test typically fall into two categories: side-by-side comparative studies and independent assessments of a device or devices on an absolute scale of merit.

Side-by-side comparison evaluations are used to rank the performance of two devices (or image-processing techniques). Unless the evaluation is related to particular elements of image display, both images should be displayed in as similar a format as possible (both printed in the same format on the same printer, for example). If one image of the comparison is screen-film and the other is digital, the images should be masked with a border and have all identifying markings masked, if at all possible, because such markings may bias observers if they know which image is film and which is digital. Images should be presented with approximately equal numbers of type A and type B displayed on the left (or right), and intermixed in random order, to avoid bias from differences in viewboxes or from first-image read. Ideally, the viewing environment should be darkened to approximate that of the ambient-lighting condition of a standard reading room.

The questions asked in the side-by-side evaluation should be as specific as possible. For example, it is preferable to ask "Which image better demonstrates the anatomy in the upper-right lung?" than "Which image do you like better in the lungs?". There are several categories of questions that are often asked in these studies. First, assessment of how well certain anatomy is visualized. Several regions may be selected that will be representative of the regions of interest in general clinical films. For example, for comparing chest films, the following anatomy might be assessed: upper right lung, lower-right lung, upper-left lung, lower-left lung, retrocardiac lung, azygo-esophageal recess, retrodiaphragmatic lung, ribs, thoracic spine, lumbar spine, hilum, etc. These regions give a good evaluation of both lucent lung and obscured lung, mediastinum, and other dense regions. A second category of question assesses image noise. Noise should be assessed in both dense and transmissive regions, being as specific as possible. A question such as "Which image has better noise (mottle) properties in the left lung?" would be appropriate. A third category assesses image sharpness. Again, evaluating sharpness in both transmissive and dense regions, or any other areas where the image processing may differ, is important. A fourth category of question compares the presence of artifacts in the two films. Last, an overall assessment is sometimes given ("Given the choice, which image would you prefer overall if only a single image were available?").

The rating scale for the side-by-side comparison should provide meaningful adjectival descriptors, and a numerical value if further fineness of scale is desired. The numerical scale may be -5 to $+5$, for example:

A much better than B		A some better than B		A and B equal	B some better than A		B much better than A	
-5	-4	-3	-2	-1	0	$+1$	$+2$	$+3$	$+4$	$+5$

There should be at least enough possible answers given to elucidate some gradation of comparison. For example, it may not be ideal to have only a three-value scale (B better than A, B same as A, A better than B). Rather, at least "some better" and "much better" should be included in possible responses. Of course, a two-alternative forced-choice study (A better than B, or B better than A) is also an option if the degree of difference between A and B is not important.

The second category of subjective observer study is the absolute-scale-of-merit test. This type of study provides more information on context than does the side-by-side study, and hence in many cases the absolute scale of merit test may be preferable. The same categories of questions may be asked in this study as in the side-by-side study (i.e., visibility of anatomy, noise, sharpness, artifacts, and overall assessment). In the absolute-scale-of-merit test, the images are displayed one at a time, and the responses are to a single image rather than a comparison of images. For this test, it is important that the images be presented in random order by patient and by image type. If the study is done in multiple readings, then images of the same patient should not be shown in the same session, in order to avoid bias from an observer remembering a previous image of a given patient. Multiple reading sessions should be separated sufficiently in time to further avoid bias from observer recall of specific patients.

The scoring for the absolute-scale-of-merit test should be both numerical and adjectival. The numerical range may go from 1 to 5 or from 1 to 10, for example. Fewer than 5 scores may not allow sufficient precision of scoring. Appropriate adjectival descriptors should be provided for at least some of the numerical scores so that the observer may calibrate himself/herself. The adjectival descriptors should be meaningful to most observers, and should cover the full range of expected responses. It is important that there be enough precision in the adjectival descriptors to discern differences in the good end of the scale where most scores will reside. For example, the following scale would be inappropriate for most tests: poor, fair, good. In such a test, virtually all responses would be good. The following scale would be better: poor, fair, good, very good, excellent. Adjectival descriptors do not have to be given for each numerical score if more than five are used (and in fact, attempting to provide too many adjectival descriptors can result in confusion for the observers, as the difference between "very, very good" and "somewhat excellent" is unclear). Observers should be instructed to use the adjectival scores that they would internally use if presented with a given image in clinical practice; they should not be asked to "use the full scoring range" in most circumstances, because one of the benefits of the absolute-scale-of-merit test is that it provides a measure of subjective ranking for interpreting the significance of any difference in scores (in other words, two devices may have a statistically significantly different score, yet both rank as "excellent").

Several general principles apply to all subjective observer studies. Patients for inclusion in this study should be selected to have as wide a range of body habitus as possible (i.e., thin, medium, and thick patients should all be included in the evaluation). If the evaluation is general (e.g., looking at visibility of anatomy) then patients with normal films and patients with as wide a range of pathology as possible should be included. Computations of the number of film pairs to present to the observers should be made based on statistical power desired, and a pilot study of a small sample of the images may be useful to determine the number of films required. As many observers as possible should be included, and should cover the range of expected competencies in the field. Most commonly, individuals board certified in the specialty are used as observers, but if a substantial number of images will be read by less experienced observers (e.g., residents or nonradiology specialists such as surgeons), then it may appropriate to include a sample of those observers in the study. If statistical power permits, reporting the outcome of the study by experience level may prove useful. Multiple devices (or image-processing algorithms) may be evaluated simultaneously using the absolute-scale-of-merit test, but one should evaluate whether sufficient statistical power is available when making multiple comparisons within the same data set.

In conclusion, the quantitative subjective observer study has a place in assessing new devices or algorithms. It should not substitute for tests of diagnostic accuracy, however, which form the last stage of device evaluation. This volume provides some excellent articles on performing tests of diagnostic accuracy, and the interested reader is referred to that text for details on those studies.

References

[1] Dobbins III JT, Ergun DL, Rutz L, Hinshaw DA, Blume H, Clark DC. "DQE(f) of Four Generations of Computed Radiography Acquisition Devices." Medical Physics 22:1581–1593, 1995.

[2] Bradford CD, Peppler WW, Dobbins III JT. "Performance Characteristics of a Kodak Computed Radiography System." Medical Physics 26:27–37, 1999.

[3] Floyd Jr CE, Chotas HG, Dobbins III JT, Ravin CE. "Quantitative Radiographic Imaging Using a Photostimulable Phosphor System." Medical Physics 17:454–459, 1990.

[4] Hillen W, Schiebel U, Zaengel T. "Imaging Performance of a Digital Storage Phosphor System." Medical Physics 14:744–751, 1987.

[5] Verdonck B, Bourel P, Coste E, Gerritsen FA, Rousseau J. "Variations in the Geometrical Distortion of X-Ray Image Intensifiers." Proc SPIE 3659, 1999, pp. 266–275.

[6] Neitzel U, Maack I, Gunther-Kohfahl S. "Image Quality of a Digital Chest Radiography System Based on a Selenium Detector." Medical Physics 21:509–516, 1994.

[7] Chotas HG, Floyd Jr CR, Ravin CE. "Technical Evaluation of a Digital Chest Radiography System that Uses a Selenium Detector." Radiology 195:264–270, 1995.

[8] Launders JH, Kengyelics SM, Cowen AR. "A Comprehensive Physical Image-Quality Evaluation of a Selenium Based Digital X-Ray Imaging System for Thorax Radiograhy." Medical Physics 25:986–997, 1998.

[9] Chotas HG, Floyd Jr CE, Ravin CE. "Memory Artifact Related to Selenium-Based Digital Radiography Systems." Radiology 203:881–883, 1997.

[10] Moy JP, Bosset B. "How Does Real Offset and Gain Correction Affect the DQE in Images from X-Ray Flat Detectors?" Proc SPIE 3659, 1999, pp. 90–97.

[11] Rose A. "The Sensitivity Performance of the Human Eye on an Absolute Scale." Journal of Optometry Society of America 38:196–208, 1948.

[12] Blackwell HR. "Contrast Thresholds of the Human Eye." Journal of Optometry Society of America 36:624–643, 1946.

[13] Bushberg JT, Seibert JA, Leidholdt Jr EM, Boone JM. *The Essential Physics of Medical Imaging*. Baltimore: Williams & Wilkins, 1994.

[14] Ergun DL, Eastgate RJ, Jennings RJ, Siedband MP. "DXSPEC, a Computer Program for Diagnostic X-Ray Spectral Filtration Studies." Univ. of Wisconsin-Madison Department of Medical Physics, 1977.

[15] Floyd Jr CE, Baker JA, Lo JY, Ravin CE. "Measurement of Scatter Fractions in Clinical Bedside Radiography." Radiology 183:857–861, 1992.

[16] Barnes GT, Brezovich IA. "The Intensity of Scattered Radiation in Mammography." Radiology 126:243–247, 1978.

[17] Neitzel U. "Grids or Air Gaps for Scatter Reduction in Digital Radiography: A Model Calculation." Medical Physics 19:475–481, 1992.

[18] Schultze Kool LJ, Busscher DLT, Vlasbloem H, Hermans J, van der Merwe P, Algra PR, Herstel W. "Advanced Multiple-Beam Equalization Radiography in Chest Radiology: A Simulated Nodule Detetion Study." Radiology 159:35–39, 1988.

[19] Vlasbloem H, Schultze Kool LJ. "AMBER: A Scanning Multiple-Beam Equalization System for Chest Radiography." Radiology 169:29–34, 1988.

[20] Barnes GT, Brezovich IA, Witten DM. "Scanning Multiple Slit Assembly: A Practical and Efficient Device to Reduce Scatter." American Journal of Roentgenology 129:497–501, 1977.

[21] Chotas HG, Floyd Jr CE, Dobbins III JT, Lo JY, Ravin CE. "Scatter Fractions in AMBER Images." Radiology 177:879–880, 1990.

[22] Barrett HH, Swindell W. *Radiological Imaging*. New York: Academic, 1981.

[23] Jenkins GM, Watts DG. *Spectral Analysis and Its Applications*. San Francisco: Holden-Day, 1968.

[24] Dainty JC, Shaw R. *Image Science*. London: Academic Press, 1974.

[25] Blackman RB, Tukey JW. *The Measurement of Power Spectra*. New York: Dover, 1958.

[26] Doi K, Loo L-N, Anderson Jr TM, Frank PH. "Effect of Crossover Exposure on Radiographic Image-Quality of Screen-Film Systems." Radiology 139:707–714, 1981.

[27] Barnes GT. "Radiographic Mottle: A Comprehensive Theory." Medical Physics 9:656–667, 1982.

[28] Braun M, Wilson BC. "Comparative Evaluation of Several Rare-Earth Film-Screen Systems." Radiology 144:915–919, 1982.

[29] Sandrik FM, Wagner RF. "Absolute Measures of Physical Image-Quality: Measurement and Application to Radiographic Magnification." Medical Physics 9:540–549, 1982.

[30] Bunch PC, Shaw R, van Metter RL. "Signal-to-Noise Measurements for a Screen-Film System." Proc SPIE 454, 1984, pp. 154–163.

[31] "Modulation Transfer Function of Screen-Film Systems." ICRU 41, 1986.

[32] Bunch PC, Huff KE, van Metter R. "Analysis of the Detective Quantum Efficiency of a Radiographic Screen-Film Combination." Journal of Optometry Society of America 4:902–909, 1987.

[33] Bunch PC. "Detective Quantum Efficiency of Selected Mammographic Screen-Film Combinations." Proc SPIE 1090, 1989, pp. 67–77.

[34] Wagner RF. "Fast Fourier Digital Quantum Mottle Analysis with Application to Rare Earth Intensifying Screen Systems." Medical Physics 4:157–162, 1977.

[35] Wagner RF, Sandrik JM. "An introduction to Digital Noise Analysis." In Haus AG (Ed.) *The Physics of Medical Imaging: Recording System Measurements and Techniques*. New York: AAPM American Association of Physicists in Medicine, 1979.

[36] Giger ML, Doi K, Metz CE. "Investigation of Basic Imaging Properties in Digital Radiography. 2 Noise Wiener Spectrum." Medical Physics 11:797–805, 1984.

[37] Giger ML, Doi K. "Investigation of Basic Imaging Properties in Digital Radiography. I. Modulation Transfer Function." Medical Physics 11:287–295, 1984.

[38] Dobbins III JT. "Effects of Undersampling on the Proper Interpretation of Modulation Transfer Function, Noise-Power Spectra, and Noise Equivalent Quanta of Digital Imaging Systems." Medical Physics 22:171–181, 1995.

[39] Fujita H, Tsai D-Y, Itoh T, Doi K, Morishita J, Ueda K, Ohtsuka A. "A Simple Method for Determining the Modulation Transfer Function in Digital Radiography." IEEE Transactions on Medical Imaging 11:34–39, 1992.

[40] Doi K, Strubler K, Rossmann K. "Truncation Errors in Calculating the MTF of Radiographic Screen-Film Systems from the Line Spread Function." Physics in Medicine and Biology 17:241–250, 1972.

[41] Cunningham IA, Fenster A. "A Method for Modulation Transfer Function Determination from Edge Profiles with Correction for Finite-Element Differentiation." Medical Physics 14:533–537, 1987.

[42] Cunningham IA, Reid BK. "Signal and Noise in Modulation Transfer Function Determinations Using the Slit, Wire, and Edge Techniques." Medical Physics 19:1037–1044, 1992.

[43] Samei E, Flynn MJ, Reimann DA. "A Method for Measuring the Presampled MTF of Digital Radiographic Systems Using an Edge Test Device," Medical Physics 25:102–113, 1998.

[44] Samei E, Flynn MJ. "Physical Measures of Image-Quality in Photostimulable Phosphor Radiographic Systems." Proc SPIE 3032, 1997, pp. 328–338.

[45] Chotas HG, Floyd Jr CE, Johnson GA, Ravin CE. "Quality Control Phantom for Digital Chest Radiography." Radiology 202:111–116, 1997.

[46] Bunch PC. "Performance Characteristics of Asymmetric Zero-Crossover Screen-Film Systems." Proc SPIE 1653, 1992, pp. 46–65.

[47] van Metter RL. "Describing the Signal Transfer Characteristics of Asymmetrical Screen-Film Systems." Medical Physics 19:53–58, 1992.

[48] Dobbins III JT, Rice JJ, Goodman PC, Patz Jr EF, Ravin CE. "Variable Compensation Chest Radiography Performed with a Computed Radiography System: Design Considerations and Initial Clinical Experience." Radiology 187:55–63, 1993.

[49] Cohen G, DiBianca FA. "The Use of Contrast-Detail-Dose Evaluation of Image-Quality in a Computed Tomographic Scanner." Journal of Computed Assisted Tomography 3:189–195, 1979.

[50] Cohen G. "Contrast-Detail-Dose Analysis of Six Different Computed Tomographic Scanners," Journal of Computed Assisted Tomography 3:197–203, 1979.

[51] Cohen G, Wagne LK, Amtey SR, DiBianca FA. "Contrast-Detail-Dose and Dose Efficiency Analysis of a Scanning Digital and a Screen-Film-Grid Radiographic System." Medical Physics 8:358–367, 1981.

[52] Cohen G, Wagner LK, McDaniel DL, Robinson LH, "Dose Efficiency of Screen-Film Systems Used in Pediatric Radiography." Radiology 152:187–193, 1984.

[53] Dobbins III JT, Rice JJ, Beam CA, Ravin CE. "Threshold Perception Performance with Computed and Screen-Film Radiography: Implications for Chest Radiography." Radiology 183:179–187, 1992.

[54] Cook LT, Insana MF, McFadden MA, Hall TJ, Cox GG. "Contrast-Detail Analysis of Image Degradation Due to Lossy Compression." Medical Physics 22:715–721, 1995.

[55] Hasegawa BH, Cacak RK, Mulvaney JA, Hendee WR. "Problems With Contrast-Detail Curves for CT Performance Evaluation." American Journal of Roentgenology 138:135–138, 1982.

CHAPTER 4
Flat Panel Detectors for Digital Radiography

John A. Rowlands
University of Toronto

John Yorkston
Eastman Kodak Company

CONTENTS

4.1 Introduction

X-ray images are formed as shadows of the interior of the body. In an x-ray department, radiologists still examine and diagnose x-ray images on illuminated view boxes, much like a century ago. Recent technological developments are revolutionizing these procedures. Because it is not yet practical to focus x rays, an x-ray detector has to be larger than the body part to be imaged. Thus a practical difficulty in making an x-ray detector is the need to image a large area. The key digital technology permitting an advance in medical x-ray applications is the flat-panel active matrix array, originally developed for laptop-computer displays.

Currently, in taking an x-ray image, a radiological technologist must load a film into a film/screen cassette; carry the cassette to the examination room; insert the cassette into the x-ray table; position the patient; make the x-ray exposure; carry the cassette back to the processor to develop the film; and check the processed film for any obvious problems to ensure that the film is suitable for making a medical diagnosis. This laborious process can take several minutes during which time the patient has to remain undressed and the x-ray room is engaged. In contrast, the ideal x-ray imaging system would, *immediately* after the patient's x-ray exposure, provide a high-quality radiograph on a video monitor. If the physical form of the detector could be similar to a film/screen cassette, it could be used with little modification of the x-ray room. Digital x-ray images would provide several advantages: less handling; more convenient patient management; immediate image viewing; computer-aided diagnosis [1, 2]; and more convenient storage on computer disks rather than in archaic film stacks. Such improvements are important, but must not reduce image quality or increase radiation exposure.

Piecemeal approaches to digital x-ray imaging have been pursued for a number of years and have highlighted an interest in the general concept of the fully digital radiology department. In this context, flat-panel imagers are of great interest as they have the potential to solve most of the problems associated with the acquisition of high-quality digital radiographs. Despite the technical issues still surrounding their implementation, they remain the only approach so far identified that has the potential to be all things to all radiologists. The rest of this chapter will describe some of the history behind their development as well as their fabrication, design, evaluation, and configuration into digital x-ray imaging systems for specific clinical tasks.

4.1.1 General requirements of x-ray imaging systems

It is important to recognize, in proposing to build a new x-ray system for medical applications, that projection imaging has been performed for over a hundred years—when Professor Roentgen first imaged Frau Roentgen's hand in the basement of their house. Since then tens of thousands of individual radiologists working empirically, but competitively, have developed and optimized the standard methods of image acquisition and interpretation. The requirements of any new imaging system will therefore be very similar to those developed by this tried and tested formula. Radiologists are justifiably unwilling to stray too far or too fast from

Table 4.1: Parameters for digital x-ray imaging systems

Clinical Task	Chest	Mammography	Fluoroscopy
Detector size	35 cm × 43 cm	18 cm × 24 cm	25 cm × 25 cm
Pixel size	$200 \times 200 \, \mu m$	$50 \times 50 \, \mu m$	$250 \times 250 \, \mu m$
Number of pixels	1750×2150	3600×4800	1000×1000
Readout time	<5 s	<5 s	1/30 s
X-ray spectrum	120 kVp	30 kVp	70 kVp
Mean exposure	$300 \, \mu R$	12 mR	$1 \, \mu R$
Exposure range	$30–3000 \, \mu R$	0.6–240 mR	$0.1–10 \, \mu R$
Noise level	$6 \, \mu R$	$60 \, \mu R$	$0.1 \, \mu R$

their usual approach. The successful identification of disease by the inspection of a projection radiograph depends heavily on the appearance of the abnormal tissue in the image. In many instances the evidence of disease can be extremely subtle. Radiologists have become expert at interpreting and diagnosing from traditional film/screen systems and any move away from this film "look" must be done very gradually if the accumulated knowledge of the field is to be maintained.

What then can past and present practices tell us about the requirements for a new imaging detector? Defining the important imaging parameters is a reasonable starting point. First, the field of view must be determined. Next, from the acceptable range of x-ray factors used to create the images, the dynamic-range requirements can be estimated. The spatial-resolution requirements determine the pixel size. Finally the level of noise which can be tolerated can be calculated from the lowest x-ray exposure required at which the system should be quantum noise limited. On this basis we can derive *a priori* requirements for our imaging systems, as shown in Table 4.1 [3, 4].

4.1.2 Digital x-ray imaging systems

There have been a number of recent reviews of digital x-ray imaging in general [3, 5, 6] and many current x-ray flat-panel imagers have been described elsewhere [7]. Consequently, only a brief review of the general concepts and approaches to digital imaging will be given here.

In a digital imaging system, at some stage, the incident x-ray image must be sampled both in the spatial and intensity dimensions. In the spatial dimension, samples are obtained as averages of the intensity over picture elements or *pixels*. These are usually square, and spaced at equal intervals throughout the plane of the image. In the intensity dimension, the signal is digitized into one of a finite number of levels or *bits*. To avoid degradation of image quality, it is important that the pixel size and the bit depth are appropriate for the requirements of the imaging task.

The dynamic range for an imaging task can be broken into two components. The first describes the ratio between the x-ray attenuation of the most radiolucent and the most radio-opaque paths through the patient appearing on the same image. The second is the precision of the x-ray signal measured in the part of the image representing the most radio-opaque anatomy. If, for example, there is a factor of 50 in attenuation across the image field and it is desired to have 1% precision in measuring the signal in the most attenuating region, then the dynamic-range requirement would be 5000. It is sometimes possible to reduce the dynamic-range requirement by using prepatient bolusing filters to increase attenuation in radiolucent areas of the image. The requirements for dynamic-range differ between imaging tasks. There are, however, some general principles for establishing the requirements of each modality. Because x rays are attenuated exponentially, an extra tenth-value layer thickness of tissue will attenuate the beam to $1/10$ of its original value. If the same tenth-value thickness is missing it will increase the x-ray fluence by a factor of 10. If a mean exposure value X_{mean} for the system is established by irradiating a uniform phantom, a range of exposure values above and below this mean value will be important. For example, in fluoroscopy using x-ray image intensifiers, XRIIs [8], it is generally established that a dynamic-range of 100:1 is useful. However, this should be distributed over $1/10$ to $10X_{mean}$ and *not* into an equal number of steps above and below X_{mean} (1–50 and 51–100) which would be $1/50\, X_{mean}$ to $2\, X_{mean}$.

One way of producing a large imaging field is to create an image receptor that is essentially one dimensional and acquires the second dimension of the image by scanning the x-ray beam and detector across the patient. In principle, a single line detector and a very highly collimated slit beam of x rays could do this. One significant advantage of this approach is the excellent rejection of scattered radiation from the resulting image. However, this approach is extremely inefficient in its utilization of the output of the x-ray tube. The collimator would remove most of the x rays and a full scan would impose an enormous heat load on the tube. To greatly improve the efficiency of such systems a multi-line or *slot* detector could be employed. Here, the x-ray beam would extend across the full image field in one dimension and be several mm wide in the other. Such systems usually use integrated detector arrays known as *charge-coupled devices* or CCDs. These are coupled optically to an x-ray phosphor that gives off light in response to stimulation by x-ray absorption. An x-ray detector for general medical applications needs to be relatively large (see Table 4.1). CCDs can only be made economically with relatively small surface areas ($\sim$4 to 16 cm^2) and thus cannot be used directly as large-area x-ray detectors. The output from the phosphor must be minified to the dimensions of the CCD using either lens systems or tapered fiber-optic bundles. If this minification is taken to extremes, poor optical coupling results in each x ray being represented on average by less than one light photon at the CCD. This leads to additional noise called *secondary quantum noise*. It is generally accepted that this **must** be avoided in a medical detector and thus most practical x-ray optically coupled sensors have optical detectors of the same or only marginally smaller size than the x-ray detector. The advent of inexpensive CMOS detectors with their potential for pixel-level electronic circuitry may remove much of the financial restriction on achieving large-area coverage by tiling many small detectors together. However, the issues of excessive fixed-pattern noise, high dark current, and concerns over the practicality of *stitching* the full image from a mosaic of smaller images remain unresolved.

A radically different approach has recently been implemented in which the geometry of the detector and source are reversed [9]. The detector is a small-area device ($\sim 5 \times 5$ cm) and the x-ray source scans across the patient. This approach holds the possibility of extremely effective scatter rejection without the use of an anti-scatter grid and may therefore result in a realistic reduction in patient dose.

Probably the most successful detectors for digital radiography to date have been photostimulable phosphors, also known as storage phosphors. These phosphors are commonly in the barium fluorohalide family, typically BaFBr:Eu. X-ray absorption mechanisms in photostimulable phosphors are identical to those of conventional phosphors. The photostimulable phosphors differ in that the useful optical signal is not derived from the light emitted in prompt response to the incident radiation as in conventional film/screen systems, but rather from subsequent stimulated light emission when electrons are released from traps in the material. The initial x-ray interaction with the phosphor crystal causes electrons to be excited. Some of these electrons produce blue light in the phosphor in the normal manner but this is not used at this point. Instead the phosphor is intentionally designed to contain electron traps that store a latent image as a spatial distribution of trapped charges. By stimulating the phosphor by irradiation with red light, these electrons are released from the traps and raised to the conduction band. This subsequently triggers the emission of shorter wavelength (blue) light. This process is called photostimulated luminescence. The digital imaging x-ray system based on this principle is *computed radiography* or CR. Early analysis of CR systems [10], a comparison with film/screen systems [11], and more recent reviews [12, 13] have been presented. In CR systems the imaging plate (a screen made using photostimulable phosphor) is positioned in a light-tight cassette or enclosure, exposed, and then read by raster scanning the plate with a laser to release the luminescence. The emitted light is collected and detected with a photomultiplier tube whose output signal is digitized to form the image. The plate is then flooded with light to erase any residual image and is then ready for reuse. CR has been implemented both in the form of portable cassettes carried between the x-ray unit(s) and a central reader, and more recently in a dedicated chest unit incorporating the plates, the reader, and an erasing light source.

There has been a separate effort to investigate readout systems based on photoconductors. X rays interact within a photoconductor producing a latent charge image. The recording of this charge distribution by the pattern of fine toner particles [14], in a process similar to photocopying, was developed into a successful system for mammography. The latent image can also be readout with a layer of liquid crystal in close proximity, which is used to modulate an incident beam of light with the x-ray image information [15]. Another novel approach is to use a scanning electron beam to readout the latent image. This has the advantage of permitting real-time readout but with the disadvantage of being a bulky vacuum device [16]. A method similar to xerography was developed for readout using a scanning laser that stimulated an optical phosphor incorporated into the toner particles deposited in an imagewise manner [17]. A very straightforward approach is to use an electrostatic probe [18, 19] held sufficiently close to the a-Se so as to couple capacitively to the latent charge image. The difficulty with this approach is getting the probes close enough to the a-Se surface to obtain adequate resolution, though it has the advantage of very low electronic noise. Optical-discharge methods using highly absorptive continuous films of photoconductor have the advantage of high resolution that is essentially limited by the laser spot size used in the laser scanners [20], because there is no scattering of light as there is in phosphors. There are, however, problems with noise sources not present in the electrometer readout method. The use of segmented readout electrodes [21] or individual electrodes [22] reduced amplifier noise by lowering the capacitance loading the preamplifier. However, no laser-discharge method has been able to eliminate the additional noise attributable to the bias charge that is necessarily read out in conjunction with the signal charge. In most laser readout methods the latent charge image was stored on the surface of the a-Se but one approach used charge trapped in the bulk of the layer [23]. Another highly novel approach was to use a gaseous imaging ion chamber to detect an image which was deposited on a plastic film and subsequently read out with a scanning electrometer [24]. All these methods have disadvantages compared to the flat-panel detectors to be discussed and thus have become less popular. Aspects of these approaches will likely be used in flat-panel detectors and provide a standard of comparison for development in the field.

4.1.3 Flat-panel detectors

In recent years the extensive financial investment in active-matrix liquid-crystal flat-panel display manufacture (AMLCD) has led to the widespread availability of this technology for a number of applications. The unique technology underlying active-matrix flat-panel displays is large area integrated circuits called *active-matrix arrays*. These have facilitated the development of a new class of medical imaging device that may solve many of the limitations inherent in the current methods of acquiring a digital projection radiograph. Active-matrix technology allows the deposition of semiconductors, most commonly amorphous silicon, across large-area substrates in a well-controlled fashion such that the physical and electrical properties of the resulting structures can be modified and adapted for many different applications. Coupling traditional x-ray detection materials such as phosphors or photoconductors with a large-area active-matrix readout structure forms the basis of flat-panel x-ray imagers.

The creation of an x-ray image may conceptually be divided into three separate stages. The first stage is the interaction of the x ray with a suitable detection medium to generate a measurable response. The second stage is the storage of this response with a recording device. The third stage is the measurement of this stored response. An example of this division is the generation of visible-light photons when an x ray interacts in a phosphor material, the subsequent creation of a latent image in the photographic film by these photons, and finally the development of the fixed photographic image. Another example is the creation of a distribution of electrical charges when x rays interact within a photoconductor. Their movement to the surface of the photoconductor forms a stored latent charge image that can finally be recorded by its effect on the distribution of charged toner particles [14]. This conceptual division of x-ray image formation into the detection, storage, and measurement stages allows an insight into the function played by active-matrix technology in modern medical imaging. In essence, active-matrix technology provides a new, highly efficient, real-time method for electronically storing and measuring the product of the x-ray interaction stage whether the product is visible wavelength photons or electrical charges.

4.1.3.1 Direct and indirect approaches

A distinction is currently made between flat-panel x-ray imaging devices that incorporate a phosphor to produce visible wavelength photons on detection of an x ray, (*indirect detection*) and those that incorporate a photoconductor to produce electrical charges on detection of an x ray (*direct detection*) [25].

In the indirect-detection approach shown in Figure 4.1(a), a phosphor layer (e.g., a screen such as Gd_2O_2S:Tb, or a structured scintillator such as CsI:Tl) is placed in intimate contact with an active-matrix array. The intensity of the light emitted from a particular location of the phosphor is a measure of the intensity of the x-ray beam incident on the surface of the detector at that point. The active-matrix arrays used for this indirect approach are similar in design to those used for document-scanning applications where visible-light is also being detected. Each pixel on the active matrix has a photosensitive element that generates an electrical charge whose magnitude is proportional to the light intensity emitted from the phosphor in the region close to the pixel. This charge is stored in the pixel until the active-matrix array is read out. The magnitude of the signal charge from the different pixels contains the imaging information inherent in the intensity variations of the incident x-ray beam. The detection process is *indirect* in that the image information is transferred from the x rays to visible-light photons and then finally to electrical charge.

In direct detection, shown in Figure 4.1(b), the x-ray detection is performed with a thick layer of photoconductor material. The application of thick amorphous silicon layers to particle and x-ray detection has been investigated [26–28] but the technical difficulties of controlling the fabrication of sufficiently thick, stable layers over large areas remain unsolved. The low atomic number, $Z = 14$, of Si also

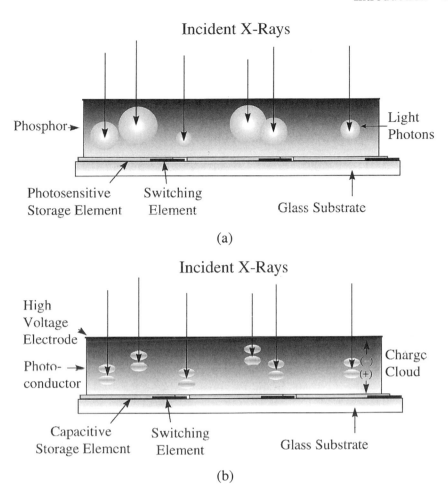

Figure 4.1: Cross section of the two major kinds of flat-panel x-ray imaging systems: (a) indirect conversion (b) direct conversion.

means that even a thick (1 to 2 mm) layer of amorphous silicon is not a particularly efficient method for direct detection of diagnostic x rays ($\sim$100 keV). More successful has been the application of thick ($\sim$0.5 to 1 mm) a-Se photoconductive layers ($Z = 34$) in direct electrical contact with an underlying flat-panel array [29, 30]. The pixels incorporate a conductive electrode to collect the charge and a capacitor element to store it (rather than a photosensitive element as in the indirect approach). Interacting x rays produce charge in the photoconductor which is then shared between the inherent capacitance of the photoconductive layer and the pixel-storage capacitance. The active-matrix arrays used in this approach are similar to those used in display applications where charge on a capacitor plate controls the light transmission through the liquid crystal in AMLCDs. The detection process is *direct* in that the image information is transferred from x rays directly to electrical charge with no intermediate stage.

The terms direct and indirect are therefore more attributable to the nature of the initial x-ray detection mechanism rather than the details of the flat-panel array design. In both approaches the flat-panel detector integrates the incoming signal over a finite period of time, therefore acting as an x-ray fluence detector rather than an individual x-ray photon detector.

Although the design of the active-matrix depends upon the response being measured (i.e., light or electrical charge) there are a number of common features shared by both types of array. Current flat-panel detectors invariably incorporate a two-dimensional array of imaging pixels. Each pixel is typically configured from a switching element and a sensing/storage element. In addition there are various metallic lines used to control the readout of the imaging information from the array of pixels. The imaging system is completed with peripheral circuitry that amplifies, digitizes, and synchronizes the readout of the image and a computer that manipulates and distributes the final image to the appropriate soft- or hard-copy device. A schematic diagram of a complete flat-panel x-ray imaging system is shown in Figure 4.2.

4.1.3.2 General operation

In Figure 4.3 the layout of a group of pixels on an active-matrix array is shown. All the switches along a particular row are connected together with a single control line. This allows the external circuitry to change the state of all the switching elements along the row with a single controlling voltage. Each row of pixels requires a separate switching control line. The signal outputs of the pixels down a particular column are connected to a single signal line. Each column of pixels has its own read out amplifier. This configuration allows the imager to be read out one horizontal line at a time. Unlike the charge-transfer read out method used in many modern

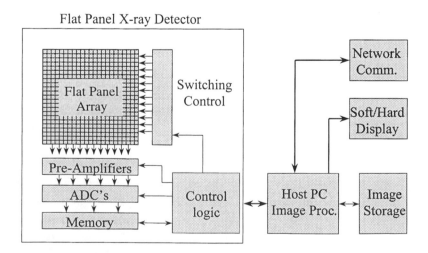

Figure 4.2: Diagram illustrating the configuration of a complete flat-panel x-ray imaging system.

CCDs, active-matrix arrays *do not* transfer signal from pixel to neighboring pixel but from the pixel element directly to the read out amplifier.

To acquire and read out a radiographic image, the active-matrix is put into an initialization state ready for an incoming signal. The external controlling circuitry holds all the switches on the array in their nonconducting (*off*) state while the x-ray exposure is made. When the exposure is finished, the switches on the first row of the array are put in their conducting (*on*) state and the signals from the pixels on this row are transferred down the appropriate signal lines to the external electronics where they are digitized and stored. The switches on this row are then returned to their *off* state and the next row is similarly addressed. The complete image is read out from the array in this sequential, self-scanning, line-by-line manner. In fluoroscopic applications, this sequence continues while the x-ray exposure is occurring, allowing real-time images such as those currently obtained from an x-ray image intensifier (XRII) to be acquired. It is important to realize that even when a particular line of pixels is being read out, the other pixels on the surface of the array are still sensitive to radiation and can combine to acquire imaging information. Even though the array is read out in a sequential self-scanning manner, the detector acquires data in a full two-dimensional manner. An important, but very challenging possibility, is the configuration of an x-ray imaging panel that could instantaneously switch between fluoroscopic and radiographic acquisition modes.

The remainder of this chapter will describe: the different types of x-ray detection media typically used with active-matrix arrays; the individual components that comprise the different designs of flat-panel x-ray imaging systems currently being developed; methods of characterizing the performance of these systems; and the imaging requirements of a number of the different medical imaging applications where they will probably find use in the future.

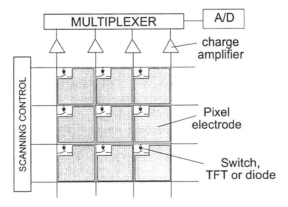

Figure 4.3: Schematic diagram of an active-matrix array and the peripheral electronics used to control the scanning and multiplex the readout.

4.2 X-ray detection media

Flat-panel x-ray detectors are typically configured from an active-matrix array coupled to one of two kinds of solid-state detection media—a photoconductor or a phosphor. Condensed state materials are used because of their high density (and thus high absorption per unit thickness) compared to gases. Solids are usually preferred to liquids as they do not require a container to hold them.

Figure 4.4 shows the electronic band structure of photoconductors and semiconductors compared to that for phosphors. There is in fact very little difference. In each case a conduction band is separated by a forbidden energy gap, E_g from the valence band. Phosphors are insulators with even larger E_g than photoconductors. The band structure for semiconductors and photoconductors differs only in the band-gap energy, E_g. Semiconductors have $E_g \sim 1$ eV; photoconductors have $E_g \sim 2$ eV. The purpose of the detection media is to absorb x rays and then produce a localized response at their surface. This is a representation of where the x ray was absorbed, in other words, an image. As shown in Figure 4.5 there are resolution losses or blurring effects that are common to all media (intrinsic effects) as well as effects specific to photoconductors and phosphors. The three intrinsic effects are geometrical, electron range, and K-fluorescence re-absorption. (a) Geometrical blurring arises when x rays are obliquely incident and, because they may be absorbed at different depths, give a different response at the surface and thus depends on the angle of incidence and the absorption of the layer and its thickness. (b) Electron-range blurring results from the energetic electron freed by radiation interaction that moves through the medium depositing energy. The range is dependent on its energy and the density of the material and is ~ 1–3 μm at 10–30 keV; ~ 10–30 μm at 50–100 keV in typical x-ray detection media. (c) K-fluorescent x rays are often released after interaction of an x ray with the K shell of an atom. The mean absorption distance of x rays of a given energy in the diagnostic energy range in x-ray detection media is greater than the range of charged particles and is typically ~ 50–200 μm.

Both photoconductors and phosphors have been studied and developed for many years for application in x-ray imaging systems such as xeroradiography [14], conventional film/screen combinations, and x-ray image intensifiers (XRII) [8]. Their current level of performance has reached a high level of optimization. The next sections will discuss some of the considerations for photoconductors and phosphors relevant to the flat-panel medical imaging applications.

4.2.1 Photoconductors

In a metal, there are already so many free carriers that the additional few released by the interaction of incident radiation cannot be easily detected. Therefore the state of matter required in a solid-state detector is one with few naturally occurring carriers, i.e., semiconductors or insulators. Detectors based on insulators or semiconductors are solid-state analogs of the gaseous ionization chamber. The free carriers generated by the action of ionizing radiation are collected and used to indicate the position of the absorption of energy from the incident-radiation field.

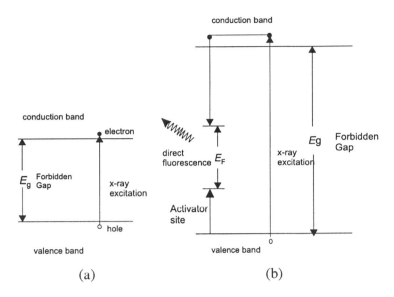

Figure 4.4: Energy band diagrams for (a) photoconductors/semiconductors and (b) activated phosphors.

As shown in Figures 4.5(d)–(f) the electric charge of the secondary particles is used to collect and guide them to the surface by applying an electric field normal to the surface. The field is applied using biasing electrodes at the top of the detector and the image is formed on the other electrodes, which must be discrete to prevent lateral spread of the image. The greater the electric field, the quicker the released charges traverse the collection volume resulting in less time for lateral diffusion and consequently a sharper final image. The charge released by the incident radiation is guided to the surface along the internal electric field lines before it can diffuse laterally and reduce the spatial resolution. This results in an MTF that is, at normal incidence, essentially independent of a-Se thickness as shown in the experimental data plotted in Figure 4.6(a). The intrinsic x-ray effects causing blurring are therefore dominant. As a first approximation the MTF of a-Se does not drop significantly with frequency, although at high energies there is some loss attributable to electron range and at low energies loss resulting from to K fluorescence. There are losses resulting from oblique incidence of x rays but it is minimized at low energies because of the high absorption. In Figure 4.6(b) is plotted a theoretical calculation for the energy dependence based on these effects [31]. An important advantage of a-Se is that it is uniform in imaging properties to a very fine scale (an amorphous material is entirely free from granularity), and can be easily and cheaply made in large areas by a low-temperature process.

In a semiconductor, with $E_g \sim 1$ eV, only a few thermally generated free carriers are present and in insulators, with $E_g \sim 2$ eV, there are essentially no free carriers at room temperature. Another requirement is that carriers released by radi-

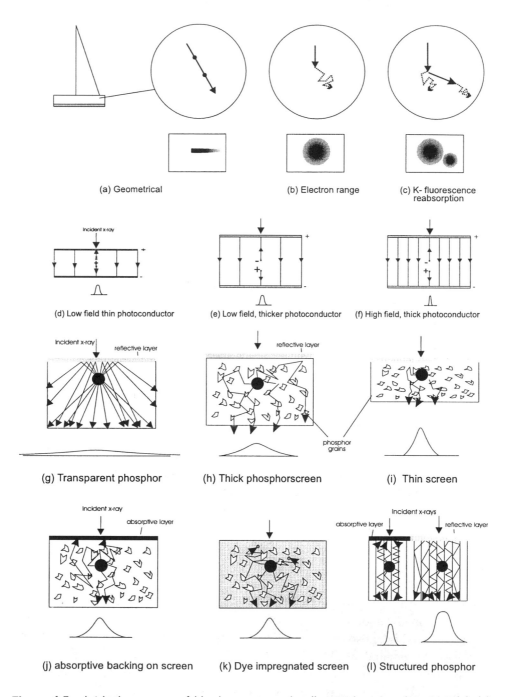

(a) Geometrical

(b) Electron range

(c) K- fluorescence reabsorption

(d) Low field thin photoconductor

(e) Low field, thicker photoconductor

(f) High field, thick photoconductor

(g) Transparent phosphor

(h) Thick phosphorscreen

(i) Thin screen

(j) absorptive backing on screen

(k) Dye impregnated screen

(l) Structured phosphor

Figure 4.5: Intrinsic sources of blurring common in all x-ray imaging detectors (a)–(c). Those sources of blurring specific to photoconductors (d)–(f), and those specific to phosphors (g)–(l). For details see text.

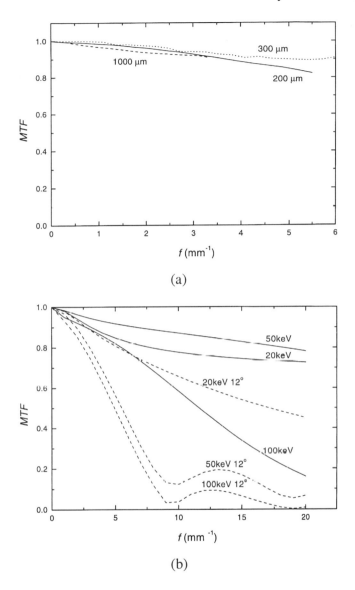

(a)

(b)

Figure 4.6: Modulation transfer functions for several x-ray media. (a) Measured MTF(f) of a-Se plotted for thicknesses of 200 μm [149], 300 μm [89], and 1000 μm [116]. (b) Theoretical dependence of MTF(f) on incident x-ray energy, calculated for a layer thickness of 500 μm. In the following phosphor curves only the optical blurring effects are shown (i.e., ignoring the intrinsic x-ray effects). (c) Swank's universal plot for MTF of phosphor screen where the curves A, B, C, D, E are defined in the text and differ in their optical properties. F is the line for a perfect fiber optic. (d) MTF of conventional powder phosphor screens with a reflective backing and no bulk dye or absorber (I [212], II and III [7], IV [190], V and VI [80]). (e) Data from (d) replotted on Swank's universal curve and compared to screen design C. (f) Measured MTF of structured CsI:Tl screen with reflective or absorptive backing redrawn from data in Hamamatsu brochure. (g) MTF of structured CsI screens all with reflective backing but differing in screen thickness (I [Hamamatsu], II [57] (i) 32, (ii) 59.5 and (iii) 38 keV, III [58], IV [19]). (h) data from (g) replotted on the universal curve compared to screen designs C and D.

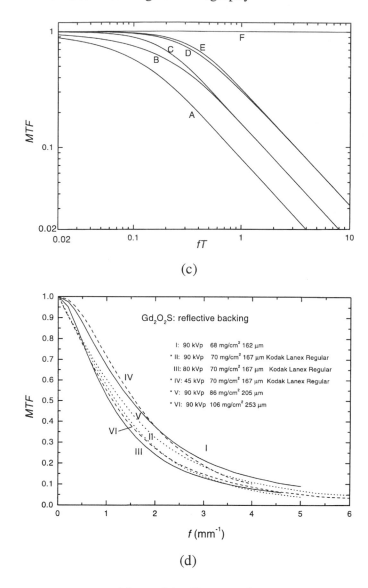

(c)

(d)

Figure 4.6: (Continued).

ation have a sufficient lifetime to reach the surface of the detection volume and be collected by the attached electrodes. Such insulators are called *photoconductors*.

In the band structure for a photoconductors shown in Figure 4.4(a) an optical photon with energy E_g can excite an electron from the valence band to the conduction band leaving behind a *hole* in the valence band (*internal photoelectric effect*). Diagnostic x rays have energy thousands of times larger than E_g. The high atomic number Z of most detection materials means that the absorption of diagnostic x rays is dominant by means of the photoelectric effect where a very energetic photoelectron is released. This energetic electron, as it passes through the solid-

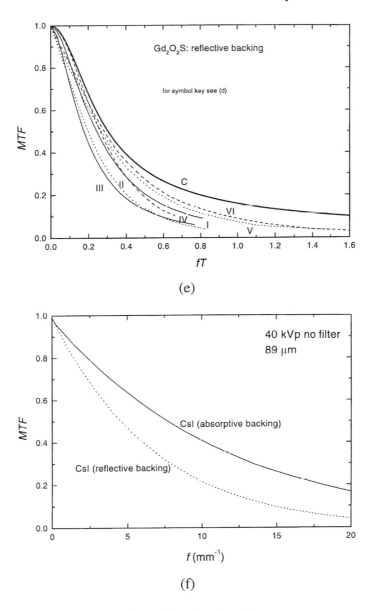

Figure 4.6: (Continued).

state detection material, causes further ionization. Under these circumstances, the amount of energy, W, necessary to create an electron-hole pair (e-h pair) is not simply E_g. Klein [32] showed that, for many semiconductors and insulators used as radiation detectors, W as a function of E_g fits a straight line with a small intercept. The slope of the line is approximately three. There is thus a requirement for an energy of $W \sim 3\,E_g$ on average, to release an e-h pair. An energy-independent loss usually ascribed to phonons is invoked to explain the intercept. Almost all photoconductors and semiconductors fit Klein's curve, provided the electric field

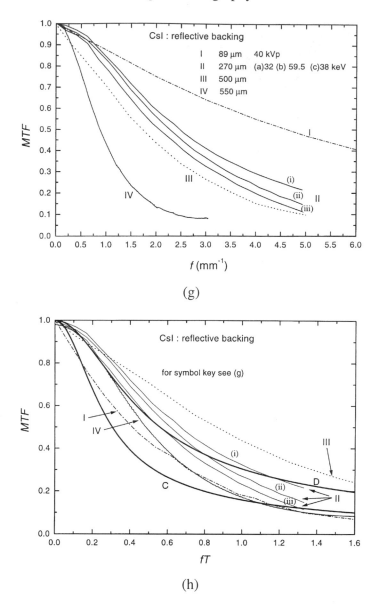

Figure 4.6: (Continued).

applied to the material is large enough to collect all the charge carriers generated by the interaction.

An important exception to Klein's rule is a-Se, the most commonly used solid-state photoconductor in medical x-ray imaging. It has a high value of W, at fields where other photoconductors show saturation ($10 \ V \, \mu m^{-1}$). This is probably because of the initial recombination of e-h pairs [33, 34]. Such recombination occurs if e-h pairs dwell too closely together before they are swept apart by the applied electric field. It has been a matter of controversy as to which kind of recombination is dominant: *geminate*, between the same e-h pair which were created together, or *non-geminate (or columnar)*, between others in the dense region of ionisation caused by the same x ray.

The literature on the development of *a*-Se is mostly concerned with optical applications [35, 36]. The first x-ray application of *a*-Se was in xeroradiography, which is no longer medically viable because of deficiencies in the toner read out method, rather than any problem with the properties of *a*-Se [37, 38] which still remains the most practical large-area photoconductor for medical imaging.

The layer of *a*-Se is deceptively simple, just an evaporated uniform layer. Each surface of the *a*-Se must have an electrode attached to permit collection of charge from the detection volume. This contact must simultaneously prevent charge from the electrodes entering into the *a*-Se. This is called a blocking contact, which must be maintained even under very high electric fields. Finally the surface of the *a*-Se at which the image is formed must have very small transverse conductivity; otherwise the image charge could migrate laterally and destroy the spatial resolution. This poor surface conductivity is achieved by introducing a high density of traps close to the *a*-Se surface.

The material used as the x-ray photoconductor is not the pure form of *a*-Se. Pure *a*-Se is not thermally stable and tends to crystallize over time (e.g., over a few months to a few years, depending on the storage temperature and ambient conditions [39]). However, the crystallization of *a*-Se can be prevented by alloying *a*-Se with about 0.5% As, denoted *a*-Se:0.5%As.

This alloy has a substantial number of hole traps so that typically the hole lifetime τ_h (or deep trapping time) is shorter than τ_h in pure *a*-Se. Doping with a halogen in the ppm range (e.g., Cl) compensates this adverse effect of adding As. The final material, *a*-Se:0.5%As + 10–20 ppm Cl, has both good hole and electron transport and is termed *stabilized a*-Se. Stabilized *a*-Se has the further advantage of showing smaller variations in its charge-transport properties than pure *a*-Se.

An important requirement of any x-ray photoconductor is that both holes and electrons should have Schubwegs (S_h and S_e) that are much longer than the photoconductor thickness (T), that is, S_h and $S_e \gg T$. The Schubweg is the mean distance traversed by a charge carrier before it is trapped and is given by the expression:

$$S = \mu\tau E, \qquad (4.1)$$

where μ is the drift mobility, τ is the carrier lifetime, and E is the applied field. The hole-drift mobility in *a*-Se is remarkably reproducible ($\mu_h = 0.13 \text{ cm}^2 \text{ V}^{-1} \text{ s}^{-1}$) whereas the electron mobility is more variable ($\mu_e = 0.003\text{–}0.006 \text{ cm}^2 \text{ V}^{-1} \text{ s}^{-1}$). However, the carrier lifetimes depend very strongly on many parameters, such as the source material, impurities, and the preparation method, for example, $\tau_h = 50$ to $500\,\mu s$ and $\tau_e = 100$ to $1000\,\mu s$. At an applied field of $E = 10 \text{ V}\,\mu m^{-1}$ these translate to $S_h \sim 6.5$ to 65 mm and $S_e \sim 0.3$ to 3 mm. From the closeness of the latter to radiological thicknesses of *a*-Se (0.2 to 1 mm) the importance of electron lifetime (and hence impurities) in controlling the x-ray photoconductivity can be appreciated.

In the past, the typical value of the electric field used in a-Se devices was $\sim 10\,\mathrm{V}\mu\mathrm{m}^{-1}$ where the value of W is 42 eV. W is known to decrease with electric field, E at a rate somewhat less than linearly [73]. Natural blocking contacts used in the early work on a-Se limited the maximum field strength to $\sim 10\,\mathrm{V}\,\mu\mathrm{m}^{-1}$. The recent development of improved blocking layers permit the electric field to be increased beyond this value [40]. A significant increase in signal should therefore be possible in future devices utilizing these new blocking contacts. A field of 30 to $80\,\mathrm{V}\,\mu\mathrm{m}^{-1}$ is high enough to increase the signal, but low enough to avoid the potential complications of the avalanche region (i.e., increased dark current and absorption depth dependent gain).

Avalanche gain can however be beneficial and is achieved when the charges released by the incident x rays are accelerated under the action of the applied electric field to velocities high enough to cause further ionization within the a-Se layer. This occurs above $\sim 100\,\mathrm{V}\,\mu\mathrm{m}^{-1}$ and can dramatically increase the measured signal response from the detector. Gains of forty have been demonstrated for x-ray irradiation (compare to gains of eight hundred for optical irradiation [41]). This would be a significant advantage in overcoming the problem of additive electronic noise in situations of low signal level such as fluoroscopy. To be of value in medical applications however, thick a-Se layers are required. It is unlikely that a straightforward increase in electric field to $100\,\mathrm{V}\,\mu\mathrm{m}^{-1}$ (even assuming proper blocking contacts) will produce controlled gain. As the a-Se is made thicker, the avalanche gain versus electric field rises very sharply. For thick x-ray layers of a-Se it may not be practically possible to control the gain uniformly across a large area. Furthermore, because x-ray photons are absorbed at different depths in the a-Se layer, each photon would have a different gain resulting in considerable gain fluctuation noise similar to Swank noise in a phosphor.

A possible approach, previously applied to silicon avalanche photodiodes, is to have separate collection and avalanche regions. The collection region constitutes the majority of the thickness of the layer and has an internal electric field below the threshold for avalanche. Carriers generated in the collection region are brought to the relatively thin high field avalanche region where the number of carriers is multiplied. The difference in electric field in the two regions could be achieved by appropriate doping.

The major disadvantage of the direct approach using a-Se is the very high voltage needed to activate the a-Se layer. Under fault conditions, this voltage could possibly damage the active-matrix array. Another disadvantage is that the atomic number, $Z = 34$, for a-Se is rather low and requires very thick layers for high quantum efficiency at diagnostic energies (~ 100 keV). For fluoroscopy it is desirable to have the highest possible quantum gain, and materials with a lower W would have a distinct advantage. The investigation of other possible photoconductor materials to replace a-Se is therefore an active area of research. Shown in Table 4.2 are some possible inorganic x-ray photoconductors with relevant radiographic parameters compared with those for a-Se.

Table 4.2: Physical properties of x-ray photoconductor layers

Material	Z	ρ $(\mathrm{g\,cm^{-3}})$	E $(\mathrm{V\,\mu m^{-1}})$	E_{g} (eV)	W (eV)	S_{h} (mm)	S_{e} (mm)	I_{dark} $(\mathrm{nA\,cm^{-1}})$
a-Se	34	4.27	10	2.2	42	6–65	0.3–3	0.01
			30		20	18–195	0.9–9	0.1
PbI$_2$	82/53	6.2	2	2.3	5*	0.04	1.6	2
PbO	82	9.8	4	1.9	9–20	—	—	1
TlBr	81/35	7.56	1	2.7	6.5*	0.15	1.6	10

The properties of the best thick-film materials have been quoted and if not available then * represents single-crystal values. Z is the atomic number of the radiological relevant elements in the material, ρ is the material density, E is the applied electric field here listed as the values typically used, E_g is the energy of the forbidden band, W is the absorbed energy in the phosphor necessary to release a single electron-hole pair, S_{h} and S_{e} are the hole and electron Schubwegs respectively, and I_{dark} is the dark current all at the value of E given. Error bars have not been given, but S and I_{dark} values are highly variable and subject to rapid improvement. All these materials have shown good charge-transport properties (i.e., $S_{\mathrm{h}}, S_{\mathrm{e}} \gg T$) for single crystals. The properties of evaporated thin films of all these materials (with the exception of a-Se) are generally less well known than those for single crystals.

Single-crystal PbI$_2$ was first investigated for nuclear radiation detectors and to permit the first imaging experiments using a vidicon structure [42]. More recently thin layers have been deposited onto active-matrix arrays to form an x-ray imaging system [43]. It shows an adequate Schubweg provided relatively high biasing fields ($2\,\mathrm{V\,\mu m^{-1}}$) are used. PbO has also been used as an imaging photoconductor for some time. The first application (in 1954) was in an optical vidicon [44] and a large-area x-ray vidicon was made in 1956 [45]. The tube was 8″ in diameter and had a 150-μm-thick layer of PbO in a p-i-n structure. The p and n regions were obtained by doping the PbO; the intrinsic region was obtained by making the PbO porous. Klein [32] reports that $W = 8$ eV for crystalline PbO and in Table 4.2 are shown representative values for evaporated layers [46]. It is difficult to manufacture because it reacts immediately with ambient air, causing both its dark resistance and its x-ray sensitivity to decrease. A more serious problem with thick layers is the degradation with use characterized by: image persistence, non-uniformity, white spots, and decreasing sensitivity [47]. It has also been used for the construction of prototype flat-panel imaging systems [46]. TlBr is a crystalline semiconductor with [48] a high ionic conductivity that gives rise to a large dark current. However, sufficiently good films have been made that it has been used as the photoconductor for large-area vidicons where it is cooled with a Peltier cooler [49] to reduce the ionic current to negligible levels.

There is a host of other materials under investigation as potential photoconductors for medical x-ray imaging including CdZnTe, CdTe, and HgI$_2$ [50, 51]. In the coming years, it is likely that many of these will be combined with active-matrix arrays to investigate their potential for diagnostic radiology. New engineered materials known as nanocomposite organic photoconductors [52, consisting of nanoparticles of heavy metals in an organic photoconductor matrix], are also being investigated and hold promise.

4.2.2 Phosphors

Many current x-ray imaging detectors employ a phosphor in the initial stage to absorb x rays and produce light. As shown in Figure 4.4(b), phosphors work by exciting electrons from the valence band to the conduction band where they are free to move a small distance within the phosphor. Some of these electrons will decay back to the valence band without giving off any radiant energy, but in an efficient phosphor, many of the electrons will return to the valence band through a local state (created by small amounts of impurities called activators) and in the process emit light. Thus, phosphors can be relatively efficient converters of the large incident energy of the x ray into light photons. Because light photons each carry only a small ($\sim$2–3 eV) energy, many light photons are created from the absorption of a single x ray.

This *quantum amplification* is the *conversion gain* of the phosphor. For example, in Gd_2O_2S:Tb, an x-ray photon energy of 60 keV is equivalent to that of 25,000 green-light quanta ($E = 2.4$ eV). However, because of competing energy loss processes, only $\sim$3600 light quanta **on average** are released per fully absorbed 60-keV x ray. A list of physical quantities for several x-ray phosphors is given in Table 4.3. The phosphors most commonly used in flat-panel imagers are Gd_2O_2S:Tb and CsI:Tl. These two materials have approximately the same conversion efficiency and will therefore produce about the same number of light photons from the absorption of equal-energy x rays. However, the physical structure of the

Table 4.3: Physical properties of inorganic phosphors

Type	Z	K-edge Energy (keV)	Density ρ (g cm^{-3})	λ (nm)	W (eV)	Γ (keV^{-1})
CaWO$_4$	74	69.5	6.06	480 ± 100	33	30
Gd$_2$O$_2$S:Tb	64	50.2	7.34	550 ± 20	17	60
CsI:Na	55/53	36/33	4.51	415 ± 50	25	40
CsI:Tl	55/53	36/33	4.51	560 ± 80	18	55

Where: symbols previously defined retain the same meaning and Γ is the number of light photons of wavelength λ released per keV of absorbed x-ray energy, W is its inverse, the absorbed energy in the phosphor necessary to release a single light photon. In comparing these values with W for the direct method, it is necessary to make some assumptions on the efficiency and fill factor of the photodiode and the efficiency of escape of light photons from the phosphor layer. If, for example, the optical quantum efficiency of the photodiode is 50%, its geometrical fill factor is 50%, and the optical conditions on the layer are such that only 50% of the created light escapes the phosphor layer, the effective value of W would be increased to eight times the value given above.

detection media constructed using each of these phosphors is very different, and has a significant effect on the resulting image quality. This will be discussed in more detail in the next sections.

4.2.2.1 X-ray screens

To create an x-ray image, a transparent phosphor would not be very effective because light could move large distances within the phosphor and cause blurring as shown in Figure 4.5(g). Instead, x-ray screens are made highly scattering or *turbid*. These screens consist of a layer of phosphor, usually of high refractive index, in the form of very fine powder, incorporated within a nonradiative but optically transparent binder layer that is coated on the surface of a plastic substrate. The x rays interacting with the phosphor emit light near their point of incidence on the screen. The light quanta must successfully escape the phosphor and be as close as possible to their point of emission when they are detected. Because of the mismatch between the index of refraction of the binder and the phosphor grains, once a light photon exits a grain it tends to reflect off the neighboring grain surfaces rather than passing through them. Thus the lateral spread of the light is confined, which helps maintain the spatial resolution of the phosphor layer. Figures 4.5(h) and 4.5(i) illustrate schematically the effect of phosphor thickness and the depth of x-ray interaction on spatial resolution of a turbid phosphor screen. There is a trade-off between phosphor thickness, and hence x-ray interaction efficiency and limiting spatial resolution. Thus, for example, screens designed for high-resolution applications are usually much thinner than general-purpose phosphor screens.

The detailed design of a phosphor screen can also affect its imaging performance. For example, factors such as phosphor grain size, size distribution, bulk absorption, and surface reflectivity, as well as material purity, can have significant effects on the image quality. The thickness of the protective overcoat layer can also affect the spatial resolution of the screen. Optical effects are used to change the imaging properties of the screen. For example, as shown in Figure 4.5(j), an absorptive backing helps reduce blurring but at the cost of reducing the amount of light escaping the front of the screen. Typically, with an absorptive backing, less than one-half of the created light quanta escapes the phosphor and is potentially available to be recorded. Light-absorbing dye can also be added to the screen to enhance the resolution as shown in Figure 4.5(k). All these factors were accumulated in a comprehensive model of screen optics attributable to Swank [53]. In this model, the resolution is the same for all screens of a given type if the resolution is expressed in terms of the dimensionless quantity fT where T is the thickness of the screen. Figure 4.6(c) shows Swank's results of the loss of resolution for five prototype screen designs (A–E) compared to an idealized system F, which has no optical effects degrading resolution. For a complete MTF of screens, the intrinsic x-ray effects also have to be included, in principle, but rarely are in practice, because the optical effects are usually dominant in turbid screens. The critical factors are therefore the thickness and the basic design of the screen. The worst, as far as resolution is concerned, is the transparent screen with a reflective backing (A); followed by a transparent screen with an absorptive backing (B). A highly scattering (diffusion limit) screen with a reflective backing (C) is better though similar to (B). Finally the best are (D) and (E) that are calculated for diffusion-limited screens with 50% light absorption in bulk and absorptive backing respectively. Thus based on Swank's model, and noting that it is important to have high light collection, which implies no absorption and reflective backing, all screens for flat-panel detectors are likely to be considered as type (C). In Figure 4.6(d) is plotted the MTF of several screens of type (C) with different mass loadings and physical thicknesses and in Figure 4.6(e) these have been plotted on Swank's universal curve.

Screens are most commonly used in conjunction with film sandwiched in a cassette. The probability of x-ray interaction with depth into the phosphor is exponential, so that the number of interacting quanta and the amount of light created will be proportionally greater near the x-ray entrance surface. High-resolution film/screen systems are therefore generally configured from a single screen placed such that the x rays pass through the film before impinging on the phosphor. This *back-screen* configuration improves the spatial resolution of the final image compared to the alternative *front-screen* configuration. Because of the thickness ($\sim$0.7 mm) of the standard glass substrate currently used for active-matrix fabrication, flat-panel x-ray systems which utilize a phosphor are all configured in the less desirable front-screen orientation.

Screens can also be used in conjunction with a fiber optic or a lens to couple the image to other optical devices, such as a CCD or a video camera. Because of the Lambertian nature of the screen emission, these methods have significant problems in maintaining good noise properties. This is because the collection efficiency of the light from the screen by the imaging device is usually rather poor and only a few light photons represent the interaction of each x ray. This transfer of light from the screen to the detector can become the limiting stage in the imaging chain and can determine the overall performance of the complete system. One of the main advantages of a flat-panel detector (in an indirect detection configuration) is that, because of its large area, it can be placed in direct contact with the emission surface of the screen. Its collection efficiency for the emitted light is consequently much higher than with most other approaches.

4.2.2.2 *Scintillators and structured phosphors*

One of the main issues with the design of powdered phosphor screens is the balance between spatial resolution and x-ray detection efficiency. As the phosphor is made thicker to absorb more x rays, the emitted light can spread further from the point of production before exiting the screen. This conflict is significantly eased by the use of a structured phosphor such as CsI. When evaporated under the correct conditions, a layer of CsI will condense in the form of needle-like closely packed crystallites. In this form, the resolution is better than for a powder phosphor screen. However, it may be enhanced by fracturing into thin pillar-like structures ($\sim$10 μm diameter) by exposure to a thermal shock. This has the effect of reducing the effective density of the structured layer to about 80 to 90% that of a single CsI crystal. This pillar or columnar structure is illustrated in Figure 4.5(l). These columns, in principle, act like fiber-optic light guides because of the difference in refractive index n between CsI ($n = 1.78$) and the air ($n = 1$), which fills the gaps between the pillars. Light photons produced by the absorption of an incident x ray will be guided toward either end of the pillar if they are emitted within the range of angles that satisfy conditions for total internal reflection. Theoretical calculations predict that 83% of the isotropically emitted light will undergo internal reflection within a perfectly uniform pillar [54]. The other 17% will scatter between pillars and cause a reduction in the spatial resolution. Actual layers of CsI have a somewhat reduced light-collimating capability caused by the unavoidable nonuniformity of the surface of the pillars and possible defects in the cracking. However, they maintain significantly higher resolutions for a given thickness of phosphor than powder screens as shown conceptually in Figures 4.5(h) and 4.5(i).

To increase the light-collection capabilities of the layer, a reflective backing can also be added to the x-ray entrance surface of the CsI to redirect the light photons emitted in this direction back toward the exit surface. This significantly increases the light output of the layer but at the cost of a reduced spatial resolution [121]. MTFs of practical layers of CsI are shown in Figure 4.6(f) for a single-layer thickness but differing by whether there is a reflective or absorptive backing or dye, Figure 4.6(g) is CsI with a reflective backing but for various layer thicknesses. These data show a considerable loss of MTF as thickness increases and this is summarized in Figure 4.6(h) which are the data of (g) replotted on Swank's universal curve. Note that all these CsI screens are better than comparable designs of powder screen, that is, Swank's type C, when plotted on the universal curve. CsI is used in all modern XRIIs and its manufacture has reached a high level of sophistication. Growth of the CsI layer onto a patterned substrate can also allow more precise control of the geometrical properties of the pillar structure [54] and the spatial resolution of the CsI layer [55].

The type of activator impurity introduced into the CsI layer controls the emission spectrum of the light. A sodium activator produces a layer that emits in the blue ($\sim$450 nm) which is well matched to the response of photocathodes used in XRII. Thallium doping produces light peaked more in the green region of the spectrum ($\sim$550 nm) which is better suited for absorption in a-Si:H layers (see Figure 4.13 later). As shown in Table 4.3 CsI:Tl also produces more light photons per absorbed x ray ($\sim$50 to 60 keV^{-1} absorbed) than almost any other x-ray phosphor. The combination of the feasibility of thick structured layers with good spatial resolution, well matched emission spectrum and high light production efficiency make CsI:Tl a natural choice for use in conjunction with an active-matrix flat-panel detector [56].

The advantages of the columnar structure of CsI have been known for many years but its somewhat hygroscopic nature and practical drawbacks such as toxicity and lack of mechanical robustness have so far limited its medical imaging applications to the input phosphor of XRIIs [57]. Here the CsI is protected from external mechanical abrasion; unlike in a conventional film cassette where the phosphor screens must have a rugged overcoat to prevent damage in everyday use. The situation with a flat-panel detector is similar to that of an XRII in that the CsI layer is well protected from external forces. Many of the practical issues limiting the use of CsI layers for more general radiography are therefore potentially solved in a flat-panel detector configuration [58].

Other interesting approaches to structured phosphors currently being investigated include fiber optic faceplates made with either glass [59] or plastic [60] loaded with scintillation impurities. Thin fibers of these materials can be packed together to produce thick layers with high x-ray absorption efficiency and excellent spatial resolution properties. The spatial-resolution of these plates to normally incident x rays can be made independent of their thickness through the use of cladding glass of lower refractive index surrounding each individual fiber and/or absorptive glass layers called extra mural absorber (EMA). Geometric spatial spreading of x-ray signal becomes the dominant source of resolution loss at the edge of the detection area where obliquely incident x rays traverse more than a single fiber. A drawback of this approach is the low efficiency for energy transfer between the incident x ray and the light photons emitted from the fiber. This is currently ~ 0.1–0.3% [60, 61] (c.f. Gd_2O_2S and CsI at about 15%) but may be improved with further research. The capability of fabricating a reasonable-cost large-area face plate suitable for general radiography has also yet to be demonstrated. Other researchers have proposed the packing of a high-efficiency scintillator (specifically Gd_2O_2S) into a thick micro-channel grid with reflective walls [62]. This would theoretically reduce the trade-off between phosphor thickness and spatial resolution. However this approach also currently suffers from a similar lack of light output resulting from absorption by the grid walls.

Table 4.3 lists properties of inorganic phosphors that were derived from the literature [63–66]. The assumptions made in the literature are not always consistent, as there are many issues related to the output of light. These include reflection and absorption within the screen, matching of the light of the phosphor to the detector, the fill-factor of the detectors, and the nature of the phosphor surface furthest from the sensor (i.e., whether it is reflecting or absorptive). Table 4.3 includes (where available) information on pure single crystals of the phosphor. Corrections are then necessary to convert these values to practical values relevant to optically coupled sensors as discussed in the table caption.

4.2.3 Noise sources in x-ray detection media

The noise in x-ray images is related to the x-ray exposure to the detector. However, the noise can be degraded by lack of absorption of the x rays, as well as by fluctuations in the response of the detector to those x rays, which are absorbed.

The initial image-acquisition operation is identical in all x-ray detectors. In order to produce a signal, the x-ray quanta must interact with the detector material. The probability of interaction or quantum detection efficiency A_Q for an x ray of energy E is given by

$$A_Q = 1 - \exp[-\mu(E, Z)T], \tag{4.2}$$

where μ is the linear attenuation coefficient of the detector material and T is its thickness. Because all practical x-ray sources for radiography are polyenergetic, that is, emit x rays over a spectrum of energies, A_Q must either be specified at each energy or as an *effective* value over the spectrum of x rays incident on the detector. This spectrum will be influenced by the filtering effect of the patient which is to *harden* the beam, in other words to make it more energetic and therefore more penetrating.

The value of A_Q can be increased by making T greater or by using materials that have higher values of μ because of increased Z or density. A_Q is plotted against x-ray energy in Figure 4.7 for some radiologically important photoconductors and phosphors at relevant thicknesses. The A_Q will in general be highest at low energies, gradually decreasing with increasing energy. If the material has an atomic absorption edge in the energy region of interest, then quantum efficiency increases dramatically above this energy, causing a local minimum in A_Q for energies immediately below the absorption edge.

There are unavoidable fluctuations in the signal produced in the detection medium even when x rays of identical energy interact and produce a response. These fluctuations are caused by the statistical nature of the competing mechanisms that occur as the x-ray deposits energy in the medium. Together these effects give rise to a category of noise known as *gain-fluctuation noise*. The first discussion of gain-fluctuation noise and estimates of its magnitude, in the context of x-ray detection with phosphors, was given by Swank [67]. The gain-fluctuation noise is experimentally determined using the *pulse-height spectrum*, or PHS, obtained using mono-energetic x-ray sources as shown in Figure 4.8 for both phosphors and photoconductors. Monoenergetic x rays are incident on the detector, one at a time, and the quantity of charge e released directly by a photoconductor or indirectly (by interaction of the released light with a photocathode of a photomultiplier) by a phosphor is measured. This is performed using a pulse-shaping circuit which has the property of integrating the charge from the photoconductor (or photomultiplier if using a phosphor) into a pulse whose height is proportional to the integrated charge. The multichannel analyzer [Figure 4.8(d)] then digitizes the pulse height and increments a counter corresponding to that height. This creates a histogram called a PHS. This can be interpreted, and if necessary calibrated using a *charge terminator* as shown in Figure 4.8(c), in terms of charge or deposited x-ray energy.

Prototypical pulse-height spectra are shown in Figure 4.8. In (e) is the ideal spectrum—all x rays give rise to equal amounts of charge, resulting in a delta function. This, as shown in the caption, has a value of the Swank factor $A_S = 1$. Other possible shapes resulting from statistical broadening, K-fluorescence escape, and optical broadening [68] caused by absorptive bulk dye or backing will have the form shown, and the corresponding, approximate value of A_S is given in the

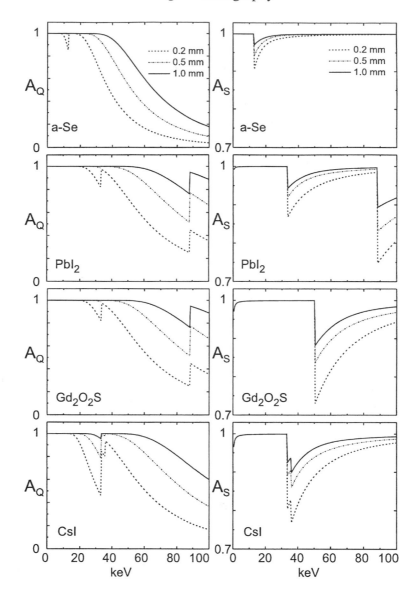

Figure 4.7: Quantum efficiencies, A_Q, and gain fluctuation (Swank) factors, A_S, for two representative photoconductors, a-Se and PbI$_2$, and two phosphors Gd$_2$O$_2$S (typical screen phosphor) and CsI (structured scintillator). The curves are calculated using the photoelectric attenuation coefficient only (graphs courtesy of D Hunt).

caption to Figure 4.8. Such measurements and related theoretical estimates have been performed for a range of detection media including the phosphors Gd$_2$O$_2$S:Tb [69, 70], CsI:Na [71], and for layers of stabilized a-Se [42, 43, 72, 73]. Examples are shown in Figure 4.9 for CsI:Na obtained from a complete XRII which, however, is dominated by the effects in the CsI:Na layer, a Gd$_2$O$_2$S with reflective backing; CaWO$_4$ with and without a reflective backing and a-Se layers. The noise caused

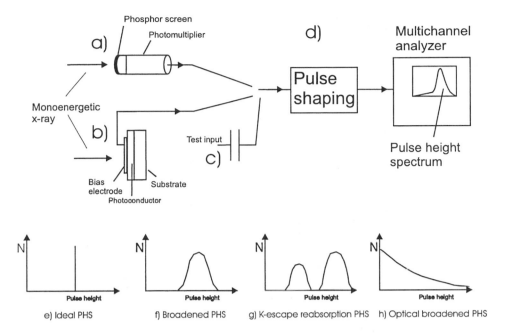

e) Ideal PHS   f) Broadened PHS   g) K-escape reabsorption PHS   h) Optical broadened PHS

Figure 4.8: Experiments methods to measure pulse-height spectra PHS for (a) phosphor layers, (b) for photoconductors, (c) test input for calibration of system in terms of charge, and (d) electronics to shape pulses from individual x-ray absorption to have a height proportional to charge deposited per x ray. The last row of the figure shows example PHS that may be observed and the corresponding value of the Swank information factor A_S. (e) Ideally, a single delta function giving Swank factor $A_S = 1$. (f) A single peak broadened by statistical processes in the screen or phosphor layer $A_S{\sim}0.95$. (g) Extra (lower energy) peak caused by K-fluorescence escape giving $A_S{\sim}0.75$. (h) Extreme broadening of peak to extent that it is exponential which can arise because of absorptive dye in phosphor layer or backing layer giving $A_S{\sim}0.5$.

by both quantum-absorption inefficiency and gain fluctuations can be combined to create the *zero-spatial-frequency detective quantum efficiency* DQE(0) that is given by

$$DQE(0) = A_Q A_S, \tag{4.3}$$

where A_S is the correction due to gain-fluctuation noise and can be expressed in terms of the first three of the i moments of the PHS, that is, the histogram of $N(\varepsilon)$ plotted against ε:

$$M_i = \Sigma N(\varepsilon)\varepsilon^i, \tag{4.4}$$

as a combination of the zeroth, first, and second moments:

$$A_S = M_1^2/(M_0 M_2). \tag{4.5}$$

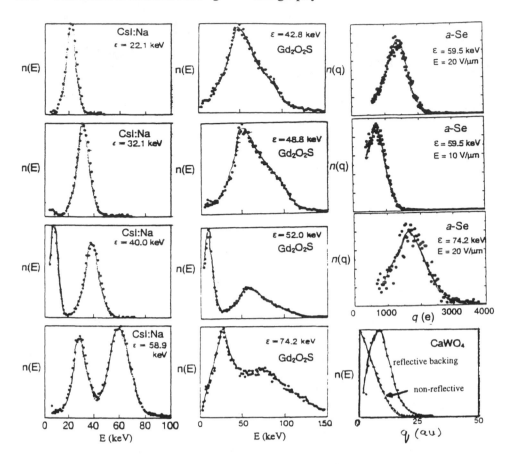

Figure 4.9: Measured pulse-height spectra for several radiologically important detection media. CsI:Na with a reflective backing measured using an XRII [71], Gd_2O_2S:Tb screen with a reflective backing measured using a photomultiplier [68] and a-Se measured using a low noise charge preamplifier [73] plotted for several x-ray energies. The curve for $CaWO_4$ is measured with and without a reflective backing.

Representative *calculated* values for the magnitude of the Swank factor A_S are plotted in Figure 4.7 for common phosphors and photoconductors. These calculations include only the broadening effects of the intrinsic x-ray phenomena, not the losses resulting from light absorption (phosphors) or charge trapping (photoconductors). They thus represent an upper limit on A_S. The energy of the incident x ray is important because above the K edge of the material, K-fluorescence escape can significantly affect the distribution of measured signals and reduces the Swank factor, representing an increase in Swank noise. Higher-Z materials with K edges in the range of energies present in a diagnostic x-ray beam will exhibit more image degradation because of this mechanism than lower-Z materials whose K edge is at lower energies. However, changes in the absorption coefficient across the K edge can also make these higher-Z materials less sensitive, on average, to

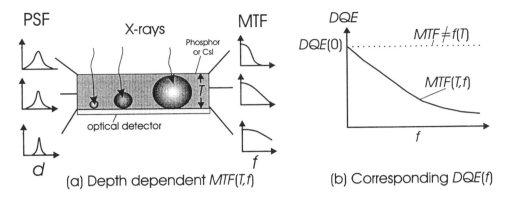

(a) Depth dependent MTF(T,f)   (b) Corresponding DQE(f)

Figure 4.10: Lubberts effect (a) showing how a depth-dependent modulation transfer function MTF(L, f) arises in a scattering phosphors layer by requiring a larger distance for light to travel (and hence scatter more) if the x ray is absorbed in an upper layer of the screen compared to a shorter path distance (and less blurring) for an x ray absorbed closer to the optical sensor in, for example, the flat-panel imager. (b) The DQE(f) drop resulting from Lubberts effect arising when the depth dependence is large [as in (a)] but if there is no T dependence of MTF then DQE is independent of f.

the lower-energy scattered radiation produced in the patient [74]. This scattered radiation can act as an additional source of noise, reducing the quality of the final image. Optical effects in the phosphor screen, or trapping in the photoconductor, can make a considerable difference to the shape of the PHS and thus to the value of A_S. Therefore PHS measured for some representative phosphors and photoconductors are shown in Figure 4.9. Note the broadening of the spectral lines and the marked change in spectrum when the reflective backing is removed.

Lubberts [75] described another important aspect of noise generation. He realized that x rays deposited at various depths within the sensor layer (phosphor or photoconductor) could have different amounts of spreading before they reached the surface of the detector. This would affect the propagation of signal and noise differently. He showed that this mechanism, now known as the Lubberts effect, decreases DQE as f increases. The concept is shown in Figure 4.10. It has long been accepted that there is a very significant loss in DQE(f) in conventional screens because of the Lubberts effect [75–80]. However, it has been implicitly assumed and in fact demonstrated in experiments using XRII, that this effect would not be important in CsI phosphors because of their high resolution [81, 82]. However, there has been a trend over time for continually increasing the thickness of the CsI phosphor in order to increase DQE(0). It may be that the Lubberts effect is therefore beginning to be important in CsI-based flat-panel detectors.

4.3 Flat-panel array technology

The history of x-ray flat-panel imagers can be traced back to the development of the optical vidicon, which was the first video tube to use a photoconductor. Previous tubes had relied on the *external photoelectric effect* (i.e., photoionization of an electron in a solid to the vacuum) which has an ultimate sensitivity limit much lower than the *internal photoelectric effect* (i.e., photoionization of an electron in a solid from the valence band to the conduction band within the same material). Albert Rose, a pioneer in understanding the quantum limits of imaging, and Paul Wiemer was closely involved with the development of the vidicon. This tube satisfied the essential requirement of being sensitive to radiation at all times but permitted read out one point at a time. The vidicon is still important in medical imaging in conjunction with XRII, though it is gradually being replaced by solid-state imaging devices such as CCDs. The first vidicon used *a*-Se as the photoconductive layer [83] and subsequent vidicons used other photoconductors such as CdSe and PbO. Wiemer [84] was one of the first to recognize the advantages of a solid-state optical detector, these being increased: "... *reliability, compactness and (reduced) cost ... and ... in the early 1960s, started the first investigations of a thin film* [85] *photoconductive approach to image sensors before the silicon integrated circuit technology had become established. This project therefore represented the development of a new thin-film technology* [86] *as well as a study of image sensors.*" (References from Wiemer [84].)

Wiemer based his new approach on the photoconductive and semiconducting films that had been used in the vidicon. These films were used as the photoconductor to convert light to charge, to make diodes which were used at each pixel for switching, and finally as TFTs which were used in the peripheral circuitry integrated onto the sensor for reading out the array line by line. One of these materials was CdSe, which was used in 1968 to make a self-scanned sensor of 12.8 mm × 12.8 mm and 256 pixels by 256 pixels of 50-μm pitch [84]. The TFT approach to *small* optical sensors soon faded to high-purity single-crystal silicon (CCDs and recently complementary metal oxide silicon or CMOS detectors). However, it was realized that the TFT technology was more suitable than single-crystal silicon for constructing large-area devices such as displays.

The first active-matrix flat-panel *display* was demonstrated by Brody [87] in 1973, and was fabricated using CdSe as the semiconductor. An x-ray sensor array using CdSe TFTs was first proposed in 1992 and subsequently demonstrated for both radiography and fluoroscopy using *a*-Se as the x-ray photoconductor [88–90]. However, the majority of today's flat-panel arrays are fabricated from *hydrogenated amorphous silicon* (a-Si:H). Research into the properties of a-Si grew from the interest in chalcogenide amorphous semiconductors pursued in the 1950s and 60s. The discovery of the beneficial effects of introducing hydrogen into the crystal lattice structure to occupy many of the dangling bonds [91] present in raw a-Si and the ability to control the electrical properties of the material by doping [92] led to the development of photo-voltaic devices in the late 1970s. The demonstration of complex electrical structures such as field effect transistors (FETs or TFTs) configured from this doped a-Si:H in the early 1980s [93] led to the development [94] of the current large-area active-matrix devices which have electrical properties suitable for numerous display and sensor applications.

The concept of coupling an a-Si:H photodiode with an overlying phosphor to detect x rays was under investigation as early as 1985 [95]. Early papers reported the use of linear a-Si:H arrays coupled with ceramic Gd_2O_2S:Tb for applications in computerized tomography [96, 97]. The formation of quasi 2D detectors configured using fiber-optic bundles to remap a 2D Gd_2O_2S screen onto a 1D a-Si:H linear sensor [98, 99] and the scanning of 1D linear sensors to achieve full 2D coverage [100]. However, the availability of a true 2D array of pixels was required before the a-Si:H approach to x-ray detection became a realistic possibility for medical imaging applications.

Only in the late 80s and early 90s did reports of true 2D x-ray detectors formed from a-Si:H and overlying phosphor screens begin to appear in the literature [25, 101–112]. The ease with which a commercially available Gd_2O_2S screen can be coupled to an a-Si:H flat-panel detector meant that much of the early work was performed with this approach. However, it was also realized at an early stage that other approaches incorporating different scintillators and photoconductors (specifically CsI:Tl and a-Se) would have advantages for particular applications [25, 90, 110, 112, 113]. More recently, papers have started to appear in the literature that describe active commercial interest in the clinical implementation of these devices [114–121, 190]. Investigators have also started probing the clinical significance of the image quality provided by these flat-panel x-ray detectors [122–125]. This signifies the evolution of the technology out of the research laboratory into the clinical environment. This next phase will determine their utility for mainstream diagnostic medical imaging. It will also answer the question of whether or not this general approach is the long-awaited enabling technology that will usher in the widespread adoption of picture archiving and communications systems (PACS) within hospital departments, as well as teleradiology between remote hospitals and clinics. The following sections will review the current technology and science behind the fabrication and application of today's active-matrix arrays in the field of medical x-ray imaging.

4.3.1 Active-matrix-array fabrication

Large-area, a-Si:H flat-panel detectors are deposited onto a glass substrate from silane gas (SiH_4) in a plasma reactor at temperatures $\sim 250°C$. The most common approach is plasma-enhanced chemical vapor deposition (PECVD). The crystal morphology of layers fabricated in such a manner is one of short-range order and long-range disorder; hence the use of the term amorphous. This disordered structure is responsible for the exceptional radiation damage tolerance that a-Si:H exhibits [126]. It is also the source of many of the problems, such as charge trapping and image lag, associated with the so-called "metastable states" created by this morphology. Such amorphous materials may exhibit many similarities to perfect crystals, for instance the presence of states throughout the material, such as the existence of bands and, more surprisingly, the presence of a forbidden band. The long-range disordered nature of a-Si:H results in the creation of states in this band-gap that would be forbidden in a perfect crystal. These band-gap states control many of the electrical properties of a-Si:H. Variation of the deposition parameters (e.g., temperature or plasma frequency) can change the morphology of the material and the defect density in the band gap. This results in a variety of materials such as nano, micro, and polycrystalline silicon which differ in the range over which the crystallite structure remains ordered before breaking down into the disordered structure characteristic of amorphous materials. These morphological differences greatly affect the electrical properties of the final material. One of the main distinguishing properties of these different crystal morphologies is the ease with which electrical charges can travel through them. This determines the mobility of the charge carriers when an external electric field is applied. Good quality amorphous silicon has carrier mobilities of ~ 1 and 0.003 cm^2 V^{-1} s^{-1} for electrons and holes respectively. Typical microcrystalline Si has mobilities that are an order of magnitude higher and polycrystalline Si is an order of magnitude higher again. However, these are still significantly less than the mobilities (~ 1300 and 500 cm^2 V^{-1} s^{-1}) typically obtained with crystalline Si. Other properties, such as the creation of metastable states under illumination and current flow, can also cause temporal variations in the electrical behavior of the amorphous layers. During the deposition process, different gases may be introduced into the plasma to control the level of doping in the a-Si:H layer in much the same way doping impurities control the electrical properties of standard crystalline-silicon components. This allows accurate control of the electrical properties of the final material. (For more details on this and other aspects of amorphous-silicon science and technology, refer to the monographs by Street [127] and Kanicki [128, 129].)

The process of forming the active-matrix array is similar to techniques developed for crystalline-silicon integrated circuits. It entails deposition and photolithographic etching of layers of a-Si:H with different doping concentrations. Other layers include dielectric insulators and conductive metals which form the other components and connections comprising the fully functional array. Depending on the complexity of the pixel design, as few as four or as many as a dozen different layers may be required to complete an array. A simplified outline of the photolithographic procedure for a single layer is shown in Figure 4.11.

The required intrinsic properties of the sensing and switching elements on an array designed specifically for medical imaging can be determined from the details of the intended application. A number of these can have a conflicting, or at least competing, effect on the array design. Factors other than imaging performance can also play a significant role in the decision of which approach to use. Perhaps the most important of these non-imaging factors are fabrication *yield* (the fraction of useful devices obtained in the overall process divided by the total number of devices made) and availability of fabrication facilities and technology. The desire to increase the fabrication yield, and hence reduce the cost of the array, pressures the designer to reduce the complexity of the pixel elements, the number of pixel elements, and the number of mask layers required for fabrication. This provides impetus to compromise the individual elements by fabrication of both the switching and sensing/storage elements at the same time even if this yields sub-optimal performance. While these modifications may improve device yield, it can be at the cost of reduced imaging performance of the final detector. Intellectual property

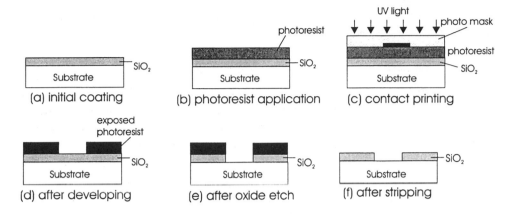

Figure 4.11: Principle of photolithography used to pattern layers of active matrix array (example shows a single layer of SiO$_2$ being patterned).

considerations can also influence the pixel design, as can experience with a particular fabrication process. For example, flat-panel display manufacture typically does not require p$^+$ deposition or thick (i.e., 2 μm) intrinsic layer processes. These additional processes make the fabrication of a p-i-n, photo- or switching diode difficult at foundries designed specifically for display manufacture. Consequently, in practice, optimal imaging performance of the pixel elements may not be the ultimate consideration in the design of the array for use as a flat-panel x-ray detector.

One significant advantage of flat-panel active-matrix fabrication methods, and the main reason it is ideally suited to medical imaging devices, is that the layers of a-Si:H can be deposited over extremely large areas. State-of-the-art a-Si:H foundries for displays use substrates exceeding 1 × 1 m. For sensors, there are foundries using device substrates ∼50 × 50 cm with 60 × 72 cm substrates becoming available in the foreseeable future. Single substrate (41 × 41 cm) imaging devices with areas larger than a traditional x-ray film (35 × 43 cm) are already being developed.

4.3.2 Active-matrix-array components

The next sections will discuss some of the different sensing/storage elements and switching elements currently being pursued. The sensing/storage elements are photodiodes for the indirect approach and electrode capacitor elements for the direct approach. Thin-film switching elements used for arrays can be divided into two distinct groups: (a) two-terminal devices, for example, diodes, metal-insulator-metal devices (known as MIMs), or metal-semi-insulator devices (known as MSIs) whose resistance is controlled by the polarity and magnitude of the voltage applied across the two contacts; (b) Three-terminal devices, for example, TFTs, where a voltage applied to the first contact (the gate) controls the resistance between the other two (the source and drain) contacts. Within these two subdivisions there are numerous approaches for design and fabrication which produce devices with different electrical properties.

4.3.2.1 Sensing/storage elements for indirect-detection

The sensing element of the indirect pixel is designed to detect visible wavelength light emitted from the overlying phosphor (for a discussion on the physics of photoconductivity see Crandall) [130]. The intrinsically disordered nature of a-Si:H has the effect of relaxing the momentum selection rules. As a consequence, the absorption coefficient of a-Si:H ($\sim 10^4$ to $\sim 10^6$ cm^{-1}) for light in the visible wavelength range is an order of magnitude higher than that for crystalline silicon ($\sim 10^3$ to $\sim 10^5$ cm^{-1}) [131, 132] even though the effective optical band gap of a-Si:H (~ 1.7 eV) is larger than that in crystalline silicon (~ 1.1 eV). The absorption coefficient depends on many factors including the defect density of states in the band gap, the morphology of the material, and the level of doping. Generally however, a ~ 0.5-μm-thick layer of undoped (i.e., intrinsic) a-Si:H is sufficient to absorb most visible wavelength photons entering the layer. However, often layer thicknesses of the order of 1 to 2 μm may be used to reduce pixel capacitance.

There are a number of ways intrinsic a-Si:H layers can be configured into a device sensitive to incident light. One distinguishing feature of these approaches is whether the device operates in a primary or secondary photoconductive mode. In the latter case, ohmic contacts to the a-Si:H layer allow a charge to be injected into the a-Si:H when a bias voltage is applied. If the recombination lifetime of the photogenerated charge carriers produced in the a-Si:H layer is longer than their transit time across the layer, there exists the possibility for *photoconductive gain*. This is a consequence of the requirement to maintain charge neutrality within the a-Si:H layer. When a photogenerated charge is collected at an electrode, a charge carrier of the same sign is injected into the layer by the other electrode to maintain charge neutrality. This injection continues until all the charge carriers of the opposite polarity reach an electrode or are lost to recombination. A single photogenerated carrier can thus effectively make a number of transits through the a-Si:H layer, giving rise to a photoconductive gain of $\sim \times 10$ to $\times 1000$. However, the required ohmic contacts also increase the dark current significantly, reducing the dynamic-range of the device. The temporal response is slowed and the magnitude of the gain is sensitive to many factors, for example, deposition parameters and details of the defect density in the band gap. This makes it difficult to fabricate devices with uniform behavior. Consequently, despite many years of development [84], secondary photoconductor mode sensors have been mostly confined to low dynamic-range applications (e.g., fax machines) [133].

There has recently been a resurgence of interest in providing gain at the pixel level to reduce the effects of additive electronic noise on the quality of the final image. One recent approach [134] describes a sensing element that incorporates a storage capacitor and a photosensitive TFT operated in photoresistive mode which produced a photoconductive gain of $\sim \times 17$. The use of a transistor structure for the sensing element simplifies the fabrication of the array because the photosensitive

TFT can be made with the same process, at the same time as the switching TFT. However, the magnitude of the signal photocurrent is dependent on the voltage across the drain source of the phototransistor. This changes as the storage capacitor integrates the photogenerated current and results in a highly nonlinear response of the pixel to varying intensities of incident light. Other more complex approaches incorporating sophisticated pixel-level amplification circuitry utilizing phototransistor sensing elements have also been reported [135] but as yet have not been applied to medical imaging.

Of greater importance for medical imaging are those devices that operate in a primary photoconductive mode. In this configuration the electrical connections to the intrinsic a-Si:H layer are blocking contacts. These prevent the injection of charge from the contacts into the a-Si:H layer while simultaneously permitting the signal charge to pass from the photoconductor to the contact. Thus the dark current and its associated noise are reduced. However, the inherent photoconductive gain for this mode of operation is limited to unity. Photodiodes are the most common example of this type of structure and will be discussed in detail.

An a-Si:H photodiode can be configured in a number of different ways, depending on the type of blocking contact to the $\sim$1 to 2-μm-thick intrinsic a-Si:H layer that absorbs the incident visible-wavelength photons. The most common approach is to use homo or hetero-junctions (i.e., junctions made from the same or different types of a-Si:H respectively) incorporating p- and n-type doped layers of amorphous or microcrystalline (μc-Si:H) silicon. These doped layers may also be alloyed with other elements such as carbon or germanium to adjust their optical properties [136, 137].

Figure 4.12(a) shows a cross section of an n-i-p photodiode made using microcrystalline silicon, μc-Si. This is only one example of the many possible designs but it will illustrate the pertinent features. The bottom metallic contact is chromium. This is followed by a $\sim$10 to 50-nm-thick n+ blocking layer, an $\sim$1.5-μm thick intrinsic a-Si:H layer, a $\sim$10 to 20-nm-thick p+ μc-Si$_{1-x}$C$_x$:H blocking layer, a $\sim$50-nm layer of transparent indium tin oxide (ITO), and finally a surface passivation layer of oxy-nitride which is very important in keeping the properties of the array stable. Sensors are usually oriented such that the p+ layer is towards the incoming light. This allows the movement of electrons, which have the higher mobility in a-Si:H, to be the main contributor of signal charge.

Light enters the intrinsic layer through the passivation layer, the ITO, and the p+ layer. Each of these layers absorbs some light, thereby reducing the absorption in the intrinsic layer and hence the signal measured in the photodiode. To lessen this detrimental effect, the passivation and ITO layers are made as thin as possible and the μc-Si:H in the p+ layer is alloyed with carbon to increase its optical band gap and hence transparency, and improve the diode reverse leakage current properties [138]. Photocharge generated in the p+ and n+ layers does not contribute to the signal charge because of the very short drift lengths of carriers in these heavily doped layers. An externally applied reverse bias voltage of $\sim$–5 V applied to the ITO, creates a depletion layer [139] across the thickness of the intrinsic a-Si:H.

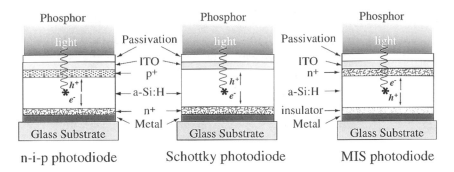

n-i-p photodiode   Schottky photodiode   MIS photodiode

Figure 4.12: Cross section of possible a-Si:H photodiode structures: (a) n-i-p, (b) Schottky, and (c) metal-insulator-semiconductor, MIS.

Each light photon absorbed in the depletion layer generates a single e-h pair. The electron moves towards the n+ layer and the hole towards the p+ layer under the action of the applied electric field. Because of the thin nature of the intrinsic a-Si:H layer and the relatively low intensities of incident photons from the overlying phosphor, geminate and non-geminate recombination [140] of the charge carriers in the bulk of the sensor are minimal. The majority of the photogenerated charge in the intrinsic layer is transferred to the n+ and p+ contacts. Some loss of charge may result from back diffusion of carriers at the p+/i-layer interface, but this is minimal at the low intensities typical of medical imaging applications.

Figure 4.13 shows the absolute quantum efficiency as a function of photon wavelength in the visible range for an ~ 1.5-μm thick n-i-p photodiode at –5V reverse bias. (Interference effects in the top passivation layer cause the pronounced periodicity.) The quantum efficiency drops at higher wavelengths because of increased penetration of the intrinsic layer and at lower wavelengths due to increased absorption in the p+ layer. Also in Figure 4.13 are the emission spectra for typical x-ray phosphors. It can be seen that the absorption range of a-Si:H is well matched to the emission from these phosphors.

The photodiode also acts as a capacitor to store the photogenerated charge. The intrinsic capacitance of the n-i-p structure is described by the parallel-plate capacitor formula:

$$C_{\mathrm{pd}} = \varepsilon_{\mathrm{r}} \varepsilon_{\mathrm{o}} A / d, \qquad (4.6)$$

where ε_{r} is the relative dielectric constant of the intrinsic semiconductor (for a-Si:H ~ 12), ε_{o} is the permittivity of free space (8.85×10^{-14} F cm^{-1}), A is the geometric area, and d the thickness of the photodiode. Thus a $100\,\mu$m $\times 100\,\mu$m, 1-μm-thick photodiode has a capacitance of ~ 1 pF. The total charge stored on the photodiode is its capacitance multiplied by the applied reverse bias voltage (e.g., ~ 5 pC at –5V-bias).

Another approach [Figure 4.12(b)] for creating an a-Si:H photodiode is a Schottky barrier diode formed when an appropriate metal is used as an electrical contact

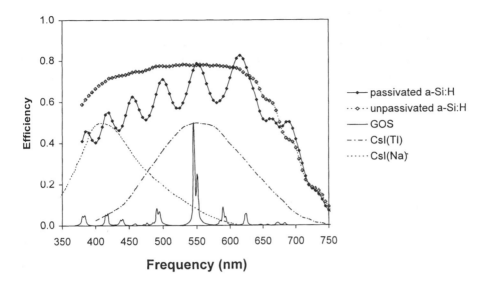

Figure 4.13: Quantum efficiency of intrinsic a-Si:H n-i-p photodiode compared to emission from various x-ray phosphors (a-Si:H efficiency data from Dr. R. Weisfield, dpiX, CsI(Tl) spectrum from Ref. [115], CsI(Na) spectrum from Bicron product guide).

to the intrinsic a-Si:H layer [129, 141, 142]. Photons interacting in the intrinsic a-Si:H layer generate e-h pairs and a reverse bias is applied to create a depletion layer for collection of this photogenerated charge. The signal charge is stored in the intrinsic self-capacitance of the photodiode also given by Eq. (4.6). The absence of a p+ layer in a Schottky diode permits a somewhat higher optical quantum efficiency than for an n-i-p diode [143]. It also means that their fabrication is more compatible with the processes used for the switching element of the pixel. Theoretically Schottky photodiodes are easier to fabricate in arrays but have an intrinsically higher dark current [144] ($\sim 10^{-9}$A cm^{-2}) than n-i-p diodes [145] ($\sim 10^{-11}$A cm^{-2}). Fabrication issues surrounding the dark-current stability and uniformity over large areas have also limited the application of these devices to medical imaging [141] with most investigators preferring to use n-i-p photodiodes.

Another a-Si:H photodiode has been reported [117] using an insulating dielectric layer in place of the p+ doped layer in a reversed (i.e., p-i-n) configuration. This is termed a MIS structure (metal-insulator-semiconductor) and is shown in Figure 4.12(c). Incident light passes through the n+ layer resulting in the movement of holes as the main component of the signal charge generated in the reverse biased depletion layer. These holes collect at the interface between the insulator and the a-Si:H layer, inducing a charge in the lower metal electrode. A refresh cycle is necessary with this design to remove the photogenerated holes present at this interface after the signal has been read out. This is achieved by reversing the polarity of the bias voltage applied to the upper metal contact. The front n+ blocking contact is placed in a forward biased condition and electrons are injected into the a-Si:H layer to neutralize the photogenerated holes. This design has the advantage of not requiring a p+ doping capability and is completely compatible with the process technology required for thin-film a-Si:H TFTs that only require n+ doping. In addition, the dielectric layer in the diode can be made from the same dielectric material used in the TFT. This allows both the sensor and TFT to be fabricated at the same time resulting in fewer processing steps.

4.3.2.2 Sensing/storage elements for direct detection

In the direct detection approach, the incoming signal has already been converted into charge by the interaction of the x rays with the overlying photoconductor. Consequently, in contrast to the myriad of designs for the photosensitive element in the indirect approach, the sensing element used in the direct approach is typically a simple charge storage capacitor and collection electrode requiring only dielectric and metal layers to construct. The storage capacitor is electrically connected to the overlying photoconductor by means of a pixel electrode. The pixel electrode acts as the foundation for the deposition of the thick layer of photoconductor that serves as the primary x-ray detection material. Finally, a continuous electrode is applied to the upper surface of the photoconductor to allow the application of an external bias voltage. Figure 4.14(a) illustrates this configuration. The choice of the top electrode metal of the active-matrix depends upon the type of electrical connection (e.g., blocking) to the photoconductive layer required [146]. With suitable choice of the metals and dielectric used in the capacitor and top electrode, the fabrication of this element can be made compatible with standard a-Si:H TFT manufacturing processes thus simplifying production and cost [147].

The operational requirements of the photoconductive layer are similar to those of the photodiode in the indirect approach in that a bias voltage must be applied across the thickness of the photoconductor to facilitate the separation and collection of the x-ray induced charges. To maintain an internal field of ~ 10 V μm^{-1} within a 500-μm-thick layer of a-Se, a bias voltage of ~ 5000 V must be applied. This high voltage has consequences for the design of the photoconductive layer, its surfaces and contacts, and the storage element. Blocking contacts to a-Se are not fully understood. However, the mechanism shown in Figure 4.14(b) that of a high density of traps within the a-Se layer close to the interface probably plays an important role. These traps, when filled, permit a rapid decrease in the field within the a-Se layer as the metal contact is approached resulting in minimal charge injection from the contact.

Without careful design it would be possible for almost the full 5000 V to appear across the switching and storage elements of the pixel in situations of high signal. This would result in failure and significant permanent damage to the performance of the array. When high voltage is first applied to the panel, the voltage drop is distributed between the pixel-storage capacitance and the a-Se pixel capacitance, which are in series, as shown in Figure 4.14(e). This configuration is a potential divider with the larger potential occurring across the smaller capacitance. Fortunately the capacitance of a ~ 500-μm-thick layer of a-Se is small (~ 5 pF cm^{-2}), so that an individual pixel of 200μm $\times 200 \mu$m has a capacitance of 0.002 pF. If

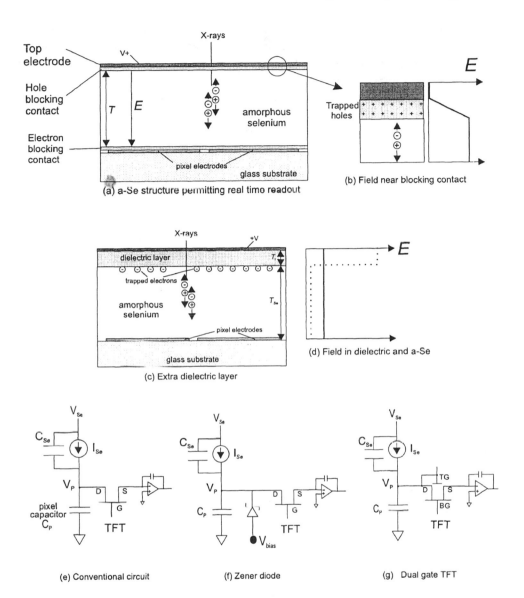

Figure 4.14: Several methods for high voltage protection of the active matrix in direct conversion flat panel imagers have been identified. In (a) a cross section of a layer of a-Se shows the functional layers in a simple direct conversion system. (b) Electric field in the region of the a-Se close to the top biasing electrode showing layer of hole traps filled with holes, creating a transition region from zero at the electrode up to the full field within the a-Se layer. (c) Dielectric layer added to trap charges and collapse field during excessive irradiation as shown in (d) Full line—field before irradiation, dotted line—after irradiation. (e) Basic circuit showing a passive immunity to an applied voltage V_{Se}. (f) Addition of a Zener diode as a safety element permits excess signal to bleed away at an exposure level controlled by the bias potential V_{bias}. (g) Second (top) gate on TFT to turn device *on* when potential V_p rises beyond a safe level controlled by the top gate dielectric layer thickness.

the storage capacitance is designed to be ~ 1 pF, the potential at the pixel electrode is only ~ 10 V with the other 4990 V being dropped across the a-Se layer. Thus, the components on the active-matrix panel can be protected in a purely passive manner from the application of the high potential.

However, this is not the only possible problem arising from the high voltage bias. If the panel is left without scanning, dark current or signal current from x-ray irradiation will cause the potential on the pixel electrode to rise towards the applied bias voltage. In the unusual event that this voltage increase is allowed to progress unchecked, the active matrix will eventually be damaged unless other means are taken to prevent the voltage at the pixel electrode reaching potentially damaging values. Two general approaches shown in Figure 4.14 have been proposed to solve this problem. The first, Figure 4.14(c), is to include an extra dielectric layer between the a-Se layer and the biasing electrode [114]. In this approach the potential drop is redistributed across the dielectric layer rather than in the storage capacitor as the potential across the a-Se layer collapses. However this protection results in increased read out complexity which must eliminate the trapped image at the a-Se/dielectric layer before subsequent exposures. This is achieved by removal of the applied bias voltage and flooding the detector with light to generate photocharge in a-Se that flows in the opposite direction to that generated by the x ray. The requirements of a refresh cycle make this approach to high-voltage damage protection incompatible with fluoroscopic (i.e., real-time read out) applications.

The second general approach is to maintain the real-time capability and also provide high-voltage protection. These methods incorporate a means of draining away the potential on the pixel if it exceeds a predetermined safe design value. Three suggestions in the literature are: (i) to include an extra component in parallel with the storage capacitor which has the desired characteristic (e.g., a Zener diode) as shown in Figure 4.14(f). A separate line biases this diode and provides a path to bleed excess charge from the pixel electrode [116]. (ii) To modify the TFT [148] by incorporation of a second gate connected to the pixel electrode as shown in Figure 4.14(g) to ensure that its channel current will increase to drain away the excess charge when the pixel potential approaches damaging levels. Because the excess charge is bled away along the read out lines, there is the potential for corruption of image information of pixels sharing the same read out line with overexposed pixels. (iii) To reverse the a-Se structure to permit a negative bias on the top electrode to ensure that the ordinary TFT will start to conduct when the pixel potential reaches the threshold value [149]. Then the circuit is as Figure 4.14(e), where the pixel potential V_p drops (becomes more negative) as exposure increases. Thus before V_p reaches damaging levels the TFT will turn *on*, draining charge away along the data line. Again, this approach has the disadvantage that excess charge from a single pixel could potentially corrupt the data from all the pixels along this particular data line. However, prototype systems have shown the ability to overcome this problem, at least for radiographic though not yet for fluoroscopic operation [149]. The simplicity of this array design makes it an attractive option.

As can be seen, although the basic design of the sensing/storage element for a direct detector is very simple, other issues surrounding the control of the high voltages required when using *a*-Se complicate the final design of the pixel. In the future, as experience with array design increases and fabrication yield improves, these issues will become less important. Other methods to overcome these problems will be developed; the use of different photoconductor materials operating satisfactorily with lower applied bias voltages and the fabrication of switching elements able to withstand higher voltages will improve the overall systems.

4.3.2.3 Switching elements: diodes

The other main component of the pixels on an active-matrix array is the switching element. As with the sensing element there are a number of different possibilities for its design. On active-matrix arrays fabricated using diodes for both the sensing and switching elements, the diodes are usually of the same type, (i.e., either all Schottky or all n-i-p diodes). Fabricating both diodes at the same time reduces the number of mask levels and consequently improves the device yield. Thus a complete array can be configured with as few as four mask steps. The general cross-sectional details of a switching diode are the same as that of the diode-sensing elements shown in Figure 4.12(a) and (b). The switching diodes are usually significantly smaller in area ($\sim$5%) than the sensing diode and are covered with a metallic light shield to prevent incident light increasing their reverse bias leakage current when they are in their *off* state. Modern diodes can achieve reverse bias current levels of $\sim10^{-11}$ A cm^{-2} at reasonable reverse bias voltages ($\sim$−3V) [145]. This gives the pixels excellent charge-retention capabilities in their unaddressed state that prevents signal loss during the signal integration period and signal sharing during the read out period. The forward bias *I–V* characteristic of the diode is also important. It determines the speed with which the image charge can be read out from the sensing element. For a diode, the forward bias current density J_f can be described by

$$J_f = J_0 \exp(e/nkT^*V), \tag{4.7}$$

where J_0 is the diode saturation current density [138] ($\sim10^{-12}$ A cm^{-2}), e is the charge of an electron, n is the diode ideality factor ($\sim$1.3–1.8) [150], k is Boltzmann's constant, T is the absolute temperature, and V the applied forward bias voltage. A drawback of a diode switch implied by this relationship is the exponential increase of the forward bias resistance with decreasing applied voltage. This intrinsic property of the diode structure affects the efficiency of charge-transfer between the sensing element and the external electronics and is a significant source of image lag in arrays utilizing diode switches. This problem can be somewhat alleviated by manipulation of the switching voltage to introduce offsets into the signal charge [115]. Another disadvantage of switching diodes is their higher capacitance (compared to TFT switches) resulting in greater signal cross talk between neighboring pixels and greater charge transients during switching. Nevertheless, their ease of fabrication makes the use of diode-switching elements attractive and a number of different pixel designs incorporating them have been reported [151–153, 171].

4.3.2.4 Switching elements: TFTs

The switching device with the best properties for the majority of medical imaging applications is the a-Si:H thin film transistor (TFT). Reviews of the basic physics [129, 154] of these devices, their fabrication [128], and theoretical modeling [155] are in the literature so only a brief discussion of their structure and the operational parameters specifically related to medical x-ray imaging will be given.

Figure 4.15 shows a cross-section of an a-Si:H TFT. This TFT is fabricated in the inverted staggered configuration with the gate as the first element deposited onto the substrate. Silicon nitride (a-Si$_3$N$_4$:H) is the usual gate insulator ($\varepsilon \sim 6.5$) and is $\sim$0.3–0.4 μm thick. The undoped a-Si:H layer is kept thin ($\sim$0.1 μm) to minimize the photosensitivity of the TFT [156]. The other layers are the n+ a-Si:H and metal source and drain contacts, the top a-Si$_3$N$_4$:H dielectric, and a final passivation layer. It should be noted that there is no p+ layer in the structure of an a-Si:H TFT. This has consequences for the sensing-element design on indirect-detection arrays because of the desire for compatibility between the process for fabricating the switching element and the sensing element. TFT switches used in indirect arrays also include a metallic light shield to prevent light affecting the *off* leakage current of the switch. The n+ a-Si:H layers control the contact between the intrinsic a-Si:H layer and the metal contacts of the drain and source. The distance between the drain and source contacts (known as the *channel length, L*) is $\sim$5 to 10 μm. TFTs are characterized by their W/L ratio where W is the width of the channel and can vary between $\sim$8 to as much as 128 μm.

Usually a-Si:H TFTs are configured to operate in the n-channel accumulation mode because of the higher field effect mobility of electrons compared to holes. This requires a positive gate voltage ($\sim +10$ to $+15$ V) to switch the device *on* and a negative voltage (~ -5 to -10 V) to switch it *off*. In the *off* condition the drain source current can be extremely small ($\sim 0.1 - 1 \times 10^{-15}$ A per μm channel width) for reasonable values of the drain-source voltage ($\sim$10 V) [157]. For a sensor array, this *off* current is particularly important because the leakage signal from all the unaddressed pixels along a data line is integrated into the signal from the pixel

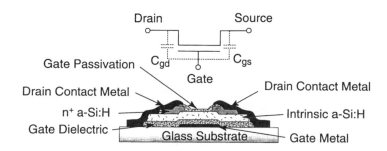

Figure 4.15: Details of the construction of a thin-film transistor, or TFT, showing a schematic cross section compared to its equivalent circuit. Also illustrated is the location of the overlap capacitance intrinsic to this type of TFT design.

being read out. Poly-silicon TFTs with a ~10 to 100× larger value of field-effect mobility for the electrons in the TFT channel [158] (~20 to 600 cm² V⁻¹ s⁻¹ and hence faster switching properties compared to standard a-Si:H TFTs), have not been applied as switching elements to medical imaging applications because of the accompanying increase in their leakage current in their *off* state. They may find a use in high-frame-rate devices for fluoroscopy and for multiplexing and amplifying circuitry to reduce the number of peripheral connections to the array. The issue of efficient fabrication of high-quality poly-Si and a-Si:H on the same substrate is an area of active research [159, 160].

In the *on* condition the drain source current, I_{ds}, through the TFT can be calculated from the expression developed for crystalline MOSFETs[161] given by

$$I_{ds} = \mu_{FE}\Gamma(W/L)(V_g - V_T - V_{ds}/2)V_{ds}, \qquad (4.8)$$

where μ_{FE} is the field-effect mobility of the electrons in the channel (~0.75 to 1 cm² V⁻¹ s⁻¹), Γ is the gate capacitance (~20 nF cm⁻²), W/L is the TFT width-to-length ratio, V_g is the gate voltage (~10 to 15 V), V_T is the threshold voltage of the TFT (~1 to 2 V), and V_{ds} is the drain-source voltage (<5 V). For values of $V_{ds} \ll (V_g - V_T)$ the TFT is in its linear range of operation and for a W/L ratio of ~10 the *on* resistance of the TFT is ~1 MΩ. This resistance, R_{on}, combined with the pixel capacitance C_{pixel} determines the RC time constant to read the signal charge from the sensing element. In contrast to the diode switch, the value of R_{on} for a TFT is essentially independent of the drain-source voltage.

The characteristic curve of a typical TFT (i.e., value of I_{ds} for different applied gate voltage V_g) is shown in Figure 4.16. The *on* to *off* ratios for the current through this device is extremely high (>10¹⁰), that is, they have excellent switching properties. It should be remembered that if the drain-source voltage approaches V_g in

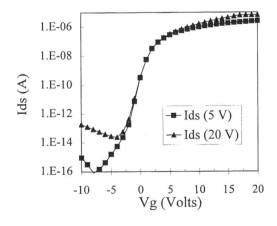

Figure 4.16: Electrical transfer characteristic where I_{ds} is the channel current and V_{gs} is the gate voltage of a typical a-Si:H TFT with $W = 16\,\mu m$ and $L = 8\,\mu m$ (courtesy of Dr. R. Weisfield, dpiX).

the *off* condition, the leakage current can increase significantly as the TFT effectively starts to turn *on*. For the direct approach, this can be used to advantage to avoid damage to the TFT. However, for the indirect method it has implications for the relative magnitudes of the photodiode reverse bias voltage and the TFT gate voltage. To prevent leakage of signal from pixels close to their saturation level, the source and drain contacts must remain at least V_T more positive than the gate voltage.

A problem in the operation of a TFT is the coupling capacitance between the gate line and the source and drain contacts of the TFT. One component of this coupling is the physical overlap ($\sim$1 to 4 μm [157, 162]) between the gate metal and the drain and source metal contacts. This is inherent in the fabrication approach currently used and results in a coupling capacitance of $\sim$10 to 15 nF cm^{-2} between the gate contact and the drain and source contacts for a TFT in its *off* condition. When the TFT is *on*, the coupling capacitance is determined by the gate capacitance of $\sim$20 nF cm^{-2} [190]. Improvements in TFT fabrication are, however, reducing the overlap capacitance to negligible values [163]. Another source of charge coupling in certain array designs is the crossover capacitance between the different metallic lines such as the data and gate control lines at each pixel. Theoretically this can contribute $\sim$1 to 2 nF cm^{-2} to the overall capacitance between the gate and data lines, depending on the dielectric material used for the array passivation (e.g., $\varepsilon_r \sim$3 to 4) [147]. However, fringing field effects can increase the value of this crossover capacitance substantially. Reducing the width of the control and signal lines at the crossover points can help reduce this capacitance. In array designs which necessitate the use of separate bias voltage supply lines, there is also capacitive coupling between these and the gate and data lines. This is mainly through the fringing fields of the photodiode contact layers. The magnitude of this coupling capacitance depends on the exact details of the array design but can be a significant contributor to the total data line capacitance seen by the external electronics.

As a result of the gate/data-line-coupling capacitance, charge is injected into the sensor and onto the data line whenever the gate voltage is switched. The polarity and magnitude of this charge must be considered when designing the charge capacity of both the sensor and the external amplification electronics because it can amount to a significant fraction of the total signal capacity of the pixel. Small changes in the gate voltage of the unaddressed TFTs along a data line can also result in *line-correlated noise* in the final image resulting from the related charge injection. Fluctuations in the bias voltage are also coupled into the data line by these mechanisms and can be an additional source of image noise.

Voltage stressing is another issue of concern for stable TFT operation [164]. It has been found that the threshold voltage, V_T in Eq. (4.8), can change with time when the TFT is subjected to sustained gate voltages. This in turn affects the TFT resistance and consequently the TFT leakage current and the time required to read the signal charge from the pixel. For the level of voltages used in typical x-ray imaging arrays ($\sim -$ 10 to +15 V_g) this effect is small and can be taken into account by appropriate choice of the read out integration time and the TFT operating voltages [165].

4.3.3 Array design

As can be appreciated from the variety of switching and sensing elements described above, the design of an active-matrix x-ray imaging array requires many decisions and compromises. Some, such as pixel size, are dictated by the application the array is to serve; others, such as the specific design of the pixel elements, are dependent on factors such as availability of technology, ease of fabrication, and intellectual property considerations. There is a continuous struggle between pixel-performance optimization and the desire for fabrication simplicity to increase yield and hence reduce the overall cost. This section will discuss some general considerations of pixel properties such as size and read out speed, as well as the configuration and general operation of various approaches to array design currently being pursued.

Detectors for digital radiography are composed of discrete elements, generally of constant size and spacing. The dimension of the *active* portion of each detector element defines an *aperture*. The aperture determines the spatial frequency response of the detector. For example, if the aperture is square with dimension, a, then its intrinsic modulation transfer function (MTF) will be of the form $\mathrm{sinc}(f)$, where f is the spatial frequency along the x or y directions. The MTF will have its first zero at the frequency $f = a^{-1}$, expressed in the plane of the detector. Thus, a detector with $a = 200\,\mu\mathrm{m}$ will have a sinc function MTF with its first zero at $f = 5$ cycles mm^{-1}.

The sampling interval, p, of the detector, that is, the pitch in the detector plane between sensitive elements, is also of considerable importance. The sampling theorem states that only spatial frequencies in the image below $(2p)^{-1}$ (the Nyquist frequency) can be faithfully imaged. If the image contains higher frequencies, then *aliasing* occurs. Here, the frequency spectrum of the image beyond the Nyquist frequency is mirrored or folded about that frequency and added to the spectrum of lower frequencies, becoming indistinguishable from them. In a detector composed of discrete non-overlapping elements, the smallest sampling interval in a single image acquisition is $p = a$. The Nyquist frequency is $(2p)^{-1}$ which, our example of $p = a = 200\,\mu\mathrm{m}$, is 2.5 cycles mm^{-1} while the aperture response falls to zero at 5 cycles mm^{-1} (twice the Nyquist frequency). The limit of the aperture response can be even higher if the dimension of the sensitive region of the detector element is *smaller* than p. This aliasing is inherent in all such detectors at the photodiode or electrode plane.

Aliasing in such detectors can be avoided by *band limiting* the image, in other words, attenuating the higher frequencies until there is no appreciable content beyond the Nyquist frequency. The blurring associated with the focal spot may serve this purpose. Alternatively, the sampling frequency of the imaging system can be increased. One method for achieving this, *dithering,* involves multiple acquisitions with a physical motion of the detector by a fraction of the pixel pitch between successive acquisitions. The subimages are then combined to form the final image. This effectively reduces p, which results in a higher Nyquist frequency. However, the most satisfactory method is one that unlike the previous examples reduces the

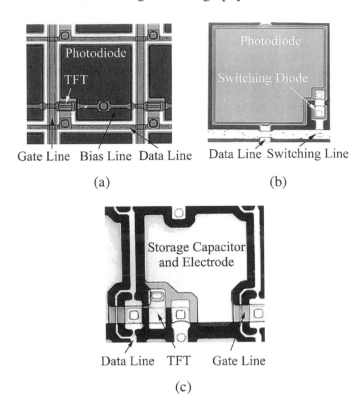

Figure 4.17: Photomicrographs of pixel arrays: (a) indirect approach using n-i-p photodiode (courtesy of Dr. R. Weisfield, dpiX);(b) indirect conversion method, diode readout switch and photodiode (courtesy of Jacky Dutin, Thomson-CSF); (c) direct method with ITO pixel electrodes [89].

response of the system both to signal (as above) and noise. This can be achieved by incorporation of blurring in the detector structure prior to sampling. This is called pre-sampling blurring.

The most fundamental decision for a digital imaging system is the size of the pixel. Detailed knowledge of the intended application is essential for this determination but array design constraints can also have significant impact. One of the main considerations, from an array design perspective, is a property known as *geometrical fill factor*, which is the fraction of the pixel area sensitive to the incoming signal. In the indirect detection approach this is just the fractional area of the sensing element which is photosensitive. In the direct detection approach the definition is more complicated as there may be electric field dependent changes in fill factor. Thus the *effective* fill factor and geometrical fill factor have to be differentiated. Figure 4.17 consists of photomicrographs of some flat-panel arrays. The active region of the photodiodes, electrodes, the switching FET, and the various control lines are all clearly visible, illustrating the fact that the geometric fill factors are not 100%.

Several factors affect the magnitude of the geometrical fill factor. These include: the alignment tolerances of the step-and-repeat technique used to photolithographically pattern the full surface area of the array from a smaller reticle mask; the precision with which a layer can be etched so as to avoid *shorts* between separate array elements; the resistance of the metal lines on the array; and the parasitic capacitance between neighboring structures. These factors are summarized for the use of the array designer as the *design rules* of a particular fabrication process. The design rules govern, among other things, the width of metallic lines ($\sim 10\,\mu$m) and the gaps between neighboring structures ($\sim 5\,\mu$m). For a particular fabrication process, the design rules are usually independent of pixel size. Consequently, the nonsensitive components of the pixel occupy a larger and larger fraction of the pixel area as the pixel pitch reduces. Figure 4.18(a, b) illustrates this dependence of fill factor with pixel pitch for a simplified design rule example (i.e., neglecting the area occupied by the switching element). Because there are irreducible elements for any particular set of design rules there will be a threshold below which the fill factor drops precipitously. This is a major issue confronting the design of arrays for applications that require high spatial resolution such as mammography (~ 50 to $100\,\mu$m pixels).

One solution that can maintain fill factor for smaller pixel sizes has been incorporated into the design of direct detection arrays as shown in Figure 4.18(c). The top electrode of the capacitive structure is extended over the top of the switching element. This *mushroom* electrode design [114] allows a high geometrical fill factor to be maintained ($\sim 85\%$) even with high-resolution array designs (~ 139-μm pitch). It has been shown theoretically that in most cases an effective fill factor of $\sim 100\%$ can be achieved in direct detectors by appropriately controlling the collection fields as shown in Figure 4.18(c) [166]. Research into methods of improving effective pixel fill factor with indirect detection approaches include the use of more aggressive design rules [7, 167], photodiodes formed from continuous layers of a-Si:H [168, 169] [Figure 4.18(d)] or optically sensitive a-Se[170] and the development of 3D structures that let the photodiode extend over the top of the switching element [145]. This is similar to the mushroom approach described above but requires a much thicker dielectric layer ($\sim 5\mu$m) between the overlying photodiode and the TFT to avoid excessive capacitive coupling effects between the two.

An important design consideration of an indirect sensing element is the thickness of the intrinsic a-Si:H layer. The compromise is between increased absorption of the incident light with thicker layers but increased charge holding capacity for thinner layers. Most contemporary photodiodes have i-layer thicknesses ~ 1.5 to $2\,\mu$m giving pixel capacitances of ~ 5 to $7\,$nF cm^{-2}. This capacitance also controls the speed with which signal charge can be extracted from the pixel and therefore affects the maximum frame rate achievable with a particular pixel design. If the switching diode and sensing diode are fabricated at the same time, the thickness of the two diodes will be the same. A thinner layer improves the forward bias current of the switch but increases its intrinsic capacitance. Therefore a compromise must be reached between the conflicting requirements of sensor optimization and switch performance [171]. This compromise may be avoided if the diodes are fabricated in separate steps but this increases the complexity and cost [172]. The pixel capacitance in the direct method can be selected independently of sensing requirements. It does however affect read out speed, saturation charge holding capacity, noise, and is also related to high-voltage damage protection.

Frame-rate considerations affect the choice of switching element design. In general, physically larger switches tend to have lower *on* resistance which improves read out speed but correspondingly lower *off* resistance which affects charge leakage from the pixel in its *off* state. Larger switches also use up more space on the panel that can reduce the pixel fill factor. Modern switching diodes are typically

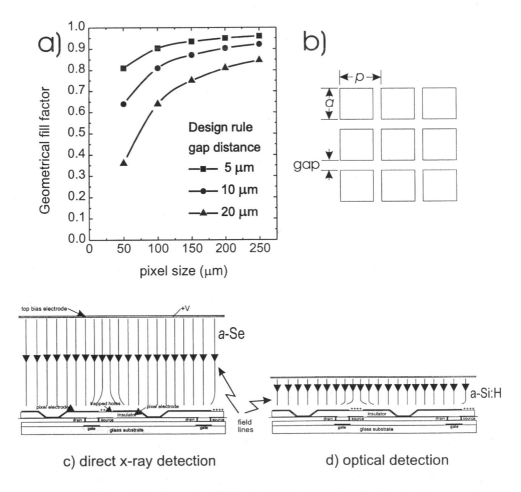

c) direct x-ray detection   d) optical detection

Figure 4.18: Plot of (a) geometrical fill factor versus pixel pitch for the simple array shown in (b) assuming the design rules limit only the gap distances between electrodes or photodiodes. Means to increase the effective fill factor are shown for the direct conversion approach by use of (c) mushroom electrodes, and for the indirect conversion approach (d) continuous photodiodes.

$\sim 10 \times 10$ to $20 \times 20 \, \mu m^2$ while current TFT designs have W/L ratios of $\sim$1:1 to 10:1 (with $L \sim$5 to $10 \, \mu m$).

One final consideration is the kind of metals used for the gate and data lines. Chromium has advantageous fabrication properties but rather high resistivity ($\sim 12 \, \mu\Omega$ cm) while aluminum has lower resistivity ($\sim 3 \, \mu\Omega$ cm) but can form spikes which cause electrical shorts in the array. Combinations of different metal layers such as Al capped with Cr result in low resistance with fewer fabrication problems [163]. On large panels the resistive and capacitive loading associated with these lines can be large enough to affect pixel switching times [173] and noise levels [174]. Increasing the line width reduces their resistance but has an adverse effect on fill factor and data line coupling capacitance.

Figure 4.19 shows cross-sectional details of several different pixel configurations currently under development. The first three are indirect detection approaches while the fourth is one example of a direct detection approach incorporating an a-Se layer and an insulator layer for high-voltage protection. An equivalent electrical circuit is also shown for each design. Electrically the greatest difference is between those using a TFT switching element and those using a diode switch. This will be discussed in more detail in Section 4.4.2.

Other pixel configurations incorporate three diodes arranged such that two form the switching element and the third the sensing photodiode [152, 153]. This design has the potential advantage of transient charge cancellation but is more complicated to fabricate and control.

4.3.4 Noise sources intrinsic to array

There are a number of noise sources intrinsic to the different components on an active-matrix array. These cause fluctuations in signal in addition to those from the noise sources inherent to the x-ray detection media described in Section 4.2.3. An understanding of their origin, nature, and magnitude can help in determining strategies to reduce their degrading effect on the final image.

The noise sources from the array can be divided into those that originate on the active-matrix itself, and those that are generated by the electrical components connected to the array. This latter type, associated with external voltage fluctuations and intrinsic amplifier noise, will be discussed in Section 4.4.3.

The noise sources inherent to the switching and sensing elements and the distributed resistances of the metallic connection lines have been discussed by a number of authors. They result from many factors ranging from the familiar thermal generation of charge carriers in resistive elements to less well known sources such as charge partition noise and trapping noise in the pixel switching elements. Many are similar to those arising in the equivalent crystalline silicon components and consequently their modeling has drawn heavily on the analysis of noise sources in MOSFETs and CCD structures [176]. Figure 4.20 shows the origin of noise sources arising on or near to the array.

An unavoidable noise source from the array, shown in Figure 4.20(a), is kTC switching noise associated with the thermal noise in the switching element

[121, 175]. This arises because the operation of a switch amounts to changing the value of a resistor. Thus kTC noise is another manifestation of Johnson noise, and in effect traps a charge of magnitude $\sqrt{(kTC)}$ on the capacitor for every operation of the switch where T is the absolute temperature and C is the pixel capacitance of the sensing/storage element of the pixel. For the flat-panel detector, this noise appears twice, in the charge trapped on the capacitor on the previous read out of the pixel and again when it is discharged. Thus for the flat-panel detector, switching noise takes the form $\sqrt{(2kTC)}$. For a 1-pF pixel capacitance at room temperature this is $\sim$560 electrons. The TFT channel resistance gives rise to another two kinds of noise while the TFT is *on*; these are Johnson noise (or thermal noise) shown

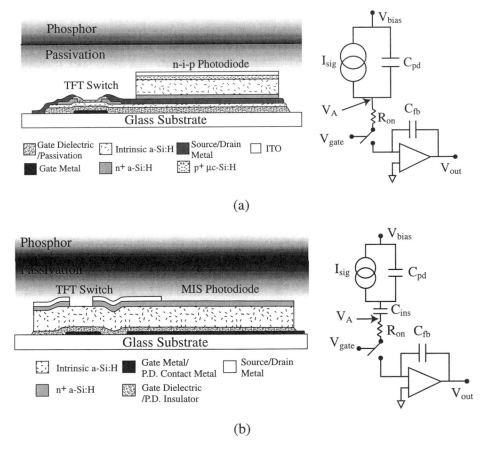

(a)

(b)

Figure 4.19: Cross section of pixel configurations and schematic circuit diagrams for various flat-panel x-ray detector concepts: (a)–(c) indirect conversion (d) one particular direct conversion approach. (a) TFT readout and n-i-p photodiode, (b) TFT readout and MIS photodiode, (c) Diode readout of n-i-p photodiode, (d) TFT readout of a photoconductor layer showing mushroom structure and high voltage protection provided by a layer of insulator below the top electrode. This demonstrates only one of the many different possible direct detection structures.

in Figure 20(b) and flicker noise (or $1/f$ noise) in the channel resistance. Both of these components are modified by the bandwidth of the read out circuit and the method of read out, for example, whether or not double correlated sampling is used, and therefore cannot be calculated until all the components of the read out chain are analyzed.

Another source of noise is the shot noise and $1/f$ noise associated with the thermally generated dark current in the photodiode or photoconductor. The magnitude of the dark current decreases as the temperature decreases. However, the signal strength also reduces as the temperature decreases because thermal excitation of photogenerated charge from traps is an important mechanism in determining charge collection efficiency. An optimal temperature for operation of the array probably exists but to date only limited investigation of it has been reported [141].

More recently, attention has turned to the effect of the distributed resistance of the metallic lines on the array [174, 176]. This is shown schematically in Figure 4.20(c). These act as a source of thermally generated noise as well as a high-frequency transmission-line noise filter when combined with the distributed cou-

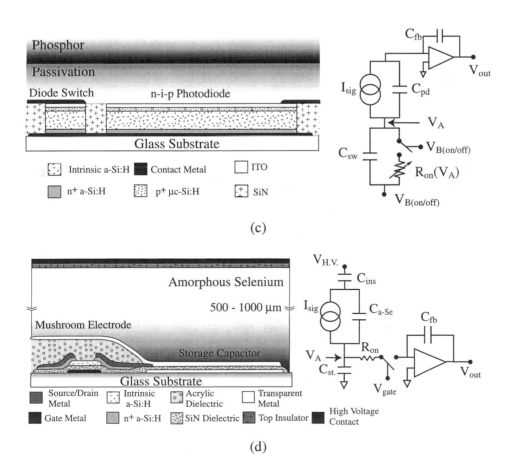

(c)

(d)

Figure 4.19: (Continued).

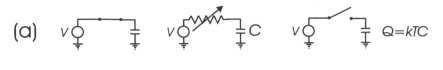

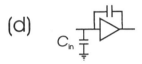

Figure 4.20: Sources of noise in flat-panel imager readout: (a) switching or kTC noise resulting from operation on pixel switch, (b) thermal noise in the TFT channel resistance R_{on}, (c) distributed resistance and capacitance along the readout data lines, and (d) capacitance loading of the input amplifier.

pling capacitance along a data, bias, or switching control line. Detailed calculations [176] show that, for values of data-line resistance ~ 2.5 kΩ and data-line coupling capacitance ~ 50 pF, this noise source can approach that of the best designed pre-amplifier. It therefore must be carefully investigated when analyzing the anticipated noise from any proposed array design. Most other noise sources from the array components such as the dark current noise, charge partition noise, and TFT trapping noise are of the order of ~ 100 to 200 electrons [176], which is negligible compared to the switching and resistance noise sources described above. Care should be taken before dismissing sources that cause correlated noise on the pixels along a particular row or column of the image. The sensitivity of the human visual system to line-correlated noise of this type can put severe constraints on the acceptable magnitude of such a source.

As the noise level and design of external electronics improves and the capabilities for fabricating arrays with lower line capacitance and resistance develop, the intrinsic noise sources from the pixel components will become more important in the optimization of the system performance.

4.4 Configuration and operation of a flat-panel x-ray imager

Up to this point we have described separately the details of the x-ray detection media and the pixel components on the different designs of active-matrix arrays currently being pursued. In this section we will discuss briefly the coupling of the x-ray detection media and the active-matrix array into a complete x-ray imaging system, and give a more detailed description of the basic operational behavior of the system. The general requirements of the external electronics and the image processing necessary to make the resulting images diagnostically useful will also be outlined.

4.4.1 X-ray imager configuration

The process of coupling the x-ray detection media to the underlying active-matrix array ranges from the relatively simple step of laying a commercially available powdered phosphor screen on top of the array and ensuring reasonably good optical contact between both, to the technologically demanding evaporation of highly specialized layers of a-Se photoconductor or CsI:Tl phosphor onto the array surface under extremely well controlled conditions. The ease with which the first approach can be achieved perhaps explains why much of the early investigative work into the imaging performance of active-matrix arrays was performed with this configuration. It is also commercially attractive because the coupling of the array and phosphor can be done with little or no risk of inducing damage in the active matrix structure.

Although it is extremely technically demanding, the control of the intrinsic properties of the different layers of a-Se has reached a level close to that of crystalline silicon [177–179]. The evaporation of the thick layers required for diagnostic energy x-ray imaging is therefore feasible as long as one takes the appropriate measures to ensure efficient blocking contacts with the underlying array electrodes [40, 146, 149].

The process of evaporating high-quality columnar-structured CsI has also been perfected for many years in association with the development of the high-performance XRII tubes common in today's radiology departments. Coupling the layer of CsI to the active-matrix array can be done in one of two ways. (a) The evaporation may be done directly onto the surface of the array where appropriate patterning of the top layer of the array can enhance the columnar structure of the CsI. (b) The CsI can be evaporated onto a separate substrate (e.g., Al) and subsequently mated to the surface of the active matrix. Both these approaches are the subject of research and development efforts in a number of different laboratories.

4.4.2 Operation of a flat-panel x-ray detector

Figure 4.19 shows simplified equivalent circuits and cross sections for a number of different pixel designs. These will help to elucidate the similarities between the operation of the different designs. Figure 4.19(a, b, and d) represent pixels with a TFT as the switching element while (c) is a double diode structure. The sensing element is represented as a capacitor and current generator whose current is dependent on the intensity of the incident x rays. The dark current of the sensing element is neglected in this analysis. The switching element has been represented as a resistor R_{on} connected to a perfect switch. The state of this switch is controlled by the voltage V_{gate}. This configuration has either resistance R_{on} (i.e., its

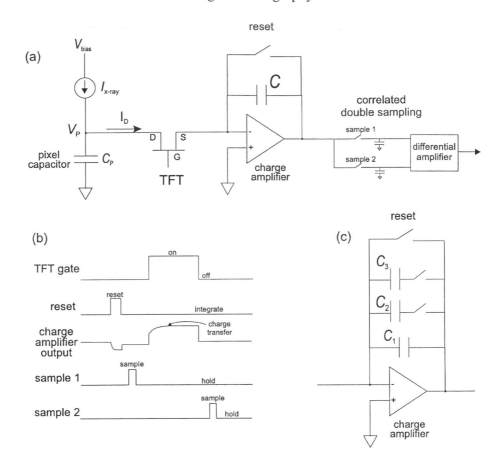

Figure 4.21: Readout electronics: in (a) the readout circuit is shown with the facility for correlated double sampling, or CDS, and in (b) readout timing diagram including operation of the reset switch and CDS, (c) variable gain preamplifier to accommodate operation at different input exposure levels without overloading.

on state) or infinitely high resistance (i.e., its *off* state). The external circuitry used with x-ray flat-panel detectors is almost invariably a charge-sensitive preamplifier configuration, which maintains its input at virtual ground. Figure 4.21 shows other more detailed aspects of the read out circuitry.

The operation of these circuits can be described by examining the voltage at the connection point between the switching element and the sensing element, V_A. In the TFT switch designs in Figure 4.19(a, b, and d), with the array in its initialized state just prior to the x-ray exposure, the switch is in its high-resistance *off* state. Then, V_A is close to ground and there is no charge present on the storage capacitor in Figure 4.19(d). When x rays are incident on the array, both indirect [Figure 4.19(a, b)] and direct designs [Figure 4.19(d)] generate a current in the sensor, I_{sig} which is integrated onto the inherent capacitance of the sensor and the storage capacitor (if present). Because of the high resistance of the switch in its *off* condition, the current integrates quicker than it can escape through the switch. This causes the voltage V_A to move towards the applied voltage V_{bias} or $V_{H.V}$. This discharges the inherent capacitance of the sensing element in Figures 4.19(a) and (b), and at the same time charges the storage capacitor in Figure 4.19(d). When the x-ray exposure is terminated, the current I_{sig} drops to zero and V_A becomes stationary. The magnitude of the change in V_A during the exposure is thus proportional to the number of absorbed x rays. During the read out cycle, the switch is put in its low-resistance *on* state. A current then flows from the external circuitry to re-establish the voltage V_A at its initial value. This current is integrated on the feedback capacitor of the preamplifier. The output voltage from the preamplifier is proportional to the magnitude of the integrated charge and therefore related to the intensity of the incident x rays. This output voltage is then finally routed to an analog to digital converter or ADC for digitization.

The process is essentially the same with the diode switch [Figure 4.19(c)]. The main difference is that V_B is varied during read out to control the state of the switching, that is, V_{Bon} and V_{Boff} at different stages of the image acquisition cycle. The initialized state has V_A close to the voltage applied to put the switching diode in its forward biased condition, V_{Bon} ($\sim$−5 V). With the control voltage set to V_{Boff} ($\sim$0 V), x-ray-generated current causes V_A to move toward ground as it discharges the inherent capacitance of the photodiode and the switching diode simultaneously. The image information is again contained in the amount of charge required to re-establish V_A to its initial value when the pixel is addressed by changing V_B to V_{Bon}.

The rate of signal transfer from the pixel to the preamplifier is determined by the discharge rate of a capacitor through a resistor. For switches whose resistance remains constant, this is characterized by the *on* resistance, R_{on}, of the switch ($\sim$1–2 MΩ for a TFT) and the effective capacitance, C_{sen}, of the sensing element ($\sim$1 to 2 pF for $\sim$100-μm pixels), giving time constants in the region of 1 to 4 μs. This read out behavior has been verified for a TFT + photodiode design [180]. For diode switches, the situation is somewhat more complex because the *on* resistance increases as the voltage across the diode switch reduces.

From this analysis, the process of reading out the information from the different designs of pixel elements is shown to be very similar. However, putting the detector into an initialization state suitable for a subsequent exposure is where the major differences between designs become manifest. The simplest situation is with TFT switch approaches where reading out the pixel information also serves as the initialization of the pixel, provided the TFT is switched *on* for a sufficient number of pixel *RC* time constants to read out all the signal charge (typically $\sim$7–10$\times R_{on}C_{sen}$) [101]. In contrast, the resistance of the diode switch increases exponentially as the voltage V_A approaches the value V_{Bon} (i.e., the closer to the true initialization condition). This variable *on* resistance of the switching diode results in excessively long time constants for the read out of small signals. This can be ameliorated using an offset voltage and optical reset cycle to move the zero signal level of V_A out of the high-resistance regime of the switching diode [172]. The

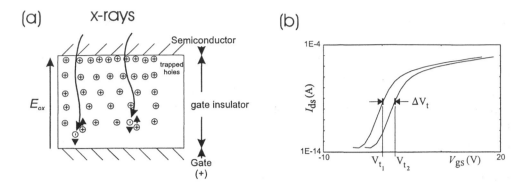

Figure 4.22: Schematic diagram of the effects of trapped charge in the gate dielectric created by irradiation causing a shift in the characteristic curve of a TFT. In (a) the trapped charge (holes) building up in the gate dielectric layer due to irradiation. (b) The shift of the threshold voltage of the TFT (i.e., the potential at which the device switches *on*) due to the permanently trapped charge, which will typically be of the order of 0.1–10% of the total charge released by irradiation.

optical reset pulse has the beneficial effect of filling many of the metastable forbidden band states in the a-Si:H sensor that can cause image lag and charge trapping in the pixel.

The pixel designs which incorporate additional capacitive structures [e.g., C_{ins} in Figures 4.19(b) [181] and (d)] also require an additional reset cycle, but for a somewhat different reason. Because of the nature of the multiple-capacitor structure, after the pixel has been read out, it is necessary to redistribute the charges in the central capacitive element to their initialization configuration before another image can be acquired. This can be achieved by manipulation of the applied bias voltage, which causes charge to flow in the direction opposite to that during image acquisition [114, 182]. This process can be facilitated by the application of optical reset pulse(s) [183]. There have also been a number of direct approaches suggested and demonstrated using *a*-Se which have configurations suitable for operation without the requirement of a reset cycle [3, 116]. It can be seen from this discussion that rather than a significant difference existing in the read out protocols of indirect and direct detectors, the differences are more associated with the details of the electrical structure of the pixel.

The situation in a real imaging device is complicated by factors not discussed in the simple model outlined above. These include: the charge-coupling transients present whenever the switching element is changed from one conduction state to another; the small but finite leakage current through the switch in its *off* state; the dark leakage current of the sensing element; and the effect of charge trapping and release from the metastable states in the sensing element.

The concept of a flat-panel detector mandates that a considerable part of the detector is directly in the radiation beam. Because the detection media will probably never absorb all of the radiation impinging on it, a considerable amount of radiation is inevitably incident directly onto the active matrix. Thus for a practical system, it is absolutely required that the array be radiation hard, at least to the dose levels anticipated during the lifetime of an array. This dose depends upon the application but has been estimated at 5000 cGy for a diagnostic detector [4, 184] and perhaps two to three orders of magnitude larger for therapy imaging [126]. It has been shown that the primary effect of radiation on a-Si:H TFTs arises in the insulator layer. Trapped charge in this layer (usually holes) can compromise the switching behavior of the TFT. The schematic of this mechanism is shown in Figure 4.22. The problems which arise if the threshold voltage changes is that the TFTs on the panel may not switch completely *on* or *off* under the control of the gate line voltage. Thus, the critical factor is that the threshold voltage should not change by an amount comparable to the actual gate voltage swing. For example the threshold change should usually be less than 5 V. It has been shown that this can be achieved even for therapy doses encountered during portal imaging [102, 126]. The radiation damage threshold for other components of flat panel imagers is also required to be high. Research has shown that the radiation damage that results in charge trapping centers in the a-Se layer, is annealed in a few hours at room temperature [178]. Similar observations have also been made with a-Si:H devices for dose levels appropriate for diagnostic imaging applications while annealing at elevated temperatures repaired the damage experienced at even higher exposures [126]. The damage in the phosphor layer at very large doses can also be a concern as irradiated phosphors will eventually accumulate trapped charge, which acts to make the material less transparent. This causes a gradual loss of light output with extended radiation exposure [64]. However, this effect is unlikely to be an issue at the dose levels experienced in normal radiographic environments.

4.4.3 Peripheral electronics requirements

The electronic and computing requirements of a flat-panel x-ray imaging system can be divided into two distinct areas. The first, the peripheral electronics, is the circuitry that supplies the required voltages to the active-matrix elements and amplifies and digitizes the signals from the pixels. This includes the logic that synchronizes the image acquisition and the read out and transfer of the image to the external computer. This part of the system must be carefully tailored to each particular detector and can have a significant effect on the imaging performance of the system. The second is the computer that controls the overall operation of the system. The software must be developed and adapted to a specific application. In real-time fluoroscopy, custom-built high-speed hardware has to be developed [174, 185] to permit real-time manipulation and transfer of images. This section will discuss issues surrounding the peripheral circuitry and how it affects the imaging performance of the complete flat-panel imaging system.

All the peripheral electronics attached to an active-matrix array can potentially act as sources of noise tending to reduce the quality of the final image. The most critical component is the preamplifier that accepts the signal from the pixels data line when they are addressed. The standard configuration is a charge-integrating design where the signal charge from the pixel is transferred to the feedback capacitor of the preamplifier. The magnitude of this feedback capacitor determines the electronic gain (mV/pC). The reset switch is used to remove the charge on the feedback capacitors before the next pixel is addressed as shown in Figure 4.21(a) with the timing diagram shown in Figure 4.21(b).

The performance of charge-sensitive preamplifiers shown in Figure 4.21(a) is usually specified by a noise floor level and a noise slope given in electrons per unit of input capacitance. Values of ~300 to 500 e for the noise floor and slopes of ~3 to 6 e pF^{-1} have been reported [115, 119]. A typical large-area flat-panel detector will present ~50 to 100 pF of input data line capacitance to the preamplifier resulting in a noise contribution of ~500 to 2000 e. Splitting the data lines to permit read out from both ends halves this input capacitance but requires double the number of preamplifiers. Calculations have shown that the preamplifiers can often be the limiting noise source [121, 186, 187]. For the zero-frequency DQE situation, this level of noise has minimal effect on systems for general radiographic and mammographic applications but becomes more important as spatial frequency increases [187] and for the low exposures encountered in fluoroscopy. In order to match the signal level to subsequent stages, it is sometimes necessary to permit variable gain preamplifiers, achieved with a switching network of feedback capacitors on each preamplifier as shown in Figure 4.21(c).

Because each data line requires its own preamplifier and there may be 2000 or more, the preamplifiers are configured into an application-specific integrated circuit (ASIC), so that many channels (usually ~64 to 128) can be fabricated on the same piece of crystalline silicon. For high-resolution arrays, where the distance between data lines becomes very small, making the circuitry at the same pitch as the pixels becomes difficult because of the large area on the ASIC required for the capacitive elements. In the future, analog multiplexers fabricated directly on the active-matrix array, probably made using poly-Si, will address this problem.

Readout configurations incorporate multiple sampling techniques such as correlated double sampling [119, 188] which can be used for various purposes. In principle it is used to measure the output of the panel twice, before and after an event, to correct for a factor that is unchanged. One approach [3] is sampling the signal from the pixel immediately before and after the image charge has been transferred to the preamplifier. This is shown in Figure 4.21(a, b) which has the feature of correcting for the kTC charge trapped on the amplifier feedback capacitor after it is reset. This specific technique does not remove the effect of low-frequency noise fluctuations. A similar noise-reduction technique can be used in which a dummy sample is obtained which will remove line frequency pick-up noise from the signal. It should be remembered that subtraction techniques increase uncorrelated noise sources by a factor of ~$\sqrt{2}$ and this must be compared against the magnitude of any reductions obtained by using these techniques.

A powerful approach to reduce the effect of the electronic noise is to increase the size of the signal from the pixel. This could be achieved by pixel-level amplification [111, 135, 189] or by increasing the amount of charge produced by the incident x-ray. This stimulates interest in alternative photoconductors such as PbI_2, PbO, and TlBr, which require less energy than a-Se (Table 4.2) or CsI:Tl (Table 4.3) to generate an e-h pair. There is also the possibility of using avalanche multiplication [41] which can be applied both to direct and indirect detectors.

The other main components of array-level circuitry are the bias voltage lines to the individual sensing elements in the indirect approach and the lines to control voltages to the switching elements. These all act as sources of image noise in flat-panel detectors. Fluctuations in their voltages can couple charge into the signal being addressed as the fluctuation occurs. This is manifest as *line-correlated noise* and is present in all the pixels along a particular control line. For example, consider a data line with 2000 pixels on an array incorporating a 32:8 ratio TFT switch with a 3-μm overlap. Each switch has a coupling capacitance between the data line and the gate line of $\sim$20 fF attributable to the intrinsic overlap and fringing fields between the gate and source/drain metallization layers. This results in a total coupling capacitance from this source of 30 pF. If the charge coupled into a preamplifier is desired to be approximately equal to the amplifier noise level ($\sim$1000 e), the *off* voltage on the remaining 1999 un-addressed pixels must remain constant to better than 5 μV between the start and end of the pixel integration time ($\sim$10 to 50 μs). This requires careful design of the components and circuit boards supplying these voltages. Because human vision is extremely sensitive to such correlated noise, the requirements on the voltages supplied to the pixels can be even more demanding.

One method to correct for line-correlated noise requires blanking off a number of columns along the edge of the array from incoming x rays. Their signal (presumed to comprise only the offset charge) is then subtracted from the other pixels along the same row [190]. This can reduce the line-correlated noise significantly. Other sources of correlated signal sharing between neighboring channels on external ASIC chips that can also cause image artifacts have also been identified [191]. Resolution of this problem requires detailed knowledge of ASIC fabrication and careful design of the chip, the associated circuit boards, and driving circuitry.

The operation of the switching diodes or TFTs requires the application and removal of voltages (typically $\sim$10 V) to the gate control lines. Because all the control lines have to pass over or under the data read out lines, as shown in Figure 4.3, and there is also coupling capacitance inherent in the switching devices, there is typically a total of $\sim$0.01 to 0.1 pF coupling capacitance per intersection. Hence, there will be $\sim$0.1 to 1 pC of charge injected into each of the data lines at every operation of a gate line. This injected charge can be of the same order of magnitude as the signal and, in the case of fluoroscopy, much larger than the signal. The one saving grace is that, in principle, the total charge injected into each line is zero when summed over the complete switch on and switch off cycle of each row of pixels. The consequences of this large charge injection are that the read out amplifiers must be extremely linear to cope with such large non-signal charges. They may also use a considerable part of their dynamic-range just to absorb this charge. This makes the design of low-noise amplifiers for fluoroscopy more difficult. There are methods to inject charge onto the array to balance the control line injection. This issue will undoubtedly be investigated further in the future as lower noise levels are attained.

4.4.4 Image processing and manipulation

The image information acquired from the current generation of flat-panel detector systems is unsuitable for immediate image display. It must be processed to remove a number of artifacts and adjust the appearance of the image information to obtain a diagnostic-quality radiograph. These corrections are either necessary to account for limitations in the performance of the flat-panel array or to allow optimal presentation of the digital data on a particular soft/hard copy display medium.

The latter type of image manipulation is a general requirement for all types of digital images and its implementation continues to be developed for currently available digital acquisition modalities, in particular storage phosphor systems [192–196]. Robust, automated tone scaling of the digital information to reliably provide an optimally presented image to the viewer has proven difficult and continues as an area of active research [197].

Other image corrections are necessary to circumvent shortcomings in the technology of flat-panel arrays and their peripheral circuitry. Because of the limited tolerances achievable in controlling the thickness and quality of the different layers on large-area flat-panel x-ray imagers, the sensitivity of the pixels to radiation and their offset signals (from dark current integration and switching transients) vary from pixel to pixel. This includes variations resulting from the thickness and quality of the photoconductor or phosphor layers coupled to the arrays. Tolerance issues in the fabrication of the peripheral amplification and controlling circuitry also add variations in pixel sensitivity and offset. The most powerful method for removal of these distracting effects is called *flat fielding*. It is implemented by application of individual pixel correction factors derived from analysis of images obtained from the array to be corrected [108, 198]. Variations in pixel and electronic offsets are corrected using *dark-field* images acquired with no x-ray exposure. Pixel sensitivity and electronic gain variations are corrected using *flood-field* images taken with a constant intensity of x-ray exposure across the full area of the detector. The linear response of the flat-panel detectors over most of their operating range means that a two-point linear technique provides an adequate correction if the system response is temporally invariant. Temporal drift in the pixel leakage currents [119, 162] and thermal drift of electronic gain and offsets can mandate periodic updating of the relevant correction factors. Most modern flat-panel detectors allow monitoring of the dark signals between patient exposures which facilitates continuous modification of the offset corrections. Measured drifts of pixel sensitivity are extremely small, even over extended periods of time [119], so acquisition of flood field data is not needed as frequently as offset correction.

Flat fielding image correction itself can generate image noise if not done carefully. Many frames should be averaged together to determine noise-free dark and flood-field values for the individual pixel corrections. Nonlinear three (or more) point corrections can also be applied to the data. The determination of the relative sizes of the two (or more) radiation flood fields must be done more accurately than the level of nonlinearity being corrected if the process is not to introduce additional artifacts into the final image. Other factors such as non-uniformities in the x-ray field attributable the x-ray anode heel effect, which are intrinsically incorporated into the flood field corrections, can cause artifacts in the corrected image if, for example, the array is rotated or moved from the exact geometrical configuration used for acquisition of the flood fields. Different modes of operation of the imaging system such as radiographic and fluoroscopic acquisition may also require independent correction factors and even time-dependent correction factors when the system is rapidly changed from one mode to another. A final point is that a flat-fielding correction is only strictly valid for independent pixels. If, for example, there is fixed pattern noise in the phosphor layer then the correction is not image independent and can potentially reappear in images even after a flat fielding has been applied.

During fabrication, defects can cause a number of different failure modes for elements on the active-matrix array. This can result in image information being lost from individual pixels or from partial or complete lines [143]. Even with a 0.1% defect rate, an array with $\sim 5 \times 10^6$ pixels will have ~ 5000 bad pixels. Methods for correcting these problems include fault-tolerant designs to allow for individual element failures by incorporating redundancy in the pixel elements. Laser ablation of individual pixel elements to remove electrical shorts between gate, data, and bias lines [128, 151] is also possible. Fault-tolerant designs, however, can have a significant effect on pixel fill factor. Furthermore, the increased complexity of fabrication can cause more problems than they solve. Their use in sensor-array fabrication is less important than in display manufacture because post-acquisition software processing of the image information is possible.

One of the main challenges for software processing of defects is in the identification of those pixels that need correction. Pixels that are completely nonfunctional can be identified easily by, for example, setting limits on the ranges of acceptable offset and gain factors obtained by the dark/flood-field techniques described above. However, pixels that are partially functional or have nonlinear response, may be missed by this procedure. Alternatively if the gain/offset limits defining a bad pixel are set too stringently, pixels which have valid data may be erroneously identified as defective. Either of these situations is undesirable. Identification of defective pixels can also be based solely on the statistics of the final processed image. A pixel whose data value is outside a threshold range determined from an analysis of its immediate neighbors can be flagged for correction. Again, a precise discrimination between defective and functional pixels based on the setting of this threshold limit is challenging.

Software processing of a digital image to remove the bad lines and *salt-and-pepper* noise generated by pixel failures discussed above, is an extensively researched topic [199]. The most common method for removal of these image defects is a median filter [200] that can be used to replace a defective pixel value with the median value of its neighbors. Satisfactory results can be obtained if single pixels or lines are being corrected but visible artifacts can arise when clusters of bad pixels or several adjacent bad lines are corrected. This is illustrated in Figure 4.23, which demonstrates different stages in the image processing chain. Figure 4.23(a) shows the raw unprocessed data obtained from an active-matrix array incorporating a layer of phosphor. Numerous bad pixels and lines are obvious, as well as artifacts arising from defects in the overlying phosphor layer; variations in pixel offset and response; and correlated line noise due to electronic offsets and charge coupling variations. In Figure 4.23(b) the appropriate gain offset corrections have been applied and the data have been converted to log exposure space for display. In Figure 4.23(c) the defective pixels and lines have been identified with a gain/offset threshold technique and corrected with a median filter. Most of the bad lines and pixels have completely disappeared but the magnified view of the index finger shows an example of the persistent artifacts that can arise when a number of neighboring lines are defective. Figure 4.23(d) shows the improvements in visibility possible when appropriate tone scale and edge enhancement are applied to the image. It also demonstrates however, that care should be taken with any image manipulation because the residual artifacts seen in the magnified view Figure 4.23(c) appear to have been somewhat enhanced by the unsharp masking technique used in preparing Figure 4.23(d).

A correction for image *carry over* or *lag* or *ghosting* may sometimes be necessary. These phenomena may be observed after large exposures to the imager or when the imager is used in mixed mode (i.e., combined fluoroscopic and radiographic imaging) and the system is moved to fluoroscopy after a large radiographic exposure. This effect has been seen in indirect detectors but not so far in direct detectors. The source of ghosting in indirect detectors has been identified as charge trapping and dynamic effects in the a-Si:H photodiodes [185, 201, 202]. Image processing schemes with controlled digital lag have been proposed to correct for these effects [202, 203].

A particularly disturbing effect, which is to be avoided at all costs, is Moiré fringing arising from spatial interference between the periodic structure of flat-panel detectors and a stationary grid. Moving the grid perpendicularly to the grid lines during the exposure using a Potter-Bucky grid arrangement should eliminate these problems.

It should be remembered that even traditional medical x-ray films inevitably suffer from artifacts caused by mechanical abrasion, mishandling, and *pick-off* in day-to-day use. The specific visual signature of these artifacts has long been recognized by radiologists and they are accepted as an unwanted but unavoidable characteristic of the imaging modality. Although completely defect free flat-panel arrays is the ultimate goal, it may be that with experience the level of acceptable artifacts in digitally produced images may be relaxed as it has been with film.

4.5 Methods of evaluating performance

During the design and development of new imaging systems there are many components and measurements which are essential to the understanding and optimization of the device. However, once the system has been made and perfected,

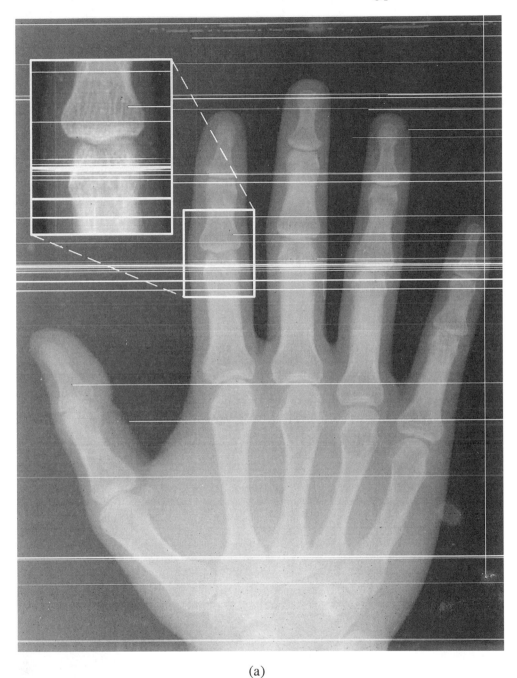

(a)

Figure 4.23: Images obtained from flat-panel imaging systems showing various common artifacts and the results of correcting them. (a) Raw unprocessed data obtained from an indirect conversion active-matrix array. (b) After the appropriate gain offset corrections and logarithmic transform have been applied. (c) The defective pixels and lines have been identified with a gain/offset threshold technique and corrected with a median filter, (d) appropriate tone scale and edge enhancement are applied to the image.

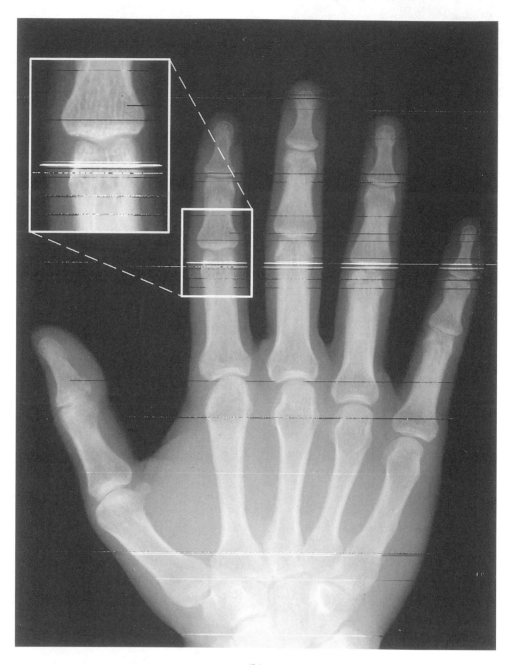

(b)

Figure 4.23:   (Continued).

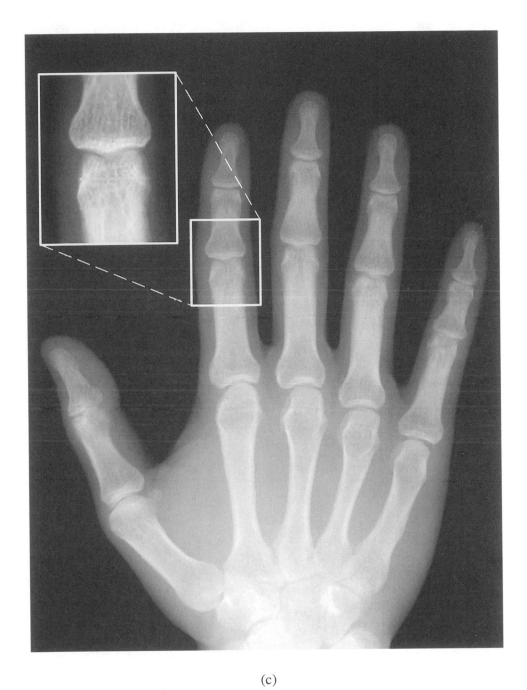

(c)

Figure 4.23: (Continued).

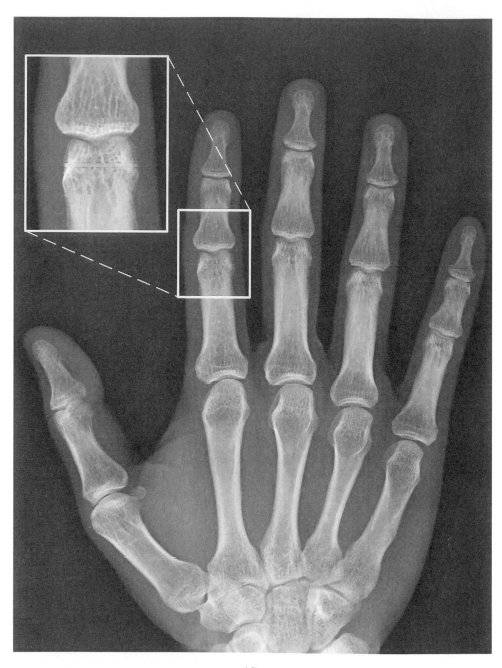

(d)

Figure 4.23: (Continued).

a new category of measurements are possible based on the imaging performance. The old saying, "The proof of the pudding is in the eating" is appropriate because, for the end user, it does not matter how the imaging system is designed it just matters how it works. For most practical applications, the spatial-frequency-dependent detective quantum efficiency, $DQE(f)$, is the appropriate metric of system performance. This test, measured over the desired operating range of exposures is the single most important benchmark for x-ray imaging systems in the field of applied medicine (see Chapter 3 for full details of these evaluation methods and practical approaches to measuring them). For system designers and those users interested in investigating improved detector design, unique opportunities arise when a complete imaging system is available. For example, arguably the best way to measure the intrinsic MTF of the x-ray detection layer (e.g., phosphor or photoconductor) is in the actual operating conditions for which they were designed, for example, as part of the flat-panel imager. Furthermore, imaging tests that require viewing of actual images can be performed. These can range from the anecdotal "I like what I see" to the semiquantitative evaluation of appropriately designed contrast-detail phantoms that test the limits of object detectability under a number of different conditions. Anthropomorphic phantoms can also be used as an initial basis for evaluating clinical acceptance. Figure 4.24 shows a set of images demonstrating the immense dynamic range of flat-panel active-matrix x-ray systems. Figure 4.24(a) shows a series of images of a skull phantom taken at various exposure levels expressed either as mAs applied to the x-ray tube or the speed S, given by the expression

$$S = 100 \times 1 \text{ mR}/X, \tag{4.9}$$

where X is the exposure incident on the detector in mR. Note that these images as first produced appear strongly dependent on the exposure level used. Of course images are normally not presented to the physician in this manner and Figure 4.24(b) shows the same series of images after appropriate windowing and leveling to restore them all to the same mean intensity and contrast. The fact that at first glance the images are identical testifies to the immense practical exposure range over which flat-panel detectors can operate. A closer look reveals, as expected, that the quantum noise is clearly visible in the lowest-exposure images, and gradually becomes less apparent as the exposure is increased.

Other important system parameters to consider are: the number and severity of artifacts in the image; freedom from lag or persistence of images; and radiation-damage resistance. Most of these factors can be established simply by access to complete imaging systems and a general knowledge of how such devices are put together. It would be very difficult for a manufacturer to conceal the most important factors of how their system is constructed because the concept of flat-panel systems is inherently so simple that it makes the analysis of their operation practically transparent. This is facilitated by the output of the imaging system being in

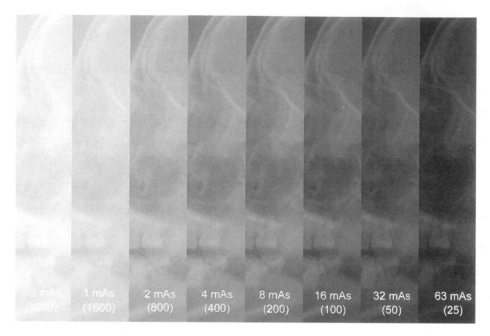

(a)

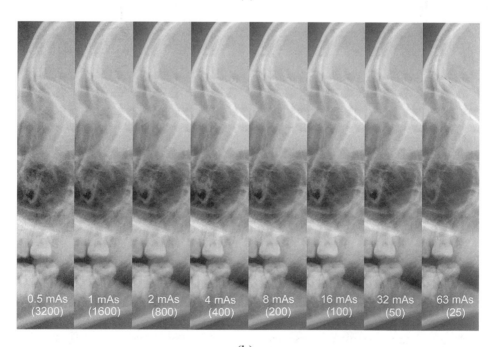

(b)

Figure 4.24: Images obtained from an indirect conversion flat-panel imaging system showing the very large dynamic range possible. (a) Uncorrected, and (b) windowed and leveled to optimize for viewing. (Images courtesy of Dr. U Neitzel, Philips Medical Systems.)

digital form and related to the input exposure. Putting this to the practical test, any user can readily obtain full response information about their panel. This allows, as a minimum, on-site verification of the manufacturer's specification. At best, it permits the ability to optimize the performance of the complete imaging chain of which the flat-panel detector is only a part.

One exception to this is the determination of the radiation-damage tolerance of the system. This cannot usually be performed nondestructively, although annealing can repair most of the radiation damage induced in the flat-panel array itself. Only by understanding the radiation sensitivity of the individual components can a realistic estimate of the overall radiation-sensitivity threshold of the system be reliably estimated. The most radiation-sensitive components are not necessarily an inherent part of the flat-panel array. For example, the crystalline silicon chips used for the analog amplification prior to digitization, may double their noise after exposure to dose levels in the range of ~ 10–100 kRads, depending on their design. Different designs of flat-panel array may also exhibit different sensitivities to radiation damage.

4.5.1 System imaging performance

Detective quantum efficiency will be defined in terms of parameters measurable from an imaging system. The resolution, expressed as the modulation transfer function or MTF(f), is combined with the spatial-frequency-dependent normalized noise power spectrum $W(f)$ [i.e., the NPS normalized by the signal squared] and the x-ray fluence Φ to obtain DQE(f):

$$\text{DQE}(f) = \text{MTF}^2(f)/[W(f)\Phi]. \qquad (4.10)$$

Plots of MTF(f), $W(f)$ and DQE(f) for direct [89] and indirect [119] conversion detectors are shown in Figure 4.25 for several exposure levels. Many clinical and pre-clinical, prototype flat-panel detectors have been designed and built and in some cases evaluated by more than one group of investigators. The choice of the particular detectors favored for this comparison was made on the completeness of the published results, which allow ease of comparison, rather than the "best" published results of a specific detector type. The MTF, NPS, and DQE from these systems will now be discussed using these data as a basis to determine the physical principles involved, not the ultimate limits that may be attained by each detector type.

The MTF of the direct and indirect systems show a distinct qualitative difference. The overall MTF of each system is the product of the MTF of the x-ray detection medium and the pixel aperture function. The intrinsic spatial resolution of a photoconductor is extremely high, which means that the system MTF for a direct detector will be dominated by the pixel aperture function. This is shown in Figure 4.25(a), where the MTF is practically identical to the pixel electrode aperture function (i.e., a sinc function). In a system that utilizes a phosphor as the x-ray detection medium, the spatial response of the phosphor is typically poorer than the

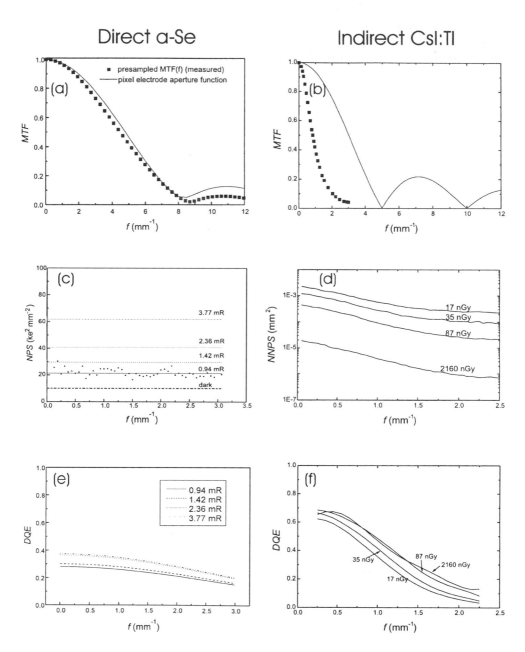

Figure 4.25: Experimentally measured plots of modulation transfer function, MTF(f); Wiener noise power spectrum, NPS(f); detective quantum efficiency, DQE(f); for direct [89] and indirect [185] conversion detectors.

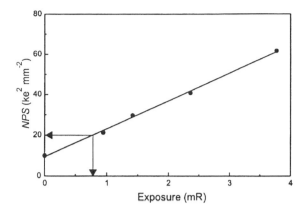

Figure 4.26: Plot of NPS(0) versus x-ray exposure obtained from data of Figure 4.25(c) at $f = 0$. The arrow indicates the additional exposure necessary to produce x-ray noise equal to the system noise (e.g., amplifier noise). The level of noise in this system can then be expressed as this exposure which can in turn be directly compared with the system design requirements given in Table 4.1.

aperture response of the pixel. The MTF of this combination will then be smaller than the MTF of the pixel aperture. This is demonstrated in Figure 4.25(b). In other words, for the a-Se system it is the pixel electrode size which defines the presampling MTF whereas for phosphor-based system (even columnar CsI) the phosphor response dominates and defines the MTF. Furthermore, for the parameters usually chosen in practical medical systems the MTF at the Nyquist frequency is ∼60% for the direct system and closer to 10% for the indirect system. This implies that noise aliasing will be severe for the direct and almost negligible for the indirect detection approach, in general. The degree of aliasing permitted by the system designer can be established from an evaluation of the pre-sampled MTF and a measurement of the area above the Nyquist frequency compared to the area below.

The NPS of direct and indirect detectors are shown in Figure 4.25(c, d) and also demonstrate striking differences. The direct detector, because of its minimal spatial filtration prior to sampling, combined with aliasing of the frequencies above the Nyquist frequency is *white* (i.e., is independent of spatial frequency). In contrast the indirect detector shows a marked drop in NPS with increasing frequency, because of the greater presampling blurring inherent in the phosphor layer demonstrated by comparing the MTFs in [Figure 4.25(a) and (b)]. Both NPS show a marked exposure dependence, but note that two conventions for the units for the ordinates have been used (*vis.* $ke^2 mm^{-2}$ and mm^2) which correspond to the unnormalized and normalized (by signal) NPS, respectively. The details of the exposure dependence are difficult to identify except in the case of the former definition where by plotting the NPS at zero spatial frequency as a function of x-ray exposure, the system noise in unit of exposure to the detector can be obtained as described in the caption to Figure 4.26.

The DQEs of the two systems are qualitatively similar: dropping by factors of $\sim \times 2$ to $\times 4$ from $f = 0$ to $f = f_{NY}$ and increasing at all f as exposure to the detector is increased. A plateau is finally reached where further increase in exposure makes no difference to the DQE. This change with exposure is attributable to additive electronic noise. The value of electronic noise can be obtained from the dependence of DQE on exposure. Of the two systems demonstrated in Figure 4.25, the electronic noise is greater in the direct detector. However the two detectors demonstrated in Figure 4.25 represent systems at different stages of development and more recent direct detection systems have reported lower noise levels. At the limit of sufficient exposure the amplifier noise level will not affect DQE. This limit is assumed in the following discussion. Closer examination reveals some typical differences. While DQE(0) of the CsI detector is larger that for the a-Se detector; DQE(f_{NY}) is larger for the a-Se detector. In other words the a-Se detector starts off with a worse DQE than CsI but drops less with spatial frequency so that at the Nyquist frequency the a-Se detector DQE is better than that of the CsI based detector. Now, the value of DQE(0) of both systems could be increased by increasing the thickness T of the x-ray sensitive layer, and undoubtedly in most of the diagnostic energy range (the exception being for mammography) the largest value will be for CsI because of its considerably larger Z and ρ. However, the decrease in DQE with frequency is probably the result of either the Lubberts effect or K-fluorescence reabsorption, both of which would be made worse by increasing T.

Unfortunately, implementing even minor modifications to the design of the different components of a flat panel x-ray imaging detector is both difficult and extremely expensive. This suggests that valuable information on system optimization can be obtained from a realistic model of the system performance. First order consequences of specific design changes can then be investigated with minimal risk. This will be examined in more detail in Section 4.5.3.

4.5.2 Component performance

Let us imagine being presented with a fully operational flat-panel x-ray detector. How much could we find out about its structure and components? Starting from the beginning and taking nothing for granted, how do we discover what a system consists of? The first and most basic measurements are to determine the field of view and the pixel pitch. The field of view is established by imaging a grid of wires of known separation x and by counting the number of wires in the image n, thus the field of view $V = (n - 1)x$. Together with a count of the number N of pixels in the image, the pixel pitch p immediately follows from $p = V/N$. Next, it is necessary to establish that the system is operating linearly. For this the characteristic curve is measured. This is a plot of signal response (sometimes called *pixel value*) as a function of exposure to the system. Most flat-panel systems will have a response close to linear. However, a manufacturer may limit access to this linear data such that only data sent through some transform (e.g., a logarithmic transform) might be available. Thus the first task would be to reverse this operation. Then MTF and NPS can be measured and DQE calculated as described in Chapter 3.

The effective fill factor F_E of direct detectors (or any detector with high resolution of the x-ray detection layer compared to the active-matrix array) can be immediately isolated from the MTF by noting the frequency of the first zero f_1 of the sinc function. Then $F_E = (f_1 p)^{-2}$ for a symmetrical pixel design where p is the pixel pitch defined previously.

The MTF of the x-ray sensing layer MTF_S can usually be obtained from the MTF_T of the total system by making reasonable assumptions about the other MTF components. For example, by making the assumption that the array MTF_A can be approximated as a sinc function with its first zero at the effective aperture size [204] and using the fact that components of MTF in a system are multiplicative:

$$MTF_T = MTF_S \times MTF_A. \tag{4.11}$$

The data for x-ray sensitive layers of a-Se, CsI:Tl and Gd_2O_2S given earlier in Figure 4.6(a, g, h) were in fact mostly computed in this manner. Considerable care must be taken to ensure that all the other important contributors to MTF loss have been corrected before the results can be considered completely reliable. However this approach has the advantage over measuring the components independently, in that the configuration is exactly the same as in actual use. For example, if the MTF of a CsI detector is measured with a microscope, differences in the actual system MTF may be introduced because the acceptance angle was different for a microscope objective than for a detector layer operating in contact. Such issues are made moot by the procedure described above based on the evaluation of an actual flat-panel system.

Measurement of DQE(0) can be used to establish the important radiological elements in the detector, their atomic number Z, and its mass loading or thickness. The quantum efficiency η requires some reasonable correction for the Swank factor and attenuation of the front of the cassette. Because the cassette front will be designed for minimal absorption, its effective Z will be much smaller than that of the detector. Thus, the contribution of the low Z input window and high Z detector layer will have different x-ray energy dependencies that can be recognized by dual energy decomposition techniques [205].

4.5.3 System-performance modeling

Chapter 2 of this book provides a detailed introduction to linear-systems analysis and the modeling of complete imaging systems. Based on such models of signal and noise propagation in a cascaded imaging system [206], theoretical analyses of indirect Gd_2O_2S:Tb and CsI:Tl based detectors [207] and direct a-Se detectors have been performed [187]. Using these models limitations of the flat-panel detector designs discussed in connection with the results of Figure 4.25 can be more critically evaluated to determine if and by how much each design can be improved.

4.5.3.1 DQE enhancement by maximization of fill factor

It has been shown that the effect of reduced fill factor has a markedly different effect on direct and indirect detectors [208]. Because charge moves directly to the pixel in the direct conversion detector, then sub-unity effective fill factor reduces the DQE(0) by the same factor. This is not the case for indirect detectors where the effect of the blurring in the phosphor layer is to provide a presampling filter which forces the sharing of signal from each x ray with many pixels, and thus even when fill factor is less than ideal there is no loss of DQE(0). Fortunately, in a photoconductor, there is the possibility of making an effective fill factor of unity even when there is a sub-optimal geometrical fill factor as the field lines can be shaped as shown in Figure 4.18(c), and (d). By utilizing an insulator layer between pixel electrodes on which a potential can build up and repel lines of electric force, a 100% fill factor can be established automatically [166].

4.5.3.2 Aliasing reduction techniques

Depending upon the resolution of the x-ray detection layer compared to the pixel size, undersampling of the image and hence aliasing may occur. Aliasing is always present regardless of the pixel size in direct detectors based on a-Se because of its high intrinsic resolution. There are however, practical means to reduce its effect on the image, albeit at the cost of reducing the overall resolution. Averaging of nearby pixels can be performed using simple or weighted averaging to accomplish effective apertures of different sizes [209].

The aliasing can in principle, be reduced or even eliminated by blurring prior to pixel sampling. Possible techniques are shown in Figure 4.27 for both the direct and indirect methods. The aim is to reduce the overall MTF sufficiently that there is essentially zero noise power above f_{NY} to be folded below and DQE becomes almost perfect nearly up to f_{NY}. However, blurring also has deleterious effects: by reducing the high-frequency components of the signal, the imaging system becomes much more susceptible to external noise (e.g., that arising in the charge amplifiers or secondary quantum statistics). Summing up, more filtering makes the system more susceptible to amplifier noise while eliminating aliasing of both signal and noise. Thus determining the ideal level of presampling blurring (i.e., the presampling modulation transfer function) is not straightforward.

4.5.3.3 DQE(f) losses

Two effects will be discussed which have both been invoked to explain loss of DQE as a function of spatial frequency. These are the Lubberts effect and K-fluorescence reabsorption.

The origin of the Lubberts effect was described earlier in connection with Figure 4.10. If an x-ray detection layer has different effective MTFs for x rays absorbed at different depths, then the Lubberts effect will be present. It appears that all commonly used phosphors, even those based on columnar CsI, exhibit this behavior to some degree or other. One could imagine however that the fiber-optic faceplates discussed earlier, with their extramural absorbers and other accoutrements which make them act as true fiber optic layers, could avoid this problem completely. In this case the MTF of the detection layer would be near unity at all relevant spatial frequencies, which is the situation with a-Se. This ensures that the

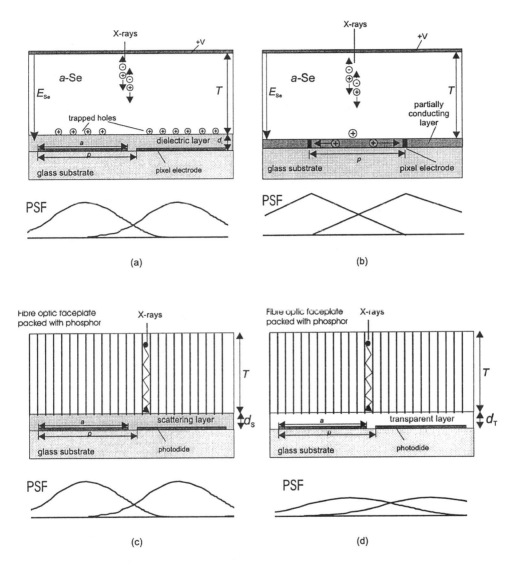

Figure 4.27: Methods for achieving blurring after the image is collected at the image plane shown with the resulting point spread function of the post detection but presampling point spread function introduced by the techniques. Methods (a) and (b) for direct conversion detectors (a) Using an insulating layer to trap the latent charge image at the thickness d_i from the pixel readout plane. (b) Using a partially conducting layer in the image plane to force the sharing of the image charge between pixels. Methods (c) and (d) for indirect conversion detectors and assuming a perfect MTF input stage e.g., a phosphor in a fiber optic matrix. (c) Interposing a diffusion layer whose MTF can be calculated by the method outlined by Swank [53] as can the MTF for a transparent layer as in (d).

MTF(L, f) is independent of depth, L, as required to avoid the Lubberts effect, but apparently also excludes the possibility of avoiding signal and noise aliasing, because it forces the MTF to be independent of frequency, f. In other word it prevents the application of the beneficial effects of blurring. How to avoid this impasse?

One concept that may circumvent this problem is the use of "perfect" MTF in the x-ray detection layer followed by a layer that produces sufficient blurring before the sampling stage to eliminate the aliasing of noise. Possible methods are shown in Figure 4.27 for direct and indirect detectors. In Figure 4.27(a) and (b) the sharing of charge landing intermediately between pixel electrodes is forced by an insulator layer on which the image is trapped so inducing a controlled blurring depending on the thickness of the insulator layer. Alternatively, a partially conducting layer can cause a sharing between small pixel electrodes with the triangular point spread function shown. A conceptual solution for the indirect detector is to use a fiber-optic-like phosphor layer then a diffuser immediately above the active-matrix array. These could take the form of a ground-glass screen or thin, highly scattering layer as shown in Figure 4.27(c), or simply an optical gap as shown in Figure 4.27(d).

K-fluorescence escape from the site of initial interaction in the x-ray detection layer and subsequent reabsorption at a remote position in this layer gives rise to substantial blurring and noise [210]. This mechanism has recently been evaluated for a series of possible x-ray detector layers by Monte Carlo modeling and shown to be quite a significant effect [211]. A related, but conceptually easier to avoid effect, is the K-fluorescence emitted from high Z impurities in the glass substrate [212].

Ironically, efforts to increase DQE(0) by increasing thickness of the sensor layer causes increased problems from both effects described in this section. Depending on the particular frequency range of interest, it may be that the efforts to increase DQE(0) by making very thick layers have been overdone and a better compromise may be achieved by reducing DQE(0) to gain DQE at higher frequencies. This is well known in the traditional film-screen world where thin layers of phosphor are used for high-resolution applications such as mammography even although thicker layers would produce higher DQE(0).

4.6 Clinical applications of complete systems

The medical applications for which flat-panel detectors are being developed and the new opportunities made possible with this technology will now be discussed in the context of the procedures currently used in clinical practice. All clinical applications will benefit from the general features of flat-panel detectors. These include: their compactness; their ability to be read out immediately after the radiation exposure to verify patient position and appropriate image exposure; to permit digital storage and communication within the hospital and beyond; to facilitate computer-aided diagnosis and second opinions; and, perhaps most importantly, the possibility of improving image quality without increasing patient x-ray exposure because of their enhanced DQE(f). Another less widely recognized benefit of flat-panel detectors arises from their inherent computer control and the fact that the majority of modern x-ray machines are also microprocessor controlled. This allows the possibility of complete synchronization of the delivery of the x-ray exposure, the acquisition and read out of the image, and the movement of the x-ray tube and other mechanical devices such as filter holders, as well as computer control of the x-ray energy. This level of integration makes the use of complex imaging procedures, such as dual-energy and conventional tomographic data acquisition, significantly more practical in a busy clinical environment. The use of these and other well known but traditionally time consuming protocols may therefore see a revival in clinical practice because of the integration of computer-controlled flat-panel detectors and modern x-ray sources. In the following there will be a description of the requirements of important clinical imaging tasks and the special opportunities for improvement made possible by digital x-ray imaging and flat-panel x-ray detectors in particular.

4.6.1 Chest radiography

Radiography of the chest is technically difficult because the required information is contained in both very radio-lucent (lung fields) and very radio-opaque (mediastinum) regions. In the past the problem was eliminated by not attempting to visualize detail in the mediastinum (which contains the heart and spinal regions). More recently it was found that by using very highly penetrating x-ray beams (130–150 kVp), both these regions could be visualized simultaneously. This was possible because the higher-energy x rays effectively reduced the contrast range of the image.

4.6.1.1 Film/screen radiography

In conventional radiography, the H&D curve of the film/screen system is designed such that the signal level in the lung region falls on the high part of the curve just before the shoulder and the signal level in the mediastinum falls on the toe of the curve. This is less than ideal and almost every x-ray room has to be set up individually to obtain acceptable images. A novel concept is to use two separate film/screens in the same cassette. This is made possible by the use of opaque blocking layers between the two film emulsions on opposite sides of the film base. This layer is removed during film processing but permits the use of radically different speed *films* and *screens* at the front and back of the cassette. The front film/screen pair is slow, with high spatial resolution and is used to image the lung fields, the back film/screen pair is faster but with lower resolution and is matched to the requirements of the signal from the mediastinum. When the film is developed the two emulsions are viewed simultaneously and their images merge to produce a characteristic unobtainable with the normal arrangement of identical front and back screens and film emulsions [213].

4.6.1.2 Radiographic equalization

The purpose of scanned equalization radiography, SER, is to reduce the dynamic-range of the aerial x-ray image **before** it is incident on the film/screen x-ray receptor. This is achieved by modulating the intensity of the x rays emitted from the source. This procedure ensures that almost all information is presented at the optimal (steepest) part of the H&D curve and consequently enhances the contrast of the image. The cost is a loss of broad-area contrast that makes the image appear rather abnormal and requires considerable physician re-education.

This equalization effect is achieved by scanning the incident x-ray beam (formed by an aperture in the collimator) and modulating the intensity of the beam entering the patient by monitoring and controlling the exit exposure. The appearance of the image is critically dependent on the size of the x-ray aperture. An appropriately-sized aperture results in a region of equalization equivalent to a digital high-pass filter, reducing or eliminating large-area variations of transmitted intensity and thus fitting the x-ray information better into the limited dynamic-range of film [214, 215]. Flat-panel x-ray detectors have an extremely wide dynamic-range and may not necessarily require such equalization to permit correct representation of the image. However, it may still be beneficial to perform equalization because it increases the signal level in the mediastinum as well as equalizing the signal-to-noise ratio in the different regions of the image.

4.6.1.3 Dual energy

The goal of dual-energy imaging in the chest is to isolate the bony details (i.e., the spine and ribs) from the soft tissues. The removal of the complex background detail can help in visualization of soft tissue abnormalities. This is achieved by obtaining two images at different x-ray energies. Then by appropriate manipulation, separation into two different basis sets is possible. The two basis sets can be recombined in a multitude of ways but the most useful is as bone and soft tissue [205]. An example pair of bone and soft-tissue images obtained with this approach is shown in Figure 4.28 compared to a normal presentation of a chest image of the same patient. As previously mentioned, the development of flat-panel imaging systems capable of easily synchronizing the rapid acquisition of multiple images at different beam energies and filtrations, will remove many of the practical obstacles that have limited the widespread use of this technique with more standard imaging modalities. It is a good example of how this new technology can facilitate the development of older ideas whose implementation was hindered by purely practical issues of image acquisition.

4.6.1.4 Digital imagers for chest radiography

A recently introduced digital chest radiography system uses electrometers to read out a latent image charge formed on the surface of a charged a-Se drum [19]. There have also been investigations of CR systems optimized for chest radiography. These images can then be post processed using, for example, unsharp masking (subtraction of a blurred version of the same image) [3, 5]. Flat-panel active-matrix x-ray imagers have also been configured for chest imaging. The foremost requirements are (see Table 4.1) a very large field of view, a reasonably high spatial resolution (100 to 200 μm pixels) and a very large dynamic-range to accommodate

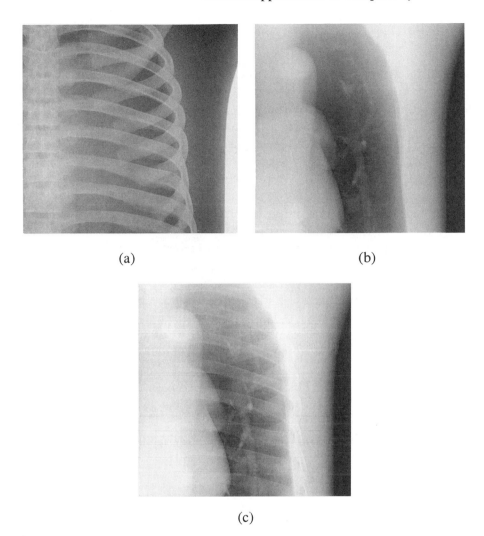

(a)   (b)

(c)

Figure 4.28: Example images of chest taken using a flat-panel detector with dual energy approach (i.e., two basis images were obtained shortly after each other) and processed to make (a) bone only and (b) soft tissue only images. The original images were acquired at the usual diagnostic exposure to the detector at 60 kVp and 120 kVp under normal and +0.5 mm Cu added filtration respectively. The latter image is shown as (c). (Images courtesy of Dr. JT Dobbins III, Duke University Medical Center.)

the different penetration of the lungs and mediastinum. Digital image processing can be used to mimic (though not exactly reproduce) the effects of beam equalization, and other techniques such as dual energy could be performed, provided rapid enough read out can be achieved.

4.6.2 Fluoroscopy

Perhaps the most demanding potential application for flat-panel imaging systems is in fluoroscopy. Very high patient doses can be delivered because of the length of some interventional fluoroscopic procedures. To reduce patient exposure during these procedures, low-radiation exposure rates are typically used. This sets a stringent limit on the system performance since the image quality must still be adequate for visualization of the surgical equipment and anatomy of interest. Therefore, the imaging system must be x-ray quantum limited even at extremely low exposure levels. The XRII is the key component of current systems that provide sufficient gain to permit x-ray quantum-limited imaging at these low exposure levels. The resulting real-time images are usually displayed using a video system (conventional or CCD) optically coupled to the XRII. The need for radiographs or stored-image sequences during fluoroscopic procedures has previously been satisfied with optical attachments to the XRII such as small format (or photofluorographic) and ciné cameras. Recently, *instant* radiography [216] and *instant replay* ciné have been made possible by digitization of the video signal.

Digital systems based on the use of XRII have several disadvantages. First, the bulky nature of the intensifier often impedes the clinician by limiting access to the patient and prevents the acquisition of some important radiographic views. Second, losses of image contrast occurs because of x ray and light scatter within the XRII tube, that is, *veiling glare* [8]. Last, but not least, geometric (pincushion) distortion of the image occurs largely because of the curved input phosphor and *S* distortion which is attributable to the Earth's magnetic field.

In contrast, an active-matrix panel is a significantly more compact device permitting better access to patients than XRIIs. It is flat, largely free from veiling glare (see Figure 4.29 which shows veiling glare measurements [217] from an indirect detector compared to published data for a typical XRII [218]) and is geometrically uniform. This facilitates quantitative image analysis; registration and clinical comparison of images from other modalities; 3D reconstruction (e.g., *volume computerized tomography*); and use in conjunction with magnetic resonance imaging (i.e., MRI). This last benefit is possible because, unlike XRIIs, flat-panel detectors are intrinsically immune to magnetic fields. Another task normally expected of a fluoroscopic system is to permit *pulsed fluoroscopy* that permits shorter x-ray pulses than conventional approaches and hence sharper images in the presence of motion. The output of the flat-panel imager should also be compatible with real-time image processing systems that can optimize the image appearance by modifying the temporal and contrast response of the system. In principle, image quality can be improved using real-time digital processing by [219]: (a) increasing the signal-to-noise ratio by averaging in either the spatial or temporal domain; and (b) modifying the display contrast to better represent the information in the image. Because of the speed of operation required, specialized hardware is necessary to implement real-time image processing [174, 224].

More efficient use of radiation in fluoroscopy can be achieved by giving normal exposures to regions most vital to the procedure while simultaneously reducing ex-

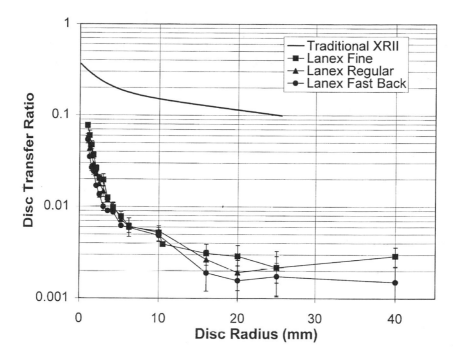

Figure 4.29: Comparison of the veiling glare measured with a $127\,\mu m$ pixel pitch indirect detector utilizing various thicknesses of Gd_2O_2S phosphors [217] with that from a standard XRII [218].

posure in the periphery that mainly gives spatial perspective and context. Such region of interest (ROI) fluoroscopy has been demonstrated using a mask subtraction method, in which the mask is either pre-computed or calculated on the fly on the simple assumption that the ROI is a circle. Another method has been proposed in which dynamic response to imaging parameters such as zoom mode or kVp change is possible without *a priori* information about the exposure profile except that the profile changes gently. The concept is to use digital processing to equalize the image, in other words, eliminate low-frequency components of the image including the ROI filter. Using any of these methods, the area exposure product and hence radiation dose to the patient can be reduced by as much as a factor of four. The ROI method is not yet in general usage but nevertheless represents one of the most promising methods for reducing radiation doses during fluoroscopy [220, 221].

Thus, the ideal flat-panel fluoroscopic system should be able to perform all current fluoroscopic procedures at a reduced dose because of its improved DQE(f). The physical form would be similar to a film/screen cassette (except for the addition of an umbilical cord) which would permit more compact C-arm design. Two major problems remain to be solved. The first is how to reduce the noise of flat-panel systems to that achievable with an XRII to permit quantum-noise limited operation at the low end of fluoroscopic exposure rates [121, 222] (i.e., $0.1\,\mu R\,s^{-1}$). The second problem is to reduce the image *carry over* or lag which often corrupts the fluoroscopic image sequence taken directly after a radiographic exposure [203, 223]. Both these issues are areas of active research and improvements in system performance and image handling bring the "perfect" system closer each year [116, 118, 174, 224].

4.6.2.1 Gastrointestinal imaging

Gastrointestinal (GI) fluoroscopy is the most common fluoroscopic procedure. Most GI fluoroscopic examinations are now performed using *double contrast*. In this technique, a patient drinks contrast material, (an aqueous suspension of an inert compound of barium in powder form), and then swallows a quantity of gas pills. The stomach acid activates the pill, generating gaseous CO_2. The gas inflates the GI tract and allows the GI walls to be separated and uniformly coated by the contrast material. Through the 2D x-ray projection of the contrast coated GI tract, the outline of the GI walls and the internal folds and crevices are made visible in the fluoroscopic image.

Motion is the essence of fluoroscopic GI studies. During the examination, the radiologist must be able to view the motion of relevant organs. Therefore, there is a need to carefully select the temporal lag of the imaging system. Combined with the motion present in the GI examination, the temporal lag causes image blurring, the degree of which depends on the velocity of motion. In GI fluoroscopy velocities up to the order of 10 to 30 mm s^{-1} are commonly seen [225]. However, the temporal lag inherent in the imaging components reduces noise. If additional digital temporal averaging, (averaging consecutive images in the image sequence) with a large averaging parameter is used to reduce noise appreciably, it causes unacceptable motion blurring. The ability of motion detection circuits to detect motion in low contrast regions is limited since they only operate on a pixel by pixel basis [219]. A clinically useful balance between the degradation attributable to motion blurring and the improvement from noise reduction is very difficult to achieve.

4.6.2.2 Digital subtraction angiography (DSA)

Digital systems for subtraction angiography based on XRII and video systems are now in widespread clinical use. The principle used in DSA is that iodine contrast media partially replaces blood in the vessels, resulting in considerable extra attenuation making it possible to image the circulating blood. Initially dual and even triple energy schemes based on the presence of the iodine K-absorption edge at ~33 keV were used but were found to have problems maintaining low enough noise. Thus, it is more practical to make images immediately before and just after the injection of iodine and *subtract* (actually a log subtraction equivalent to a division is used) away the first image (called the *mask*), ideally leaving an image of just the iodinated blood. This image is enhanced in contrast (or *windowed*) and leveled to show the vessels clearly [226]. The blood moves quickly through the body and thus it is necessary to capture the images very rapidly. Simultaneously, it is necessary to have low-noise images to permit the significant contrast enhancement required. Thus the requirements for DSA are quite different from fluoroscopy.

While images may be required at 30 s^{-1}, the mean exposure level to the detector per image will be one (coronary arteries – 10 μR) to two or three (peripheral and neuro – 100 to 1,000 μR) orders of magnitude larger than for fluoroscopy ($\sim$1 μR).

4.6.3 Mammography

Mammography is the only projection x-ray imaging modality that attempts to visualize soft-tissue contrast. The photoelectric effect is used to achieve soft-tissue contrast and this requires the use of very low kVp [227]. The geometrical situation in mammography is also unusual in that only one half of the field of the x-ray tube is used. The purpose of this arrangement is to ensure that the central ray grazes the chest wall, eliminating the possibility of missing breast tissue close to the chest wall. This also requires the detector to be sensitive as close as possible to the chest wall [3, 5].

Originally, mammograms were obtained using film with no intensifying screen. This produced excellent images albeit with very large radiation doses. This dose was reduced to some degree by the introduction of xeromammography [14], the first large-scale medical application of a-Se, which used only minor modifications of the conventional electrophotographic (i.e., photocopier) process. It was a technical and commercial success in its day. It had a huge dynamic-range because the toner development process greatly enhanced edge detail making microcalcifications more conspicuous. However, with the introduction of mammographic film/screen systems, xeromammography is no longer competitive. Film/screen has a much smaller dynamic-range than non-screen film or xeromammography. Therefore it requires an extreme amount of breast compression to equalize the x-ray path length to the point that the whole breast can be visualized. The standard procedure is film/screen with a single screen, in back screen configuration with the film facing the radiation. The very highly absorbed radiation used in mammography is preferentially absorbed close to the screen surface ensuring the highest possible image resolution. Digital mammography is starting to be important to clinical practice, but is still undergoing development. Its potential advantages are increased dynamic-range; possibly permitting reduced breast compression, and the ability to visualize dense breasts. Small field-of-view digital systems are available to guide needle biopsies and full field-of-view systems are undergoing clinical trials. The first full-field systems are either limited field-of-view systems, which make a full field by scanning, or area systems made of tiled arrays of CCDs [5]. Active-matrix systems are under development [149] and clinical evaluation [228], and the challenge is to make pixels small enough, with high enough fill factor, sensitive all the way to the chest wall, and at an affordable cost. The current consensus is that 100-μm pixels may not be quite small enough but 50 μm will be more than adequate. Both clinical and scientific studies are necessary to resolve this resolution problem. The intrinsically high resolution of a-Se [31] combined with the relative simplicity of the active-matrix array design used for direct conversion and the possibility of using electrostatic focusing to ensure an essentially 100% effective fill factor suggest that this may be the optimal approach for mammography [229]. There are problems associated with making connections to an array at this small pitch that are exacerbated by the requirement that the detector be sensitive right to the edge on the side close to the chest wall. It has been suggested to make a multiplexer using the a-Si:H semiconductor to reduce the number of external wiring connections [7] to alleviate this problem.

4.6.4 Tomography

Tomography blurs out the shadows of superimposed structures to allow better isolation of the structures of interest than is possible in conventional projection radiography. Conventional tomography uses a rigid connecting rod linking the x-ray tube and an x-ray film/screen cassette. Thus when the tube moves in one direction, the film moves in the opposite direction. The plane of interest within the patient is positioned by the operator to lie at the fulcrum, and is thus the only plane that remains at a sharp focus in the image. All points above and below this focal plane are blurred. In the simplest systems the tube path is a straight line, consequently *linear tomography*. Other paths are possible. The more the tomographic motion differs from the shape of the object being examined, the less likely it is to produce artifacts. Thus tomographic units have been designed to operate with a wide variety of curvilinear motions. The width of the blurring out of the plane is controlled by the tomographic angle—the effective section thickness is reduced as the tomographic angle increases.

4.6.4.1 Digital tomosynthesis

If the x-ray tube moves but the digital sensor capable of being read out many times is kept stationary, then tomograms can be synthesized at any desired level within the patient by digital post-processing. The advantage of this approach is that it reduces the patient's dose as multiple tomograms can be obtained at the same total dose as a single conventional tomogram. Recent application of a 100-μm pixel pitch CsI:Tl flat-panel detector to digital tomosynthesis in mammography has been reported [230]. It can be expected that the approach will be extended to other clinical applications, as suitable flat-panel images become available.

4.6.4.2 Computerized area tomography

The availability of flat-panel detectors is expected to reinvigorate the concept of using area detectors in computerized tomography (i.e., cone beam CT). Such approaches have been used for angiography and other specialized applications where the advantages of the interventional simplicity of a conventional x-ray room is preferable to the confining situation of a conventional CT scanner [231] yet there was also the need for fully 3D images. Flat-panel detectors offer the benefit of mechanical simplicity because full 3D information can be acquired in a single rotation. With the use of an area detector, the z-direction spatial resolution is significantly improved over more traditional techniques, although the consequences of the increased level of scatter are still to be fully investigated. The application of

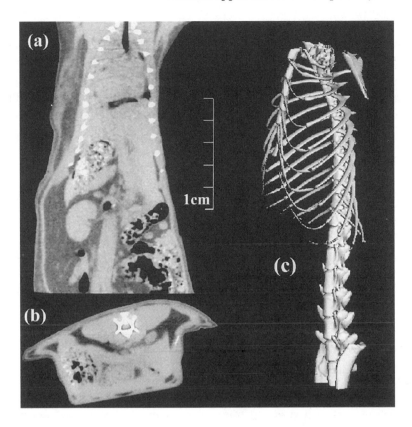

Figure 4.30: Cone beam CT reconstructed images of a rat obtained at 100 kVp using an indirect flat-panel x-ray imager. (a) Coronal slice (voxel dimensions: $x = 0.5$ mm (horizontal); $z = 0.25$ mm (vertical); slice thickness $= 0.5$ mm). (b) Axial slice (voxel dimensions: $x - y - 0.1$ mm; slice thickness $= 2.0$ mm). (c) Volume rendering of rat skeleton (voxel dimensions: $x = y = 0.5$ mm; slice thickness $= 0.25$ mm). (Images courtesy of Dr. J Siewerdsen, William Beaumont Hospital.)

both direct [232] and indirect [233] conversion flat-panel imagers to cone beam CT have been reported. The contrast and spatial resolution of the latter system have been shown to be at least comparable to that obtained with a conventional CT device. Example images are shown in Figure 4.30 that demonstrate a number of different reconstructions of a rat from 300 projections acquired at 100 kVp with a prototype system [233]. The images exhibit excellent soft-tissue delineation, good spatial resolution of the bony features, and demonstrate the excellent resolution in the z direction. However, production of such images requires detailed attention to many factors to ensure linearity and freedom from lag [234].

4.6.5 Portal imaging

During radiation therapy there is a need to obtain images to confirm the correct positioning of the patient in the output *portal* of the therapy machine. Conventionally these portal images are obtained with a film in contact with a metal build-up layer usually made of 1-mm Cu plate [235]. A problem with this approach is that it is necessary to retrieve the film from the treatment room for development and so it is not practical to use that day's portal image to control or adjust that day's treatment. This is the reason for interest in digital portal imaging, to permit the imaging of the patient in the portal remotely and immediately after an initial small positioning exposure is made ($\sim$2 to 4 cGy *c.f.* to total daily treatment dose of the order of 100 cGy). There is a further problem with portal images; it is often very difficult to see the details of interest which are typically bony landmarks. It is not possible to see soft-tissue contrast with high-energy beams, and even bones can be difficult to visualize because of inadequate contrast and/or resolution. One improvement possible with conventional systems is the use of high-contrast films that have very high gammas approaching those of lithographic films. In combination with a metal plate and phosphor screen, these enhance the weak inherent contrast to an acceptable level [236].

Many approaches to digital portal imaging have been tried [235] and the results have generally been disappointing and thus the acceptance of the concept has been slow. The most commonly used approach is to optically couple a phosphor screen (with metal build-up layer) to an optical video camera. Because the camera and its electronics are rather sensitive to radiation-damage, they are typically located at a distance from the main beam axis. This, coupled with the fact that the camera tube or CCD has a small size, inevitably leads to poor optical coupling that gives rise to two problems. The first is the emergence of an unwanted secondary quantum sink where each absorbed x ray is represented on average by less that a single light photon. The second is the dominance of electronic noise [237]. Because these two image-quality problems arise from the poor optical coupling between the phosphor screen and the detector, it is to be expected that a flat-panel solution will eliminate this problem entirely as the screen and active-matrix array are in direct contact. This significantly improves the capture efficiency of the pixels for light emitted from the phosphor and is possible because of the excellent radiation damage tolerance of the a-Si:H material. The issue of the radiation tolerance of the peripheral electronics (typically crystalline Si) is yet to be solved. Shielding them from the direct beam is impractical at megavoltage energies, while moving them further back from the edge of the array would increase the size of the detector housing. In certain treatment configurations this may cause problems with collisions between the housing and the patient or the table and would therefore diminish one of the most important benefits of a flat-panel detector over the camera mirror systems, that is, their significantly reduced bulk.

The flat-panel approach has been investigated using both indirect [106] and direct detectors [238] and from both a theoretical and experimental perspective. Example portal images of head phantoms taken with both direct and indirect conversion detectors are shown in Figure 4.31. Not only can flat-panel imagers be used to obtain images but can also in principle be used for transit dosimetry if the detector is designed to respond to radiation in the same manner as tissue. This requires

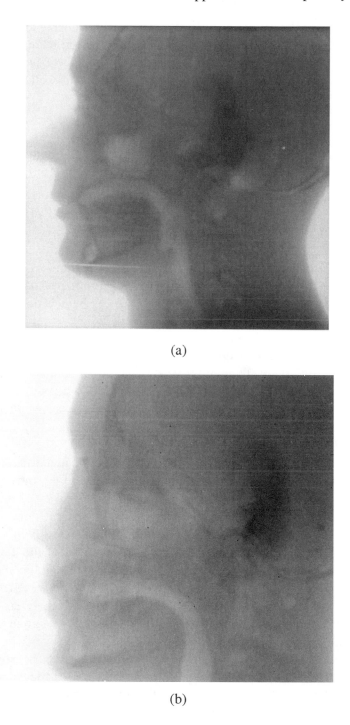

(a)

(b)

Figure 4.31: Portal images of head phantoms taken with high energy beam from a therapy machine using (a) a direct conversion detector. (Image courtesy of Dr. G Pang, Toronto Sunnybrook Regional Cancer Center) and (b) an indirect conversion detector. (Image courtesy of Dr. J Siewerdsen, William Beaumont Hospital.)

the detector to be tissue equivalent and investigation of the degree to which various designs of portal imager can be tissue equivalent have been undertaken recently [239]. It was shown that a direct conversion panel in which the a-Si:H photodiodes were used to directly convert the incident x rays to charge was well matched to this requirement.

4.7 Future prospects

The field of flat-panel x-ray detectors is still relatively new and there will undoubtedly be many advances in system design and improvements in system performance in the years to come. Improvements to watch for include: increased numbers of active elements per pixel, perhaps allowing an amplifier at every pixel, and integrated read out electronics to make an *x-ray imager on glass*; increased x ray to charge conversion gain either by use of improved photoconductors with intrinsically lower W or avalanche gain. However, the main features of future systems will probably remain similar to those of today unless new materials are developed or there are advances in other fields such as nano-science, which are just beginning to be explored.

It is humbling to recognize that even before the advent of high-purity-silicon integrated circuits, thin-film techniques essentially similar to those used for flat-panel x-ray sensors described here were used to construct complete optical video cameras on glass. It is encouraging that this work was done so early and with what would now be regarded as unsophisticated equipment, as it underscores the essential simplicity and robustness of the technological approach now being used for large-area flat-panel x-ray imagers.

The study of amorphous materials has been the scientific underpinning of much of the work described, but as forcefully pointed out by Mort [35], the development of successful amorphous materials greatly outstripped the ability of theory to explain their behaviors. In the case of flat-panel imagers at least three amorphous materials are of great importance. The first, whose discovery was in antiquity, is optical glass; the second, which was discovered at the end of the 19th century, was the photoconductivity of amorphous selenium, and the last in the 1970s is the dopable semiconductor, amorphous silicon. It is difficult to imagine flat-panel imagers without the use of amorphous materials and the developments in understanding and production of these materials will continue to be of great importance to the field.

As fabrication techniques and device yields improve, more sophisticated switching structures with reduced coupling capacitance, lower leakage currents, smaller physical area, and more robust operating characteristics will undoubtedly continue to be developed. These advances will help improve the imaging performance of today's active-matrix arrays to the point where the dominant factor will be the properties of the x-ray detection medium, even for the most demanding low signal level and high-resolution applications such as fluoroscopy and mammography.

The investigation of large-area flat-panel sensors presents us with a large variety of previously unexplored problems in detector physics. These new problems and indications of how they may be resolved have been discussed which will, we believe, eventually provide the understanding to permit an ideal x-ray imaging detector to be constructed. At present there is still a tension between the manufacture of sensors for medicine by processes which were designed for mass-production applications versus highly specialized cottage-industry approaches. Flat-panel foundries optimized for medical imaging are needed but their establishment and ongoing running expenses present a problem because of the huge capital investments needed compared to the relatively small number of panels which will be required each year to keep the medical market satisfied, combined with a limit on the acceptable cost to the end user. The initial investment for flat-panel detectors will be high but over time it is believed that their quality will justify the cost and perhaps eventually cost will decrease.

Will one kind of detector eventually dominate and in that case which one? The issues have been raised many times. The first issue favors the direct approach: it is probably more economical to produce a direct panel, at least while there are many foundries mass producing essentially identical panels for active-matrix displays. In contrast, the indirect panels have the requirement for photodiodes which mandates special facilities devoted to medical applications. A second issue that seems to favor the indirect approach is that it is more practical to make a highly absorbing detector layer from the high-density phosphor than for the lower density and atomic number a-Se. There are however some unresolved issues as to the desirability of using very thick phosphor screens. However, taking into consideration that there is not only one requirement for a medical x-ray imager, but a huge range depending on the clinical task that it has to accomplish, it seems likely that for the foreseeable future there will be a place for both approaches.

It is our opinion that flat-panel detectors are **the** unifying concept in medical imaging. Flat-panel detectors will be here for as long as x-ray imaging remains a viable imaging modality. How long will that be for? Only time will tell.

Acknowledgments

The National Cancer Institute of Canada (NCIC) financially supports this work through a Terry Fox Program Project Grant "Imaging for Cancer." We would like to acknowledge useful discussion and comments on the text by Dr. Wei Zhao and Dr. Richard Weisfield.

References

[1] Chan HP, Doi K, Galhotra S, Vborny CJ, MacMahon H, Jokich PM, "Image Feature Analysis and Computer-Aided Diagnosis in Digital Radiography. 1. Automated Detection of Microcalcifications in Mammography." Med Phys 14:538–548, 1987.

[2] Giger ML, Ahn N, Doi K, MacMahon H, Metz CR, "Computerized Detection of Pulmonary Nodules in Digital Chest Images: Use of Morphological Filters in Reducing False-Positive Detections." Med Phys 17:861–865, 1990.

[3] Rougeot H, "Direct X-Ray Photoconversion Processes." In Hendee W, Trueblood J (Eds.) *Digital Imaging*. AAPM Monograph 22, Medical Physics Publishing, 1993, pp. 9–96.

[4] Zhao W, Rowlands JA, "X-Ray Imaging Using Amorphous Selenium: Feasibility of a Flat Panel Self-Scanned Detector for Digital Radiology." Med Phys 22:1595–1604, 1995.

[5] Yaffe MJ, Rowlands JA, "X-Ray Detectors for Digital Radiology." Phys Med Biol 42:1–39, 1997.

[6] Cowen AR. "Digital X-Ray Imaging." Meas Sci Technol 2:691–707, 1991.

[7] Antonuk LE, El-Mohri Y, Hall A, Jee KW, Maolinbay M, Nassif SC, Rong X, Siewerdsen JH, Zhao Q, Weisfield RL. "A Large Area 97 mm Pitch Indirect-Detection, Active-Matrix, Flat Panel Imager (AMFPI)." Proc SPIE 3336, 1998, pp. 2–13.

[8] Vosburg KG, Swank RK, Houston JM. "X-Ray Image Intensifiers." Advances in Electronic and Electron Physics 43:205–244, 1977.

[9] Solomon EG, Wilfley BP, Van Lysel MS, Joseph AW, Heanue JA. "Scanning-Beam Digital X-Ray (SBDX) System for Cardiac Angiography." Proc SPIE 3659, 1999, pp. 246–257.

[10] Hillen W, Schiebel U, Zaengel T. "Imaging Performance of a Digital Storage Phosphor System." Med Phys 14:745–751, 1987.

[11] Sanada S, Doi K, Xu X-W, Yin F-F, Giger ML, MacMahon H. "Comparison of Imaging Properties of a Computed Radiographic System and Screen-Film Systems." Med Phys 18:414–420, 1991.

[12] Kato K. "Photostimulable Phosphor Radiography Design Considerations." In *Specification, Acceptance Testing and Quality Control of Diagnostic X-Ray Imaging Equipment*. AAPM, 1994, pp. 731–769.

[13] Dobbins III JT, Ergun DL, Rutz L, Hinshaw DA, Blume H, Clark DC, "DQE(f) of Four Generations of Computed Radiography Acquisition Devices." Med Phys 22:171–181, 1995.

[14] Boag JW. "Xeroradiography." Phys Med Biol 18:3–37, 1973.

[15] Rieppo PM, Rowlands JA. "X-Ray Imaging Using Amorphous Selenium: Theoretical Feasibility of the Liquid Crystal Light Valve for Radiography." Med Phys 24:1279–1292, 1997.

[16] Luhta R, Rowlands JA. "Feasibility of a Large Area X-Ray Sensitive Vidicon for Medical Fluoroscopy: Signal and Noise Factors." Med Phys 24:621–631, 1997.

[17] May JW, Lubinski AR. "High Resolution Computed Radiography by Scanned Luminescent Toner Radiography." Proc SPIE 1896, 1993, pp. 292–312.

[18] Jeromin LS, Klynn LM, "Electronic Recording of X-Ray Images." J Appl Photo Engin 5:183–189, 1979.

[19] Neitzel U, Maack I, Gunther-Kohfahl S. "Image Quality of a Digital Chest Radiography System Based on a Selenium Detector." Med Phys 21:509–516, 1994.

[20] Zermeno A, Kirby T, Cowart R, Marsh L, Ong P. "Laser Readout of Electrostatic Images." Proc SPIE 173, 1979, pp. 81–87.

[21] Korn DM, Johnson SP, Nelson OL, Ziegler RJ. "A Method of Electronic Readout of Electrophotographic and Electroradiographic Images." J Appl Photo Engin 4:178–182, 1978.

[22] Rowlands JA, Hunter DM, Araj N. "X-Ray Imaging Using Amorphous Selenium: A Photoinduced Discharge Method for Digital Mammography." Med Phys 18:421–431, 1991.

[23] DeMonts H, Beaumont F. A New Photoconductor Imaging System for Digital Radiography.'' Med Phys 16:105–109, 1989.

[24] Moores BM, Dovas T, Pullan B, Booler R. "A Prototype Digital Ionographic Imaging System." Phys Med Biol 30:11–20, 1985.

[25] Drewery JS, Cho G, Fujieda I, Jing T, Kaplan SN, Perez-Mendez V, Wildermuth D, Street RA. "Amorphous Silicon Pixel Arrays." Nucl Inst Methd A310:165–170, 1991.

[26] Perez-Mendez V, Morel J, Kaplan SN, Street RA. "Detection of Charged Particles in Amorphous Silicon Layers." Nucl Inst Methd A252:478–482, 1986.

[27] Equer B, Karar A. "Amorphous Semiconductors for Particle Detection: Physical and Technical Limits and Possibilities." Nucl Inst Methd A275:558–563, 1989.

[28] Hatanaka Y, Chang ZB, Mimura H. "Soft X-Ray Image Sensor Using Hydrogenated Amorphous Silicon." Jap J Appl Phys 24:L129–L130, 1985.

[29] Brauers A, Conrads N, Frings G, Schiebel U, Powell MJ, Glasse C, "Charge Collection in a Se Photoconductor on a Thin Film Transistor Array During X-Ray Imaging." Mat Res Soc Proc 467:919–924, 1997.

[30] Rowlands JA. "Imaging with Amorphous Selenium." AJR 167:409–411, 1996.

[31] Que W, Rowlands JA. "X-Ray Imaging Using Amorphous Selenium: Inherent Spatial Resolution." Med Phys 22:365–374, 1995.

[32] Klein C. "Bandgap Dependence and Related Features of Radiation Ionisation Energies in Semiconductors." J Appl Phys 39:2029, 1968.

[33] Pai DM, Enck RC. "Onsager Mechanism of Photogeneration in Amorphous Selenium." Phys Rev B11:5163, 1975.

[34] Que W, Rowlands JA. "X-Ray Photogeneration in Amorphous Selenium: Geminate Versus Columnar Recombination." Phys Rev B51:10,500–10,507, 1995.

[35] Mort J. *The Anatomy of Xerography—Its Invention and Evolution*. Jefferson, NC: McFarland, 1989.

[36] Wang Y, Champness CH. "Xerographic Properties of Chlorine-Doped Amorphous Selenium." In *Proceedings of the Fifth International Symposium on the Uses of Selenium and Tellurium*. Belgium: STDA, 1995, pp. 175–186.

[37] Brodie I, Gutcheck RA. "Radiographic Information Theory and Application to Mammography." Med Phys 9:79–95, 1982.

[38] Brodie I, Gutcheck RA. "Minimum Exposure Estimates for Information Recording in Diagnostic Radiology." Med Phys 12:362–367, 1985.

[39] Shukri Z, Caron M, Rougeot H. "Selenium Alloys with Improved Thermal Stability for Digital X-Ray Detector Applications." Proc SPIE 3659, 1999, pp. 48–55.

[40] Polsichuk B, Shukri Z, Legros A, Rougeot H. "Selenium Direct Converter Structure for Static and Dynamic X-Ray Detection in Medical Imaging." Proc SPIE 3336, 1998, pp. 494–504.

[41] Tanioka K, Shidara K, Hirai T, "A Highly Sensitive Camera Tube Using Avalanche Multiplication in an Amorphous Selenium Photoconductive Target." Proc SPIE 1656, 1992, p. 2.

[42] Shah KS, Bennett P, Klugerman M, Moy LP, Entine G. "Lead Iodide Films for X-Ray Imaging." Proc SPIE 3032, 1997, pp. 395–404.

[43] Shah KS, Bennett P, Cirignano L, Dmitriyev Y, Klugerman M, Mandal K, Moy LP, Street RA. "Characterization of X-Ray Imaging Properties of PbI_2 Films." Mat Res Soc Symp Proc 487:351–326, 1998.

[44] Heijne L, Schagen P, Buining H. "An Experimental Photoconductive Camera Tube for Television." Philips Tech Rev 16:23, 1954.

[45] Jacobs J, Berger H. "Large-Area Photoconductive X-Ray Pickup-Tube Performance." Electrical Engineering 75:158, 1956.

[46] Brauers A, Conrads N, Frings G, Schiebel U, Powell MJ, Glasse C. "X-Ray Sensing Properties of a Lead Oxide Photoconductor Combined with and Amorphous Silicon TFT Array." Mat Res Soc Proc 507:321–326, 1998.

[47] Weiss J. "Large Field Cineradiography and Image Intensification Utilising the TVX System." Radiology 76:264, 1961.

[48] Shah KS, Lund JC, Olschner F, Moy L, Squillante MR. "Thallium Bromide Radiation Detectors." IEEE Trans Nucl Sci 36:199, 1989.

[49] Ouimette DR, Nudelman S, Aikens R. "A New Large Area X-Ray Image Sensor." Proc SPIE 3336, 1998, pp. 470–476.

[50] Squillante MR, Zhang J, Zhou C, Bennett P, Moy L. "New Compound Semiconductor Materials for Nuclear Detectors." Mat Res Soc Proc 302:319–328, 1993.

[51] Bencivelli W, Bertolucci E, Bottigli U, Del Guerra A, Messineo A, Nelson WR, Randaccio P, Rosso V, Rosso P, Stefanini A. "Evaluation of Elemental and Compound Semiconductors for X-Ray Digital Radiography." Nucl Inst Methd A310:210–214, 1991.

[52] Wang Y, Herron N. "X-Ray Photoconductive Nanocomposites." Science 273:632–634, 1996.

[53] Swank RK. "Calculation of Modulation Transfer Function of X-Ray Fluorescent Screens." Appl Opt 12:1865–1870, 1973.

[54] Stevels ALN, Schrama-de Paw ADM. "Vapor-Deposited CsI:Na Layers, II. Screens for Application in X-Ray Imaging Devices." Philips Res Repts 29:353–362, 1974.

[55] Jing T, Cho G, Drewery J, Fujieda I, Kaplan SN, Mireshghi A, Perez-Mendez V, Wildermuth D. "Enhanced Columnar Structure in CsI Layer by Substrate Patterning." IEEE Trans Nucl Sci 39:1195–1198, 1992.

[56] Nagarkar VV, Gupta TK, Miller SR, Klugerman Y, Squillante MR, Entine G. "Structured CsI(Tl) Scintillators for X-Ray Imaging Applications." IEEE Trans Nucl Sci 45:492–496, 1998.

[57] Hillen W, Eckenbach W, Quadfleig P, Zaengel T. "Signal-to-Noise Performance in Cesium Iodide X-Ray Fluorescent Screens." Proc SPIE 1443, 1991, pp. 120–131.

[58] Moy J-P. "Image Quality of Scintillator Based X-Ray Electronic Imagers." Proc SPIE 3336, 1998, pp. 187–194.

[59] Boone JM, Duryea J, Seibert JA. "Imaging Performance of a Terbium-Doped Fiber Optic Screen for Diagnostic Imaging." Proc SPIE 2163, 1994, pp. 64–72.

[60] Shao H, Miller DW, Pearsall CR. "Scintillating Fiber Optics for X-Ray Radiation Imaging." Nucl Inst Meth A299:528–533, 1990.

[61] Choi WY, Walker JK, Jing Z. "A High Resolution Digital X-Ray Imaging System Based on the Scintillating Plastic Microfibre Technology." Proc SPIE 2163, 1994, pp. 150–157.

[62] Sabol JM, Boone JM. "Monte Carlo Simulation of Photon Transport within a Hybrid Grid-Detector System for Digital Mammography." Proc SPIE 3032, 1997, pp. 266–274.

[63] Arnold BA. "Physical Characteristics of Screen-Film Combinations." In *The Physics of Medical Imaging: Recording System Measurements and Techniques*. AAPM Medical Physics Monograph 3, 1979, pp. 30–71.

[64] Blasse G, Grabmaier BC. *Luminescent Materials*. Berlin: Springer-Verlag, 1994.

[65] Holl I, Lorenz E, Mageras G. "A Measurement of the Light Yield of Common Inorganic Scintillators." IEEE Trans Nucl Sci 35:105–109, 1988.

[66] Valentine JD, Wehe DK, Knoll GF, Moss CE. "Temperature Dependence of CsI(Tl) Absolute Scintillation Yield." IEEE Trans Nucl Sci 40:1267–1274, 1993.

[67] Swank RW. "Absorption and Noise in X-Ray Phosphors." J Appl Phys 44:4199–4203, 1973.

[68] Drangova M, Rowlands JA. "Optical Factors Affecting the Detective Quantum Efficiency of Radiographic Screens." Med Phys 13:150–157, 1986.

[69] Trauernicht DP, Van Metter R. "The Measurement of Conversion Noise in X-Ray Intensifying Screens." Proc SPIE 914, 1988, pp. 100–116.

[70] Ginzburg A, Dick CE. "Image Information Transfer Properties of X-Ray Intensifying Screens in the Energy Range from 17 to 320 keV." Med Phys 20:1013–1021, 1993.

[71] Rowlands JA, Taylor KW. "Absorption and Noise in Cesium Iodide X-Ray Image Intensifiers." Med Phys 10:786–795, 1983.

[72] Fahrig R, Rowlands JA, Yaffe MJ. "X-Ray Imaging Using Amorphous Selenium: Detective Quantum Efficiency of Photoconductive Image Receptors for Digital Mammography." Med Phys 22:153–160, 1995.

[73] Blevis IM, Hunt DM, Rowlands JA. "X-Ray Imaging Using Amorphous Selenium: Determination of Swank Factor by Pulse Height Spectroscopy." Med Phys 25:638–641, 1998.

[74] Yip KL, Whiting BR, Kocher TE, Trauernicht DP, Van Metter RL. "Understanding the Relative Sensitivity of Radiographic Screens to Scattered Radiation." Med Phys 23:1727–1737, 1996.

[75] Lubberts G. "Random Noise Produced by X-Ray Fluorescent Screens." J Opt Soc Amer 58:1475–1483, 1968.

[76] Nishikawa R, Yaffe MJ. "Effect of Finite Phosphor Thickness on Detective Quantum Efficiency." Med Phys 16:773–780, 1989.

[77] Nishikawa R, Yaffe MJ. "Effects of Various Noise Sources on the Detective Quantum Efficiency of Phosphor Screens." Med Phys 17:887–893, 1990.

[78] Nishikawa R, Yaffe MJ. "Model of the Spatial-Frequency-Dependent Detective Quantum Efficiency of Phosphor Screens." Med Phys 17:894–904, 1990.

[79] Van Metter R, Rabbani M. "An Application of Multivariate Moment-Generating Functions to the Analysis of Signal and Noise Propagation in Radiographic Screen-Film Systems." Med Phys 17:65–71, 1990.

[80] Trauernicht DP, Yorkston J. "Screen Design for Flat-Panel Imagers in Diagnostic Radiology." Proc SPIE 3336, 1998, pp. 477–484.

[81] Drangova M, Rowlands JA. "Measurement of the Spatial Wiener Spectrum of Nonstorage Imaging Devices." Med Phys 15:151–157, 1988.

[82] Fu T, Roehrig H. "Noise Power Spectrum, MTF and DQE of Photoelectronic Radiographic Systems." Proc SPIE 454, 1984, pp. 377–386.

[83] Weimer PK. "Television Camera Tubes: A Research Review." Advances in Electronics and Electron Physics, 13:387–437, 1960.

[84] Weimer PK. "Image Sensors for Solid-State Cameras." Advances in Electronics and Electron Physics, 37:181–262, 1975.

[85] Weimer PK, Sadasiv G, Meyer Jr JE, Meray-Horvath L, Pike WS. Proc IEEE 55:1591, 1967.

[86] Wiemer PK, Borkan H, Sadasiv G, Meray-Horvath L, Shallcross FV. Proc IEEE 52:1479, 1964.

[87] Brody TP, Asrars JA, Dixon GD. "A 6″ × 6″ 20 Lines per Inch Liquid Crystal Display Panel." IEEE Trans Electronic Devices ED-20:995–1001, 1973.

[88] Zhao W, Blevis I, Germann S, Rowlands JA, Waechter DF, Huang ZS. "A Flat Panel Detector for Digital Radiography Using Active-Matrix Readout of Amorphous Selenium." Proc SPIE 2708, 1996, pp. 523–531.

[89] Zhao W, Blevis IM, Waechter DF, Huang Z, Rowlands JA. "Digital Radiology Using Active-Matrix Readout of Amorphous Selenium: Construction and evaluation of a Prototype Real-Time Detector." Med Phys 24:1834–1843, 1997.

[90] Zhao W, Rowlands JA. "A Large Area Solid-State Detector for Radiology Using Amorphous Selenium." Proc SPIE 1651, 1992, pp. 134–143.

[91] Chittick RC, Alexander JH, Sterling HF. "The Preparation and Properties of Amorphous Silicon." J Electrochem Soc 116:77–81, 1969.

[92] Spear WE, LeComber PG. "Substitutional Doping of Amorphous Silicon." Solid State Comm 17:1193–1196, 1975.

[93] Snell AJ, Mackenzie KD, Spear WE, LeComber PG, Hughes AJ. "Application of Amorphous Silicon Field Effect Transistors in Addressable Liquid Crystal Display Panels." Appl Phys 24:357–362, 1981.

[94] Yamano M, Takesada H. "Full Color Liquid Crystal Television Addressed by Amorphous Silicon TFTs." J Non-Cryst Solids 77–78:1383–1388, 1985.

[95] Guang-Pu W, Okamoto H. "Amorphous Silicon Photovoltaic X-Ray Sensor." Jap J Appl Phys 24:1105–1106, 1985.

[96] Takahashi T, Itoh H, Shimada T, Takeuchi H. "Design of Integrated Radiation Detectors with a-Si Photodiodes on Ceramic Scintillators for Use in X-Ray Computed Tomography." IEEE Trans Nucl Sci 37:1478–1482, 1990.

[97] Itoh H, Matsubara S, Takahashi T, Shimada T, Takeuchi H. "Integrated Radiation Detectors with a-Si Photodiodes on Ceramic Scintillators." Jap J Appl Phys 28:L1476–L1479, 1989.

[98] Mochiki K, Hasegawa K, Namatame S. "Amorphous Silicon Position-Sensitive Detector." Nucl Inst Meth A273:640–644, 1988.

[99] Hasegawa K, Mochiki K, Takahashi H, Namatame S, Satow Y. "Imaging System with an Amorphous Silicon Linear Sensor." Rev Sci Instr 60:2284–2286, 1989.

[100] Takahashi H, Harada K, Nakazawa M, Hasegawa K, Mochiki K, Hayakawa Y, Inada T. "Development of a New Radiography System with 16 Amorphous Silicon Linear Sensors." In *IEEE Nucl Sci Symp Med Imag Conf*, Vol. 2, 1992, pp. 1336–1337.

[101] Antonuk LE, Boudry J, Kim CW, Longo M, Morton EJ, Yorkston J, Street RA. "Signal, Noise and Readout Considerations in the Development of Amorphous Silicon Photodiode Arrays for Radiotherapy and Diagnostic X-Ray Imaging." Proc SPIE 1443, 1991, pp. 108–119.

[102] Antonuk LE, Boudry J, Yorkston J, Wlid CF, Longo MJ, Street RA. "Radiation Damage Studies of Amorphous-Silicon Photodiode Sensors for Applications in Radiotherapy Imaging." Nucl Inst Meth A299:143–146, 1990.

[103] Antonuk LE, Yorkston J, Boudry J, Longo MJ, Jimenez J. "Development of Hydrogenated Amorphous Silicon Sensors for High Energy Photon Radiotherapy Imaging." IEEE Trans Nucl Sci 37:165–170, 1990.

[104] Street RA, Nelson S, Antonuk L, Perez-Mendez V. "Amorphous Silicon Sensor Arrays for Radiation Imaging." Mat Res Soc Symp Proc 192:441–452, 1990.

[105] Antonuk LE, Yorkston J, Boudry J, Longo MJ, Street RA. "Large Area Amorphous Silicon Photodiode Arrays for Radiotherapy and Diagnostic Imaging." Nucl Inst Meth A310:460–464, 1991.

[106] Antonuk LE, Boudry J, Wang W, McShan D, Morton EJ, Yorkston J, Street RA. "Demonstration of Megavoltage and Diagnostic X-Ray Imaging with Hydrogenated Amorphous Silicon Arrays." Med Phys 19:1455–1466, 1992.

[107] Yorkston J, Antonuk LE, Morton EJ, Boudry J, Huang W, Kim CW, Longo MJ, Street RA. "The Dynamic Response of Hydrogenated Amorphous Silicon Imaging Pixels." Mat Res Soc Symp Proc 219:173–178, 1991.

[108] Antonuk LE, Yorkston J, Kim CW, Huang W, Morton EJ, Longo MJ, Street RA. "Light Response Characteristics of Amorphous Silicon Arrays for Megavoltage and Diagnostic Imaging." Mat Res Soc Symp Proc 219:531–536, 1991.

[109] Fujieda I, Nelson S, Street RA, Weisfield RL. "Characteristics of a-Si Pixel Arrays for Radiation Imaging." Mat Res Soc Symp Proc 219:537–542, 1991.

[110] Perez-Mendez V, Cho G, Fujieda I, Kaplan SN, Qureshi S, Street RA. "The Application of Thick Hydrogenated Amorphous Silicon Layers to Charge Particle and X-Ray Detection." Mat Res Soc Symp Proc 149:621–630, 1989.

[111] Cho G, Conti M, Drewery JS, Fujieda I, Kaplan SN, Perez-Mendez V, Qureshi S, Street RA. "Assessment of TFT Amplifiers for a-Si:H Pixel Particle Detectors." IEEE Trans Nucl Sci 37:1142–1148, 1990.

[112] Perez-Mendez V, Cho G, Drewery J, Jing T, Kaplan SN, Qureshi S, Wildermuth D. "Amorphous Silicon Based Radiation Detectors." J Non-Cryst Solids 137–138:1291–1296, 1991.

[113] Fujieda I, Cho G, Drewery J, Gee T, Jing T, Kaplan SN, Perez-Mendez V, Wildermuth D, Street RA. "X-Ray and Charged Particle Detection with CsI(Tl) Layer Coupled to a-Si:H Photodiode Layers." IEEE Trans Nucl Sci. 38:255–262, 1991.

[114] Lee DL, Cheung LK, Jeromin LS. "A New Detector for Projection Radiography." Proc SPIE 2432, 1995, pp. 237–249.

[115] Chabbal J, Chaussat C, Ducourant T, Fritsch L, Michailos J, Spinnler V, Vieux G, Arques M, Hahm G, Hoheisel M, Horsachek H, Schulz R, Spahn M. "Amorphous Silicon X-Ray Image Sensor." Proc SPIE 2708, 1996, pp. 499–510.

[116] Tsukamoto A, Yamada S, Tomisaki T, Tanaka M, Sakaguchi T, Asahina H, Suzuki K, Ikeda M. "Development and Evaluation of a Large Area Selenium-Based Flat-Panel Detector for Real-Time Radiography and Fluoroscopy." Proc SPIE 3659, 1999, pp. 14–23.

[117] Kameshima T, Kaifu N, Takami E, Morishita M, Yamazaki T. "Novel Large Area MIS-Type X-Ray Image Sensor for Digital Radiography." Proc SPIE 3336, 1998, pp. 453–462.

[118] Colbeth RE, Allen MJ, Day DJ, Gilblom DL, Klausmeier-Brown ME, Pavkovich J, Seppi EJ, Shapiro EG. "Characterization of an Amorphous Silicon Fluoroscopic Imager." Proc SPIE 3032, 1997, pp. 42–51.

[119] Jung N, Alving PL, Busse F, Conrads N, Meulenbrugge HM, Rutten W, Schiebel U, Weibrecht M, Wieczorek H. "Dynamic X-Ray Imaging System Based on Amorphous Silicon Thin-Film Array." Proc SPIE 3336, 1998, pp. 396–407.

[120] Chaussat C, Chabbal J, Ducourant T, Spinnler V, Vieux G, Neyret R. "New CsI/a-Si $17'' \times 17''$ X-Ray Flat-Panel Detector Provides Superior Detectivity and Immediate Digital Output for General Radiography Systems." Proc SPIE 3336, 1998, pp. 45–55.

[121] Schiebel U, Conrads N, Jung N, Weibrecht M, Wieczorek H, Zaengel T, Powell MJ, French ID, Glasse C. "Fluoroscopic X-Ray Imaging with Amorphous Silicon Thin-Film Arrays." Proc SPIE 2163, 1994, pp. 129–140.

[122] Volk M, Strotzer M, Gmeinwieser J, Alexander J, Frund R, Seitz J, Manke C, Spahn M, Feuerbach S. "Flat-Panel X-Ray Detector Using Amorphous Silicon Technology: Reduced Radiation Dose for the Detection of Foreign Bodies." Invest Radiology 32: 373–377, 1997.

[123] Strotzer M, Gmeinwieser J, Spahn M, Volk M, Frund R, Seitz J, Spies V, Alexander J, Feuerbach S. "Amorphous Silicon, Flat-Panel, Detector Versus Screen-Film Radiography: Effect of Dose Reduction on the Detectability of Cortical Bone Defects and Fractures." Invest Radiology 33:33–38, 1998.

[124] Kump KS, Shi S. "Clinical Comparison of a New Digital X-Ray Detector System with a Conventional Screen Film System." Proc SPIE 3659, 1999, pp. 464–470.

[125] Shaber GS, Lee DL, Bell J, Powell G, Maidment ADA. "Clinical Evaluation of a Full Field Digital Projection Radiography Detector." Proc SPIE 3336, 1998, pp. 463–469.

[126] Boudry JM, Antonuk LE. "Radiation Damage of Amorphous Silicon, Thin-Film, Field Effect Transistors." Med Phys 23:743–754, 1996.

[127] Street RA, *Hydrogenated Amorphous Silicon.* Cambridge: Cambridge University Press, 1991.

[128] Kanicki J. *Amorphous and Microcrystalline Semiconductor Devices: Volume I Optoelectronic Devices.* Boston: Artech House, 1991.

[129] Kanicki J. *Amorphous and Microcrystalline Semiconductor Devices: Volume II Materials And Device Physics.* Boston: Artech House, 1992.

[130] Crandall RS. "Photoconductivity". In *Semiconductors and Semi-Metals.* New York: Academic Press, 1984, Vol. 21, Part B, Chapt. 8.

[131] Cody GD, Abeles B, Wronski C, Stephens CR, Brooks B. "Optical Characterization of Amorphous Silicon-Hydride Films." Solar Cells 2:227, 1980.

[132] Borsenberger PM, "Spectral Sensitization of Amorphous Silicon by Bromoindium Phthalocyanine." J Appl Phys 62: 2942–2945, 1987.

[133] Kagawa T, Matsumoto N, Kumabe K. "Amorphous Silicon Photoconductive Sensor." Jap J Appl Phys 21:251–256, 1981.

[134] Yamaguchi M, Kankeo Y, Tsutsui K. "Two-Dimensional Contact-Type Image Sensor Using Amorphous Silicon Photo-Transistor." Jap J Appl Phys 32:458–461, 1993.

[135] Hack M, Lewis AG, Bruce RH, Lujan R. "Optically Addressable Input Circuit for Two-Dimensional Image Sensing." Mat Res Soc Symp Proc 219: 167–172, 1991.

[136] Street RA, Biegelsen DK. "The Spectroscopy of Localized States." In *Topics in Applied Physics 56*. New York: Springer Verlag, 1984, p. 242.

[137] Sussmann RS, Ogden R. "Photoluminescence and Optical Properties of Plasma Deposited Amorphous Si_xC_{1-x} Alloys." Phil Mag B44:137–158, 1981.

[138] Weisfield RL, Tsai CC. "The Role of Carbon in Amorphous Silicon nip Photodiode Sensors." Mat Res Soc Symp 192:423–428, 1990.

[139] Street RA. "Measurement of Depletion Layers in Hydrogenated Amorphous Silicon." Phys Rev B 27:4924–4932, 1983.

[140] Carasco F, Spear WE. "Photogeneration and Geminate Recombination in Amorphous Silicon." Phil Mag B 47: 495–507, 1983.

[141] Munro P, Boulus DC. "X-Ray Quantum Limited Portal Imaging Using Amorphous Silicon Flat-Panel Arrays." Med Phys 25:689–702, 1998.

[142] Drake DG, Jaffray DA, Wong J. "A Prototype Amorphous Silicon Array Based Radiotherapy Portal Imager." Proc SPIE 3023, 1997, pp. 32–41.

[143] Powell M, French ID, Hughes JR, Bird NC, Davies OS, Glasse S, Curran JE. "Amorphous Silicon Image Sensor Arrays." Mat Res Soc Symp Proc 258:1127–1137, 1992.

[144] Hoheisel M, Brutscher N, Oppolzer H, Schild S. "The Interfaces a-Si:H/Pd and a-Si:H/ITO: Structure and Electronic Properties." J Non-Cryst Solids 97:959–962, 1987.

[145] Powell MJ, Glasse C, French ID, Franklin AR, Hughs JR, Curran JE. "Amorphous Silicon Photodiode-Thin Film Transistor Image Sensor with Diode on Top Structure." Mat Res Soc Symp Proc 467:863–868, 1997.

[146] Johanson RE, Kasap SO, Rowlands JA, Polischuk B. "Metallic Electrical Contacts to Stabilized Amorphous Selenium for Use in X-Ray Image Detectors." J Non-Cryst Solids 227–230:1359–1362, 1998.

[147] Den Boer W, Aggas A, Byun YH, Gu T, Zhong JZZ, Thomsen SV, Jeromin LS, Lee DLY. "Thin Film Transistor Array Technology for High Performance Direct Conversion X-Ray Sensors." Proc SPIE 3336, 1998, pp. 520–528.

[148] Zhao W, Law J, Waechter D, Huang Z, Rowlands JA. "Digital Radiology Using Active-Matrix Readout Amorphous Selenium: Detectors with High-Voltage Protection." Med Phys 25:539–549, 1998.

[149] Polischuk B, Rougeot H, Wong K, Debrie A, Poliquin E, Hansroul M, Martin JP, Trong T-T, Choquette M, Laperriere L, Shukri Z. "Direct Conversion Detector for Digital Mammography." Proc SPIE 3659, 1999, pp. 417–425.

[150] Van Berkel C, Powell MJ, Franklin AR, French ID. "Quality Factor in a-Si:H nip and pin Diodes." J Appl Phys 73:5264–5268, 1993.

[151] Graeve T, Huang W, Alexander SM, Li Y. "Amorphous Silicon Image Sensor for X-Ray Applications." Proc SPIE 2415, 1995, pp. 177–181.

[152] Cho G, Drewery JS, Hong WS, Jing T, Lee H, Kaplan SN, Mireshghi A, Perez-Mendez V, Wildermuth D. "Utilization of a-Si:H Switching Diodes for Signal Readout From a-Si:H Pixel Detectors." Mat Res Soc Symp Proc 279:969–974, 1993.

[153] Graeve T, Li Y, Fabans A, Huang W. "High-Resolution Amorphous Silicon Image Sensor." Proc SPIE 2708, 1996, pp. 494–498.

[154] Powell MJ. "The Physics of Amorphous-Silicon Thin-Film Transistors." IEEE Trans Elect Dev 36:2753–2763, 1989.

[155] Shur MS, Slade HC, Ytterdal T, Wang L, Xu Z, Hack M, Aflatooni K, Byun Y, Chen Y, Froggatt M, Krishnan A, Mei P, Meiling H, Min B-H, Nathan A, Sherman S, Stewart M, Theiss S. "Modeling and Scaling of a-Si:H and Poly-Si Thin Film Transistors." Mat Res Soc Symp Proc 467:831–842, 1997.

[156] Tsukada T. "Amorphous Silicon Thin-Film Transistors." J Non-Cryst Solids 164–166:721–726, 1993.

[157] Hack M, Mei P, Lujan R, Lewis AG. "Integrated Conventional and Laser Re-Crystallized Amorphous Silicon Thin Film Transistors for Large Area Imaging and Display Applications." J Non-Cryst Solids 164–166:727–730, 1993.

[158] Sameshima T. "Status of Thin Film Transistors." J Non-Cryst Solids 227–230:1196–1201, 1998.

[159] Mei P, Boyce JB, Hack M, Lujan R, Ready SE, Fork DK, Johnson RI, Anderson GB. "Grain Growth in Laser Dehydrogenated and Crystallized Polycrystalline Silicon for Thin Film Transistors." J Appl Phys 76:3194–3199, 1994.

[160] Mei P, Boyce JB, Fork DK, Anderson G, Ho J, Lu J, Hack M, Lujan R. "Hybrid Amorphous and Polycrystalline Silicon Devices for Large Area Electronics." Mat Res Soc Symp Proc 507:3–12, 1998.

[161] Hofstein SR. In *Field Effect Transistors*. Englewood Cliffs: Prentice-Hall, 1966, Chap. 5.

[162] Antonuk LE, El-Mohri Y, Siewerdsen JH, Yorkston J, Huang W, Scarpine VE, Street RA. "Empirical Investigation of the Signal Performance of a High Resolution, Indirect-Detection, Active-Matrix Flat-Panel Imager (AMFPI) for Fluoroscopic and Radiographic Operation." Med Phys 24:51–70, 1997.

[163] Powell MJ, Glasse C, Curran JE, Hughes JR, French ID, Martin BF. "A Fully Self-Aligned Amorphous Silicon TFT Technology for Large Area Image Sensors and Active-Matrix Displays." Mat Res Soc Symp Proc 507:91–96, 1998.

[164] van Berkel C, Powell MJ. "The Resolution of Amorphous Silicon Thin Film Transistor Instability Mechanisms Using Ambipolar Transistors." Appl Phys Lett. 51:1094–1096, 1987.

[165] Brunst G, Harms H, Ashworth J, Rosan K, Kemper K. "a-Si:H TFTs and Their Application in Linear Image Sensors." J Non-Cryst Solids 97–98:1343–1346, 1987.

[166] Pang G, Zhao W, Rowlands JA. "X-Ray Imaging Using Amorphous Selenium: Maximization of Effective Fill Factor." Med Phys 25:1636–1646, 1998.

[167] Antonuk LE, El-Mohri Y, Huang W, Jee KW, Maolinbay M, Scarpine VE, Siewerdsen JH, Verma M, Yorkston J, Street RA. "Development of a High Resolution Active-Matrix, Flat-Panel Imager with Enhanced Fill Factor." Proc SPIE 3032, 1997, pp. 2–13.

[168] Street RA, Wu XD, Weisfield R, Ready S, Apte R, Nguyen M, Nylen P. "Two Dimensional Amorphous Silicon Image Sensor Arrays." Mat Res Soc Symp Proc 377:757–766, 1995.

[169] Rahn JT, Lemmi F, Weisfield RL, Lujan R, Mei P, Lu J-P, Ho J, Ready SE, Apte RB, Nylen P, Boyce JB, Street RA. "High-Resolution, High Fill Factor a-Si:H Sensor Arrays for Medical Imaging." Proc SPIE 3659, 1999, pp. 510–517.

[170] Jean A, Laperriere L, Legros A, Mani H, Shukri Z, Rougeot H. "A New Cesium Iodide-Selenium X-Ray Detector Structure for Digital Radiography and Fluoroscopy." Proc SPIE 3659, 1999, pp. 298–306.

[171] van Berkel C, Bird NC, Curling CJ, French ID. "2D Image Sensor Arrays with Nip Diodes." Mat Res Soc Symp Proc 297:939–944, 1993.

[172] Chabbal J, Chaussat C, Ducourant T, Fritsch L, Michailos J, Spinnler V, Vieux G, Arques M, Hahm G, Hoheisel M, Horbaschek H, Schulz R, Spahn M. "Amorphous Silicon X-Ray Image Sensor." Proc SPIE 2708, 1996, pp. 499–510.

[173] Yorkston J, Antonuk LE, Seraji N, Boudry J, Huang W, Morton EJ, Street RA. "Comparison of Computer Simulations with Measurements from a-Si:H Imaging Arrays." Mat Res Soc Symp Proc 258:1163–1168, 1992.

[174] Colbeth RE, Allen MJ, Day DJ, Gilblom DL, Harris R, Job ID, Klausmeier-Brown ME, Pavkovich J, Seppi EJ, Shapiro EG, Wright MD, Yu JM. "Flat Panel Imaging System for Fluoroscopy Applications." Proc SPIE 3336, 1998, pp. 376–387.

[175] Fujieda I, Street RA, Weisfield RL, Nelson S, Nylen P, Perez-Mendez V, Cho G. "High Sensitivity Readout of 2D a-Si Image Sensors." Jap J Appl Phys 32:198–204, 1993.

[176] Huang Z, DeCrescenzo G, Rowlands JA. "Signal and Noise Analysis Using a Transmission Line Model for Large Area Flat-Panel X-Ray Imaging Sensors." Proc SPIE 3659, 1999, pp. 76–89.

[177] Haugen C, Kasap SO, Rowlands JA. "Charge Transport and Electron-Hole Pair Creation Energy in Stabilized a-Se X-Ray Photoconductors." J Phys D: Appl Phys 32:200–207, 1999.

[178] Haugen C, Kasap SO, Rowlands JA. "X-Ray Irradiation Induced Bulk Space Charge in Stabilized a-Se X-Ray Photoconductors." J Appl Phys 84:5495–5501, 1998.

[179] Kasap SO. "Photoreceptors: The Selenium Alloys." In Diamond ASD (Ed.) *Handbook of Imaging Materials*. New York: Marcel Dekker, 1991, pp. 329–377.

[180] Antonuk LE, Yorkston J, Huang W, Boudry J, Morton EJ, Longo MJ, Street RA. "Radiation Response Characteristics of Amorphous Silicon Arrays for Megavoltage Radiotherapy Imaging." IEEE Trans Nucl Sci 39:1069–1073, 1992.

[181] Kobayashi I, Funakoshi A, Tago A, Kaifu N, Takeda S, Takami E, Morishita M, Hayashi S, Mochizuki C, Endo T, Tamura T, Tashiro K, "Photoelectric Conversion Apparatus and X-Ray Image Pickup Apparatus." US Patent No. 5,793,047 (1998).

[182] Lee DLY, Cheung LK. "Method and Apparatus for Acquiring an X-Ray Image Using a Solid-State Device." US Patent No. 5,319,206 (1994).

[183] Lee DLY, Cheung LK. "Apparatus and Method for Eliminating Residual Charges in an Image Capture Panel." US Patent No. 5,563,421 (1996).

[184] Zhao W, Waechter DF, Rowlands JA. "Digital Radiology Using Active-Matrix Readout of Amorphous Selenium: Radiation Hardness of Cadmium Selenide Thin Film Transistors." Med Phys 25:527–538, 1998.

[185] Bruijns TJC, Alving PL, Baker EL, Bury R, Cowen AR, Jung N, Luijendijk HA, Meulenbrugge HJ, Stouten HJ. "Technical and Clinical Results of an Experimental Flat Dynamic (Digital) X-Ray Image Detector (FDXD) System with Real-Time Corrections." Proc SPIE 3336, 1998, pp. 33–44.

[186] Siewerdsen JH, Antonuk LE, Yorkston J. "Theoretical Performance of Amorphous Silicon Imagers in Diagnostic Radiology." Proc SPIE 2708, 1996, pp. 484–493.

[187] Zhao W, Rowlands JA. "Digital Radiology Using Active-Matrix Readout of Amorphous Selenium: Theoretical Analysis of Detective Quantum Efficiency." Med Phys 24:1819–1833, 1997.

[188] Buttler W, Hosticka BJ, Lutz G. "Noise Filtering for Readout Electronics." Nucl Inst Meth A288:187–190, 1990.

[189] Matsuura N, Zhao W, Huang Z, Rowlands JA. "Digital Radiology Using Active-Matrix Readout: Amplified Pixels for Fluoroscopy." Med Phys 26:672–681, 1999.

[190] Weisfield RL, Hartney MA, Street RA, Apte RB. "New Amorphous Silicon Imager Sensor for X-Ray Diagnostic Medical Imaging Applications." Proc SPIE 3336, 1998, pp. 444–452.

[191] Weisfield Rl, Hartney M, Schneider R, Aflatooni K, Lujan R. "High Performance Amorphous Silicon Image Sensor for X-Ray Diagnostic Medical Imaging Applications." Proc SPIE 3659, 1999, pp. 307–317.

[192] Lee H, Daly S, Van Metter RL. "Visual Optimization of Radiographic Tone Scale." Proc SPIE 3036, 1997, pp. 118–129.

[193] Freedman M, Mun SK, Pe E, Lo SCB, Nelson M. "Image Optimization Procedures for the Fuji AC-1." Proc SPIE 1897, 1993, pp. 480–502.

[194] Vuylsteke P, Schoeters E. "Multiscale Image Contrast Amplification (MUSICA^{TM})." Proc SPIE 2167, 1994, pp. 551–560.

[195] Barski L, Van Metter RL, Foos D, Lee H, Wang X. "New Automatic Tone Scale Method for Computed Radiography." Proc SPIE 3335, 1998, pp. 164–178.

[196] Vuylsteke P, Dewaele P, Schoeters E. "Optimizing Computed Radiography Imaging Performance." In *The Expanding Role of Medical Physics in Diagnostic Imaging*. Madison: Advanced Medical Publishing, 1997, pp. 107–151.

[197] Van Metter R, Foos D. "Enhanced Latitude for Digital Projection Radiography." Proc SPIE 3658, 1999, pp. 468–483.

[198] Moy JP, Bosset B. "How Does Real Offset and Gain Correction Affect the DQE in Images from X-Ray Flat Detectors?" Proc SPIE 3659, 1999, pp. 90–97.

[199] Hu J, Yan H, Hu X. "Removal of Impulse Noise in Highly Corrupted Digital Images Using a Relaxation Algorithm." Opt Eng 36:849–856, 1997.

[200] Dougherty ER, Astola J. *An Introduction to Nonlinear Image Processing*. Bellingham: SPIE, 1994.

[201] Antonuk LE, Yorkston J, Huang W, Boudry J, Morton EJ, Longo MJ, Street RA. "Factors Affecting Image Quality for Megavoltage and Diagnostic X-Ray a-Si:H Imaging Arrays." Mat Res Soc Symp Proc 258:1069–1074, 1992.

[202] Wieczorek H. "Measurement and Simulation of the Dynamic Performance of a-Si:H Image Sensors." J Non Cryst Solids 164–166:781–784, 1993.

[203] Pairjavid S, Granfors PR. "Compensation for Image Retention in an Amorphous Silicon Detector." Proc SPIE 3659, 1999, pp. 501–509.

[204] Yorkston J, Antonuk LE, Seraji N, Huang W, Siewerdsen J, El-Mohri Y. "Evaluation of the MTF for a-Si:H Imaging Arrays." Proc SPIE 2163, 1994, pp. 141–149.

[205] Macovski A, In *Medical Imaging Systems*. Englewood, Cliffs: Prentice-Hall, 1983, Chap. 11.

[206] Cunningham IA, Westmore MS, Fenster A. "A Spatial Frequency Dependent Quantum Accounting Diagram and Detective Quantum Efficiency Model of Signal and Noise Propagation in Cascaded Imaging Systems." Med Phys 21:417–427, 1994.

[207] Siewerdsen JH, Antonuk LE, El-Mohri Y, Yorkston J, Huang W, Cunningham IA. "Signal, Noise Power Spectrum, and Detective Quantum Efficiency of Indirect Detection Flat Panel Imagers for Diagnostic Radiology." Med Phys 25:614–628, 1998.

[208] Cunningham IA. "Degradation of the Detective Quantum Efficiency Due to a Non-Unity Fill Factor." Proc SPIE 3032, 1997, pp. 22–31.

[209] Ji WG, Zhao W, Rowlands JA. "Digital X-Ray Imaging with Amorphous Selenium: Reduction of Aliasing." Med Phys 25:2148–2162, 1998.

[210] Cunningham IA, "Linear Systems Modeling of Parallel Cascaded Stochastic Processes: The NPS of Radiographic Screens with Reabsorption of Characteristic X Radiation." Proc SPIE 3336, 1998, pp. 220–230.

[211] Boone JM, Seibert JA, Sabol JM, Tecotzky M. "A Monte Carlo Study of X-Ray Fluorescence in X-Ray Detectors." Med Phys 26:905–916, 1999.

[212] Yorkston J, Antonuk LE, El-Mohri Y, Jee K-W, Huang W, Maolinbay M, Rong X, Siewerdsen JH, Trauernicht DP. "Improved Spatial Resolution In Flat Panel Imaging Systems." Proc SPIE 3336, 1998, pp. 556–563.

[213] Gray JE, Stears JG, Swenson S, Bunch PC. "Evaluation of Resolution and Sensitometric Characteristics of an Asymmetric Screen-Film Imaging System." Radiology 188:537–539, 1993.

[214] Plewes DB. "A Scanning System for Chest Radiography with Regional Exposure Control: Theoretical Considerations." Med Phys 10:646–654, 1983.

[215] Plewes DB, Vogelstein E. "A Scanning System for Chest Radiography with Regional Exposure Control: Practical Implementation." Med Phys 10:655–663, 1983.

[216] Rowlands JA, Hynes DM, Edmonds EW. "System for Digital Acquisition of Gastrointestinal Images." Med Phys 16:553–560, 1989.

[217] Yorkston J, Antonuk LE, El-Mohri Y, Huang W, Lee KW, Scarpine VE, Siewerdsen JH. "Measurements of Flare with an a-Si:H Imaging Array." Med Phys 23(6):1076, 1996 (abstract).

[218] Luhta R, Rowlands JA. "Origins of Flare in X-Ray Image Intensifiers." Med Phys 17(5):913–921, 1990.

[219] Rowlands JA. "Real-Time Digital Processing of Video Image Sequences for Videofluoroscopy." Proc SPIE 1652, 1992, pp. 294–303.

[220] Rudin S, Bednarek DR. "Region of Interest Fluoroscopy." Med Phys 19: 1183–1189, 1993.

[221] Labbe MS, Chiu MY, Rzeszotarski MS, Bani-Hashemi AR, Wilson DL. "The X-Ray Fovea, a Device for Reducing X-Ray Dose in Fluoroscopy." Med Phys 21:471–481, 1994.

[222] Hunt DC, Zhao W, Rowlands JA. "Detective Quantum Efficiency of Direct, Flat Panel Detectors for Fluoroscopy." Proc SPIE 3336, 1998, pp. 195–201.

[223] Granfors PR. "Performance Characteristics of an Amorphous Silicon Flat Panel X-Ray Imaging Detector." Proc SPIE 3659, 1999, pp. 480–490.

[224] Jung N, Gipp T, Jacobs, Paul H. "Real-Time Image Processing Platform for the Correction of X-Ray Detector Related Artifacts." Proc SPIE 3659, 1999, pp. 974–985.

[225] Nguyen TC, Rowlands JA. "A Study of Motion in Gastro-Intestinal X-Ray Fluoroscopy." Med Phys 16:569–576, 1989.

[226] Mistretta CA. "Digital Radiography—A Search for Better Images." In *Recent Developments in Digital Imaging*. AAPM Medical Physics Monograph 12, New York: AIP, 1985.

[227] Fahrig R, Rowlands JA, Yaffe MJ. "X-Ray Imaging Using Amorphous Selenium: Optimal Spectra for Digital Mammography." Med Phys 23:557–567, 1996.

[228] Venkatakrishnan V, Yavuz M, Niklason LT, Opsahl-Ong B, Han S, Landberg C, Nevin R, Hamberg L, Kopans DB. "Experimental and Theoretical Spectral Optimization for Digital Mammography." Proc SPIE 3659, 1999, pp. 142–149.

[229] Zhao W, Rowlands JA, Germann S, Waechter DF, Huang Z. "Digital Radiology Using Self-Scanned Readout of Amorphous Selenium: Design Considerations for Mammography." Proc SPIE 2432, 1995, pp. 250–259.

[230] Niklason LE, Venkatakrishnan V, Hamberg LM, Christian BT, Opshal-Ong B, Kopans DB. "Digital Breast Imaging: Tomosynthesis and Digital Subtraction Angiography." Radiology 205(P):742, 1997.

[231] Fahrig R, Holdsworth DW, Lownie S, Fox AJ. "Computed Rotational Angiography: System Performance Assessment Using *In Vitro* and *In Vivo* Models." Proc SPIE 3336, 1998, pp. 305–315.

[232] Ning R, Tang X, Yu R, Zhang D, Conover D, Zhang D. "Flat Panel Detector Based Cone Beam Volume CT Imaging: Detector Evaluation." Proc SPIE 3659, 1999, pp. 192–203.

[233] Jaffray DA, Siewerdsen JH, Drake DG. "Performance of a Volumetric CT Scanner Based upon a Flat-Panel Imager." Proc SPIE 3659, 1999, pp. 204–214.

[234] Siewerdsen JH, Jaffray DA. "A Ghost Story: Spatio-Temporal Response Characteristics of an Indirect-Detection Flat-Panel Imager." Med Phys 26:1624–1641, 1999.

[235] Boyer AL, Antonuk LE, Fenster A, VanHerk M, Meertens H, Munro P, Reinstein LE, Wong J. "A Review of Electronic Portal Imaging Devices (EPIDs)." Med Phys 19:1–16, 1992.

[236] Haus AG, Dickerson RE, Huff KE, Monte S, Atanas M, Matloubieh A. "Evaluation of a Cassette-Film-Screen Combination for Radiation Therapy Portal Localization Imaging with Improved Contrast." Med Phys 24:1605–1608, 1997.

[237] Mah D, Rowlands JA, Rawlinson JA. "Measurement of Quantum Noise Sources in Fluoroscopic Systems for Portal Imaging." Med Phys 23:231–238, 1996.

[238] Mah D, Rowlands JA, Rawlinson JA. "Portal Imaging Using Amorphous Selenium: Sensitivity to X Rays from 40 kVp to 18 MV." Med Phys 25:444–456, 1998.

[239] El-Mohri Y, Antonuk LE, Yorkston J, Jee K-W, Lam KL, Siewerdsen JH. "Relative Dosimetry Using Active-Matrix Flat-Panel Imager (AMFPI) Technology." Med Phys 26:1530–1541, 1999.

CHAPTER 5
Digital Mammography

Martin J. Yaffe
University of Toronto

CONTENTS

5.1 Introduction

5.1.1 Breast cancer

Breast cancer is a major killer of women. Approximately 179,000 women were diagnosed with breast cancer in the U.S. in 1998 and 43,500 women died of this disease [1]. Breast cancer is a disease in which there is a loss of control of the proliferation of the epithelial (glandular) cells. The breast is structurally organized as shown in Figure 5.1. It is composed of several lobes, each of which drains into a major duct and these converge at the nipple. Each lobe contains lobules composed of the glandular tissue which, in lactation, delivers milk to the ducts. Breast cancer occurs in the terminal ductal lobular unit, usually within the ductules. As long as the cancer cells remain within the duct (ductal carcinoma *in situ* or DCIS) the probability of a cure is very high. Once the cancer becomes invasive, the cells have the potential to migrate away from their site of origin. Commonly, they enter the lymphatic system and cancer cells may lodge in the axillary lymph nodes in the armpit or spread further (metastasize) to more distant sites in the body such as the liver or brain. Most frequently, it is metastatic cancer which causes death from breast cancer.

The causes of breast cancer are largely still unknown, although in the last few years, two genes, which in a mutated form carry a high risk of breast cancer, have been identified. This likely only accounts for about 4% of breast cancer incidence and most breast cancer is of unknown etiology (cause).

Because we are uncertain of the cause of most breast cancer, we do not yet know how to prevent it and currently, the most effective means demonstrated to prevent death from breast cancer is detection when the cancer is *in situ* or minimally invasive and before metastasis has occurred to the point that treatment is

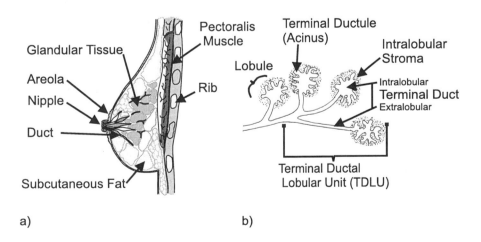

a)   b)

Figure 5.1: Schematic anatomy of the breast. a) lateral view, b) terminal ductal lobular unit, where most breast cancers arise (adapted from Wellings).

ineffective [2, 3]. The most effective means currently available for accomplishing this is mammography: that is x radiography of the breast.

Mammography is used both for investigating symptomatic patients (diagnostic mammography) and for screening of asymptomatic women in selected age groups. It is also used for pre-surgical localization of suspicious areas and in the guidance of needle biopsies.

Breast cancer is *detected* on the basis of four types of signs on the mammogram:

(a) the characteristic morphology of a tumor mass,

(b) certain presentations of mineral deposits as specks called microcalcifications,

(c) architectural distortion of normal tissue patterns caused by the disease, and

(d) asymmetry between corresponding regions of images of the left and right breast.

After a suspicious abnormality is detected, a further set of criteria is applied to the image to increase the radiologist's level of confidence that the abnormality does or does not represent cancer. This process is referred to as radiological diagnosis and may entail the production of additional specialized images. A positive *radiological diagnosis* is confirmed by tissue sampling (biopsy) which can be done surgically or with a less-invasive needle core sampling procedure.

5.1.2 Challenges in imaging the breast

An imaging system for detection or diagnosis of breast cancer must provide visualization of the key signs of disease listed above. In order to allow visualization of the subtle changes in tissue x-ray attenuation associated with breast cancer, the imaging system must precisely measure the transmitted x-ray intensity through all regions of the breast and must amplify the small contrast to produce visible signals that exceed the perceptual threshold of the viewer. Much of the important information in the mammogram is contained in the fine detail associated with microcalcifications and thin fibers radiating from the tumor mass and, therefore, the spatial resolution of the imaging system must be very high. Because of these requirements, mammography is one of the most technically demanding radiological imaging techniques.

5.1.3 Screen-film mammography

5.1.3.1 Strengths

In discussing the development of digital mammography, it is critical that the value of conventional screen-film mammography is not undermined. Screen-film mammography is and will continue to be a valuable tool for detection and radiological diagnosis of breast cancer and is the only tool that has been demonstrated to have a role in reducing mortality from this disease through early detection as part of a routine screening program. In fact, screen-film mammography has several distinct advantages and these become particularly evident when one attempts to develop an alternate, improved technology. Among others, these advantages are:

(a) the technology is relatively inexpensive,

(b) the image receptor is capable of achieving very high limiting spatial resolution —in excess of 20 line-pairs/mm,

(c) images are conveniently displayed using view-box technology. In particular, the ability to display multiple images simultaneously is very important,

(d) film performs an inherent logarithmic compression of dynamic range onto the available optical densities of the film. This often provides an acceptable rendition of information acquired in the mammogram in a single presentation, without the need to adjust display parameters.

5.1.3.2 Limitations

In screen-film mammography the film must act as an image-acquisition detector as well as a storage and display device. In these roles, it performs very well in providing excellent spatial resolution of high-contrast structures and is an efficient medium for long term storage of image data. As in any situation, however, where many jobs must be done simultaneously, certain compromises result and these are discussed below.

5.1.3.2.1 Contrast/latitude. Breast tumors and microcalcifications, which are an important early indicator of cancer, are visualized in the mammogram due to differential x-ray attenuation between these structures and normal breast tissue. The overall displayed contrast of structures on the mammogram is actually a result of the combination of this "attenuation contrast" and the photographic (optical density) gradient of the mammographic film.

Figure 5.2 shows measured x-ray attenuation coefficients of fibroglandular breast tissue, fat and breast carcinoma versus x-ray energy [4]. Subject contrast is related to the difference in attenuation coefficients between these tissues, and the very small differences between these curves illustrate why mammography is such a challenging imaging task, particularly when the tumor is surrounded by fibroglandular tissue. As shown in Figure 5.3, attenuation contrast decreases rapidly with increasing x-ray energy. To maximize attenuation contrast, mammography is conventionally carried out with low-energy x-ray spectra, typically using a molybdenum anode x-ray tube operated at a potential of approximately 26 kVp with additional molybdenum beam filtration. The breast attenuates x rays very strongly at these energies, and, therefore, to obtain adequate signal from the image receptor, a relatively high dose compared to general radiography (>1 mGy mean glandular dose per image) is received by the breast.

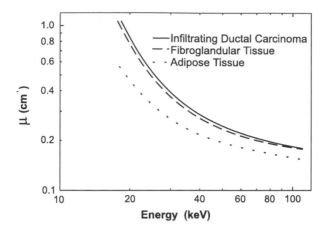

Figure 5.2: X-ray linear attenuation coefficients of fat, fibroglandular tissue and ductal carcinoma plotted versus energy. (From Johns and Yaffe [4].)

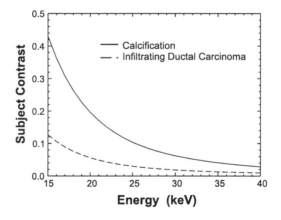

Figure 5.3: Dependence of subject contrast in mammography on x-ray energy (monoenergetic case).

The display contrast properties of the radiographic film are described by the gradient of its characteristic curve. A typical curve for a mammographic screen-film combination is shown in Figure 5.4(a). Because of its sigmoidal shape, the range of x-ray exposures over which the film display gradient is significant (i.e., the image latitude) is limited to a factor of about 25, as shown in Figure 5.4(b) where the display gradient is plotted versus exposure to the imaging system. This may be a problem because, depending on the composition of the breast, the maximum range of transmitted exposures can be 100:1 or more. If a tumor is located in either a more lucent or more opaque region of the breast, then even though the attenuation contrast provided by the x-ray beam is significant, the final contrast displayed to the radiologist may be considerably reduced because of the low gradient of the film

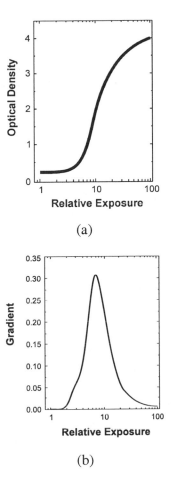

Figure 5.4: (a) Typical characteristic curve for a mammographic screen-film combination, (b) gradient of the characteristic curve plotted versus log relative exposure.

over that part of the range. This is particularly a concern in patients whose breasts contain large amounts of fibroglandular tissue, the so-called dense breast [5, 6].

5.1.3.2.2 Noise.   All radiological images contain random fluctuation due to the statistics of x-ray quantum absorption. This noise can limit the reliability of detection of small or subtle structures. In addition, other sources of noise, due to the structure of the fluorescent screen and the granularity of the film emulsion used to record the image, compound this problem. An ideal imaging system will be "x-ray quantum limited," meaning that x-ray quantum noise is the dominant source of random fluctuation. When a system is x-ray quantum limited, further reduction in relative noise requires an increase in the number of x rays incident on the imaging system, that is an increase in patient dose. Generally, existing mammographic screen-film systems are not quantum limited, because at high spatial frequencies, noise in the imaging system is dominated by film granularity and screen structure, not by the number of x-ray quanta recorded.

An imaging system can be made quantum limited by reducing intrinsic noise sources and by using more x rays to form the image. For a fixed system speed, the latter is best accomplished by increasing the x-ray interaction efficiency of the screen.

5.1.3.2.3 Compromise between resolution and efficiency.

Another possible limitation of screen-film mammography is the tradeoff between spatial resolution and detector x-ray interaction (detection) efficiency. In a fluorescent screen used with film, spatial resolution is determined mainly by the amount of blur attributable to diffusion of light travelling from the point of x-ray interaction in the screen to the film. Screen blur increases as the thickness of the screen is increased. To maintain high spatial resolution, mammographic screens must be kept relatively thin. Although there have been some recent developments in high-density phosphor materials, which could allow high interaction efficiency for thin screens [7], the detection efficiency of many of the currently available systems is typically only 60–70%, necessitating increased radiation dose.

5.1.3.2.4 Inefficiency of scatter rejection.

Even at the low x-ray energies used in mammography, Compton x-ray scattering is an important process of interaction between the x-ray beam and the breast. The magnitude of singly and multiply-scattered x-ray quanta impinging upon the imaging system is generally comparable to the intensity of directly transmitted primary radiation. By adding a "uniform," noisy background to the image, detection of scattered quanta reduces image contrast, signal-to-noise ratio, and the dynamic range available for recording useful information.

Most mammography is performed using a radiographic grid which discriminates geometrically against scattered radiation. Although the scattered radiation does not carry useful information, it does generate light from the screen which exposes the film, helping to achieve the required optical density. The loss of this scattered radiation, and inefficiency of the grid in transmitting the desired primary radiation to the screen, results in a requirement of increased radiation dose to the patient. Typically, this increase is on the order of a factor of 2–3 compared to imaging without a grid [8].

5.2 Digital mammography

Digital mammography replaces the screen-film image receptor with a detector which provides an electronic signal proportional to the intensity of x rays transmitted by the breast. When digitized and stored in computer memory, the image can be processed and displayed on a soft copy or hard copy device. By separating the image acquisition from the storage and display functions, each can be optimized. Potentially this allows the limitations of screen-film mammography to be overcome and facilitates improved detection or diagnosis of breast cancer.

5.2.1 Technical requirements of the detector

Important detector properties for digital mammography are: field coverage, geometrical characteristics, quantum efficiency, sensitivity, spatial resolution, noise characteristics, dynamic range, uniformity, acquisition speed, and cost. For dynamic studies (breast angiography, tomosynthesis), the rate at which sequential images can be acquired is also important.

5.2.1.1 Field coverage

The imaging system must be able to record the transmitted x-ray signal over the entire projected area of the breast. Mammography can be accommodated by a receptor of dimensions 18 cm × 24 cm for small and average-size breasts, however, an imaging field of 24 cm × 30 cm may be required to image larger breasts in a single exposure.

5.2.1.2 Geometrical characteristics

Some of the factors to be considered here are the "dead regions" that may exist within and around the edges of the detector. In an electronic detector used for digital radiography, these might be required for routing of wire leads or placement of auxiliary detector components such as buffers and clocks. Dead regions can also result when a large-area detector is produced by abutting together smaller detector units (tiling). For detectors composed of discrete detector elements or "dels" (as distinguished from displayed picture elements or pixels), we can define the *fill-factor* as the fraction of the area of each detector element that is sensitive to the incident x rays. Any dead area within the detector results in inefficient use of the radiation transmitted by the patient. In mammography, it is important that the active area of the detector extends as close to the patient's chest wall as possible to avoid excluding breast tissue from the image. Most screen-film mammography systems lose no more than 3-mm coverage at the chest wall.

Another geometrical factor which must be considered is distortion. A high-quality imaging system will present a faithful spatial mapping of the input x-ray pattern to the image output. The image may be scaled spatially, however the scaling factor should be constant over the image field. Distortion will cause this mapping to become nonlinear. It may become spatially or angularly dependent. This may be the case when lens, fiber, or electron optics are used in the imaging system and give rise to "pincushion" or "barrel" distortion.

Digital detectors can be of two general types, captive sensors or replaceable cassettes. In the former, the receptor and its readout are integrated into the x-ray machine. While this requires a specially-designed machine with higher capital cost, it also eliminates the need for loading, unloading, and carrying of cassettes to a separate reader and the labor costs involved. As well, the use of a single or a limited number of receptors simplifies the task of correction for non-uniformities of the receptors (see below). On the other hand, a reusable cassette system has the advantage of being compatible with existing mammography units and a single readout system can serve multiple mammography machines.

5.2.1.3 Quantum efficiency

In all x-ray detectors, to produce a signal, the x-ray quanta must interact with the detector material. The probability of interaction or *quantum efficiency* for quanta of energy $E = hv$ is given by:

$$\eta = 1 - e^{-\mu(E)T}, \tag{5.1}$$

where μ is the linear attenuation coefficient of the detector material and T is the active thickness of the detector. The quantum efficiency must be specified at each energy in the spectrum or must be expressed as an "effective" value over the spectrum of x rays *incident on the detector*. This spectrum will be influenced by the filtering effect of the patient which is to "harden" the beam, that is, to make it more energetic and, hence, more penetrating.

The quantum efficiency can be increased by making the detector thicker or by using materials which have higher values of μ because of increased atomic number or density. The quantum efficiency versus x-ray energy for various thicknesses of some detector materials considered for digital mammography is plotted in Figure 5.5. The quantum efficiency generally decreases with increasing energy. If the material has an atomic absorption edge in the energy region of interest, then quantum efficiency increases dramatically above this energy, causing a local minimum in η for energies immediately below the absorption edge.

5.2.1.4 Spatial resolution

Spatial resolution in mammography is only partially determined by the receptor characteristics. Resolution also depends on factors unrelated to the receptor such as penumbra due to the effective size of the x-ray source and the magnification between the anatomical structure of interest and the plane of the image receptor as well as relative motion between the x-ray source, patient, and image receptor during the exposure. Detector-related factors arise from its effective aperture size, spatial sampling interval between measurements, and any lateral signal-spreading effects within the detector or readout.

Detectors for digital radiography are often composed of discrete dels, generally of constant size and spacing. The dimension of the active portion of each del defines an aperture. The aperture determines the spatial-frequency response of the detector. For example, if the aperture is square with dimension, d, then the modulation transfer function (MTF) of the detector will be of the form sinc (f), where f is the spatial frequency along the x or y directions, and the MTF will have its first zero at the frequency $f = d^{-1}$, expressed in the plane of the detector (Figure 5.6). A detector with $d = 50\,\mu$m will have an MTF with its first zero at $f = 20$ cycles/mm. Because of magnification, this frequency will be slightly higher in a plane within the breast.

Also of considerable importance is the sampling interval, p, of the detector, that is, the pitch in the detector plane between sensitive elements or measurements. The sampling theorem states that only spatial frequencies in the pattern below $(2p)^{-1}$

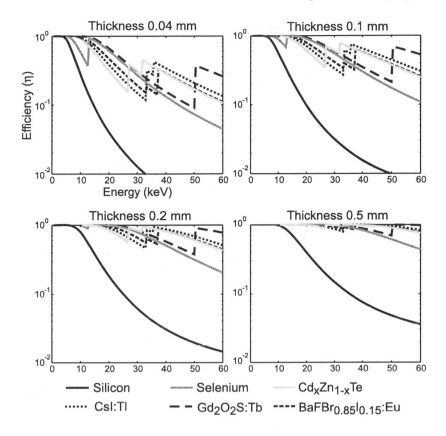

Figure 5.5: X-ray quantum efficiency versus energy for different thicknesses of materials used for detectors for digital radiographic systems.

(the Nyquist frequency) can be faithfully imaged. If the pattern contains higher frequencies, then *aliasing* occurs, wherein the frequency spectrum of the image pattern beyond the Nyquist frequency is mirrored or folded about that frequency and added to the spectrum of lower frequencies, increasing the apparent spectral content of the image at these lower frequencies [9]. In a detector composed of discrete elements, the smallest sampling interval in a single image acquisition is $p = d$, so that the Nyquist frequency is $(2d)^{-1}$ while the aperture response falls to 0 at twice that frequency (higher if the dimension of the sensitive region of the detector element is smaller than d, for example, when the fill factor of the detector element is less than 1.0). Thus, such detectors are susceptible to aliasing.

Aliasing of signal can be avoided by "band limiting" the image, in other words, attenuating the higher frequencies such that there is no appreciable image content beyond the Nyquist frequency. The blurring associated with a phosphor may serve this purpose. Note that this does not prevent the aliasing of high spatial frequency noise. Alternative methods that reduce aliasing effects of both signal and noise require the sampling frequency of the imaging system to be increased. One method

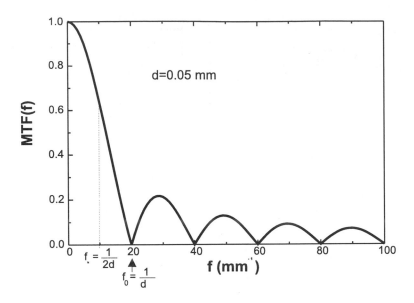

Figure 5.6: Spatial frequency response of a rectangular aperture indicating the first 0 of the response at d^{-1} and the Nyquist frequency of $(2p)^{-1}$. Typically $p \geqslant d$.

for achieving this, known as *dithering*, involves multiple acquisitions accompanied by a physical motion of the detector by a fraction of the pixel pitch between successive acquisitions. The subimages are then combined to form the final image. This effectively reduces p, thereby providing a higher Nyquist frequency.

Some detectors are not pixellated at the x-ray absorption stage, but rather d and p are defined in their readout mechanism. This is the case for the photostimulable phosphor detector system described below, where the phosphor plate is continuous, but the laser readout samples the plate at discrete locations. This can provide some flexibility in independently setting the sampling interval (scanning raster) and effective aperture size (laser spot size) to avoid aliasing. Issues of sampling in digital radiographic systems have been reviewed by Dobbins [10].

In the design of the digital mammography system, it is important that other physical sources of unsharpness be considered when the aperture size and sampling interval are chosen. If, for example, the MTF is limited by unsharpness due to the focal spot, it would be of little value to attempt to improve the system by designing the receptor with smaller detector elements. Currently, however, all digital mammography systems are limited by the detector resolution.

5.2.1.5 Noise

All images generated by quanta are statistical in nature, that is, although the image pattern can be predicted by the attenuation properties of the patient, it will fluctuate randomly about the mean predicted value. The fluctuation of the x-ray intensity follows Poisson statistics, so that the variance, σ^2, about the mean number of x-ray quanta, N_0, falling on a detector element of a given area, is equal to N_0. Interaction with the detector can be represented as a binomial process with probability of success, η, and it has been shown [11] that the distribution of interacting quanta is still Poisson distributed with standard deviation

$$\sigma = (N_0\eta)^{1/2}. \qquad (5.2)$$

If the detection stage is followed by a process that provides a mean gain $\overline{g}$, then the "signal" becomes

$$q = N_0\eta\overline{g}, \qquad (5.3)$$

while the variance in the signal is

$$\sigma_q^2 = N_0\eta(\overline{g}^2 + \sigma_g^2), \qquad (5.4)$$

where σ_g^2 represents the variance in the gain factor.

In general, the distribution of q is not Poisson even if g is Poisson distributed. The effect of additional stages of gain (or loss) can be expressed by propagating this expression further [12, 13]. It is also possible that other independent sources of noise will be contributed at different stages of the imaging system. Their effect on the variance at that stage will be additive and the fluctuation will be subject to the gain of subsequent stages of the imaging system.

In screen-film systems, contrast depends on the actual optical density achieved on the film and, therefore, on exposure. Inappropriate exposure can result in a degradation in image quality due to lack of contrast. Because the contrast in the digital system is adjustable it is more relevant to quantify the signal-to-noise ratio and use this in determining the exposure required in producing an image. Continuing the simplified analysis given above, the SNR can be expressed as

$$\text{SNR} = (N_0\eta)^{1/2}\left[\frac{\sigma_g^2}{g^2} + 1\right]. \qquad (5.5)$$

In a well-designed detector, the number of quanta incident on the detector and η should be the main factors influencing SNR. However, it is also important that the fluctuation in the gain is small compared to g^2. This is one reason why a fairly high value of g is desirable.

A complete analysis of signal and noise propagation in a detector system must take into account the spatial frequency dependence of both signal and noise. Signal transfer can be characterised in terms of the modulation transfer function, $\text{MTF}(f)$, where f is the spatial frequency, while noise is described by the noise power or Wiener spectrum $W(f)$. Methods for calculating the Wiener spectral properties of a detector must correct for nonlinearities in the detector and must properly take into account the spatial correlation of signal and statistical fluctuation (see Chapter 3).

A useful quantity for characterizing the overall signal and noise performance of imaging detectors is their spatial frequency-dependent detective quantum efficiency, $DQE(f)$. This describes the efficiency in transferring the signal-to-noise ratio (squared) contained in the incident x-ray pattern to the detector output. Ideally, $DQE(f) = \eta$ for all f, however, additional noise sources will reduce this value and often cause the DQE to decrease with increasing spatial frequency. $DQE(f)$ can be treated as a sort of quantum efficiency, in that when it is multiplied by the number of quanta incident on the detector, one obtains $SNR_{out}^2(f)$, also known as the number of noise-equivalent quanta, $NEQ(f)$, used to form the image. Typically DQE for a screen-film detector has a value on the order of only 0.2 to 0.3 at a spatial frequency of 0 cycles/mm, and this may fall to 0.05 at a few cycles/mm [14, 15].

As will be discussed in Section 5.3.1, it is important that the number of secondary quanta or electrons at each stage of the detector is somewhat greater than $N_0\eta$, to avoid having the detector noise being dominated by a "secondary quantum sink."

5.2.1.6 Sensitivity

The final output from the detector is an electrical signal, so that sensitivity can be defined in terms of the charge produced by the detector (before any external amplification) per incident x-ray quantum of a specified energy. The sensitivity of any imaging system depends on η and on the primary conversion efficiency (the efficiency of converting the energy of the interacting x-ray to a more easily measurable form such as optical quanta or electric charge). Conversion efficiency can be expressed in terms of the energy, w, necessary to release a light photon in a phosphor, an electron–hole pair in a photoconductor (or semiconductor), or an electron–ion pair in a gaseous detector. Values of w for some typical detector materials are given in Table 5.1. The limiting factor is related to the intrinsic band structure of the solid from which the detector is made. In Figure 5.7(a), the basic band structure of a crystalline material is shown. Normally the valence band is fully populated with electrons and the conduction band is empty. The energy gap governs the scale of energy necessary to release an electron hole pair, that is, to promote an electron from the valence band to the conduction band. However, though this energy is the *minimum* permitted by the principle of conservation of energy, this can be accomplished only for photons of energy exactly equal to the energy gap. For charged particles releasing energy (e.g., through the slowing down of high-energy electrons created by an initial x-ray interaction), requirements of conserving both energy and crystal momentum as well as the presence of competing energy-loss processes, require, on average, at least three times as much energy as the band gap to release an electron-hole pair [16]. In Figure 5.7(b) the situation for a phosphor is shown. In this case, the first requirement is to obtain an electron hole pair. Subsequently, the electron returns to the valence band by means of a luminescence center created by an activator added to the host material. This requires that the energy E_F of the fluorescence light be less than the band gap energy E_G,

Table 5.1:

Material	Z	E_K (keV)	W (eV)	ω_K (approx.)
Gd_2O_2S	64	50.2	13	0.92
CsI(Tl)	55/53	36.0/33.2	19	0.87
BaFBr (as photostim. phosphor)	56/35	37.4/13.5	50–100	0.86
High purity Si	14	1.8	3.6	<0.05
Amorphous selenium	34	12.7	50 (at $10V/\mu m$)	0.6
PbI_2	82/53	88/33.2	4.8	0.95/0.85
$Cd_{0.8}Zn_{0.2}Te_1$	48/30/52	26.7/9.7/31.8	~5	0.85/0/0.85

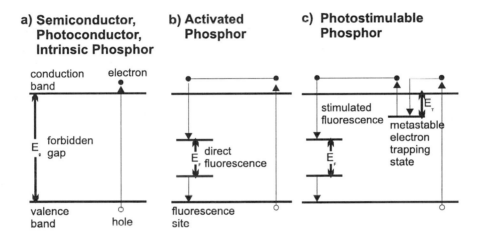

Figure 5.7: Schematic energy level diagrams for a) semiconductor detector, b) phosphor, c) photostimulable phosphor.

and therefore further inevitable inefficiencies exist in a phosphor compared to a photoconductor of the same E_G.

5.2.1.7 Dynamic range

The dynamic range can be defined as

$$DR = \frac{X_{\mathrm{max}}}{X_{\mathrm{noise}}}, \qquad (5.6)$$

where X_{max} is the x-ray fluence providing the maximum signal that the detector can accommodate and X_{noise} is the fluence that provides a signal equivalent to the quadrature sum of the detector noise and the x-ray quantum noise.

While this definition describes the performance of the detector on an individual pixel basis, it is less useful for predicting the useful range of detector operation for a particular imaging task. This is because, at the bottom of this range, the signal-to-noise ratio (SNR) is only 1, which is seldom acceptable. Also, it is rare to base a medical diagnosis on a single image pixel and therefore, for most objects, the SNR is based on the signal from multiple pixels. For a large object, the noise on a pixel-by-pixel basis can be large; however, if there is integration over the object, the effective SNR will improve approximately as the square root of the area (with some correction for correlation effects caused by unsharpness of the imaging system). We have, therefore, offered a second definition of "effective dynamic range" which we have found useful:

$$DR_{\text{eff}} = \frac{k_2 X_{\text{max}}}{k_1 X_{\text{noise}}}. \tag{5.7}$$

Here, the constant k_1 is the factor by which the minimum signal must exceed the noise for reliable detection. Rose [17] has argued that k_1 should be on the order of 4 or 5 depending on the number of elements in the image and the imaging task. The constant k_2, which is dependent on the imaging task and the system MTF, reflects the improvement in SNR due to integration over multiple pixels. Effectively, this causes the dynamic range of the imaging system to increase even though the maximum signal level and the single pixel noise level have not changed. Maidment et al. [18] and Neitzel [19] have analyzed this problem for the case of digital mammography.

In practice, the required dynamic range for an imaging task can be decomposed into two components. The first describes the ratio between the unattenuated beam and the x-ray attenuation of the most radio-opaque path through the breast to be included on the same image. The second is the precision of x-ray signal to be measured in the most radio-opaque part of the image. In mammography, for an effective energy of 20 keV and a breast composed of 50% adipose tissue and 50% fibro-glandular tissue, 6 cm thick, the attenuation factor is approximately 42. If it is required to have 1% precision in measuring the signal in the most attenuating region, then the dynamic range requirement would be 4200.

In defining the range of operation for a detector, one must consider both the need for adequate x-ray fluence to achieve the desired quantum counting statistics at the low end of the range as well as detector phenomena such as saturation or "blooming" that can occur with large signals. The dynamic range of the detector can also be reduced by operations to correct for nonuniformity, as discussed in the next section.

5.2.2 Uniformity

It is important that the digital mammographic imaging system provide uniformity, that is, the sensitivity must be constant over the entire area of the image. Otherwise patterns that disrupt the effective interpretation of the image may result. These patterns are sometimes referred to as "fixed pattern noise." In an analog imaging system, great pains must be taken in the design and manufacture of detectors to ensure that they provide uniform response.

In a digital system, the task is much easier because, at least over a considerable range, differences in response from element to element can be corrected. This is accomplished by imaging an object of uniform x-ray transmission, recording the detector response, and using this as a "correction mask." This process is called "flat fielding." If the detector has linear response to x rays, then the correction involves two masks, one with and one without radiation, to provide slope and intercept values for the correction of each element. To avoid increasing image noise in the flat-fielding correction process, it is important that the correction masks have very low noise. This can be most easily accomplished by averaging several acquired flat-field images together to create the final mask.

It is often observed that slight nonlinearities exist in detectors and the degree of nonlinearity varies among dels. When such differential nonlinearity exists, flat-fielding may be effective in correcting images produced at detector signals near the intensity used for calibrating the flat-field correction; however, nonuniformity over the image will become apparent for other intensity levels, depending on how much they differ from the flat-fielding condition. If the detector response is nonlinear, then measurements must be made over a range of intensities and a nonlinear function fit to the response of each element to obtain the correction coefficients.

In some detectors, nonuniformities might exist only over rows and columns of the detector rather than over individual elements. This greatly reduces the number of coefficients that must be stored.

Flat fielding causes the original detector signals to be altered. It is important to recognize that if signal values are restricted to a fixed scale, for example, 0 to 4095, then the flat-fielding correction may reduce the dynamic range of the detector if there is significant nonuniformity of response among dels.

5.3 X-ray detectors for digital mammography

5.3.1 Phosphor-based detector systems

Most x-ray imaging detectors employ a phosphor in the initial stage to absorb the x rays and produce light, which is then coupled to an optical sensor (photodetector). The use of relatively high-atomic-number phosphor materials causes the photoelectric effect to be the dominant type of x-ray interaction. The photoelectron produced in these interactions is given a substantial fraction of the energy of the x-ray. This energy is much larger than the bandgap of the crystal (Figure 5.7(b)) and, therefore, in being stopped, a single interacting x-ray has the potential to cause the excitation of many electrons in the phosphor and thereby the production of many light quanta. We describe this "quantum amplification" as the *conversion gain*, g_1. For example, in a Gd_2O_2S phosphor, the energy carried by a 25-keV x-ray quantum is equivalent to that of 10,400 green-light quanta ($E_g = 2.4$ eV). Because of competing energy-loss processes and the need to conserve momentum, the *conversion efficiency* is only about 15%, so that, on average, it requires approximately 13 eV per light quantum created in this phosphor (Table 5.1). The conversion gain is then approximately 1560 light quanta per interacting x-ray quantum.

The energy-loss process is stochastic and, therefore, g has a probability distribution, with standard deviation, σ_g, about its mean value as illustrated in Figure 5.8(a). Swank [20] described this effect and the "Swank factor," A_s, characterizes this additional noise source. The Swank factor is calculated in terms of the moments of the distribution of g as

$$A_s = \frac{M^2}{M_0 M_2},\qquad(5.8)$$

where M_i indicates the ith moment of the distribution.

The number of light quanta produced when an x-ray interacts in a phosphor depends both on its incident energy and the mechanism of interaction with the phosphor crystal. The most likely type of interaction, the photoelectric effect, will result in both an energetic photoelectron and either a second (Auger) electron or a fluorescent x-ray quantum being produced. The energy of fluorescence depends on the shell in which the photoelectric interaction took place. The threshold K-shell energy for these interactions is shown for some detector materials in Table 5.1. Also in the table is the K-fluorescence yield, ω_K the probability of emission of x-ray fluorescence given that a K-shell photoelectric interaction has occurred. The fluorescent quanta are either reabsorbed in the phosphor or escape. In either case, if they are not absorbed locally, the apparent energy deposited in the phosphor from the x-ray quantum is reduced, giving rise to a second peak in the distribution with a lower value of g. The effect of fluorescence loss is to broaden the overall distribution of g (Figure 5.8(b)), thus decreasing A_s and causing an increase in σ_g. For many detector materials (e.g., Gd_2O_2S), their K-shell interactions lie above the energy range used for mammography and therefore, K fluorescence effects are not an issue.

There are both advantages and disadvantages in imaging with an x-ray spectrum that exceeds the K edge of the phosphor. Clearly, the value of η increases, however the "Swank noise" does also. In addition, deposition of energy from the

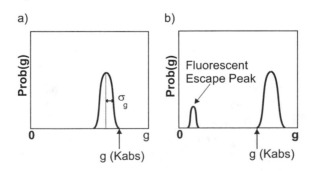

Figure 5.8: Distribution of initial gain of a detector stage. The Swank factor characterizes the distribution in terms of its moments: a) energy below K edge of detector, b) energy above K edge results in K fluorescence escape peak.

fluorescence at some distance from the point of initial x-ray interaction causes the point spread function of the detector to increase, resulting in decreased spatial resolution.

After their formation, the light quanta must successfully escape the phosphor and be effectively coupled to the next stage for conversion to an electronic signal and readout. It is desirable to ensure that the created light quanta escape the phosphor efficiently and as near as possible to their point of formation.

Figure 5.9 illustrates the effect of phosphor thickness and the depth of x-ray interaction on spatial resolution of a phosphor detector. The probability of x-ray interaction is exponential so that the number of interacting quanta and the amount of light created will be proportionally greater near the x-ray entrance surface.

While travelling within the phosphor, the light will spread—the amount of diffusion being proportional to the path length required to escape the phosphor. X rays interacting close to the photodetector give rise to a sharper (less blurred) optical signal than those which interact more distantly. The paths of most optical quanta will be shortest if the photodetector is placed on the x-ray entrance side of the phosphor. It is often only possible, however, to record the photons which exit on the opposite face of the phosphor screen, that is, those which have had a greater opportunity to spread. If the phosphor layer is made thicker to improve quantum efficiency, the spreading becomes more severe. This imposes a fundamental compromise between spatial resolution and η. Methods to channel the optical photons out of the phosphor without spreading can significantly improve phosphor performance. This is accomplished, in part, with the use of CsI phosphors in detectors for digital mammography.

Figure 5.10 illustrates the propagation of signal through the various energy-conversion stages of an imaging system. In the diagram, N_0 quanta are incident on a specified area of the detector surface (Stage 0). A fraction of these, given by the quantum detection efficiency, η, interact with the detector (Stage I). In a perfect imaging system, η would be equal to 1.0. The mean number, N_1 of quanta interacting represents the "primary quantum sink" of the detector. The fluctuation about

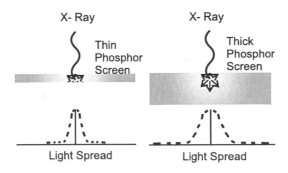

Figure 5.9: Effect of the thickness of a conventional phosphor layer on spatial resolution (line-spread function).

N_1 is $\sigma_{N1} = (N_1)^{1/2}$. This defines the signal-to-noise ratio, SNR, of the imaging system which increases as the square root of the number of quanta interacting with the detector.

Regardless of the value of η, the maximum possible SNR of the imaging system will occur at this point and if the SNR of the imaging system is essentially determined there, the system will be x-ray quantum limited in its performance. However, the SNR will, in general, become reduced in passage of the signal through the imaging system because of losses and additional sources of fluctuation.

To avoid losses that can occur at subsequent stages, it is important that the detector provide adequate quantum gain, g_1, directly following the initial x-ray interaction. Stages II and III illustrate the processes of creation of many light photons from a single interacting x-ray (conversion gain) and the escape of quanta from the phosphor with mean probability g_2. Here, light absorption, scattering and reflection processes are important.

Further losses occur in the coupling of the light to the photodetector which converts light to electronic charge (Stage IV) and in the spectral sensitivity and optical quantum efficiency of the photodetector (Stage V). If the conversion gain of the phosphor is not sufficiently high to overcome these losses and the number of light quanta or electronic charges at a subsequent stage falls below that at the primary quantum sink, then a secondary quantum sink is formed. In this case the statistical fluctuation of the light or charge at this point becomes an additional important noise source. Even when an actual secondary sink does not exist, a low value of light or charge will cause increased noise. This becomes evident in a spatial-frequency-dependent analysis of SNR as a reduction of the detective quantum efficiency with increasing spatial frequency. Figure 5.11 illustrates the effect of optical coupling efficiency of light from a phosphor to a photodetector on DQE(f) for an optically-coupled system [21].

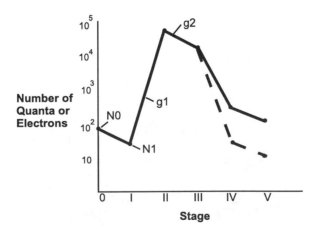

Figure 5.10: Quantum accounting diagram can be used to identify quantum sinks in a multi-stage imaging system.

Figure 5.12 illustrates two approaches for coupling a phosphor to a photodetector. In Figure 5.12(a) a lens is used to collect light emitted from the surface of the phosphor material. Because the size of available photodetectors such as CCDs is limited by manufacturing considerations to a maximum dimension of only 2 to 5 cm, it is often necessary to demagnify the image from the phosphor to allow coverage of the required field size in the patient. The efficiency of lens coupling is determined largely by the solid angle subtended by the collecting optics. For a single lens system, the coupling efficiency is given by [22, 23]

$$\xi = \frac{\tau}{4F^2(m+1)^2},\tag{5.9}$$

where τ is the optical transmission factor for the lens, F is the f-number of the lens (ratio of the focal length to its limiting aperture diameter), and m is the demagnification factor from the phosphor to the photodetector. For a lens with $F = 1.2$, $\tau = 0.8$ and $m = 10$, ξ will be 0.1%.

Because of this low efficiency, the SNR of systems employing lens coupling is often limited by a secondary quantum sink, especially where the demagnification factor is large and/or g_1 is small.

It is also possible to use fiber optics to affect the coupling. These can be in the form of fiber-optic bundles (Figure 5.12(b)), where optical fibers of constant diameter are fused to form a light guide. The fibers form an orderly array so that there is a one-to-one correspondence between the elements of the optical image at the exit of the phosphor and at the entrance to the photodetector. Where demagnification is required, the fiber-optic bundle can be tapered by drawing it under heat. While

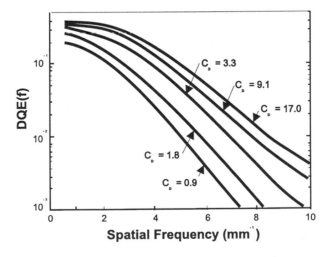

Figure 5.11: Effect of coupling efficiency on spatial-frequency dependent DQE. Numbers on each curve represent the coupling efficiency in terms of the number of electrons produced at the photodetector per x-ray quantum interacting in the phosphor.

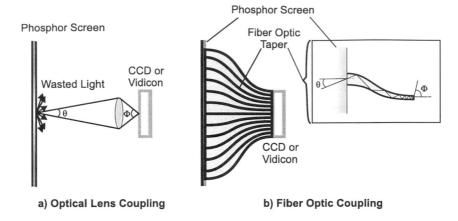

Figure 5.12: Methods to achieve coupling with demagnification between a phosphor and a photodetector (a) lens, (b) fiber-optic.

facilitating the construction of a detector to cover the required anatomy in the patient, demagnification by tapering also reduces coupling efficiency by limiting the acceptance angle at the fiber-optic input. A simplified expression for the coupling efficiency of a fiber optic taper is

$$\xi = \alpha \tau (\theta) \frac{NA^2}{m^2}, \tag{5.10}$$

where α is the fraction of the entrance surface that comprises the core glass of the optical fibers, $\tau(\theta)$ is the transmission factor for the core glass, NA is the numerical aperture of the untapered fiber, and m is the demagnification factor caused by tapering. For example, a taper with 2 times demagnification ($m = 2$), with $\alpha = 0.8$, $\tau = 0.9$, and $NA = 1.0$, has an efficiency of 18%, about seven times higher than a lens with $F = 1.2$ with the same demagnification factor and about 2.5 times higher than a lens with $F = 0.7$. It should be noted that for both lenses and fiber optics, the transmission efficiency is dependent on the angle of incidence, θ of the light and, therefore, a complete analysis involves an integral of the angular distribution of emission of the phosphor over θ. A comparison of the efficiency of lens versus fibreoptic coupling is shown in Figure 5.13 [24].

Fiber-optic bundles are subject to geometric distortion which must be minimized. To maintain high resolution, the crosstalk of signal between fibers must be controlled and this is accomplished, in part, by the use of an extramural absorber (EMA), i.e., an optically attenuating material incorporated between individual fibers in the bundle to absorb light that escapes from the fibers or that directly enters the fiber cladding material on the entrance surface of the bundle.

Both fiber-optic and lens designs are used in small-field-of-view cameras for digital mammography to couple a phosphor to a full-frame CCD photodetector [25]. These systems are used for guiding needle biopsy and for localization of

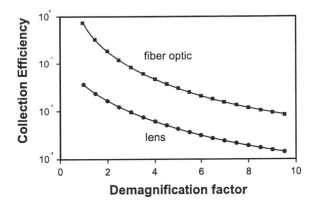

Figure 5.13: Efficiency of coupling with lenses and fiber-optics. In coth cases, efficiency falls as the demagnification factor between the input and output increases.

suspicious lesions. Typically only about $2\times$ demagnification is employed, resulting in acceptable coupling efficiency.

5.3.2 Full-area digital mammography detector systems

5.3.2.1 Demagnifying phosphor/fibreoptic/CCD system

Although it is possible to extend the approach described above to create a full-area detector, Eq. (5.9) indicates that the large demagnification factor that would be required would result in unacceptably low coupling efficiency and a secondary quantum sink. This problem can be circumvented by designing the detector as a mosaic of smaller modules. One manufacturer, Trex, uses a mosaic of 3×4 detectors, each one employing a demagnification on the order of $2\times$. This system produces a full-size image of the breast with approximately 40 micron pixels (Figure 5.14).

The x-ray absorbing phosphor in this system is composed of thallium-activated cesium iodide (CsI:Tl). The advantage of utilizing CsI as the x-ray absorber is that it can be grown in columnar crystals which act as fiber optics. When coupled to the photodiode pixels, there is little lateral spread of light and, therefore, high spatial resolution can be maintained. In addition, unlike conventional phosphors in which diffusion of light and loss of resolution become worse when the thickness is increased, CsI phosphors can be made thick enough to ensure a high value of η while maintaining high spatial resolution.

5.3.2.2 Amorphous silicon phosphor flat-panel detectors

Active matrix LCDs (AMLCDs) have been made using amorphous (hydrogenated amorphous silicon [26, 27]. The active matrix is a large-area integrated circuit consisting of a large number of thin-film field-effect transistors (TFTs) connected to individual photodetector elements in a matrix.

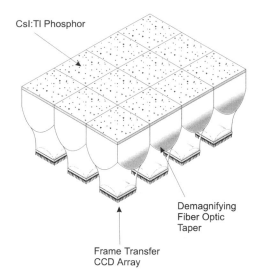

CsI:Tl Phosphor

Demagnifying
Fiber Optic
Taper

Frame Transfer
CCD Array

Figure 5.14: Full field detector formed as a mosaic of small-field devices. Each of the 12 modules consists of a demagnifying fiber-optic taper which couples light from a CsI:Tl phosphor layer to a full frame CCD.

The potential advantages of such self-scanned, compact readout systems include their compactness, freedom from veiling glare, geometric uniformity, and immunity to stray magnetic fields. To produce an x-ray detector, CsI:Tl is evaporated directly onto the active matrix [28, 29].

The principle of operation of an amorphous silicon detector is shown schematically in Figure 5.15. The dels are configured as photodiodes (Figure 5.15(a)) which convert the optical signal from the phosphor to charge and store that charge on the capacitance of the element. Being low-noise devices, the photodiodes provide a very large dynamic range, on the order of 40,000:1. A typical thin-film transistor readout array is shown in Figure 5.15(b). The signal is read out by activation of scanning control lines for each row of the device, connected to the gates of TFTs located on each detector pixel. An entire row of the detector array is activated simultaneously and the signal is read on lines for each column in the array which connect all the TFT sources in that column to a low-noise charge amplifier. The amplified signals from the columns are then multiplexed and digitized. This allows fast detector readout and requires a number of electronic channels equal to the number of columns of the array.

Alternatively, instead of TFT readout various diode switching schemes can be used [30, 31]. The advantage of the diode approach is that, because the photodiode has to be made anyway, the switching diode can be made at the same time without increase in the number of material-processing steps. The disadvantages of diode readout is a strong nonlinearity and large charge injection.

The area allocated to each pixel of the array must contain the photodiode, switching device, and control and signal lines so that the fill factor is less than

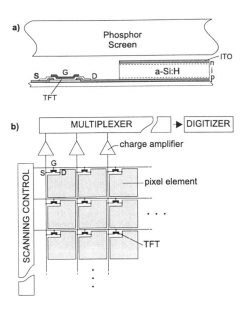

Figure 5.15: Amorphous silicon full-field detector. a) Light from a CsI:Tl layer is direct coupled to a photodiode on each del. b) The readout array on an amorphous silicon plate uses thin film transistor switches to multiplex the charge stored on the capacitance of each del to readout lines.

100%. This potential loss of x-ray utilization efficiency becomes proportionately greater as the pixel size is decreased and provides a challenge for the application of this technology to very high resolution applications. Currently dels of $100\,\mu$m have been produced and new techniques [32] should allow sizes down to 50 or $60\,\mu$m.

General Electric has produced a system using CsI on a-Si with a del of $100\,\mu$m. The detector assembly fits onto a modified GE conventional mammography unit.

5.3.2.3 Photostimulable phosphors

Probably the most widespread detectors for digital radiography to date have been photostimulable phosphors, also known as storage phosphors. These phosphors are commonly in the barium fluorohalide family, typically $BaFBr:Eu^{2+}$, where the atomic energy levels of the europium activator determines the characteristics of light emission. X-ray absorption mechanisms are identical to those of conventional phosphors. They differ in that the useful optical signal is not derived from the light that is emitted in prompt response to the incident radiation, but rather from subsequent emission when electrons and holes are released from traps in the material [33, 34] The initial x-ray interaction with the phosphor crystal causes electrons to be excited (Figure 5.7(c)). Some of these produce light in the phosphor in the normal manner, however, the phosphor is intentionally designed to contain traps which store the charges. By stimulating the crystal by irradiation with

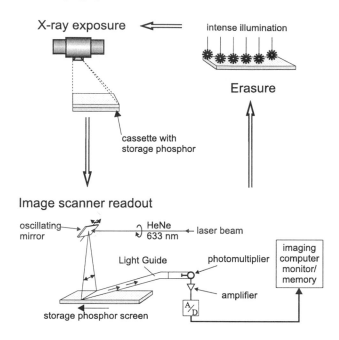

Figure 5.16: Digital mammography system based on a photostimulable phosphor with laser raster readout.

red light, electrons are released from the traps and raised to the conduction band of the crystal, subsequently triggering the emission of shorter wavelength (blue) light. This process is called photostimulated luminescence. The physics of photostimulable phosphor imaging has been reviewed in more detail elsewhere [35, 36].

In the digital radiography application, the imaging plate is positioned in a light-tight cassette or enclosure, exposed and then read by raster scanning the plate with a laser to release the luminescence (Figure 5.16). The emitted light is collected and detected with a photomultiplier tube whose output signal is digitized to form the image.

The energy levels in the crystal are critical to the effective operation of the detector (Figure 5.7(c)). The energy difference between the traps and the conduction band E_T must be small enough so that stimulation with laser light is possible, yet sufficiently large to prevent random thermal release of the electron from the trap. The energetics should also provide for wavelength of the emitted light that can be efficiently detected by a photomultiplier and for adequate wavelength separation between the stimulating and emitted light quanta to avoid contaminating the measured signal. The electrons liberated during irradiation either produce light promptly or are stored in traps. Because the "prompt" light is not of interest in this application, the efficiency of the storage function can be improved by increasing the probability of electron trapping. On the other hand, when these electrons are released by the stimulating light during readout, the probability of their being retrapped instead of producing light would then be higher, thus reducing the efficiency the readout. The optimum balance occurs where the probabilities of an excited electron being retrapped or stimulating fluorescence are equal. This causes the conversion efficiency to be reduced by a factor of 4 compared to the same phosphor without traps, that is, a factor of 2 from the prompt light given off during x-ray exposure and another factor of 2 from unwanted retrapping of the electrons during readout.

In addition, the decay characteristics of the emission must be sufficiently fast that the image can be read in a conveniently short time while capturing an acceptable fraction of the emitted energy. In practice, depending on the laser intensity, the readout of a stimulable phosphor plate yields only a fraction of the stored signal. This is a disadvantage with respect to sensitivity and readout noise, however, it can be helpful by allowing the plate to be "pre-read," in other words, read out with only a small part of the stored signal to allow automatic optimization of the sensitivity of the electronic circuitry for the main readout.

The photostimulable phosphor is a convenient detector for digital radiography in that, when placed in a cassette, it can be used with conventional x-ray machines. Large-area plates are conveniently produced, and because of this format, images can be acquired quickly. The plates are reusable, have linear response over a wide range of x-ray intensities, and are erased simply by exposure to a uniform stimulating light source to release any residual traps.

One limitation of this type of detector is that because the traps are located throughout the depth of the phosphor material, the laser beam providing the stimulating light must penetrate into the phosphor. Scattering of the light within the phosphor causes release of traps over a greater area of the image than the size of the incident laser beam. This results in loss of spatial resolution, which is aggravated if the plate is made thicker to increase η. An ideal solution to this problem would be a phosphor which was nonscattering for the stimulating light and both non-scattering and nonabsorbing for the emitted light. Limitations can arise in the readout stage, where efficient collection of the emitted light requires great attention to design. This can result in a secondary quantum sink, especially at high spatial frequencies, causing a reduction of $DQE(f)$. Fuji is currently performing clinical evaluation of a photostimulable phosphor plate system for use in digital mammography. The system is designed to provide data at a sampling interval of 100μm.

5.3.3 Scanned-beam acquisition

In these systems, the detector is in the form of a multilinear array of dels and the image is acquired by scanning the detector assembly across the breast in synchrony with a fan beam of x rays. This design limits the required number of dels, while allowing high spatial resolution (small detector aperture and pitch) to be achieved. This is an important cost factor when expensive detector technologies are employed. Another advantage is the inherent high efficiency rejection of scattered radiation afforded by slot-beam systems, where the detector can be collimated to match the pre-patient fan beam. This can be accomplished without the need for interspace material in the beam.

One disadvantage of scanning systems is the longer overall time to acquire the image. Although this may preclude some dynamic studies, it does not result in blurring because each portion of the image is acquired in a very short time. If there is significant motion in the breast, then a misregistration artifact is more likely to occur. Another disadvantage is that because most of the x-ray beam is removed by the fan-beam collimation, there is inefficient use of x-ray tube heat loading. This requires that the x-ray tube used in this application be designed with an increased heat capacity. To mitigate against both of these effects, the number of rows in the detector (and the width of the x-ray slot beam) can be increased. The system design then involves a tradeoff between the shorter imaging time and improved use of heat loading afforded by a wide slot detector system and the improved scatter rejection and less critical mechanical alignment available with a narrower slot.

Scanned slot systems have been built using the phosphor/fiberoptic taper/CCD concept described in 5.3.2.1. We have used such a design to construct a digital mammography system [37, 38]. The detector consists of a strip of CsI(tl) phosphor material, coupled to three fiberoptic tapers which are abutted with mitre joints at their input surfaces as shown in Figure 5.17(a). Their taper ratio of 1.58:1 provides demagnification with acceptable light-collection efficiency for this application while creating a space between the tapers at the output to accommodate the outer non-active regions of 3 CCD arrays, which are bonded directly on the tapers. The detector slot is approximately 3.5 mm wide.

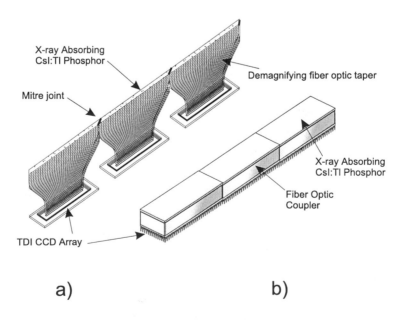

a)   b)

Figure 5.17: Scanned slot digital mammography detector based on CsI:Tl coupled to a TDI CCD via a) demagnifying fiber-optic taper, b) straight coupling (Fischer system).

In scanning systems it is useful to acquire the image in time-delay-integration (TDI) mode, in which the x-ray beam is activated continuously during the image scan and charge collected in pixels of the CCDs is shifted down CCD columns at a rate equal to but in the opposite direction of the motion of the x-ray beam and detector assembly across the breast. The collected charge packets remain essentially stationary with respect to a given projection path of the x rays through the breast and the charge is integrated in the CCD column to form the resultant signal. When the charge packet has reached the final element of the CCD, it is read out on a transfer register and digitized. The CCD array can be cooled using thermoelectric devices to reduce noise and increase the dynamic range of the image receptor as necessary. In such systems the spatial resolution is dependent on accurate alignment of the signal-gathering columns of the detector with the scan direction and on correct synchronization with charge clocking in the CCDs with the scan motion. Fischer Imaging Inc. is currently evaluating a scanning system at several clinical sites (Figure 5.17b). The Fischer system differs from the one described above in that it employs a non-tapered fiber-optic coupling and a wider slot ($\sim$14 mm). In addition, the inherent del is 25 μm, allowing a limited-area, high-resolution "spot" mode. For normal resolution, the signals from adjacent dels are summed to provide an effective 50 μm del.

5.3.4 Solid-state electrostatic systems

5.3.4.1 Amorphous selenium

In phosphor systems, absorbed x rays release light which must escape to the surface to create an image. Lateral spread of light is determined by diffusion, resulting in a point spread function whose width is comparable to the thickness of the phosphor. The loss of high-spatial-frequency information can be alleviated by using a phosphor such as CsI, which can be produced in the form of columnar structures, such that it behaves like a fiber optic. However, the channelling of light is not perfect [39].

There are several advantages in the use of solid state electrostatic systems rather than phosphors [40]. A detector based on a structureless electrostatic layer is shown in Figure 5.18. X rays interacting in the photoconductor plate release electrons and holes which, because they are charged, can be guided directly to the surfaces of the photoconductor by the applied electric field. The latent charge image on the photoconductor surface is, therefore, not blurred significantly even if the plate is made thick enough to absorb almost all of the incident x rays [41]. In addition, the efficient collection of the signal from each interacting quantum eliminates problems associated with secondary quantum sinks. Bulky and expensive optical coupling elements are not required.

Amorphous selenium (a-Se) is the most highly developed photoconductor for x-ray applications. Its amorphous state makes possible the maintenance of uniform imaging characteristics to almost atomic scale (there are no grain boundaries) over large areas. The primary function of the a-Se layer is to attenuate x rays, generate free electron-hole pairs (in proportion to the intensity of the incident x rays), and

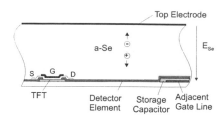

Figure 5.18: Direct conversion detector system based on amorphous selenium photoconductor.

collect them at the electrodes. To achieve a high value of η, the detector must be of adequate thickness (Figure 5.5). High conversion efficiency in converting absorbed x-ray energy into free electron-hole pairs requires high electric fields. Finally, the number of bulk traps in the layer must be small, so that virtually all the freed carriers reach their appropriate electrode. Each surface must have an electrode attached to permit collection of charge from the a-Se while preventing entry of charge from the electrodes into the a-Se. This is called a *blocking contact*. Finally the surface of the a-Se at which the image is formed must have a very small transverse conductivity. Otherwise the image charge could migrate laterally and destroy the resolution. The small transverse conductivity is achieved by introducing a high density of traps in the a-Se very close to the image interface [42].

Flat panel detectors for digital radiography, based on the use of an active matrix readout method for a-Se have been described by Lee *et al.* [43] and Zhao and Rowlands [44, 45]. The potential features of this method are: high image quality, real-time readout rate, and compact size. During x-ray exposure, energy is absorbed by the a-Se layer and the charge created is drawn by the internal electric field E_{Se} to the surfaces (Figure 5.18). The image charge is collected by the del electrode and accumulated onto its capacitance. On each del, the electrode and storage capacitor are connected to a TFT switch. The readout device can be similar to that used with the CsI(Tl)/amorphous silicon system (Figure 5.15b), where, in this case, the photodiode elements are replaced by electrodes. The external scanning control circuit generates pulses to turn on all the TFT switches on a row of the array and transfers charge from the del capacitors to the readout lines (columns). The charge is then collected and amplified by an amplifier on each line and the data for the entire row is multiplexed out. This sequence is repeated for each row of the array. The readout can be in real time, thus facilitating dynamic procedures. Fahrig *et al.* [46] have analyzed the factors influencing DQE in a-Se x-ray detectors. Polischuk et al. have recently described an a-Se detector with 85-μm dels for digital mammography [47].

5.3.4.2 *Other direct-conversion systems*

Other direct-conversion detector materials are becoming available. These may have advantages compared to selenium in terms of higher atomic number and density for improved η at higher energies, their values of w, the ability to be operated

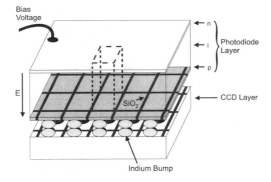

Figure 5.19: Hybrid detector consisting of an x-ray absorbing photoconductor or photodiode on one substrate coupled via indium bump bonding to a separate readout CCD. Such detectors have been designed for slot scanning systems.

at relatively low collection bias fields, cost, ease and reliability of manufacturing, etc. These materials include zinc cadmium telluride, thallium bromide, [48] and PbI_2 [49].

For scanning digital mammography systems, it is possible to form the detector as a hybrid between an x-ray absorber formed as an array of photodiodes or photoconductive dels and a TDI CCD readout formed on a separate substrate (Figure 5.19). The two matrices are joined on a del-by-del basis by a series of microscopic indium "bumps." Thus charge liberated in the detection layer is transferred via the indium to be collected and integrated down CCD columns and finally digitized. Detectors of this design were initially used for imaging in the infrared spectrum and have been shown to provide very high spatial resolution and other desirable imaging characteristics when modified for use with x rays [50]. In some cases, it may also be possible to evaporate the detector material directly onto a pickup electrode surface on the readout device.

5.4 Display of digital mammograms

One of the potential advantages of digital mammography is the extended dynamic range compared to screen-film. The increased amount of information recorded in the image, however, imposes a major challenge in developing an effective and practical means for image display [51].

The two most practical display technologies currently available are laser film printers and cathode-ray-tube (CRT) monitors. Neither has sufficient latitude or dynamic range to accommodate the data available in a digital mammogram in a single display representation. High-resolution laser film printers are able to provide an adequately small pixel size to allow all of the image elements of the digital mammogram to be recorded on the film, however, the single-emulsion film used for printing provides a smaller range of optical densities than is available with conventional mammography film. As a result, unless multiple versions of the image are printed with different display parameters, some or all of the image is likely to be displayed at reduced contrast, making it difficult to detect the extremely subtle differences between cancers and the surrounding normal tissue.

Similarly, "soft copy" devices such as CRT monitors do not have sufficient dynamic range to display all of the intensity information at one setting, however they allow interactive adjustment of display while viewing the image. The radiologist can then explore the acquired information with different display settings. While this is not difficult to do, it is time consuming and not practical for routine work in a busy radiology department.

Of equal importance, for several of the digital mammography systems, even state-of-the-art CRT monitors are not able to display a full digital mammogram at more than half its spatial resolution. This problem can be partially overcome using a combination of image roam and local zoom features, however, once again, this is a labor-intensive process and there is the risk that the radiologist, in performing these operations, will lose the gestalt of the image.

Therefore, unless effort is spent in developing new display technologies or improving existing technologies to create a practical method for presenting digital mammograms to radiologists, some of the advantages of digital mammography will be lost. Indeed, the clinical acceptance of digital mammography will be seriously compromised.

One way to overcome some of the limitations of display technology is to use image processing techniques to enhance lesion visibility. Current efforts in this area by various investigators include the use of wavelet transformations, image filtering, and grey-level enhancements [52–59]. Preliminary results from these studies have shown two important points. First, with image processing, the image lesions become more detectable. Second, these studies indicate that different types of mammographic lesions (masses, microcalcifications, architectural distortions, etc.) need different types of enhancements (either different algorithms or a different set of parameters). Because it is not known *a priori* what type of lesion is present in an image, a series of different techniques would need to be applied, creating several images from each mammogram. This is costly if film is the display medium; in addition, potentially longer viewing times would be required if the radiologist routinely had to scroll through a series of image-processing parameters. Our current experience indicates that this is not acceptable to the radiologist in clinical practice. Furthermore, although application of the enhancement technique may make a lesion more conspicuous, this process may severely distort the image and impair detection of other possible lesions. Possibly, this problem can be solved by the use of artificial intelligence to determine the most appropriate processing based on detected patterns in the mammogram.

5.4.1 Peripheral equalization

One drawback of using local enhancement is that the dynamic range of the image is still large, greater than the latitude of laser printers and CRT monitors. The large dynamic range requirement comes about because of two factors, the varying thickness of the breast and variations in tissue composition. This is illustrated in

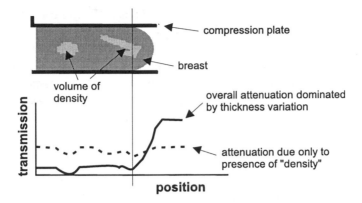

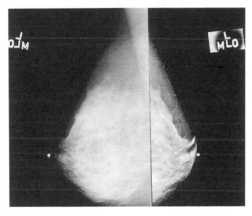

Figure 5.20: The dynamic range requirement in digital mammography is due to the variation in composition of the breast as well as variation in thickness of the tissue across the image.

Figure 5.21: Peripheral equalization can be used to reduce the effective dynamic range of the image by suppressing the effect of thickness variation. Left—unequalized mammogram, Right—mammogram that has been processed with peripheral equalization.

Figure 5.20. The thickness variations take place mainly in the periphery, where it is difficult to accomplish uniform mechanical compression of the breast.

It is possible to reduce the dynamic range requirement of the display medium by suppressing the effect of the thickness variations. This can be accomplished by traditional image processing techniques such as unsharp masking, or by using a more spatially selective peripheral equalization technique [60, 61].

The technique involves low-pass filtering of the digital mammogram and automated identification of a transition region where the thickness of the breast decreases from the value in the region of uniform compression to zero at the edge of the breast.

Once this region has been identified, the low-pass image can be used to create a compensation function. A correction algorithm is then applied in which the uniformly compressed region of the image requires no correction whereas in the transition region the image is multiplied by a smoothly increasing function that essentially equalizes the apparent thickness of the breast in the image (Figure 5.21). Because the correction is based only on the low spatial frequency components of the image, local variations attributable to composition are maintained without distortion, providing an image which preserves fine and intermediate detail, but which encompasses a lower dynamic range than the original image.

5.5 Clinical status of digital mammography

As noted above, currently four digital mammography systems are being evaluated in the clinical environment. Each of the manufacturers is conducting studies to attempt to satisfy USFDA requirements on equipment performance. In addition, there are two major multi-institutional clinical studies in progress. In one, being conducted at seven institutions, using three machine types, the accuracy of digital versus screen-film mammography is being compared in women who require breast biopsy. These women all have greater than 33% of the area of the breast on the mammogram containing dense tissue. Biopsy results will allow the imaging performance to be compared with the true disease state in this selected population.

The second study, involving two institutions and only the GE system, is being carried out in a screening environment, where, in the population being imaged, there is no a priori reason to expect that the participants have breast disease. The results of these studies are not available at this time, however preliminary reports indicate similar sensitivity to screen-film mammography with improved specificity [62]. Anecdotally, radiologists in these studies note that while the spatial resolution of the images is not as high as in screen-film mammography, the contrast, and the ability to visualize structures surrounded by dense tissue is often better.

5.6 Applications of digital mammography

The most obvious benefit expected from digital mammography is an improvement in sensitivity and specificity brought about by improved quality of image acquisition and by the ability to manipulate the digital image while it is being viewed. In addition, digital mammography can facilitate the introduction of powerful imaging applications which were largely impractical until the images were available in digital form. These include computer-aided detection and diagnosis, contrast-uptake imaging, telemammography, tomosynthesis, and quantitative image analysis.

5.6.1 Computer-aided detection and diagnosis

Even with high-quality modern mammography, some breast cancers may be missed on initial interpretation yet are visible in retrospect [63]. Double reading of screening mammograms by a second radiologist has been shown to improve the cancer detection rate by 9–10% [64, 65]. Computer analysis of the mammogram can be used to emulate a second reader and may detect lesions that are missed by the radiologist to increase detection sensitivity [66, 67]. The terms "computer-aided detection" and "computer-aided diagnosis," both generically abbreviated as "CAD," refer to detection or diagnosis by a radiologist who considers the results of pattern analysis performed by a computer as well as statistical information that is presented regarding the probability of malignancy. These provide a "second opinion" that the radiologist can take into consideration in making his/her final interpretation. Computers are not subject to fatigue or distraction, and CAD results for a particular algorithm should be free of intra-observer variation.

It is widely anticipated that digital mammography will greatly facilitate the use of CAD methods, because elimination of the need for prior digitization of images will result in a saving of time and effort [68]. Moreover, any improvement in image quality of digital mammography over film-screen mammography in terms of improved dynamic range or signal-to-noise ratio should allow better performance of CAD.

In a digital mammography CAD system, suspicious locations would be indicated to the radiologist by arrows or some other marking on the display screen. After a lesion is detected, artificial intelligence could be used to estimate the likelihood of malignancy (computer-aided diagnosis) to reduce the number of false positive biopsies and thereby increase diagnostic specificity. A comprehensive review of computer-aided diagnosis in mammography is provided by Giger in *Handbook of Medical Imaging, Vol. 3, Display and PACS.*

5.7 Telemammography

Telemammography is the transmission of mammographic images from one location to another in digital format. These locations can be within a particular facility, such as the mammography clinic and the operating room. Alternatively, the images can be sent over much longer distances, such as between a mammography unit in a remote facility, lacking a specialized trained mammographic radiologist, and a center of expertise where interpretation or consultation would be provided [69–71].

Although teleradiology is commonly used in many areas of radiology, adequate telemammography systems are only now appearing [62, 72].

A practical telemammography system requires that the images be in digital form. This can be accomplished by film digitization, but it is much more desirable and convenient if they are acquired directly on a digital system. An important requirement of a telemammography system is adequate communication bandwidth. This is most appropriately matched to the speed of image production and/or the acceptable delay time between the examination and when the image is interpreted. Other important issues relate to the performance of the image management system, in providing effective and convenient image retrieval, and the mechanism for remote consultation [73]. The need for image compression to reduce the amount of data that must be transmitted is not clear and depends on the cost of the communications modality, the size of the images, and the overhead involved in compressing and decompressing the data.

It is critical that the telemammography system not degrade the diagnostic quality of the mammograms. This requires that any data coding, compression, and display strategies maintain the high intrinsic quality of the images and introduce no unacceptable artifacts.

A telemammography system can be considered at two levels: (1) the basic network compression and transmission hardware and software and (2) a user application with which the radiologist interacts. Because the technology of image communication is likely to undergo rapid change and improvement, it is important to provide this separation so that the system will appear more or less the same to the user even though drastic modifications may occur over time at the network level to enhance performance.

If image compression is performed to reduce transmission costs and increase speed, it can be either lossless (no information is deleted from the image) or "lossy." Although the latter can provide greater compression ratios, such as reduction of the amount of data in an image by a factor of 10 or more, the more moderate gains (a factor of 2 to 3) obtained with lossless compression may be preferable for legal reasons, and with high-speed transmission, may be completely satisfactory. In either case, mechanisms for automatic correction of transmission errors will be necessary.

The transmission speed and cost depend on the type of network technology that is employed. The requirements for speed depend on whether the images are to be sent as a batch, perhaps overnight, or to be sent and interpreted in real time. For batch transmission, networks of modest speed may be acceptable. For real-time applications, slight delays of even several seconds may be disturbing to the radiologist.

Depending on needs and budget, image transmission could be carried out over standard T1 telephone links [74] (up to 1.544 Mbits/s) or higher speed such as asynchronous transfer mode (ATM) links. For more remote locations where the infrastructure for these may not exist, satellite communication may be more appropriate, despite the higher initial setup cost, because it can provide arbitrarily high speed and can be operated virtually anywhere, including mobile van sites.

Several possible applications of telemammography can be anticipated. At present, when diagnostic mammography is performed in the absence of an on-site expert radiologist, patients may require a second appointment to receive supplementary views so that their breast problem can be adequately evaluated. Telemammography would allow radiologists to monitor and interpret problem-solving mammography on-line for a nearby or even distant location. Screening examinations could also be read remotely, eliminating the need to transport films from the remote fixed site or mobile van to the main facility. Clinical images could be remotely monitored for technical quality as they are performed so that patients would not have to return for repeat exposures. Radiologists at different locations could see and discuss the same case simultaneously. Interactive teaching conferences could be conducted between different sites. Finally, mammographic images could be transmitted to the offices of referring physicians, expediting patient care and eliminating the need for patients to transport and possibly misplace their own studies.

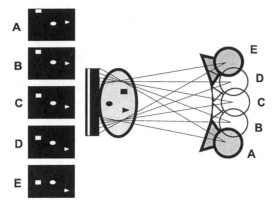

Figure 5.22: Tomosynthesis, in which digital images obtained at different x-ray tube angles are shifted and combined to suppress information from regions other than the plane of interest within the breast.

5.8 Tomosynthesis

A significant advantage of digital imaging is that image data can be readily manipulated. This advantage is particularly apparent in tomosynthesis, which is a refinement of blurring tomography, a technique that has long been performed with screen-film technology. In blurring tomography, the x-ray source and image receptor move in a linear, circular, or other more complex path during the exposure of the patient in such a manner as if they were connected to move about a fulcrum. The motion has the effect of blurring anatomical structures lying above or below the plane of the fulcrum, thereby largely obliterating their contrast. Structures in the "focal plane" are imaged sharply, giving the impression that only a slice of the patient anatomy is imaged. In digital mammography this principle can be applied by moving the x-ray source in a pattern and obtaining a series of low-dose images at different source positions. The detector remains stationary and the image data can be shifted appropriately in the computer to synthesize the tomographic image (Figure 5.22). Tomosynthesis improves the conspicuity of lesions by eliminating irrelevant contrasts and may be useful in imaging the dense breasts where fibrous tissue can obscure the visibility of a mass or other signs of cancer [75]. Because each image can be acquired at low dose, the overall examination may not require any more radiation than does a single, high-quality image. Furthermore, by increasing conspicuity of structures tomosynthesis may allow mammography to be done with less compression of the breast; in fact, reduced compression may facilitate tomosysnthesis by increasing the z-axis separation of structures.

5.9 Quantitative image analysis: Risk assessment

Following pioneering work by Wolfe [76] we have been assessing whether quantitative analysis of breast density data and textures of digitized film mammograms of asymptomatic women can allow prediction of future risk of breast cancer.

There is now good evidence that this is the case [77–79] and a relative risk of a factor of four to six has been associated with high-versus-low-density mammographic patterns. Density scores and other relevant information could be automatically extracted from digital mammograms in the future to help, for example, in defining the optimum screening interval for different risk groups or to monitor whether risk can be reduced by dietary or drug interventions [80, 81].

5.10 Dual-energy mammography

It has been suggested that even if the contrast limitations of film-screen mammography were overcome with digital mammography, some lesions would still be missed, particularly in dense breasts, because of the complexity of overlying fibroglandular structures. Unwanted contrasts caused by these structures form "clutter" noise which masks the structures of greatest interest. The availability of digital imaging facilitates the implementation of techniques to increase lesion conspicuity. One technique is dual-energy mammography [82]. By obtaining digital images with two substantially different x-ray spectra, it is possible to combine these images to produce hybrid images in which the contrast of relevant structures is preserved while the unwanted masking contrasts are largely removed. This process could be done at the viewing station so that various structures within the image can be surveyed dynamically.

5.11 Contrast-uptake imaging of the breast

Magnetic-resonance imaging of the breast with intravenous administration of GdDTPA contrast agent has shown remarkable performance in detection of small breast cancers in women with dense breasts, where mammography has not performed well and also in outlining the extent of disease [83–86]. Much of the benefit from these images likely accrues from the use of the contrast agent. Digital mammography should allow similar information to be gathered more quickly and at lower cost by providing a series of digital subtraction images which demonstrate the uptake and washout of contrast material [87]. Studies to evaluate digital breast angiography are currently underway.

5.12 Conclusion

By overcoming many of the technical limitations of screen-film mammography, digital mammography could provide images of improved contrast sensitivity and facilitate the accurate detection and diagnosis of breast cancer. There are several viable detector technologies available for image acquisition, and these provide increased DQE compared to screen-film systems. Image display and image navigation still provide challenges in the development of a practical, clinically acceptable system. There are several exciting and potentially important applications in breast imaging that will be made possible through the introduction of digital mammography. In light of the increased cost of a digital mammography unit compared to screen-film mammography, it is these that may well justify the purchase of a digital system.

References

[1] Landis SH, Murray T, Bolden S, Wingo PA. "Cancer Statistics, 1998." CA Cancer J Clin 48:6–29, 1998.

[2] Tabar L, Fagerberg G, Chen H-H *et al.* "Efficacy of Breast Cancer Screening by Age: New Results from the Swedish Two-County Trial." Cancer 75:2507, 1995.

[3] Smart CR, Hendrick RE, Rutledge JH III *et al.* "Benefit of Mammographic Screening in Women Ages 40–49 Years." Cancer 75:1619, 1995.

[4] Johns PC, Yaffe MJ. "X-Ray Characterization of Normal and Neoplastic Breast Tissues." Physics in Medicine and Biology 32:675–695, 1987.

[5] Taylor P, Hajnal S, Dilhuydy M-H, Barreau B. "Measuring Image Texture to Separate 'Difficult' from 'Easy' Mammograms." British Journal of Radiology 67:456–63, 1994.

[6] Boyd NF, O'Sullivan B, Campbell JE, Fishell E, Simor I, Cooke G, Germanson T. "Mammographic Patterns and Bias in Breast Cancer Detection." Radiology 143:671–674, 1982.

[7] Beutel J, Kitts El. "The Image Quality Characteristics of a Novel Film/ Screen System for Mammography." Proc SPIE 2708, 1996, pp. 233–240.

[8] Wagner AJ. "Contrast and Grid Performance in Mammography." In Barnes GT, Frey GD (Eds.) *Screen Film Mammography Imaging Considerations and Medical Physics Responsibilities.* Madison: Medical Physics Publishing, 1991, pp. 115–134.

[9] Bendat JS, Piersol AG. *Random Data Analysis and Measurement Techniques*, 2nd Edition. New York: Wiley, 1986, p. 338.

[10] Dobbins JT III. "Effects of Undersampling on the Proper Interpretation of Modulation Transfer Function, Noise Power Spectra, and Noise Equivalent Quanta of Digital Imaging Systems." Med Phys 22:171–181, 1995.

[11] Barrett HH, Swindell W. *Radiological Imaging.* New York: Academic Press, 1981, pp. 97.

[12] Rabbani M, Shaw R, Van Metter R. "Detective Quantum Efficiency of Imaging Systems with Amplifying and Scattering Mechanisms." J Optical Soc Am A4:895–901, 1987.

[13] Cunningham IA, Westmore MS, Fenster A. "A Spatial Frequency Dependent Quantum Accounting Diagram and Detective Quantum Efficiency Model of Signal and Noise Propagation in Cascaded Imaging Systems." Med Phys 21(3): 417–427, 1994.

[14] Bunch PC, Huff KE, Van Metter R. "Analysis of the Detective Quantum Efficiency of a Radiographic Screen-Film Combination." J Optical Society of America A4:902–909, 1987.

[15] Bunch PC. "The Effects of Reduced Film Granularity on Mammographic Image Quality." In Van Metter R, Beutel J (Eds.) *Medical Imaging. Physics of Medical Imaging.* Proc SPIE 3032, 1997, pp. 302-317.

[16] Klein CA. J Appl Phys 39:2029, 1968.

[17] Rose A. "The Sensitivity Performance of the Eye on an Absolute Scale." J Optical Society of America 38:196, 1948.

[18] Maidment ADA, Fahrig R, Yaffe MJ. "Dynamic Range Requirements of X-Ray Detectors for Digital Mammography." Med Phys 20:1621–1633, 1993 (see also letter in 21:1215).

[19] Neitzel U. "Discernable Gray Levels and Digitization Requirements in Digital Mammography." Med Phys 21:1213–1214, 1994.

[20] Swank RK. "Absorption and Noise in X-Ray Phosphors." J Appl Phys 44:4199–4203, 1973.

[21] Maidment ADA, Yaffe MJ. "Analysis of the Spatial-Frequency Dependent DQE of Optically Coupled Digital Mammography Detectors." Med Phys 21:721–729, 1994.

[22] Miller LD. "Transfer Characteristics and Spectral Response of Television Camera Tubes." In Biberman LM, Nudelman S (Eds.) *Photoelectronic Imaging Devices*, Vol. 1. New York: Plenum, 1991, pp. 267–290.

[23] Maidment ADA, Yaffe MJ. "Analysis of Signal Propagation in Optically Coupled Detectors for Digital Mammography: II Lens and Fibre Optics." Phys Med Biol 41:475–493, 1996.

[24] Hejazi S, Trauernicht DP. "Potential Image Quality in Scintillator CCD-Based Imaging Systems for Digital Radiography and Digital Mammography." In Van Metter R, Beutel J (Eds.) *Medical Imaging 1996: Physics of Medical Imaging*. Proc SPIE 2708, 1996, pp. 440–449.

[25] Roehrig H, Yu T, Schempp WV. "Performance of X-Ray Imaging Systems with Optical Coupling for Demagnification Between Scintillator and CCD Readout." Proc SPIE 2279, 1994, pp. 388-401.

[26] Piper W, Bigelow JE, Castleberry DE, Possin GE. "The Demands on the *a*-Si FET as a Pixel Switch for Liquid Crystal Displays." In *Amorphous Semiconductors for Microelectronics*. Proc SPIE 617, 1986, pp. 10–15.

[27] Powell M. "The Physics of Amorphous-Silicon Thin-Film Transistors." IEEE Trans Electron Devices 36:2753–2763, 1989.

[28] Perez-Mendez V, Cho G, Fujieda I, Kaplan SN, Qureshi S, Street RA. "The Application of Thick Hydrogenated Amorphous Silicon Layers to Charged Particle and X-Ray Detection." Mat Res Soc Symp Proc 149:621–630, 1989; (also Lawrence Berkeley Laboratories Report LBL-26998, April, 1989).

[29] Fujieda I, Cho G, Drewery J, Gee T, Jing T, Kaplan SN, Perez-Mendez V, Wildermuth D. "X-Ray and Charged Particle Detection with CsI(Tl) Layer Coupled to a-Si:H Photodiode Layers." IEEE Trans Nucl Sci 38:255–262, 1991.

[30] Chabbal J, Chaussat C, Ducourant T, Fritsch L, Michailos V, Spinnler V, Vieux G, Arques M, Hahm G, Hoheisel M, Horbaschek H, Schulz R, Spahn M. "Amorphous Silicon X-Ray Sensor." In Van Metter R, Beutel J (Eds.) *Medical Imaging 1996: Physics of Medical Imaging*. Proc SPIE 2708, 1996, pp. 499–510.

[31] Graeve T, Li S, Alexander SM, Huang W. "High-Resolution Amorphous Silicon Image Sensor." In Van Metter R, Beutel J (Eds.) *Medical Imaging 1996: Physics of Medical Imaging.* Proc SPIE 2708, 1996, pp. 494–498.

[32] Rahn JT, Lemmi F, Weisfeield RL *et al.* "High Resolution, High Fill Factor *a*-Si:H Sensor Arrays for Medical Imaging." In: Van Metter R, Beutel J (Eds.) *Medical Imaging 1999: Physics of Medical Imaging,* Proc SPIE 3659, 1999, pp. 510–517.

[33] Takahashi K, Kohda K, Miyahara J. "Mechanism of Photostimulated Luminescence in BaFX:Eu2+(X=Cl,Br)." J Luminescence 31&32: 266, 1984.

[34] von Seggern H, Voigt T, Knupfer W, Lange G. "Physical Model of Photostimulated Luminescence of X-Ray Irradiated BaFBr:Eu^{2+}." J Appl Phys 64:1405–1412, 1998.

[35] Kato K. "Photostimulable Phosphor Radiography Design Considerations." In Seibert JA, Barnes GT, Gould RG (Eds.) *Specification, Acceptance Testing and Quality Control of Diagnostic X-Ray Imaging Equipment,* American Institute of Physics. New York: Woodbury (American Association of Physicists in Medicine Monograph #20), 1994, pp. 731–769.

[36] Bogucki TM, Trauernicht DP, Kocher TE. "Characteristics of a Storage Phosphor System for Medical Imaging." Technical and Scientific Monograph No. 6, Eastman Kodak Health Sciences Division, 1995.

[37] Nishikawa RM, Mawdsley GE, Fenster A, Yaffe MJ. "Scanned Projection Digital Mammography." Med Phys 14:717–727, 1987.

[38] Yaffe MJ. "Direct Digital Mammography Using a Scanned-Slot CCD Imaging System." Medical Progress Through Technology 19:13–21, 1993.

[39] Spekowius G, Boerner H, Eckenbach W, Quadfleig P. Simulation of the Imaging Performance of X-Ray Image Intensifier/TV Camera Chains." In Van Metter R, Beutel J (Eds.) *Medical Imaging 1995: Physics of Medical Imaging,* Proc SPIE 2432, 1995, pp. 12–23.

[40] Brodie I, Gutcheck RA. "Minimum Exposure Estimates for Information Recording in Diagnostic Radiology." Med Phys 12:362–367, 1985.

[41] Que W, Rowlands JA. "X-Ray Imaging Using Amorphous Selenium: Inherent Resolution." Med Phys 22:365–374, 1995.

[42] Pai DM, Springett BE. "The Physics of Electrophotography." Rev Mod Phys 65:163–211, 1993.

[43] Lee DLY, Cheung LK, Palecki EF, Jeromin LS. "A Discussion on Resolution, Sensitivity, S/N Ratio and Dynamic Range of Se-TFT Direct Digital Radiographic Detector." Proc SPIE 2708, 1996, pp. 11–522.

[44] Zhao W, Rowlands JA. "A Large Area Solid-State Detector for Radiology Using Amorphous Selenium." In *Medical Imaging VI: Instrumentation.* Proc SPIE 1651, 1992, pp. 134–143.

[45] Zhao W, Rowlands JA. "X-Ray Imaging Using Amorphous Selenium: Feasibility of a Flat Panel Self-Scanned Detector for Digital Radiology." Med Phys 22:1595–1604, 1995.

[46] Fahrig R, Rowlands JA, Yaffe MJ. "X-Ray Imaging With Amorphous Sele-nium: Detective Quantum Efficiency of Photoconductive Receptors for Digi-tal Mammography." Med Phys 22:153–160, 1995.

[47] Polischuk B, Rougeot H, Wong K, Debrie A, Poliquin E, Hansroul M, Mar-tin J-P, Truong T-T, Choquette M, Laperriere L, Shukri Z. "Direct Conver-sion Detector for Digital Mammography." In Van Metter R, Beutel J (Eds.) *Medical Imaging 1999: Physics of Medical Imaging*. Proc SPIE 3659, 1999, pp. 417–425.

[48] Shah KS, Lund JC, Olschner F, Moy L, Squillante MR. "Thallium Bromide Radiation Detectors." IEEE Trans Nuclear Science 36:199–202, 1989.

[49] Street RA, Rahn JT, Ready SE, Shah KH, Bennett PR *et al.* "X-Ray Imaging Using Lead Iodide as a Semiconductor Detector." In Van Metter R, Beutel J (Eds.) *Medical Imaging 1999: Physics of Medical Imaging*, Proc SPIE 3659, 1999, pp. 36–47.

[50] Mainprize JG, Ford NL, Yin S, Tumer T, Yaffe MJ. "Image Quality of a Pro-totype Direct Conversion Detector for Digital Mammography." Proc SPIE 3659, 1999, pp. 398–406.

[51] Shtern F, Winfield D *et al.* "Report of the Working Group on Digital Mam-mography, Digital Displays and Workstation Design." Academic Radiology 6 (Suppl. 4): S197–218, 1999.

[52] Clarke LP, Kallergi M, Qian W, Li HD, Clark RA, Silbiger ML. "Tree-Structured Non-Linear Filter and Wavelet Transform for Microcalcification Segmentation in Digital Mammography." Cancer Letters 77:173–181, 1994.

[53] Laine A, Fan J, Schuler S. "A Framework for Contrast Enhancement by Dyadic Wavelet Analysis." In Gale AG, Astley SM, Dance DR, Cairns AY (Eds.) *Digital Mammography*. Amsterdam: Elsevier Publishing, 1994, pp. 91–100.

[54] Morrow MW, Paranjape RB, Rangayyan RM, Desautels JEL. "Region-Based Contrast Enhancement of Mammograms." IEEE Transactions on Medical Im-age Processing 11:392-406, 1992.

[55] Pisano E, Johnston RE, Pizer S, McLelland R. "Computer Enhancement of Digitized Mammograms." Radiology 181(p):5–15, 1991.

[56] Tachoes PG, Correa J, Souto M, Gonzalez C, Gomez L, Vidal J. "Enhance-ment of Chest and Breast Radiographs by Automatic Spatial Filtering." IEEE Transactions on Medical Imaging MI-10:330–335, 1992.

[57] Wei Q, Clarke LP, Kallergi M, Li G-D, Velthuizen RP, Clark RA, Silbiger ML. "Tree-Structured Nonlinear Filter and Wavelet Transform for Microcalcifica-tion Segmentation in Mammography." Proc SPIE 1905, 1993, pp. 509–520.

[58] Cowen AR, Giles A, Davies AG, Workman A. "An Image Processing Algo-rithm for PPCR Imaging." Proc SPIE 1898, 1993, pp. 833–841.

[59] Freedman M, Pe E, Zuurbier R, Katial R, Jafroudi H, Nelson M, Lo S-CB, Mun SK. "Image Processing in Digital Mammography." Proc SPIE 2164, 1994, pp. 57–554.

[60] Bick U, Giger ML, Schmidt RA, Nishikawa RM, Doi K. "Density Correction of Peripheral Breast Tissue on Digital Mammograms." RadioGraphics 16:1403–1411, 1996.

[61] Byng JW, Critten JP, Yaffe, MJ. "Thickness Equalization Processing for Mammographic Images," Radiology 203:564–568, 1997.

[62] Lewin JD, Hendrick RE, D'Orsi CJ, Moss LJ, Sisney GA, Karellas. "A Clinical Evaluation of a Full-field Digital Mammography Prototype for Cancer Detection in a Screening Setting." Supplement to Radiology 209(p):238, 1998 (Abstract).

[63] Bird RE, Wallace TW, Yankaskas BC. "Analysis of Cancers Missed at Acreening Mammography." Radiology 184:613–617, 1992.

[64] Anderson EDC, Muir BB, Walsh JS et al. "The Efficacy of Double Reading Mammograms in Breast Screening." Clinical Radiology 49:248, 1994.

[65] Thurfjell EL, Lernevall KA, Taube AAS. "Benefit of Independent Double Reading in a Population-Based Mammography Screening Program." Radiology 191:241, 1994.

[66] Jiang Y, Nishikawa RM, Schmidt RA, Metz CE, Giger ML, Doi K. "Improving Breast Cancer Diagnosis with Computer-Aided Diagnosis." Academic Radilogy 6:22–23, 1999.

[67] Kupinski MA, Giger ML. "Automated Seeded Lesion Segmentation on Digital Mammograms." IEEE Trans Med Imaging 17:510–517, 1998.

[68] Kobatake H, Takeo H, Hawano S. "Tumor Detection System for Full-Digital Mammography." In Doi K, MacMahon H, Giger ML, Hoffman KR (Eds.) *Computer Aided Diagnosis in Medical Imaging*. Amsterdam: Elsevier, 1999, pp. 87–94.

[69] Abdel-Malek A, Kopans D, Moore R et al. "Telemammographic System Development—Issues and Possible Solutions," In Gale AG (Ed.) *Digital Mammography*. Bristol: IOP Publications, 1994.

[70] Mattheus RA, Temmerman Y, Verhellen P et al. "Management System for a PACS Network in a Hospital Environment." Proc SPIE, 1991.

[71] Sund T. "Full-Scale Replacement of a Visiting Radiologist Service with Teleradiology." In *Proc. International Symposium Canadian Assoc Radiol.* Berlin: Springer-Verlag, 1991, p. 811.

[72] Fajardo LL, Yoshino MT, Seeley GW et al. "Detection of Breast Abnormalities on Teleradiology Transmitted Mammograms." Investigative Radiology 25:1111, 1990.

[73] Batnitzky S, Rosenthal SJ, Siegal EL et al. "Teleradiology: An Assessment." Radiology 177:11, 1990.

[74] Abdel-Malek A. "Experience with a Proposed Teleradiology System for Digital Mammography," Proc SPIE 2435, 1995, p. 200.

[75] Niklason LT, Christian BT, Niklason LE, Kopans DB, Castleberry DE, Opsahl-Ong BH, Landberg CE, Slanetz PJ, Giardino AA, Moore R, Albagli D, DeJule MC, Fitzgerald PF, Fobare DF, Giambattista BW, Kwasnick RF, Liu J, Lubowski SJ, Possin GE, Richotte JF, Wei CY, Wirth RF. "Digital Tomosynthesis in Breast Imaging." Radiology 205:399–406, 1997.

[76] Wolfe JN. "Risk for Breast Cancer Development Determined by Mammographic Parenchymal Pattern," Cancer 37:2486–92, 1976.

[77] Boyd NF, Byng JW, Jong RA, Fishell EK, Little LE, Miller AB, Lockwood GA, Tritchler DL, Yaffe MJ. "Quantitative Classification of Mammographic Densities and Breast Cancer Risk: Results from the Canadian National Breast Screening Study." Journal of the National Cancer Institute 87:670–675, 1995.

[78] Byrne C, Schairer C, Wolfe J, Parekh N, Salane M, Brinton LA, Hoover R, Haile R. "Mammographic Features and Breast Cancer Risk: Effects with Time, Age, and Menopause Status." Journal of the National Cancer Institute 87:1622–1629, 1995.

[79] Warner E, Lockwood G, Math M, Tritchler D, Boyd NF. "The Risk of Breast Cancer Associated with Mammographic Parenchymal Patterns: A Meta-Analysis of the Published Literature to Examine the Effect of Method of Classification." Cancer Detection and Prevention 16:67–72, 1992.

[80] Spicer DV, Ursin G, Parisky YR, Pearce JG, Shoupe D, Pike A, Pike MC. "Changes in Mammographic Densities Induced by a Hormonal Contraceptive Designed to Reduce Breast Cancer Risk." Journal of the National Cancer Institute 86:431–5, 1994.

[81] Boyd NF, Greenberg C, Lockwood G, Little L, Martin L, Byng J, Yaffe M, Tritchler D. "The Effects at 2 Years of a Low-Fat High-Carbohydrate Diet on Radiological Features of the Breast: Results from a Randomized Trial." Journal of the National Cancer Institute 89:488–96, 1997.

[82] Johns PC, Drost DJ, Yaffe MJ, Fenster A. "Dual Energy Mammography: Initial Experimental Results." Medical Physics 12:297–304, 1985.

[83] Heywang SA, Wolf A, Pruss E et al. "MR Imaging of the Breast with Gd-DTPA: Use and Limitations." Radiology 171:95–103, 1989.

[84] Kaiser WA, Zeitler E. "MR Imaging of the Breast: Fast Imaging Sequences with and without Gd-DTPA Preliminary Observations." Radiology 170:681–686, 1989.

[85] Frouge C, Guinebretiere J-M, Contesso G et al. "Correlation between Contrast Enhancement in Dynamic Magnetic Resonance Imaging of the Breast and Tumor Angiogenesis." Investigative Radiology 29:1043–1049, 1994.

[86] Harms SE, Flamig DP. "Present and Future Role of MR Imaging." In Haus A, Yaffe MJ (Eds.), *Syllabus of Categorical Course on Technical Aspects of Mammography*, Radiological Society of North America. Illinois: Oak Brook, 1994, pp. 255–261.

[87] Watt AC, Ackerman LV, Windham JP et al. "Breast Lesions: Differential Diagnosis Using Digital Subtraction Angiography." Radiology 159:39–42, 1986.

CHAPTER 6
Magnetic Resonance Imaging

David Pickens
Vanderbilt University Medical Center

CONTENTS

6.1 Introduction

Magnetic resonance imaging is one of the major computerized imaging modalities available at any large metropolitan hospital and in many facilities in smaller cities and towns. This imaging technology provides capabilities for physicians to obtain images of pathology that are different from those obtained with other modalities and are often complementary. Additionally, magnetic resonance systems can provide information unavailable by any other imaging method.

The initial clinical installations were in major research medical centers in the United States and Europe. Since these first installations of the early 1980s, systems have been commercialized by major manufacturers that are installed in all types of facilities worldwide. These include installations in dedicated separate buildings as well as in multistory hospitals. Systems that are mounted in trailers so they can be moved from location to location by truck as required with minimum setup times are equal in performance to most stationary installations. These latter systems are complete imaging facilities that can go where they are needed.

Such is the revolution in medical imaging that originated from the work of Block and his coworkers at Stanford and Purcell and his colleagues at Harvard, both of whom reported their independent discoveries of nuclear magnetic resonance in *Physics Reviews* in 1946 (Block, Hansen *et al.* 1946; Purcell, Torrey *et al.* 1946). Working independently, these researchers described nuclear magnetic resonance (NMR) in bulk matter using different descriptions of what turned out to be the same phenomenon. The Stanford researchers described the precession of nuclear magnetization in a magnetic field, which produced an electromotive force in a radio frequency coil by induction, called "nuclear induction." The Harvard group investigated the transitions of magnetic nuclei between different quantized states while in a magnetic field and the absorption of radio frequency energy at resonance, called "nuclear magnetic resonance." After publication of the work of the two groups, discussions resolved the fact that both were describing aspects of the same phenomenon. In 1952 Block and Purcell shared the Nobel Prize in physics for this discovery.

Many researchers have developed techniques that have moved these discoveries from physics into different applications. Chemists quickly found that the NMR frequency of a particular nucleus depends in part on the chemical structure of the material due to shielding effects on the nucleus from the cloud of electrons surrounding it. This causes a small shift in the frequency of the signal that became known as the "chemical shift." In situations where different parts of the molecule exist in different chemical environments, a set of small frequency changes is observed. The recording of these chemical shifts as an aid in determining molecular structure is known as NMR spectroscopy.

Early experiments in biology began about the time that the first discoveries of the NMR phenomena began to be reported. Evidently, Bloch made the first biological measurement by placing his finger into the radio frequency coil of his early instrument with the subsequent production of a strong signal due to the spin of the

hydrogen nucleus. Others began to investigate body fluids and tissues from both animals and humans in the 1950s. Instrument development brought high-performance
Fourier NMR spectroscopy into the realm of the emerging field of molecular biology where it remains a major tool in biological science research.

Part of the development of instrumentation, especially in the 1960s, led to the
production of high field magnets with bores large enough to accommodate perfused
organs. These technical advances led to extensive studies of various molecules
in vivo and preceded subsequent advances in spectroscopy of the human body.
These early developments have now led to imaging methods that provide clinical
diagnostic information unavailable by other techniques.

6.2 Basic principles

6.2.1 Macroscopic magnetization

Understanding the phenomenon of magnetic resonance can be daunting, since
it involves physical phenomena described by complex mathematical relationships.
Much of the description of magnetic resonance can be found in the seminal works
of Purcell, Block, Rabi, Hahn, and others (Purcell, Torrey *et al.* 1946; Rabi, 1939;
Block, Hansen *et al.* 1946; Hahn, 1950). These works contain detailed mathematical descriptions of the phenomena involved, which will not be repeated here. What
follows is more descriptive in nature, intended to pique the interest of the reader.

The nucleus of an atom containing neutrons and protons (or a single proton) exhibits a magnetic field associated with the protons. Since each proton and neutron
has a magnetic dipole, the nucleus exhibits a magnetic moment (μ) that depends
on the number of protons and neutrons present. In addition, the nucleus exhibits a
property called spin (short for nuclear spin angular momentum number) that is also
related to the number of protons and neutrons present. The symbol I is conventionally used to represent spin. I can have values of 0, half-integers, or whole integers.
For those nuclei with even atomic weights and even atomic numbers, $I = 0$. Such
nuclei are unaffected by a magnetic field and cannot be observed by magnetic resonance. Nuclei having either integer or half-integer spin numbers are affected by
magnetic fields and can be detected by magnetic resonance spectroscopy. Nuclei of
interest for purposes of magnetic resonance imaging have half integer spin numbers. Such nuclei can exist in $2I + 1$ discrete Zeeman energy states. Table 6.1
shows a list of some nuclei of interest in medicine and biology.

Due to the nature of its spin and its natural abundance in tissues that are largely
made of water, the hydrogen nucleus, a proton, is most often the nucleus of choice
in magnetic resonance imaging (MRI) and magnetic resonance spectroscopy.

In many descriptions of the interaction of the nuclear moment with a magnetic
field, the model that is used is that of the bar magnet. A bar magnet is characterized
by having a north and a south pole, which means that one end of the magnet will
orient itself towards the earth's north pole, while the other end points to the earth's
south pole. As most people know, bar magnets with north poles pointing toward
each other will repel and when oriented north to south, will attract. These properties
are useful in describing what happens with the nuclear moment in a magnetic field.

Table 6.1: Selected nuclei useful in magnetic resonance imaging and spectroscopy

Nucleus	I	Magnetic Moment μ	γ mHz/T	% Isotropic Abundance	Concentration in the Body
^{1}H	1/2	2.79	42.58	99.98	100
^{17}O	5/2	1.89	5.77	0.04	50
^{19}F	1/2	2.63	40.08	100.00	4×10^{-6}
^{23}Na	3/2	2.22	11.27	100.00	8.0×10^{-2}
^{31}P	1/2	1.13	17.25	100.00	7.5×10^{-2}

From [(Bushberg, Seibert *et al.* 1994), p. 292]. [(Haake, Brown *et al.* 1999), p. 27].

In a magnetic field the magnetic moment, or "magnetic dipole" will position itself so that the north pole points in the direction of the applied magnetic field. The magnetic moment (μ) in a magnetic field of strength B has a magnitude and a direction and is therefore a vector quantity.

There are many nuclei containing an odd number of protons or neutrons respectively that could be used in magnetic resonance imaging, but those listed in Table 6.1 are important biologically. Those nuclei with strong magnetic moments, μ, are better candidates for imaging than the others. Especially important and listed in Table 6.1 is the biological concentration of these nuclei. It is clear that the most likely candidate for imaging will be the single proton, the hydrogen nucleus, due to its high concentration as a component of most of the molecules in biological tissues, particularly water, its isotopic abundance, and its strong magnetic moment. Other nuclei can be imaged, but most of the descriptions that follow assume that the target species is the proton, due to its strong magnetic moment and concentration in tissues. Protons are variously referred to as "protons," "nuclei," "water," and "spins," so unless otherwise specified, these terms will refer to protons alone.

In normal biological tissues, the proton spins are randomly distributed when the tissues are not located in a magnetic field. This distribution, due to thermal agitation, results in no net magnetic vector for the protons in the tissue. However, when the tissue is placed in an external magnetic field, their angular momentum and magnetic moment cause the nuclei to begin to align with the external field. There are two energy states associated with the alignment: one in the direction of the magnetic field ("parallel") and one in the direction opposite to the magnetic field ("anti-parallel"). The parallel orientation is in a slightly lower energy state, so there are a few more nuclei oriented in this direction than in the anti-parallel direction. This difference results in a slight but detectable magnetic moment.

The nuclei can be considered symmetrical spinning objects. When the magnetic moments of the nuclei are subjected to the external magnetic field, there is a net torque or rotational force that tries to force the nuclei to align with the magnetic field. Because of their rotational angular momentum, the magnetic moment of the nuclei initiates a periodic motion around the direction of the magnetic field. This periodic motion is known as precession and the angular frequency of the precession depends on the strength of the applied magnetic field B_0.

An often-described way of demonstrating precession and the behavior of a spinning proton in a magnetic field is the analogy with a toy top (see Figure 6.1). When the top is set on its axis and is spinning, it is acted on by the force of gravity, which begins to pull on the top. This torque causes the top, due to its rotational angular momentum, to begin to rotate or wobble around the direction of the gravitational field, precessing at a frequency that is changing due to the effects of friction and the slowing of the rotating element of the top. Eventually, of course, the top falls over because the frictional forces cause the angular momentum to decrease to the point where gravity is able to pull the top over. This does not happen with nuclei because there are no frictional forces.

The frequency of precession is related to the strength of the magnetic field, B_0. The relationship is known as the Larmor equation:

$$\omega = \gamma\, B_0, \tag{6.1}$$

where ω is the angular frequency of precession in radians and γ is the gyromagnetic ratio which is an intrinsic property of each element, and B_0 is the magnetic field strength measured in Tesla, T. One T equals 10,000 gauss; the earth's magnetic field is about 0.05 gauss. This frequency can be converted to linear frequency, f, in mHz by dividing ω by 2π. The frequency of precession is a distinguishing characteristic of different elements. For protons the gyromagnetic ratio is 42.58 mHz/T. Table 6.1 lists the gyromagnetic ratios of several elements of interest in medical imaging. The unique frequency dependence for each element enables the elements to be studied on an individual basis. Thus, the frequency of precession of hydrogen nuclei at 1 T is 42.58 mHz, while that of C^{13} is 10.7 mHz. These differences in precessional frequencies can be used to advantage to detect the nuclei of different atoms in the molecules of biological tissues separately in a given magnetic field.

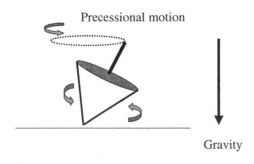

Precessional motion

Gravity

Figure 6.1: A toy top spinning on its axis is affected by friction, which slows the spin. As the top slows, the effect of gravity increases due to the resulting decrease of angular momentum and the top begins to precess about the direction of the force of gravity.

6.2.2 Reference frames

When nuclei are not in a magnetic field, there is no preferred orientation of the spins and no detectable magnetic effect. However, when placed in an external magnetic field, the nuclei tend to align themselves so that they are somewhat more oriented toward the direction of the magnetic field. The sum of all of the magnetic moment vectors of the individual nuclei yields the net magnetization vector **M**. Since **M** is a vector quantity, it represents changes in the average orientation and distribution of magnetic moments in a sample.

Two conventions are used to represent what happens when nuclei are exposed to an external magnetic field. The orientation of the static applied magnetic field, B_0, is conventionally taken to be along the z-axis of a three-dimensional Cartesian coordinate system. The z-axis, also called the "longitudinal" direction, is shown in the up position in Figure 6.2. The x- and y-axes lie in a plane perpendicular to the z-axis, forming the "transverse" x,y-plane. An observer "sees" the nuclei subjected to a magnetic field along the z-axis, precessing around the z-axis at the Larmor frequency. If a secondary magnetic field perturbs the precessing nuclei, they change position relative to the z-axis by describing complex spiral patterns until an equilibrium state is reached. The complex motion of the individual magnetic moments, averaged by the net magnetization vector **M**, in response to a perturbing secondary magnetic field is difficult to describe and understand in this static Cartesian coordinate system (Riddle, Lee, 1999).

In order to simplify the task of describing the motion of the magnetic moments, one can view the Cartesian coordinate system as if one were standing at the origin of the Cartesian coodinate system, the x,y-plane forming the surface on which to stand. In this description, the x- and y-axes rotate around the z-axis at the Larmor frequency. An example used in the literature of this rotating reference frame makes the analogy of standing on the platter of a spinning phonograph record (Fukushima, Roeder, 1981; Bushberg, Seibert *et al.* 1994). To the observer standing on the spinning record, the label is not moving, because both observer and label spin at the same speed. To an observer away from the system, the record

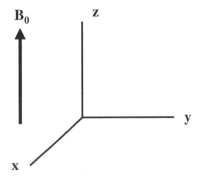

Figure 6.2: A Cartesian coordinate system is usually used when describing the effect of magnetic fields on nuclei. By convention, the static field, B_0, is oriented in the z direction.

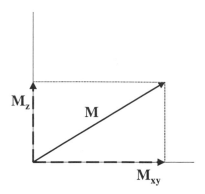

Figure 6.3: The net magnetic vector, **M**, is described by its component vectors. These component vectors are M_z along the z axis and M_{xy} in the plane of the x and y axes. When **M** is moved completely into the xy plane, $M_z = 0$.

is spinning at 33 1/3 rpm. Thus, the rotating reference frame eliminates the spin at the Larmor frequency so that one can describe small changes in the precession frequency of nuclei without having to keep up with the Larmor frequency. If the observer continues to rotate at 33 1/3 rpm, but the platter spins at 32 rpm, then the platter appears to rotate at 1 1/3 rpm in the opposite direction from the point of view of the observer.

The device of the rotating reference frame and the use of the net magnetization vector **M** provide a convenient way of describing what happens to the magnetization during magnetic resonance imaging. When all the nuclei are in an external magnetic field and an equilibrium state has been reached, then the net magnetic vector, **M**, can be said to be in alignment with the z-axis. If an external magnetic field perturbs the nuclei, then the net magnetic vector may no longer be perfectly aligned with the z-axis. By convention, the net magnetic vector is considered in terms of its component vectors, M_z and M_{xy}, shown in Figure 6.3. As the **M** vector moves away from alignment in the z-direction, the M_z or longitudinal component decreases while the M_{xy} or transverse component increases. If an external field is strong enough to cause the entire **M** vector to tip into the x, y-plane, then the M_z component is 0 and the M_{xy} component is identical to the net magnetization vector **M**.

6.2.3 Excitation and resonance

In order to perform imaging, it is necessary to perturb the nuclear magnetic moments precessing about the external field B_0. This is accomplished by applying a radio frequency (RF) energy pulse perpendicular to the z-axis about which the nuclei are precessing. The RF pulse produces a magnetic field, B_1, which, if it is of the proper frequency, will cause the nuclei to be reoriented with respect to their orientation in the z-direction. There are two ways to consider this phenomenon.

One involves a quantum mechanical approach, while the other uses a classical physics approach.

If we assume the nuclear spins are in a state of thermal equilibrium, precessing around the direction of the external magnetic field, then we know that there are some nuclei that are oriented parallel to the static external field, while a slightly smaller number are oriented antiparallel, in the higher energy state. The difference in energy between these two states is ΔE, the discrete energy gap. When the exact energy, ΔE is applied, a transition from the lower energy level to higher energy level occurs, so that more nuclei are now in the antiparallel direction, compared to the situation prior to the application of the RF pulse. For this to happen, the frequency of the RF energy has to match the Larmor frequency exactly, i.e., the RF pulse has to be in resonance with the Larmor frequency. The number of nuclei that undergo the transition from the low to the high-energy state depends on the pulse width and amplitude. As the RF energy is applied, more and more of the nuclei orient themselves antiparallel so that eventually there are more in the high-energy state than the low-energy state (Bushberg, Seibert *et al.* 1994).

The classical view of the same phenomenon describes the RF energy of the B_1 field as a waveform with sinusoidally varying electric and magnetic fields. In this description, the magnetic field consists of two vectors of equal magnitude rotating in opposite directions. These vectors come into alignment at the peak of each half cycle of the sinusoidal RF wave. For these vectors to couple magnetically to the magnetic moments of the nuclei, the angular rotation of these vectors has to occur at the Larmor frequency. This coupling is the resonance phenomenon described earlier. If one looks at what occurs from the standpoint of the rotating frame, it is evident that if the RF field is applied along the x-axis at the Larmor frequency, it appears as a stationary magnetic field. As the B_1 field is applied, the net magnetic moment rotates so that it lies in the x,y-plane. The orientation of the net magnetic moment along the x,y-plane is $90°$ ($\pi/2$) from its original position along the z-axis. If the B_1 field is applied for a longer period of time or the pulse intensity is greater, then the net magnetic moment can be rotated to $180°$ (π), $270°$ ($3/2\pi$) or back to 0 ($360°$ or 2π). Any angle can be obtained by the proper selection of timing and intensity of the RF pulse at the Larmor frequency. This angle is usually called the "tip or flip angle" and is important in the design of pulse sequences (Figure 6.4). If the RF pulse is at a different frequency, resonance will not occur, with the result that there is no effect on the net magnetic moment and it does not move from its stable state along the z-axis (Bushberg, Seibert *et al.* 1994).

It should be noted that the field produced by the RF energy is much smaller than the static field. A part of the phenomenon of resonance is that the effects of the B_1 field are cumulative, so that a B_1 field of a few gauss can cause realignment of the net magnetic vector even though the static B_0 field is measured in thousands of gauss.

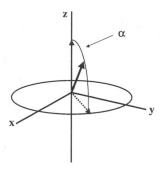

Figure 6.4: When a magnetic field whose cumulative effect is stronger than that of the static field B_0 alone is applied along the x- or y-axis, the net magnetic vector **M** is "rotated" toward the x,y-plane. This means that the M_z component becomes smaller, while the M_{xy} component grows. The angle of the rotation is called the tip or flip angle, α, and can range from a few degrees to $180°$. Many pulse sequences use a tip angle of less than $90°$.

6.2.4 Relaxation times

Relaxation refers to the return of the magnetization to a stable, unperturbed state of minimum energy after the magnetization has been perturbed by application of the RF pulse. In this equilibrium state, the component of the magnetic vector in the z-direction, M_z, is again greater than the $M_{x,y}$ component (i.e., more nuclei are in parallel than antiparallel alignment) and the nuclei precess about the z-axis at the Larmor frequency. Relaxation thus involves giving up the energy absorbed from the RF pulse during the process of resonance (Riddle, Lee, 1999; Birn, Donahue *et al.* 1999).

If one considers the relaxation process in terms of the change of the components of the net magnetization vector projected onto the z-axis and in the x,y-plane, there are two relaxation time constants that are of interest. These time constants and the ability to observe nuclei in various temporal stages of relaxation according to these time constants form the basis of magnetic resonance imaging. These two time constants are called T1 and T2.

Recall that during and immediately after the application of the $90°$ RF pulse, the net magnetization vector lies in the x,y-plane, i.e., $M_{xy} > 0$ and $M_z = 0$. Once the RF pulse terminates, as the entire system relaxes to its equilibrium state, the net magnetic moment "rises" out of the x,y-plane, while the M_z-component gradually returns to the equilibrium state in the z-direction. If one views everything from the viewpoint of the rotating framework, the M_z component increases with time or evolves as described by the following equation:

$$M_z = M_0\left[1 - e^{-t/\text{T1}}\right]. \tag{6.2}$$

Here, M_z is the magnetization in the z direction, equal to 0 immediately after a $90°$ RF pulse, M_0 is the magnetization at equilibrium in the z-direction, T1 is the time constant, called the spin–lattice relaxation time, describing the return of the

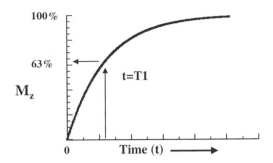

100%

63%

M_z

t=T1

0   Time (t) ⟶

Figure 6.5: T1 is the time constant describing the spin–lattice relaxation time. It represents the time required for 63% of the magnetization M_z to regrow to equilibrium after application of a 90° RF pulse.

M_z component to a stable equilibrium state, and t is time. T1 is the time required for 63% of the magnetization to grow back toward a stable state. T1 relaxation is shown in Figure 6.5. It is a measure of the interaction of nuclei with their molecular environment and is determined in part by how quickly energy can be transferred from the nuclei being observed to the environment or "lattice."

T1 can be used to characterize different materials, such as tissues or fluids. Often, changes in T1 values are observed in various disease processes that change the environment within an organ. However, the values of T1 depend on the strength of the magnetic field in which the tissue is placed. Table 6.2 shows some of the differences between low field and high field systems. The energy transfer from the excited nuclei to the lattice depends on the frequency of the translational, vibrational and rotational motions of the molecules surrounding the excited nuclei. The closer the frequency of the molecular motion is to the Larmor frequency of the excited nuclei, the more likely it is that energy will be transferred to the lattice, resulting in a shorter time for the excited nuclei to return to equilibrium. Since many proteins in tissues have molecular motion frequencies in the range of about 1 MHz, a lower Larmor frequency implies more efficient transfer of energy from the exited nuclei to the lattice. This is the source of the field dependence of T1 measurements.

At equilibrium, in the presence of the applied static magnetic field, the precession of the nuclei about the z-axis is incoherent, i.e., the nuclei are not in phase. Application of the RF pulse at the Larmor frequency causes the nuclei to precess in phase about the center of the x, y-plane so long as the RF pulse is present. When the RF pulse is turned off, this phase coherence is gradually lost. T2 is the time constant that describes phase dispersion, the loss of phase coherence in the transverse or x, y-plane. It is also known as the spin–spin relaxation time. The equation describing the change in signal is given as

$$M_{xy} = M_0 e^{-t/T2}, \qquad (6.3)$$

where M_{xy} is the transverse magnetic moment at the time t and M_0 is the initial transverse magnetization at $t = 0$, when the RF pulse has been turned off. T2 represents the time required for the transverse magnetization vector to decrease to 37% of its magnitude at the time $t = 0$, as shown in Figure 6.6. T2, then, is a time constant that is important in imaging applications because it is related to the molecular structure of the biological tissues being imaged.

The T2 time constant of tissues can be strongly affected by perturbing magnetic fields. These can cause the observed T2 value to be much shorter than the actual T2 value of a particular sample. The shortening of the T2 time constant due to effects such as inhomogeneities of the magnet, applied external fields, or local fields induced in samples are described by a time constant known as T2*, which has important implications in imaging that will be discussed later in this chapter. The T2 time constant is generally shorter than the overall time required for the nuclei to return to equilibrium (T1). However, T2 and T1 are equal for pure water.

T1 and T2 form the basis for the contrast available in magnetic resonance imaging, along with T2*, blood flow, and the number of nuclei present (proton density). The values for T1, T2, and T2* are affected by the magnetic field strength, the characteristics of the tissues being imaged, the presence of internal or external perturbing magnetic fields, and in the case of T2*, localized magnetic properties of

Table 6.2: T1 and T2 relaxation times for various tissues

Tissue Type	T1 (0.5 T) (msec)	T1 (1.5 T) (msec)	T2 (msec)
CSF	1800	2400	160
White Matter	500	780	90
Gray Matter	650	900	100
Muscle	550	870	45
Liver	350	500	40
Fat	210	260	80

[From (Bushberg, Seibert *et al.* 1994), p. 308]. See also (Bottomley, Foster *et al.* 1984).

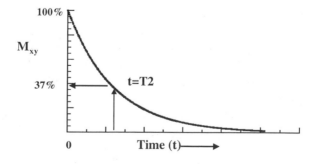

Figure 6.6: T2 is the time constant describing the spin–spin relaxation time. It represents the time required for the M_{xy} component of the net magnetization to return to zero after application of a 90° RF pulse.

the tissues themselves, e.g., the presence of paramagnetic blood degradation products, elements with unpaired electron spins (see Section 6.6.1, "Contrast agents") or ferromagnetic products.

6.2.5 Gradients

A magnetic field gradient is a magnetic field whose strength varies linearly with distance along a certain direction. This produces a linear variation in precessional frequencies along the applied direction. The change in precessional frequencies provides a means for obtaining information about the spatial location of nuclei in the body. A gradient field is produced by saddle coils placed in the core of the magnet in such a way that when electric current is applied to the coils, a magnetic field that linearly adds to or subtracts from the static field in a given direction is superimposed on the static field. The result of the presence of the gradient field is that the magnetic field imposed on nuclei in one location along the gradient differs slightly from that imposed on nuclei in a different location along the gradient. Because of these slightly different magnetic fields, the frequency of precession differs slightly for nuclei along the direction of the gradient (Figure 6.7). These differences in frequency can be used to determine the spatial locations of nuclei along the gradient and forms the basis of imaging.

In modern imagers, there are three coils of different designs that cause the imposition of a gradient field along each of the three axes of the system. By applying a current to the individual coils or to groups of these coils, a gradient along any

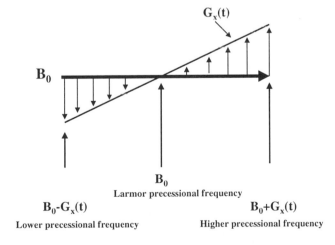

Figure 6.7: A linear gradient field, $G_x(t)$, applied along the direction of a static field, B_0, causes protons to experience different magnetic environments along the direction of the gradient. Where the gradient is slightly negative, the field is slightly lower than the static field and the precessional frequency is lower according to the Larmor equation. Where the gradient field adds to the static field, the precessional frequency is slightly higher. In the center of the range of the gradient, protons experience only the effect of the static field, so the precessional frequency is that corresponding to the static field B_0.

given direction can be created. These gradients are typically turned on at specific times, as part of pulse sequences used to excite samples in specific ways in order to obtain an image.

The magnetic fields produced by the coils are very small relative to the B_0 field. In fact, the magnetic fields generated by the coils are of the order of a few hundred gauss compared to static fields of 15,000 gauss or more. The gradient coils are energized so that these small magnetic fields subtract from the static field B_0 at one end of the gradient field, and add to the static field B_0 at the other end, passing through the static field value in the middle. This means that nuclei located in the center of the gradient precess at the nominal Larmor frequency, corresponding to the static magnetic field, whereas those on one end or the other of the range of the gradient precess at slightly higher and lower frequencies, respectively.

6.2.6 Detection and free induction decay

A 90° RF pulse causes the net magnetic vector to "flip" into the transverse plane. If one considers the behavior of the net magnetic vector from the viewpoint of the static laboratory reference frame, one realizes that, at the moment the 90° pulse is turned off, the magnetic vector is rotating about the z-axis in the x, y-plane at the Larmor frequency. If a coil is placed in the transverse plane so that its axis lies in the plane of the rotating magnetic vector (i.e., in the x, y-plane), then the lines of force of the magnetic field will pass through the coil, inducing an electromotive force (in volts) that oscillates at the Larmor frequency. This coil is essentially a radio antenna. The induced signal is proportional to the number of nuclei that resonate with the applied RF signal, the RF pulse width, the strength of the RF signal, and the number of coils used to detect the signal.

It should be noted that a signal is only detected when there is a component of the net magnetization vector in the x, y-plane, i.e., detection occurs when M_{xy} is not equal to zero. The reasons are apparent when one considers what happens in the presence of the external magnetic field alone. Recall that at equilibrium, M_z is at its maximum value and, since the magnetic moments are not in phase, $M_{xy} = 0$. The value of M_z derives from the contributions of many nuclei precessing around the z-axis; however, individual magnetic dipole moments can be found anywhere within a cone of precession around the z-axis as shown in Figure 6.8. At equilibrium, a coil positioned near the z-axis does not experience an oscillating magnetic field, so there is no induced voltage. No signal is detected.

After an RF pulse causes the magnetic moments of the nuclei to orient themselves with the RF field, the magnetic moments of the nuclei are positioned at 90° to the z-axis. At the moment the RF field is turned off, the nuclear magnetic moments are in phase and are in the x, y-plane. There is no component of the magnetization in the z-direction, i.e., $M_z = 0$. A coil placed so that its axis is in the x, y-plane senses the oscillation of the net magnetic vector as it precesses in the x, y-plane at the Larmor frequency and passes through the coil. Since the net magnetic vector has a north and south pole, the coil is exposed to a magnetic field oscillating from north to south. This produces an alternating voltage (i.e., an AC

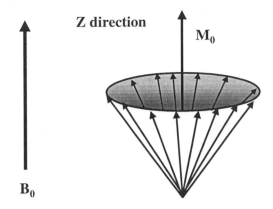

Figure 6.8: At equilibrium, the magnetic dipole moments of protons placed in a static field, B_0, precess at the Larmor frequency. The magnetic dipole moments distribute themselves around the direction of the static field with no phase coherence, describing a cone. The net magnetic moment, M_0 is the maximum longitudinal magnetization resulting from contributions by all of these magnetic dipoles.

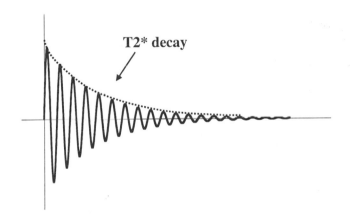

Figure 6.9: The signal measured by a detector coil in the x, y-plane immediately after a 90° RF pulse is turned off is called a free induction decay (FID) signal. It is a sine wave at the Larmor frequency that decays exponentially at a rate described by T2* due to effects of field inhomogeneities. The signal represents the loss of phase coherence and subsequent reduction of M_{xy} to 0.

signal) in the coil. As soon as the RF pulse is turned off the amplitude of this AC signal decays as shown in Figure 6.9, because of the loss of phase coherence due to T2* relaxation. This voltage is called the free induction decay (FID) signal.

In the preceding discussion, the assumption has been that the material being observed contains only hydrogen nuclei in completely identical chemical and magnetic environments, all precessing at a single Larmor frequency. All of the nuclei experience the same magnetic field and therefore produce FIDs having a single frequency. However, if some of these identical nuclei were to experience a different magnetic field, either due to some interaction within the sample or because a spatially varying magnetic field has been applied to the sample, then the signal induced in the receiver coil will be much more complex. The reason for this is that nuclei at different locations experience different magnetic fields, which in turn cause these nuclei to precess at different Larmor frequencies based on the local value of the magnetic field strength. In this circumstance, the FID signal detected by the receiving coil is a superposition of all of the individual Larmor frequencies from all of the nuclei. This signal containing many different frequencies can be decoded using the Fourier transform, which leads to a reconstruction method used in imaging.

6.3 Magnetic resonance imaging

6.3.1 Producing an image

6.3.1.1 Slice selection

In order to produce an image using magnetic resonance, one must excite the protons in a volume of interest and then find a method to distinguish the locations of a subset of these protons from the different location of all of the others. The key to the development of methods for producing images of the spatial distribution of protons, i.e., a map of proton densities, in a part of the body being imaged is to modify the Larmor equation so that the magnetic field at each location in an image or volume from which one wishes to obtain information is uniquely different. This modification to the Larmor equation has this appearance:

$$\omega(r_i) = \gamma\left(B_0 + \vec{G} \cdot \vec{r}\right), \tag{6.4}$$

where $\omega(r_i)$ is the frequency of a proton at location r_i, $\vec{G}$ is a vector quantity describing the gradient amplitude and direction, and γ is the gyromagnetic ratio. Gradient magnitude is typically expressed in milliTesla/meter (mT/m) or in gauss/cm. Note that 10 mT/m = 1 gauss/cm. This equation is the key to the imaging process, because it indicates that the frequency of precession is a function of the static field as well as the gradient field at each location (r_i). Thus, the precession frequency for each proton is uniquely defined by its position.

To collect the data necessary for obtaining images, a series of events must take place. An RF pulse must be applied to the region to be imaged, a slice or multiple slices must be specified, the signal produced by the relaxation of the net magnetic moment must be detected and gradient fields must be turned on at appropriate times to control the range of Larmor frequencies experienced by the protons. This series of events, which must be timed very precisely is known as a pulse sequence. Pulse sequences are the fundamental method by means of which image contrast is controlled, so pulse sequence design is very important and requires considerable care. It should be stated that pulse sequences can become very complex and pulse sequence design is an area of continuing innovation in magnetic resonance imaging.

Historically, many different image formation methods have been used in the development of modern MRI systems. Among the earliest approaches were the sensitive point and sensitive line methods. In the sensitive point method, a small region in a volume of interest can be selected by oscillating the gradients over time in all three directions, such that only nuclei located at a specific point, actually a volume element (voxel), experience a uniform gradient. These nuclei resonate with an RF pulse and emit a signal from that voxel, while all other nuclei do not produce a signal. To cover the entire volume of interest, the oscillating gradients are changed so that the resonating voxel moves. In this way, an image can be built on a point-by-point basis. Nuclei outside the voxel being addressed experience a different magnetic field strength, so that resonance does not occur. The line scanning method is similar to the sensitive point method except that a line is read out in the presence of a linear gradient and two oscillating gradients, using an RF pulse containing the frequencies corresponding to the precessional frequencies of the nuclei along the linear gradient field. Figure 6.10 shows these two methods for reading out the signal. The linear gradient is usually in the z-direction. Both of these methods have been replaced by more modern and efficient imaging methods because it was quickly realized that controlling the gradient switching to achieve the necessary oscillations is technically difficult and leads to long imaging times with relatively poor signal-to-noise ratios (SNR).

MRI imaging is currently designed to produce images of slices, i.e., tomographic images, throughout the body. While more recent applications and methods will permit true three-dimensional imaging, two-dimensional imaging methods predominate. The selection of the slice or slices to be imaged is a fundamental requirement of two-dimensional imaging protocols. Slice selection was initially performed by using an oscillating gradient in one direction coupled with an RF pulse containing a single frequency, the Larmor frequency, in a manner very similar to the sensitive point/sensitive line methods described earlier. In order to select a slice for imaging, the oscillating gradient applied a magnetic field across a sample so that only at the "pivot point" was at the static, unperturbed magnetic field. On either side of the selected slab, the nuclei experienced time-varying magnetic fields which eliminated the possibility of resonance with the applied RF pulse. This approach caused the excitation of a slab of tissue, the slice of interest, from which signals could be obtained to reconstruct an image. To excite a different slab, the amplitude of the oscillations was changed so the pivot point is located in a different place.

This approach to slice selection suffers from several problems. The first is that in early systems, it was technically difficult to switch the large inductive loads required to impose the oscillating gradients. However, modern gradient systems can accommodate these requirements. Second, the oscillating gradient creates a Gaussian-like slab profile containing contributions from tissues considerably beyond the nominal selected slab thickness. Third, this approach virtually eliminates

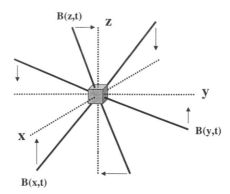

Figure 10a: The sensitive point method of imaging uses three oscillating gradients, along the x, y and z-directions respectively. Only the voxel or point at the intersection of the pivot point of all three gradients provides a signal after resonance with an RF pulse. All the protons elsewhere in the imaging field are subjected to varying magnetic fields from the oscillating gradients, so they do not resonate with the applied RF pulse. By varying the location of the pivot points, the entire volume can be scanned.

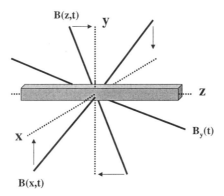

Figure 10b: The sensitive line method is similar to the sensitive point method except that one gradient is a stationary linear gradient. The other two gradients pivot as in the sensitive point method. The effect of this approach is to acquire data from a "line" in the imaging volume for each RF pulse. The x and y-dimensions are controlled by the size of the pivot point, while the z-direction is defined by the linear gradient. The line can be moved around the imaging volume by changing the location of the pivot points in the two oscillating gradients while the linear gradient remains on.

the possibility of using multislice excitation pulse sequences, which are now commonly used in MRI.

The technique currently used for slice selection employs a tailored RF pulse in the presence of a linear, non-varying magnetic field gradient. In this approach, all of the problems with oscillating gradients are eliminated at the expense of more complex RF hardware. Selective excitation slice selection makes use of the fact

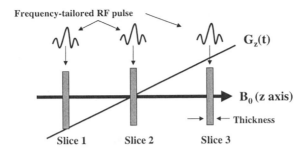

Figure 6.11: Slice selection is performed by tailoring the frequency content of an RF slice selection pulse so that the range of frequencies present corresponds to the range of Larmor frequencies produced by a linear gradient imposed in the selected direction. If the linear gradient is imposed in the z-direction as shown, then the range of frequencies can be quickly changed so that only slices at different positions (Slice 1, Slice 2, or Slice 3) will be excited, while protons at other positions do not resonate.

that with currently available equipment, in particular digitally controlled frequency synthesizers driving the transmitters, it is relatively easy to create an RF pulse containing a wide range of frequencies above and below the nominal Larmor frequency of the system. In the presence of a linear gradient field, one only needs to determine where the slice of interest should be, instruct the frequency synthesizer to produce a range of frequencies consistent with the slice position and thickness corresponding to the value of the gradient within the slice, and excite the slab. To change positions of the slab, the synthesizer produces another RF pulse of controlled bandwidth exciting a slab in another position. This is diagrammed in Figure 6.11.

The use of the linear gradient and the frequency-tailored RF pulse for slice selection has several otherwise unavailable benefits. The slice profile of the selected slice becomes dependent on the stability of the linear gradient and the accuracy of the frequency band produced by the RF transmitter, not on the switching capability of the gradient system.

Currently available digital RF systems as well as gradient drivers are very accurate, so slices of specified thickness are readily produced. Another major advantage of this approach is the speed with which slices can be excited. Since the linear gradient only has to be switched on and can be designed to stabilize very rapidly, it becomes feasible to produce multiple RF pulses in relatively rapid sequence, each selecting and exciting a different parallel slice through the body. With this capability, multislice imaging becomes a standard feature of the imager.

6.3.1.2 Frequency encoding

In the acquisition of data to create a single slice image, an RF pulse with a tailored frequency range excites a slice of the body from which information will be collected to produce the image in the presence of a slice selection gradient. After the RF pulse has been turned off, magnetic moments of the nuclei begin to relax to the equilibrium state as described above in Section 6.2.4.

It was recognized by Paul Lauterbur (Lauterbur, 1973) that linear gradients could be used to distinguish between different locations of protons in space based on the novel idea that linear gradients cause different nuclei at different locations in an object to experience different magnetic fields and, therefore, because of the Larmor equation, precess at different frequencies. In his landmark paper in *Nature*, he described the use of the Fourier transform to recover the frequency information which yields a one dimensional projection of the object of interest, where the projection represents the summation of all of the signals received from tissues perpendicular to the gradient. By rotating the object and successively applying the linear gradient followed by the tailored, multi-frequency RF pulse, a series of one dimensional projections were obtained. Lauterbur then used filtered backprojection algorithms, commonly used in computed tomography, to reconstruct the two-dimensional image of the water-filled tubes he used in his experiment.

The readout process involves the detection of signals from the nuclei in the presence of a linear gradient, the readout gradient, also called the frequency encode gradient (FEG), which encodes their position along a line into different frequencies along this line. The direction of the FEG is perpendicular to that of the slice-selection gradient which is applied during the RF pulse. Typically, the linear gradient is implemented so that the protons in the center of the line experience the static magnetic field, i.e., the gradient has no effect. On one side of the center value, the magnetic field decreases linearly to a value up to 40 gauss lower than the static field strength, while, in the opposite direction, the field increases to up to 40 gauss higher than the static field strength. The effect of the gradient is to produce a range of precessional frequencies according to Eq. (6.4). When the broad-band signal is received by the system, it is converted into digital form which is Fourier transformed to produce a frequency spectrum. The magnitude or modulus of the spectrum represents the one-dimensional profile of the imaged object.

6.3.2 *Projection reconstruction*

In Lauterbur's original paper, projection reconstruction was used to produce the images he reported. Projection reconstruction is based on concepts from computed tomography (CT) imaging that permit images to be reconstructed from one-dimensional projections. The basic idea of projection reconstruction derives from early work by Radon as described by Brooks and di Chiro (Brooks, Di Chiro, 1976). In this reconstruction approach, a collection of one-dimensional profiles (ray sums in CT) are created at a number of different angular positions around an object from which a two-dimensional image is to be reconstructed. In order to produce the reconstructed image, is it is assumed that each profile can be "projected back" along a path identical to that from which the data comprising the one-dimensional profile is assumed to have come. Then, all of these backprojected profiles can be summed to produce a representation of the structures from which the profiles were obtained. This processing is known as simple backprojection. It is not useful without modification because it produces a blurred image, making discrete structures unrecognizable [see Figure 6.12(a)].

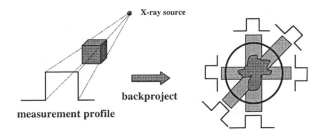

A. Simple backprojection

Figure 12a: Image reconstruction from computed tomography using simple backprojection yields an unusable blurred image due to summation of "tail" artifacts from the projections. Each profile that is summed is the response of an x-ray detector array to the attenuation of the x-ray beam as it passes through an object of interest. Once obtained, these projections are "projected back" along the direction from which they were originally recorded. All of the backprojected data are summed to produce the reconstructed image.

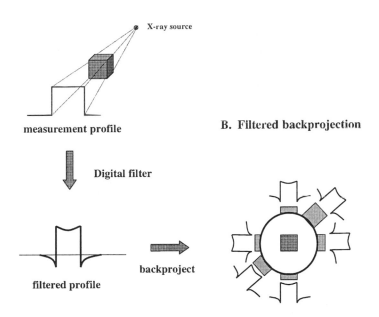

B. Filtered backprojection

Figure 12b: Each profile is obtained as before, but before performing the backprojection, each profile is filtered to limit its spatial frequency content, resulting in the alteration of the shape of each profile so that there are positive and negative components present. When these are algebraically summed, the components which cause blurring of the images in the simple backprojection example are no longer present except at the extreme periphery of the field. The object of interest is faithfully represented, while artifacts at the edges of the field are not displayed. The reconstruction is much more accurate than simple backprojection.

The blurring can be readily understood by using an intuitive example. If a series of profiles are collected of a single point and then reconstructed with simple back-projection by summing all the profiles, the reconstruction will show a "star" with the original point at the center. With an increasing number of projections, the reconstruction will begin to resemble a probability density distribution proportional to $1/r$, where r is the distance from the point, because, in the limit, superposition of these profiles through a single point is equivalent to rotating one profile through 360°. This results in a blurred image (Herman, 1980).

In order to solve the blurring problem, the method of filtering the profiles prior to backprojection is used. A ramp filter is combined with a window function to produce a convolution filter that is applied to each profile's low frequency information and high-frequency noise. The filter alters the profiles so that when the profiles are backprojected and algebraically summed, the result is a good representation of the actual object that was imaged. The star artifact from overlapping projection tails is normally outside the field of view and is not displayed. Figure 6.12(b) shows the process of filtered backprojection.

Reconstruction from projections can be performed by other methods in addition to filtered backprojection. Techniques such as the algebraic reconstruction technique (ART) or Fourier reconstruction can be used as well (Herman, 1980). These methods are all derived from work done for CT, which allowed the manufacturers of early MRI systems to simply use the reconstruction hardware and software from existing CT products to commercialize their systems more quickly. Current commercial systems do not use projection reconstruction because it has disadvantages, especially with respect to the speed of acquisition and possible artifacts. However, the use of projection reconstruction is reported in the literature from time to time in various research projects and can be useful for reducing motion artifacts (Glover, Pauly, 1992).

6.3.3 Phase-encoding and Fourier reconstruction

Fourier reconstruction uses the Fourier transform to convert information collected in frequency space to image information representing the two-dimensional distribution of spin-densities in the volume of interest. This approach was proposed by Kumar, Welti, and Ernst in 1975 (Kumar, Welti *et al.* 1975). A modification called spin-warp two-dimensional Fourier transform imaging was proposed by Edelstein *et al.* in 1980 (Edelstein, Hutchinson *et al.* 1980). In acquiring the data for a single image in two dimensions, a pulse sequence is executed to create a two-dimensional spatial map of frequencies. This spatial frequency map is related to the image by way of a two-dimensional Fourier transform and is often referred to as a "k-space" map.

Each frequency value in the two-dimensional array (k_x, k_y) contains information related to the magnetization in space, transformed by the presence of linear gradients via the following relationship:

$$S(k_x, k_y) = \int \left(M_t(x, y)e^{-i(k_x x + k_y y)} \right) dx\, dy, \qquad (6.5)$$

where S is the value at a point in the two-dimensional array in k-space, M_t is the magnitude of the magnetization at (x, y) at time t, and k_x and k_y are spatial frequencies. In this equation the substitutions

$$k_x = \gamma \int \mathbf{G}_x \, dt,$$

$$k_y = \gamma \int \mathbf{G}_y \, dt, \tag{6.6}$$

have been made. The k_x-values are collected in the direction of the frequency encoding gradient (x-direction) while the k_y-values are collected in the direction of the phase encoding gradient (y-direction). The k-space matrix is collected one row at a time, each row with a different amplitude of the phase encoding gradient (PEG).

Since k-space has Hermitian symmetry due to positive and negative phase shifts induced by the phase encoding gradient, some scanning methods make use of this property by acquiring data covering only 60% of the full matrix. This increases the acquisition speed at the price of SNR.

While projection reconstruction uses a slice-selection gradient and a perpendicular gradient, the readout gradient, to produce the projections necessary for performing reconstruction of a planar image, the Fourier method requires the additional use of a phase-encoding gradient. The additional gradient is used to add phase information to the signal, which makes it possible to include information along the the second dimension of the slice. Figure 6.13 shows a typical pulse sequence with phase-encoding gradients.

In a typical spin echo pulse sequence (or any other sequence), the order of application of gradients establishes how the information will be recorded by the system to produce the image. The slice select gradient is turned on in the presence of the first RF pulse to excite a slice at a particular location in the magnetic field. Following the slice excitation process, the phase-encoding gradient is turned on for a specific period of time at a specified amplitude. After the phase-encoding gradient is turned off, a 180° RF pulse is applied in the presence of a slice-select gradient, followed by a frequency-encoding gradient and readout of the spin echo in the x-direction. The resulting signal contains not only spatial information encoded as frequency in the x-directions as rows of the k-space matrix, but also the data are phase shifted in the y-direction (from row to row of the k-space matrix), thus providing the information necessary to reconstruct the image in the y-direction.

After the first slice select gradient has been turned off, all spins in the selected slice are precessing at the same Larmor frequency. At this point, a gradient is applied perpendicular to the readout direction. This gradient, the phase-encoding gradient, causes spins to precess at frequencies that increase linearly in the direction of the applied gradient. The gradient is on for a specific time and with a different strength for each data collection step. In the first data collection step, the PEG is at maximum strength at one end of the y-axis field, the strength of the PEG then

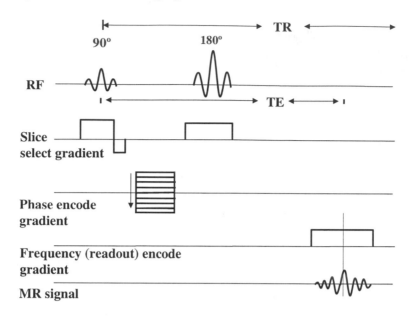

Figure 6.13: A schematic diagram of a typical spin-echo pulse sequence shows the basic components of a pulse sequence. The diagram represents one TR or repetition period between 90° pulses. During the execution of the pulse sequence, RF pulses and gradients are turned on repetitively to produce the signal, in this case the spin-echo, which will be used to reconstruct an image. The phase-encoding gradient shown in this diagrammatic representation indicates that with each execution of the pulse sequence (each TR period), a different phase-encoding amplitude is used until all of k-space has been sampled.

decreases progressively until, in the last data collection step, the PEG is at maximum strength at the opposite end of the y-axis field. During each data collection step the spins return to the Larmor frequency of the static field, but because of the previously applied phase-encoding gradient, their phase is shifted with respect to its value at the end of the slice-selection RF pulse. After the phase has been shifted, a 180° pulse is applied in the presence of another slice select gradient identical to the first, to cause the evolution of the spin echo. At the time the echo has formed, the readout gradient is turned on and the signal is recorded.

The final step of the image reconstruction process is to apply a two-dimensional Fourier transform to the k-space matrix. A similar process using a second phase-encoding gradient permits the reconstruction of three-dimensional data sets using three-dimensional Fourier reconstruction.

6.3.4 The development of contrast

The goal of magnetic resonance imaging is to produce contrast between tissue types based on differences in the way these tissues respond to different manipulations of the net magnetic field vector by means of RF energy and gradient field switching. Switching of the various parameters leading to signals being produced from anatomic structures during the imaging process is accomplished through the use of pulse sequences. The critical parameters of a pulse sequence specify the strength, temporal order, polarity, duration, and repetition rate of RF pulses and gradients. The pulse sequence is the most critical part of image acquisition, since it defines what the characteristics of the image will be. Pulse sequence design is considered by many to be a "black art," left to a few highly skilled individuals. Sometimes this description is accurate; it is difficult to develop a new pulse sequence that produces the desired contrast between tissues without introducing artifacts.

There are many different pulse sequence designs which produce useful tissue contrast. The most basic are the spin echo pulse sequence, the inversion recovery spin echo pulse sequence, and the gradient echo (sometimes called the gradient recalled echo) pulse sequence. Each of these pulse sequences has many variations that lead to improvements in some aspect of displayed contrast information. In addition, these pulse sequences can be designed to provide single images during the operation of the pulse sequence, multiple discrete images (anisotropic image sets), or true three-dimensional image sets (isotropic image sets). Typically, there are many tradeoffs between parameters ensuring that a diagnostically useful image is obtained and the need for high speed in the acquisition process.

Contrast is produced by controlling several different intrinsic parameters related to the chemical makeup of the tissues, and extrinsic parameters not specifically related to the chemistry of the tissues. Intrinsic parameters are the relaxation constants T1 and T2, the proton density (number of protons per mm^3 of tissue), the chemical shift (see Section 6.4.6), and any flow within the tissue. Extrinsic parameters include the pulse timing represented by TR, the repetition time, and TE, the time to evolution of an echo, and the flip angle, the angle to which the net magnetic vector is rotated (between very small and 180°, but usually 90° or less).

Since the goal of imaging is to differentiate between tissues having different relaxation times, it can be useful to review published data for typical tissues. The relaxation times for a variety of tissues in vivo are listed in Table 6.2. As this table indicates, the T1 values of the various tissue types depend on the magnetic field strength as well. As noted in the reference, the values in tables such as this are considered approximate (±20%) and cannot be used for accurate contrast calculations. T2 values vary much less with field strength, although there is some variation. However, over the ranges of field strengths used for medical imaging, tables of values usually show T2 for tissues as independent of field strength. A further assumption is that these values are for normal tissues. In many but not all disease processes, the values of T1 and T2 will increase, thereby altering tissue contrast in the resulting images.

6.3.5 Pulse sequences

6.3.5.1 Free induction decay

The simplest pulse sequence for nuclear magnetic resonance chemical studies is a 90° RF pulse followed by a signal from the spins tipped into the transverse plane. The next 90° pulse occurs at some subsequent time TR.

6.3.5.2 Spin echo

The spin echo pulse sequence is the basic pulse sequence of MR imaging (Figure 6.13). Spin echoes were first described by Hahn in a landmark paper in 1950 as a way to address the problem of measuring T2 decay in FID experiments (Hahn, 1950). In this paper, he described how the FID signal can be made to reappear so that it can be recorded, rather than decaying rapidly as determined by the T2* time constant. The approach he took was to apply a 90° pulse to move the net magnetization vector into the transverse plane, followed by a 180° refocusing pulse a short time later. As with the simple FID pulse sequence, the instant the 90° RF pulse is turned off, the phases of the spins whose contributions make up the net magnetic moment begin to change due to the local variations in the magnetic field. This phase dispersal is the T2* decay.

However, if a 180° pulse is applied to the spin system before the transverse component decays away, the dephasing can be reversed so that the spins come back into "focus" as if the dephasing had not taken place. The 180° pulse causes the spins to shift by 180° in the transverse plane so that instead of dephasing, the spins rephase, coming back into phase before beginning to dephase again. This rephasing increases the transverse magnetization vector so that a new echo evolves as the spins rephase. This signal is the spin echo, which decays again under the effects of T2* unless another 180° rephasing pulse is applied.

A more accessible description of what happens can be provided if one remembers that the magnetization rotated into the transverse plane is a vector sum representation of individual magnetic moment contributions. Viewed from the laboratory frame of reference this vector is actually precessing at the Larmor frequency. As T2* decay occurs the individual magnetic moment vectors distribute themselves throughout the transverse plane, i.e., they lose phase coherence and the net magnetic moment vector vanishes. However, the application of the 180° refocusing pulse shifts all of the magnetic moments in the transverse plane by 180° to the other side of the transverse plane where the faster magnetic moments now begin to rephase with the slower magnetic moments so that the magnitude of the net magnetic moment vector increases again. At some time, the magnitude of the net magnetic moment vector reaches a maximum, the center of the spin echo, and then the dephasing process begins again.

A train of 180° RF pulses causes successive rephasing by repeatedly shifting the magnetization 180° across the transverse plane after each 180° RF pulse. This pulse sequence is known as the Carr–Purcell–Meiboom–Gill (CPMG) sequence. The maximum value of the spin echo following each 180° pulse constitutes a point on the exponential decay describing spin–spin relaxation. The T2 time constant is measured at the point on this decay curve where the signal is 37% of the maximum amplitude of the first echo. Thus, a 90° RF pulse followed by carefully timed 180° RF pulses gives an envelope of the T2 decay in the presence of T2*, as shown in Figure 6.14.

If a sequence of 90° pulses is applied and the *time of repetition* (TR) is insufficient to allow complete recovery of the longitudinal magnetization, the amount of

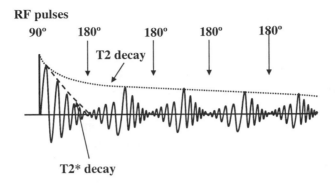

Figure 6.14: A pulse sequence consisting of a 90° pulse followed by carefully timed 180° pulses produces a series of spin-echoes of decreasing amplitudes. Each individual echo decays with a time constant given by T2*, but the decaying peak echo amplitudes are fit to an exponential decay curve to obtain T2. This special pulse sequence makes it possible to compute parametric T2 images, rather than the T2-weighted images obtained normally.

magnetization tipped into the transverse plane by the second 90° pulse will be less than that after the first 90° pulse. The result is that the magnitude of the second spin echo will be less than that of the first spin echo. After the third 90° pulse the amplitude of the spin echo is even smaller, but at this point the system enters a steady state condition where there is no additional loss of echo magnitude due to continuing loss of transverse magnetization, i.e., where the system is saturated and the available longitudinal magnetization is equal from pulse to pulse.

In imaging, regardless of which pulse sequences are used, combinations of the relaxation times and the proton density contribute to the image contrast. By varying the time of application of the RF pulses and gradients, the contributions of these parameters can be varied to produce an image that is said to be "T1-weighted," "T2-weighted," or "proton-density weighted." The important consideration is that the imaging sequences do not produce "pure" T1, T2, or proton density images. Pure or parametric images must be computed from multiple acquisitions with selected timing characteristics. Various parametric images can be produced from different ways of acquiring the image data, but this requires post-processing of specifically collected images.

The spin echo pulse sequence, consisting of a series of alternating 90° and 180° RF pulses, is used for a variety of imaging tasks to produce different contrasts between tissues based on varying contributions of the relaxation times, the proton density and other parameters. The basic spin echo imaging pulse sequence can be used to produce proton density weighting, T1 weighting, and T2 weighting. The key variables for achieving a particular weighting in the image are the principal timing parameters of the pulse sequence: TE, the echo time, and TR, the repetition time.

The pulse sequence is applied multiple times depending on the image size and the amount of averaging needed to attain the required SNR. The repetition time,

TR, is defined as the time from the center of a 90° RF pulse to the center of the next 90° RF pulse. The echo time, TE, is defined as the time from the center of the 90° pulse to the center of the spin echo. TE/2 is the time from the center of the 90° RF pulse to the center of the 180° rephasing RF pulse. The overall sequence timing is a product of the TR of the pulse sequence and the number of phase encoding steps required, assuming that no repetition of the sequence for noise averaging is done. Thus, for a spin echo sequence with a TR of 2 seconds and 128 phase encoding steps, the time to perform the acquisition would be 256 seconds plus a few seconds delay for cycling the sequence. If multiple acquisitions for signal averaging were done, then the time would be a multiple of 256 seconds, so the formula for the time required for acquiring an image is

$$\text{TR} \times \#\text{Steps} \times \#\text{acq}, \tag{6.7}$$

where TR is the repetition rate, # Steps are the number of phase acquisitions, and # acq is the number of times the sequence is repeated to reduce noise.

MR images often have a relatively poor SNR. Because of this, simple noise reduction by signal averaging is often needed. Effectively, signal averaging means that the image is collected multiple times so that the final image produced by the system is an average of the multiple images acquired. Since the noise is assumed to be uncorrelated from acquisition to acquisition, its amplitude does not increase as the images are summed, but the signal common to all of the acquired images increases. The increase in SNR from signal averaging is equal to the square root of the number of acquisitions. Thus, 4 acquisitions improve SNR by a factor of 2. While it is possible, in principle, to increase the SNR arbitrarily by simply increasing the number of acquisitions, practical limitations to 6–8 acquisitions are imposed by patient motion and total imaging time.

In a normal spin echo sequence, a lot of time usually elapses after the acquisition of the echo, but before the end of TR. During this "dead time," the system can select and excite other slices so that it is possible to acquire 20–30 slices during the time required for one slice, with no apparent additional total time needed for the sequence. Each slice is independently excited and acquired with conventional spin echo weighting. The system is simply using the available time to advantage to acquire the additional slices. The total number of slices that can be collected in this multi-slice acquisition is a function of TR/(TE + constant), where the constant represents overhead time.

Among the other factors contributing to a loss of contrast are effects due to motion of the tissues, effects that are a result of the flow of blood or other fluids, effects due to molecular diffusion of protons, and microscopic perfusion in tissues. Other effects such as chemical shift and magnetic susceptibility differences between tissues affect spin echo imaging less often, but can create significant changes in signal intensity with other types of pulse sequences.

The magnitude of the spin echo is related to the signal intensity I displayed in the final image after the reconstruction process is approximated by

$$I \approx M_0 f(\text{vel})\left[1 - e^{-\text{TR}/\text{T1}}\right], e^{-\text{TE}/\text{T2}}, \qquad (6.8)$$

where M_0 is the initial value for the transverse magnetization, and $f(\text{vel})$ is a flow-related signal change (Bushberg, Seibert *et al.* 1994). This equation indicates that changing the TR value of a pulse sequence will influence the T1 weighting of the image, especially when TR and T1 are approximately equal, while changing the TE will alter the T2 weighting.

6.3.5.2.1 T1-weighted spin echo.

To achieve T1 weighting, a spin echo pulse sequence is designed to reduce the contributions due to T2 and spin density. This is achieved by using a short TR, usually less than 500–600 msec, and a short TE of 20 msec or less. The short TR ensures that there will be maximum differences in the longitudinal recovery between tissues with different T1 relaxation times. The short TE ensures that transverse magnetization will not dephase and loose these differences, i.e., that the T2 decay will not have a major effect on the T1 differences encoded into the data. The selection of the TR and TE can be understood by observing that in images of the head, the shortest T1 relaxation time (at 1.5 T) is due to fat, while the longest is due to cerebrospinal fluid (CSF) (see Figure 6.15). If one looks at the longitudinal recovery curves, one observes that fat returns to equilibrium faster than white matter, which returns faster than gray matter, which returns faster than CSF. Since these differences cannot be read-out directly, because they are effects that occur in the direction of B_0, they must be read out indirectly as differences in transverse signal. In order to maintain the differences in transverse magnetization that reflects the longitudinal differences, T2 decay must be minimized. Since T2 is very small compared to T1, it is necessary to use a 180° rephasing pulse after only a short delay from the termination of the 90° pulse. Thus, a 180° pulse applied at $TE/2$ causes rephasing to occur at TE. If TE is short (20 msec or less), then the T2 dephasing does not have time to occur and the differences due to T1 are preserved in the magnitude of the signal converted to image intensities. Figure 6.16 shows how T1 weighted contrast is produced.

6.3.5.2.2 Spin density weighting.

Spin density-weighting in a spin echo image gives image intensities intended to allow tissues with large proton densities that respond strongly to the external magnetic field to be distinguished from tissues with lower proton densities. At equilibrium, the longitudinal magnetization will be greater for greater proton densities. Tissues with large numbers of protons include fats and fatty components. In this version of spin echo imaging, a long TR is used so that the longitudinal magnetization differences between tissues due to T1 are mostly eliminated because the tissues have time to nearly return to equilibrium. With a TR value of 2000–3000 msec, most differences in longitudinal magnetization are related to proton densities. When the next 90° pulse occurs, the distribution of the transverse magnetizations is mostly related to the proton densities of the tissues. To preserve this information so that T2 decay cannot strongly

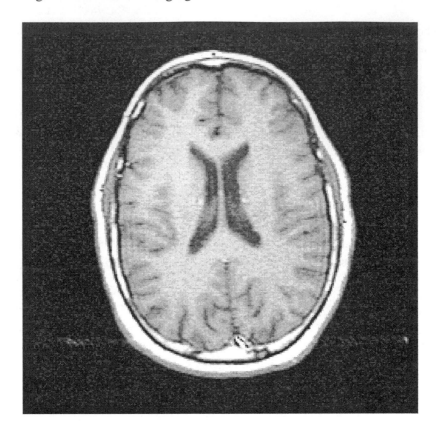

T1 - Weighted Spin Echo Image

Figure 6.15: A T1-weighted image from a spin-echo data set of the head. In T1-weighted images, the most obvious feature is that the CSF is dark. Note also that fatty tissue at the surface of the brain as well as marrow and fatty tissue outside the skull are very light. Vascular structures can be seen around the edges of the image and are also light. Gray matter is somewhat darker than white matter. These correspond to the curves seen in Figure 6.16. Also noticeable is a slight amount of Gibbs artifact.

influence the resulting image contrast, a very short TE is required, on the order of about 20 msec. The signal collected and converted to image contrast is primarily attributable to proton density. Figure 6.17 diagrams a pulse sequence for the production of proton density weighting.

6.3.5.2.3 T2-weighting. In this version of spin echo imaging, the TR is long, 2000–4000 msec, to reduce T1 effects. A long TE is used to produce contrast differences that are mostly due to differences in the T2 relaxation of the tissues. Tissues that have long T2 time constants will maintain phase coherence of the transverse magnetization, while other tissues with shorter T2 relaxation times dephase in the

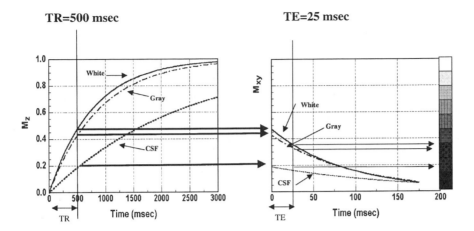

T1 Contrast

Figure 6.16: A contrast diagram demonstrates the origin of T1 contrast in reconstructed images of the head at 1.5 T from a pulse sequence having the timing that produces T1 contrast. The difference in evolution of M_z for gray and white matter on the one hand vs. the CSF signal on the other hand is noteworthy. It is also useful to note that timing is likely to be very critical to enable gray and white matter to have sufficiently different contrast to be observed as different in the images. [Redrawn from (Bushberg, Seibert *et al.* 1994.)]

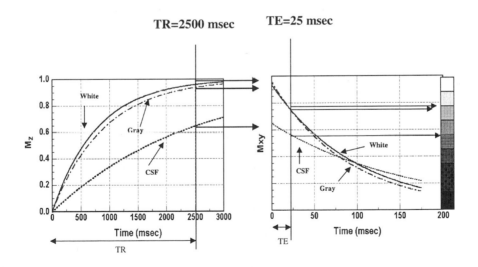

Proton Density Contrast

Figure 6.17:   Longitudinal recovery and transverse decay curves for proton density weighted images. Separation of gray and white matter requires careful timing selection, while CSF is easily separated from the other tissues. [Redrawn from (Bushberg, Seibert *et al.* 1994.)]

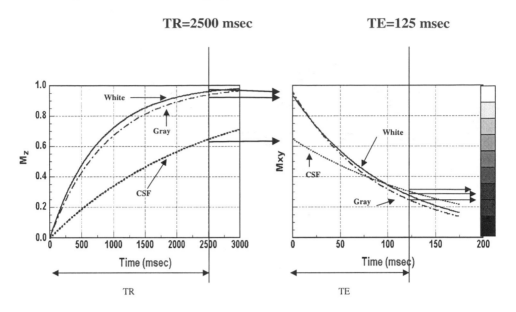

T2 Contrast

Figure 6.18: T2 contrast is obtained in head images by using a long TR to reduce T1 contributions and a long TE to obtain separation of white, gray, and CSF signals. However, the long TE reduces available signal, causing a decrease in SNR in the resulting images. [Redrawn from (Bushberg, Seibert *et al.* 1994.)]

transverse plane and loose signal intensity. The long TE of 80–150 msec permits the T2 dephasing to occur, weighting the image in favor of T2. A problem with T2-weighted images is that as one extends TE, the difference between the transverse relaxation curves of different tissues increases, leading to improved image contrast, but at the cost of a decrease in signal intensity. Thus, if one uses an excessively long TE, the SNR decreases. T2 weighted tissue contrast is shown in Figure 6.18.

6.3.5.2.4 Spin echo variations.   After the first spin echo has been read out, it is perfectly feasible to wait for another TE/2 interval and apply another 180° refocusing pulse so that another spin echo will occur at a TE of two times the first echo. The data are used to form a second image at the same location as the first. This pulse sequence is sometimes called a symmetric double echo pulse sequence because the second echo comes at two times the TE of the first. If the TE of the first and second echoes are not related by an integer factor, then the sequence is called an asymmetric double echo pulse sequence. Additional echoes can be obtained until the signal loss causes the resulting images to be unacceptable due to low SNR. In this manner, it is feasible to obtain a series of different image slices at increasing TE values. These images reflect a loss signal intensity in each successive echo due to T2 relaxation. As mentioned earlier, a fit to the amplitude of the echo describes an envelope of the T2 relaxation constant for the tissue.

Another variation of spin echo imaging is fast spin echo, also known as turbo spin echo. This pulse sequence is based on the RARE (rapid acquisition with relaxation enhancement) method described by Hennig *et al.* (Hennig, Naureth *et al.* 1986). Fast spin echo is an extension of the multi-echo spin echo sequence except that each successive 180° pulse uses a different phase encoding gradient value. In this type of pulse sequence, a series of 180° RF refocusing pulses is applied after a 90° RF pulse in the presence of a changing phase encoding gradient, so that k-space for a single image is sampled rapidly by the echo train that follows the 90° pulse. The echo train duration is the time during which the echoes are acquired, and the echo train length is defined as the number of echoes following each 90° RF pulse. Successive echoes appear at increasing TE, so the effective TE of the sequence must be determined by knowing which one of the echoes occurs when the phase encoding gradient is zero. Since a zero phase-encoding gradient defines the center of k-space, which defines the overall contrast in the image, positioning the center point early or late in the echo train can significantly affect the overall contrast in the resulting image. This pulse sequence is diagrammed in Figure 6.19. This works reasonably well because a larger number of phase encoding gradient

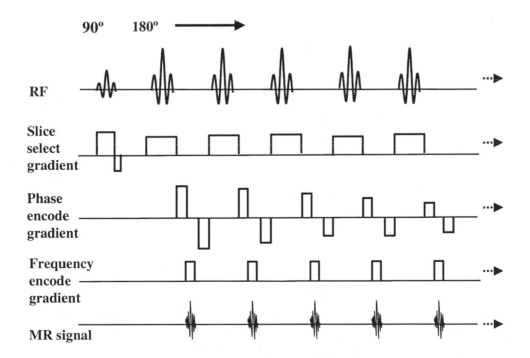

Figure 6.19: Part of a fast spin echo pulse sequence is shown in which a 90° pulse is followed by a train of 180° pulses, each with a different phase-encoding amplitude. A rewind gradient is used prior to each refocusing RF pulse. The effective TE of the sequence occurs at the time when the phase-encoding gradient is at a value of 0.

echoes increases detail rather than contrast. As each echo is produced, transverse magnetization continues to decay, so that echoes show a decaying signal intensity due to T2. This decay can cause blurring in the multi-echo images, especially if the zero phase-encoding gradient occurs early in the pulse train and the T2 of the tissues is short.

With fast spin-echo sequences, a multi-shot or a single shot approach can be used. In a multi-shot approach, several excitation pulses are used, followed by the refocused echo train, to produce a complete sampling of k-space. In the single shot pulse sequence, a single 90° excitation pulse is followed by the acquisition of enough spin echoes to completely sample k-space. Single shot approaches tend to make use of specialized acquisition methods, such as half-Fourier acquisition, and high-performance gradient systems. Names that have been given to some of these approaches include HASTE (half-Fourier acquisition single-shot turbo spin echo) and SSFSE (single-shot fast spin echo) (Semelka, Kelekis *et al.* 1996). Using these methods, half-second spin-echo image acquisition is possible.

6.3.5.3 Inversion recovery

The inversion recovery variation of the spin echo pulse sequence is used to produce image contrast related to differences in T1 relaxation by enhancing these differences. The inversion recovery pulse sequence is different from the conventional spin-echo pulse sequence in that there is an initial preparatory 180° RF pulse, followed by a delay time known as the inversion time, TI. After TI, a standard spin echo pulse sequence follows with the usual readout of the data as a spin echo. The 180° RF pulse is slice-selective, so all of the spins in the slice are inverted. Once the inverting 180° RF pules is turned off, the longitudinal magnetization begins to recover, but since it has been inverted, the recovery time is much longer than with a 90° RF pulse. While recovery of the longitudinal magnetization is underway, the application of the 90° pulse rotates those spins that have realigned from the inverted state into the transverse plane to produce a signal regardless of whether the longitudinal magnetization is positive at this point or not. This signal has an intensity given by:

$$I = M_0 f(\text{vel})\left(1 - 2e^{-\text{TR}/\text{T1}}\right), \tag{6.9}$$

where $f(\text{vel})$ is a function of motion, usually due to blood flow. The factor 2 accounts for the recovery from the 180° inverting pulse.

This pulse sequence uses a short TE, so that signal amplitude is maximized without major T2 contributions to the signal. The choice of TI changes the contributions of different tissues with different T1 relaxation times to the image contrast. With short TIs, the longitudinal magnetization can be considered to be in phase or out of phase and the inverted magnetization can start from negative 100% of the spin recovery and evolve through 0 to full recovery (100%), or it can be considered to begin at 100% after the 180° inverting pulse, decay with a T1 to 0, then begin recovering towards its starting point at 100%. This leads to two possible ways to

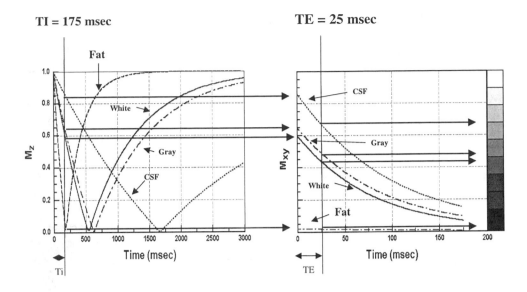

STIR Contrast

Figure 6.20: Contrast diagram for a STIR pulse sequence, which produces images in which tissue signals can be suppressed by selecting the inversion time (TI) to correspond to the null point of the tissue signal. In this diagram, fat has been "nulled out," so images of the head have greatly reduced contrast contributions from fatty tissue. Contrast in the image is similar to T2 contrast, except that the technique is inherently based on T1 contrast methods.

display the signal: a phase image that demonstrates the entire range from $-M_z$ to M_z or a magnitude image, where the portion from 0 to M_z is displayed as a loss of M_z from 100% to zero, then a recovery back to 100%.

This latter version of the inversion recovery pulse sequence is called STIR (Short Tau Inversion Recovery) and is shown in Figure 6.20. A short TI time and a magnitude display are used. With STIR, short T1 tissues produce a lower signal than other tissues and the recovery curves of all tissues pass through a zero-point (null or bounce point). By selecting this null point carefully, it is possible to selectively suppress tissue signals. This technique can be quite effective and is often used to suppress the signal emitted by fat, although the signals emitted by all other tissues are also altered by this pulse sequence. A typical TI for fat suppression is in the range of 140–170 msec.

The null point can produce an interesting artifact due to the possibility that positive longitudinal magnetization can occur in one tissue while negative longitudinal magnetization occurs in another neighboring tissue. This happens when one tissue exhibits a short T1 and the other a longer T1. If a magnitude image is used to display the contrast, these two tissues can have the same intensity in the image. If the two tissues are next to each other, the result is a loss of contrast or a signal void that can actually help outline an area that another T1 pulse sequence would display less conspicuously (Mitchell, 1999, p. 148).

Another variant on the basic inversion recovery sequence uses a very long TI to eliminate the signal emitted by a fluid such as cerebrospinal fluid. This pulse sequence is implemented by using a TI of 2000 msec or more to specifically remove the contrast due to CSF from the image. This pulse sequence is known as FLAIR (fluid-attenuated inversion recovery), which is characterized by a long TE and TR to obtain T2 weighting. This pulse sequence can become relatively time-consuming, especially if implemented as a spin echo of pulse sequence, and the overall SNR is low because of the loss of signal as the inverted spins in the tissues return to equilibrium.

Inversion recovery spin echo pulse sequences can be implemented using the same techniques used in conventional spin echo sequences, but long acquisition times often preclude their use. However, fast spin echo versions of inversion recovery are available on high-performance imagers, as are echo planar sequences. These fast techniques make inversion recovery methods much more likely to be used because of the significant improvements in the rate of acquisition.

6.3.5.4 Gradient echoes

Gradient echoes, as the name implies, are "echoes" produced by switching gradients that return dephasing protons to an in-phase state from which the signal produced in the transverse plane can be read. A principal feature of gradient echo pulse sequences is that they do not use a 180° RF refocusing pulse. Rather, they depend on reversing the polarity of a magnetic field gradient, a process called gradient reversal. Since the presence of a gradient after an RF pulse causes dephasing of the protons, a gradient that is equal in strength and duration, but opposite in polarity, brings the protons back into focus. If the reversed gradient is maintained, the spins dephase again and the signal disperses. The maximum signal occurs when the initial and the reversed gradients are balanced; that is, they are of equal amplitude and duration (Figure 6.21).

Gradient echoes, also called gradient-recalled echoes, are really FIDs rather than true echoes. Because they represent a dephasing of the protons followed by a rephasing, there are no mechanisms in these pulse sequences that result in a cancellation of the effects of magnet inhomogeneities. Effects due to tissue magnetic susceptibilities, where interfaces between different tissues can distort the magnetic field locally, somewhat like a small gradient field, also are observed. Time-varying magnetic fields due to microscopic motions and molecular diffusion can also have an effect. Thus, the gradient echo pulse sequences are affected by T2* rather than T2, resulting in a very rapid dispersion of transverse magnetization and loss of signal compared to a spin echo pulse sequence with T2 dispersal. Because of this sensitivity, gradient echo pulse sequences require more stringent instrumentation designs and careful consideration of tissue effects in order to be used effectively.

There are many advantages to gradient echo pulse sequences. Because there is no 180° rephasing RF pulse and evolution time for the spin echo, the pulse

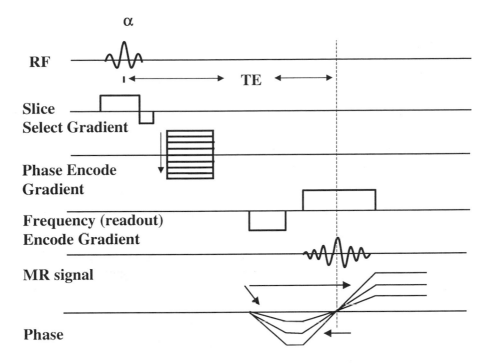

Figure 6.21: Gradient echo pulse sequences are characterized by not having a refocusing pulse. Instead, a bi-phasic gradient causes protons to initially go out of phase, then come back into phase to produce a signal that looks like an echo formed in a spin-echo pulse sequence. The dephasing occurs during the initial "on" period of the readout gradient. Following a period during which no field gradient is applied, the readout gradient is turned on with the opposite polarity, causing the dephased protons to rephase completely when the second application of the gradient exactly matches, but is opposite from, the initial application. At this point the signal is maximized and is digitized. The second lobe of the gradient remains on and the signal is lost due to continuing dephasing. Note also that, for improved signal strength, the applied RF pulse is often less than a 90° pulse.

sequence can be executed more rapidly, permitting additional slices to be obtained in the same TR period as in spin echo imaging. Also, because of the absence of 180° RF pulses, the RF power deposition in the patient is considerably lower than for a comparable spin echo pulse sequence. Other characteristics include the use of angles of less than 90° for the RF pulse, the partial flip angle. This partial flip angle, α, is used to control contrast in gradient echo sequences such that the TR can be reduced while maintaining adequate transverse magnetization to produce a signal. Because of their shorter imaging times, gradient echo pulse sequences can help to reduce motion artifacts that are a source of problems in conventional spin echo imaging and have permitted three-dimensional acquisitions to become practical for routine clinical use. Furthermore, since TE is a function of either the separation between the negative and positive gradient lobes or the reduced amplitude of one of the gradients, much shorter TE times are possible. Since the TE controls the degree of T2* weighting, different types of contrast mechanisms are possible with gradient echo imaging.

Gradient echo sequences use partial flip angles, less than 90°, for the RF pulses to control contrast in the resulting image. For a given TR, the recovery of the longitudinal magnetization is a function of the T1 value of a particular tissue. Small values of α cause only small reductions in longitudinal magnetization while still forming a substantial, measurable transverse component.

Therefore, the longitudinal magnetization can recover more quickly. For very short TR values, the partial flip angle results in more transverse magnetization and in a higher SNR than that which would result if a 90° pulse were used. Figure 6.22 shows a plot of the effects of using short TR and low flip angles. For a usable imaging sequence, multiple applications of the RF pulse are required. If there is insufficient time for the longitudinal magnetization to recover during the sequence, then the longitudinal magnetization will become progressively smaller with each pulse. This "saturation," reduces the amount of longitudinal magnetization available for tipping into the transverse plane, with a concomitant reduction in available signal.

Variations in TR, TE, and the flip angle affect the type of contrast in an image acquired with gradient echo methods. In pulse sequences where the TR is sufficiently long and a long TE is used in the presence of a large flip angle (more than 45°), the overall contrast has the appearance of a spin echo image, except that the

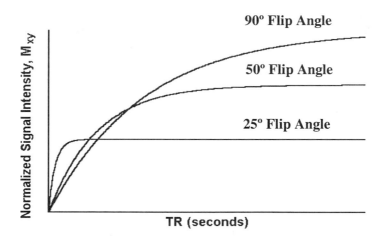

Effects of Flip Angle on M$_{xy}$

Figure 6.22: The flip angle, α, is very important in gradient echo imaging because a low flip angle can produce a larger transverse magnetization than a larger flip angle for short TR values. In the figure, a 25° flip angle initially produces more signal than either a 50° or 90° flip angle, so a fast pulse sequence would benefit from a small flip angle to maximize the available transverse magnetization.

contrast weighting is a function of T2* rather than T2. A short TE produces contrast weighting related to T1. For smaller flip angles of 30° or less, there is a relatively small amount of T1 contrast, since little transverse magnetization is flipped into the transverse plane. A proton density weighting is obtained with a short TE, while a longer TE produces T2* weighting.

When the TR is very short, less than 50 msec, an equilibrium condition known as steady state free precession (SSFP) occurs after a few RF pulses. In this situation, both longitudinal and transverse magnetization components exist at the end of each cycle. When the TR is lower than the longitudinal recovery time of the tissues, the longitudinal magnetization does not have time to recover, so the system is said to be saturated. However, the longitudinal magnetization lost at the time of application of the RF pulse has time to partially recover to the point where a steady state amount of longitudinal magnetization is available at the beginning of each RF pulse. If the TR is less than the T2* value of the tissue, then some transverse magnetization will be present as well at the end of the cycle just before the next RF pulse. Upon application of the RF pulse, some of the transverse magnetization is converted to longitudinal magnetization, while some of the longitudinal magnetization is converted to transverse magnetization. When this happens a state of dynamic equilibrium is established that exists for the remainder of the data acquisition time. Contrast then becomes a function of the TR and the flip angle used, assuming a short TE. For small flip angles and short TR, proton density weighting is predominant. For medium flip angles and short TR, a combination of T2/T1 weighting is achieved. For larger flip angles and short TR, T2* weighting is observed. These pulse sequences have been given various names by the manufacturers. GRASS (gradient recalled acquisition in the steady state) and FISP (fast imaging with steady state precession) are among the more common acronyms.

In order to achieve T1 weighting, a means of eliminating residual transverse magnetization can be employed, thus reducing T2* contributions. Long TR values can be used, but to keep the acquisition as short as possible, this approach is not as desirable as using spoiling to eliminate the transverse magnetization. Spoiling refers to a process in which, after the echo is acquired, the existing transverse magnetization is scrambled or destroyed, so that none exists at the start of the next RF pulse. Spoiling can be achieved in two ways. The first is to use additional strong gradients to dephase the transverse magnetization. The second approach is to alter the phase of the RF signal slightly for each of the transmit-receive cycles, eliminating the possible build-up of a steady state transverse component. With spoiling and a short TR, a short TE sequence with a moderate-to-large flip angle, T1 weighting is achieved. These sequences are used with MR contrast agents to exploit the greater sensitivity of the contrast agent to magnetic susceptibility effects. Common acronyms for these pulse sequences are FLASH (fast low angle shot) and SPGR (spoiled GRASS or spoiled gradient recalled acquisition in the steady state).

Another class of gradient echo pulse sequences is known as magnetization prepared rapid gradient echo (MP-RAGE) sequences (Figure 6.23). These are very rapid sequences that can produce two-dimensional images in a few hundred milliseconds. These sequences use TRs of 5–7 msec and TEs of about half of the TR.

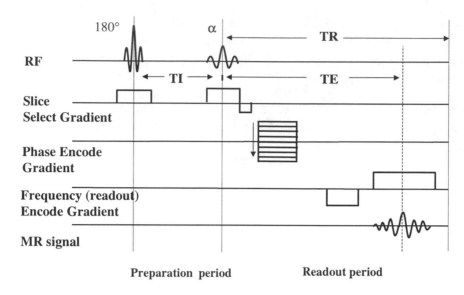

Figure 6.23: Magnetization prepared-rapid gradient echo (MP-RAGE) pulse sequence demonstrates the use of preparation of the magnetization, followed by rapid gradient echo readout of the resulting contrast. The MP-RAGE pulse sequence shown will produces T1-weighted images due to the 180° RF pulse followed by an inversion time, TI. Other preparation pulses can produce T2-weighting or chemical shift weighting.

Low tip angles (α less than 30°) are used with these sequences to reduce saturation effects. In these pulse sequences, a single or multiple pulse train is used to "prepare" the protons to produce T1, T2, or chemical shift weighting in the resulting images. After the preparation pulses, the entire image is read out using a FLASH-like sequence. These pulse sequences have been called TurboFLASH and snapshot FLASH, or TurboGRASS. For T1 weighting of the images, the preparation pulse is a single 180° inversion pulse followed by an inversion time or delay just before the readout of the slice. Because the longitudinal magnetization is continuing to evolve as the readout part of the sequence is active, the effective inversion time, T_{eff}, is defined as the inversion time plus the acquisition time divided by two, where the inversion time is the time from the start of the 180° pulse and the start of the FLASH part of the sequence. T2 weighting can be achieved as well by using a preparation pulse train of the form 90°–180°–90° separated by a time, τ, prior to the FLASH part of the sequence.

Contrast in MP-RAGE images depends on when the signal from the center of k-space is collected relative to the preparation pulses. If standard sequential phase ordering is used, the center of k-space occurs in the center of the readout of the image, so the contrast depends on the number of phase encoding steps, the TR, and one-half the number of acquisitions. If centric ordering is used, then contrast depends only on TR, since the center of k-space is read out at the beginning of the imaging portion of the sequence.

6.3.5.5 Echo planar imaging

Echo planar imaging (EPI) is a technique for obtaining an entire two-dimensional image in the period of one TR. This method was originally described by Peter Mansfield (Mansfield, Morris, 1982) in the late 1970s and allows images to be acquired in 50 msec or less. It is one of the most difficult types of pulse sequences to implement because of the constraints placed on the imaging hardware. These pulse sequences can use the same preparation pulses as those used by MP-RAGE. It is the readout part of the sequence that differs. In echo planar imaging, the readout gradient oscillates during collection so that each time the gradient makes an excursion from negative to positive, a new line of k-space is read out. The phase encoding gradient is turned on for a short time just before the readout of each echo, and hence the term "blipped" EPI is used. This is equivalent to a single phase-encoding step, except that the oscillating gradient produces all the phase encoding steps needed to read out all of the k-space. Very stable high-performance gradient driver electronics, able to produce gradient strengths of 20 to 40 mT/mm are required to switch the gradients at about 1 kHz for this type of pulse sequence.

Some of the pulse sequences acquire all of the phase encoding steps in one TR using a single RF pulse and are known as single-shot EPI sequences (Figure 6.24). Segmented EPI acquires groups of phase encoding steps with each RF pulse, giving rise to two shot or multi-shot EPI sequences. Multi-shot EPI images can show improved SNR with fewer artifacts. In addition, for multiple shots, there are multiple RF pulses, so the TR of the sequence is shorter than for single shot EPI, where TR is in fact infinite.

The images obtained from a single shot echo planar sequence are usually heavily T2 or T2* weighted. Because of the way the acquisition proceeds, there is effectively no TR, since the RF pulse is not repeated; all the necessary encoding is accomplished with a single pulse. Since all the phase-encoding information is collected in a single series of echoes, T2* decay occurs throughout the acquisition period, making the resulting echoes very susceptible to effects from magnet inhomogeneities, tissue susceptibility effects, and slight nonuniformities or nonlinearities of the gradients. Additionally, there is usually not enough time to acquire a very high resolution EPI image, so the image resolution is lower than that available with conventional imaging, typically 64 × 64 or 128 × 128 pixels.

The SNR is limited since a large number of data points are collected in a short time. With this short acquisition time, the bandwidth used during readout can be ten times greater than in a spin echo pulse sequence and the noise increases as the square root of the bandwidth. Furthermore, because the signal is decaying at a rate determined by T2* and T2, an attempt to collect additional k-space samples to improve spatial resolution may cause only noise components at the tails of the relaxation envelope to be sampled.

Among the several additional effects that contribute to degradation of echo planar images, off-resonance effects and chemical shifts are especially problematic. Off-resonance effects can be due to phase accumulations that can occur when

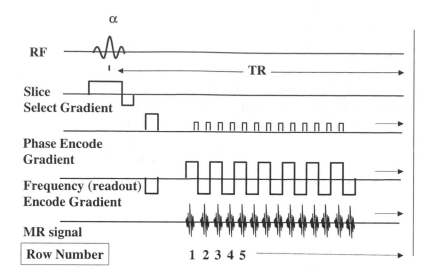

Figure 6.24: The echo planar pulse sequence is characterized by an oscillating readout gradient with an interleaved "blipped" phase encoding gradient The effective TE is normally taken as the center of the echo train. In single shot EPI, all of the echoes necessary to create an image occur after the RF pulse, so TR is effectively infinite. Multi-shot EPI uses several shorter echo trains after application of the RF pulses to collect the required data, so a TR value can be defined.

there are magnetic field inhomogeneities, differences in susceptibility between tissue and air or other materials, motion during the acquisition, and chemical shifts (Thomas, 1993). These phase additions cause a misplacement of information in the reconstructed image, since the result of the phase addition is indistinguishable from the effects of the purposely applied gradient field. Because EPI has an extended time in which no refocusing of the transverse magnetization occurs during the extended readout, it is especially likely to show many or all of these effects as distortions of the reconstructed image. Chemical shift effects may require that fat or water suppression be used during the EPI sequences to avoid the pronounced image degradation effects.

In an echo planar pulse sequence, the preparation pulses permit different types of contrast to be produced and can help reduce image distortions due to sources of magnetic susceptibility and other off-resonance effects. These preparation pulses can be spin-echo, inversion recovery, or FLASH-like in their design. The addition of a refocusing 180° pulse, timed so that it refocuses transverse magnetization at the center of the acquisition, where the oscillating phase encoding gradients are at their minimal amplitude, helps to reduce T2* contrast as well as susceptibility artifacts. The TE used is that at the center of the echo train. Multi-shot EPI images can have improved SNR and fewer artifacts. In addition, multiple shots make use of multiple RF pulses, so the TR of the sequence is shorter than the effective TR of a single shot acquisition. The $TE_{effective}$ of a single shot echoplanar pulse sequence is the time interval from the RF pulse to the center of the k-space acquisition, i.e., the center of the pulse train encoding phase information.

6.3.5.6 Multidimensional imaging and contrast

Thus far, the assumption in the foregoing descriptions has been that the images collected are two-dimensional. The frequency encoding of position produces a line of k-space and the repetition with increasing phase steps allows the additional lines in k-space to be encoded, thus making it possible to collect the entire k-space matrix needed for a two-dimensional Fourier transform for image reconstruction. This two-dimensional image can be at any angle with respect to the orientation of the static magnetic field, one of the strengths of MRI. Additionally, it is possible to collect multiple slice images that are parallel to each other, but at different positions along the selected axis perpendicular to the two-dimensional image plane. This type of multislice acquisition of two-dimensional images produces an image set that covers three dimensions of the body as a series of two-dimensional slices. This is called an anisotropic acquisition because, unlike the two dimensions in the image plane, the third dimension, the slice thickness, is implied. Typically, the slice-selection dimension, i.e., the thickness of the slice, is greater than the in-plane resolution, and slices can be separated by a considerable distance.

It is entirely possible, especially with more recently developed rapid gradient echo pulse sequences, to acquire what is known as isotropic three-dimensional volumetric data sets. These are characterized by having voxel dimensions of equal size. Three-dimensional imaging using Fourier transform reconstruction requires an additional phase encoding gradient to encode position in the third dimension. The pulse sequence performs frequency encoding of position after applying the phase encoding gradient in the in-plane direction. These gradients are preceded by a phase encoding gradient to encode position perpendicular to the plane defined by the frequency encoding gradient. The reconstruction of the three-dimensional k-space data is achieved by applying the Fourier transform sequentially. This method produces true three-dimensional volumetric images of equal resolution in all three dimensions. Unfortunately, the times required with conventional spin echo imaging sequences make three-dimensional imaging impractical. Improved gradient systems and fast receivers have made faster methods commonly available and have reduced acquisition times to a few minutes. Improvements in speed can also be achieved by acquiring true three-dimensional data, but with larger sized through-plane resolution, an anisotropic collection strategy, which serves to reduce the imaging time even more at the expense of resolution in one dimension.

6.3.6 Image characteristics and artifacts

6.3.6.1 Signal-to-noise ratios (SNR)

In the presence of excessive image noise, diagnostically important information in the image may be obscured. There are some sources of noise in MRI which can be controlled directly by means of system settings. In addition, there are sources of noise attributable to the instrument itself and to the patient. Optimization of the SNR often involves compromises, so that some consideration of the final SNR in an image must be kept in mind during the imaging process. The SNR can be estimated from the following relationship

$$\text{SNR} \propto I \times \text{Vox}(x, y, z) \times \sqrt{(\text{NEX})} \times 1/(\sqrt{(\text{BW})}) \times \\ \times f(\text{QF}) \times f(\text{B}_0) \times f(\text{gap}) \times f(\text{recon}), \tag{6.10}$$

where I is the signal intensity based on the pulse sequence, $\text{Vox}(x, y, z)$ is voxel volume, NEX is number of excitations, BW is the receiver bandwidth, $f(\text{QF})$ is a function of the quality factor of the RF coil, $f(\text{B}_0)$ is a function of the static magnetic field strength, $f(\text{gap})$ is a function of the spacing between slices, and $f(\text{recon})$ is a function of the algorithm used for reconstruction.

The most important parameter affecting the overall SNR is the strength of the magnetic field, B_0. A larger B_0 value causes more spins to participate, with a resulting increase in the size of the net magnetic vector, which leads to a larger longitudinal magnetization to be shifted into the x, y-plane during data collection. The increase in SNR scales approximately linearly with increases in the field, so a 0.5 T system will, all things being equal, produce an image having a SNR of about 1/3 of that of a system using a 1.5 T superconducting magnet. While this would lead one to believe that systems with the strongest superconducting magnets produce the best images, the increased magnetic field strength produces secondary effects, so that the expected increase in SNR is at least partially offset by increased T1 times, power deposition effects, and an increased tendency toward artifact production.

The image SNR is also affected by the number of protons contributing to each voxel value. This depends on the particular tissue being imaged, the field of view and the corresponding spatial resolution, and the slice thickness. Since the detected signal comes from a volume of tissue, the more protons the volume contains, the higher is the signal contribution. Increasing the slice thickness increases the volume of each voxel, as does specifying a coarser matrix (larger in-plane dimensions) for the acquisition. Increasing the field of view, all other things being equal, also increases the voxel size and thus increases the overall SNR, but at the price of decreased spatial resolution.

Because of the many trade-offs involved in the course of producing an acceptable image, the very best SNR may not be achievable with a single acquisition. As described in Section 6.3.5.2 on spin-echo imaging, usually two or more identical images are acquired during the pulse sequence and they are added together. Uncorrellated noise, such as thermal noise in the coils and from the patient's body, from which most of the image noise derives, will be averaged and therefore reduced in comparison with the signal. The SNR improves by a factor of $\sqrt{\text{NEX}}$ where NEX is the number of image acquisitions. Two acquisitions improve the SNR by a factor of 1.41. However, the increased time needed to acquire multiple identical images increases the possibility of patient motion, which can reduce the usability of the images.

Another aspect of the data acquisition process that can affect image noise is the sampling bandwidth or sampling rate of the analog-to-digital converter, the component of the receiver subsystem that converts the time-varying analog echo signal from the receiver coil into the digital form the computer system uses for image reconstruction. The bandwidth of the receiver is inversely proportional to the square root of the SNR, so narrowing the bandwidth available for digitizing the signal reduces the noise components digitized along with the echo signal. This is especially important in those parts of the echo where the signal is reduced due to dephasing. The use of a narrow digitizing bandwidth requires more time, so that TE increases slightly. An increased TE can present a problem for certain types of pulse sequences, especially T1-weighted high-speed sequences. Also, if a narrow bandwidth is used in a T2-weighted acquisition, where the T2 relaxation time of the tissues is less than the time required for sampling the data, additional noise may be introduced, thus decreasing the SNR. The sampling bandwidth must also take account of the field of view (FOV) and the pixel size; changing the bandwidth must reflect a change in the readout gradient strength and duration. Thus, reducing the bandwidth by half requires the readout gradient strength to be reduced by half, while the on-time of the gradient must be increased by a factor of 2. There can be increases in chemical shift artifacts as well.

A further parameter affecting the SNR is the signal from the receiving coil. Coil design, discussed in more detail in Section 6.5.5, has a significant effect on the signal received from the subject. Because the body has capacitance and inductance, it becomes a source of noise during the absorption and emission of RF energy. The body, when placed in or next to a coil, causes an effect called "loading," in which the coil couples to the body electrically. Since the body is never in exactly the same position with respect to the coil, the amount of loading differs from one imaging event to the next. Additionally, since different bodies load the coil differently, it is necessary for the system to retune the coil to the resonance frequency for each imaging task in order to maximize the SNR of the detected signal. Adjusting the coil-receiver coupling for maximum signal transfer is called "matching" or "tuning" the coil. The closer the coil is to the signal-producing tissues of interest, the better the SNR will be, so a surface coil can provide a better SNR than a body coil. However, the response of the surface coil falls off with distance from its face, so the optimum signal is obtained when the structure of interest is near the surface of the body adjacent to the coil. Quadrature coils, including surface coils, produce a higher SNR than coils of conventional linear design.

6.3.6.2 Resolution

Resolution defines the minimum distance between two separate distinguishable objects in an image. In the context of MRI, this distance is determined in part by the voxel size. Voxels have two dimensions in the plane of the slice and a third dimension, the slice thickness. The image consists of a two-dimensional array of pixels whose gray scale image density or pixel value is characteristic of the imaged tissues. Each voxel in the patient maps to a corresponding two-dimensional pixel in the image. To increase the resolution of an image, a larger number of voxels per slice needs to be acquired and a larger number of pixels needs to be displayed. These pixels then represent correspondingly smaller voxels in the tissues. The actual size of the voxels can be determined by the number of pixels in each dimension of the two-dimensional image divided into each corresponding dimension of the field of view. This gives the in-plane size of the voxel, while the slice thickness describes the other dimension.

Resolution in clinical systems is often a trade-off between various parameters of the imaging process affecting the SNR. As described in the previous discussion, the SNR depends on many factors, including the voxel volume. An increase in resolution requires additional signal to maintain the overall SNR of a corresponding lower resolution image acquisition. Thus, reducing the voxel size by a factor of 4, as when one goes from $256 \times 256 \times 5$ mm slice to a $512 \times 512 \times 5$ mm slice will degrade the SNR by a factor of 2. To compensate for this, one would have to acquire 4 identical images (NEX = 4). Another way to improve resolution is to reduce the thickness of the slice, but this reduces the volume and therefore the resulting SNR.

Because the intensity of the signal assigned to a voxel is a function of the average of all of the tissue types in the voxel, some small amounts of tissue may not be observable in a thick slice, while they would be detectable in a thinner slice. This phenomenon is called partial volume averaging. Due to partial volume averaging, the signal produced by a voxel is composed of contributions from all spins in the voxel. If the voxel is located in a part of the body where several tissue types converge, it is possible for more than one tissue to contribute to the average.

The ability to resolve two objects of interest in an image depends on the field of view (FOV), the strength of the gradients, the characteristics of the particular coil being used, the size of the image matrix in pixels, and the sampling bandwidth. In conventional clinical imaging, overall spatial resolution is similar to that obtained with a CT scanner, 0.5 mm to 1 mm when imaging objects such as the head and brain. However, what can actually be resolved depends strongly on a variety of factors. It would be theoretically possible to collect data from a 1 cm field of view with 512 sample points, yielding a resolution higher than 0.02 mm. Most likely, noise, lack of gradient capacity, or time limitations would prevent the images from being useful. In general, the theoretical limit of resolution of MRI imaging is in the range of 15 to 20 μm, limited by the molecular diffusion of protons within the tissues. This is far beyond what a clinical imaging system can produce. It is, however, nearly reached in magnetic resonance microscopy, where 50 μm resolution or better is possible (Callaghan, 1991).

6.3.6.3 Contrast

Contrast refers to the ability of the image to display differences of image intensity for tissues having different properties. A high contrast image shows a large intensity difference between two tissues whose properties differ only slightly. In a low-contrast image, two different tissues lying side by side are relatively difficult to distinguish because the intensities of the pixels are nearly equal. In general, high contrast images are limited by the resolution, while low-contrast images are limited by image noise.

Contrast in MR images is a complex function of many different factors. These include the relaxation time constants, T1 and T2 and the proton density of the tissues as discussed in Section 6.3.5 on pulse sequences, as well as flow effects, effects due to contrast agents that alter local magnetic fields (magnetic susceptibility agents which affect T2 decay), diffusion effects, and others. Regardless of the mechanism, a significant reason for using MRI is that it is capable of providing outstanding soft tissue contrast and imaging of flow effects. The parameters related to image acquisition that allow the contrast to be optimized are described throughout this section. They include the TR, TE, flip angle, slice thickness, presence of flow compensation, presence of saturation pulses, the use of additional pulses such as for diffusion weighting of the images, and the use of contrast agents.

6.4 Common artifacts

Artifacts are those parts of an image that do not reproduce the actual tissue being imaged. They can vary from being relatively localized to a small part of an image to those that render the entire image useless. Artifacts can be caused by the patient or by extraneous effects. Machine problems and radio frequency leaks can cause extraneous artifacts. Among the artifacts attributable to the patient are those resulting from either voluntary or involuntary motions, and those due to tissue interfaces that produce sudden, drastic changes in the signal intensity. It is worthwhile to understand the nature of artifacts so that a determination can be made as to whether a particular artifact has altered the image so that it is no longer diagnostically useful. Sometimes artifacts are sufficiently subtle to make such determinations difficult.

6.4.1 Magnetic field variations

The instrument itself can be responsible for several types of artifacts. Magnetic field nonuniformities can cause tissue contrast to be shifted to the wrong place in the image. Since position is determined by the local magnetic fields applied to the protons, the reconstruction software assumes that the gradients are linear and that the static magnetic field is uniform over the working volume. If the static field is not homogeneous enough, then there are likely to be observable distortions in the image. These problems were more often encountered with earlier systems that were poorly shimmed at installation or in the tuning process for each imaging acquisition. Modern systems, especially those using self-shielded superconducting magnets, are mostly immune from variations in the static field unless there is a system problem.

6.4.2 Gradient effects

Gradients are assumed to be linear and non-time varying when they are switched on. They are also assumed to have the specified amplitudes. Failure of these constraints on the operation of the gradients leads to a variety of problems. One type of distortion that can occur is observed when a gradient driver is unable to deliver the requested amplitude at the extreme positions. Since gradients normally operate in a positive–negative manner with a zero point in the center, a fall-off in amplitudes with increased field strength results in changes of voxel size at the edges of the field of view. A variant of this problem can occur when the frequency encoding gradient and phase encoding gradients do not produce the same signal levels at the maximum for a given pulse sequence. The resulting difference causes the in-plane pixels to become rectangular rather than square, leading to a distortion in the image.

6.4.3 Local field variations

Localized variations in the magnetic field can have profound effects on the re-constructed images. An example is the presence of a ferromagnetic material in the

Susceptibility Artifact - signal "blow out"

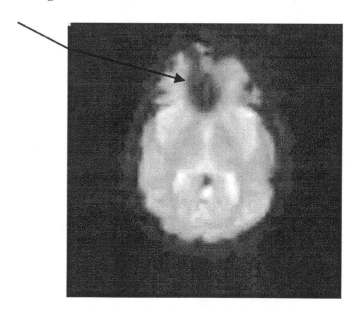

Gradient echo - echo planar acquisition

Figure 6.25: A single shot EPI image of the head. The image acquisition matrix is 64×64, so the overall appearance of the image is somewhat blurred. Additionally, there is a very large "hole" in the anterior cingulate area of the brain. This is a magnetic susceptibility artifact that occurs when the image plane is close to the air sinus and air passages of the nasal areas. The difference in effective field at the air-tissue interface causes a displacement of signal to the edges of the affected area. This artifact is quite common in EPI imaging, which is very sensitive to local susceptibility effects.

image field that causes a massive but localized susceptibility effect and subsequent loss of image information near the ferromagnetic object. Among the items that can cause this problem are steel hair pins, noncompatible prosthetic devices, some dental appliances, even certain types of eye-shadow containing magnetic materials. All of these materials cause the magnetic field lines to be distorted, producing localized changes in the field with resulting changes in the Larmor frequency, leading to mispositioning of image information. Usually, the result is a signal void with a bright rim and other positional distortions in the region. Similar effects can be produced in nonferromagnetic materials if they are conductors, due to gradient-switching-induced current flow during gradient echo imaging. In addition, some interfaces between regions having very different characteristics, such as air-tissue interfaces in the head, can cause a dramatic loss of signal in gradient echo images due to magnetic susceptibility differences. An example of such a distortion is shown in Figure 6.25.

6.4.4 Imaging coil nonuniform response

Other commonly observed artifacts related to magnetic fields are caused by nonuniform responses of imaging coils. Ordinarily, volume coils such as the head or body coil are expected to produce a uniform field across the coil and along the length of the coil. Many older coils produce a fall-off in intensity that can be seen in the images as a fall off in intensity as one moves away from the conductors. This is usually not a problem with newer designs. However, surface coils, especially linear coils, have a very characteristic nonuniform intensity response as shown in Figure 6.26. A simple circular coil can exhibit a decrease in signal response as one moves perpendicularly away from the center of the coil. Likewise, a uniform response is observed in a plane parallel to the plane of the coil, but only within the boundaries of the coil. More complex surface coils such as those used for spine imaging show signal loss as one moves away from the surface coil towards the center of the body.

The RF system can also produce artifacts. External signal sources that fall into the range of the receiver, either as primary frequencies or harmonics, can cause "discretes" or narrow bands or distortions that appear perpendicular to the direction of the frequency encoding gradients. This artifact depends on the particular imaging sequence and the operating conditions of the receiver and the coils at the time the effect occurs. The RF shielded room is supposed to eliminate external interference causing artifacts of this kind, but room integrity can fail or subtle sources of conduction can cause RF to leak into the room. Sometimes, a broad-band RF signal is detected by the imager, which leads to a uniform distribution of a "herringbone" artifact.

Other artifacts due to RF effects are related to the slice selection process. Slice selection depends on producing slice profiles that are rectangular in the reconstructed images. Rectangular slice profiles in cartesian space come from sinc $(\sin \omega / \omega)$ pulses in k-space. A slice profile refers to the appearance of the thickness of the slice with respect to a plot of thickness vs. intensity. Such a plot would

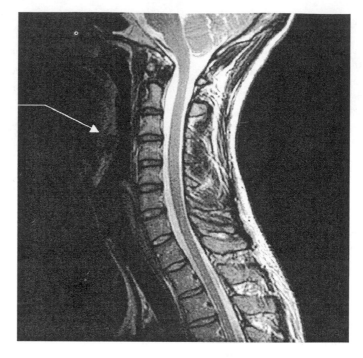

Signal Fall Off

T2 - weighted Image of Cervical Spine

Figure 6.26: T2-weighted image of the cervical spine acquired with a surface coil shows the characteristic image intensity changes seen with surface coils. The part of the body closest to the coil, in this case the back of the cervical spine area on the right of the figure, is well-represented with strong signal and good contrast. The anterior part of the neck and other anatomical areas on the left of the figure show signal loss or "fall-off" due to the nonlinear response of the surface coil: the further it is away from the active elements of the coil, the lower is the signal detected. This nonuniform response should be contrasted with the nearly perfectly uniform response of a volume coil, such as a head coil.

ideally look like a rectangular pulse. Assuming perfectly rectangular slice profiles, multislice imaging would be performed so that slices are adjacent to each other. Unfortunately, it is virtually impossible to achieve a perfect slice profile. In reality the profile takes on a somewhat curved form with "tails" that spread beyond the nominal profile width at low amplitudes. This form of slice-to-slice "cross-talk" occurs because an individual slice receives small contributions from parts of the body beyond the requested slice thickness. Contrast or SNR can suffer depending on the type of pulse sequence used. To reduce this effect, interleaved acquisitions are performed, in which every other slice is collected first, then a one-slice shift is made and the other slices are collected, based on the idea that the out-of-slice contributions will be minimized if adjacent slices are not collected sequentially.

6.4.5 Patient-related artifacts

Motion is the most likely cause of image artifacts that can be attributed to the patient. People move both voluntarily and involuntarily during the course of scans. Squirming, blinking, attempting to speak during an acquisition can cause imaging problems. Coughing, sneezing and any number of other respiratory motions, most of which are not entirely controllable by the subject, can create large motion artifacts. Additionally, the heart pumps blood, so blood flow can cause specific types of motion artifacts in the images. Secondarily, CSF flow can affect images. There are obviously many sources of artifacts, many of which can be very complex and depend on the type of pulse sequence being used.

Especially problematic are pulse sequences requiring long acquisition times. Long acquisition times increase the likelihood that the patient will move during the data collection period. Also, long acquisition times imply that multiple respiratory periods, many heart beats, and even peristalsis can create situations where part of the information about an organ or a surface is in one position during part of the study, possibly for several phase-encoding steps, then in another position for several additional phase encoding steps, then in yet other positions and so on. These types of motions, typical of respiratory motion during imaging of the liver, can be sufficiently severe to destroy the useful information in the image. Such "ghosting" effects due to motion create partial image information that is mispositioned, yielding light-dark artifacts that are characteristic of motion in the phase-encoding direction. Motion in the frequency encoding direction tends to create more subtle degradations in the form of blurring, because the readout of the echo is typically much faster, reducing the time when motion could cause severe misplacement of information.

Many ways have been devised to address motion problems. If the patient moves voluntarily, it is always possible to reacquire the images. Reversing the phase and frequency encoding directions can substantially improve images blurred by involuntary motion such as the pulsatile motion of cranial vessels. The use of cardiac gating to control the acquisitions reduces cardiac-related motion by forcing the acquisition to proceed in synchrony with the cardiac cycle. This approach also helps to reduce artifacts due to chest motion and can reduce flow artifacts due to high-velocity blood flow. Respiratory triggers have been used, but with less success, principally because their use tends to greatly increase the length of time required for the acquisition. A more elaborate approach to respiratory triggering, called ROPE (respiratory ordered phase encoding), has been used as well. However, many newer systems with high-performance gradients can produce pulse sequences that acquire the necessary information during a single breath-hold, so respiratory triggering becomes unnecessary.

Flow effects are often a source of artifacts in images of the head, but they can also occur in images where substantial vascular flow is present, such as in the aorta during some types of abdominal imaging. Flow creates artifacts by causing two principal problems. The first is the presence of what are known as "flow voids" or sections where there is loss of signal, often a total loss. These signal losses are caused by turbulent blood flow causing the spins in the blood to dephase or by rapid flow in which excited protons move out of the slice before the readout can be completed. The second artifact is a "phantom" or ghost in the phase encoding direction, the spacing of which is related to the flow rate. Various techniques are available to compensate for flow and will be described in the next sections. MR angiography, which images flow effects, is an important part of the repertoire of clinical imaging techniques.

6.4.6 Other artifacts

There are several other types of artifacts that are important, since they occur frequently in MR images: the Gibbs phenomenon, aliasing, chemical shift and partial volume effects. All of these produce a readily recognized artifact, which can be reduced or eliminated by changes in the pulse sequence.

The Gibbs phenomenon or ringing artifact is seen at bright edges, next to low signal areas such as the edge of the brain-fatty scalp boundary in a transverse image of the head (Figure 6.27). This artifact is characterized by alternating light-dark banding in the frequency encoding direction and is caused by data truncation and by undersampling in the phase encoding direction. Ringing in an area of clinical importance can cause significant problems with interpretation of the image. An easy way to reduce this effect is to use a larger collection matrix, which will reduce the artifact at the cost of additional time.

Another artifact is known as wrap-around or aliasing. This artifact is characterized by a misplacement of anatomical features. In a typical example of this kind of artifact the image of a patient's nose is wrapped around so that it is displayed overlapping the back of the head. This may occur when a portion of the head and the nose extend beyond the selected FOV. The sampling bandwidth defines the range of frequencies that can be sampled in the frequency encoding direction. According to the Nyquist theorem, the sampling frequency must exceed the highest frequency that can be represented without ambiguity by at least a factor of two. Any signal containing frequencies above the upper limit set by the Nyquist frequency will be "wrapped around" to reappear as a corresponding signal at a frequency below the Nyquist limit. The reconstruction process cannot tell that an aliased frequency that originated from beyond the Nyquist frequency does not belong at the lower frequency to which it has been wrapped around. Thus, the image of the nose in this example ends up being improperly placed at the back of the head because the frequencies originating from the nose take on the appearance of the lower frequencies associated with the back of the head. This problem can be avoided by using a larger FOV, using a finer sampling interval (collect 512 samples, but use the central 256), or in modern machines, by using a digital filter to band-limit the data.

Aliasing can occur in the phase encoding direction as well, producing an artifact in images that is often called a "zebra stripe." This artifact is caused by field heterogeneities outside the FOV, creating a phase interference that produces visible striping. If one increases the FOV so that there are no phase ambiguities, i.e., no phases that wrap back beyond 360°, then the artifact is removed. Only that part of the FOV that is of interest is displayed. Another way to avoid this problem is to oversample in the phase direction, which can be accomplished without an increase in imaging time in situations where $NEX \geqslant 2$ would otherwise be used. By sampling at twice the desired interval in the phase direction, phase wrap around is avoided and the SNR remains the same as if $NEX = 2$. Yet another way to avoid phase encoding direction aliasing is to use saturation pulses just outside of the FOV, effectively removing any potential signal aliasing from those structures whose signal is eliminated.

Chemical shift affects the Larmor frequency of nuclei. Ideally, all nuclei of a given type would precess at exactly the same frequency. When a spatially variant magnetic field of known characteristics is applied, then the precession frequencies can be derived from the local magnetic field strength. However, the magnetic field of a nucleus is shielded by the electrons forming chemical bonds in the immediate vicinity of the nucleus. This shielding causes a shift of the Larmor frequency called the chemical shift. The result is that the there can be a small but noticeable effect due to screening. The screening constant, σ, is much less than 1 and causes a small

Gibbs Artifact

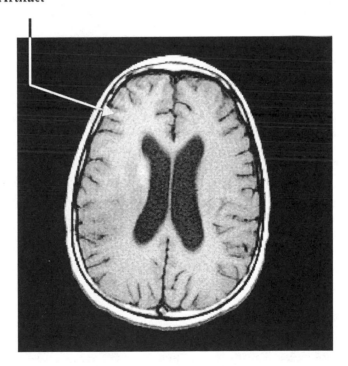

Figure 6.27: T1-weighted image of the head demonstrates a Gibbs or truncation artifact. The artifact is characterized by light and dark bands near the edges of high contrast structures, here the fat-skull-brain interface, oriented in the frequency encoding direction. The artifact can be reduced or eliminated by acquiring a larger data matrix.

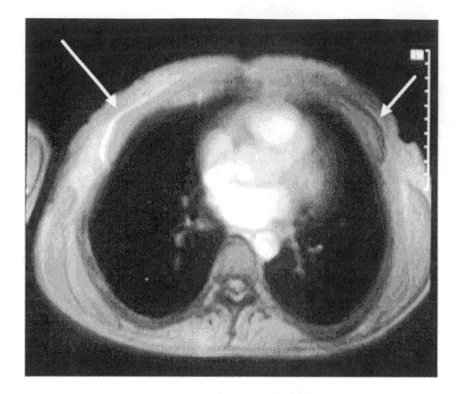

Chemical Shift Artifact in Chest Wall

Figure 6.28: Chemical shift artifacts can be relatively subtle or very obvious, depending on the pulse sequence and the types of tissues being imaged. In this example, the characteristic light artifact is seen on one side of the chest wall, while the corresponding dark area is seen on the other.

change in the Larmor frequency. This small change is the cause of certain types of artifacts in imaging (Riddle, Lee, 1999).

Chemical shift artifacts are an important class of artifacts observed in many imaging situations. These artifacts are typically more obvious at 1.5 T than at lower field strengths, since the difference between fat and water increases linearly with field strength. Chemical shift artifacts occur because the chemical environment of protons bound to carbon in fat causes these protons to resonate at a frequency which is lower by about 220 Hz (3.5 PPM) than the resonant frequency of protons in water molecules. This difference in resonance causes a misplacement of fat with respect to water in the frequency encoding direction that is readily detectable in the images at the transition from water to fatty tissues, as shown in Figure 6.28. It has the appearance of an artificial decrease in signal on the side of the image where two tissues meet and an increase in signal where the two tissues overlap.

The displacement depends on the FOV and is a function of the frequency difference (Δf), the number of pixels, and the receiver bandwidth.

$$\text{shift(pixels)} = \Delta f \times \text{number of pixels/bandwidth.} \qquad (6.11)$$

The chemical shift artifact is less of a problem with a higher bandwidth. In practice, this means that using a stronger gradient in the frequency encoding direction will produce a greater bandwidth per pixel, with the result that the chemical shift is contained within a single pixel and is not seen in the image. However, this approach can cause a loss of SNR, since SNR is proportional to the square root of the bandwidth. An exchange of the phase encoding and frequency encoding directions can move these artifacts so that they are less of a problem in some cases.

Partial volume effects, discussed in Section 6.3.6.2, are another source of artifacts. These effects are not unique to MR imaging and can also be seen in computed tomographic and other images. If an interface between two kinds of tissue occurs within a voxel, the resulting image pixel simply displays a gray level proportional to the weighted average of the signals deriving from these tissues. Thus, phase boundaries may be shifted by as much as the width of a single image pixel.

6.5 Hardware and software components

The typical magnetic resonance imaging system consists of a number of subsystems that together are able to perform MR imaging. These subsystems are highly refined and relatively complex in modern imagers. They include a magnet, a radio frequency transmitting system, a radio frequency receiving system, a gradient control system, and a computer system to control all of these components. A significant part of the configuration is the software that supervises and controls the operations of all of the various subsystems.

6.5.1 Magnetic fields

Of necessity, a magnet of some type is needed. The function of the magnet is to produce a uniform magnetic field, B_0, within which data acquisition for imaging occurs. The more uniform the field in the working volume, the more likely the imager is to produce images of superior quality, since the spatial resolution and SNR are determined in part by the uniformity of the magnetic field. The larger and more homogeneous the field in the working volume, the more expensive the magnet and the larger the physical dimensions it is likely to have. In addition to magnetic field homogeneity, the magnet must be stable over time. Since field strength is a contributor to image SNR, the strength of the permanent magnetic field is important as well. Other important considerations include patient access, which depends on the diameter of the opening in the magnet, and the extent of the magnetic field beyond the magnet's structure.

The homogeneity of a magnet is most often expressed as the diameter of the spherical volume (DSV in cm) that can be used for imaging. In order to be able to image as much of the body as possible, one wishes to achieve the highest uniformity of the magnetic field in the largest possible volume. For very high-performance imaging systems capable of spectroscopy, one might expect to have specifications of a 50 cm DSV at 1 part per million (PPM) or better. Non-imaging systems are typically 2–3 orders of magnitude better than this over much smaller volumes.

For high quality images to be obtained, the magnet must be able to produce a temporally very stable magnetic field. High quality images cannot be obtained from a system whose static field drifts during imaging. Superconducting systems are the most stable of the magnet designs and once they have attained stability, they can maintain a field change of less than 0.1 PPM/hr. Other designs require careful design and configuration to avoid problems of temporal stability.

The field strength available for imaging ranges from 0.02 T to more than 4 T. Installed systems used in clinical imaging have field strengths up to 3.0 T, while research imaging systems with field strengths as high as 11 T are being planned. There is an adequate natural abundance of protons for imaging at very low fields, but as the field strength is increased, the number of protons that transition from low to high-energy states increases. This translates to higher SNRs in the images, other things being equal. However, there are effects of increased T1 relaxation at increasing field strength that can reduce image contrast, effects of reduced RF penetration at higher operating frequencies required by high field strengths, increased chemical shift artifacts, and increased costs for constructing the magnet and siting it.

Other considerations of magnet design include access of and to the patient. To be of practical use the system must accommodate a range of patient sizes. Superconducting magnet designs currently available use a solenoid configuration which can have a patient access bore of up to about 60 cm and a length of 1.6–1.8 m for compact magnets and 2.6–2.8 m for conventional systems. Some systems are designed for head-only use and have smaller bores. In all of these designs, the comfort of the patient and the necessary access to the patient for contrast agent injection and other interactions is important. With specialized designs, such as those intended for use during surgical procedures, many trade-offs are made in order to provide the needed access. One configuration has the appearance of two donuts with a space between them for a surgeon to operate on the patient while imaging is performed. Other specialized systems using either superconducting or permanent fields are oriented so that the pole pieces are above and below the patient. These low field systems have very good access characteristics, useful for claustrophobic patients and very young children.

A final consideration is the extent to which the magnetic field extends beyond the useful structure of the system. This field is known as the fringe field of the magnet. Since the magnetic field cannot be entirely contained within the magnet's structure, it is often necessary to use designs that tend to confine the lines of force. Many types of electrical equipment including monitors and image intensifiers are very sensitive to magnetic fields and do not work properly in fields extending from an imaging magnet. Pacemakers can be affected by small fields as well. Permanent magnet systems have iron or steel return paths with vertical pole pieces that tend to do a good job of confining the magnetic field, reducing the fringe field to almost nothing. In addition, these are relatively low field strength magnets, which helps to reduce the fringe fields. Solenoid magnets, superconducting systems of 1 T and up, can exhibit fringe fields that extend outward by many meters if no action is taken to reduce the field. Two approaches are used. The first is to surround the magnet structure with high permissivity iron shields, which tend to draw in the lines of force. Some of these shields weigh in excess of 40 tons, limiting placement of the magnet. The other, more modern approach is to use an additional set of coils wound around the main magnet structure that opposes the field outside of the bore of the magnet while having minimal effect on the field within the bore. These coils are known as bucking coils. They reduce the fringe field distances considerably without the use of massive amounts of steel. The object of all the shielding is to reduce the distance of the 5 gauss field line away from the magnet to the smallest value possible.

6.5.2 Magnet systems

Three basic designs, shown in Figure 6.29, have been used for imaging systems. These are resistive magnets, permanent magnets, hybrid systems that combine elements of both, and superconducting systems. Resistive magnets are designed to use electrical power to supply the energy for creating the static field, B_0. Usually the design of these magnets involves multiple coils of wire or conductive strips arranged to produce a uniform field in the center of the magnet structure. The coils can be wound in air ("air core magnets") or around ferromagnetic formers, where the iron provides a return path for the magnetic flux. Since these magnets depend

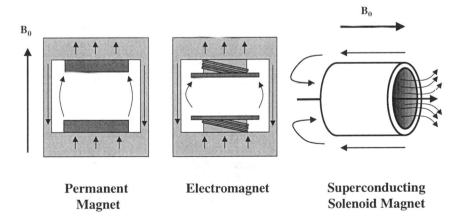

Permanent   **Electromagnet**   **Superconducting**
Magnet   **Solenoid Magnet**

Figure 6.29: Permanent magnet systems and many electromagnet systems use iron or steel return paths and a vertical orientation for the B_0 field. Many of these systems are actually hybrids incorporating permanent magnet elements and electric coils to improve the field homogeneity. Superconducting magnets are usually solenoid designs with a horizontal B_0 field whose return path extends away from the magnet, although newer systems use active shielding to help confine the field.

on current passing through a wire, there are resistive effects, which lead to heating when the field is activated. In order to remove heat, resistive magnets are usually water-cooled. Thus, there is an ongoing expense for electricity, often in the 50 kW range, and for cooling water. Resistive magnets are no longer made for whole body applications, but can be practical for imagers designed for specific parts of the body such as joints. They tend to have relatively low field strengths due to engineering considerations concerning heating and power consumption. Additionally, field uniformity is usually several orders of magnitude lower than in the best superconducting systems, which limits these designs to specific imaging applications.

Permanent magnet systems have a number of potential advantages when compared to resistive systems. The designs lend themselves to vertical orientation of the field, with iron or steel return paths for the magnetic lines of force. This can be a substantial advantage for machines that reduce the feeling of claustrophobia. Additionally, the vertical orientation of the field and the return paths limit the fringing fields so that the 5 gauss line is very close to the magnet structure. Furthermore, there are advantages in the design of the RF coils used with these systems. There are no cryogens required for the system. Disadvantages include limits on field strength and relatively low field uniformity. It should be noted that while clinically usable images can be produced on low field systems, high-performance imaging techniques and MR spectroscopy may not be available due to the limitations of the system design. Another disadvantage for some machines has been the weight of the machine, but more modern designs have lessened this concern.

Some systems that have been developed use permanent magnets to produce most of the static field along with electromagnetic coils to make the field more uniform. The concept of this design is that poor uniformity of the field can be compensated for by the use of resistive coils to "shim" the field, making it more uniform. This approach is similar to the design of superconducting systems and has made it possible to develop low field hybrid systems that produce excellent images.

Superconducting magnets make use of the properties of some compounds such as niobium-titanium alloys which, when maintained at liquid helium temperatures, allow electric current to flow with no resistance. Wire made of these materials is used to wind solenoidal magnets used for imaging systems. With superconductivity, once current flows in the magnet windings, it continues to flow without an external power source. While the magnetic field from such a system eventually decays to zero, the rate of this decay, measured in parts per million of the original field strength, is on the order of less than 0.05 PPM/hour. Superconducting magnets are used in high-performance systems, where excellent field uniformity, great temporal stability, and high field strengths are required. Echo-planar image acquisitions and spectroscopy require superconducting magnets.

Superconducting magnets are designed differently from others in part because of the requirements to keep the superconducting wires at liquid helium temperatures. The magnet structure is designed as a cryostat to contain the wire bathed in liquid helium (LHe). There usually are many layers of heat-reflecting plastic film and one or more vacuum chambers to insulate the LHe. Some earlier designs use chambers of liquid nitrogen to help in reducing heat flow to the LHe. All of these steps are necessary to reduce the rate at which helium, which is relatively expensive in the quantities needed to fill an imaging magnet, boils off. Modern designs are able to maintain adequate levels of LHe for several months or more. Many of the newest magnets incorporate refrigeration systems as part of the magnet to condense gaseous helium back to liquid, further reducing boil-off.

With superconducting magnet systems there is the possibility of a "quench." Quenching refers to the situation when part of the superconducting magnet structure, which includes superconducting switches and junctions, becomes non-superconducting. At that point, the high current in the wire (200–400 A) causes the wire to heat up, leading to subsequent vaporization of the LHe. Once this starts, the energy in the magnet is dumped into heat and the LHe boils off rapidly. Modern magnets are very stable and are designed to prevent any hazard to personnel in the area. However, a quench can be dramatic, causing a loud noise as the escaping gaseous helium is routed to an outside vent. Ordinarily, no damage is done to the magnet, but it must be checked prior to any attempt to return it to operation. Safety systems installed with superconducting magnets ("emergency magnet shutdown" systems) initiate a controlled quench to bring the field down rapidly, but not destructively.

6.5.3 Shimming

All magnets require shimming in order to produce the most uniform field possible in a spherical volume that is sufficiently large to permit imaging or spectroscopy. Shimming requires combinations of small pieces of metal to be placed around the magnet structure during installation (passive shims) and coils of wire through which current is passed during operation (active shims) to produce small gradients in the B_0 field which improve the uniformity of the field in the selected volumes. Typical superconducting magnets have both room temperature shim coils and superconducting shim coils oriented in the x, y, and z-directions allowing combinations of coils to be activated with different amounts of current to produce the required uniformity. Properly shimmed superconducting magnets can achieve better than ± 0.15 PPM uniformity over a 24 cm DSV and better than ± 2 PPM over a 45 cm DSV. For spectroscopy and other specialized applications, local shimming can often be accomplished for volumes of interest that are smaller than that provided by static active or passive shims so as to optimize the uniformity of the local field.

6.5.4 Siting, shielding, and safety

Siting a magnet is a task requiring careful attention to a number of details related not only to the magnet and its associated equipment, but also to the access by people and equipment to the area where the magnet is located. Environmental considerations are important. These include the availability of power, cooling water (some gradient systems are water-cooled), access, facility vibration, and air conditioning. In addition, the site must be magnetically shielded to keep fringe fields below levels that could interfere with magnetically sensitive instruments such as pacemakers. Radio frequency shielding will also most likely be required. The signals detected by the system's radio receiver are very small. Consequently, it is usually necessary for the imager to be surrounded by a properly designed radio frequency shield, called a "screen room," which eliminates RF interference from outside sources and confines the machine's RF transmitter signal to the shielded room.

Large masses of moving metal can affect the operation of an imager, so it is necessary to survey an area to make sure that large objects such as moving vehicles or elevators are located far enough away from the system to preclude any affect on the magnetic fields. Additionally, it is necessary to ensure that untrained people do not have ready access to the magnet room. Accidents have occurred when cleaning crews rolled equipment toward a magnet, not knowing the effect of a strong magnetic field on a ferrous object.

6.5.5 Radio frequency systems

The signal necessary to induce nuclei to absorb RF energy during resonance and to subsequently produce a detectable signal that can be processed to form an image comes from the radio frequency system. The RF system consists of two major parts, the transmitter section and the receiver section. The transmitter system is a series of components consisting of a frequency synthesizer and modulator, a high-power amplifier, and a coil. These components are used to produce a radio frequency pulse having a specific carrier frequency with a modulation or envelope containing multiple frequencies above and below the carrier frequency consistent with the Larmor equation in the presence of a gradient field.

The frequency synthesizer, under control of the supervisory computer, produces the carrier frequency and can control the phase of the RF pulse. The carrier is mixed with a signal from the modulator, which produces an envelope based on digital functions stored in the system. This envelope is generated from a set of complex numbers (512 is typical of some systems) stored on disk and converted to an analog signal during the modulation process to produce an RF pulse having the desired phase and frequency bandwidth characteristics. Different stored functions have different applications during imaging. A narrow bandwidth envelope produces a frequency selective or "soft" RF pulse characterized by having a bandwidth in which the amplitudes of the frequencies are not equal. This results in a narrower band of frequencies over a longer transmitter duty cycle (on-period). These pulses are used with gradients to determine the slice thickness and slice profiles. A non-frequency selective pulse ("hard" pulse) is characterized by having a short duration with frequencies of equal amplitude with a bandwidth of ± 20 kHz. The envelope used is a square wave. Such pulses are used for determining resonant frequencies and for use in generating composite pulses for fat suppression.

The transmitter is a high power radio frequency amplifier that drives the transmit RF coil to produce the excitation of the protons. Transmitters vary in design and capabilities, but usually have peak power output capabilities of several thousand watts at higher fields, since the power requirements increase with the square of the field strength. These outputs are available with solid state or vacuum tube designs. Part of the careful design of the transmitter is to couple the signal from the transmitter output to the particular transmit coil being used. Since the transmitter has substantial power output capabilities, the system design incorporates features to avoid the possibility of causing RF burns in patients or operators. Additionally, the system contains components designed to monitor the power deposition into the patient or the object being imaged.

The U.S. Food and Drug Administration (FDA) has established guidelines on the deposition of RF energy in the body. The MR system monitors the specific absorption rate (SAR) for energy deposition to ensure that there is no significant heating due to the applied RF energy. SAR has units of watts/kilogram of body weight. The goal of SAR limits is to prevent the patient from experiencing heating over 1°C. All clinically used systems (FDA-approved for clinical use) restrict the availability of transmitter power by monitoring many different parameters to make sure that this threshold is not exceeded.

The transmitter is coupled to a specialized antenna, called an RF coil, that is designed to broadcast the radio frequency signal from the transmitter to the protons in the patient. The goal of the coil's design is to provide a uniform distribution of the RF energy in the patient and to produce a magnetic field, B_1, perpendicular to the B_0 field. There are many different ways such coils can be designed, from simple closed loops of wire to coils designed to surround the patient's body. The shape and design of the coils depends on the specific application. Common to all of the coils are the capacitive and inductive elements that cause the coil to resonate at the appropriate (Larmor) frequency, so that the transmitter energy is efficiently coupled to the coil and the patient.

Often, the same coils are used to receive the signal from the patient during the evolution of an echo. The important parameters are the RF uniformity of the coil and the signal sensitivity (SNR) associated with the coil. Since the coil does not need to both transmit and receive a signal simultaneously, a switching network can be used to couple the transmit/receive coil alternately to the transmitter output during RF transmission and to the receiver after the transmitter has been turned off.

Most imaging systems have several coils available, including a whole body coil, a head coil, and other special purpose coils. The body coil is a transmit/receive coil designed for a large uniform excitation volume. For superconducting magnets with the static field along the bore, the design of the body coil must be such that it creates a B_1 field perpendicular to the bore of the magnet. One design is known as a saddle coil, which is essentially a pair of Helmholz coils wrapped on a cylindrical former. This is a linearly polarized coil, which means that the RF excitation applied to the coil causes an oscillating B_1 field to be applied across the coil perpendicular to the static field. The usual design for this is known as a "birdcage," since the conductors form a cage-like structure (Figure 6.30). In contrast, permanent magnet systems with a vertical field can use a solenoid coil, which has some advantages in performance over the birdcage design (Schenck, 1993).

Additional uniformity of excitation is achieved by using a phase splitter to produce a 90° phase shift in the signal. When applying the standard and the phase-shifted RF signal to the coil through the phase shifter, a rotating field of constant amplitude is produced. This technique is known as quadrature excitation. It not only improves the RF uniformity of the coil during transmission at high field strengths, but it also reduces the RF power requirements compared to a conventional (linearly polarized) coil at all field strengths.

Another important consideration for RF coils is the SNR obtainable with a particular coil. In general the closer the coil is to the source of the signal, the better the SNR will be. This is why a surface coil placed near an area of interest will usually outperform a volume coil such as a body or head coil. However, the performance of the surface coil is typically limited to a distance from the coil equal to its diameter. The performance capability of a coil can be measured by the quality factor or "Q-value" which is related to the resonant performance of the coil. High values of Q indicate a highly resonant coil.

Coils are affected by proximity to the body. In fact, a body coil changes its performance characteristics considerably when a patient lies in it. The patient is said to "load" the coil, reducing its Q and therefore its performance. In order to compensate for this loading when a patient is placed in the machine, a tuning capability is provided for most coils so that the optimum Q can be reached with different patients in the coil. Tuning maximizes the energy transfer from transmitter to coil to patient and from patient to coil to receiver.

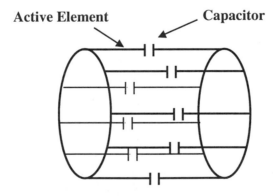

8 Element Birdcage Resonator

Figure 6.30: High-performance volume coils are often of the "birdcage" design, so named because the elements make the coil look like a cage. These coils can produce superior field uniformity within the coil structure, so they are very useful for general imaging where the body can fit in the coil. Bird cage coils can be linearly polarized or can be designed as quadrature coils. Most high-performance systems use the quadrature design.

When receiving a signal with a coil, the same principles apply as when using the coil for transmission. If the signal being received from a coil is obtained from a pair of points on the coil and electronically phase shifted to remove the 90° phase shift applied during the transmit operation and the resultant signals are added, then an increase of 2.5:1 in SNR over a conventional linear polarized coil can be realized. This operation is known as quadrature reception (MacFall, 1997).

Since proximity with a part of the body improves the SNR characteristics of a coil, receive-only designs have been produced to optimize signal detection. These coils are called surface coils and can be relatively simple in design. They are designed to lie on or under the patient and have the characteristics that the best performance occurs within the confines of the coil and no deeper than the radius of the coil. Among the considerations for using surface coils are protection of the patient from RF burns and ensuring that the RF signal transmitted during slice selection does not destroy the coil. The former is accomplished by encasing the coil in plastic, while the latter is achieved by careful design of the coupling network so that the coil is effectively non-responsive during transmission. Usually, the RF transmitter operates through the body coil, although specialized surface coils that are both transmit and receive coils are used in special applications. Quadrature surface coils have been designed as well.

Another approach to improving SNR with surface coils is the phased array coil. A phased array uses a set of coils from which a combined signal permits the collection of image information over a larger region than that covered by a single coil. The goal is to achieve better improvements in SNR than is possible with a single coil, while permitting imaging over a distance greater than that which can be imaged by a single coil. Separate electronics are required for each coil element, including separate receiver channels to reduce the pickup of correlated noise. These additional requirements and the more complex image reconstruction methods needed for the additional data can lead to superior performance for tasks such as whole spine imaging compared to conventional body coils. A significant improvement in patient throughput can result, since multiple acquisitions to cover large areas of the body are not needed.

The receiver must take the signal collected from the body by the coil, boost it through a preamplifier, and process it so that it can be used by the reconstruction system. The first thing the receiver must accomplish is to remove the carrier frequency, the Larmor frequency, while leaving intact the range of frequencies enveloping the carrier. The information used for reconstruction purposes is carried by audio frequencies on either side of the Larmor frequency. A typical maximum range is ±100 kHz. The receiver filters the signal after the demodulation step and digitizes the data so that the computer system can perform the reconstruction. Digitized data consists of real and imaginary components extracted from 0°/90° phase shifts in the early analog stages of the receiver subsystem. The resulting data is spread between positive and negative frequencies, where the maximum frequency is one-half the sampling frequency. This approach known as quadrature detection improves SNR over conventional detection because of the use of narrow band filters (Fukushima, Roeder, 1981). Careful design avoids certain types of errors that are characteristic of quadrature detection.

Digital receivers shift the frequency of the received signal and digitize the signal at $2\times$ the rate dictated by the Nyquist limit. This results in an inherent 90° phase shift. Because of this approach, phase shifting for quadrature detection makes use of digital rather than analog methods, yielding a simple, more accurate system. Any filtering that might be needed can be accomplished digitally as well. The trade-off is that the very high speed A/D converters necessary for bit resolution are more expensive and may not be as available, leading to problems with contrast resolution in some imaging situations, such as true 3D acquisitions (MacFall, 1997).

A pulse programmer is part of the system specifying the waveforms used to generate differing types of imaging sequences. The pulse programmer, under computer control, establishes how the transmitter produces the waveforms for each data collection operation by specifying the shape of the waveform and the timing of the various events necessary to collect the data. This operation includes controlling not only the RF systems, but also the gradient subsystem. Computer control of the pulse programmer implies that the user has access to different programs that produce different kinds of pulse sequences. The manufacturers provide pulse programming languages that users can employ to develop new pulse sequences for specialized applications or for research purposes. Because of the flexibility that these languages permit for controlling all aspects of the operation of the imager, the time needed to develop a mastery of pulse programming is often long.

6.5.6 Gradient system

The gradient system provides the perturbations to the static magnetic field, B_0, necessary to produce phase and frequency changes in the precession of target nuclear spins in order to encode position information. Gradient coils produce linear variations in the static field in the x, y, and z-directions. For some purposes, such as oblique imaging, gradients can be turned on in combinations so that the resultant is a vector sum of the gradient pair in operation. Gradients are implemented by supplying current to pairs of coils surrounding the direction of the B_0 field, the bore of the magnet in superconducting systems, so that the static field varies in the direction of the gradient. Gradient capability is measured in milliTesla/meter (mT/m) or Gauss/centimeter (G/cm). The current is supplied by gradient amplifiers that are controlled by the supervisory computer system so that they can be turned on and off to provide frequency and phase encoding for imaging and slice selection in a wide variety of pulse sequences.

Four characteristics of the gradient system are important to imaging. The strength of the gradient, the rise time and slew rate, the duty cycle, and the compensation for eddy currents. The strength of the gradients directly affects the resolution available in the images, as well as the imager's ability to perform certain types of imaging procedures such as echo-planar imaging. The rise time (shorter is better) influences how short the gradient duration can be and thus, how short echo times can be. Slew rate is the rate of change of current in a coil once the current has

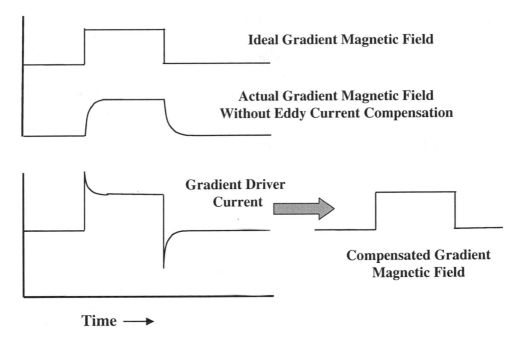

Ideal Gradient Magnetic Field

**Actual Gradient Magnetic Field
Without Eddy Current Compensation**

**Gradient Driver
Current**

**Compensated Gradient
Magnetic Field**

Time ⟶

Figure 6.31: The ideal gradient magnetic field should rise to a specified level instantaneously, hold this level for the specified time, then return to baseline instantaneously. Real systems, however, ramp up to a level, hold the level, then ramp down. However, changing magnetic fields, called eddy currents, are induced in the cryostat during the ramp up period. These alter the effective magnetic field produced by the gradient coils. A preemphasis circuit is used in the gradient drivers to compensate for the effects of the eddy currents. The combination of the preemphasis and the eddy current produces a gradient field closer to the ideal. When preemphasis is combined with a shielded gradient coil set, the gradient magnetic field is improved even more, especially for very high gradient fields with rapid switching, such as those used in EPI imaging.

been switched on. Both of these are important in echo-planar imaging. The duty cycle refers to the amount of time a gradient system is actually operating. The gradient currents in a coil can be high enough to cause considerable heating. While both water cooling and forced air cooling are used to stabilize the temperature of the gradient coils and gradient amplifiers, the duty cycle is often less than 100%, which means that the gradients cannot be on continuously in most systems.

The gradient systems are designed to produce a linear gradient field in the selected direction. This system is also designed to switch very rapidly and this switching can induce eddy currents (Thomas, 1993; MacFall, 1997). Eddy currents are due to induced currents in surrounding components such as the cryostat, shields, other coils, and other components. These time-varying induced currents in turn have magnetic fields associated with them that combine with the desired gradients to produce a combination that would differ from the desired wave shape if it were not for eddy current compensation built into the gradient system. Electronic compensation or pre-emphasis alters the shape of the waveform so that the combined gradient wave and eddy current have a shape closer to the ideal than without compensation. However, the compensation itself induces eddy currents that are not corrected.

Another approach to reducing eddy currents now used successfully in many high-performance systems is the shielded gradient set. In this design, additional coils are constructed as part of the gradient set that serve to cancel the components that would induce eddy currents in the first place. These coils are designed so that the inner field of the gradient set is minimally affected by outer shielding gradients. The best overall approach combines pre-emphasis in the waveform with gradient shielding to produce the gradient waveform (Figure 6.31).

Most clinical systems are designed so that the coils that create the x, y, and z-gradients are permanently mounted within the structure of the system. For superconducting systems, the bore tube contains the coils that produce the gradients. The same gradient set is used for all operations of the system and it is not removable. Vertical systems using permanent magnets use fixed coils mounted in the housing structure of the system. For very high-performance, special gradient inserts are available, often from third party suppliers. These have special characteristics that are superior for some imaging applications. An example of such an insert is a high-performance head-only gradient insert for functional magnetic resonance. With such an insert installed, the fixed gradient sets would not be operational.

6.5.7 Computer systems

MR imaging systems, especially those intended for high-performance applications, use multiple computers to control and operate the imager. A typical arrangement is to use a general purpose workstation as the supervisory computer on which the operator's console runs. The operator interacts with an application control program that permits her/him to control the functions of the imager. The console usually has one or two monitors, so that the functions for running the machine are displayed on one monitor while the images are displayed on the other. There are numerous ways to implement this, but the goal is to provide the operator with the flexibility to image patients rapidly and efficiently.

When the operator executes a function, the application control program initiates a series of events that leads to data acquisition. This includes communications with different subsystems in the imager that are controlled by individual small computer systems dedicated to that subsystem. Software for all of the dedicated subsystems resides on hard disks and is downloaded to the dedicated subsystems at startup and during setup for imaging.

The many subsystems acquire the data and store it, usually in a specialized storage memory for processing into images. This storage memory is connected to one or more array processors that execute the Fourier transform and filter operations much more quickly than the general purpose computer would be capable of doing. Array processors are dedicated to producing images as rapidly as possible by parallelizing the image processing tasks. Multiple array processors provide additional parallelism.

Display systems are dedicated to assisting the operators in running the imager. However, clinical systems often have additional associated consoles designed to permit physicians or others to review images efficiently without preventing the operators from continuing to scan. These consoles can be dedicated computers networked to the main control computer or they can be specific satellite computers that operate in the background as the system collects data. In circumstances where image information is recorded on transparency film, the display stations can be used for filming. They can also be used for specialized processing such as three-dimensional volume rendering or the production of parametric images resulting from a specialized data acquisition. Current display technologies use conventional high resolution color and/or monochrome CRT monitors, but high-performance active matrix liquid crystal displays are becoming available for clinical systems.

Interaction with the system is by means of a keyboard and a pointing system. Some user interfaces have used touch screen technology effectively to allow the operators to set up scan protocols and parameters with minimal conventional keyboard interactions. Usually, a pointing device that interacts with the screen displaying the processed images augments these controls. Trackballs and mouse devices are the usual pointing devices. Newer systems use workstation-like window systems, using one large monitor for virtually all interactions and displays.

Data are stored on high speed media. Current technology for image storage, software to run the imager, pulse sequences, RF waveforms, and other information is the hard disk drive. Archiving of image information can be on one of several different types of media including digital audio tape (DAT) and magneto-optical disks (MO). Other storage systems that may be used, especially in low volume environments such as low field systems installed in some outpatient clinics, may include a recordable compact disk (CD-R). Higher end systems can be configured for local backup, but might also use standard communications protocols to move images to a medical archive system for storage and viewing access. The current standard for these protocols is called Digital Imaging and Communications in Medicine, version 3.0 (DICOM 3.0), which is an evolving standard that has done a reasonable job of defining connectivity issues for vendors, so that systems can communicate with each other.

Some of the ancillary systems associated with the imager include cardiac gating/monitoring systems and respiratory triggering systems. These systems are designed to permit using the selected physiological signal to trigger pulse sequence acquisitions in order to reduce motion artifacts due to involuntary, physiological motion. Additional equipment, from third party vendors, might include a pulse oximeter for patient monitoring and possibly an audio/video system to both communicate with the patient during scans and provide comforting, distracting music or movies.

6.6 Current techniques and areas of research

This section covers some of the areas that have been particularly important in MR imaging in the last few years. Several of these techniques are research tools, while others have recently been adopted by clinical imaging specialists as part of the toolbox for evaluating disease processes. For these techniques to move from research to clinical utility requires that they be approved by the FDA as having clinical utility. Each of these areas has been described extensively in the literature, so the subsequent discussion is, of necessity, rather brief.

6.6.1 Contrast agents

Contrast between tissues requires that there be a difference in the relaxation times, T1 and T2, so that the image intensities assigned to the tissues derives from a pulse sequence that enhances T1 or T2 contributions to image intensity. When tissues are significantly different and the correct pulse sequence is chosen, then contrast differences based on the tissue relaxation times alone can be observed in the images. However, when the goal is to image a tumor surrounded by normal tissues, their relaxation times may be sufficiently similar that little or no contrast is developed, thus making identification of the abnormality very difficult. When properly used, contrast agents can enhance the relaxation time differences between two similar tissues so that they can be distinguished in the resulting images. However, the contrast agents themselves are not observed in the images. Rather, their effect on nearby protons produces the increase in contrast between tissues.

Most contrast agents are used to enhance T1 relaxation. These agents typically use metal chelates of gadolinium, such as gadopentetate dimeglumine, and are considered to be extracellular space agents, which disperse relatively rapidly from vascular system to interstitial spaces by diffusion across capillary walls in most tissues except the brain. In the brain, the blood-brain barrier ordinarily excludes these agents unless there is a pathologic process resulting in blood-brain barrier disruption. While they are considered extracellular agents, with the proper timing and selection of pulse sequences, these agents can be used for arterial imaging as well. Some gadolinium chelates, such as gadobenate dimeglumine, have been used as hepatocyte imaging agents, where the contrast agent is transported across the cell membrane (Mitchell, 1999).

Three phases follow the injection of any contrast agent. The arterial phase lasts a short time, about 20–30 sec. During this time, imaging produces bright arterial contrast with little contrast enhancement in veins. The contrast agent is distributed in the blood pool, the blood vessel system including veins and capillary beds, after about a minute. This phase is useful for imaging the liver because the liver vessels are enhanced; whereas hypovascular liver tumors are less enhanced. After two or more minutes, the agent has crossed capillary walls and has begun to distribute in tissue interstitial spaces. Hyperintensities are observed in abnormal tissues with large interstitial spaces such as some metastatic tumors. During this time, the agents is filtered by the kidney, beginning the excretion process. Renal

MR imaging is greatly enhanced at this point. Because of the extended time required for the contrast agent to be filtered from the blood, fast imaging is not nearly as critical in this last phase. Figure 6.32 shows an example of the use of contrast agents.

The gadolinium-based agents can be especially useful in brain imaging. Because the normal blood-brain barrier excludes blood and contrast agents, normal brain tissue is not enhanced in the presence of gadolinium. Arteries and veins become bright while the contrast agent passes through. However, injuries or disease processes disrupt the blood-brain barrier, permitting the gadolinium contrast agents to penetrate the abnormal area. This results in a a clinically very useful enhancement. The best results are obtained when imaging is performed several minutes after injection.

There are other contrast agents with very different properties than gadolinium chelates. Among the most interesting are superparamagnetic iron oxide particles, which are taken up by the reticulo-endothelial system. These agents contain

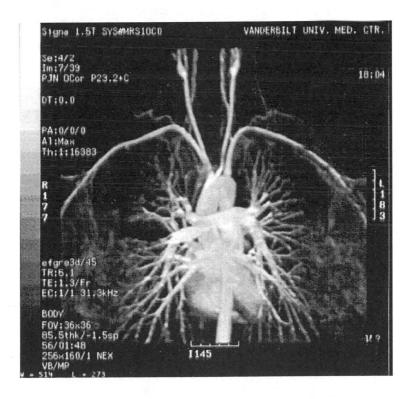

Early Phase Contrast-enhanced Image

Figure 6.32: Example of an early phase contrast study in which the arterial system in the chest is especially well demonstrated. In addition to the heart, the pulmonary arterial system is very prominent in this T1-weighted image. Other images acquired later in time demonstrate tissue and venous phases more prominently.

both ferric (Fe^{3+}) and ferrous (Fe^{2+}) iron and oxygen in a core surrounded by polysaccaride. When injected, these agents create a T2 or T2* enhancement in T2-weighted and T2* weighted images, which is especially useful in evaluating liver tumors. In liver imaging, these agents cause a loss of signal in the liver, with the result that certain types of tumors, which do not take up the contrast agent, remain bright and are readily observed in the images. Much smaller particle sizes are used to create T1, T2, and T2* enhancements, resulting in increased signal in T1-weighted images and decreased signal in T2-weighted images (Mitchell, 1999).

6.6.2 Angiography/flow

Moving body fluids create complex motion artifacts that interfere with some types of imaging. However, over the time that magnetic resonance imaging has been developed in the clinical environment, many investigators have worked to develop pulse sequences that reduce or eliminate flow artifacts, as well as pulse sequences to enhance specific types of flow for the purpose of providing qualitative and quantitative angiographic information. There is considerable interest in arterial and venous blood flow, but some work has been done in imaging CSF flow as well. There is a substantial literature of techniques and methodologies for implementing magnetic resonance angiography (MRA) without the use of externally supplied contrast agents. Similarly, there are many articles discussing the use of contrast agents for angiography. The latter studies were described in Section 6.6.1.

Flow imaging can produce a wide variety of contrasts for moving protons, compared to surrounding stationary tissues. Depending on the requirements and the particular pulse sequences, one may have rapidly moving blood produce a very bright, angiography-like signal. Other techniques, so-called "black blood" sequences, produce a total absence of signal in the arterial system. Many of these techniques lend themselves to three-dimensional acquisitions and resulting three-dimensional display techniques. These post-processing algorithms produce pseudo-three-dimensional presentations of the arterial or venous segments in a form where depth and position can be readily perceived. These approaches often serve to alleviate some of the problems associated with flow imaging related to turbulence and artificially distorted diameters of vascular structures.

Enhanced imaging of flow can occur under several circumstances. In spin echo imaging, when a blood vessel is perpendicular to the slices selected for multislice imaging, an increase in intensity is observed where the flow is directed into the slice. This enhancement is caused by unsaturated blood from outside the selected slices flowing into the field during imaging. The presence of additional longitudinal magnetization from the fresh blood is detected as additional signal. Because blood in the center of the slices remains at a steady state saturation level, this effect decreases with slice depth. Venous flow can be imaged more easily because the flow rate of arterial blood is so high that there is hardly enough signal to detect. Some pulse sequences use saturation pulses that are applied outside the selected slices, so that the blood flowing into the selected slices is fully saturated. Without longitudinal magnetization, the saturated blood does not contribute to the signal.

When a multi-echo spin echo sequence is used, another mechanism for producing an increase in signal utilizes rephasing of even echoes. Every second echo produces an enhancement of the intensity of the blood because the transverse magnetization comes back into phase. This effect works particularly well for relatively slow venous flow.

Gradient echo pulse sequences produce substantial signal enhancements for flowing blood and CSF. With the short TRs used in gradient echo imaging, unsaturated blood or CSF produces a greatly enhanced signal in the next excitation, the amount of which depends on the slice thickness or volume for 3D imaging, the flow velocity, and the particular TR used. Unfortunately, the moving spins can create artifacts in the form of ghosts as mentioned in Section 6.4.5. There are some ways to correct for these artifacts while maintaining the bright blood image for purposes of enhancing visualization of the vessels.

Gradient echo imaging is generally performed with the assumption that the tissues being imaged are not moving. The pulse sequences are designed to induce dephasing in the readout direction, followed by rephasing and the production of an echo. In static tissues, the bipolar gradient causes an evolving change in phase as long as it is on. Once turned off, the phase accumulated for nonmoving tissues is maintained. When the gradient of opposite polarity is turned on sometime later, the phase accumulated by the previous gradient is removed so that all nuclei come into phase when the second gradient is turned off. As long as the areas under the gradient waveform are identical, all nuclei will come back into phase and can produce an echo. However, in order to read out the signal, the second lobe of the bipolar readout gradient must remain on. Thus, the second lobe exhibits about twice the area of the first part of the echo and forces the spins to go out of phase by the end of the readout period. Figure 6.33 shows a diagram of this. If spins are moving during the first part of the bipolar readout pair, they will accumulate phase. When the second part of the readout pair is applied, the moving spins will come into focus more rapidly than the stationary spins and continue to dephase at the time when the stationary spins are focused. These out of phase components can produce ghosting in the images, so it is necessary to correct for these moving spins in some fashion.

An approach to eliminating the out-of-phase components is provided by gradient moment nulling. In this technique for flow compensation in gradient echo images, a third gradient pulse of the same polarity as the initial pulse is used to force all the spins into focus at the same time. This approach works as long as the sum of the areas of these gradients equals zero. This form of gradient moment nulling is called first order flow compensation or velocity compensation because it removes the velocity component of flow from the signal. The first-order compensation assumes that the velocity is constant during the pulse sequence. Otherwise, higher order compensations would be needed, but they would require additional gradient lobes and be rather cumbersome to use.

Two of the most often used techniques for angiography without the use of contrast agents are time of flight imaging pulse sequences and phase contrast imaging. Time of flight (TOF) methods use the phenomenon of enhancement of the imaged

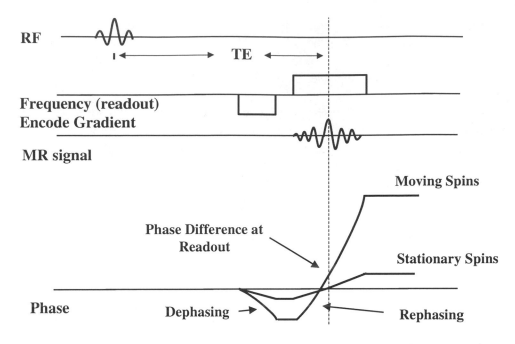

Figure 6.33: In the presence of a gradient echo pulse sequence moving spins dephase at a rate that increases while the initial readout gradient lobe is present. Stationary spins dephase during the gradient-on period and are then rephased by the initial part of the oposite gradient (See Figure 6.21). During the second lobe of the readout gradient, the moving spins rephase faster than the stationary spins, so at the time of maximum signal amplitude for the stationary spins, the moving spins have passed through zero phase and are continuing to accumulate additional phase. The effect is to produce ghosting artifacts that are characteristic of motion, either from flow or from body motion such as respiration.

blood when partially saturated blood is replaced by unsaturated blood from outside the slice. Two different forms of TOF are usually available: a two-dimensional and a three-dimensional version. In this method, the protons in blood are "tagged" or altered magnetically so that when blood "washes" into the slice or volume, it has different signal characteristics than the tissues surrounding the vessels. This is a technique that works for vessels that are perpendicular (or very close to perpendicular) to the slice. If the spins within the slice are saturated, then fresh unsaturated blood flowing into the slice produces a brighter signal. However, this signal depends on the T1 value, the velocity, and the direction of the blood flow. It is useful to use stacks of thin slices along an arterial or venous segment of interest, followed by maximum intensity projection (MIP) post-collection processing to assemble an image of the bright vascular structures surrounded by less conspicuous tissues. The MIP image is formed from the stack of flow-enhanced images perpendicular to the collected slices. Both arteries and veins will appear bright unless a presaturation region is applied outside of the slices of interest to select one set of vessels or the other. Vessels that are not perpendicular or whose direction with respect to

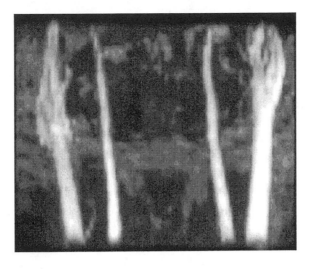

3D-TOF Images of Vessels in the Neck

Figure 6.34: 3D-Time of Flight (3D-TOF) image of the vessels of the neck. This acquisition used no contrast enhancement, yet it provides an especially good visualization of the carotid arteries.

the imaging slices varies lose intensity as they move away from the perpendicular orientation. The pulse sequences usually used are gradient echo with a short TE, a TR of 20–50 msec, thin slices, and gradient moment nulling for velocity compensation. Complex flow patterns such as those occurring in aneurysms and near stenotic regions are often not visualized well by MIP images from 2D TOF acquisitions.

Three-dimensional TOF permits visualization of tissue volumes with improved in plane resolution compared to 2D methods. Usually, the SNR is improved as well. With three-dimensional TOF, contrast agents that shorten T1, such as gadolinium, can be used to compensate for loss of longitudinal magnetization caused by the large numbers of excitation pulses needed for definition of the imaging volume. A non-contrast-enhanced example of 3D TOF is shown in Figure 6.34.

Phase contrast methods display phase changes resulting from the flow of blood in vessels. This results in reduced contributions from non-moving tissues and possible quantitation of the blood velocity and flow direction. Two sets of images, acquired as an interleaved set, are used to present images of phase change due to motion. One image set is motion-compensated and the other is not, so the complex difference between them is the motion of blood recorded as phase changes, assuming the stationary tissues remain stationary. The phase change is produced by varying the time between lobes of the bipolar readout gradient waveform velocity encoding variable, V_{enc}, so that a velocity that produces a 180° phase shift in one direction is encoded. The pulse sequence is useful and quantitative over a range of zero to V_{enc}. Velocities higher than this value will wrap phase and be indistinguishable from slower velocities because they will be assigned the same gray scale in the images. This is a form of aliasing of the velocity information. It is however important to select the V_{enc} value carefully, because very slow flow can be lost if V_{enc} is too high. Quantitative composite images of blood velocity can be produced from phase contrast images in three directions, but the acquisition times can be long.

6.6.3 Diffusion/perfusion imaging

6.6.3.1 Diffusion imaging

Diffusion refers to the random movement of water molecules. In pure water, this movement is unrestricted and depends on temperature. At 37°C, the diffusion coefficient of water is $2.2 - 2.5 \times 10^{-3}$ mm²/sec. However, motion in tissues is more complex and is restricted by various permeable or impermeable boundaries such as cell membranes and capillary walls. In tissues, the diffusion coefficient will therefore be different from that of pure water and highly dependent on the particular environment being imaged, and the direction of the measurement. This process is also time-dependent, since longer diffusion times increase the likelihood that the water will contact a boundary. Because of these dependencies, it is possible to use diffusion measurements in tissues to obtain information about the structure and permeability of the tissues (Le Bihan, Basser, 1995).

MR imaging methods can provide the only direct measurement of diffusion coefficients in living tissues by producing images in which the major contribution to contrast is from diffusion coefficients. The means of achieving this was originally proposed for chemical NMR by Stejskal and Tanner (Stejskal, Tanner, 1965), who inserted two additional pulsed, motion-sensitizing gradients on either side of the 180° pulse in a spin echo sequence. These two added gradients have a specific amplitude and duration and are defined by a "b" value, which is used to describe the degree of echo attenuation induced by the gradients. Without the added gradients, the pulse sequence would produce T2 weighting. However, in the presence of diffusion and the added gradients, additional attenuation of the signal occurs. Several research groups pioneered the development of diffusion-weighted imaging using the approach initially proposed by Stejskal and Tanner (Wesby, Moseley *et al.* 1984; Merboldt, Hankicke *et al.* 1985; Hennig, Naureth *et al.* 1986; Le Bihan, Breton *et al.* 1986).

A technique originally proposed by Le Bihan (Le Bihan, Breton *et al.* 1986), called the intravoxel incoherent motion (IVIM) method is based on signal attenuation due to dephasing of the transverse magnetization as a result of random motion of the protons within a magnetic field gradient. In the IVIM model, the attenuation in an image, S_1, is a function of T2 decay, the diffusion coefficients (D and D^*) and the gradient factor, b, which is a function of the strength and duration of the added gradients. The coefficient D is the pure self-diffusion coefficient, D^* is the effective diffusion coefficient due to protons moving through capillary beds during perfusion, and f is the fraction of moving protons within a voxel. Both D and D^* have units of mm^2/sec and f is unitless.

$$S_1 = S_0 e^{-TE/T2} e^{-b \cdot D} \left[(1 - f) + f \cdot e^{-b \cdot D^*} \right]. \qquad (6.13)$$

In this equation, $b = \Sigma G^2 \gamma^2 d^2 (2d/3 + I)$ (summed over all gradients and all directions), where G is the amplitude of each added gradient pulse (mT/m), d is the duration of each gradient pulse (sec), I is the time interval between the two paired gradient pulses (sec), γ is the gyromagnetic ratio, S_0 is proportional to proton density, TE is the echo time, and T2 is the transverse relaxation time.

The IVIM technique defines diffusion as random motion of the water molecules and assumes that perfusion, by Le Bihan's definition, can be thought of as "macroscopic" diffusion, because of the random geometry of the capillary bed and/or the random flow directions. Thus, capillary flow manifests itself as a dephasing of the transverse magnetization with no net shift in phase; that is, there would be as many negative shifts as positive shifts with a mean of zero and no preferred directionality.

In Le Bihan's original work, no attempt was made to separate diffusion and capillary flow effects. With this assumption, if two images are acquired, one standard image with no added gradients (b_0) and a second image with added gradients (b_1), an apparent diffusion coefficient (ADC) can be calculated by taking a pixel-by-pixel log-ratio of the two images to cancel T2 effects. In this model the ADC contains both diffusion and flow effects. Since the computation of the diffusion parameters from the IVIM method requires complex fitting of a model to the attenuation curve produced from multiple acquisitions at increasing b values, most approaches to diffusion-weighted imaging use ADC and phase images, because they can provide useful information without the problems associated with fitting a model (see Figure 6.35). Diffusion tensor imaging resolves the issue of directional components in the ADC by ensuring that data from all 3 directions are collected. Then, the diffusion tensor equation is solved to produce the directionally independent trace of the tensor for a particular capillary bed (van Geldereen, de Vleeshouwer et al. 1994; Jones, Horsfield et al. 1999).

Diffusion imaging can be used to demonstrate restricted diffusion abnormalities. These abnormalities occur very quickly, usually within minutes, after the onset of an acute embolic stroke. Interruption of normal cell-wall activities, such as the sodium-potassium pump system, occurs in stroke and shows up in diffusion weighted images as an increase in diffusion restriction, a signal increase. Additionally, changes in interstitial volume and cell swelling prior to the onset of edema can also be demonstrated in these images. Conventional T2 weighted images often do not show any abnormalities until as late as 4 to 6 hours after the event, when edema has occurred. By most accounts, diffusion weighted imaging is the most sensitive available method for demonstrating acute stroke. Thus, diffusion imaging provides a means for evaluating stroke during the six-hour window when clot-dissolving drugs can be used effectively for embolic strokes. Diffusion imaging and image processing is now available on many commercial scanners.

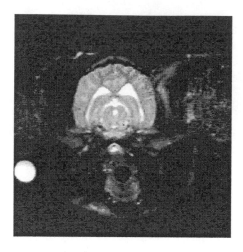 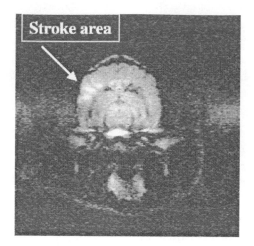

T2-weighted Image   **Diffusion-weighted Image**

Acute Stroke in an Animal Model

Figure 6.35: A T2-weighted image of the brain of an animal model with acute stroke is shown on the left side of the figure. The T2-weighted image is relatively normal in appearance. In the right image, diffusion weighting shows an enhanced area, indicative of disrupted blood flow and resulting changes in diffusion within the affected area. Diffusion imaging demonstrates changes within minutes after a stroke, several hours before the defect is observable on conventional MR images or with computed tomographic studies.

Very little work has been done with diffusion weighted imaging outside the brain. Since this technique depends on sensitizing the image acquisition to very small amounts of motion, it is very difficult to image other organs that tend to undergo significant motion. Some work has been done with animals, on organs other than the brain, such as the kidneys, but clinical imaging is currently confined to the brain. The demonstration of cerebro-vascular events is important clinically and the head can be restrained reasonably well to ensure that movement does not contaminate the images.

A variety of different pulse sequences can be used to produce diffusion-weighted contrast. Much work has been done with two-dimensional spin-echo imaging using diffusion gradients with b values approaching 1000 or more. The strength of these gradients is usually limited by the hardware gradient system. Additionally, eddy currents can be especially severe with large, long duration gradients, so unshielded gradient systems generally do not perform well for diffusion imaging. Current imagers are able to use EPI acquisitions, which avoid problems associated with patient motion, a serious issue when using spin-echo sequences. In addition, EPI allows many images to be collected with increasing b-values, so that a mathematical fit of signal attenuation in an area of the image can be performed. Half-Fourier turbo spin echo (HASTE) sequences are also among the pulse sequences that have been demonstrated. HASTE avoids the susceptibility artifacts that are often problematic with EPI. With rapid acquisitions of many b-value images, parametric determination of the diffusion coefficient is possible using a model-fitting approach. Otherwise, the ADC or "apparent diffusion coefficient" is determined from the multiple measurements at increasing b-values. From these diffusion-weighted images, parametric ADC maps can be computed rapidly.

6.6.3.2 Dynamic contrast perfusion imaging

Perfusion of tissues in the brain can be studied by using the high speed imaging capabilities of currently available imaging systems coupled with short, rapid arterial injections of a contrast agent, typically one of the gadolinium-based agents, to perform first-pass imaging of tissue capillary perfusion (Baird, Warach, 1998). Fast T1-weighted gradient echo imaging, which provides a signal increase, can be used. T2* weighted gradient echo or EPI imaging (susceptibility imaging) can be used to provide a drop in signal as the bolus of contrast agent passes through the tissue being studied. In one study, investigators acquired data with a T2-weighted high speed imaging sequence enabling them to obtain data with a temporal resolution of one second (Rosen, Belliveau *et al.* 1990). Using injections of dysprosium-DTPA (Dy-DTPA) at 0.2 mmole/kg, they were able to obtain an intensity vs. time curve showing a sudden loss of signal, followed by a return to baseline and start of recirculation, after passage of the bolus through the brain of a dog. They converted the area under these curves to relative concentration vs. time using the following approach: they assumed that a decrease in intensity with increasing concentration follows a single exponential function, related to the T2 rate change for signal decay:

$$-\ln(S(t)/S_0)/\text{TE} = \text{concentration}(t) \cdot k \cong R2^* \cong (1/T2^*), \qquad (6.14)$$

where k is a constant depending on the tissue, the pulse sequence used and the field strength they determine empirically, $S(t)$ is the time dependent intensity, and S_0 is the base-line signal intensity. The area under the concentration-time curve is proportional to blood volume in the organ. If the arterial function is known, the volume can be found. Additionally, if the mean transit time (MTT) can be found, also using the arterial function, then the flow can be computed according to the classic Stewart equation:

$$\text{Flow} = \text{Volume}/\text{mean transit time.} \qquad (6.15)$$

There are numerous problems with computing mean transit time and blood volume in the brain. The bolus spreads after injection, requiring deconvolution of the arterial input function to properly determine mean transit time. The proportionality constant relating relaxation rate to concentration must be known. The fractional tissue volume must also be known. Because of the difficulties of computing flow, Rosen *et al.* and Gore and Majumdar have addressed the simpler problem of blood volume determination and have shown that it is possible to determine regional relative blood volumes proportional to cerebral blood volume (Gore, Majumdar, 1990; Rosen, Belliveau *et al.* 1990).

6.6.4 Magnetization transfer contrast

Most of the protons that participate in MR imaging are considered to be free water protons whose T2 relaxation is slow enough that it can be readily observed. These protons are observed during standard MR imaging. However, there are other protons that are bound to macromolecules and cell membranes in what are considered "solid" tissues such as muscle and cartilage. Fat-containing tissues do not contain such bound protons. Bound protons exhibit a very broad range of resonant frequencies compared to those in unbound water molecules, and a short T2, making it difficult to directly image them by conventional means. In tissues, an equilibrium state in which magnetization is transferred from one state to the other exists between these two components. Because of the exchange of magnetization between pools, a perturbation of one affects the other.

If these macromolecular protons are excited by RF signals at several kHz above or below the resonant frequency of unbound water, these macromolecular protons transfer their magnetization to nearby water protons in the form of saturation. This transfer of saturation causes a reduction of available signal that can be used to enhance the imaging of certain tissues. Since this is a relatively slow phenomenon, the offset RF pulse is applied for a long time, sometimes several seconds, saturating transverse magnetization. During this time, as an equilibrium state of magnetization transfer is reached, the longitudinal magnetization of free water containing tissues is reduced. The result is a loss of signal intensity, which can be exploited for imaging certain tissues. In multislice imaging, there is a partial saturation of macromolecular hydrogen, which reduces overall contrast. This occurs because these macromolecular protons can be partially saturated throughout the selected volume during each excitation pulse, since they exhibit a broad range of resonant frequencies.

Several areas of clinical utility have been identified for magnetization transfer (MT) techniques where the tissue suppression is useful. Early work was done for MR angiography of the brain (Adkinson, 1994). In these studies, MT imaging methods were used to suppress protein-bound brain tissue so that the contrast between it and non-signal suppressed blood was increased. Other work in the brain has shown increases in SNR by using MT to enhance visualization of gray matter by suppressing white matter signals. This has been demonstrated to be of use in multiple sclerosis (MS) where the inflammatory process of the disease causes water to be less tightly bound to the protein rich myelin, reducing the signal that would normally be seen in MT images of the brain. Thus, one can compare T1-weighed images without MT with those made with MT, demonstrating changes in the MT ratio (MTR) given by $1 - M_{MT}/M_0$. Areas of demylination are displayed as a decrease in MTR (Bradley, 1999).

6.6.5 Functional MRI

Functional MRI (fMRI) has been developed as a tool that makes it possible to observe the brain as it performs various tasks. It makes use of the so-called "BOLD" effect, where BOLD stands for "blood oxygen level difference". In the current theory of this technique, blood is normally in an equilibrium state, with equal amounts of oxyhemoglobin and deoxyhemoglobin present in the capillaries when the brain is not engaged in a specific task. However, when called upon to perform a task, the neurons needed to perform the task increase their metabolic rates and require additional oxygen to function. The vascular system responds by providing much more oxygenated blood than required at equilibrium, so the deoxyhemoglobin is partly displaced by oxyhemoglobin. Deoxyhemoglobin is paramagnetic, while oxyhemoglobin is diamagnetic, an important difference, because deoxyhemoglobin causes the signal from blood to be lower than if there were only oxyhemoglobin. Thus, a reduction in the amount of deoxyhemoglobin present in the vessels causes the signal to increase slightly in images acquired during the activation (Ogawa, Lee *et al.* 1990). This happens because the extraction of oxygen from the blood does not change very much. The effect is generally very small, yielding increases in signal on the order of 1 to 3% at 1.5 T, or twice as much at 3.0 T.

In order to visualize these changes, a heavily T2*-weighted pulse sequence is used. It is typically implemented as an EPI pulse sequence, so that the entire brain can be imaged at relatively high speed. Multiple volumes of images are acquired over time, during which a stimulus and a rest period are used to evaluate a particular part of the brain. The resulting image sets, often a few thousand images, are postprocessed using a statistical threshold applied to ensemble averages of pixels over time to produce a series of maps that can be overlaid on the images to indicate which areas of the brain have experienced increases in blood flow related to the task being performed (Figure 6.36). This technique provides a tool for high resolution investigations of specific areas of the brain involving carefully developed stimuli.

Numerous kinds of studies have been initiated by physicians, neuroscientists, psychologists, and others who study functional pathways in the brain. Because of its ability to visualize an area of the brain being activated while the subject performs a prescribed task, fMRI is a very powerful tool for both research and clinical applications. However, it has a number of associated problems. The first is that it is very difficult to have even cooperative subjects stay completely still during acquisitions that may last the many minutes required to obtain a usable SNR. Head movements cause motion artifacts that obscure subtle changes in brain response. A second problem is that small blood vessels in areas of interest can produce enough signal for the post-processing algorithms to mistake vascular artifacts as activation, thereby diluting the value of the information obtained. Another problem is that this technique is an indirect measure of the activation of groups

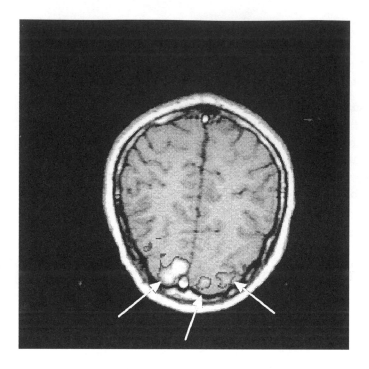

**Binocular Vision Activation Map
Overlaid on T1-Weighted Anatomical Image**

Figure 6.36: This figure shows an overlay onto the optic centers of activation maps acquired during a task involving visual stimulation. The overlay comes from an EPI acquisition collected over 5.4 minutes, processed to find the statistical correlation of signal changes with the alternating task-rest cycle, which is overplayed on the corresponding T1-weighted anatomical image.

of neurons, not a direct measure, such as in positron emission tomography (PET) where a radiopharmaceutical is taken up by the metabolic pathways in the neurons. Since fMRI is an indirect measure of brain activity, the dynamics of blood flow may not be as closely matched to neuronal activity as would be desired. Also, fMRI suffers from poor temporal response, on the order of seconds/volume of information acquired, compared to techniques such as magnetoencephalography or electroencephalography, which have millisecond resolving capability, but with poor spatial resolution.

Both cognitive and motor/sensory studies have been performed. Many different evaluations of how people interpret motion, understand words, move fingers, experience pain, and view images have been performed. Numerous examples of these and other types of studies are described in the literature (Braver, Cohen *et al.* 1997; Desmond, Gabrieli *et al.* 1997; Mattay, Callicott *et al.* 1998; Menon, Luknowsky *et al.* 1998; Cramer, Finklestein *et al.* 1999; Ishai, Ungerleider *et al.* 1999).

6.6.6 Hyperpolarized gas imaging

Among the more interesting developments in MR imaging are techniques involving the use of hyperpolarized gases. The noble gas isotopes ^{3}He and ^{129}Xe can be processed to have a large nonequilibrium nuclear spin polarization via a collision-spin exchange mechanism with an alkali-metal vapor, typically rubidium, in a special pressurized cell that permits pumping the system with a high-power laser. A mixture of rubidium, nitrogen, and ^{3}He or ^{129}Xe is exposed to circularly polarized laser light in a heated glass chamber which is placed in a magnetic field. Depending on the available laser power, 8 to 20 hours of operation is required to produce sufficient hyperpolarized ^{3}He at about 10 to 50% of the total amount. Considerably less ^{129}Xe is produced by similar means. During this time, the angular momentum of the laser light is transferred to the rubidium, which in turn transfers some of the polarization to the ^{3}He nuclei. Once polarized, cooled, and transferred to a delivery system, ^{3}He can be used for a variety of research purposes (Middleton, Black et al. 1995).

Hyperpolarized gases have interesting properties that are considerably different from protons in an equilibrium state. Firstly, the hyperpolarization of the gases outside the imaging magnet implies that the magnetic field strength of the imager is relatively unimportant to SNR, since it does not polarize the gas. Secondly, each application of an RF pulse to the hyperpolarized spin system represents a reduction in polarization by a certain amount, so there must be sufficient hyperpolarized gas present to survive multiple applications of RF pulses that are used for imaging. However, since there is no time required for repolarization by the static field, rapid imaging methods can be used. Thirdly, ^{3}He is a totally inert gas that is not soluble in blood, making it useful for ventilation studies, but not for angiography. ^{129}Xe, on the other hand, is soluble in blood, but is more difficult to polarize and very expensive. Fourthly, rapid diffusion in the gas phase tends to reduce the available image resolution.

Hyperpolarized ^{3}He and ^{129}Xe can have a nonequilibrium nuclear polarization that is substantially larger than the equilibrium polarization of protons in water in the body. This polarization has been described as being in the range of 10^4 to 10^5 larger, more than compensating for the greatly reduced spin density of the gases (Black, Middleton et al. 1996). The possibility of producing a SNR that is an order of magnitude larger than that expected with conventional imaging has been demonstrated in numerous studies. Additionally, the T1 of hyperpolarized gas is in the tens of seconds, permitting transport, manipulation, and delivery of these gases to subjects.

Typically, ^{3}He has been used in imaging lung tissues, which are exceedingly difficult to visualize with conventional MR imaging methods. The use of ^{3}He provides a major increase in available signal and has been demonstrated in structural images of lungs in animals and humans. These images have the spatial resolution of magnetic resonance imaging with the sensitivity of radioisotope ventilation scintigraphy, without the disadvantages of the latter. Hyperpolarized gas imaging eliminates or reduces many of the problems associated with lung imaging, including weak MR signals due to low tissue proton density, local susceptibility variations that result in very short T2* times and blurring due to physiological motion. Recently, dynamic imaging of lung function has been demonstrated that takes advantage of the superior SNR of ^{3}He in the lungs, while using innovative methods of data collection and controlled ventilation of animals to achieve an excellent demonstration of respiratory function (Viallon, Cofer et al. 1999). Lung air spaces have been studied with ^{3}He in humans to evaluate small airway disease in people who smoke or have allergies, while EPI has been evaluated for use in dynamic imaging of the lungs (de Lange, Mugler et al. 1999; Saam, Yablonskiy et al. 1999).

^{129}Xe work has been directed toward using this gas as both a lung ventilation agent and as an angiographic contrast agent, especially for neurovascular imaging. Due to its solubility in blood, dissolved ^{129}Xe produces a substantial chemical shift. This could provide the possibility of producing gas-phase images and soluble-phase ^{129}Xe images (Mugler, Driehuys et al. 1997). A difficulty with ^{129}Xe has been the delivery of enough polarization to the tissues to produce satisfactory images. However, more efficient polarization methods have been developed which overcome this problem, producing polarizations of 60% in a few hours. An additional consideration is that Xe has an anesthetic effect, so some subjects have experienced side effects similar to those found in persons recovering from surgical anesthesia.

6.6.7 Cardiac imaging

Cardiac MR imaging has been an area of active and continuous development since the inception of practical clinical MRI imaging. It is also one of the most challenging, both for system and technique development and for clinical interpretation. It has only been relatively recently, with improved imaging techniques, that considerable clinical interest in cardiac MRI has occurred. This has led equipment manufacturers to produce specially enhanced versions of their scanners that are optimized for high speed acquisition and processing needed to image the heart in a clinical setting. An example of a cardiac image is shown in Figure 6.37.

The heart is a complex moving organ, which presents great challenges to imaging with magnetic resonance methods. Additionally, many of the patients who are evaluated have sufficiently compromised cardiac and respiratory function that they cannot hold their breath for long, imposing another constraint on obtaining usable images.

Cardiac imaging has great appeal for answering important questions about cardiac function. The user wishes to know if coronary arteries are patent, if the cardiac muscle is adequately perfused, and if the tissue contracts properly in order to supply the needed amount of blood. In the case of ischemia, where the blood supply to the cardiac muscle has been reduced or cut off for a period, the clinician wants to know how much of the tissue is still alive and can be expected to function once the blood supply is restored. Other available imaging methods such as cardiac

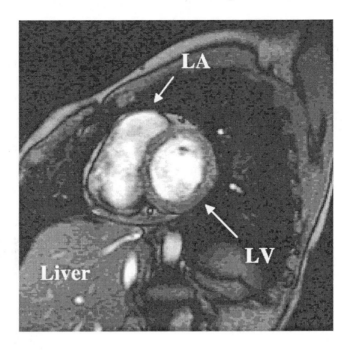

Thin-slice Oblique Gradient Echo Image

Figure 6.37: Cardiac image in an oblique orientation is positioned to demonstrate the left atrium and ventricle. This is part of a series collected using rapid gradient echo methods to produce a cine presentation, which shows the heart's contractions when played back as a movie. This image is heavily T1-weighted and was acquired without a contrast agent.

catheterization have associated limitations and risks that are mostly eliminated by using magnetic resonance imaging (McVeigh, 1997).

Coronary artery imaging is an often-sought goal of cardiac imaging. Because of the size and location of the coronary arteries, this aspect of cardiac imaging has been difficult to implement with a satisfactory clinical presentation. Many investigators have demonstrated coronary artery segments in images, but without any real clinical utility of the images. Coronary arteries are small, sinuous, and embedded in a layer of fat next to a large muscle mass. Furthermore, they are constantly moving, due to the mechanical motion of the heart as well as respiratory motion. Thus, thin sections taken in multiple oblique positions with fat suppression at high speeds are required for successful imaging along sections of the vessel (Axel, 1993).

Motion of the heart is typically addressed in one of two ways: cardiac gating and high speed imaging. With cardiac gating, the electrocardiogram is monitored and used to trigger acquisition during a phase of the cardiac cycle during which motion is minimized. The sequence acquires part of an image with each detected beat. Quiescent time periods during the sequence can be used to acquire data from other slices of the heart. This approach is called prospective gating and has been used with spin echo pulse sequences to produce images of the heart at various stages of the cardiac cycle. Retrospective gating, where gradient echo imaging is performed without regard to the cardiac cycle, has also been used. With this technique, cardiac timing information is also recorded. After collection of all of the image data, post-processing software is used to produce images computed from the original data, reflecting the position of the cardiac chambers at particular parts of the cardiac cycle. While the approach using cardiac gating provides good images, it can extend the acquisition time significantly. Extended acquisition times provide greater opportunities for the patient to move.

Current cardiac MRI is able to make use of high speed imaging techniques that are available on many commercial systems. These techniques include EPI sequences and turboFLASH methods, where whole images are collected during quiescent phases of the cardiac cycle during a single heartbeat (Slavin, Riederer *et al.* 1998). Other widely used methods employ gradient echo sequences so that a few lines of k-space are collected for several heart beats until enough information for image reconstruction is collected. This approach has been called the segmented k-space technique, first introduced in the early 1990s (Adkinson, Edelman, 1991). Collection of the data occurs at diastole to minimize motion and ensure that the heart is in nearly the same position during each collection. Since a relatively small number of beats produces enough information for reconstructing images, the collection can occur during a single breath-hold. Three-dimensional data sets can be acquired using a multiple breath-hold approach, although not all patients can tolerate holding their breath.

Another approach to rapid acquisition for cardiac work uses spiral scanning methods (Kerr, Pauly *et al.* 1997). Here, the gradient system is used to scan k-space in a spiral fashion for each RF pulse so that all of k-space is represented along a path that begins in the center of k-space and spirals out. Multiple acquisitions of RF over several heartbeats provide enough spiral k-space trajectories to describe k-space adequately. The biggest problem with this approach is that the data are in non-Cartesian coordinates, so reconstruction requires regridding of the data into an x, y-coordinate system prior to application of the conventional Fourier transform. The great advantage of this method is that it is very efficient in covering k-space, so it is very useful for cardiac imaging (Axel, 1993). Newly reported techniques move from multiple image 2D methods to fully three dimensional acquisitions that improve on the through-plane resolution (cross-talk) suffered by 2D methods. Segmented k-space 3D spiral sequences using gradient echo methods with innovative spherical stacking of spiral trajectories can produce excellent images of the coronary blood vessels using multiple breath-holds or motion compensation techniques (Thedens, Irarrazaval *et al.* 1999).

Other approaches to cardiac imaging are aimed at providing a quantitative evaluation of cardiac function by monitoring cardiac wall motion. The methods used (McVeigh, 1996) depend on presaturation tagging in patterns imposed on the heart or velocity encoded phase maps for defining the motion of the ventricular walls.

With these techniques, resting and stress evaluation of regional wall motion abnormalities is feasible and clinically useful.

Cardiac motion determination by cardiac tagging uses a three-stage process. The tissue is "marked" by placement of saturation bands using spatially selective RF pulses. Numerous saturation patterns have been developed and are described in the literature. This is followed by acquisition of a sequence of images in which the motion of the saturation bands is apparent. The motion of the saturation bands is used to compute the motion of the myocardium, leading to evaluation of the stress on the muscle at various times during the cardiac cycle. These bands are typically matched to the type of motion that is to be studied. The tagged images can provide estimates of the strain tensor at each point in the myocardium for each point in time during the cardiac cycle, yielding a wealth of quantitative information about the local behavior of the myocardium during contraction (McVeigh, 1996).

Cardiac motion can also be followed using velocity encoding methods. The velocity of the transverse magnetization is followed and encoded as phase changes obtained using bipolar motion-encoding gradient pulses. These methods are more susceptible to motion artifacts compared to tagging, but do not suffer from tag fading due to T1 recovery, as can occur with tagging sequences. In this approach at least four different acquisitions are required from which the 3D velocity vector at each pixel in the image can be found. Four acquisitions are needed because this approach uses image differences to compute velocity gradients in the myocardium after the removal of bulk translations and rotations, which cause significant phase shifts in the velocity-encoded images. Analysis is by means of the 3D trajectory of each point in the heart obtained by integrating the observed velocities or by directly finding the strain tensor from spatial gradients in the velocity field (McVeigh, 1996).

Functional cardiac studies produce information that is used to create models of the heart during the cardiac cycle. Among the parameters related to ventricular function that can be found are radial thickening and circumferential shortening. These changes can be formed into processed maps showing reconstructions of the left ventricle indicating thinning of the wall in the presence of infarct damage. Other types of maps and presentations are possible along with computation of eigenvectors and eigenvalues of the strain tensor (McVeigh, 1996).

6.7 Conclusions: What does the future hold?

The future uses of MRI are likely to be many and varied. As equipment improves, pulse sequences and acquisition techniques that were not possible previously will move into routine clinical use. Many of these techniques will be based on ultra-fast imaging methods such as EPI, which can provide near-real-time imaging. fMRI techniques will be refined for use not only as a tool to study the brain, but also for clinical purposes. Cardiac MRI will see continuing refinements, so that it will become the study of choice for many types of qualitative and quantitative evaluations of ventricular function. Additionally, improvements in coronary angiography will approach the goal of completely noninvasive evaluation of blood flow to the heart. Vascular imaging techniques will provide greater accuracy along with noninvasive quantitative flow measurements for clinical use. A very exciting area is the increasing use of MRI to guide probes during surgical procedures, as well as to provide imaging for biopsies. The integration of MR imaging and MR spectroscopy in clinical instruments will continue to gain acceptance for clinical applications, especially for the evaluation of tumors and of the results of treatment. New techniques such as the use of hyperpolarized gases for imaging will become valuable aids to clinical protocols for the evaluation of lungs and for perfusion studies.

While many of the advances and future uses of MR imaging are likely to be refinements of ongoing developments, there are strong possibilities that totally new developments will further enhance the capabilities of MRI. As the CT scanner before it, MRI is increasingly a required and highly important imaging capability for hospitals of all sizes. Newer instruments will be easier to install and operate and will have capabilities that equal or exceed the best currently available equipment. The availability of higher fields and high-performance gradient systems associated with the high field systems is likely to bring new and exciting areas of research due to SNR improvements. Low field systems for specialized applications will continue to provide new capabilities to sites that cannot afford or don't need high-performance superconducting systems. Accompanying all of these developments are the improvements in computer processing. Real-time rendering of three-dimensional images with interaction capabilities and new display paradigms are likely to be among the developments that will become available in this exciting field of medical imaging (Glover, Herfkens, 1998).

References

Adkinson D. "Improved MR Agiography: Magnetization Transfer Suppression with Variable Flip Angle Excitation and Increased Resolution." Radiology 190:890, 1994.

Adkinson DJ, Edelman RR. "Cineagiography of the Heart in a Single Breathhold with a Segmented TurboFlash Sequence." Radiology 178:357–360, 1991.

Axel L. "Cardiac Imaging." In Bronskill M, Sprawls P (Eds.) *The Physics of MRI: 1992 AAPM Summer School Proceedings*. Woodbury, NY: American Institute of Physics, Inc., 1993, pp. 371–382.

Baird AE, Warach S. "Magnetic Resonance Imaging of Acute Stroke." Journal of Cerebral Blood Flow and Metabolism 18(6):583–609, 1998.

Birn RM, Donahue KM *et al.* "Magnetic Resonance Imaging: Principles, Pulse Sequences, and Functional Imaging." In Hendee WR (Ed.) *Biomedical Uses of Radiation*. Weinheim, NY: Wiley-VCH, 1999, Part A, pp. 481–548.

Black RD, Middleton HL *et al.* "In Vivo He-3 MR Images of Guinea Pig Lungs." Radiology 1999:867–870, 1996.

Block F, Hansen WW *et al.* "Nuclear Induction." Phys Rev 69:127, 1946.

Bottomley PA, Foster TH *et al.* "A Review of Normal Tissue Hydrogen NMR Relaxation Times and Relaxation Mechanisms from 1–100 MHz: Dependence on

Tissue Type, NMR Frequency, Temperature, Species, Excision, and Age." Med Phys 11(4):425–448, 1984.

Bradley WG. "Optimizing Lesion Contrast without Using Contrast Agents." J Magn Reson Imaging 10:442–449, 1999.

Braver TS, Cohen JD *et al.* "A Parametric Study of Prefrontal Cortex Involvement in Human Working Memory." Neruoimage 5:49–62, 1997.

Bronskill MJ, Graham S. "NMR Characteristics of Tissue." In Bronskill M, Sprawls P. (Eds.) *The Physics of MRI: 1992 AAPM Summer School Proceedings.* Woodbury, NY: American Institute of Physics, Inc., 1999, Monograph 21.

Brooks RA, Di Chiro G. "Principles of Computer Assisted Tomography (CAT) in Radiographic and Radioisotopic Imaging." Physics in Medicine & Biology 21(5):689–732, 1976.

Bushberg, JT, Seibert JA *et al. The Essential Physics of Medical Imaging.* Baltimore: Williams & Wilkins, 1994.

Callaghan PT. *Principles of Nulcear Magnetic Resonance Microscopy.* Oxford: Clarendon Press, 1991.

Cramer SC, Finklestein SP *et al.* "Activation of Distinct Motor Cortex Regions During Ipsilateral and Contralateral Finger Movements." J Neurophysiol 81:383–387, 1999.

de Lange EE, Mugler JPI *et al.* "Lung Air Spaces: MR Imaging Evaluation with Hyperpoloarized 3He Gas." Radiology 210:851–857, 1999.

Desmond JE, Gabrieli JDE *et al.* "Lobular Patterns of Cerebellar Activation in Verbal Working-Memory and Finger-Tapping Tasks as Revealed by Functional MRI." J Neuroscience 17(24):9675–9685, 1997.

Edelstein WA, Hutchinson JMS *et al.* "Spin-Warp NMR Imaging and Applications to Human Whole-Body Imaging." Phys Med Biol 25:751–756, 1980.

Fukushima E, Roeder SBW. *Experimental Pulse NMR: A Nuts and Bolts Approach.* Reading, MA: Addison-Wesley Publishing Company, Inc., 1981.

Glover GH, Herfkens RJ. "Research Directions in MR Imaging." Radiology 207:289–295, 1998.

Glover GH, Pauly JM. "Projection Reconstruction Techniques for Reduction of Motion Effects in MRI." Magn Reson Med 28:275–289, 1992.

Gore JC, Majumdar S. "Measurement of Tissue Blood Flow Using Intravascular Relaxation Agents and Magnetic Resonsonance Imaging." Magn Reson Med 14:242–248, 1990.

Haake EM, Brown RW *et al. Magnetic Resonance Imaging: Practical Principles and Sequence Design.* New York: Wiley-Liss, 1999.

Hahn EL. "Spin Echos." Physical Review 80(4):580–594, 1950.

Hennig J, Naureth A *et al.* "RARE Imaging: A Fast Imaging Method for Clinical MR." Magn Reson Med 3:823–833, 1986.

Herman GT. *Image Reconstructions from Projections: The Fundamentals of Computerized Tomography.* New York: Academic Press, 1980.

Ishai A, Ungerleider LG *et al.* "Distributed Representation of Objects in the Human Ventral Visual Pathway." Proc Natl Acad Sci USA 96(August):9379–9384, 1999.

Jones DK, Horsfield MA *et al.* "Optimal Strategies for Measuring Diffusion in Anisotropic Systems by Magnetic Resonance Imaging." Magn Reson Med 42:515–525, 1999.

Kerr AB, Pauly JM *et al.* "Real-Time Interactive MRI on a Conventional Scanner." Magn Reson Med 38:355–367, 1997.

Kumar A, Welti D *et al.* "NMR Fourier Zeugmatography." J Magn Reson 18:69–83, 1975.

Lauterbur P. "Image Formation by Indued Local Interactions: Examples Employing Nuclear Magnetic Resonance." Nature 242(March 16):190–191, 1973.

Le Bihan D, Basser PJ. "Chapter 1: Molecular Diffusion and Nuclear Magnetic Resonance." In Le Bihan D (Ed.) *Diffusion and Perfusion Magnetic Resonance Imaging: Applications to Functional MRI.* New York: Raven Press, 1995.

Le Bihan D, Breton E *et al.* "MR Imaging of Intravoxel Incoherent Motions: Application to Diffusion and Perfusion in Neurologic disorders." Radiology 161:401–407, 1986.

MacFall JR. *Hardware and Coils For MR Imaging.* Categorical Course in Physics: The Basic Physics of MR Imaging. Chicago: Radiological Society of North America, 1997.

Mansfield P, Morris PG. *NMR Imaging in Biomedicine.* New York: Academic Press, 1982.

Mattay VS, Callicott JH *et al.* "Hemispheric Control of Motor Function: A Whole Brain Echo Planar fMRI Study." Neuroimaging 83:7–22, 1998.

McVeigh ER. "MRI of Myocardial Function: Motion Tracking Techniques." Magnetic Resonance Imaging 14(2):137–150, 1996.

McVeigh ER. *Cardiac MR Imaging.* Categorical Course in Physics: The Basic Physics of MR Imaging. Chicago: Radiological Society of North America, 1997.

Menon RS, Luknowsky DC *et al.* "Mental Chronometry Using Latency-Resolved Functional MRI." Proc Natl Acad Sci USA 95:10902–10907, 1998.

Merboldt KD, Hankicke W *et al.* "Self-Diffusion NMR Imaging Using Stimulated Echos." J Magn Reson 64:479–486, 1985.

Middleton H, Black RD *et al.* "MR Imaging with Hyperpolarized 3He Gas." Magn Reson Med 33:271–275, 1995.

Mitchell DG. *MRI Principles.* Philadelphia: W. B. Saunders Company, 1999.

Mugler JP, Driehuys B *et al.* "MR Imaging and Spectroscopy Using Hyperpolarized ^{129}Xe Gas: Preliminary Human Results." Mag Res Med 37:809–815, 1997.

Ogawa S, Lee TM *et al.* "Oxygenation Setnsitive Contrast in Magnetic Resonance Imaging of Rodent Brain at High Magnetic Fields." Magn Reson Med 14:68–78, 1990.

Purcell EM, Torrey HC *et al.* "Resonance Absorption by Nuclear Magnetic Moments in a Solid." Phys Rev 69:37, 1946.

Rabi II. "The Molecular Beam Resonance Method for Measuring Nuclearmagnetic Moments." Phys Rev 55:526, 1939.

Riddle WR, Lee H. "Magnetic Resonance: Principles and Spectroscopy." In Hendee WR (Ed.) *Biomedical Uses of Radiation.* Weinheim, NY: Wiley-VCH, 1999, Part A, pp. 421–476.

Rosen BR, Belliveau JW *et al.* "Perfusion Imaging with NMR Contrast Agents." Mag Res Med 14:249–265, 1990.

Saam B, Yablonskiy DA *et al.* "Rapid Imaging of Hyperpolarized Gas Using EPI." Magn Reson Med 42:507–514, 1999.

Schenck JF. "Radiofrequency Coils: Types and Characteristics." In Bronskill MJ, Sprawl P (Eds.) *The Physics of MRI: 1992 AAPM Summer School Proceedings.* Woodbury, NY: The American Institute of Physics, Inc., 1993, pp. 98–134.

Semelka RC, Kelekis NL *et al.* "HASTE MR Imaging: Description of Technique." J Magn Reson Imag 6(4):698–699, 1996.

Slavin GS, Riederer SJ *et al.* "Two-Dimensional Multishot Echo-Planar Coronary MR Angiography." Mag Res Med 40:883–889, 1998.

Stejskal E, Tanner J. "Spin Diffusion Measurements: Spin Echos in the Presence of Time-Dependent Field Gradient." Journal of Chemical Physics 42:288–292, 1965.

Thedens DR, Irarrazaval P *et al.* "Fast Magnetic Resonance Coronary Angiography with a Three-Dimensional Stack of Spirals Trajectory." Magn Reson Med 41:1170–1179, 1999.

Thomas SR. "Magnets and Gradient Coils: Types and Characteristics." In Bronskill MJ, Sprawls P (Eds.) *The Physics of MRI: 1992 AAPM Summer School Proceedings.* Woodbury, NY: The American Institute of Phyiscs, Inc., 1993, pp. 56–97.

van Geldereen P, de Vleeshouwer MHM *et al.* "Water Diffusion and Acute Stroke." Magn Reson Med 31:154–163, 1994.

Viallon M, Cofer GP *et al.* "Functional MR Microscopy of the Lung Using Hyperpolarized 3He." Magn Reson Med 41:787–792, 1999.

Wesby GE, Moseley ME *et al.* "Translational Molecular Self-Diffusion in Magnetic Resonance Imaging: Effects and Applications." Investigative Radiology 19(6):391–498, 1984.

CHAPTER 7
Three-Dimensional Ultrasound Imaging

Aaron Fenster, Donal B. Downey
The John P. Robarts Research Institute and
the University of Western Ontario

CONTENTS

7.1 Introduction

The discovery of x rays over 100 years ago heralded a new way of visualizing the human body. The use of x rays produces a radiographic shadow in a two-dimensional image of the three-dimensional (3D) structures within the body. Although this imaging approach is extremely useful and is still in use today, all three-dimensional information is lost to the physician. Many attempts have been made to develop imaging techniques in which three-dimensional information within the body was preserved in a recorded image. In the early 1970s, the introduction of CT revolutionized diagnostic radiology. For the first time, three-dimensional information was presented to the physician as a series of tomographic, two-dimensional (2D) image slices of the body. In addition, for the first time in radiology, computers became central in the processing and display of the images. The availability of true 3D anatomical information stimulated the field of 3D visualization for a variety of applications in diagnostic radiology [1–3].

The history of ultrasound imaging is much more recent than x-ray imaging. Following the pioneering work of Wild and Reid [4] in the 50's, the medical use of ultrasound progressed slowly. A-mode systems, producing oscilloscope traces of acoustic reflections, preceded systems producing B-mode grey-scale images of the anatomy, which was followed by systems producing real-time tomographic images of the anatomy and blood flow. The image quality of medical ultrasound has advanced from low-resolution, bi-stable images to images with much greater detail, making ultrasound an important and often indispensable imaging modality in disease diagnosis and obstetrics. Because it is not invasive and because of the improved image quality, and the addition of blood flow and perfusion information by means of the Doppler effect, ultrasonography is progressively achieving a greater role in radiology, cardiology, and in image-guided surgery and therapy. The major advantages of ultrasound imaging are:

- The ultrasound transducer is small and easily manipulated, allowing the generation of real-time tomographic images at orientations and positions controlled by the user.

- The ultrasound image has sufficient resolution (0.2 mm to 2.0 mm) to display details of many structures within the body.

- The ultrasound imaging system is inexpensive, compact, and mobile.

- Ultrasound imaging can provide real-time images of blood velocity and flow, allowing the physician to map vascular structures ranging in size from arteries to angiogenic tumour vessels.

In spite of these very important advantages, ultrasound imaging still suffers from several limitations, which academic investigators and imaging companies are addressing. In this chapter, we discuss a recent technological advance in ultrasonography achieving rapid growth—the development of 3D ultrasound imaging.

7.2 Limitations of ultrasonography addressed by 3D imaging

Many limitations of ultrasound imaging relate to fundamental physical aspects of the interaction of ultrasound with tissues and the detection of the ultrasound echoes. The development of ultrasound contrast agents addresses these limitations. Limitations related to resolution and noise are being addressed with improved transducers and image speckle reduction approaches. These advances will significantly improve ultrasound imaging, making it useful in treatment planning. Three-dimensional ultrasonography development discussed below will also be enhanced by these two areas of advancement and will have a wide range of clinical applications.

The development of 3D ultrasound addresses the subjectivity of the conventional ultrasound exam. In conventional 2D ultrasonography, an experienced diagnostician manipulates the ultrasound transducer, mentally transforms the 2D images into a lesion or anatomical volume, and makes the diagnosis or performs an interventional procedure. This approach is suboptimal primarily because a spatially flexible 2D imaging technique is used to view 3D anatomy/pathology. This is particularly important in interventional procedures such as brachytherapy, cryosurgery, or biopsy, as the process of quantifying and monitoring small changes during the procedure is severely limited by the 2D restrictions of conventional ultrasound imaging. Specifically, 3D ultrasound imaging addresses the following limitations:

- Conventional ultrasound images are two-dimensional. Therefore, the diagnostician must mentally transform multiple tomographic images to form a 3D impression of the anatomy/pathology during the diagnostic examination, or during an image guided interventional procedure. This process is not only time-consuming and inefficient, but more important, variable and subjective, which may lead to incorrect decisions in diagnosis, planning, and delivering the therapy.

- Diagnostic (e.g., obstetrics) and therapeutic decisions (staging and planning) often require accurate estimation of organ or tumor volume. Current ultrasound volume measurement techniques use only simple measures of the width in two views and assume an idealized shape to calculate volume. This practice potentially leads to inaccuracy and operator variability.

- It is difficult to place the 2D image plane at a particular location within an organ, and even more difficult to find the same location again later. Thus, 2D ultrasound is ill-suited for planning or monitoring therapeutic procedures, or for performing quantitative prospective or follow-up studies.

- Because of the restrictions imposed by the patient's anatomy or position, it is sometimes impossible to orient the 2D transducer to the optimal image plane. Visualization of the anatomy is hindered, preventing accurate diagnosis of the patient's condition and monitoring of interventional procedures.

The goal of 3D ultrasound imaging is to overcome these limitations. Three-dimensional imaging will provide the diagnostician or therapist a more complete view of the anatomy, thereby reducing the variability of conventional ultrasound techniques.

Medical ultrasound imaging is inherently tomographic, providing information that is necessary for reconstructing and visualizing 3D images. However, unlike CT and MR imaging, in which the images are usually acquired at a slow rate as a stack of parallel slices, ultrasound provides tomographic images at a high rate (15–60 images per second), and the orientation of the images is arbitrary and under the user control. The high rate of image acquisition, the arbitrary orientation of the images, and the unique problems imposed by ultrasound image speckle, shadowing, and distortions, provide unique problems to overcome, and opportunities to be exploited in extending ultrasound imaging from its 2D presentation of images to 3D and time varying 3D (or 4D).

Over the past two decades, many investigators have focused their efforts on the development of various types of 3D imaging techniques by taking advantage of ultrasound imaging positioning flexibility and data acquisition speed [5–11]. These approaches have focused on reconstructing a 3D image by integrating transducer position information with the 2D ultrasound image. However, because of the enormous demands on the computers needed to produce near-real-time and low-cost systems, most attempts did not succeed. It is only in the last few years that computer technology and visualization techniques have progressed sufficiently to make 3D ultrasound imaging viable. Review articles describing progress in the development of 3D ultrasound imaging for use in radiology and echocardiology have been published in the past few years [6, 8, 11–16]. These articles provide extensive lists of references and show that there have been numerous attempts at producing 3D ultrasound systems by many investigators.

In this chapter, we review the various approaches that investigators have pursued in the development of 3D ultrasound imaging systems. We describe the systems and their operation, show example images demonstrating their use, and report on the performance of these systems.

7.3 Three-dimensional ultrasound scanning techniques

7.3.1 Introduction

Except for the development of 2D arrays for direct 3D ultrasound imaging, all the approaches made use of conventional 1D ultrasound transducers producing 2D ultrasound images. However, the major differences in the various 3D ultrasound imaging approaches came from the specific methods used to locate the position of ultrasound image slice within the volume under investigation. Producing high-quality 3D images without distortions requires that the ultrasound transducer's position is known accurately and precisely. Clearly, the choice of the technique used to locate the transducers's position for 3D imaging is crucial in producing an accurate representation of the anatomy.

In general, current 3D ultrasound imaging systems are based on commercially available transducers whose position is accurately controlled by a mechanical device or monitored by a position sensing device. Position data may be obtained from stepping motors in the transducer's scan head, a translation or rotation mechanical device, or a position and orientation sensor that may be electromagnetic, acoustic, or mechanical. Depending on the type of scanning technique used, the 2D images may be arranged in the pattern of a wedge, a series of parallel slices, a cone obtained by rotation around a central axis, or in arbitrary orientations. These approaches are discussed in detail in the subsequent sections.

To produce 3D images without distortions, three factors must be considered and optimized. First, the scanning technique must be rapid or gated to avoid artifacts that result from involuntary, respiratory, or cardiac motion. Second, the locations and orientations of the acquired 2D images must be known accurately and the devices used must be calibrated correctly to avoid geometric distortions and measurement errors. Third, the scanning technique must be easy to use so that it does not interfere with the patient exam or be inconvenient to use. Four different approaches have been pursued: mechanical scanners, free-hand scanning with location sensing, free-hand scanning without location sensing, and 2D arrays.

7.3.2 Mechanical scanning devices

In this scanning approach, a series of 2D images is recorded rapidly while the conventional transducer is moved over the anatomy using a variety of mechanical motorized techniques. Because mechanical means are used to move the conventional transducer over the anatomy in a precise predefined manner, the relative position and angulation of each 2D image can be accurately known, avoiding geometric distortions and inaccuracies. Thus, when the transducer is moved, the 2D images generated by the ultrasound machine are acquired at predefined spatial or angular intervals.

Before efficient, high-speed computer-based image digitizers were readily available, the 2D images were stored on videotape for later processing. However, with current computer technology, the images are either stored in their original digital format in the ultrasound system's computer memory, or the video output from the ultrasound machine is digitized immediately and stored in an external computer memory. Either the ultrasound machine's computer or an external computer reconstructs the 3D image using the predefined geometric information, which relates the digitized 2D images to each other. The angular or spatial interval between the digitized 2D images is pre-computed and is usually made adjustable to minimize the scanning time while optimally sampling the volume.

Various mechanical scanning approaches are available, requiring that the conventional transducer be mounted in a special mechanical assembly and made to rotate or translate by a motor. Mechanical assemblies used in 3D scanning can vary in size from small integrated 3D probes that house the mechanism within the transducer housing, to ones employing an external fixture to house the ultrasound transducer.

The integrated mechanical scanning 3D probes are usually easy for the operator to use. However, they are larger and heavier than conventional probes, and require the purchase of a special ultrasound machine that can interface to them. The external fixtures are generally bulkier than the integrated probes, but they can be adapted to any conventional ultrasound machine's transducers, obviating the need to purchase a special purpose 3D ultrasound machine. Thus, improvements in image quality and developments of new imaging techniques (e.g., Doppler power) by the ultrasound machine manufacturers can also be achieved in 3D. In addition, because the external fixture can house a transducer from any ultrasound machine, the 3D capability is available in conjunction with most ultrasound machines in a department.

Investigators and commercial companies have developed different types of mechanical assemblies used to produce 3D images. These can be divided into three basic types of motion, as shown schematically in Figures 7.1, 7.3, 7.4 and 7.6: linear, tilt, and rotation.

7.3.2.1 Linear 3D scanning

In this approach, the transducer is translated linearly over the patient's skin, so that the 2D images are parallel to each other. This is accomplished by mounting the conventional transducer in an assembly that houses a motor and drive mechanism as shown in Figure 7.1(a). When the motor is activated, the drive mechanism moves the transducer with a motion that is parallel to the skin surface. The 2D images are acquired at regular spatial intervals that sample the anatomy appropriately. Alternatively, the 2D images can be acquired at regular temporal intervals (e.g., 30 images per second), so that a regular spatial interval will be obtained when the linear translation velocity is constant. The ability to vary the sampling interval is necessary to allow imaging of the anatomy in 3D with a sampling interval that is appropriate for the particular elevational resolution of the transducer.

Because the set of 2D images are parallel to each other (see Figure 7.1(b)) with a known spatial sampling interval, many of the parameters required for the reconstruction can be pre-computed and the reconstruction time can be shortened. A 3D image can be obtained immediately after performing a linear scan [17].

Although the resolution in the 3D image is not isotropic, the simplicity of the scanning motion makes interpretation of the 3D image more easily understood. In the planes of the 3D image corresponding to the original 2D images, the resolution will be unchanged. Because of the poor elevational resolution of the transducer, the resolution in the scanning direction will be worst. Thus, for optimal resolution, a transducer with good elevational resolution should be used.

Vascular ultrasound imaging relies on the Doppler effect to measure the velocity of blood. This technique has been extended to imaging of flowing blood in the vasculature by either color coding the velocity or the reflected power in the Doppler signal. Three-dimensional imaging using the linear scanning approach has been used successfully in many vascular imaging applications using B-mode, color Doppler imaging of the carotid arteries [18–23], tumor vascularity [24–27],

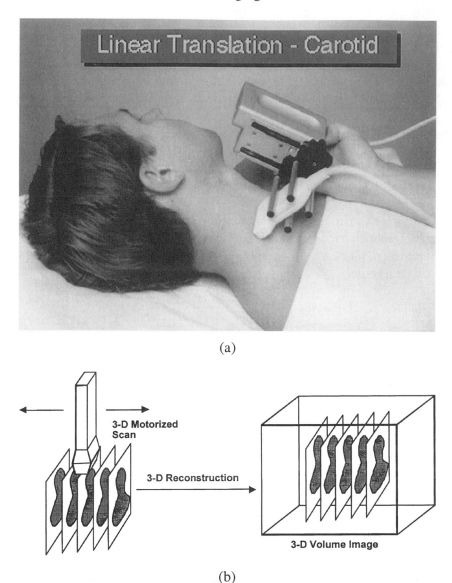

(a)

(b)

Figure 7.1: (a) Photograph of a linear scanning mechanical assembly being used to image the carotid arteries. (b) Schematic diagram showing the linear scanning approach, in which a series of parallel 2D images are collected and used to reconstruct the 3D image.

test phantoms [20, 28], and Doppler power imaging [18, 20, 26]. For a detailed discussion of ultrasound imaging techniques see an example of the linear scanning approach with an external fixture is shown in Figure 7.2. Beyond these applications, the utility of linear scanning in echocardiology has also been proved in cardiology using a transesophageal approach with a horizontal scanning plane and pull-back of the probe [29–31].

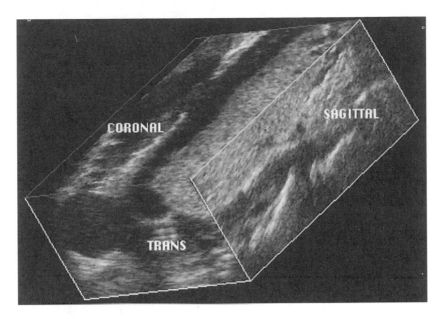

Figure 7.2: 3D image of a patient's thyroid. The image has been "sliced" to reveal the coronal, sagittal, and transaxial views of the thyroid using the multi-planar reformatting visualization approach.

7.3.2.2 Tilt 3D scanning

In this scanning geometry, the transducer is tilted by the mechanical assembly about an axis that is parallel to the face of the transducer as shown in Figure 7.3(a). The tilting axis can be either at the face of the transducer, producing a set of 2D images that intersect at the face, or above the transducer axis, causing the set of 2D planes to intersect above the skin. This type of motion has been carried out with an external fixture as well as an integrated 3D probe approach. In either case, this approach allows the transducer face or the 3D probe housing to be placed at a single location on the patient's skin. In the external fixture approach, motor activation causes the transducer to pivot on the point of contact of the skin (Figure 7.3(b)). The integrated 3D probe approach allows the housing to be placed against the skin, while the transducer is tilted and slides against the housing to produce an angular sweep (Figure 7.3(c)).

This process of acquiring the 2D images at constant angular intervals during the tilting motion, results in the storage of a set of 2D image planes arranged in fan-like geometry. This approach can sweep out a large region of interest with variable predefined angular separation as shown in the 3D image of the prostate in Figures 7.4 and 7.5, and other imaging applications [19, 32–36].

The 3D tilting scanning approach lends itself to compact designs for both integrated 3D probes and external fixtures. Kretztechnik (Zipf, Austria) and Aloka (Korea) have developed special 3D ultrasound systems with integrated 3D probes for use in abdominal and obstetrical imaging. Life Imaging Systems Inc. (Lon-

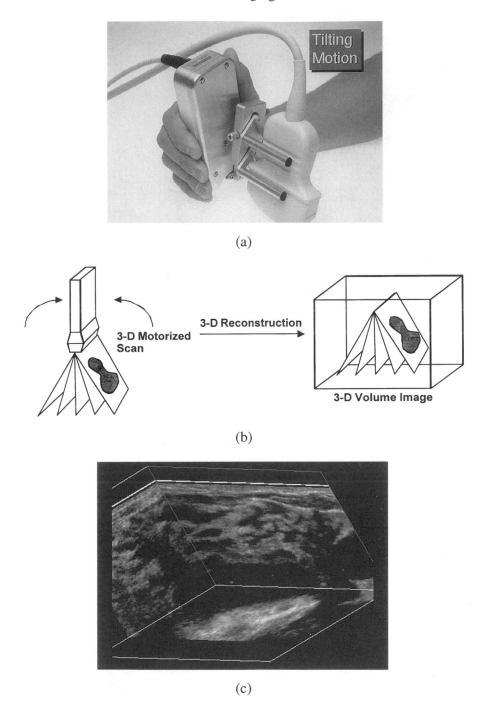

Figure 7.3: (a) Photograph of a tilt scanning mechanical assembly with a curvilinear transducer in place. (b) Schematic diagram showing the tilting scanning approach, in which a
series of 2D images are collected as the transducer is tilted and then reconstructed into a
3D image. (c) 3D image of a patient with a poly-cystic breast. The image was obtained using
the tilt scanning approach.

don, Canada) has demonstrated an external fixture assembly for use in abdominal imaging that can couple to any manufacturer's ultrasound machine.

The tilt scanning approach can also be used with endocavity transducers, such as transesophageal (TE) and transrectal (TRUS) transducers (Figure 7.4). In this approach, a side-firing linear transducer array is used with either the external fixture or integrated 3D probe. When the motor is activated, the transducer rotates about its long axis while 2D images are acquired. After a rotation of about 80° to 110°, the

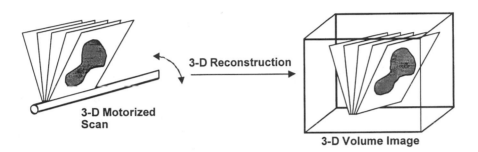

Figure 7.4: Schematic diagram of the tilt scanning approach used with a side-firing transrectal transducer. This approach is being used to produce 3D images of the prostate.

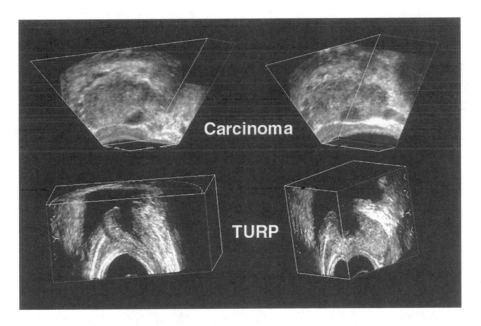

Figure 7.5: Three-dimensional images of the prostate. The top two images were obtained with the tilt scanning approach using a side-firing transrectal transducer. The image has been "sliced" to reveal a tumor (dark lesion) and its relationship to the seminal vesicle. The bottom two images were obtained with the rotational approach using a end-firing transrectal transducer. The 3D prostate image has been "sliced" to display the TURP (trans-urethral resection procedure) deficit.

acquired 2D images are arranged in fan-like geometry similar to that obtained with the tilting scan used for abdominal imaging. This approach is successful in prostate imaging (see Figure 7.5) [18, 19, 26, 37, 38] and 3D ultrasound guided cryosurgery [17, 39–41] and has been commercialized by Life Imaging Systems Inc. (London, Canada). TomTec Inc. (Munich, Germany) has demonstrated application of this approach in echocardiology by using a TE transducer, in which the imaging plane is vertical (i.e., parallel to the axis of the probe). The probe was rotated by an external motor assembly with the axis of rotation along the central axis of the probe [12, 42].

The main advantage of the tilt scanning approach is that the scanning mechanism can be made compact to allow easy hand-held manipulation. In addition, using a suitable choice of scanning angle and angular interval, the scanning time can be made short. With reduced resolution, Aloka has exhibited the acquisition of three volumes per second. However, with a typical angular interval of 1° or less and a scanning angle of about 90°, the scanning time can range from three seconds to nine, depending on the number of focal zones and depth of the imaging field. Because the set of planes is acquired in a predefined geometry, again, many of the geometric parameters can be precalculated, allowing immediate 3D reconstructions.

As with the tilt scanning approach, the resolution will not be isotropic. Because of the fan-like geometry of the acquired 2D images, the distance between acquired planes will increase with depth. Near the transducer, the sampling distance will be small, while far from the transducer the distance will be large. The change in sampling distance with depth can be made to match approximately the elevational resolution degradation of 2D ultrasound transducers with depth. Nonetheless, the resulting resolution in the 3D image will be worse in the scan (tilting) direction, because of the combined effects of elevational resolution and sampling, and will degrade with distance from the transducer because of beam divergence.

7.3.2.3 Rotational 3D scanning

In this scanning geometry, a motor rotates the transducer array by more than 180° around an axis that is perpendicular to the array and bisects it as shown in Figure 7.6. The rotational scanning approach allows the axis of rotation to remain fixed as the transducer rotates, causing the acquired images to sweep out a conical volume in a propeller-like fashion. As with the tilting mechanical scanning approach, the angular rotational interval between acquired 2D images is adjustable and remains fixed during the scan, resulting in a set of acquired 2D images arranged as shown in Figure 7.6. Also similar to the tilting scanning approach, rotational scanning can be implemented using both the external fixture, and the integrated 3D probe approach.

The rotational scanning approach causes the images to intersect along the central rotational axis, with the highest spatial sampling near this axis and the poorest away from it. The combined effects of the changing sampling with distance from the axis of rotation and the changing elevational resolution with depth will cause

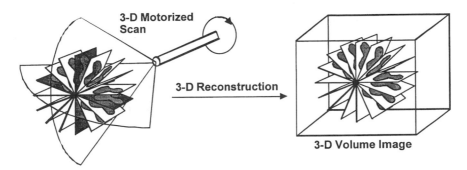

Figure 7.6: Schematic diagram of the rotational scanning approach used with a end-firing transrectal transducer. This approach has been used in gynaecological imaging and to produce 3D images of the prostate.

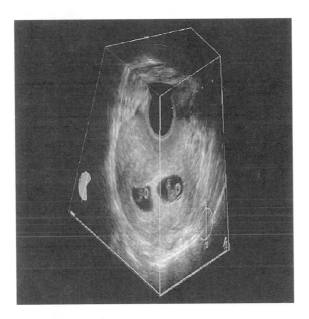

Figure 7.7: Three-dimensional image of a pregnant uterus with twins. The image has been "sliced" to reveal the two gestational sacs. This image was obtained by means of the rotational scanning approach using an end-firing endovaginal transducer.

the resolution in the 3D image to vary in a complicated manner. The resolution will be highest nearer to the transducer, and will degrade farther from the transducer because of both axial and elevational resolution degradation in the original 2D images. In addition, improper angular sampling may impose additional resolution degradation away from the central scanning axis.

This approach has been used successfully for transrectal imaging of the prostate and endovaginal imaging (Figure 7.7). Downey reported on the use of rotational scanning for imaging the prostate with 200 images (320×320 pixels each) acquired in 13 seconds over a 200° angular sweep [26]. Imaging of the heart, using a multiplane transesophageal transducer, has been demonstrated by other investigators [7, 43, 45].

Because the acquired images intersect along the rotational axis in the center of the volume, any motion of the axis of rotation or of the patient during the acquisition will cause artefacts in a reconstructed 3D image. For example, if motion were to occur, the images acquired at 0° and 180° will not be mirror images of each other, requiring acquisition of images beyond 180° and that the reconstruction uses these images to compensate for the motion artifacts. In addition to the sensitivity to motion, the relative geometry of the acquired images must be accurately known. Thus, if the transducer array is placed into its housing in a way that causes an image tilt or offset from the rotation axis, then 3D image distortions will occur. These geometrical non-idealities must be known and the reconstruction must compensate for these to avoid artifacts in the center of the 3D image.

7.3.3 Sensed free-hand scanning

The mechanical scanning approach to 3D ultrasonography offers speed and accuracy, however, the bulkiness and weight of the scanning mechanisms hinder the examination at times. In addition, because of the restricted scanning geometrics, complete large structures are difficult to scan. To overcome this problem, many investigators have attempted to develop various free-hand scanning techniques that do not require a motorized fixture. In this approach, a position and orientation sensor is attached to the transducer, which is held by the operator and manipulated in the usual manner over the anatomy to be imaged. While the transducer is being manipulated, conventional 2D images generated by the ultrasound machine are recorded by a computer together with their position and angulation. Thus, the operator is free to manipulate the transducer and select the optimal orientation, which best displays the anatomy and accommodates complex surfaces of the patient. Because the scanning geometry is not predefined, as with the mechanical scanning approaches, the relative positions and angulation of the digitized 2D images must be accurately known. This information is then used to reconstruct the 3D image in a manner that avoids distortions and inaccuracies. In addition, because the relative locations of the acquired 2D images are not predefined, the operator must scan the anatomy by ensuring that the sampling is appropriate and that the set of 2D images has no significant gaps. This can generally be achieved by training operators to scan the anatomy in a constant velocity that is appropriate for the acquisition frame rate. Over the past two decades, several free-hand scanning approaches have been developed which use four basic position sensing techniques: articulated arm, acoustic, magnetic field, and image-based.

7.3.3.1 Articulated arm 3D scanning

The simplest free-hand scanning approach can be achieved by mounting the ultrasound transducer on a multiple jointed mechanical arm system. Potentiometers, located at the joints of the movable arms, provide the information necessary to calculate the relative position and angulation of the acquired 2D images. This arrangement allows the operator to manipulate the transducer and scan the desired patient anatomy, while the computer records the 2D images and the relative angulation of all the arms. Using the position and angulation of the transducer and hence of each recorded 2D image, the 3D image can be reconstructed. To avoid distortions and inaccuracies in the reconstructed 3D image, the potentiometers must be accurate and precise and the arms must not flex. Sufficient accuracy can be achieved by keeping individual arms as short as possible and reducing the number of movable joints. Thus, increased precision and accuracy in the reconstructed 3D image can be achieved at the expense of reduction in scanning flexibility and reduction in the size of the scanned volume.

7.3.3.2 Acoustic free-hand 3D scanning

One of the first free-hand scanning methods used to produce 3D ultrasound images made use of acoustic ranging. In this approach, three sound-emitting devices, such as spark gaps, were mounted on the transducer, and an array of fixed microphones were mounted above the patient. To produce a 3D image of a volume of interest, the operator moved the transducer freely over the patient's skin. While the transducer was moved and 2D ultrasound images were recorded, the sound-emitting devices were activated and the microphones continuously received sound pulses. The position and orientation of the transducer, and hence the recorded images, were then determined from knowledge of the speed of sound in air and the time-of-flight of the sound pulses from the emitters on the transducers to the fixed microphones. The fixed microphones needed to be placed over the patient in providing unobstructed lines-of-sight to the emitters and sufficiently close to allow detection of the sound pulses with good signal-to-noise. Because the speed of sound varies with temperature and humidity, corrections were required to avoid distortions in the 3D image [5, 46–52].

7.3.3.3 Three-dimensional scanning with magnetic field sensors

The most popular and successful free-hand scanning approach makes use of a six-degree-of-freedom magnetic-field sensor, which measures the ultrasound transducer's position and orientation. This approach (Figure 7.8) uses a transmitter, which produces a spatially varying magnetic field, and a small receiver containing three orthogonal coils to sense the magnetic-field strength. By measuring the strength of three components of the local magnetic field, the ultrasound transducer's position and angulation can be detected.

Magnetic field sensors are small and unobtrusive allowing for less constraining tracking of position and orientation than the previously described approaches. However, their accuracy can be compromised by electro-magnetic interference from sources such as CRT monitors, AC power cabling, and some electrical signals from ultrasound transducers. In addition, ferrous and highly conductive metals will distort the magnetic field causing errors in the recorded geometric information.

These effects can combine to produce distortions in the reconstructed 3D images. This approach is also susceptible to errors in the determination of the location of the moving transducer if the magnetic field sampling rate is not sufficiently high, and the transducer is moved too quickly. This image "lag" artefact can be overcome with a sampling rate of about 100 Hz or higher. By ensuring that the environment

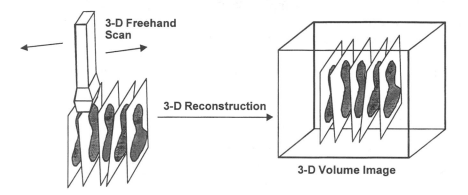

Figure 7.8: Schematic diagram showing the free-hand scanning approach. The 2D images are arranged without a regular geometry. For accurate 3D reconstruction, the position and orientation of each plane must be known.

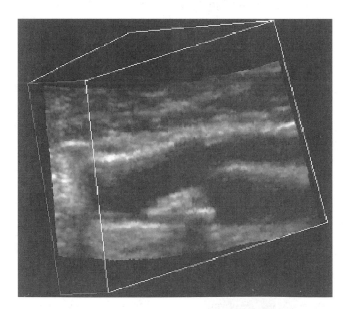

Figure 7.9: Three-dimensional B-mode image of the carotid arteries obtained with the free-hand scanning approach using a magnetic portioning and orientation device. The 3D image has been "sliced" to reveal an atherosclerotic plaque at the entrance of the internal carotid artery. The plaque is heterogenous with calcified regions casting a shadow in the common carotid artery.

of the scanned volume is free of electrical interference and metals, and with the appropriate sampling rate, high-quality 3D images can be obtained as shown in Figure 7.9.

Two companies are currently producing magnetic positioning devices of sufficient quality for 3D ultrasound imaging: the Fastrack by Polhemus and Flock-of-Birds by Ascension Technologies. Investigators have used these devices successfully in many diagnostic applications, such as: echocardiography, obstetrics and vascular imaging [19, 53–63].

7.3.3.4 *Three-dimensional tracking by speckle decorrelation*

The free-hand scanning techniques described above require a sensor to measure the relative positions of the acquired images. Measurement of the relative positions can also be accomplished using the well-known phenomenon of speckle decorrelation. When a source of coherent energy interacts with scatterers, the reflected spatial energy pattern will vary and appear as a speckle pattern. Image speckle is characteristic of ultrasound images and is used in making images of the velocity of moving blood. In this situation, two sequential signals generated by scattering of ultrasound from stationary red blood cells will be correlated, i.e., the speckle pattern will be identical. However, the signal from moving red blood cells will be decorrelated, and the degree of decorrelation is proportional to the distance the cells moved between acquisition of the signals.

The same principle can be used in 3D ultrasound. If two images are acquired from the same location, then the speckle pattern will be the same with maximum correlation. However, if one of the images is moved with respect to the first, then the degree of decorrelation will be proportional to the distance between the two images [64]. The exact relationship relating the degree of decorrelation to distance will depend on many transducer parameters including the number of focal zones, the degree of focusing, and the tissue depth. Thus, obtaining accurate determination of the separation between two images will require careful determination of the relationship between distance and various transducer parameters.

In free-hand scanning, it is not possible to guarantee that the motion will generate images that are parallel to each other. Thus, to determine if the transducer has been tilted or rotated, a more complicated strategy must be adopted. Typically, the acquired images are subdivided into smaller regions, and similar regions in adjacent images are cross correlated. In this manner, a pattern of decorrelation values is generated, and used to generate a pattern of vectors. These are then analyzed to give not only the relative position but also the orientation between adjacent images, which are used in the reconstruction algorithm.

7.3.4 *Free-hand scanning without position sensing*

Although the sensed free-hand scanning approach allows the transducer to be manipulated in the usual manner, it nevertheless requires that a device be added to the transducer to sense the position and orientation. An alternative 3D scanning approach involves manipulating the transducer over the patient without any sensing

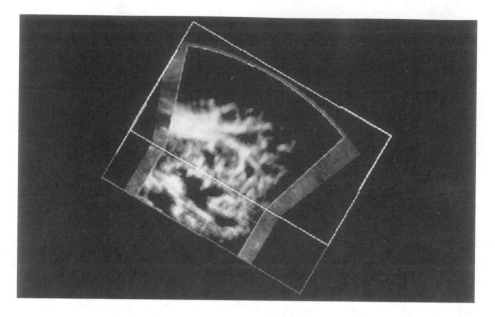

Figure 7.10: Three-dimensional power Doppler image of a kidney. The image was obtained with the free-hand scanning approach without any positioning sensing. The image has been "sliced" to demonstrate that excellent 3D reconstructions can be obtained of vascular structures. However, the geometry may not be correct and measurements should not be made with images obtained with this approach.

device and reconstructing the 3D image assuming a predefined scanning geometry. Because no geometrical information is recorded during the transducer's motion, the transducer must be moved in a constant linear or angular velocity so that the acquired images are obtained with a regular spacing. For example, the transducer may be moved over the skin in a linear motion, while the 2D images are recorded at regular temporal intervals. If the transducer's motion is uniform and steady, then, with the knowledge of the transducer's velocity and scanning distance, a very good 3D image may be reconstructed as shown in Figure 7.10 [18]. However, this approach does not guarantee that the image geometry or image distances are correct. Therefore, 3D images obtained using this approach should not be used for measurements.

7.3.4.1 Two-dimensional arrays

The use of conventional 1D arrays for 3D imaging requires that a planar beam of ultrasound be swept over the anatomy using either a mechanical or free-hand approach. A better approach would be to keep the transducer stationary but use electronic scanning to sweep the ultrasound beam over the volume. This has been accomplished with the use of 2D arrays, which produce a broad ultrasound beam covering the entire volume under examination. Investigators have described a number of 2D array designs, but the one developed at Duke University for real-time 3D echocardiography is the most advanced and has been used for clinical imaging [65–71].

The transducer used in real-time 3D imaging is composed of a 2D phased array of elements, which are used to transmit a broad beam of ultrasound diverging away from the array and sweeping out pyramidal volumes. The returned echoes are detected by the 2D array and then processed to display in real-time multiple planes from the volume. These planes can be manipulated interactively to allow the user to explore the whole volume under investigation.

The use of 2D arrays is being tested for real-time echocardiographic 3D imaging by producing about 20 3D views per second of the beating heart. However, before this approach becomes widespread in diagnostic imaging, some problems must be overcome. These problems are related to cost and low yield resulting from the manufacture of numerous small elements and the connection and assembly of many electronic leads. This can be alleviated with the use of sparse arrays, which have already produced useful images. Because the 2D arrays are small, measuring about 2 cm by 2 cm in size, the volume imaged is relatively small and suited for cardiac imaging, but not yet for larger organs.

7.4 Reconstruction of the 3D ultrasound images

The reconstruction process refers to the generation of a 3D representation of the anatomy by placing the acquired 2D images at their correct relative position. After the 2D ultrasound images have been acquired and their relative position and orientation recorded from either a predefined scanning geometry (mechanical scanners) or from a free-hand scanning approach, the 3D image can be reconstructed using two distinct methods: feature-based and voxel-based reconstruction.

7.4.1 Feature-based reconstruction

In this method, the 2D images are first analyzed and desired features in each acquired 2D image are identified and classified. For example, in echocardiographic or obstetrical imaging, the boundaries of the fluid-filled regions may be outlined manually or by using an automated computerized method. The boundaries of different structures may be assigned different colors and other structures are eliminated, generating solid mesh representations of the desired structures. This approach has been used extensively in echocardiographic imaging to identify the boundaries of the ventricles either manually or automatically. From the 3D surface model descriptions of the heart chambers, the complex motion of the left ventricle can be viewed with a computer workstation. A similar approach has been also used to reconstruct the vascular lumen in 3D using intravascular ultrasound imaging (IVUS).

The main advantage of this approach is that the 3D image has been reduced to describe the surfaces of a few structures, enabling the use of computer workstations optimized for viewing surfaces. In addition, this approach increases artificially the contrast between different structures by the manual or automatic classification step,

leading to improved visualization of the 3D anatomy. It also enables efficient manipulation of the image, including "fly-through," using inexpensive computer display hardware.

However, this approach also has major disadvantages. Because the classification process identifies and stores simple descriptions of anatomical boundaries,
important image information, such as subtle features and tissue texture, is lost at
the initial phase of the reconstruction. The boundary identification step is tedious
and time consuming if done manually or is subject to errors if done automatically
by a computer. In addition, the classification process also artificially accentuates
the contrast between different structures, again distorting or misrepresenting subtle image features.

To avoid image artifacts and generation of false information, the classification
process must be accurate and reproducible. When the image contrast is high, as
found between soft tissues and fluid-filled regions, the classification stage can be
accurate. However, the classification is very difficult in situations where the image contrast is small, as found between tumors and tissue or different soft tissues.
Because of the tedious and potentially erroneous aspects of the boundary identification process, this method for reconstruction of 3D ultrasound images is not often
used. It is useful though in situations where volume measurements of fluid-filled
regions is needed.

7.4.2 Voxel-based 3D ultrasound reconstruction

The more popular approach to the 3D ultrasound image reconstruction is based
on the use of the set of acquired 2D images to build a voxel-based volume (i.e., 3-
dimensional grid of picture elements). Reconstruction is accomplished by placing
each pixel in the acquired 2D images in its correct location in the three-dimensional
gridded volume, using its location in the 2D image and the relative orientation and
position of that 2D image with respect to the other acquired images. If a particular
voxel in the volume is not sampled by the scanning process, i.e., no 2D acquired
image intersects it, then its value (color or grey scale) is calculated by interpolation using the values from neighboring voxels in the same acquired image and/or
neighboring 2D images [38].

Both rotational and tilting mechanical scanning approaches require a reconstruction method that transforms the acquired data from cylindrical coordinates to
Cartesian. If the ultrasound transducer axis, and hence the rotation axis, is designated as the z-axis; the reconstruction of every x–y plane is the same and consists
of mapping the source image pixel values $P(r, \theta, z)$ in cylindrical coordinates to
the reconstructed image pixel values $P'(x, y, z)$ in Cartesian coordinates. For each
value of z, this is done by computing the polar coordinates (r, θ), where:

$$r = \sqrt{(x^2 + y^2)}$$
$$\theta = \arctan(x/y),$$

(7.1)

of each Cartesian grid point. The image values of $P'(x, y)$ are obtained by bilinear interpolation from the values $P(r, \theta)$ of its nearest neighbors in the appropriate source image. Therefore, the pixel value of each reconstructed 3D image point is a weighted average of four source image pixel values from the same x–y plane. By using a pre-computed lookup table of interpolation weights, which is applied repeatedly for each successive z value, the 3D image can be rapidly reconstructed from the set of 2D images [38].

This voxel-based reconstruction approach preserves all the original information so that the original 2D images can always be generated as well as new views not found in the original set of acquired images. However, if the scanning process does not sample the volume properly, leaving gaps between acquired images with a distance greater than about half the elevational resolution, the interpolation process will fill the gap with information that does not represent the true anatomy. In this situation, erroneous information is introduced and the resolution in the reconstructed 3D image will be degraded.

To sample the volume properly and to avoid gaps, large data files will be generated, requiring efficient 3D viewing software. Typical data files can range from 16 Mb to 96 Mb depending on the application. For example, data files of 96 Mb have been reported in 3D TRUS imaging of the prostate for cryosurgical guidance [17, 72].

Because the voxel-based reconstruction approach maintains all the image information, the 3D image can be reviewed repeatedly using a variety of rendering techniques. For example, the operator can scan through the data (i.e., view the complete 3D image) and then choose the rendering technique that best displays the desired features. The operator may then use segmentation and classification algorithms to measure volumes, segment boundaries, or perform various volume-based rendering operations. If the process has not achieved the desired results, then the operator can return to the original 3D image and attempt a different procedure.

7.5 Effects of errors in 3D ultrasound image reconstruction

Except for systems using 2D arrays, 3D ultrasound images are reconstructed from multiple 2D images using knowledge of their relative positions and orientations. Any errors in position and orientation of the 2D images will lead to 3D image distortion and measurement errors.

7.5.1 Mechanical linear scanners

The acquired 2D images are constrained to be parallel in the mechanical linear scanning approach. To avoid 3D image distortions, two geometrical parameters must be known accurately: the distance d and the tilt angle θ between the acquired 2D images, and the scanning direction. From Figure 7.11 we can then estimate the error ΔA in an arbitrary area A and the error ΔV in an arbitrary volume V due to errors Δd in d and $\Delta \theta$ in θ.

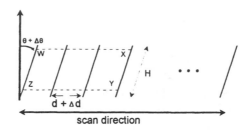

scan direction

Figure 7.11: Schematic diagram of: a linear 3D scanning approach showing the edge view of multiple 2D images used in the 3D reconstruction. Also shown are: the tilt angle, θ, and distance, d, between acquired 2D images; as well as the error in the tilt angle, $\Delta\theta$, and error in the distance, Δd, between acquired images.

In their book on 3D ultrasound, Nelson *et al.* showed that the errors ΔA and ΔV are [73]:

$$\frac{\Delta A}{A} = \frac{\Delta V}{V} = \left(1 + \frac{\Delta d}{d}\right)\left(1 + \frac{\tan\Delta\theta}{\tan\theta}\right)\cos\Delta\theta - 1$$

$$\cong \frac{\Delta d}{d} + \frac{\Delta\theta}{\tan\theta} - \frac{(\Delta\theta)^2}{2}, \tag{7.2}$$

for $\Delta\theta \ll 1$ (radian), so that $\tan\Delta\theta \approx \Delta\theta$ (radians) and $\cos\Delta\theta \approx 1 - (\Delta\theta)^2/2$.

The relative volume error $\Delta V/V$ in an arbitrary volume V will be the same as the relative area error $\Delta A/A$ in an arbitrary area for the following reason. The measurement of volume from a 3D image is made by summing the cross-sectional areas in multiple parallel image slices, and then multiplying by the interslice distance. Because this separation is known accurately, the errors will sum as the volume is summed.

To estimate the error in the volume we consider that the tilt angle is known exactly (or equal to 90° with respect to the scan direction). Thus, the percentage error in volume or area will be equal to that in d. Then, to ensure that the error in volume measurements is less than 5% (for $d = 1$ mm), the systematic error in the distance between acquired images, Δd, must be less than 0.05 mm.

7.5.2 Mechanical tilting scanners

Tong *et al.* [74] have performed an analysis of the linear, area, and volume measurement errors for a mechanical tilting transducer approach (Figure 7.12), which was described in Section 7.3.2.2. In this scanning approach, the transducer is tilted through a total scan angle Θ about its face, by mechanically rotating the probe about its axis, while a series of N 2D images is digitized at equally spaced angular intervals. If the region digitized in each 2D image is of size X by Y (Figure 7.12), the reconstructed 3D image will be in an annular sector of a cylinder with an average radius of R, subtending an angle Θ about the rotation axis with inner radius R_0, which is the distance from the rotation axis to the top of the digitized region.

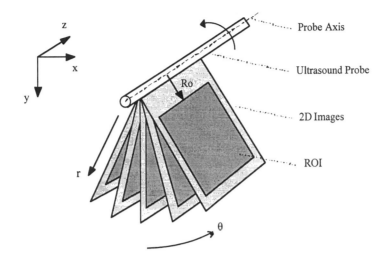

Figure 7.12: Schematic diagram illustrating the geometry used for 3D scanning using the tilt scanning approach with a transrectal transducer. A region-of-interest (ROI) is digitized in each of a series of conventional 2D images that are acquired while the side-firing transducer is rotated about its axis through an angle θ. The ROI is shown as the shaded area with an inner radius is R_0.

Thus, correct reconstruction of the 3D image requires that the two geometrical parameters R_0 and Θ must be known accurately.

If the 3D image was (erroneously) reconstructed with the parameters $R_0 + \Delta R$ and $\Theta + \Delta\Theta$ instead as of R_0 and Θ, then the average radius of the annular sector (mean of inner and outer radii) would be $R + \Delta R$, with an area $A + \Delta A$. Using these parameters, Tong *et al.* [74] showed that the relative error in area, $\Delta A/A$, in the x–y plane of Figure 7.12, is exactly:

$$
\begin{aligned}
\frac{\Delta A}{A} &= \left(1 + \frac{\Delta R}{R}\right)\left(1 + \frac{\Delta\Theta}{\Theta}\right) - 1 \\
&= \frac{\Delta R}{R} + \frac{\Delta\Theta}{\Theta} + \frac{\Delta R}{R}\frac{\Delta\Theta}{\Theta}.
\end{aligned}
\tag{7.3}
$$

The error in a volume measurement can be estimated by considering that a 3D volume measurement is made by summing the cross-sectional organ areas in multiple parallel image slices, and then multiplying by the interslice separation. Because this separation is known accurately, the relative volume error $\Delta V/V$ in an arbitrary volume V will be the same as the relative area error $\Delta A/A$ in an arbitrary area A:

$$
\frac{\Delta V}{V} = \frac{\Delta A}{A} = \frac{\Delta R}{R} + \frac{\Delta\Theta}{\Theta} + \frac{\Delta R}{R}\frac{\Delta\Theta}{\Theta},
\tag{7.4}
$$

where R is now the mean radius of the measured volume from the axis of rotation.

To estimate the required accuracy in the geometrical parameters, we consider that the location of the axis of rotation is known exactly. Then, the percentage error in volume will equal that in Θ. To ensure a volume error of less than 5% for a scanning angle of $\Theta = 80°$, $\Delta\Theta$ must be less than 4°, so that, for a scan containing $N = 100$ 2D images, the angular interval between images must be accurate to 0.04°. Similarly, if the scan angle, Θ, is known exactly, the percentage error in volume will equal that in R. Then, to ensure a volume error of less than 5% for $R = 10$ mm requires that ΔR be less than 0.5 mm.

The reader is referred to the publication by Tong *et al.* [74] for a detailed analysis of the shape, distance, area, and volume distortions that arise from these errors in the mechanical tilting approach, a calibration method for virtually eliminating them, and the method for calculating the mean radius R of a volume.

7.5.3 *Tracked free-hand scanners*

In the free-hand scanning approach, the movement of the ultrasound transducer is not constrained. Therefore, accurate 3D reconstructions require that the position and orientation of each digitized 2D image be known accurately. The required geometrical information can be obtained using a variety of techniques, discussed in detail in Section 7.3, such as mechanical arms [61], spark gaps [48], and magnetic sensors [6, 15, 54, 57, 58].

To obtain 3D images free of distortions, both random and systematic errors must be avoided. Random errors are avoided by ensuring that the position and orientation measurements are obtained with good SNR. However, accurate calibration of the position and orientation sensing devices is the most important requirement for distortion-free reconstructions and measurement accuracy. Random errors are important is they relate to image quality, but they will tend to "average out" over the distances and volumes to be measured. However, systematic errors will not, leading to distortions and measurement errors.

A number of investigators have addressed the issues involved in calibrating free-hand scanners. Detmer *et al.* [54] describe a calibration technique that makes use of a small bead and cross-wire calibration method. This approach was used to investigate the accuracy of a magnetic positioning device (Flock of Birds, Ascension Technology Corp., Burlington, Vermont), and demonstrate that the RMS error at a tissue depth of 60 mm ranged from 2.1 mm to 3.5 mm. This error depended on the distance from the transmitter to the small receiver, which was mounted on the ultrasound transducer. Leotta *et al.* [58] reported on two calibration methods for magnetic positioning devices, and found an RMS calibration error of about 2.5 mm. In a later paper, Leotta *et al.* [58] examined an upgraded version of the magnetic positioning devices, and found an RMS calibration error ranging from 0.5 mm to 2.5 mm, depending on tissue depth.

These reports demonstrated that free-hand systems using the magnetic positioning device have errors greater then that exhibited by mechanical scanners. However, their size and ease of use makes the free-hand approach an attractive alternative to the bulkier mechanical-scanning approach.

7.6 Viewing of 3D ultrasound images

Once reconstructed, the 3D image can be viewed interactively using any 3D visualization software. Image acquisition characteristics of a 3D ultrasound system are crucial in determining the quality of the final image. Nevertheless, the rendering technique chosen also plays an important, and at times, dominant role in determining the information transmitted to the operator by the 3D ultrasound image display. Numerous techniques for displaying 3D images are still being actively investigated by many investigators and commercial companies. Display techniques for 3D ultrasound imaging can be divided into three broad classes: surface-based, multi-planar, and volume-based rendering. The optimal choice of the rendering technique is generally determined by the clinical application, and often under the control of the user.

7.6.1 Surface-based rendering (SR)

The most common 3D display technique is based on visualization of surfaces of structures or organs. In this approach, a segmentation and classification step precedes rendering. In the first step, the operator or the algorithm analyzes each voxel in the 3D image and determines the structure to which it belongs [75]. Boundaries of anatomical structures can be identified by the operator using manual contouring [76–78], or by algorithms that can use simple thresholding, or more complex statistical and geometric properties of parts of the 3D image. Although segmentation of boundaries in 2D and 3D images is still a very active area of research, the optimal method for 3D ultrasound imaging has not been found. Once the tissues or structures have been classified and their boundaries identified, the boundary is represented by a wire-frame or mesh and the surface is texture mapped with an appropriate color and texture to represent the anatomical structure.

The wire-frame rendering approach was used first in 3D ultrasound imaging because it is the simplest and does not require advanced computer workstations. In this approach, the boundaries between structures are represented by a network of lines, which can be viewed in 3D perspective. This approach has been used for displaying the fetus [46, 79–81], various abdominal structures [82–84], the endocardial and epicardial surface of the heart [50, 77, 85–89], and septal defects [90].

The wire-frames or other more complex representations of the surfaces can be texture-mapped, shaded, illuminated, and depth cues added, so that both topography and 3D geometry are more easily comprehended. Automatic rotation, or user-controlled motion, is generally useful to allow the operator to view the anatomy from different perspectives. This approach has been used successfully by many investigators in rendering of echocardiographic [8, 16, 30, 32, 91–94] and obstetrical 3D images [10, 95].

7.6.2 Multi-planar viewing (MPR)

This technique requires that either a 3D voxel-based image be reconstructed first, or an algorithm be developed that extracts any arbitrarily oriented plane from

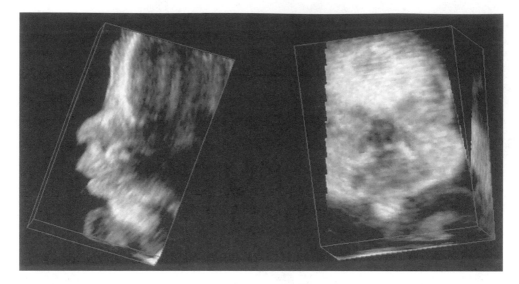

Figure 7.13: Three-dimensional image of a fetal face displayed using the multi-planar viewing approach. The 3D image is presented as a polyhedron with the faces painted with the appropriate 2D image. The polyhedron can be sliced and the faces tilted to reveal the appropriate 2D image in relation to the other faces. In this figure, the 3D image has been sliced and oriented to display a profile and a face view of the fetal face.

the originally acquired images [94]. Two approaches have been developed to view the 3D image information. In the first approach, computer user-interface tools are provided to the operator to allow selection of single or multiple planes, including oblique from the 3D. With appropriate interpolation, these planes may appear similar to the images that would be obtained by conventional 2D ultrasound imaging. Often, three perpendicular planes are displayed on the screen simultaneously, with cues providing relative orientation information. This method presents 2D images to the operator that are familiar and allows the operator to orient the planes optimally for the examination [10, 96–99].

A second approach is based on multi-planar visualization with texture mapping. In this technique, the 3D image is presented as a polyhedron representing the boundaries of the reconstructed volume. Each face of the polyhedron is rendered, using a texture-mapping technique with the appropriate ultrasound image for that plane [100]. User interface tools are provided, allowing the polyhedron to be rotated to obtain the desired orientation of the image. The faces of the polyhedron can be moved in or out parallel to the original, or reoriented obliquely, while the appropriate ultrasound data are texture-mapped in real time on the new face. In this way, the operator always has three-dimensional image-based cues relating the plane being manipulated to the rest of the anatomy [11, 19, 22, 38]. Figure 7.13 shows examples of the use of this approach in 3D displaying of anatomy.

7.6.3 Volume rendering (VR)

Both the surface-based and multi-planar rendering techniques reduce the display of three-dimensional information to a display of 2D information in the form of complex or planar surfaces. Because our visual senses are best suited for surface viewing and interpretation, these two approaches are easily understood by the operator. However, surface- or planar-based display techniques present only a small part of the complete 3D image at one time.

An alternative approach is the volume-rendering technique, which presents to the viewer a display of the entire 3D image after it has been projected onto a 2D plane. The most common approach used in 3D ultrasound imaging is based on the ray-casting techniques [101–103], which project a 2D array of rays through the 3D image (see Figure 7.14). Each ray intersects the 3D image along a series of voxels. The voxel values along each ray are examined and weighted to achieve the desired rendering result. If the structures in the 3D image have been segmented and classified, the voxels can be weighted and/or colored appropriately to achieve a translucent representation. Another common approach is to display only the voxels with the maximum (minimum) intensity along each ray to form a "maximum (minimum) intensity projection" (MIP) image as shown in Figure 7.15.

The most common approach used in 3D ultrasound imaging is the translucency/opacity rendering approach. In this approach, the voxels along each ray are weighted according to Eq. (7.5):

$$C_{out} = C_{in}(1 - a(i)) + c(i)a(i), \tag{7.5}$$

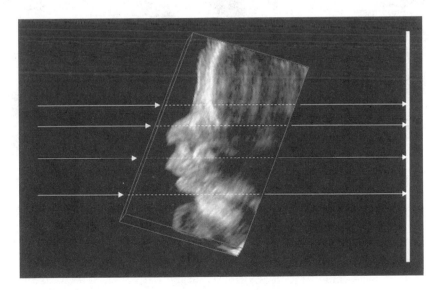

Figure 7.14: Image showing the ray-casting approach. An array of rays are cast through the 3D image projecting the 3D image onto a plane producing a 2D image. The rays can be made to interact with the 3D image data in different ways to produce different types of renderings.

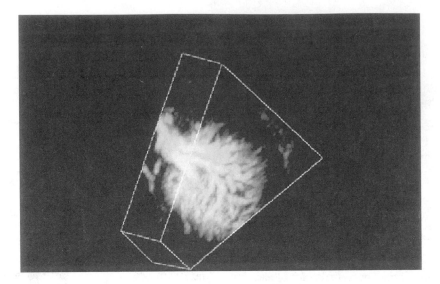

Figure 7.15: The 3D image of the kidney has been rendered using a MIP (maximum intensity projection) algorithm with the ray-casting approach.

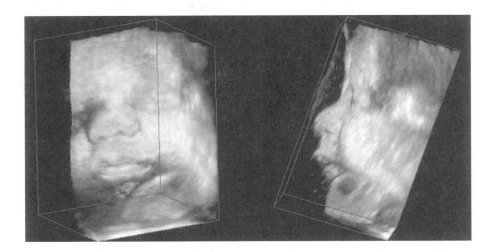

Figure 7.16: The 3D image of the fetal face has been rendered using a translucency-rendering algorithm with the ray-casting approach. In this image, the amniotic fluid has been made transparent, and tissues have been made transparent or opaque depending on the voxel intensity as described in Eq. (8.5).

where C_{out} is the value of the ray exiting from the ith voxel, and C_{in} is the value of the ray entering the ith voxel. The parameters c and a are chosen to control the specific desired rendering result, where a controls the opacity and c is a modified voxel shade value that can be based on the voxel value or local gradient, and chosen to control the luminance of the voxel. For example, if $a(i) = 0$, then the ray will be transmitted through ith voxel, as if it were transparent; if $a(i) = 1$, then the voxel is considered to be opaque or luminescent depending on the value of c. Typically, the values of a are added along each ray and when the sum reaches 1, the value C_{out} is displayed.

Volume-based techniques, which display the anatomy in a translucent manner, preserve all the 3D information, but project it (after nonlinear processing), onto a 2D plane for viewing. Although depth cues can be added (e.g., stereo viewing), this approach results in images that are difficult to interpret. Thus, this approach is best suited for simple anatomical structures in which clutter has been removed or is not present. Investigators have demonstrated success, particularly in displaying fetal [10, 15, 60, 62, 104, 105] and vascular anatomy [18, 106]. An example of the translucency rendering approach is shown in Figure 7.16. In this example, the values of c and a have been chosen to make the voxel values in the amniotic fluid transparent and the values in the soft tissues nearly opaque.

In general, ray casting techniques are computational intensive, requiring a very large number of rays to be used to generate satisfactory results. However, with current personal computers and efficient implementation of the algorithms, real-time manipulation of the 3D image with continuous ray-casting is possible.

7.7 Three-dimensional ultrasound system performance

7.7.1 Introduction

Ultrasound imaging provides an important non-invasive modality for measuring anatomical and pathological structures. The role of quantitative measurements in ultrasound imaging has progressed with advances in ultrasound technology. With the ongoing developments and improvements in technology, ultrasound imaging is being relied upon for making measurements of internal anatomical structures and blood flow.

An important part of the patient imaging with 3D ultrasound is to provide image data of sufficient quality to measure the length, area or volume of organs and to follow their temporal changes. While qualitative visual assessment is valuable, quantitative data provides a more accurate basis for decision making and comparisons against previous studies or reference data bases. 3D ultrasound imaging is ideally suited for providing quantitative measurements such as volume, area and distance in complex anatomical structures [15, 37, 50–52, 56, 57, 107–111].

7.7.2 Measurement accuracy

In most applications, measuring the organ or lesion volume, rather than its diameter or perimeter, is the goal. However, conventional ultrasound imaging provides only 2D images, from which the 3D structure must be estimated. Over the years, techniques have been developed that provide useful estimates of organ volume using 2D ultrasonography. Many studies have been published on the accuracy and reproducibility of these techniques for various applications, such as the estimate of gestational age, the effects of growth retardation, or prostate volume.

Although these techniques have proven to be valuable, the estimation of the volume of an organ or anatomical structure suffers from many deficiencies that 3D ultrasound addresses. The main deficiency relates to the fact that direct measurement of volume is not possible with 2D methods, because information is not available to connect adjacent 2D images.

The accuracy of a measurement technique reflects its ability to measure the "truth," for example, how close the measured volume is to the actual organ volume. Because 3D ultrasound imaging provides a complete view of the structure rather then just a few selected planes, it is anticipated that 3D ultrasound should provide more accurate estimates of volume, especially for complex structures. In addition, 3D ultrasound promises to provide volume measurements with reduced variability because the whole structure is available rather than two or three user-selected planes.

7.7.2.1 Distance measurement

Because ultrasound images are tomographic in nature, measurement of length within the 2D image has always been possible. The accuracy and precision of the measurement depends on the frequency of the transducer, field-of-view, and the resolution of the ultrasound machine. Distance measurement requires that the operator select two points. Because the 3D image is available, these points need not lie on the same original acquired image. They can instead be located on two different acquired images, which have been geometrically located relative to each other by the 3D reconstruction process. Thus, for the distance measurement to be accurate, the reconstruction process must not distort the geometry.

Tong *et al.* have evaluated the accuracy of distance measurements by imaging a 3D wire phantom of known dimensions and then measured the distances between the wires [112]. The phantom was composed of four layers of 0.25-mm-diameter surgical wires, with eight parallel wires per layer. Each layer was separated from its neighbor by 10.00 ± 0.05 mm, and each wire was also separated from its neighbours in the layer by 10.00 mm. The wire phantom was immersed in a bath com-

Table 7.1: Measurements of distances between adjacent wires obtained with a wire phantom made of four layers of wires 10.00 mm apart and four wires in each layer also 10.00 mm apart

Direction of Wire Axis	Direction of Measurement	Measured Distance, Mean $\pm$ Std. dev. (mm)
Z	Δx	10.11 ± 0.11
Z	Δy	10.10 ± 0.06
X	Δy	10.12 ± 0.17
X	Δz	10.07 ± 0.29

posed of a 7% glycerol solution (1540 m/s speed of sound) and then imaged with a 3D TRUS system.

The 3D system made use of a mechanical tilting scanning mechanism, which rotated a TRUS transducer with a side firing linear array (Figure 7.4) around its long axis. The wire phantom was scanned first with the wires placed parallel to the axis of rotation of the probe (the z axis), and then with the wires oriented parallel to the x axis. The 3D images were reconstructed using 100 2D images, which were collected over 60°.

The separations between wire layers were then measured in the 3D images of the phantom and the results are tabulated in Table 7.1. The results of this study showed that, with proper calibration of the scanning geometry and using a mechanical scanning approach, a 3D ultrasound imaging system can provide distance measurements with an error of about 1.0%.

7.7.2.2 Cross-sectional area measurement using 3D ultrasound

Because the 3D image can be "sliced" in any orientation (Figure 7.13), any desired cross section of the organ may be obtained. For measurement of cross-sectional area, the optimal "slice" can be found by using a multi-planar reformatting technique and the desired area can then be outlined either manually, using planimetric techniques [112, 113], or automatically, using segmentation algorithms. The area of the region is measured by counting the pixels in the outlined region and multiplying by the pixel area.

7.7.2.3 Volume measurement in 3D images of balloons

The volume of an organ may be measured by either manual or automated techniques using a 3D image. Automated techniques for segmenting an anatomical structure and measuring its volume are still under development in many laboratories. An alternative manual technique, called manual planimetry, makes use of the multi-planar viewing technique to "slice" the 3D image into a series of uniformly-spaced parallel 2D images. In each 2D image, the cross-sectional area of the organ is manually outlined on the computer screen using a mouse, trackball, or other pointing device. The areas on these slices are then summed and multiplied by the interslice distance to obtain an estimate of the organ volume.

An important application of 3D ultrasound imaging is the measurement of prostate volume for normalizing the PSA (prostate specific antigen) value. To evaluate the accuracy of volume measurements using 3D ultrasound, Tong *et al.* used a 3D TRUS system to image five balloons filled with different known volumes of 7% glycerol solution, and compared the measured volumes obtained from the 3D images, to the true volumes [112]. As for the distance accuracy experiment described above, each image data set consisted of 100 2D images, scanned through 60°. The volume of the ballons were then measured using manual planimetry by slicing the 3D image in steps of 0.2 mm (Table 7.2).

The volume measurements shown in Table 7.2 have a root-mean-square (rms) error of 0.9% and an rms precision of 1.7%. Also, a least-squares regression of

Table 7.2: Volume measurement accuracy obtained by imaging balloons filled with different volumes of water/glycerol solution

True Volume (cm^3)	Measured Volume, Mean $\pm$ Std. dev. (cm^3)	True-Measured (cm^3)	Error (%)
23.14	22.81 $\pm$ 0.33	0.33	1.4
35.79	35.49 $\pm$ 0.72	0.3	0.8
41.69	41.27 $\pm$ 0.65	0.42	0.1
49.66	49.84 $\pm$ 0.62	−0.18	0.4
65.84	66.31 $\pm$ 1.29	−0.47	0.7

measured versus true volume resulted in a best-fit line with a slope of 1.0004 ± 0.0039 and a correlation coefficient of 0.99997.

7.7.2.4 *Volume measurements of prostates in vitro*

Volume measurement of water filled balloons using 3D ultrasound images produces idealized and presumably the most accurate measurements. To determine the accuracy of volume measurement in a more realistic situation, Elliot *et al.* compared the measurement of prostate volume using 3D TRUS to their true volumes [113]. For this study, six prostates, with seminal vesicles and some periprostatic fat attached, were harvested from fresh cadavers, fixed and imaged with a 3D TRUS system, while immersed in a solution of 7% glycerol in distilled water [113].

The prostate volumes were measured by manual planimetry using a similar technique to the balloon volume measurements. Each prostate was "sliced" into 20–30 transaxial slices 2–5 mm apart and the boundary of the prostate in each slice outlined. The volume was obtained by summing the area-thickness products of each slice. A linear regression of measured versus true volume yielded a slope of 1.006 ± 0.007. The accuracy (rms deviation from the line of identity) of the measurements was 2.6%, and the precision (rms deviation from the best fit line) was 2.5%.

The volume of one cadaveric prostate was measured 10 times to obtain an estimate of the precision of volume estimation using manual planimetry from a 3D image. This resulted in a mean prostate volume of 25.32 cm^3, and a standard deviation of 0.43 cm^3, or 1.7% of the mean.

These *in vitro* studies using balloons and cadaveric specimens clearly show that, by using a properly calibrated 3D ultrasound imaging system under ideal laboratory conditions, the accuracy of 3D volume estimates can be very good, with errors of less than 5%.

7.7.2.5 *Volume measurements in vivo*

A number of investigators have shown that 3D ultrasound can be used successfully for volume measurements in a variety of organ systems. Brunner *et al.* [114]

showed an increased accuracy in follicular volume measurements. Chang *et.al.* [115] have shown good volume measurement results for fetal heart volumes across a range of gestational ages. Riccabona *et al.* [116] showed good accuracy between voided urine volumes and measured bladder volumes pre-void. Hughes *et al.* [57] measured a variety of organ volumes and found that the errors ranged from 2% to 6%. Favre *et al.* [108] reported that in measuring fetal arm and thigh circumference using 3D ultrasound for fetal weight estimation, the mean error was—1.4% for macrosomic fetuses. Lee *et al.* [117] measured thigh and abdomen volume for birth weight prediction, compared the results to 2D ultrasound, and found that the mean systematic error using 3D ultrasound was $0.03\% \pm 6.1\%$ while the results for 2D ultrasound were $0.60\% \pm 8.8\%$.

7.7.2.6 *Choice of inter-slice distance for volume measurements*

Volume estimation requires that the 3D image of the organ be "sliced" into individual parallel slices and the boundary of the anatomical structure outlined in every slice. The question arises as to what is the maximum inter-slice distance that still provides accurate volume estimates, since the choice of inter-slice distance will affect the volume measurement accuracy. As the inter-slice thickness is reduced, the accuracy will increase, but the length of time needed for the manual planimetry will also increase because more 2D image slices must be outlined for each volume measurement. While a large interslice distance will be less time consuming, the volume estimate may be in error if the structure is complex. Thus, it is important to determine the largest interslice thickness that still results in accurate volume measurements.

Usually, irregular or complex structures require the use of smaller interslice distances. However, using an interslice distance less than the spacing of the original 2D images used to reconstruct the 3D image (i.e., less than the elevational resolution) will not result in increased accuracy. Because of varying sizes and geometries of different organs, use of different transducers, and imaging of structures at different depths, it is difficult to generalize the choice of interslice distance.

To examine the effect of the choice of the interslice distance in a specific application (3D TRUS), Elliot *et al.* repeatedly measured the volume of one cadaveric prostate in a 3D TRUS image by manual planimetry in the transaxial, sagittal, and coronal planes [113]. Interplane distance ranged from 1 mm to 15 mm. The results showed that the measured prostate volume was constant (within the precision of the volume estimation) up to an interslice distance of 8 mm. An interslice distance greater than 8 mm resulted in an underestimation of the prostate volume.

Other reports addressing this issue have recommended interslice distances ranging from 2 mm to 5 mm for measuring prostate volume using 2D ultrasound and serial planimetry [118, 119].

7.7.3 *Intra- and inter-observer variability*

Currently, volume estimation with 2D ultrasound is done by measuring the diameter of the structure from one or more images and assuming a particular organ or tumor shape. For prostate volume measurements, the height H, width W, and length L of the prostate from two selected orthogonal views, and estimation of the prostate volume V as that of the corresponding ellipsoid, $V = (\pi/6)HWL$ is used [118]. Because the prostate is not ellipsoidal, choosing the appropriate orthogonal views and which three chords to use in measuring H, W, and L in the selected views is largely dependent on observer preference, leading to high inter-observer variability in volume estimation. Even for a single observer with a single set of images, the choice remains arbitrary, leading to high intra-observer variability.

However, with 3D ultrasound, the entire prostate is available for volume measurement. Thus, any arbitrarily shaped volume can be measured and the only observer variability is in deciding the boundary of the anatomical structure.

To determine whether 3D based volume measurements are less variable than 2D based volume measurements, Tong *et al.* carried out an intra- and inter-observer variability study to measure prostate volume [120]. They used eight observers in the study and compared the variability of prostate volume measurements made with 2D and 3D techniques. Four observers were experienced radiologists and four were technicians or graduate students. The prostates of fifteen patients were scanned *in vivo*, reconstructed, and then measured. The volume of each prostate was measured four times by each observer:

(i) twice by means of the HWL method, using transverse and sagittal cross sections of the 3D image to measure H, W, and L; and,

(ii) twice by means of the 3D US method, using manual planimetry with an inter-slice spacing of 4 mm.

The analysis of variance (ANOVA) was then used to assess the intra- and inter-observer variability of prostate volume measurements made using the HWL and 3D US methods [121, 122]. The intra- and inter-observer standard errors of measurement SEM_{intra} and SEM_{inter} were used to characterize the variability of volume measurements, which were also expressed in terms of the minimum volume changes ΔV_{intra} and ΔV_{inter} that can be detected with a given confidence level in successive measurements.

The ANOVA results are shown in Table 7.3, showing that prostate volume measurement using 3D TRUS provides results that are less variable. Using the 3D method, the intra-observer SEM is reduced by about a factor of three, and the inter-observer SEM by about a factor of two. However, by doing similar analyses on subsets of prostates classified by volume, it was found that the SEM values varied with the average volume of the subset. Thus, for each method, the volume of each prostate was normalized by its average value for that method, and the ANOVA was repeated. The results are also tabulated in Table 7.3 (as SEM/prostate volume) and show similar improvements in the use of 3D ultrasound [120].

Because SEM values are abstract, they are often interpreted in terms of the minimum volume change that can be confidently detected between successive measurements at the 95% level of confidence, which is given by $\Delta V = 2.77$ SEM.

Table 7.3: Results of the intra- and inter-observer study comparing prostate volume measurements using 3D ultrasound and the conventional HWL method

	SEM (cm^3)		SEM/Volume (%)	
	3D	HWL	3D	HWL
Intra	3.6	12.2	5.1	15.5
Inter	9.6	16.6	11.4	21.9

Table 7.4: Values of the minimum relative prostate volume change that can be detected between successive prostate volume measurements at the 95% level on confidence. These values are given by $\Delta V = 2.77$ SEM

	ΔV/Mean (%)	
	3D	HWL
Intra	14	43
Inter	32	61

The values for minimum-detectable prostate volume change are tabulated in Table 7.4. The intra-observer variability values show that if one observer measures the prostate volume, and the same observer makes a follow-up measurement, then the volume must change by 43% before it can be confidently detected by the HWL method. However, the volume must change by only 14% before it can be confidently detected by the 3D ultrasound method. The inter-observer variability values show that if one observer measures the prostate, and another observed makes a follow-up measurement, then the prostate must change by 61% before it can be confidently detected by the HWL method, but by only 32% by the 3D method.

This increase in sensitivity could be clinically beneficial, particularly in the nonsurgical management of prostate cancer. In these patients, the normalized PSA value is followed carefully. Thus, to be able to interpret changes in the normalized PSA value, the prostate volume must be measured with a technique that provides the minimum variability. These results indicate that using the 3D ultrasound method instead of the HWL method significantly reduces the variability of prostate volume measurements, making patient PSA-level monitoring more reliable.

Chang *et al.* [115] also reported on a comparison of the reproducibility of 3D ultrasound with the HWL method in the assessment of fetal liver volume, and demonstrates that both the intra- and inter-observer reproducibility are improved with 3D ultrasound. Their volume measurements had an intra-observer standard deviation of 8.46 cm^3 for the HWL method and 2.15 cm^3 for 3D ultrasound.

7.8 Trends and future developments

7.8.1 Summary

Scientific and technological advances in the past five years have enabled the development of clinically useful 3D ultrasound systems. Current ultrasound systems now allow real-time or fast 3D acquisition, real-time reconstruction, and real-time 3D image manipulation. With these powerful new imaging tools, we are now entering a new phase focusing on demonstrating clinical utility.

Investigators have already demonstrated that useful 3D ultrasound images can be acquired quickly without interfering with the clinical exam. It has also been demonstrated that the 3D image can be examined either at the site where the image was generated or at a remote site with equal clinical results. A number of investigators have evaluated the utility of quantitative measurements with 3D ultrasound and have clearly demonstrated that volume measurements are both more accurate and less variable than measurements performed with 2D ultrasound. This has particular importance in applications involving measurements of prostate volume for normalization of the PSA value and for planning prostate therapy; and fetal organ volume monitoring for diagnosis of fetal growth retardation. Other useful applications have been demonstrated such as left ventricular volume measurement for ejection fraction estimation, fetal face rendering for improved abnormality diagnosis, renal vasculature demonstration, and tumor vascularity detection and quantification with ultrasound contrast agents.

Although 3D ultrasound has already been demonstrated to be useful, progress still must be made for this technique to become a routine tool. The following sections describe some of the future trends and needed developments in 3D ultrasonography.

Table 7.5: Standard error of measurements and minimum detectible change or determining the coordinates of brachytherapy seeds in 3D ultrasound images of an agar phantom

Coordinate	SEM_{inter} (mm)	SEM_{intra} (mm)	Δ_{inter} (mm)	Δ_{intra} (mm)
X	0.30	0.28	0.82	0.78
Y	0.35	0.33	0.97	0.91
Z	0.36	0.29	0.98	0.79

7.8.2 Use of 3D ultrasound in brachytherapy

It is now recognized that 3D ultrasound imaging has an important role to play in ultrasound-guided brachytherapy. Its role could be greatly expanded if brachytherapy seeds could be accurately detected and their locations determined. Consequently, a study was conducted to determine the variability of measuring the location of brachytherapy seeds in 3D ultrasound images using a tissue mimicking phantom.

The ultrasound phantom was made of 3% by weight agar gel to which was added to 7% solution of glycerol containing 50-μm cellulose particles [123]. To simulate the rectum and accommodate the transrectal ultrasound transducer, a 2.5-cm-diameter acrylic rod was suspended in the molten mixture, which was allowed to solidify. When the rod was removed, the resulting channel simulated the rectum.

Twenty gold brachytherapy seeds, approximately 1 mm in diameter and 3 mm long, were inserted into the phantom in a fan pattern at varying depths. After all the seeds were inserted, 3D ultrasound images of the phantom were acquired using a 3D TRUS system with a tilting scanning approach as shown in Figure 7.3(a). Seven observers measured the Cartesian coordinates of all the seeds in the 3D image, and an analysis of variance (ANOVA) was performed to determine the standard error of measurement and the minimum detectible change in the coordinates.

The results are shown in Table 7.5. These results indicate that under ideal conditions, such as those found when imaging agar phantoms, the location of the seeds

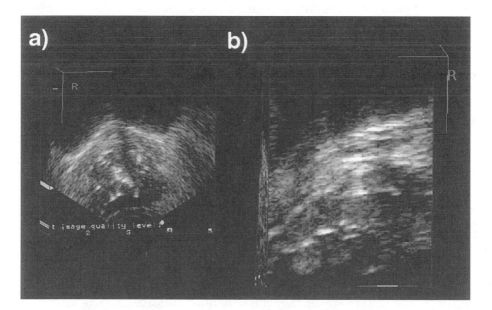

Figure 7.17: Three-dimensional image of a patient's prostate after a brachytherapy procedure. a) shows a transverse view with the radioactive seeds seen as bright structures; b) shows a longitudinal view of the same prostate with the seeds seen as the 3-mm-long bright structures.

can be detected at the 95% confidence level to better than 1 mm. Two factors affect the measurement of the seed localization. The first is the size of the seed, resulting in uncertainty in identifying the center of the seed. The second is the loss of resolution caused by the poor elevation resolution of the ultrasound transducer. This affects the appearance of the seeds in the rotational direction, causing the seeds to smear with increasing depth.

The above results demonstrate that brachytherapy seeds can be identified in 3D images of a phantom without specular reflectors generating image clutter. Images of prostates *in vivo* show clutter, which may make identification of seeds more difficult. Figure 7.17 shows two views of the prostate in a patient who has undergone a brachytherapy procedure. The 3D ultrasound images show that all the seeds are difficult to distinguish, and that image proccessing techniques or improvements in the echogenicity of the seeds must be achieved before all seeds could be reliably identified.

7.8.3 Automated or semi-automated measurements

Currently volume measurements require that the user "slice" the 3D image in serial parallel sections and then outline the visible structure using manual planimetry. This approach is time consuming and subject to errors caused by fatigue. Automated or semi-automated methods need to be developed to segment desired structures.

These techniques must be fast and accurate, and require that the user initiate the process easily. Because it has been already demonstrated that 2D techniques are highly variable, a useful 3D segmentation technique would have important applications in both diagnosis and treatment planning.

7.8.4 Fast and accurate free-hand scanning

Currently, free-hand scanning techniques have already been developed making use of magnetic positioning devices or speckle decorrelation. These techniques are still subject to potential artefacts and inaccuracies. Further progress must be made for these techniques to become routine tools producing high-quality images under all circumstances. In addition, improvements in 2D arrays are still required to produce images of the quality produced by conventional 1D arrays. Nevertheless, 2D arrays producing 3D images directly are already useful when real-time 3D imaging is required as in echocardiography.

7.8.5 Visualization

Visualization tools useful for 3D ultrasound imaging are already available and used in 3D systems. However, they still require complicated user interfaces and an array of tools to manipulate the 3D ultrasound images. For 3D ultrasound imaging to become widely accepted, intuitive tools are required to manipulate the 3D image allowing the user to view any section of the anatomy in relation to other sections. In addition, the user requires intuitive and real-time tools to produce volume-rendered images. Currently, production of volume-rendered images requires manipulation of multiple parameters. Techniques are needed that provide immediate optimal rendering based on both image data and the organ being viewed, without significant user intervention.

7.9 Conclusions

Clinical experience with 3D ultrasound has already demonstrated clear advantages in both disease diagnosis and in image guidance for minimally invasive therapy. Technical advances will improve 3D imaging even further, making this new tool routine in the hands of the ultrasound imaging user. To achieve wide-spread use, advances in both 3D visualization software and instrumentation are required, and the potential for innovations is clearly present. Based on the pace of development in the past five years, we anticipate major advances in the next five years, leading to new and improved application in a wide variety of medical disciplines.

References

[1] Fishman EK, Magid D, Ney DR *et al.* "Three-Dimensional Imaging." Radiology 181:321–337, 1991.

[2] Robb RA, Barillot C. "Interactive Display and Analysis of 3D Medical Images." IEEE Trans Med Imaging 8:217–226, 1989.

[3] Vannier MW, Marsh JL, Warren JO. "Three-Dimensional CT Reconstruction for Craniofacial Surgical Planning and Evaluation." Radiology 150:179–184, 1984.

[4] Wild JJ, And Reid JM. Application of Echoranging Techniques to the Determination of the Structure of Biological Tissues." Science 115:226–230, 1952.

[5] Brinkley JF, Muramatsu SK, McCallum WD, Popp RL. "*In Vitro* Evaluation of an Ultrasonic Three-Dimensional Imaging and Volume System." Utrasonic Imaging 4:126–139, 1982.

[6] Fenster A, Downey DB. "3D Ultrasound Imaging: A Review." IEEE Engineering in Medicine and Biology 15:41–51, 1996.

[7] Ghosh A, Nanda NC, Maurer G. "Three-Dimensional Reconstruction of Echocardiographic Images Using the Rotation Method." Ultrasound in Med & Biol 8:655–661, 1982.

[8] 8. Greenleaf JF, Belohlavek M, Gerber TC, Foley DA, Seward JB. "Multidimensional Visualization in Echocardiography: An Introduction." Mayo Clin Proc 68:213–219, 1993.

[9] King DL, Gopal AS, Sapin PM, Schroder KM, Demaria AN. "Three Dimensional Echocardiography." Am J Card Imaging 3:209–220, 1993.

[10] Nelson TR, Pretorius DH. "Three-Dimensional Ultrasound of Fetal Surface Features." Ultrasound Obstet Gynecol 2:166–174, 1992.

[11] Rankin RN, Fenster A, Downey DB, Munk PL, Levin MF, Vellet AD. "Three-Dimensional Sonographic Reconstruction: Techniques and Diagnostic Applications." AJR 161:695–702, 1993.

[12] Belohlavek M, Foley DA, Gerber TC, Kinter TM, Greenleaf JF, Seward JB. "Three- and Four-Dimensional Cardiovascular Ultrasound Imaging: A New Era for Echocardiography." Mayo Clin Proc 68:221–240, 1993.

[13] Fenster, A. "3D Sonography-Technical Aspects." In Bogdahn U, Becker G, Schlachetzki F (Eds.) *Echoenhancers and Transcranial Color Duplex Sonography.* Berlin, Vienna, Oxford, Edinburgh, Boston, London, Melbourne, Paris, Tokyo: Blackwell Science, 1998, pp. 121–140.

[14] Spaulding KA, Kissner ME, Kim EK *et al.* "Three-Dimensional Gray Scale Ultrasonographic Imaging of the Celiac Axis: Preliminary Report." J Ultrasound Med 17:239–248, 1998.

[15] Nelson TR, Downey B, Pretorius DH, Fenster A. *"Three-Dimensional Ultrasound.* Philadelphia: Lippincott, Williams and Wilkins, 1999.

[16] Ofili EO, Nanda NC. "Three-Dimensional and Four-Dimensional Echocardiography." Ultrasound in Med & Biol 20:669–675, 1994.

[17] Downey DB, Chin JL, Fenster A. "Three-Dimensional US-Guided Cryosurgery." Radiology 197(P):539, 1995.

[18] Downey DB, Fenster A. Vascular Imaging with a Three-Dimensional Power Doppler System." AJR 165:665–668, 1995.

[19] Fenster A, Tong S, Sherebrin S, Downey DB, Rankin RN. "Three-Dimensional Ultrasound Imaging." SPIE Physics of Medical Imaging 2432, 1995, pp. 176–184.

[20] Guo Z, Fenster A. "Three-Dimensional Power Doppler Imaging: A Phantom Study to quantify Vessel Stenosis." Ultrasound in Med & Biol 22:1059–1069, 1996.

[21] Picot PA, Rickey DW, Mitchell R, Rankin RN, Fenster A. "Three Dimensional Color Doppler Imaging of the Carotid Artery." SPIE Proc: Image Capture, Formatting and Display 1444, 1991, pp. 206–213.

[22] Picot PA, Rickey DW, Mitchell R, Rankin RN, Fenster A. "Three-Dimensional Color Doppler Imaging." Ultrasound in Med & Biol 19:95–104, 1993.

[23] Pretorius DH, Nelson TR, Jaffe JS. "3-Dimensional Sonographic Analysis Based on Color Flow Doppler and Gray Scale Image Data: A Preliminary Report." J Ultrasound Med 11:225–232, 1992.

[24] Bamber JC, Eckersley RJ, Hubregtse P, Bush NL, Bell DS, Crawford DC. "Data Processing for 3D Ultrasound Visualization of Tumor Anatomy and Blood Flow." Proc SPIE 1808, 1992, pp. 651–663.

[25] Carson PL, Li X, Pallister J, Moskalik A, Rubin JM, Fowlkes JB. "Approximate Quantification of Detected Fractional Blood Volume and Perfusion from 3D Color Flow and Doppler Power Signal Imaging." In *1993 Ultrasonics Symposium Proceedings.* Piscataway, NJ: IEEE, 1993, pp. 1023–1026.

[26] Downey DB, Fenster A. "Three-Dimensional Power Doppler Detection of Prostatic Cancer." AJR 165:741, 1995.

[27] King DL, King DLJ, Shao MY. "Evaluation of *In Vitro* Measurement Accuracy of a Three-Dimensional Ultrasound Scanner." J Ultrasound Med 10:77–82, 1991.

[28] Guo Z, Moreau M, Rickey DW, Picot PA, Fenster A. "Quantitative Investigation of In Vitro Flow Using Three-Dimensional Color Doppler Ultrasound." Ultrasound in Med & Biol 21:807–816, 1995.

[29] Pandian NG, Nanda NC, Schwartz SL, Fan P, Cao Q. "Three-Dimensional and Four-Dimensional Transesophageal Echocardiographic Imaging of the Heart and Aorta in Humans Using a Computed Tomographic Imaging Probe." Echocardiography 9:677–687, 1992.

[30] Ross Jr JJ, D'Adamo AJ, Karalis DG, Chandrasekaran K. "Three-Dimensional Transesophageal Echo Imaging of the Descending Thoracic Aorta." Am J Cardiol 71:1000–1002, 1993.

[31] Wollschlager H, Zeiher AM, Geibel A, Kasper W, Just H. "Transesophageal Echo Computer Tomography of the Heart." In Roelandt JRTC, Sutherland GR, Iliceto S, Linker DT (Eds.) Cardiac Ultrasound. London: Churchill Livingstone, 1993, pp. 181–185.

[32] Delabays A, Pandian NG, Cao QL et al. "Transthoracic Real-Time Three-Dimensional Echocardiography Using a Fan-Like Scanning Approach for Data Acquisition: Methods, Strengths, Problems, and Initial Clinical Experience." A Jrnl of CV Ultrasound & Allied Tech 12:49 59, 1995.

[33] Downey DB, Nicolle DA, Fenster A. "Three-Dimensional Orbital Ultrasonography." Can J Ophthalmol 30:395–398, 1995.

[34] Downey DB, Nicolle DA, Fenster A. "Three-Dimensional Ultrasound of the Eye." Administrative Radiology Journal 14:46–50, 1995.

[35] Gilja OH, Thune N, Matre K, Hausken T, Odegaard S, Berstad A. "In Vitro Evaluation of Three-Dimensional Ultrasonography in Volume Estimation of Abdominal Organs." Ultras in Med & Biol 20:157, 1994.

[36] Sohn C, Stolz W, Kaufmann M, Bastert G. Die Dreidimensionale Ultraschalldarstellung Benigner und Maligner Brusttumoren—Erste Klinische Erfahrungen." Geburtsh u Frauenheilk 52:520–525, 1992.

[37] Elliot TL, Downey DB, Tong S, Mclean CA, Fenster A. "Accuracy of Prostate Volume Measurements In Vitro Using Three-Dimensional Ultrasound." Academic Radiology 3:401–406, 1996.

[38] Tong S, Downey DB, Cardinal HN, Fenster A. "A Three-Dimensional Ultrasound Prostate Imaging System." Ultrasound in Med & Biol 22:735–746, 1996.

[39] Chin JL, Downey DB, Onik GM, Fenster A. "Three-Dimensional Ultrasound Imaging and Its Application to Cryosurgery for Prostate Cancer." Techniques in Urology 2:187, 1997.

[40] Chin JL, Downey DB, Onik GM, Fenster A. "Three Dimensional Transrectal-Quided Cryoablation for Prostate Cancer: Techniques and Initial Results." J of Urology 159:910–914, 1998.

[41] Onik GM, Downey DB, Fenster A. "Three-Dimensional Sonographically Monitored Cryosurgery in a Prostate Phantom." J Ultrasound Med 15:267–270, 1996.

[42] Martin RW, Bashein G. Measurement of Stroke Volume with Three-Dimensional Transesophageal Ultrasonic Scanning: Comparison with Thermodilution Measurement." Anesthesiology 70:470–476, 1989.

[43] Ludomirsky A, Silberbach M, Kenny A, Shiota T, Rice MJ. "Superiority of Rotational Scan Reconstruction Strategies for Transthoracic 3-Dimensional Real-Time Echocardiographic Studies in Pediatric Patients with CHD." J Am Coll Cardiol 169A, 1994 (Abstract).

[44] McCann HA, Chandrasekaran K, Hoffman EA, Sinak LJ, Kinter TM, Greenleaf JF. "A Method for Three-Dimensional Ultrasonic Imaging of the Heart *In Vivo*." Dynamic Cardiovasc Imaging 1:97–109, 1987.

[45] Roelandt JRTC, Ten Cate FJ, Vletter WB, Taams MA. "Ultrasonic Dynamic Three-Dimensional Visualization of the Heart with a Multiplane Transesophageal Imaging Transducer." Journal of the American Society of Echocardiography 7:217–229, 1994.

[46] Brinkley JF, McCallum WD, Muramatsu SK, Liu DY. "Fetal Weight Estimation from Lengths and Volumes Found by Three-Dimensional Ultrasonic Measurements." J Ultrasound Med 3:163–168, 1984.

[47] King DL, King Jr DL, Shao MYC. "Three-Dimensional Spatial Registration and Interactive Display of Position and Orientation of Real-Time Ultrasound Images." J Ultrasound Med 9:525–532, 1990.

[48] King DL, Harrison MR, King Jr DL, Gopal AS, Kwan OL, Demaria AN. "Ultrasound Beam Orientation During Standard Two-Dimensional Imaging. Assessment by Three-Dimensional Echocardiography." J Am Soc Echocardiogr 5:569–576, 1992.

[49] Levine RA, Handschumacher MD, Sanfilippo AJ *et al.* "Three-Dimensional Echocardiographic Reconstruction of the Mitral Valve, with Implications for the Diagnosis of Mitral Valve Prolapse." Circulation 80:589–598, 1989.

[50] Moritz WE, Pearlman AS, McCabe DH, Medema DH, Ainsworth ME, Boles MS. "An Ultrasonic Technique for Imaging the Ventricle in Three Dimensions and Calculating Its Volume." IEEE Trans Biomed Eng BME-30:482–491, 1983.

[51] Rivera JM, Siu SC, Handschumacher MD, Lethor JP, Guerrero JL. "Three-Dimensional Reconstruction of Ventricular Septal Defects. Validation Studies and *In Vivo* Feasibility." J Am Coll Cardiol 23:201, 1994.

[52] Weiss JL, Eaton LW, Kallman CH, Maughman WL. "Accuracy of Volume Determination by Two-Dimensional Echocardiography: Defining Requirements under Controlled Conditions in the Ejecting Canine Left Ventricle." Circulation 67:889–895, 1983.

[53] Bonilla-Musoles F, Raga F, Osborne NG, Blanes J. "Use of Three-Dimensional Ultrasonography for the Study of Normal and Pathologic Morphology of the Human Embryo and Fetus: Preliminary Report." J Ultrasound Med 14:757–765, 1995.

[54] Detmer PR, Bashein G, Hodges T *et al.* "3D Ultrasonic Image Feature Localization Based on Magnetic Scanhead Tracking: *In Vitro* Calibration and Validation. Ultrasound in Med & Biol 20:923–936, 1994.

[55] Ganapathy U, Kaufman A. "3D Acquisition and Visualization of Ultrasound Data. Visualization in Biomedical Computing." Proc SPIE 1808, 1992, pp. 535–545.

[56] Hodges TC, Detmer PR, Burns DH, Beach KW, Strandness Jr DE. "Ultrasonic Three-Dimensional Reconstruction: *In Vitro* and *In Vivo* Volume and Area Measurement." Ultrasound in Med & Biol 20:719–729, 1994.

[57] Hughes SW, Arcy TJD, Maxwell DJ *et al.* "Volume Estimation from Multiplanar 2D Ultrasound Images Using a Remote Electromagnetic Position and Orientation." Ultrasound in Med & Biol 22:561–572, 1996.

[58] Leotta DF, Detmer PR, Martin RW. "Performance of a Miniature Magnetic Position Sensor for Three-Dimensional Ultrasound Imaging." Ultrasound in Med & Biol 23:597–609, 1997.

[59] Gilja OH, Detmer PR, Jong JM *et al.* "Intragastric Distribution and Gastric Emptying Assessed by Three-Dimensional Ultrasonography." Gastroenterology 113:38–49, 1997.

[60] Nelson TR, Pretorius DH. "Visualization of the Fetal Thoracic Skeleton with Three-Dimensional Sonography: A Preliminary Report." AJR 164:1485–1488, 1995.

[61] Ohbuchi R, Chen D, Fuchs H. "Incremental Volume Reconstruction and Rendering for 3D Ultrasound Imaging." SPIE Visualization In Biomedical Computing 1808, 1992, pp. 312–323.

[62] Pretorius DH, Nelson TR. "Prenatal Visualization of Cranial Sutures and Fontanelles with Three-Dimensional Ultrasonography." J Ultrasound Med 13:871–876, 1994.

[63] Raab FH, Blood EB, Steiner TO, Jones HR. "Magnetic Position and Orientation Tracking System." IEEE Transactions on Aerospace and Electronic Systems AES-15:709–717, 1979.

[64] Tuthill TA, Krucker JF, Fowlkes JB, Carson PL. "Automated Three-Dimensional US Frame Positioning Computed from Elevational Speckle Decorrelation." Radiology 209: 575–582, 1998.

[65] Shattuck DP, Weinshenker MD, Smith SW, Von Ramm OT. "Explososcan: A Parallel Processing Technique for High Speed Ultrasound Imaging with Linear Phased Arrays." J Acoust Soc Am 75:1273–1282, 1984.

[66] Smith SW, Pavy Jr HG, Von Ramm OT. "High-Speed Ultrasound Volumetric Imaging System. Part I. Transducer Design and Beam Steering." IEEE Trans Ultrason Ferroelec Freq Contr 38:100–108, 1991.

[67] Smith SW, Trahey GE, Von Ramm OT. "Two Dimensional Arrays for Medical Ultrasound." Ultrason Imaging 14:213–233, 1992.

[68] Snyder JE, Kisslo J, Von Ramm OT. "Real-Time Orthogonal Mode Scanning of the Heart. I. System Design." J Am Coll Cardiol 7:1279, 1986.

[69] Turnbull DH, Foster FS. "Beam Steering with Pulsed Two-Dimensional Transducer Arrays." IEEE Trans Ultrason Ferroelec Freq Contr 38:320–333, 1991.

[70] Von Ramm OT, Smith SW. "Real Time Volumetric Ultrasound Imaging System." Proc SPIE 1231, 1990, pp. 15–22.

[71] Von Ramm OT, Smith SW, Pavy Jr HG. "High-Speed Ultrasound Volumetric Imaging System. Part II. Parallel Processing and Image Display." IEEE Trans Ultrason Ferroelec Freq Contr 38:109–115, 1991.

[72] Chin JL, Downey DB, Onik G, Fenster A. "Three-Dimensional Prostate Ultrasound and Its Application to Cryosurgery." Tech Urol 2:187, 1996.

[73] Nelson *et al.*

[74] Tong S, Cardinal HN, Downey DB, Fenster A. "Analysis of Linear, Area, and Volume Distortion In 3D Ultrasound Imaging." Ultrasound in Med & Biol 24(3):355–373, 1997.

[75] Bezdek JC, Hall LO, Clarke LP. "Review of MR Segmentation Techniques Using Pattern Recognition." Med Phys 20:1033–1048, 1993.

[76] Neveu M, Faudot D, Derdouri B. "Recovery of 3D Deformable Models from Echocardiographic Images." Proc SPIE 2299, 1994, pp. 367–376.

[77] Coppini G, Poli R, Valli G. "Recovery of the 3D Shape of the Left Ventricle from Echocardiographic Images." IEEE Trans Med Imaging 14:301–317, 1995.

[78] Lobregt S, Viergever MA. "A Discrete Dynamic Contour Model." IEEE Trans Med Imaging 14:12–24, 1995.

[79] Sohn C, Grotepab J, Swobodnik W. "Moglichkeiten der 3 Dimensionalen Ultraschalldarstellung." Ultraschall 10:307–313, 1989.

[80] Sohn C, Rudofsky G. "Die Dreidimensionale Ultraschalldiagnostik—Ein Neues Verfahren fur die Klinische Routine?" Ultraschall Klin Prax 4:219–224, 1989.

[81] Brinkley JF, McCallum WD, Muramatsu SK, Liu DY. "Fetal Weight Estimation from Ultrasonic Three-Dimensional Head and Trunk Reconstructions. Evaluation *In Vitro*." Am J Obstet Gyn 144:715, 1982.

[82] Sohn C, Grotepass J. "Representation Tridimensionnelle par Ultrason." Radiologie J CEPUR 9:249–253, 1989.

[83] Sohn C, Grotepab J, Schneider W *et al.* "Erste Untersuchungen zur Dreidimensionalen Darstellung Mittels Ultraschall." Z Geburtsh u Perinat 192:241–248, 1988.

[84] Sohn C. "A New Diagnostic Technique: Three-Dimensional Ultrasound Imaging." In *Ultrasonics International 89 Conference Proceedings*, 1989, pp. 1148–1153.

[85] Fine DG, Sapoznikov D, Mosseri M, Gotsman MS. "Three-Dimensional Echocardiographic Reconstruction. Qualitative and Quantitative Evaluation of Ventricular Function." Computer Methods and Programs in Biomedicine 26:33–44, 1988.

[86] Nixon JV, Saffer SI, Lipscomb K, Blomqvist CG. "Three-Dimensional Echoventriculography." Am Heart J 106:435–443, 1983.

[87] Martin RW, Bashein G, Detmer PR, Moritz WE. "Ventricular Volume Measurement from a Multiplanar Transesophageal Ultrasonic Imaging System. An *In Vitro* Study." IEEE Trans Biomed Eng 37:442–449, 1990.

[88] Linker DT, Moritz WE, Pearlman AS. "A New Three-Dimensional Echocardiographic Method of Right Ventricular Volume Measurement: In Vitro Validation." J Am Coll Cardiol 8:101–106, 1986.

[89] Sawada H, Fujii J, Kato K, Onoe M, Kuno Y. "Three Dimensional Reconstruction of the Left Ventricle from Multiple Cross Sectional Echocardiograms *Value For Measuring Left Ventricular Volume.*" Br Heart J 50:438–442, 1983.

[90] Belohlavek M, Foley DA, Gerber TC, Greenleaf JF, Seward JB. "Three-Dimensional Ultrasound Imaging of the Atrial Septum: Normal and Pathologic Anatomy." J Am Coll Cardiol 22:1673–1678, 1993.

[91] McCann HA, Sharp JC, Kinter TM, McEwan CN, Barillot C, Greenleaf JF. "Multidimensional Ultrasonic Imaging for Cardiology." Proc IEEE 76:1063–1073, 1988.

[92] Wang XF, Li ZA, Cheng TO *et al.* "Clinical Application of Three-Dimensional Transesophageal Echocardiography." American Heart Journal 128:381–389, 1994.

[93] Belohlavek M, Foley DA, Gerber TC, Greenleaf JF, Seward JB. "Three-Dimensional Reconstruction of Color Doppler Jets in the Human Heart." J Am Soc Echocardiogr 7:553–560, 1994.

[94] Fenster A, Dunne S, Chan TK, Downey D. "Method and System for Constructing and Displaying Three Dimensional Images." US Patent No. 5,454,371, Oct 3, 1995.

[95] Lees WA. "3D Ultrasound Images Optimize Fetal Review." Diagnostic Imaging (March):69–73, 1992.

[96] Zosmer N, Jurkovic D, Jauniaux E, Gruboeck K, Lees C, Campbell S. "Selection and Identification of Standard Cardiac Views From Three-Dimensional Volume Scans of the Fetal Thorax." J Ultrasound Med 15:25–32, 1996.

[97] Gerscovich EO, Greenspan A, Cronan MS, Karol LA, McGahan JP. "Three-Dimensional Sonographic Evaluation of Developmental Dysplasia of the Hip. Preliminary Findings." Radiology 190:407–410, 1994.

[98] Kuo HC, Chang FM, Wu CH, Yao BL, Liu CH. "The Primary Application of Three-Dimensional Ultrasonography in Obstetrics." Am J Obstet Gynecol 166:880–886, 1992.

[99] Kirbach D, Whittingham TA. "3D Ultrasound—The Kretztechnik Voluson Approach." European Journal of Ultrasound 1:85–89, 1994.

[100] Robb RA. *Three-Dimensional Biomedical Imaging. Principles and Practice.* New York: VCH Publishers, Inc., 1995.

[101] Lichtenbelt B, Crane R, Naqvi S. *Introduction To Volume Rendering.* Upper Saddle River NJ: Prentice Hall, 1998.

[102] Levoy M. "Volume Rendering, a Hybrid Ray Tracer for Rendering Polygon and Volume Data." IEEE Computer Graphics and Appl 10:33–40, 1990.

[103] Levoy M. "Efficient Ray Tracing of Volume Data." ACM Transactions on Graphics 9:245–261, 1990.

[104] Nelson TR, Pretorius DH, Sklansky M, Hagen-Ansert S. "Three-Dimensional Echocardiographic Evaluation of Fetal Heart Anatomy and Function: Acquisition, Analysis, and Display." J Ultrasound Med 15:1–9, 1996.

[105] 105. Pretorius DH, Nelson TR. "Fetal Face Visualization Using Three Dimensional Ultrasonography." J Ultrasound Med 14:349–356, 1995.

[106] Fine D, Perring S, Herbetko J, Hacking CN, Fleming JS, Dewbury KC. "Three-Dimensional (3D) Ultrasound Imaging of the Gallbladder and Dilated Biliary Tree. Reconstruction From Real-Time B-Scans." The British Journal of Radiology 64:1056–1057, 1991.

[107] Geiser EA, Ariet M, Conetta DA, Lupkiewicz SM, Christie Jr LG, Conti CR. "Dynamic Three-Dimensional Echocardiographic Reconstruction of the Intact Human Left Ventricle. Technique and Initial Observations in Patients." Am Heart J 103:1056–1065, 1982.

[108] Favre R, Bader AM, Nisand G. "Prospective Study on Fetal Weight Estimation Using Limb Circumferences Obtained by Three-Dimensional Ultrasound." Ultrasound Obstet Gynecol 6:140–4, 1995.

[109] Gilja OH, Smievoll AI, Thune N et al. "In Vivo Comparison of 3D Ultrasonography and Magnetic Resonance Imaging in Volume Estimation of Human Kidneys." Ultrasound in Med & Biol 21:25–32, 1995.

[110] Riccabona M, Nelson TR, Pretorius DH. "Three-Dimensional Ultrasound: Accuracy of Distance and Volume Measurements." Ultrasound Obstet Gynecol 7:429–434, 1996.

[111] Sivan E, Chan L, Uerpairojkit B, Chu GP, Reece A. "Growth of the Fetal Forehead and Normative Dimensions Developed by Three-Dimensional Ultrasonographic Technology." J Ultrasound Med 16:401–405, 1997.

[112] Tong S, Downey DB, Cardinal HN, Fenster A. "A Three-Dimensional Ultrasound Prostate Imaging System." Ultrasound Med Biol 22:735, 1996.

[113] Elliot TL, Downey DB, Tong S, Mclean CA, Fenster A. "Accuracy of Prostate Volume Measurements In Vitro Using Three-Dimensional Ultrasound." Acad Radiol 3:401–406, 1996.

[114] Brunner M, Obruca A, Bauer P, Feichtinger W. "Clinical Application of Volume Estimation Based on Three-Dimensional Ultrasonography." Ultrasound Obstet Gynecol 6:358–361, 1995.

[115] Chang FM, Hsu KF, Ko HC et al. "Fetal Heart Volume Assessment by Three-Dimensional Ultrasound." Ultrasound Obstet Gynecol 9:42–48, 1997.

[116] Riccabona M, Johnson D, Pretorius DH, Nelson TR. "Three-Dimensional Ultrasound: Display Modalities in the Fetal Spine and Thorax." Eur J Radiol 22:141–145, 1996.

[117] Lee F, Bahn DK, McHugh TA, Kumar AA, Badalament RA. "Cryosurgery of Prostate Cancer. Use of Adjuvant Hormonal Therapy and Temperature Monitoring—A One Year Follow-up." Anticancer Res 17:1511–1515, 1997.

[118] Terris MK, Stamey TA. "Determination of Prostate Volume by Transrectal Ultrasound." The Journal of Urology 145:984–987, 1991.

[119] Aarnink RG, Wijkstra H. "Errors in Transrectal Ultrasonic Planimetry of the Prostate. Computer Simulation of Volumetric Errors Applied to a Screening Population." Ultrasound in Med & Biol 21:1083–1084, 1995.

[120] Tong S, Cardinal HN, Downey DB, Fenster A. "Inter- and Intra-Observer Variability and Reliability of Prostate Volume Measurement via 2D and 3D Ultrasound Imaging." Ultrasound in Med & Biol 24:673–681, 1997.

[121] Eliasziw M, Young SL, Woodbury MG, Fryday-Field K. "Statistical Methodology for the Concurrent Assessment of Interrater and Intrarater Reliability: Using Goniometric Measurements as an Example." Physical Therapy 74:777–788, 1994.

[122] Mitchell JR, Karlik SJ, Lee DH, Eliasziw M, Rice GP, Fenster A. "The Variability of Manual and Computer Assisted Quantification of Multiple Sclerosis Lesion Volumes." Med Phys 23:85–97, 1996.

[123] Rickey DW, Picot PA, Christopher DA, Fenster A. "A Wall-Less Vessel Phantom for Doppler Ultrasound Studies." Ultrasound in Med & Biol 21:1163–1176, 1995.

CHAPTER 8
Tomographic Imaging

David J. Goodenough
George Washington University

CONTENTS

8.1 Introduction

The first clinically useful computed-tomography (CT) system was pioneered by Godfrey Hounsfield of EMI Ltd. in England. This system was installed in 1971 in the Atkinson Morley Hospital near London [1]. In fact, Hounsfield shared the Nobel Prize for Medicine in 1979 with Alan Cormack from Tufts University. This introduction of computed tomography (CT) into the commercial market for radiological imaging in the mid 1970s had profound effects on the subsequent developments in medical imaging. Both the "computer" (C) attribute and the "Tomography" (T) attribute became firmly established in the radiological armamentarium.

Until the advent of CT, computer and digital imaging had only minimal success in penetrating the medical-imaging department. With the possible exception of nuclear medicine, most computer-based systems were met with apprehension because of aspects of cost, reliability, and siting complexity. The EMI scanner arrived on the scene with an impact not unlike that of x-ray systems following Roentgen's discovery in 1895. In fact, the dissemination was so rapid that CT brought with it a less distinguished legacy of Certificate of Need and other regulatory review processes. These processes were designed, in part, to limit the dissemination and perceived cost of CT scanners and related CT procedures.

From a preliminary image-analysis assessment, the success of early CT scanners seems surprising, even in retrospect. Why, for example, should a modality that only scanned heads and took several minutes to acquire an image of a 13-mm slice, in matrices of only 80×80 (3 mm $\times$ 3 mm pixels) meet with such keen reception from neuroradiologists? Until this time, these same neuroradiologists found image-quality improvements primarily in the area of ever-increasing spatial resolution (at the $100\text{-}\mu$-levels or better). The answer to the question is actually complex, and perhaps best understood by those diagnosticians who had been working in the often information-starved (statistically speaking) field of nuclear medicine, where spatial resolution was also measured in the cm range. The answer lies in two concepts, namely: (1) what is now called CONTRAST RESOLUTION; and (2) reduced complexity of competing anatomical patterns, sometimes called STRUCTURE NOISE [2].

ADVANTAGES OF CT

⇑ Improved Contrast Resolution and
⇓ Decreased Structure Noise

8.2 Overview of CT as an image device

Computed tomography (CT) is the term generally used to characterize the imaging technique in which transmission measurements of a narrow beam of x rays, made at several different angles or projections around a given object, may be used with an appropriate computer program or algorithm to re-synthesize particular slices of interest within the object.

Computed tomography differs from the more conventional x-ray tomography in that one uses digital or computer techniques to restore the slice of interest rather than the analog (conventional tomographic) techniques of deliberately casting unwanted information into "out-of-focus" planes on a film moving in a complex prescribed geometrical pattern with the x-ray tube. One problem with the older conventional tomographic techniques was that the unwanted information is reduced to a general scatter or fog level on the film-thus reducing inherent contrast. Both older analog and newer digital tomographic techniques have in common the desire to isolate a given plane (actually a thin section) of information from the sometimes confusing information arising from the rest of the three-dimensional object found superimposed on the relevant information. Similar superposition of unwanted information is found, for example, when a single projection (e.g., A.P.) is obtained on a standard two-dimensional image receptor such as a radiograph. The failure of the older analog techniques to clearly separate a slice from the rest of the object was another major limitation.

CT, radiography, and nuclear medicine are fundamentally limited by the Poisson statistics of the number of detected quanta. Given the typical radiation dose levels and quantum detection efficiency (QDE) of CT and competing radiographic modalities, it is not difficult to predict the signal-to-noise ratio of a given small signal in a uniform surround. In fact, for a simple model of CT and radiographic screen film imaging, it has been shown that for certain signal sizes, intrinsic detectability can be somewhat similar between the two modalities. In general, the relationship will depend on many physical variables of the imaging systems, as well as the size of the signal (target) [3].

However, the simple models of detection (e.g., a simple sphere in a uniformly filled water bath), as will be discussed later in this chapter, will not describe the complex perceptual task of finding a signal in a highly structured projection radiograph such as a chest x ray, wherein many anatomical planes (or thin slices) may be considered superimposed upon each other presenting potentially competing anatomic patterns which can distract the viewer from a small lesion or fracture. Thus, the "tomos" interest, whereby one "slice" may be separated from the rest of the object.

8.3 Scanner design

Various types of CT systems have been developed (Table 8.1). These scanners use various combinations of motion(s), geometric design, and detector types. Each design must focus on how to get an adequate number of rays (or x-ray attenuation lines of sight), within a given view or angle, as well as the need to obtain an adequate number of views or angles around the object being scanned.

The first generation used a single scanning beam which first translated across the object, before rotating 1° and repeating the process (Figures 8.1(a) and (b)).

The pencil beam scanner design of the EMI Mark I head scanner, shown in Figure 8.1(b), used a single detector and single x-ray source assembly to generate the narrow beam x-ray attenuation coefficient data used for each slice (actually two

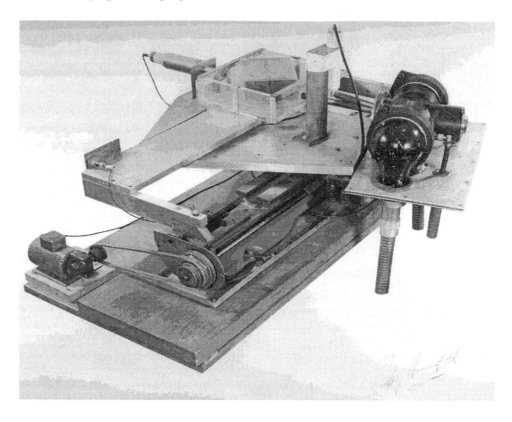

Figure 8.1(a): Lithograph of Hounsfield Original Test Lathe, signed and presented to the author in the late 1970s.

slices were acquired simultaneously by using two crystals placed end to end, much like today's multislice scanners). The pencil beam scanners were typically characterized by both rotate and translate motions with a total rotation angle ranging from 180° to 240°. The type of x-ray tube was typically of continuous emission design. This design use d a combination of linear and rotational motions to generate a series of x-ray transmission profiles. This type of design, although originally slow (several-minute scans), offered some built in redundancy of sampling that makes the reconstruction problem somewhat easier. The initial design suffered from long scan time, allowing the possibility of patient motion. Although some ingenious pneumatic drives were designed to produce dual motion acquisition in several seconds, it became clear that there was a need for single motion machines. In addition, the original EMI scanner used a water bath to surround the patient's head. A water bath provided a constant path length of attenuation, and thus a number of practical advantages such as reducing the extent of (spectral) beam hardening resulting from transmission through varying distance, as well as reduced dynamic range requirements on the detector system. Because the original scanners utilized a scanning pattern of only about 180°, one encountered an uneven deposition of energy throughout the patient's head according to well known depth-dose distribu-

Table 8.1: Scanner types

Dual Motion	*Pencil Beam*—(1st Generation)
Dual Motion	*Hybrid*—Multiple Pencil Beam (2nd Generation)
Single Motion	*Fan Beam*—(Rotating detector and x-ray source) (3rd Generation) Single slice, or multi-slice
Single Motion	*Fan Beam*—(Rotating source only) (4th Generation)
No Mechanical Motion	*Fan Beam*—(Scanning Electron Beam) (5th Generation)

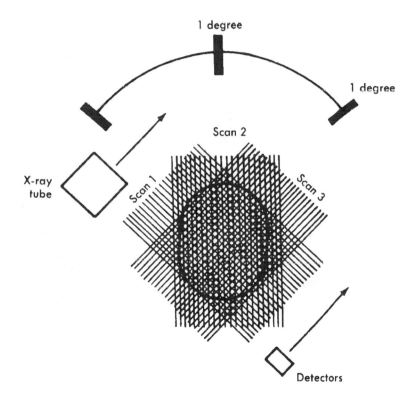

Figure 8.1(b): EMI scan pattern (first-generation geometry). Linear sweeps to obtain rays, followed by angular rotation to obtain views.

tion with maximum dose at about 90° on the x-ray tube side of the scan. Partial scans (180°+ fan angle) are still used today to obtain faster scans.

The second-generation systems (so-called hybrid machines) used multiple detectors instead of a single detector monitoring a single x-ray source, such a detector source configuration might be described as a limited fan beam (note, however, that the rotate and translate motions were preserved).

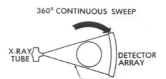

Figure 8.2(a): Early third-generation geometry (courtesy, General Electric Corporation). Detectors and x-ray tubes rotate in synchrony.

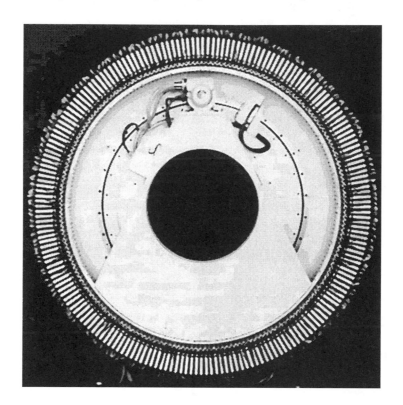

Figure 8.2(b): Early fourth-generation geometry (courtesy, American Science & Engineering). Only tube rotates on inscribed circle of continuous ring of detectors.

In the hybrid system, multiple detectors were used to enable the system to rotate a larger angular increment than for a single-detector system. By increasing the number of detectors, the same number of rays as the pencil scanner could be obtained in 10 to 20 seconds. This type of machine was usually still characterized by a continuous-emission x-ray source.

Single-motion machines include third- and fourth-generation designs. The so-called third generation system (see Figure 8.2(a)) utilizes a fan-beam geometry involving a large number of detectors designed to rotate in synchrony with the x-ray tube moving in a single continuous rotational motion. The bank of detectors, arranged in an arc, look back at the x-ray source which moves synchronously with

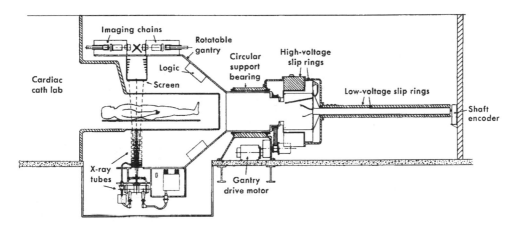

Figure 8.3(a): Dynamic spatial reconstructor (adapted from [4]).

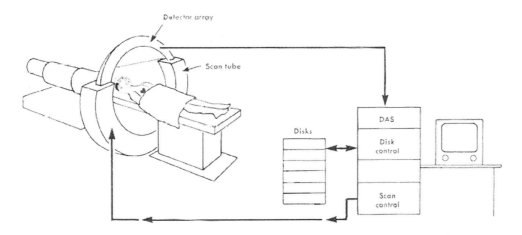

Figure 8.3(b): Imatron—electron beam scanner (adapted from [5]).

the detector. In addition, one encountered pulsed-emission x-ray sources. A variant of the single-motion design was partially funded by the NIH and became the American Science and Engineering (AS&E) scanner. This scanner was considered fourth-generation geometry in which several hundred detectors were kept fixed on a stationary ring while the x-ray source itself moved on an inscribed circle within the detector ring (see Figure 8.2(b)). Third- and higher-order generation systems were advocated because the data may be acquired in times on the order of five seconds or less, opening up the possibility of significant decreases in motion artifacts. Another variation on this fourth-generation design, was a source which rotated outside a continuous detector ring, which at the correct moment, rocked (or nutated) the near-sided detectors aside, allowing the source to emit x rays unimpeded to the far-side detectors. This approach was developed by EMI and later marketed by Toshiba. As technology improved, third- and fourth-generation geometry achieved full 360° scan rotations in 1 second or less, considerably reducing problems of patient motion.

One important area of development was the potential for heart scanning. In terms of the temporal constraints of the beating heart, and the needs for adequate spatial and density discrimination levels, it is clear that one either needs to develop high dose (photon fluence) rates to be delivered in about 50 ms by single or multiple sources, or, perhaps develop adequate "gating" of the cardiac and respiratory cycles in synchrony with the data acquisition scheme. An important early development in this area was the work on the dynamic spatial reconstructor (DSR) performed at the Mayo Clinic using multiple (28) x-ray sources and image intensifiers to achieve "dynamic" reconstructions of the heart [4]. A slightly later competing approach to heart scanning utilized a scanning electron beam system (EBS) scanned across a row(s) of scattering foils emitting x rays upwards to a semicircular arc of detectors. The source position needed no mechanical motion, only electronic steering [5]. This device, which also offered multislices by adding more rows of scattering foils, developed by Douglas Boyd and colleagues at the University of California at San Francisco (UCSF), was licensed to the Imatron Corporation and has enjoyed fairly wide-spread use more recently to rapidly scan and quantify or "score" calcified vessels as a possible risk factor in heart disease. Similar "scoring" algorithms have been developed for use with subsecond third- and fourth-generation scanners.

One area of early interest that was promoted for scanners was the possibility of developing the quantitative aspects of CT. The term "tomochemistry" was used to describe the general attempt to unfold the energy-dependent contributions of the compton and photoelectric contributions of the CT number. Although only minimally developed, there remain possibilities for filtering the polychromatic x-ray spectrum and/or utilizing monoenergetic sources and photon-counting devices for CT reconstructions aimed at unfolding electron density and atomic number contributions [6].

A significant development for third- and fourth-generation scanners was the development of so-called helical or spiral scanners (Figure 8.4). This approach incorporated a moving table during the rotation of the x-ray tube. The net effect is that the x-ray path describes a helical (spiral or corkscrew) pattern around the scanned volume of the patient. The major advantage of spiral scanning is the volume of coverage for a given rotation of x-ray exposure. The gain in coverage is described by the pitch which describes the number of slice thicknesses the table moves during one revolution. Typical pitches range up to 2 or more in single slice systems, and N times that in multislice scanners with N slices (N is currently about 4).

The "tomos," or slice, is ideally an infinitely thin plane separated from the other planes above or below its location. In reality, the tomos ranges from perhaps 0.5 mm in a current multislice CT scanner to the original EMI levels of several mm (e.g., 13-mm in EMI Mark I head scanner) still used today. A single slice CT scanner, with a well-collimated x-ray beam may produce a rather distinct slice, where for example, the slice sensitivity may be well defined and reasonably constant across the CT slice. With the introduction of spiral scanning, the slice is not so simply defined by the x-ray collimation; rather, the nature of the moving table (slice) requires interpolation schemes to provide estimates of information within a given slice. This information is, in fact, acquired in an acquisition which includes information from the slice above and below the slice of interest and then interpolates the data to establish an effective slice at a given position.

An important positive feature of the multislice scanner is the way in which spiral information can be better restored to a slice of interest compared to the complication of single-slice spiral interpolators used with a single moving slice (table); this is particularly a problem for high pitch ratios. In fact, even though the original EMI Mark I scanner was actually the original multislice scanner with juxtaposed A and B dual slices, the field rather rapidly adopted a single-slice acquisition approach for about twenty years until the rediscovery of twin-beam CT scanners by Elscint Ltd.

It should be noted that CT scanners have traditionally been CAT scanners in that, by geometric design and patient orientation, scanners produced intrinsically AXIAL planes. Other planes of interest (particularly *sagittal* and *coronal*, and even *oblique planes*) could only be generated by first acquiring a series of axial slices, and then reformatting the acquired data into a set of other planes. This process was generally called multi planar reconstruction, or MPR (Figure 8.5).

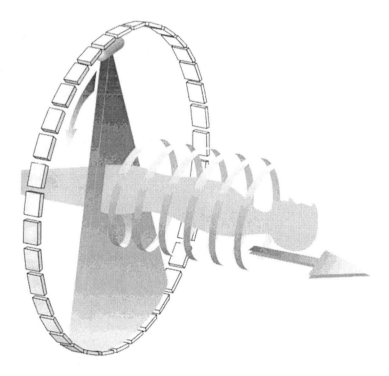

Figure 8.4(a): Helical scanning. The table moves continuously while the x-ray tube rotates (courtesy of Picker International).

SINGLE-SLICE HELICAL RECONSTRUCTION

360⁰ Linear Interpolation   **180⁰ Linear Interpolation**

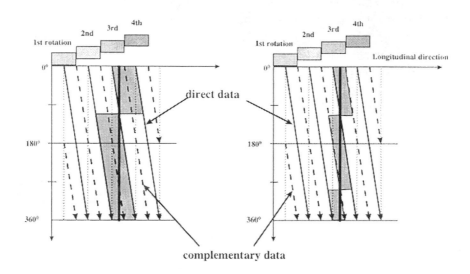

Figure 8.4(b): Two types of Interpolating schemes of single-slice CT (adapted from [18]).

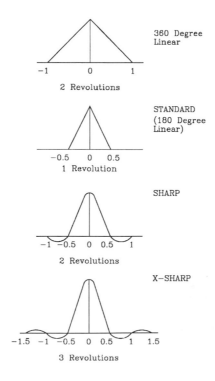

Figure 8.4(c): Spiral interpolation filters (courtesy of Picker International).

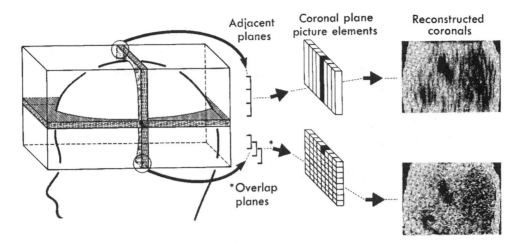

Figure 8.5(a): Original multiplanar reconstruction as developed by William Glenn (adapted from [7]).

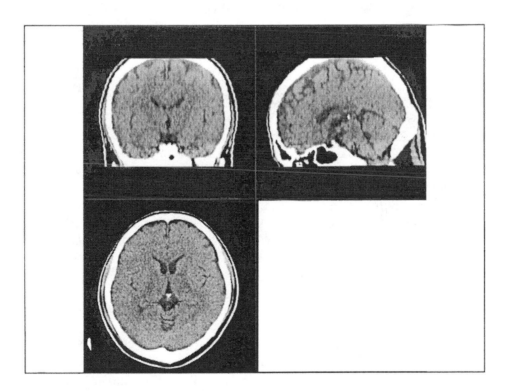

Figure 8.5(b): Modern multislice CT MPR. Note significantly improved image quality (courtesy, Toshiba Medical Systems).

Several factors limit the utility of the MPR process. First, as mentioned previously, each slice of the axial tomos has finite thickness, often several millimeters.

This finite slice thickness for a series of contiguous axial slices immediately imposes a requirement of interslice interpolation. Thus, in MPR approaches, the resolution in the z-axis direction (i.e., normal to the acquired axial slices) is limited by the interslice spacing and interpolation scheme. Moreover, the problem is not readily solved by acquiring thinner and thinner slices. In practice, there are many potential problems for acquiring thin slices with single-slice scanners; namely the finite focal spot size limits not only the in-plane $x-y$ resolution; but also the z-axis resolution. It is also often difficult to collimate thin slices and this fact complicates the dose profile along the z-axis, particularly measured at central locations. The results tend to produce deleterious dose buildup factors for thin slices as scattered radiation becomes an increasing contribution to nearest neighbors. Additionally, the acquisition of more and more thin slices to cover a given volume with single-slice scanners usually involves greater patient scanning time because the per slice axial slice acquisition is usually already scanned at the minimum scan time (about 1 second per slice). Thus, motion unsharpness and patient dose may both be negatively affected by thin-slice acquisition, single-slice CT scanners in that to cover a given volume takes more slices and therefore more time.

CONVENTIONAL THIN-SLICE SCANNING

⇓ Improved (less) Partial Volume
⇑ Increased Scan Time
⇑ Increased Dose Buildup

The advent of spiral CT certainly helped the patient motion issue in that the spiral process offers greater volume coverage for a given scan time. Although, as mentioned previously, the complex nature of spiral interpolators and high pitch ratios can lead to degenerate slice profiles, during which the ideally uniform square wave slice sensitivity profiles (which are fairly well matched in modern nonhelical scanners) become more and more Gaussian-like. This interpolation process tends to create slices where the full width at half maximum (FWHM) is often matched to the nominal slice width, but the extra tails of the slice extend the sensitivity profile significantly into the neighboring slices, and much beyond the normal slice width (Figure 8.6). Although MPR techniques from spiral scanning may at first order appear seamless, the accuracy and continuity of the information may be compromised by the spiral process.

Against this backdrop of volume scanning and MPR techniques for conventional single-slice scanning and spiral scanning is seen the recent introduction of multislice CT scanners. Such scanners offer two distinct advantages for volume scanning: (1) a potentially thinner slice that can be achieved by physical and/or electronic collimation and (2) a better defined sensitivity profile. One may, however, encounter challenges of a need for increased beam stability in the x-ray slice (z) direction, particularly at the edges of the detectors; or, risk the potential of increased dose buildup from using a beam of considerably larger size to avoid penumbra effects. These topics will be re-addressed later in this chapter.

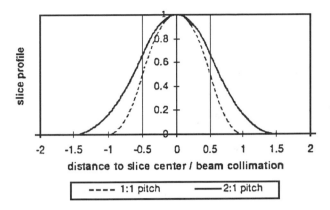

slice profiles: single slice CT

Figure 8.6: Spiral Slice Sensitivity Profile (SSP) of single-slice CT in Spiral Mode. The pitch describes the number of slice widths the table moves during a single rotation. As the pitch increases, SSP curves deviate more and more from an ideal square wave (−0.5 to 0.5) more similar to "step and shoot" conventional (non-spiral) CT.

8.4 Reconstruction techniques

The mathematical basis of the reconstruction of an object from the data obtained in a number of views around the object was developed as early as 1917 by Radon. In 1956, Bracewell developed practical techniques for measuring microwave radiation emitted by the sun by using a series of strip measurements. In 1975, Gordon cited over 1500 references, including those mentioned above, related to image reconstruction [8].

The first published attempt at medical application of reconstruction was carried out by Oldendorf in 1961 using a method called "spin migration." Important experiments were also carried out in 1963 by Kuhl and colleagues at the University of Pennsylvania utilizing a tomographic image scanner for radionuclide imaging and developing the concepts of single-photon computed emission tomography (SPECT). Terpogossian *et al.*, also exploited many of the same reconstruction methods for positron emission tomograph (PET) scanners [9].

Consider the nature of the signals one might expect from examining an isolated pin or needle (impulse source) as one moves around the periphery and generates views or profiles around the pin. If one only had the profile data from views around an object, how might it be used to estimate the original object distribution? The first tendency would probably be to literally throw back (or back project) the given data for each profile across the whole x/y plane (Figure 8.7(a)). If one does this, one will generate a crude estimate of the object of interest, but one also generates some background information which is not in the original object. This spurious information will tend to obscure or diminish the contrast and true nature of the real object of interest. Such a simple operation is usually called *back projection* [10].

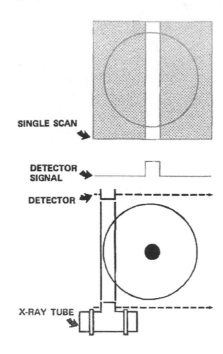

Figure 8.7(a):   Reconstruction concepts. The concept of signal reading of rays during linear sweeps.

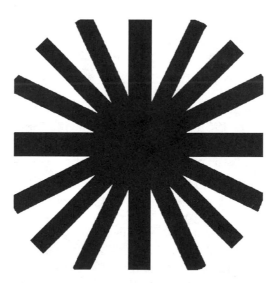

Figure 8.7(b):   Reconstruction concepts. Simple back projection renders a crude central image but the process also generates radial spokes leading to a $1/r$ dependence.

If one considers what happens when one back projects several of the profiles obtained from scans around the periphery of an isolated central pin, one obtains a

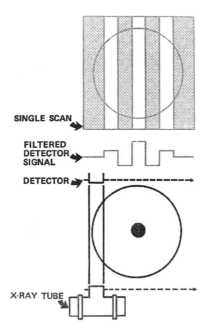

SINGLE SCAN

FILTERED
DETECTOR
SIGNAL

DETECTOR

X-RAY TUBE

Figure 8.7(c):   Reconstruction concepts. The radial spokes can be removed by back projecting a modified or "filtered" version of the profile. The negative lobes lead to cancellation of the spokes. The process is called filtered back projection.

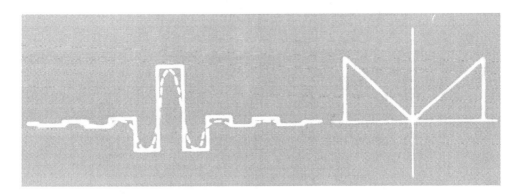

Figure 8.7(d):   Reconstruction concepts. The process of reconstruction can be accomplished in the spatial domain with filtered back projection using the real space deconvolution filter on left; or simple multiplicative operation in spatial frequency domain using the Fourier transform of the deconvolution filter, which is a RAMP filter shown truncated to reduce high frequency noise components.

hot central region somewhat resembling the pin, but one also has an accompanying characteristic star-type artifact with "spokes" radiating from the point of interest, obviously greatly degrading the spatial information concerning the point of interest (Figure 8.7(b)).

From information theory and linear-system analysis, if it is known how each point is blurred or degraded by a system then, under certain conditions of linearity and isoplanacity and in the absence of statistical noise, it is possible to exactly characterize or predict the resulting output image $o(r)$ based on amount of degradation introduced in real space (r), by the point spread function, $\mathrm{psf}(r)$ to the original input distribution $i(r)$. This process is called convolution [11]. In an analogous way, if it is known how each individual point is blurred by an image-forming operation (such as a simple back-projection operation), one might hope to "deconvolve" or deblur the deleterious effect of simple back projection and return to the original object. The correction for the blurring function (or deconvolution) can be carried out on each projection by filtered back projection wherein each profile data is corrected for the effect of the simple back-projection operations (Figure 8.7(c)). Such complicated spatial convolution operations reduce to simple multiplicative relationships of Fourier transforms in the Fourier spatial domain. Thus, another way of dealing with the CT reconstruction is to take the profile data generated from the scanning and data-acquisition system and generate the corresponding Fourier transform for each projection and work with multiplicative operations of the input spatial frequency content $I(\nu)$, and modulation transfer function (MTF) in Fourier

$$o(r) = i(r) * \mathrm{psf}(r), \tag{8.1}$$

$$O(\nu) = I(\nu)\mathrm{MTF}(\nu), \tag{8.2}$$

space to predict the output frequency spectrum $O(\nu)$.

Each different angle or view will give a separate Fourier transform which may be multiplied by the Fourier transform (in its noiseless limit a ramp function) representing the correction function. In this manner, a series of one-dimensional Fourier array transforms may be built up to establish a two-dimensional Fourier array. One may then interpolate between sampled points in the Fourier plane and inverse Fourier transform to return to the (now deconvolved) object of interest. Under certain conditions and in the absence of noise, this resynthesis can become exact. Interestingly enough, these so-called analytic or potentially exact types of mathematical reconstructions by means of filtered back projection or Fourier multiplicative techniques were not applied in the first CT scanners, namely the EMI head scanner. Rather, the original reconstruction techniques involved iterative computer techniques in which the profiles are taken, back projected, and then successively modified or iterated until the modified data are consistent to within predefined limits of all their x-ray profiles. Successive approximations and changes occur after each iteration to make the profile converge to a solution. There continues to be some discussion about the efficacy of the various analytic and iterative (arithmetic) techniques (especially in the presence of noise) [8].

8.5 CT image quality

It is well known that a beam of monoenergetic x rays traversing matter is attenuated exponentially according to the well-known formula:

$$I = I_o \exp(-\mu x). \tag{8.3}$$

One can note that the attenuation is affected by the composition of the material as represented by the local linear x-ray attenuation coefficient μ, as well as the distance x through which the beam traverses. Figure 8.8(a) shows the relative mass attenuation coefficients of some substances of biological interest, as well as a typical CT x-ray energy spectrum (Figure 8.8(b)). (The mass attenuation coefficients are obtained from the linear attenuation coefficients by dividing by density.) In the diagnostic energy range, attenuation is determined primarily by the photoelectric effect and Compton effect [6].

Equation (8.4) shows how the output of an original EMI machine was related to the effective linear attenuation coefficient μ, characterizing a local region of interest as compared to the linear attenuation coefficient of water, μ_w.

$$\text{EMI} - \text{CT\#} = 500 \frac{(\mu - \mu_w)}{\mu_w} \doteq 2530(\mu - \mu_w). \tag{8.4}$$

This local region or volume of interest in a CT scan is often called the voxel, ΔV the volume element represented by the product of the matrix of pixel size— $\Delta x \Delta y$, times Δz—the slice thickness, ($\Delta V = \Delta x \Delta y \Delta z$); thus, for the EMI head scanner, the EMI number found in the original reconstruction matrix of 80×80 corresponded to voxel elements of 3 mm $\times$ 3 mm $\times$ 13 mm. The numbers found in these voxels are theoretically linearly related to the difference between the attenuation coefficient of the region of interest and the attenuation coefficient of water (approximately $0.190\,\text{cm}^{-1}$). This differential attenuation was amplified by a factor of approximately 2530 (which is essentially 500 divided by the linear attenuation coefficient of water, μ_w, at the typical effective energy ((approximately 70 keV)) of the scanner) for the original EMI scanner. When this EMI $-$ CT scaling is applied to attenuation coefficients encountered within tissues, one arrives at the original EMI $-$ CT scale where $+500$ is bone, 0 is water, and -500 is air, and where most tissue is found between approximately -50 and $+50$. Note parenthetically that this original EMI scale is now routinely expanded by a factor of 2, in which case $+1000$ would represent bone and -1000 would represent air, but 0 still represents water. This ± 1000 scale is considered the Hounsfield (H) scale (although interestingly, exactly double that developed by Hounsfield). In the current Hounsfield scale, a change of 10 H CT units represents a 1% change in the attenuation (or density) of a water-like tissue. One finds that, for example, gray and white matter are separated by only a few H numbers, and thus a CT system must have noise or precision levels of only a few H, to offer an extremely fine x-ray "probe" to distinguish between very small fractional per cent changes in attenuation corresponding to small differential changes in tissue density or tissue composition.

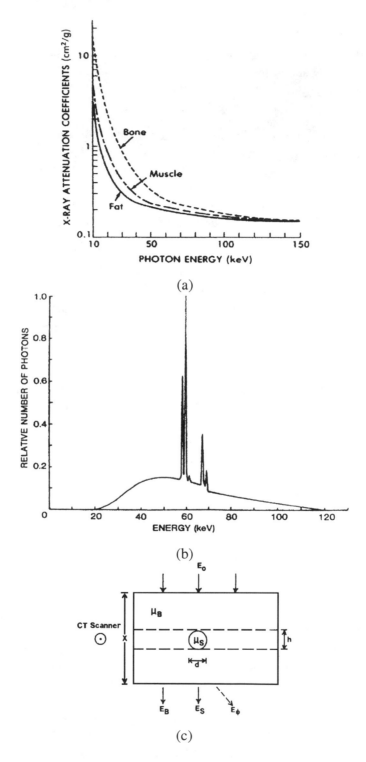

(a)

(b)

(c)

Figure 8.8:   Linear attenuation coefficients 8(a) and typical CT x-ray spectrum 8(b). A model of detection is shown in Figure 8(c).

Consider a simple model, wherein a homogeneous material characterized by a linear attenuation coefficient μ_B has an embedded signal of diameter d characterized by μ_S (Figure 8.8(c)). If one were to image, from the top, using a radiograph, with some incident exposure and some exit exposure corresponding to the primary radiation E_B, and some exit exposure attributable to the scattered radiation, $E_\emptyset$, then for fairly large signals (where the spatial resolution or MTF would not be expected to be a limiting parameter), one may generate the radiographic contrast or film density difference ΔD between the signal and the background which ultimately limit the corresponding change in light photons reaching the eye. For signals of small or low contrasts, the visual contrast encountered in radiography may be given by the product of the difference between the attenuation coefficient of the signal (that is μ_S) and the background (μ_B), multiplied by the size of the signal d and the film gradient G of the relative x-ray response curve of the screen/film combination used in obtaining the radiograph. If we introduce the x-ray scatter component $E_\emptyset$, then the contrast is even further degraded by the ratio of E_B to E_B plus $E_\emptyset$ [12].

Similarly,

$$C_r = G(\mu_S - \mu_B)d \quad \text{(without scatter)}, \tag{8.5}$$

$$C_{rs} = G(\mu_S - \mu_B)d\frac{E_B}{E_B + E_\emptyset} \quad \text{(with scatter)}. \tag{8.6}$$

When one performs a similar analysis for computed tomography to determine the contrast reaching the eye from the signal region and the background region, then one must introduce the appropriate parameters into the general CT equation given by Eq. (8.4), but modified for Hounsfield scale. Assume that the luminance display function is to a first approximation a linear function, then, in this case the contrast is given by the difference between signal and background attenuation coefficients divided by the difference between the background μ_B and the lower window-setting attenuation coefficient. (The window is usually considered a subset of attenuation values μ_L or CT numbers. Below the lower window setting, all values are displayed black, while those above the upper setting are displayed white with linear shades of gray scale (or intensity) applied between the lower and upper setting.)

$$C_{ct} = \frac{\mu_S - \mu_B}{\mu_B - \mu_L}. \tag{8.7}$$

This term in the denominator of the above-mentioned CT equation ($\mu_B - \mu_L$), is an extremely important parameter in CT imaging because, whereas the normal contrast latitude loop of a radiographic screen film is invariable after photographic development, within a CT system, the contrast-latitude loop is left variable and subject to operator selection by the choice of viewing "window" to examine some given subregion of the continuum of attenuation values found between air and bone. One is really allowing the viewer to choose, for example, a high-contrast and low-latitude or a low-contrast and a wide-latitude view of the same object.

Note also, that the density-exposure relationship of a given screen film is quite limiting of latitude or dynamic range. Given a G-gradient value of about 2, one is really limited to a dynamic range of about 100 between viewing regions of the film where the film is underexposed (the toe) and too light, and the film is too dark to read in the shoulder region. CT, in comparison, can offer a dynamic range of 12 bits or 4096 (or more) in the image display. It does this not only by offering sufficient signal-to-noise ratio as discussed below but also by limiting scatter to a few percent in collimated detectors that approach narrow beam geometry conditions.

There seems to be no question that freeing the viewer from the limited contrast-latitude range of film is an important attribute in CT systems. If one examines the relationship between the visual contrast in CT versus radiography from this simple type of model, one sees that the contrast given by CT is approximately equal to the contrast given by radiography divided by $G(\Delta\mu)d$:

$$C_{ct} = C_r / G(\mu_B - \mu_L)d. \tag{8.8}$$

Thus, according to this fairly simple model, computed tomography contrast is greater than the radiographic contrast whenever the product of G times $(\mu_B - \mu_L)$ and d is less than unity. Because $\mu_B - \mu_L$ is often on the order of 200 H, or 0.02 cm^{-1}, this equation shows that radiographic signals will have to have extremely large diameters (several centimeters), or have high differential attenuation coefficients to try to compete with computed tomography. In fact, it is probable that this high-contrast (display or windowing) property of CT systems enabling it to show very small differential changes in the attenuation coefficient of tissue is one way in which CT systems, by means of electronic image display, have made a significant breakthrough in the diagnostic arena. However, let us note that the parameter $\mu_B - \mu_L$ which is involved in the so-called window settings (choice of contrast and latitude in the CT system) is obviously being used to increase the relative performance of CT versus radiography. If we were to use similar means of expanding the contrast scale in radiography, such as certain contrast stretching techniques, one might then, under certain conditions, hope to decrease the imaging advantage of CT. We may then ask what limits our ability to do this? Well, essentially any image-processing technique including those used in computed tomography and those that we might hope to apply to radiography will be ultimately limited by the signal-to-noise ratio limits that are an intrinsic property of the acquired information. Thus, if the noise level is very large then it probably makes no sense to augment or stretch the contrast of objects within the image because we will essentially be increasing or blowing up the noise fluctuations as fast as the signal contrast.

The question to then ask is whether CT has an inherent advantage over radiography in terms of signal-noise ratio. For fairly large areas, the noise in radiography may be described by Eq. (8.9), which relates the fluctuations in optical density to the light transmission (T) reaching the eye. The relative noise fluctuations in light transmitted through the radiograph is

$$\frac{\sigma(T)}{T} \sim \frac{G}{(\bar{n}_x d^2)^{1/2}}. \tag{8.9}$$

One again encounters the parameters G (the film gradient), and d (the signal diameter), as well as the inherent photon flux limits of the x-ray beam used or effectively detected in the radiograph, $\bar{n}_x$ [12].

Consideration of the noise in computed tomography shows that the fluctuations in terms of light transmission reaching the eye $[\sigma(T)]/T$ is approximated by Eq. (8.10), which shows an inverse square-root dependence on the dose D (i.e., proportional to n_x) used in the CT scan, the pixel dimension w, the slice thickness h, and the area of the signal under consideration a.

$$\frac{\sigma(T)}{T} \approx \frac{(Dwha)^{-1/2}}{\mu_B - \mu_L}. \tag{8.10}$$

Note: when "a" equals the nominal *pixel* area—w^2, this relationship will show a cubic dependence on w^3; this gives rise to the early claim that improvements in spatial resolution require a cubic increase in dose in CT systems. This dependence is *only* true if one requires a constant noise per pixel; for a constant noise per unit area, the dependence is more to the first power.

It should be kept in mind that these approaches are overly simplistic because they ignore important questions of correlation properties or power spectrum properties of the noise, involving the mottled appearance of noise fluctuation [13].

If one now looks at the comparison of the signal-to-noise ratios for CT versus radiography, one finds some interesting relationships reflecting the important image parameters: G, the gradient of the radiograph screen film combination, d, the diameter of the signal, $\bar{n}_x$, the photon flux, and the differential attenuation between the signal and background ($\mu_S - \mu_B$). If one assumes the same x-ray spectrum used in CT and radiography (actually, radiographs are usually recorded at lower kVp), then one arrives at a fairly interesting relationship between the signal-to-noise ratio of CT, SNR_{ct}, compared to that of radiography, SNR_r, where, in the absence of significant scatter,

$$\frac{SNR_r}{SNR_{ct}} \sim \frac{2}{d(cms)}. \tag{8.11}$$

This relationship is reached by assuming a photon information level in radiography of approximately 10^7 photons per centimeter square [12]. It is rather interesting that the relationship predicts that the advantage of computed tomography will increase as the diameter of the signal *decreases*. Thus, at a diameters of a few cm, signals might be detected equally in radiography and CT; however, when signal diameters get down to the order of a cm or so, the signal-to-noise ratio of CT might be appreciably better than that of radiography. However, it should be noted that there is a practical limit to how small a signal one might hope to find with CT systems because of the volume-averaging effect (the slice width as well as the pixel) and the realization that the spatial resolution of CT systems is often far inferior to that of radiography. In addition, as mentioned earlier, improvements in spatial resolution place demands on dose, (e.g., to have the same pixel noise level in a pixel of one half size, one might need an eight-fold increase in dose). In light of the present dose levels of CT scanners (10–50 m gray) there is obviously some need to pay attention to changes in the upper end of this scale. Thus, for small objects where the contrast (in particular the edge perception) is strongly influenced by the spatial resolution (MTF), (i.e., related approximately to the integral of the MTF squared), the contrast in CT and radiography will be weighted by the square of the MTF of the imaging system [14]. MTF's for some CT and radiographic systems are shown (Figure 8.9). One can note that intrinsic spatial resolution of radiographs is still severalfold (lp/mm vs lp/cm) that of CT.

Thus, as one tries to detect very small higher-contrast signals, such as microcalcifications, radiography may indeed again offer higher signal detectability then CT. One must also keep in mind the important differences presented by the two modalities in terms of pattern recognition and anatomical noise as well as the influence of other parameters of CT image-quality as shown in Table 8.2.

In terms of CT sensitometry or CT number linearity (the relationship between the CT numbers and underlying x-ray attenuation coefficient), one should note that it is not surprising that two different types of CT machines, encompassing different design features that impose differing spectral quality of the x-ray beam (such as presence or absence of beam shaping filters), might produce different CT numbers for the same nominal object. Although, by and large, there is good correlation of H numbers among CT systems, there is some small variation, and in particular, objects showing high atomic number properties can be expected to show fairly different results when modulated by the different x-ray energy spectra because of the cubic dependence on the atomic number of the photoelectric component of the attenuation. The exact relationship between CT number and attenuation coefficient is complicated by the fact that the CT system uses a polychromatic spectrum of x-ray energies (for example, an x-ray tube typically operating at 100 kVp, 120 kVp, or 140 kVp). Because the x-ray photons in the energy spectrum are subject to both photo-electric (μ_{pe}) and Compton (μ_c) interactions, the total attenuation coefficient will be given by: $\mu = \mu_{pe} + \mu_c$. Then, because μ_{pe} is strongly dependent on atomic number (e.g., Z^3) as well as electron density (N_e), and μ_c is primarily dependent on electron density (N_e), the calculated values of CT numbers (i.e., μ) will represent a complicated dependence on both the atomic number and the electron density of the material attenuating the x-ray spectrum. This subject has been discussed in an article where the CT values were examined for correlation with physical density and atomic number cubed (Z^3) [16]. Likewise, the actual energy distribution is an important factor because the photoelectric effect is inversely proportional to E^3, whereas the Compton effect is only weakly dependent on energy.

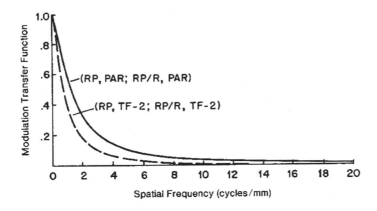

Figure 8.9(a): MTF's of Screen films versus CT, shown here, a medium speed (PAR) and faster TF-2 calcium tungstate screens.

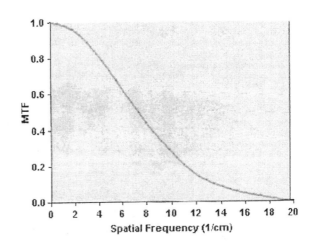

PSF (average)

FWHM : 0.66 mm
FWTM : 1.14 mm

MTF	Frequency (1/cm)
50%	7.3
10%	13.3
5%	15.5
2%	18.0

PSF Roll-off option : On
Pixel Size Degradation : On
Bead Size Correction : On

Figure 8.9(b): MTF's of Screen films versus CT, shown here, a medium CT scanner high-resolution MTF.

The CT x-ray reconstruction process assumes that each volume element or voxel acts independently in terms of its x-ray attenuation properties. That is to say, the CT number or x-ray attenuation coefficient for each voxel is generally assumed to be the value obtained if one could physically excise each voxel from its surround and then calculate its effective x-ray attenuation properties. Although this assumption will be relatively correct for homogenous volume elements (after appropriate corrections for beam hardening scatter, reconstruction filters, etc.), it can be shown to be distinctly incorrect for stratified volume-averaging substances with finite spatial extent, particularly when the two substances being averaged have significantly different x-ray attenuation properties [15, 16].

It has been demonstrated both theoretically and experimentally that the computed tomographic values have *nonlinear* dependence on the relative fractional

Table 8.2: Image quality factors in CT

Dose	—Surface, Central, Single or Multiple Slice
Sensitometry (*CT Number Scale*)	—kVp, Beam Hardening, Post Processing
Spatial Resolution	—Detector Size, Focal Spot Size, Geometry, Pixel Size, Reconstruction Algorithms
Noise Level	—Standard deviation, power spectrum
Artifacts	—Mechanical Alignment of Tube and Detectors
	—Patient Movement
	—Detector Imbalance, Non-linearity, or Instability
	—Generator Regulation (Variation in kVp or mA)
Slice Sensitivity and Thickness	—X-ray Collimation, Detector Width, Number of Slices, Geometry, Pitch, Interpolation, Reconstruction Algorithms
Field Uniformity	—Calibration, Beam Hardening, Scatter Correction
Display System	—CRT-Brightness, Contrast
	—TV-Brightness, Contrast
	—Multiformat Camera Gray Scale, Processing
	—Laser Camera Gray Scale, Processing (look up tables)

content *as well as* the spatial distribution of the stratified substances, particularly if bone and/or air, and/or contrast agents are involved. It was shown, for example, that the CT value of the same stratified partition of 70% Teflon and 30% air could vary by as much as several hundred Hounsfield numbers, depending on whether the partitioned volume had a diameter of 6 cm or 1 cm [15].

As mentioned earlier, this result is contrary to the basic reconstruction assumption, that each voxel is characterized by an x-ray attenuation value independent from the x-ray attenuation properties of its neighbors. In a systems-analysis sense, the volume-averaging phenomenon can be considered to lead to "nonlinear" and "nonstationary" conditions, in that the output of a particular volume-averaged voxel depends on its surrounding values [16]. It was shown that the composite or averaged x-ray attenuation value produced by a beam traversing two stratified or layered substances, is analogous to the problem of characterizing the composite decay curve of a mixture of the two isotopes, one with a fast decay rate (short half-life), the other with a long decay rate (long half-life). The initial decay is dominated by the rapid decay of the short-lived component, whereas the latter decay is dominated by the longer-lived component, because the short-lived component has essentially decayed away.

The physical equations that describe the composite linear x-ray attenuation of an x-ray beam in space by two stratified substances and the composite decay characterizing a mixture of two isotopes in time are identical equations, following substitution of decay rate (λ) and time (t) for x-ray attenuation coefficient (μ) and spatial extent (d), respectively. In continued analogy to this more familiar case of the composite decay curve from a mixture of radioisotopes, it is known that the effective decay rate of the mixture of two isotopes depends on the point in time under consideration. Similarly the effective linear attenuation of an x-ray beam traversing a volume-averaged voxel, situated in a surround of other volume-averaged voxels, depends on the location in space of the voxel under consideration, as well as the attenuation history of the beam in traversing the other volume-averaged voxels, along the x-ray beam passage.

It may be of interest to note that the volume averaging does not have to occur only in the slice thickness (or z direction), but could just as readily take place across pixels in the x or y direction, depending on the aperture width of the source and detector, and their coincidence with an edge or interface of volume-averaged pixels across rows or columns along their "line of sight." The resulting artifacts have been called the edge-gradient effects [17]. It is straightforward to realize that the correction approaches are actually independent of any particular coordinate choice (x, y, or z), and will thus work to correct artifacts produced by averaging across the z, x, or y directions, when applied appropriately.

When both the identity of the two substances being volume averaged and the spatial distribution or dimension over which the averaging takes place are known, then, the effective CT value in each voxel is totally predicted, outside of other nonlinear effects such as beam hardening and scatter.

Consider the case where two substances characterized by respective linear x-ray coefficients μ_1 and μ_2 exist as volume-averaged, partitioned, stratified regions which are averaged over spatial extent d. The slice thickness is denoted by h, the fraction of μ_1 is Z/h, the fraction of μ_2 is $1 - Z/h$. Then the effective attenuation coefficient μ_{eff} is given by [16]:

$$\mu_{\text{eff}} = \mu_2 - \frac{1}{d} \log_e \left\{ 1 + \frac{Z}{h} [\exp(\mu_2 - \mu_1)d - 1] \right\}. \tag{8.12}$$

The limiting cases of the above equation yield the expected values in that for

$$\text{Case 1} \quad Z = 0, \quad \mu_{\text{eff}} = \mu_2, \tag{8.13}$$

$$\text{Case 2} \quad Z = h, \quad \mu_{\text{eff}} = \mu_1, \tag{8.14}$$

and for Case 3 $\quad (\mu_2 - \mu_1)d \rightarrow 0$, then
$$\mu_{\text{eff}} \rightarrow \mu_1 Z/h + \mu_2(1 - Z/h). \tag{8.15}$$

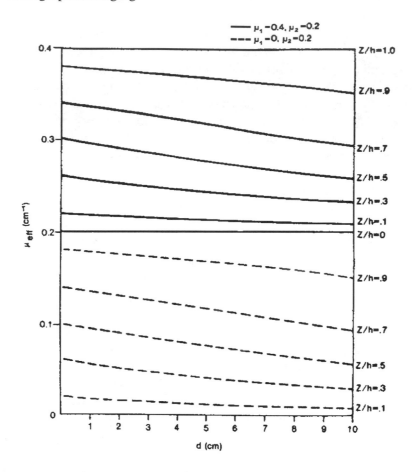

Figure 8.10: Influence of spatial extent of volume averaging on effective attenuation value. Top: Bone like substance averaged with water. Bottom: Air like substance averaged with water.

Cases 1 and 2 obviously correspond to the situation of no volume averaging. Case 3 corresponds to the often assumed first-order linear equation for simple volume averaging. This linear equation will only be true when the product of the difference in μ values $(\mu_2 - \mu_1)$ and the spatial extent (d) of the differing regions is small. The exact solution indicates a nonlinear dependence not only on $(\mu_2 - \mu_1)$, but also on the spatial extent (d) or distribution of the volume averaging (Figure 8.10).

The knowledge of the actual nature of volume averaging can lead to post-processing correction approaches. One approach taken is to use a priori information to estimate μ_1 and μ_2, to obtain estimates of d from the reconstruction and to predict the nature of volume averaging in a particular CT scan. A correction algorithm can be used to reconstruct the data back to the "true" independent voxel values [16].

8.6 Other artifacts in CT

There are many types of artifacts encountered in CT machines depending on the particular generation and design of CT scanner. Indeed, artifacts may be extremely visually disturbing. Perhaps the most commonly encountered artifact in the original EMI scanners were vertical streaks, which were caused by problems of movement of the patient, problems of misalignment or faulty timing of the CT system, or over-ranging, that is, the values lying outside the dynamic range of the detector system. One also found radiating streaks coming from foreign or very dense substances, herringbone artifacts which may arise from a combination of dense objects, algorithm, or disk problems.

Concentric circle (rings or bands) artifacts were seen in early third-generation scanners, particularly related to nonlinearity of detector response of early xenon gas detectors. Circular artifacts are still seen in water bath scans of certain third-generation scanners; however they are rather subtle in appearance and often subclinical in that they can not usually be seen in scans of complex anatomy. These usually result from detector or, perhaps more correctly, electronic detector imbalance in third-generation scanners.

Other artifacts result from failure to correctly compensate for beam hardening or scatter. A particularly insidious artifact is the partial volume artifact explained in the previous section, which is a fundamental problem in single-slice scanners, but may perhaps be reduced by interpolation of information from multi-slice scanners.

8.7 Multislice CT

A multislice CT system permits multiple (typically up to four) slices to be acquired in a single rotation. Such scanners may significantly reduce the scanning time for acquiring volume data and for improving longitudinal spatial or z-axis resolution. The key factor is that the x-ray collimation allows simultaneous radiation of several adjoining z-axis slices at the same time. This significantly enhances x-ray tube utilization.

A selectable-slice-thickness multi-row detector (SSMD) is a 2D detector which permit the slice thickness to be varied (Figure 8.11). The principle of detection is the same as that of conventional single-slice detectors typically using a solid-state detector incorporating a scintillator and a photodiode. Several thousand detector elements are placed in a 2D array in the radial arc direction as well as in several rows (up to 34) in the longitudinal (z) axis direction. The minimum slice thickness can be as low as 0.5 mm, depending on the detector size (in z direction) as well as the collimation used. The multiple detector elements in the slice direction and a data-acquisition system (DAS) can be multiplexed so that the slice thickness for data acquisition can be varied, for example, data for 4 slices can be output to the DAS. Typically, slice thicknesses can be selected in the range from 0.5 mm to 10 mm [18]. Different manufacturer's multislice detector designs are listed in Figure 8.11(c).

One potential problem for the multislice system is that a wider area is scanned at one time, and therefore more scattered radiation per slice is generated affecting

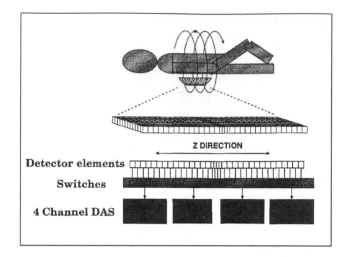

Figure 8.11(a):   Aspects of multislice CT. Concept of how multiple small detectors may be grouped into four distinct channels (courtesy of Toshiba Medical Systems, [18]).

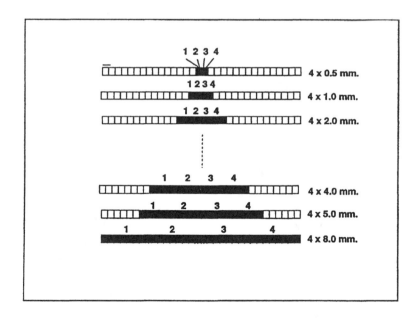

Figure 8.11(b):   Aspects of multislice CT. Examples of grouping to achieve four slices of indicated slice width (courtesy of Toshiba Medical Systems, [18]).

deleteriously both image-quality and radiation dose. Therefore, the collimator and detector design must be optimized for multislice CT detectors and may need to compensate for x-ray beam movements in the longitudinal direction by allowing a wider beam than the actual slice thickness, thus impacting deleteriously on dose buildup from neighboring slices (Figure 8.11(d)).

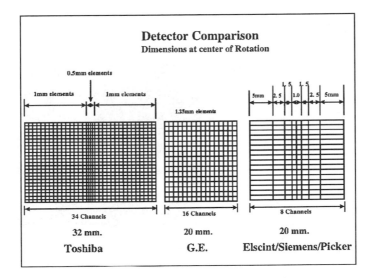

Figure 8.11(c): Aspects of multislice CT (courtesy of Toshiba Medical Systems, [18]). Examples of different manufacturer's approach to constant or variable detector sizes, and total beam coverage.

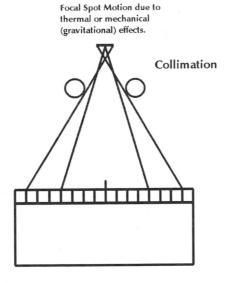

Figure 8.11(d): Aspects of multislice CT, [18]. Hypothetical example of how beam width at detector may include beam movement from focal spot movement (similar to umbra/penumbra of finite focal size).

Current technology is capable of scanning at 0.5 s per rotation, with multislice detectors which permit simultaneous 4-slice acquisition. Such designs subject the rotating gantry and heavy x-ray tube to 10s of normal gravitational force levels.

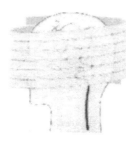

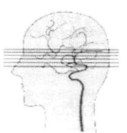

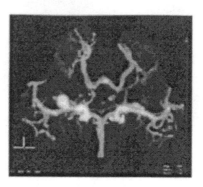

Figure 8.12:   CTA with Multislice (courtesy of Toshiba Medical Systems [18]).

The data acquisition system (DAS) and a high-speed image reconstruction system must provide for multislice CT reconstruction.

In conventional single-slice CT scanner, the helical pitch is typically 1 to 2.0, which reflects the table movement distance per rotation in terms of the slice width. The multislice CT system permits simultaneous M-slice acquisition, therefore, the helical pitch is often stated as M times that of single-slice helical scanning [18].

One of the clinical advantages of multislice CT is the possible use for CT angiography (CT-A) whereby arterial and venous phases can be separated in repeated multislice helical scanning (Figure 8.12). The time from the injection of contrast medium to enhancement of the lesion differs from patient to patient. Techniques have been developed for monitoring the flow of contrast medium and automatically triggering scanning exactly when the contrast medium reaches the lesion. This significant improvement in x-ray utilization reduces the load on the x-ray tube, permitting helical scanning to be performed for a longer period without the need to wait for x-ray tube cooling. This is an important feature in modern CT scanners because the tube is often operating near its limit [18].

Multislice helical scanning also permits the slice thickness of images to be selected in a different manner than single-slice collimation. The slice thickness in multislice helical scanning can be determined not only by the slice width and the pitch (P), but also the shape and the width of the interpolating filter in the longitudinal (z) direction [18].

It is important to optimize the sampling density in the z direction. The helical scan data can be tracked as a vertical axis which shows the rotation angle, and the horizontal axis shows the longitudinal position. If the conventional helical pitch is simply extended for regularly spaced multislice detectors, the complementary data

MULTI-SLICE HELICAL: Simple Extension
of single-slice reconstruction

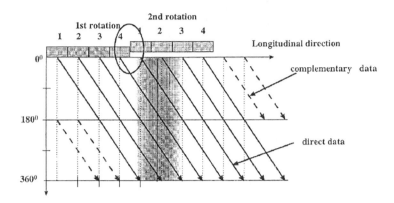

Figure 8.13(a): Multislice CT z-axis sampling [18]. Integral pitch leads to redundant data.

MULTI-SLICE HELICAL: Optimized Sampling

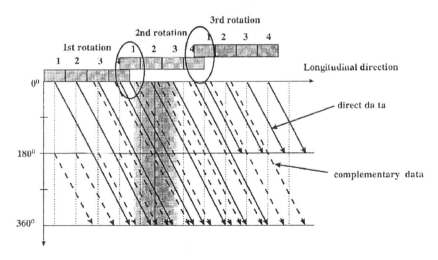

Figure 8.13(b): Multislice CT z-axis sampling [18]. Offset from integral pitch leads to improved sampling.

are redundant, resulting in non-optimal sampling. In a manner somewhat analogous to satisfaction of Nyquist criteria by quarter-offset sampling techniques of third-generation CT, scanning methods have been developed that achieve superior longitudinal (z) sampling by offsetting the z-axis data trails. The conventional $1/4$ offset (actually $1/2$ detector spacing) of third-generation scanners helps sampling in the $x-y$ direction [10], whereas offset sampling to achieve non-integral pitch helps z-axis sampling [18] (Figure 8.13).

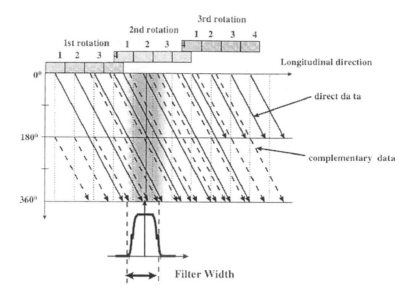

Figure 8.13(c): Multislice CT z-axis sampling [18]. Filtering along the z-axis.

slice profiles: Multislice CT

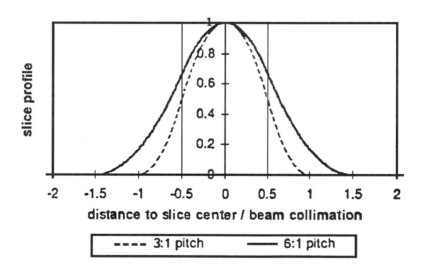

Figure 8.14: SSPs for spiral multislice. Fractional pitch of multislice leads to better approximation of conventional "step-and-shoot" single-slice CT, more similar to ideal square wave (-0.5 to 0.5) (also see Figure 8.6).

In the filter interpolation method, a filter with a certain width is set in the longitudinal direction and optimized sampling data are filter processed. This method is based on the concept of multi point weighted interpolation. By changing the shape

Table 8.3: Slice profile and noise comparison (1 vs 4 slice CT)

Helical Pitch*	Single Slice CT			4 Slice CT		
	FWHM Ratio	FWTM Ratio	Noise Ratio	FWHM Ratio	FWTM Ratio	Noise Ratio
0	1.00	1.00	1.00	1.00	1.00	1.00
1	1.00	1.56	1.15	1.00	1.56	0.57
2	1.27	2.23	1.15	1.27	2.23	0.57
3	1.75	3.00	1.15	1.00	1.56	1.05
4	2.25	3.82	1.15	1.27	2.23	0.81
6	3.25	5.52	1.15	1.27	2.23	1.05
8	4.25	7.27	1.15	1.27	2.23	1.15

* Note, pitch of M-slice scanner, is usually denoted M × pitch of single slice scanner. Thus, a pitch of 1 for a single slice scanner, is effectively 4 for a 4 slice multislice scanner. Conversely, a pitch of 1 for a 4 slice multislice scanner is effectively a pitch of 0.25 for a single slice scanner

and width of this filter, it is possible to freely adjust the slice profile configuration, the effective slice width, and the image noise characteristics [18].

In terms of slice sensitivity profiles, multislice helical CT provide a slice profile (Figure 8.14) at the midpoint between 180° LI and 360° linear interpolation (360° LI) of single-slice helical scanning (Figure 8.4(c)).

The relationships between z-axis filter width and helical pitch influence the standard deviation (SD) of the image noise in multislice CT. The SD values decrease with a decrease in pitch and with an increase in filter width. The SD values for multi-helical CT have been reported with optimal z-axis sampling to be 20% smaller than those for single-slice helical CT [18].

Similar results have recently been reported in an independent study of single versus multislice CT [19]. The results of this study, shown in Table 8.3, reveal that with judicious selection of multislice pitch (i.e., obtaining 1/4 slice shifts in the z-axis), not only can slice width (FWHM) be improved (i.e., more congruent with nominal square wave), but also, noise can be reduced! It is particularly important to remember that noise reduction in CT corresponds to reductions in *the square of Dose* (assuming strictly Poisson x-ray statistics determine noise, i.e., no other noise sources) for the same nominal image-quality—all other factors staying constant [14].

8.8 CT scanner performance

It has already been mentioned in this chapter that CT scanners have evolved from the earliest scanners operating at scan times of several minutes, with iterative reconstructions of several minutes, and reconstruction matrices of 80×80 (i.e., 3 mm × 3 mm pixels) to the current situation of scanners operating at scan times of one or sub-second complete rotations, with virtually instantaneous (hard wired or fast array processors) reconstructions 512×512 or 1024×1024 matrices of even several simultaneous thin slices from multiple detector banks. Such advances in scan time and/or spatial resolution levels have become more and more demanding

Standard Head Imaging

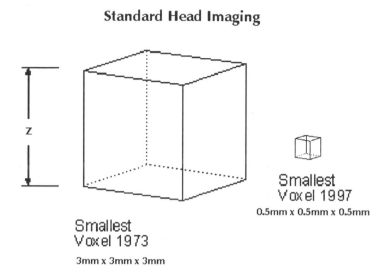

Figure 8.15: Changes in Voxel size over time for Head-Scan Field of View. One can note the improvement in 3D resolution, and the movement towards smaller (and more isotropic) volumes.

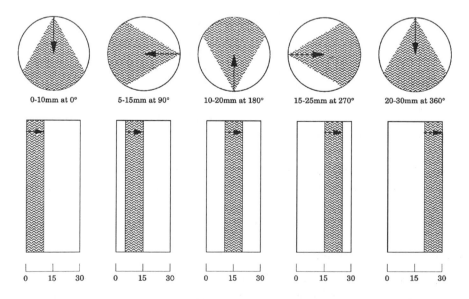

Figure 8.16: Schematic Representation of Spiral Scanning produces images that contain information from the 10 mm slice above and below the 10 mm slice of interest. Total travel is 30 mm for pitch of 2.

on state-of-the-art electronic circuitry, x-ray tube technology, detector technology, and mechanical engineering (Figure 8.15).

A major challenge of understanding spiral image-quality for both single slice and multislice is that the CT image of the slice of interest is actually influenced by the content of the slice immediately above and below it (Figure 8.16). This influence may be enhanced or diminished depending on the pitch (the number of slice thicknesses the table moves per 360° tube rotation), and the spiral interpolator (the weighting function of the 3D data set of attenuation measurements acquired during the spiral acquisition).

There are several areas of measurement of CT scanners that are important in spiral and multislice spiral scanners, including the concept of slice thickness and spatial resolution.

8.8.1 Slice thickness or sensitivity profile

A test object such as a line, thin strip, or series of small heads may be angled through the z-axis of the intended scan volume so that the axial slice produces a trigonometric projection of the angled test object onto the axial (x, y) plane. It is important to use thin objects (or a series of small discrete objects) so that the phenomenon of nonlinear partial voluming artifacts do not perturb the slice thickness result [20]. A shallow ramp angle affords a trigonometric enlargement factor in the axial scan plane. For example, the use of the 23° ramp angle in this CATPHAN® phantom produces a 2.4-fold enlargement of the ramp in the scan plane (Figure 8.17(a)). This enlargement is helpful in increasing the accuracy and precision of the slice width measurement and minimizing the effects of the finite axial spatial resolution of the scanner on the slice thickness measurement. It is also useful in simultaneously measuring several slice profiles from a multi-slice CT scanner (Figure 8.17(b)). A slice thickness profile may be generated from the

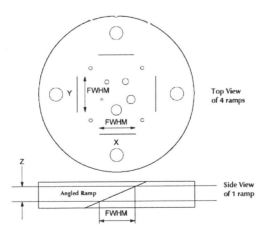

Figure 8.17(a): Shallow-angled slice ramp in z-axis produces a magnified version of the $(x-y)$ plane (courtesy, The Phantom Laboratory, Salem, NY).

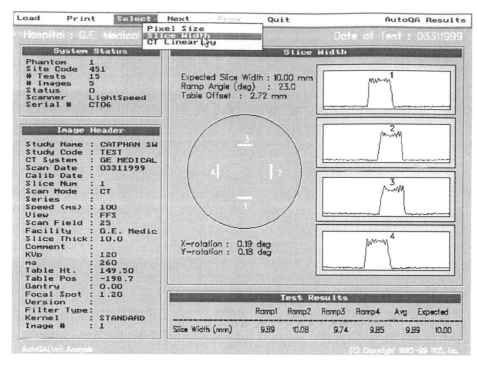

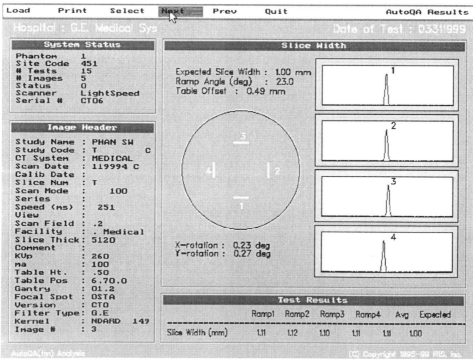

Figure 8.17(b): Use of angled ramps with GE lightspeed multislice scanners, to test slice thickness and position (top 10 mm slice, bottom 1 mm slice) (software courtesy of The IRIS, Inc., Frederick, Maryland).

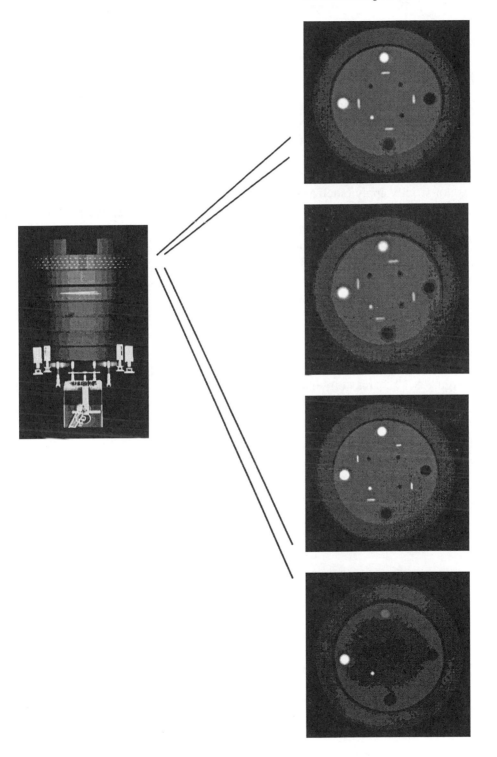

Figure 8.17(c): Example of testing of 4–5 mm slices on Picker MX 8000 scanner. Only 3 of the slices actually intercept the slice ramps.

CT scan of the angled test object, and metrics such as the full width half maximum (FWHM) and/or the full width at tenth maximum (FWTM) can be determined.

8.8.2 Spatial resolution (Point spread function (PSF)

The basic properties of a linear isoplanatic imaging system can be characterized by the manner in which each point in the object plane is spread or blurred in the image plane as a point spread function [11, 14]. Although a CT scanner may not be strictly linear nor isoplanatic, it is reasonably well behaved over a considerable range of inputs and spatial extent. Even when isoplanaticity (position invariance) does not strictly apply (such as the differences in radial and tangential response in the scan plane attributable to ray sampling and view sampling), the response may be characterized in certain isoplanatic regions (such as annuli at varying radii).

An isolated small bead is placed in the phantom as a point source. The bead dimension must be chosen small enough (in this case, approximately $250\,\mu m$) so that it effectively constitutes a point source, or provisions can be made to correct or deconvolve the finite spatial extent or size of the point source.

The point source is an attractive method of characterizing the CT scanner because the point spread function (PSF) from the bead can be used to describe the spreading in the conventional axial (x, y) plane of the CT scanner psf (x, y) and the spreading of the point in the slice thickness or z domain SSP(z), as illustrated in (Figure 8.18). This combination of information from the x, y, and z axes, essentially describes the 3D point spread function PSF (x, y, z). The SSP (z) can be conveniently obtained by spiral scanning the isolated bead and creating a multi-

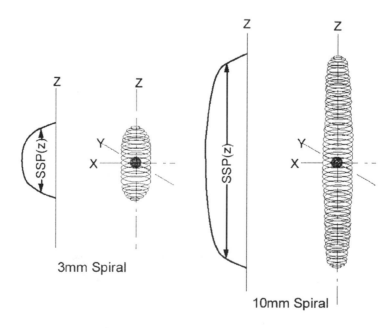

Figure 8.18: Concept of 3D PSF—the 2D PSF (x, y) is combined with the SSP (z).

planar or 3D image set in which a z-axis profile can be generated from a stack of planes through a given point location in the x, y plane [21].

In addition, as mentioned earlier, for linear isoplanatic systems, the 2D Fourier transform can be applied to the point spread function to yield the modulation transfer function (MTF) of the CT scanner (Figure 8.9(b)). The MTF describing the transfer or modulation of contrast as a function of spatial frequency, can also be related to high-contrast resolution of periodic patterns such as sine wave patterns or square wave patterns [14].

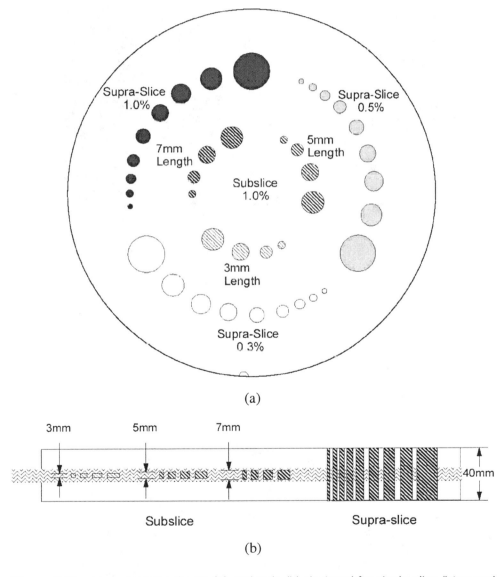

Figure 8.19: Low-contrast spheres (a) and rods (b) designed for single slice "step and shoot," as well as spiral CT scanners (c) (courtesy, The Phantom Laboratory, Salem, NY).

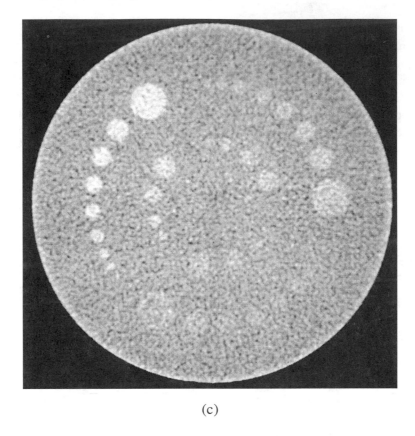

(c)

Figure 8.19:   (Continued).

The ultimate test of a CT scanner is its diagnostic efficacy in detecting disease. Although a number of test objects ranging from high-contrast (tumor like) spheres and cylinders are offered in phantoms (Figure 8.19), the true complexity of anthropomorphic shapes, motions, and biological composition remains very challenging to simulate (Figure 8.20).

8.9 Developments in other modalities

Much success has been obtained in terms of reconstruction of the distribution of radioactive emission sources. In particular, commercial instruments have been produced for reconstruction using single-photon emission sources SPECT (single-photon emission computed tomography) following the pioneering work of Kuhl *et al.* [22]; as well as PET reconstruction of positron coincidence photons following the work of Ter Pogossian and Phelps [9]. Such developments are important in medicine because of the opportunity to study quantitatively physiological processes, *in vivo*. Challenges in nuclear medicine modality remain in working with relatively low photon fluence levels (e.g., a typical administered activity of 1 mCi$= 3.7 \times 10^7$ dps $= 37$ MBq), attenuation in the body, and limiting geomet-

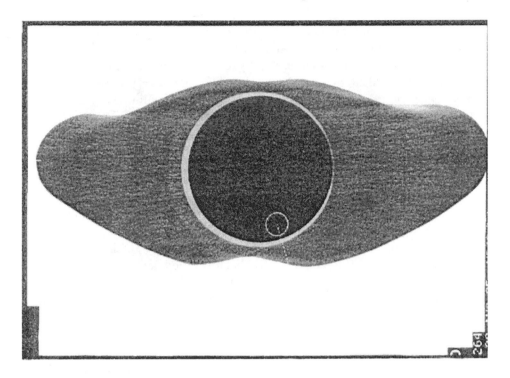

Figure 8.20: Anthropomorphic shell for phantom modules, designed to better simulate human imaging (courtesy, The Phantom Laboratory, Salem, NY).

rical detecting systems which yield very low overall efficiency for detection of gamma rays. Scan times are thus usually of many minutes duration and record counts of only 100–1,000 counts per square cm, thousands of time lower than radiographs and CT images. Much recent interest has been generated from the idea of using coincidence detection (CD) with dual-headed SPECT camera devices in coincidence mode or even in single counting mode for detecting 511 keV gamma rays from positron emissions [23]. Again, counting statistics and limited spatial resolution limit performance.

Other modalities in various stages of development and investigation in terms of reconstruction potential include ultrasound and heavy particle beams. Each of these modalities holds its own diagnostic promise.

MRI, in particular, has encountered huge scientific and commercial success in generating excellent contrast resolution without the use of ionizing radiation. MRI differs from CT in many ways, including the fact that mechanical movement is not utilized to acquire rays and views around the object. Rather, ingenious combinations of magnetic field gradients and radio frequency resonances at the Larmor frequency of NMR are used to stimulate and spatially encode the RF excitation from changing orientation of magnetic moments of spinning protons (or occasionally other nuclei). MRI has the ability to produce exquisite contrast differences not only between the proton density differences of tissues (analogous to CT exploiting electron density differences), but also the magnetic-resonance relaxation properties (T1 and T2). In addition, the potential for spectroscopic and functional imaging remain of interest if still somewhat limited by signal-to-noise ratios obtainable with current magnetic field strengths and the noise levels of the very sensitive electronic circuits needed to process the extremely small signal amplitudes of some of the MRI phenomena [24].

8.10 Conclusions

To fully explore the anatomy and physiology of the human body, it would be very useful to have a 3D data set that would provide selection of arbitrary planes and subvolumes of information within the body. In the absence of direct 3D acquisition (as at least theoretically possible for MRI), the next best hope is for the re-synthesis of highly accurate "Tomos" slices to make up a 3D data set.

The quest for true "Tomos" in CT has been pursued actively for almost three decades. Finer and finer in-plane (x, y) resolution (now about 0.25 mm or 2 lp/mm-approaching some practical radiographic procedures, particularly with significant patient magnification technique) has been accompanied by finer spatial resolution (e.g., 0.5 mm) in the z-axis, as denoted by the slice thickness or sensitivity profile, particularly with the recent (re) introduction of multislice CT.

Of course, these resolution levels are of little value if patient movement of several mm is associated with long acquisition times. Thus, the advent of very fast, subsecond scanners with multislice capabilities offers great promise for rapid volume acquisition of CT data. In addition, the increased utilization of the x-ray output (by greater solid angle use) helps reduce the limitation of tube overheating in sustained acquisition(s) of large volumes of data. The current multislice scanners are probably only the beginning of improved 3D CT acquisition because as the beam coverage improved from only 2–3 cm at present, to probably severalfold larger regions of large-area detectors, one should see even more improvement. Such methods will still need to contend with issues of scatter and carefully monitor the level of patient dose, however. An interesting future for CT still remains.

Acknowledgements

The author would like to acknowledge the help, perseverance and diligence of Arlene Corby in the preparation of the manuscript, and James Tyeryar in the preparation of the figures used in the chapter.

References

[1] Bull J. "History of Computed Tomography." In Newton TH, Potts, DG (Eds.) *Radiology of Skull and Brain. Technical Aspects of Computed Tomography.* St. Louis, MO: The C. V. Mosby Company, 1981, Vol. 5, Chapter 108, pp. 3835–3849,

[2] Kundel HL. "Peripheral Vision, Structured Noise and Film Reader Error." Radiology 114:269–273, 1975.

[3] Goodenough DJ, Weaver KE, David DO. "Comparative Aspects of Radiology and CT." Investigative Radiology 17:510–523, 1982.

[4] Ritman EL, Robb RA, Johnson SA, Chevalier PA, Gilbert BK, Greenleaf JF, Sturm RE, Wood EH. "Quantitative Imaging of the Structure and Function of the Heart, Lungs, and Circulation." Mayo Clinic Proc 53:3–11, 1978.

[5] Boyd DP, Gould RG, Quinn JR, Sparks R, Stanley JH, Hermannsfeldt WB. "A Proposed Dynamic Cardiac 3-D Densitometer for Early Detection and Evaluation of Heart Disease." IEEE Trans Nuclear Science NS-26:2724–2727, 1979.

[6] Pullan BR, Ritchings RT, Isherwood I. "Accuracy and Meaning of Computed Tomography Attenuation Values," In *Radiology of Skull and Brain. Technical Aspects of Computed Tomography*. St. Louis, MO: The C. V. Mosby Company, 1981, Vol. 5, Chapter 111, pp. 3904.

[7] Glenn Jr WR, Davis, KR, Larsen GN *et al.* "Alternative Display Formats for Computed Tomography (CT) Data." In Potchen EJ (Ed.) *Current Concepts in Radiology.* St. Louis, MO: The C. V. Mosby, 1977, Chapter 5, pp. 88–124.

[8] Gordon R, Herman GT, Johnson SA. "Image Reconstruction from Projections." Scientific American, October: 56–58, 1975.

[9] Ter-Pogossian M. "Physical Aspects of Emission Computed Tomography." In *Radiology of Skull and Brain. Technical Aspects of Computed Tomography*. St. Louis, MO: The C. V. Mosby Company, 1981, Vol. 5, Chapter 131, pp. 4372–4388.

[10] Brooks RA, Di Chiro G. "Theory of Image Reconstruction in Computed Tomography." Radiology 117:561–572, 1975.

[11] Rossmann K. "Point Spread-function, Line Spread-function, and Modulation Transfer Function: Tolls for the Study of Imaging Systems." Radiology 93:257–272, 1969.

[12] Rossmann K. "Spatial Fluctuations of X-Rays Quanta and the Recording of Radiographic Mottle." American Journal of Roentgenol, Radium Ther Nuclear Medicine 90:863–869, 1963.

[13] Hanson KM, Boyd DP. "The Characteristics of Computed Tomographic Reconstruction Noise and Their Effect on Detectability." IEEE Trans Nuclear Science NS-25:160–173, 1978.

[14] Goodenough DJ. "Psychophysical Perception of Computed Tomography Images." In Newton, TH and Potts, DG.: *Radiology of Skull and Brain. Technical Aspects of Computed Tomography*. St. Louis, MO: The C. V. Mosby Company, 1981, Vol. 5, Chapter 115.

[15] Goodenough DJ, Weaver KE, Davis DO, LaFalce S. "Volume Averaging Effects in Computerized Tomography." American Journal of Roentgenology, February, 1982; and American Journal of Neuro Radiology (AJNR) 2:585–599, 1981.

[16] Goodenough DJ, Weaver KE, Costaridou H, Eerdmans H, Huysmans P. "A New Software Correction Approach to Volume Averaging Artifacts in Ct." Computerized Radiology 10(2/3):87–98, 1986.

[17] Joseph P. "Artifacts in computed tomography." In Newton TH, Potts DG (Eds.) *Radiology of Skull and Brain. Technical Aspects of Computed Tomography*. St. Louis, MO: The C. V. Mosby Company, 1981, Vol. 5, Chapter 114.

[18] Saito Y. "Multislice X-Ray CT Scanner." Medical Engineering Laboratory, Toshiba Corporation Medical Review No. 66.

[19] Hu H. "Multislice Helical CT: Scan and Reconstruction." Medical Physics 26:5–18, January, 1999.

[20] Goodenough DJ, Weaver KE, Davis DO. "Development of a Phantom for Evaluation and Assurance of Image Quality in CT Scanning." Optical Engineering 16:52–65, 1977.

[21] Goodenough DJ, Levy JR, Kasales C. "Development of Phantom for Spiral CT." Computerized Medical Imaging and Graphic 22:247–255, 1998.

[22] Kuhl DE, Edwards RQ. "Image Separation Radioisotope Scanning." Radiology 80:653–661, 1963.

[23] Shreve P, Steveneton R, Deters E *et al.* "FDG Imaging of Neoplasms Using a SPECT Camera Operating in Coincidence Mode." European Journal of Nuclear Medicine 24:80, 1997.

[24] Bushong SC. *Magnetic Resonance Imaging, Physical and Biological Principles*. St. Louis, MO: The C. V. Mosby Company.

Part II. Psychophysics

Introduction to Part II

Human observers are an integral part of any imaging system. Image quality can be described in purely physical terms, but optimal image quality can only be described with reference to the performance of an imaging task. The relation between physical image quality and diagnostic performance is the borderland between physics and psychology known as psychophysics. The first three chapters in the perception section deal with the current state of the art in the development and testing of psychophysical models for predicting human observer performance. Myers provides an overview of ideal observer models, Abbey and Buchod describe linear models, Eckstein, Abbey and F. O. Buchod provide an overview of available models and a roadmap for future model development. The chapter by Wilson, Jabri, and Manjeshwar shows how human observer models can actually be used to improve the design of dynamic fluoroscopic imaging systems. The chapter by Samei, Eyler and Baron on the effect of anatomical backgrounds on perception provides a bridge between the hardcore psychophysics and the softer studies of human image perception by considering the problems of moving from statistically defined images to real images of real people. Rolland summarizes the progress in the simulation of realistic yet mathematically definable backgrounds for use in the models.

The methodology for assessing human performance is very important because there is wide variability both within and between human observers even when they perform relatively simple visibility and detection tasks. The receiver operating characteristic (ROC) analysis has emerged as one of the major statistical analytical tools available to characterize human performance. It can correct for variability in the application of decision criteria. It is an active area of research in imaging. The chapter by Metz updates this very important methodology and elaborates its strengths and weaknesses, while the chapter by Chakraborty describes some of the variants of classical ROC analysis and their application to special problems in diagnostic imaging. There is also a need to go beyond the limitations imposed by the use of the ROC analysis. One approach is to evaluate observer agreement rather than the accuracy. The chapter by Polansky reviews the classical method for measuring agreement in imaging and describes an alternative methodology based on mixture distribution analysis.

Human performance even on simple tasks such as detecting tumors or fractures is complicated by the need to locate abnormalities embedded in the complex patterns of anatomical details on images. The chapter by Kundel deals with the role of

visual search in detection tasks. Human performance also depends upon expertise-
the combination of talent, training, and experience. Nodine and Mello-Thoms review the status of studies of expertise in radiology and stress the implications for
training and certifying radiologists.

In the final chapter Krupinski reviews the contributions that have been made by
image perception research to the field of medical imaging.

It is the hope of the editor that these chapters mark just the beginnings of our
knowledge about the perception of medical images. They provide summaries, reviews, and comprehensive bibliographies. What a place to start learning.

Harold L. Kundel

CHAPTER 9
Ideal Observer Models of Visual Signal Detection

Kyle J. Myers
Food and Drug Administration

CONTENTS

9.1 Introduction

The objective evaluation of imaging systems requires three important components: (1) identification of the intended use of the resulting images, which we shall refer to as the *task*; (2) specification of the *observer*, who will make use of the images in order to perform the task; and (3) a thorough understanding of the statistical properties of the objects and resulting images. With these components, a *figure of merit* can be determined for evaluating the performance of the observer on the specified task [1]. In the next sections we consider each of these elements more fully.

9.1.1 The task

Medical imaging tasks can be broadly categorized as either *classification* or *estimation* tasks. In a classification task a decision is made regarding from which class of underlying objects the data are derived. In this chapter we shall concentrate on the binary decision task, where the image is to be classified into one of two possible alternatives, truth state 1 (T_1) or truth state 2 (T_2). When the states represent signal present (abnormal) versus signal absent (normal), the task is referred to as signal detection. The determination of whether a lesion or tumor is present in an image is a signal-detection task. More generally the two states are differentiated by whatever properties of the objects in class 2 distinguish them from objects in class 1.

An estimation task involves the quantitation of one or more parameters that describe the object, based on the raw data. The parameter might be the size, location, or activity of a tumor, the amount of flow in a vessel, or the cardiac ejection fraction. In tomographic imaging the reconstruction step results in a discrete image that is meant to estimate the spatial distribution of some characteristic of the object, for example, the distribution of a radioactive tracer.

There is a natural relationship between classification and estimation tasks; one can think of estimation as classification where the number of classes is the number of possible values the parameters to be estimated can assume. Thus reconstruction of a 128×128 image using 128 gray levels is classification into $(128)^3$ classes! Even so, the signal-detection theory framework for analyzing classification tasks is generally applicable, although this example shows that the number of effective classes represented by an estimation task can be very large.

In present times quantitation tasks typically involve a numerical algorithm applied to an image by a computer, rather than a computation by a human. Because the purpose of this chapter is to describe ideal-observer models and discuss their relationship to human perception, we shall say little more about such estimation tasks here. However, because reconstructions from tomographic data are often interpreted by humans, we shall address ideal-observer performance on reconstructed images to some extent below.

9.1.2 Objects and images

For a digital imaging system the data consist of a set of M discrete measurements $\{g_1, g_2, \ldots, g_M\}$, where g_m represents the mth measurement. Most commonly, the data are the M pixels or gray levels of a digital image, although the data might equally well be the raw (projection) data from a tomographic system. The data values can be arranged to form a column vector $\mathbf{g}$ in an M-dimensional space which we shall call data space, where the mth component is the value detected at discrete element m. The data space can be assumed to be a Hilbert space if we impose the usual definitions of norm and scalar product.

The data are the result of an image-formation process whereby a continuous object $f(\mathbf{r})$ is mapped to the data set $\mathbf{g}$. (For a more detailed description of image formation and noise in imaging systems, see Barrett and Myers [2].) This mapping can be represented quite generally by the following expression:

$$\mathbf{g} = \mathcal{H}\mathbf{f} + \mathbf{n}, \qquad (9.1)$$

where the imaging operator $\mathcal{H}$ is an integral operator defined by

$$g_m = \int f(\mathbf{r})h_m(\mathbf{r})\mathrm{d}^2 r + n_m, \quad m = 1, \ldots, M, \qquad (9.2)$$

and $h_m(\mathbf{r})$, called the *sensitivity function*, gives the contribution to the mth measurement from the object at point $\mathbf{r}$. The M-dimensional vector $\mathbf{n}$ represents the noise in the data set.

The only assumption made in writing the imaging process as (9.2) is that the system be linear. The sensitivity function is closely related to a matrix called the crosstalk matrix, which describes how well particular Fourier coefficients of the object can be recovered from a set of discrete measurements. The crosstalk matrix is particularly useful for characterizing shift-variant imaging systems [3].

In a classification task, each truth state, often called a hypothesis, represents a single object (in the nonrandom signal problem) or a class of objects (in the random signal problem). The object is considered to be a continuous function $f(\mathbf{r})$ of two or three spatial dimensions, and it may have temporal dependence as well. In writing Eq. (9.1) we regard the object as a vector $\mathbf{f}$ in a Hilbert space, say $\mathcal{L}_2$, which we refer to as object space. The imaging operator is a mapping from object space to data space.

The fact that the noise is represented as additive does not restrict us to additive noise situations. It is understood that the noise is the difference between the expected data set in the absence of noise and the actual data set. That is,

$$\mathbf{n} = \langle \mathbf{g} \rangle - \mathbf{g}, \qquad (9.3)$$

where the angle brackets denote a statistical average over all the contributions to randomness in the data. All data are random because of measurement noise, which might be photon noise as in the case of radiographic imaging, or thermal noise as in magnetic resonance imaging. Additionally, the data might have some randomness because of underlying randomness in the objects being imaged. The mean data set under the jth hypothesis is then

$$\mathrm{T}_j: \quad \langle \mathbf{g} \rangle = \mathcal{H} \langle \mathbf{f} \rangle_j = \mathcal{H} \bar{\mathbf{f}}_j, \tag{9.4}$$

where $\bar{\mathbf{f}}_j$ is the mean object in class j. The full probabilistic nature of the data under truth state j is contained in the probability density function (PDF) on $\mathbf{g}$, that is, $\mathrm{pr}(\mathbf{g}|\mathrm{T}_j)$, where the vertical bar is read "conditioned on." (We have assumed that the data are able to take on sufficient numbers of values so as to be modeled by a continuous-valued vector described by a probability density function.) Another name for $\mathrm{pr}(\mathbf{g}|\mathrm{T}_j)$ is the *likelihood* of the data given hypothesis j.

9.1.3 The observer

Statistical decision theory [4–6] invokes the concept of a decision-maker, or observer. In the simple binary case, the decision-maker's task is to determine which of two classes the data set belongs to. In medical imaging the radiologist is usually the observer of the clinical image, although many investigators are developing computerized diagnosis systems. Generally speaking, the observer is an entity (human or algorithm) that makes use of the data to classify it into states of truth, which we have designated T_1 and T_2 in the binary decision case.

We assume that the observer's decision rule involves no guessing or randomness (the same data set always leads to the same decision) and no equivocation (every data vector leads to one decision, either class 1 or class 2). It then follows that the observer forms a scalar *decision variable*, or *test statistic*, which we shall call $t(\mathbf{g})$, in order to classify the data. In general the formulation of the test statistic involves nonlinear operations on the data set. We shall discuss the exact form of the dependence of $t(\mathbf{g})$ on the data in subsequent sections.

Once the test statistic is determined, the observer compares it to a *threshold* t_c to decide between the two hypotheses. The entire set of operations—from object

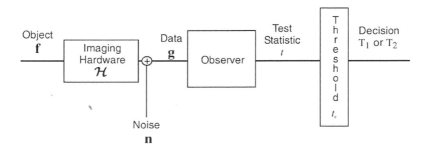

Figure 9.1: The entire set of operations—from object to data set to decision—envisioned by the statistical decision theory model for a classification task.

to data set to decision—envisioned by the statistical decision-theory model for a classification task is represented schematically in Figure 9.1.

9.1.4 Decision outcomes and ROC curves

The test statistic $t(\mathbf{g})$ is itself a random variable, because it is a functional of the multivariate random-data vector $\mathbf{g}$. The probability density function on $t(\mathbf{g})$ depends on the state of truth, and is denoted by $\text{pr}(t(\mathbf{g})|T_j)$ for state T_j. It is the fact that the density functions on $t(\mathbf{g})$ for each state overlap, as shown in Figure 9.2, that renders the decision-making process interesting. Defined in terms of classification task performance, image quality is determined by the degree of separation/overlap of these two density functions.

Figure 9.2 shows that there are four possible decision outcomes for any value of Λ_c:

1. True positive (TP): T_2 is true; observer decides T_2 is true.
2. False positive (FP): T_1 is true; observer decides T_2 is true.
3. False negative (FN): T_2 is true; observer decides T_1 is true.
4. True negative (TN): T_1 is true; observer decides T_1 is true.

Two of the above alternatives result in the observer correctly determining the underlying hypothesis, but we also see that two types of errors can be made. If the problem is to decide whether signal is present or absent, and the observer says a signal is present when it fact it is not, a type I error is made. In radar terminology this is called a *false alarm*, while in the medical literature it is called a *false positive*. When the signal is present but the observer chooses the noise-only alternative, we say a *miss*, or *false negative* has occurred. This is known as a Type II error. It follows that the *true-positive fraction* (TPF) is the probability of a true-positive decision. This is known as the *sensitivity* in the medical imaging literature. The *false-positive fraction* (FPF) is the probability of deciding in favor of the signal-present

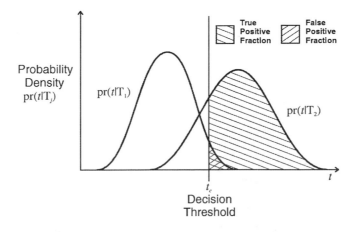

Figure 9.2: The decision theory paradigm.

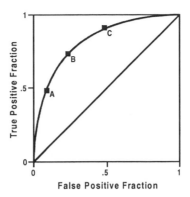

Figure 9.3: Example ROC curve showing 3 operating points: (A) conservative threshold; (B) moderate threshold; (C) lax threshold.

hypothesis when the signal is not there. In medical applications the *specificity* is often reported, which is given by (1-FPF).

The observer's threshold t_c specifies the *operating point* of the observer, that is, the (TPF, FPF) pair. By varying the threshold, a family of (TPF, FPF) points can be generated. A graph of these points is known as the *receiver operating characteristic* curve, or ROC curve, an example of which is given in Figure 9.3. Metz discusses the properties and measurement of ROC curves in Chapter 18 of this volume [6].

9.1.5 Factors that influence image quality

The degree of overlap of the density functions in Figure 9.2 is a measure of the usefulness of the system for discriminating between data from each of the two hypotheses. ("System" in this context means the entire chain of Figure 9.1, including the data-acquisition process and the observer's decision-making process.) Many factors contribute to the spread of the decision variable, as portrayed in Figure 9.4. If the discrimination task is hindered only by measurement noise, meaning the object under each hypothesis is nonrandom, it is said to be noise-limited. This is the narrowest set of density functions depicted in Figure 9.4. Biological variability (also called object variability or signal variability in the literature) adds to the randomness in the data, and hence the randomness in the decision variable, as indicated by the set of dashed functions in the figure. For images reconstructed from limited data, the decision variables are further spread by artifacts. The figure also shows what happens when the observer has an internal noise mechanism, as well as limits to the spatial area of integration, so that the density functions become spread even further.

Each of these factors can be influenced through choices available to the imaging-system designer. In the sections below, we shall describe investigations into a number of these sources of decision-variable spread, and offer observations

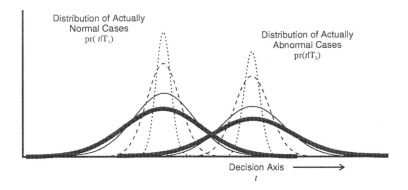

Figure 9.4: Distribution of the observer's test statistic, illustrating the factors that contribute to their spread and overlap: (1) dots = distributions from measurement noise alone; (2) dashes = distributions from noise + object variability; (3) thin solid curves = distributions when effects of artifacts are added in; (4) bold solid curves = distributions from noise, object variability, artifacts, and observer variability.

regarding the relationship between human- and machine-observer performance and the implications for system design.

9.1.6 Decision errors and costs

As we have seen, the overlap in the test-statistic density functions means every decision strategy will result in decision errors if score is kept over a large number of images. If costs are assigned to the decision outcomes, an average cost for the decision strategy can also be tallied.

Let D_i represent a decision in favor of truth state i, so that $\Pr(D_i | T_j)$ is the probability of choosing state i when state j is true. In this notation the total probability of error is written

$$P_e = \Pr(D_1 | T_2) + \Pr(D_2 | T_1). \tag{9.5}$$

Costs can be associated with every decision, both those that are correct and those that are in error. Let c_{ij} be the cost associated with choosing truth state i when truth state j is actually true. (Positive costs indicate a penalty.) The average cost or *Bayes risk* of the decision-making process is then defined as

$$\begin{aligned}\langle C \rangle = {} & c_{22}\Pr(D_2 | T_2) + c_{21}\Pr(D_2 | T_1) \\ & + c_{12}\Pr(D_1 | T_2) + c_{11}\Pr(D_1 | T_1). \end{aligned} \tag{9.6}$$

The costs include the cost of subsequent medical procedures as well as harder-to-quantify costs associated with morbidity and mortality.

An observer strategy can be designed to minimize P_e or Bayes risk. Or, one of the figures of merit described in the next section can be optimized.

9.1.7 Figures of merit

A measure of the overlap in the density functions of the test statistic is the signal-to-noise ratio defined by

$$\text{SNR}_t = \frac{\bar{t}_2 - \bar{t}_1}{\sqrt{\frac{1}{2}\sigma_{t_1}^2 + \frac{1}{2}\sigma_{t_2}^2}}, \tag{9.7}$$

where $\bar{t}_j = \langle t(\mathbf{g}) | T_j \rangle$ is the mean of the decision variable given truth state j and

$$\sigma_{t_j}^2 = \langle (t(\mathbf{g}) - \bar{t}_j)^2 | T_j \rangle, \tag{9.8}$$

is the variance of the test statistic under hypothesis j. This figure of merit should be used with caution when the test statistic is not Gaussian distributed; the widths of highly skewed density functions may not be well described by a variance.

Discrimination performance can also be indicated by the TPF at a given FPF, which does not require any special form for the probability law for the test statistic. Comparison of two observers or two imaging systems then rests on the choice of FPF relevant for the task, and determination of the system that gives higher TPF. This figure of merit is called the *Neyman-Pearson criterion* [4].

The Neyman–Pearson approach summarizes classification performance based on a single point on the ROC curve. Because the choice of operating point is somewhat arbitrary, many investigators in image quality report area under the entire ROC curve, referred to as AUC. The AUC is given by

$$\text{AUC} = \int_0^1 \text{TPF}\,d(\text{FPF}). \tag{9.9}$$

When the distributions in Figure 9.2 overlap completely, TPF = FPF at every threshold value. Thus the ROC curve for a worthless test is the 45° line and the area under the curve is 0.5. A perfect test, where there is no overlap in the density functions, gives an AUC of 1.0.

If the decision variable is normally distributed (see Section 9.2.3), the AUC is related to SNR_t by [8]

$$\text{AUC} = \frac{1}{2} + \frac{1}{2}\text{erf}\left(\frac{\text{SNR}_t}{2}\right), \tag{9.10}$$

where $\text{erf}(z)$, called the error function, is defined by

$$\text{erf}(z) = \frac{2}{\sqrt{\pi}}\int_0^z e^{-y^2}\,dy. \tag{9.11}$$

Another figure of merit, called the *detectability* and denoted d_A, is derived from the AUC by means of an inverse-error function:

$$d_A = 2 \, \mathrm{erf}^{-1}(2\mathrm{AUC} - 1). \tag{9.12}$$

The detectability represents an equivalent SNR based on the area under the ROC curve. When the test statistic is Gaussian distributed under each hypothesis, SNR_t and d_A are equivalent. In situations where the form of the test statistic is unknown, for example, when AUC is measured directly in psychophysical studies, it is common to express the experimental results in terms of d_A.

So far, we have not specified the form of the test statistic. In the next section we consider the special case of the ideal observer. As we shall see, the form of the test statistic for the ideal observer is greatly dependent on the statistics of the data sets under the two hypotheses.

9.2 The Bayesian or ideal observer

The ideal observer is defined in signal-detection theory as that observer that makes use of all available in an image, as well as any prior information, to optimize classification performance. Unlike real (human) observers, the ideal observer contributes no additional noise or uncertainty in the decision-making process. Only the actual variability in the object classes and noise in the measurement system contribute to ideal-observer decision errors. Thus the performance of this model observer provides an upper bound on the performance of any observer or decision strategy.

It can be shown [4] that the ideal observer achieves the following:

- Minimum Bayes risk

- Minimum error

- Maximum AUC

- Maximum TPF at specified FPF

9.2.1 The optimal test statistic

The secret to the ideal observer's success lies in its reliance on a test statistic of the form [4]

$$\Lambda(\mathbf{g}) = \frac{\mathrm{pr}(\mathbf{g}|T_2)}{\mathrm{pr}(\mathbf{g}|T_1)}. \tag{9.13}$$

The ideal observer calculates the likelihood of the data under each of the hypotheses, $\mathrm{pr}(\mathbf{g}|T_j)$, and compares their ratio to a threshold to determine which hypothesis to choose. Not surprisingly, then, $\Lambda(\mathbf{g})$ is known as the *likelihood ratio*. It can be shown that a likelihood-ratio test is the optimum strategy for an observer designed to minimize either decision errors or average cost. In either case the likelihood ratio is the test statistic, and the operating point (decision threshold) determines whether average cost or error is minimized.

Because monotonic transformations of the discriminant function do not change a decision, the logarithm of the likelihood ratio, or log-likelihood ratio for short, can also be used. As we shall see, the log-likelihood ratio is particularly useful in cases where the probability density function on the data under each hypothesis has an exponential form. We shall denote the log-likelihood ratio by $\lambda(\mathbf{g})$.

From Eq. (9.13) we see that computation of $\Lambda(\mathbf{g})$ and hence SNR_t requires full knowledge of the statistics of the data, including the exact form of the signal if it is nonrandom, or full knowledge of the object statistics if the objects in each class are in some sense random, as well as complete information regarding the image formation process and the measurement noise. The ideal observer must know the threshold and maintain it exactly on each decision trial. If minimum-average-cost performance is sought, the ideal observer must know all the costs of making each kind of decision. As we shall see, these rigorous requirements make calculation of ideal-observer performance difficult for clinically realistic tasks.

9.2.2 Moments of the optimal test statistic

To calculate the TPF and FPF at each threshold, and thus compute AUC, requires knowledge of the probability density functions shown in Figure 9.2. Knowledge of the moments of a random variable, or its characteristic function, are avenues for determining its PDF. Barrett et al. [8] have shown that the particular form of the ideal-observer test statistic leads to some interesting relationships between its moments under each hypothesis.

The moments of the likelihood ratio under hypothesis 1 are defined by

$$\langle \Lambda^{k+1} | T_1 \rangle = \int_{\infty} d^M g \, \text{pr}(\Lambda | T_1) \Lambda^{k+1} = \int_{\infty} d^M g \, \text{pr}(\Lambda | T_1) \left[\frac{\text{pr}(\Lambda | T_2)}{\text{pr}(\Lambda | T_1)} \right]^{k+1}$$

$$= \int_{\infty} d^M g \, \text{pr}(\Lambda | T_2) \left[\frac{\text{pr}(\Lambda | T_2)}{\text{pr}(\Lambda | T_1)} \right]^k = \langle \Lambda^k | T_2 \rangle, \qquad (9.14)$$

where the expectation integrals are over the M-dimensional data space and we have dropped the explicit dependence of Λ on the data $\mathbf{g}$. We see that the moments of the likelihood ratio under truth state 1 are easily expressed in terms of the moments under state 2. This is true for *any* task, regardless of the form of the PDF on Λ, simply by virtue of the special form of the ideal decision variable.

In particular, the mean of Λ under T_1 is

$$\langle \Lambda | T_1 \rangle = \int_{\infty} d^M g \, \text{pr}(\Lambda | T_1) \left[\frac{\text{pr}(\Lambda | T_2)}{\text{pr}(\Lambda | T_1)} \right] = \int_{\infty} d^M g \, \text{pr}(\Lambda | T_2) = 1, \qquad (9.15)$$

by the normalization of probability density functions. The variance of Λ under T_1 is given by

$$\sigma_{\Lambda_1}^2 = \langle \Lambda^2 | T_1 \rangle - (\bar{t}_1)^2 = \bar{t}_2 - 1. \qquad (9.16)$$

Thus only two free parameters must be determined to find the SNR associated with the likelihood ratio: its mean and variance under one of the hypotheses.

The log-likelihood ratio is defined by $\exp(\lambda) \equiv \Lambda$, from which we can see immediately by Eq. (9.14) that

$$\langle \exp[(k+1)\lambda] | T_1 \rangle = \langle \exp(k\lambda) | T_2 \rangle. \qquad (9.17)$$

But the moment-generating function of a random variable x is defined by

$$M(x) = \langle \exp(xs) \rangle. \qquad (9.18)$$

Hence Eq. (9.17) relates $M_1(k+1)$, the moment-generating function of λ under hypothesis 1 evaluated at $(k+1)$, to $M_2(\lambda)$, the moment-generating function of λ under hypothesis 2 evaluated at k. This relationship hold for all k. Swensson and Green [9] have shown that the only statistic satisfying this special relationship is the log-likelihood ratio.

Either the moment-generating function of a random variable, or its close cousin the characteristic function, can be used to generate moments of the random variable [10]. Because the characteristic function of a random variable uniquely determines its PDF, it shouldn't be too surprising from Eq. (9.14) that the PDFs of λ under each hypothesis are tightly related. See Barrett *et al.* [8] for a more in-depth exploration of these relationships.

9.2.3 When the log-likelihood ratio is normal

Equation (9.14) states that the moments of $\Lambda(\mathbf{g})$ under T_1 can always be written in terms of its moments under T_2. In particular, knowledge of both the mean and variance of $\Lambda(\mathbf{g})$ under T_2 is sufficient to specify the means and variances of $\Lambda(\mathbf{g})$ under both hypotheses. It follows that the same can be said of $\lambda(\mathbf{g})$. When the argument can be made that the log-likelihood is normally distributed under one hypothesis, Barrett *et al.* have shown that it is necessarily normally distributed under the other hypothesis [8]. It is then possible to express the means and variances of $\lambda(\mathbf{g})$ under each hypothesis in terms of a single parameter, the mean of $\lambda(\mathbf{g})$ under T_1.

When can the assumption be made that the decision variable is normally distributed under at least one of the hypotheses? Often this assumption is justified by the assumption that the test statistic is a linear functional of the data $\mathbf{g}$, and if the data are normally distributed, then so must be the test statistic. Such is the case for the ideal-observer decision variable for nonrandom signals and Gaussian noise. As we shall see in Section 9.3.1, the calculation of ideal-observer SNR is straightforward in that simple case.

Of greater interest is the situation where the signals are random and/or the noise is non-Gaussian, for in that case the ideal observer may well be a nonlinear functional of the data. Nevertheless, $\lambda(\mathbf{g})$ may still be approximately or asymptotically normal. Barrett *et al.* adopt an argument to this effect from standard statistics texts and give it an imaging twist. In statistics it is common to consider a data set $\mathbf{g}$ that consists of many independent observations $\{\mathbf{g}_k\}$. The independence of the samples allows the statistician to write the density function on the entire data set as a product of the densities of the independent samples (a trick we shall use in the independent, additive noise examples of Section 9.3.1.1):

$$\text{pr}(\mathbf{g}|T_j) = \prod_{k=1}^{K} \text{pr}(\mathbf{g}_k|T_j), \tag{9.19}$$

in which case the log-likelihood ratio is given by

$$\lambda(\mathbf{g}) = \sum_{k=1}^{K} \left\{ \log\left[\text{pr}(\mathbf{g}_k|T_2)\right] - \log\left[\text{pr}(\mathbf{g}_k|T_1)\right] \right\}. \tag{9.20}$$

This expression, a sum of random variables, is asymptotically normal as the number of sample vectors K becomes large, because of the central-limit theorem. To put Eq. (9.20) in an imaging context, imagine that an image $\mathbf{g}$ is made up of K statistically independent subimages $\mathbf{g}_k$. Then $\lambda(\mathbf{g})$ is asymptotically normal as long as there are enough subimages contributing to the sum in Eq. (9.20) for the central-limit theorem to work its magic.

Because normality of $\lambda(\mathbf{g})$ under one hypothesis implies normality under the other, just showing normality under one hypothesis means the SNR expression of Eq. (9.7) can be used with confidence. Moreover, only one parameter, the mean of the likelihood ratio under hypothesis 2, must be determined to compute AUC.

9.2.4 The likelihood generating function

As we shall see in the examples of Section 9.3 below, the brute-force determination of ideal-observer performance for tasks with object variability can be quite tedious. An alternative approach was recently presented by Barrett *et al.*, who have derived a general theory of the ROC curve that is applicable to any arbitrary discriminant function [8]. For the special case of the ideal observer, where the discriminant function is known to be the log-likelihood ratio, it can be shown that there are strong constraints on the form of the probability density functions $\text{pr}(\lambda(\mathbf{g})|T_j)$. These constraints enable one to determine bounds on AUC using an entity called the *likelihood-generating function*. The likelihood-generating function, or LGF, contains all that is needed to derive all moments of the log-likelihood ratio under both hypotheses. Recall that as originally presented, Eq. (9.10) was valid only for normally-distributed decision variables. The essence of the contribution of these authors is the extension of the range of validity of Eq. (9.10) so that, using the LGF and one mild approximation, AUC can be determined for non-Gaussian log-likelihood ratios.

Additional bounds on AUC have been reported by Shapiro [11]. Combining these with the results of Barrett *et al.* enable one to give both upper and lower bounds on AUC in order to bracket ideal-observer performance quite tightly. The calculation of AUC is still not a fait accompli with this formalism; it remains a difficult calculation for complex tasks. Clarkson has investigated the LGF approach for a variety of signal detection tasks [12].

9.3 Calculation of ideal-observer performance: examples

We shall begin our exploration of ideal-observer performance calculations with the oft-used example in which the signal and background is assumed to be known exactly. From there we'll progress to the calculation of ideal-observer performance for more realistic objects, incorporating object variability. The latter is an area of active research by investigators in the field today.

9.3.1 Nonrandom signals

Consider the stylized binary classification task in which the form of the object is nonrandom and known exactly under each hypothesis. This special case is referred to as the signal-known-exactly/background-known-exactly (SKE/BKE) task.

9.3.1.1 Uncorrelated Gaussian noise

Initially let us assume that the data consist of M independent samples, each corrupted by zero-mean, additive Gaussian noise. Under each hypothesis the data components are given by

$$T_j: \quad g_m = [\mathcal{H}\mathbf{f}_j]_m + n_m, \quad m = 1, 2, \ldots, M, \tag{9.21}$$

where $[\mathcal{H}\mathbf{f}_j]_m$ is the expected value in the mth detector in the absence of noise when hypothesis j is true.

Let $\overline{g}_{mj} = [\mathcal{H}\mathbf{f}_j]_m$ and let σ^2 be the noise variance in each detector channel. The probability density function on the mth detector output can then be written as

$$pr(g_m \mid T_j) = (2\pi\sigma^2)^{-1/2} \exp\left[\frac{-(g_m - \overline{g}_{mj})^2}{2\sigma^2}\right]. \tag{9.22}$$

Because the noise samples are statistically independent, the probability density function for the data vector $\mathbf{g}$ is the product of the densities of the g_m's:

$$pr(\mathbf{g} \mid T_j) = \prod_{m=1}^{M} (2\pi\sigma^2)^{-1/2} \exp\left[\frac{-(g_m - \overline{g}_{mj})^2}{2\sigma^2}\right]. \tag{9.23}$$

We can use Eq. (9.23) to write the likelihood ratio (Eq. (9.13)) as:

$$\Lambda(\mathbf{g}) = \frac{\displaystyle\prod_{m=1}^{M}(2\pi\sigma^2)^{-1/2}\exp\left[\frac{-(g_m - \bar{g}_{m2})^2}{2\sigma^2}\right]}{\displaystyle\prod_{m=1}^{M}(2\pi\sigma^2)^{-1/2}\exp\left[\frac{-(g_m - \bar{g}_{m1})^2}{2\sigma^2}\right]}$$

$$= \prod_{m=1}^{M}\exp\left[\frac{(\bar{g}_{2m} - \bar{g}_{1m})g_m}{\sigma^2} - \frac{\bar{g}_{2m}^2 - \bar{g}_{1m}^2}{2\sigma^2}\right], \qquad (9.24)$$

where the second form follows by canceling common terms in the numerator and denominator. Taking the log of this expression, the decision rule is to compare

$$\log[\Lambda(\mathbf{g})] = \lambda(\mathbf{g}) = \sum_{m=1}^{M}\exp\left[\frac{(\bar{g}_{2m} - \bar{g}_{1m})g_m}{\sigma^2} - \frac{\bar{g}_{2m}^2 - \bar{g}_{1m}^2}{2\sigma^2}\right], \qquad (9.25)$$

to a new threshold $\lambda_c = \log(\Lambda_c)$. The second term in the last expression, which is proportional to the difference in expected signal energies under each hypothesis, is independent of the data and can therefore be incorporated into the decision threshold. Let $\Delta\bar{g}_m = (\bar{g}_{2m} - \bar{g}_{2m})$ be the expected difference data in the mth channel. We can then write the following equivalent decision rule:

$$\text{Choose } T_2 \text{ when } \sum_{m=1}^{M}[\Delta\bar{g}_m g_m] > \lambda_c, \text{ else choose } T_1, \qquad (9.26)$$

or

$$\text{Choose } T_2 \text{ when } \Delta\bar{\mathbf{g}}'\mathbf{g} > \lambda_c, \text{ else choose } T_1. \qquad (9.27)$$

The ideal observer performs a matched-filter operation, correlating the received data with the expected difference data in each channel. Implementing this strategy for a variety of λ_c settings yields the ideal observer's ROC curve.

9.3.1.2 Correlated Gaussian noise

In the more general case where the additive noise is still assumed to be independent of hypothesis but now characterized by a covariance matrix $\mathbf{K_n}$, the density function on the data is written

$$\text{pr}(\mathbf{g}|T_j) = \left[(2\pi)^M \det(\mathbf{K_n})\right]^{-1/2}\exp\left[-\frac{1}{2}(\mathbf{g} - \bar{\mathbf{g}}_j)' \mathbf{K_n}^{-1}(\mathbf{g} - \bar{\mathbf{g}}_j)\right], \qquad (9.28)$$

where $\det(\cdot)$ indicates the determinant of the matrix.

The ideal decision function is determined by forming the ratio of this expression for hypotheses 1 and 2, canceling common terms in the numerator and denominator, and taking the log, much as what was done to derive Eq. (9.25). When the crank is done turning, the ideal decision rule can be found to be

$$\text{Choose T}_2 \text{ when } \Delta\bar{\mathbf{g}}^t \mathbf{K_n}^{-1}\mathbf{g} > \lambda_c, \text{ else choose T}_1. \tag{9.29}$$

Now the ideal observer makes use of the known noise correlations to decorrelate or "whiten" the noise in the data before correlating with the expected difference in each channel.

It is now possible to calculate a figure of merit for the ideal observer for this problem by calculating the mean and variance of the $\lambda(\mathbf{g})$ under each hypothesis. The difference in means in the numerator of Eq. (9.7) turns out to be identical to the variance, and we find that

$$\text{SNR}_I^2 = \Delta\bar{\mathbf{g}}^t \mathbf{K_n}^{-1} \Delta\bar{\mathbf{g}}, \tag{9.30}$$

where the subscript "I" on the SNR indicates that this is the figure of merit for the ideal observer.

For stationary noise $\mathbf{K_n}^{-1}$ is a Toeplitz (or block Toeplitz) matrix, which is often well approximated by a circulant matrix. Such matrices are diagonalized by a discrete Fourier transform, making the calculation of Eq. (9.30) quite easy in the Fourier domain. Wagner and Brown [13] gave Fourier-domain expressions for the ideal-observer SNR of Eq. (9.30) for all the major medical imaging modalities, all in the form:

$$\text{SNR}_I^2 = \int d\boldsymbol{v} |\Delta\tilde{\bar{\mathbf{g}}}(\boldsymbol{v})|^2 \text{NEQ}(\boldsymbol{v}), \tag{9.31}$$

where the tilde indicates that $\Delta\tilde{\bar{\mathbf{g}}}(\boldsymbol{v})$ is a Fourier-domain quantity which depends on the two- or three-dimensional spatial frequency $\boldsymbol{v}$, and $\text{NEQ}(\boldsymbol{v})$ can be interpreted as the frequency-dependent density of quanta at the input of a perfect detector that would yield the same output noise as the real detection system under evaluation [14]. Equation (9.31) is valid as long as the objects to be discriminated are nonrandom and known exactly, and the noise is stationary and Gaussian.

9.3.1.3 Poisson noise

Now consider the case where the ideal observer is faced with the task of discriminating between two exactly-specified signals in Poisson noise. The likelihood of the data under hypothesis j is then given by

$$\text{pr}(\mathbf{g}|\text{T}_j) = \prod_{m=1}^{M} \frac{e^{-\bar{g}_{mj}} \bar{g}_{mj}^{g_m}}{(g_m)!}, \tag{9.32}$$

from which the ideal observer's test statistic can be shown to be [14]

$$\lambda(\mathbf{g}) = \sum_{m=1}^{M} g_m \ln \frac{\overline{g}_{m2}}{\overline{g}_{m1}}. \tag{9.33}$$

We see that when the image contains Poisson noise the optimum operation on the data is again a linear filtering operation, only now the filter is a nonlinear functional of the expected signals under the two hypotheses.

The signal-to-noise ratio associated with this test statistic is:

$$\text{SNR}_{\text{I}}^2 = \frac{\left[\sum_{m=1}^{M} (\overline{g}_{m2} - \overline{g}_{m1}) \ln \frac{\overline{g}_{m2}}{\overline{g}_{m1}} \right]^2}{\frac{1}{2} \sum_{m=1}^{M} (\overline{g}_{m2} + \overline{g}_{m1}) \ln \frac{\overline{g}_{m2}}{\overline{g}_{m1}}}. \tag{9.34}$$

Note what happens when locations in the image have expected values known to be nonzero for one hypothesis and zero for the other. The test statistic becomes infinite when the data is nonzero at that location. This implies an infinite SNR_I as well, and Eq. (9.34) bears this out. This effect is attributable to the power of the *a priori* information regarding the expected values in a particular pixel in the image.

Expressions of the form Eq. (9.33) and Eq. (9.34) are relevant when the image contains Poisson noise of sufficiently low count level that it is not appropriate to approximate its behavior with a Gaussian density function. When the number of counts in each detector is greater than about 10, a Gaussian approximation can be made [16].

9.3.2 Random signals

In the previous section we presented all that is needed for the assessment of imaging systems based on SKE/BKE classification tasks. One needs an accurate model of the signals to be discriminated and a characterization of the measurement system in order to form the likelihood of the data under each hypothesis. If imaging systems could be rank ordered for all tasks on the basis of their performance on SKE/BKE tasks, we could conclude this chapter now. The hard truth is that not only are systems that perform well for estimation tasks not necessarily optimized for detection tasks (see Section 9.6) but a system designed for optimal SKE/BKE classification performance can be woefully outclassed (!) when the objects have some randomness.

Consider the problem of determining the optimal trade-off between resolution and collection efficiency in a gamma-ray imaging system. Early attempts in this direction focused on the calculation of the mean and variance of the reconstructed image, both of which in general depend on the object and on the position in the image. A formalism called the noise kernel was developed from which these quantities, as well as the noise autocorrelation function, could be calculated. (For a review, see Barrett and Swindell [16].) Results of these calculations are frequently given in terms of a position-dependent signal-to-noise ratio or pixel SNR. The noise-kernel formalism yields a complete statistical description of the reconstructed images through second-order statistics, but it is nevertheless an incomplete statement of image quality. The difficulty is that the noise kernel and pixel SNR are not directly related to task performance. (See Burgess for a nice illustration of this shortcoming of pixel SNR [17].

Tsui *et al.* [18] and Wagner *et al.* [15] performed early task-based assessments of apertures for planar emission imaging systems. Tsui *et al.* [18] considered an SKE/BKE detection task. Wagner *et al.* based their investigation on the so-called Rayleigh task, where the observer is asked to decide if the object consists of one Gaussian blob or two, on a uniform background. In each case there was no uncertainty in either the object structure or the background, so the only randomness in the task was attributable to measurement noise. Both studies found that the largest possible open aperture gave superior performance for the specified task and the ideal observer; optimal performance was obtained when spatial resolution was sacrificed entirely for photon-collection efficiency.

This surprising result indicates that there is no tradeoff between resolution and counts after all, because spatial resolution is not required. Yet, great gaping apertures are not the norm in clinical practice. Tsui *et al.* [18] recognized that if another task were considered, one in which the background is uniform but random, resolution would be required for optimal task performance. A subsequent series of theoretical and simulation studies demonstrated that this discrepancy between clinical practice and theoretical analysis is indeed a characteristic of the exactly-specified tasks that were considered [19–21]. In essence, more complex tasks put more stringent requirements on the deterministic properties of the imaging system.

This cautionary tale is a clear mandate for evaluating imaging systems on the basis of ideal-observer performance for more realistic tasks in which the assumptions of known signal and/or known background are relaxed. The catch is that, as we shall see, the Bayesian observer is almost always nonlinear in such cases, and determination of SNR_I may require lengthy numerical calculations and/or Monte Carlo simulations.

9.3.2.1 *Gaussian object class*

One "toy" problem incorporating object variability where the ideal-observer strategy is determinable is the case where the objects under each hypothesis are random and described by a Gaussian probability density function. While this example would not be a realistic model of most imaging situations, it serves to illustrate how such uncertainty in the object impacts the ideal decision function.

Let the object under hypothesis j be a Gaussian random process with mean $\langle \mathbf{f} | T_j \rangle = \bar{\mathbf{f}}_j =$ and autocovariance function $\mathcal{K}_{\mathbf{f}_j}$. For additive zero-mean Gaussian noise, the data are Gaussian distributed with mean

$$\bar{\mathbf{g}}_j = \mathcal{H}\bar{\mathbf{f}}_j, \tag{9.35}$$

and covariance matrix

$$\mathbf{K_{g_j}} = \mathcal{H}\mathcal{K}_{f_j}\mathcal{H}^\dagger + \mathbf{K_n}, \tag{9.36}$$

under hypothesis j, where $\mathcal{H}^\dagger$ represents the adjoint of the operator $\mathcal{H}$. Similar algebra to what yielded Eq. (9.29) can be used to show that the ideal observer compares the test statistic below with a threshold to determine which hypothesis is most likely [22]:

$$\lambda(\mathbf{g}) = -1/2\,\mathbf{g}^t\left(\mathbf{K_{g_2}^{-1}} - \mathbf{K_{g_1}^{-1}}\right)\mathbf{g} + \left(\mathbf{\bar{g}}_2^t\mathbf{K_{g_2}^{-1}} - \mathbf{\bar{g}}_1^t\mathbf{K_{g_1}^{-1}}\right)\mathbf{g}. \tag{9.37}$$

Computing this test statistic requires the observer to perform a nonlinear operation on the data vector $\mathbf{g}$, as can be seen by studying the first term of $\lambda(\mathbf{g})$. This term represents a prewhitened autocorrelation of the data with itself. The second term in the expression resembles the prewhitened matched filter we are accustomed to finding in a signal-known-exactly task. This generalized linear term is now the difference between the prewhitened matched filter outputs for the average signal under each of the hypotheses.

When the variances under each of the hypotheses are equal, the quadratic term disappears and a linear test is optimum. If, however, the mean signal is zero under both hypotheses, the linear term drops out and the ideal observer does a purely quadratic test. In such a task a linear observer, such as a Hotelling observer (see Chapter 11 in this volume), would have no discrimination ability.

If the ideal observer is faced with a detection task in which hypothesis 2 is that a random signal is present and hypothesis 1 is that no signal is present, and the observer has no information regarding the randomness of the object under T_2, the object covariance function $\mathcal{K}_{f_2}$ in Eq. (9.36) effectively approaches infinity. We can write down the test statistic for this case:

$$\lambda(\mathbf{g}) = \mathbf{g}^t\mathbf{K_n^{-1}}\mathbf{g}. \tag{9.38}$$

The ideal observer forms a quadratic test statistic normalized by the noise covariance. If the data give rise to a sufficiently high test statistic, the observer decides that the data represent a signal-present state. Barrett et $al.$ [23] and Wagner and Barrett [24] have discussed this detection problem in detail and have shown that the ideal observer's decision variable follows the χ^2 probability law.

Myers and Wagner [22] showed that the optimal quadratic tests represented by Eq. (9.37) and Eq. (9.38) may be represented as a sequence of two linear operations: first estimate the object, then match filter to detect. As Wagner and Barrett have pointed out, the ideal observer does not supply information regarding which signal is present when deciding that the hypothesis "signal present" is true in these detection tasks with signal variation, even though the ideal observer can be thought of as having formed an estimate of the signal. Rather, the output of the ideal observer is a single response: "signal present" or "signal absent."

9.3.2.2 Background uncertainty

Perhaps a more realistic model for a class of random objects is obtained by considering the object to be the sum of two independent components, the signal to be detected or discriminated, and a background [25]. Let us presume for now that the signal under hypothesis j is nonrandom and known, so we denote it by $\mathbf{s}_j$. The background will be denoted $\mathbf{b}$. The signal is derived from whatever aspect(s) of the objects in class 2 distinguishes it in the detection or discrimination task from class 1. For example, the signal might be a nodule to be detected in a detection task. The background is whatever is left that makes up the object, for example, the ribs and other "non-nodule" structures in a chest film. We have taken the liberty of writing the signal and background here as vectors in data space. They are therefore the outcome of the measurement process acting on the object-space signal and background quantities in the absence of noise. The measurement noise $\mathbf{n}$ is a characteristic of the imaging system; it is what makes the data random when a particular signal and background is imaged. The statistics of $\mathbf{n}$ may be independent of $\mathbf{b}$ and $\mathbf{s}_j$ if the noise can be modeled as additive. For Poisson noise, though, the statistics of the noise would depend on the mean data vector, which is a function of the signal and background.

The assumption that the signal and background are additive is a slight loss of generality, in that it disallows obscuring signals. For radiological imaging with penetrating radiation, this additive assumption is not unreasonable.

The randomness in the background is characterized by the probability density function $\mathrm{pr}_{\mathbf{b}}(\mathbf{b})$, which describes the ensemble of possible backgrounds. We assume this ensemble is the same under each hypothesis. (Previously the only probability density function we encountered was that which described the randomness in the data attributable to measurement noise. When additional randomness from the objects is to be incorporated, we need to subscript the probability density functions to clarify which random variable they characterize.)

Consider a simple detection problem where T_1 represents a signal-absent condition. For a particular realization of the random background, the noise is just $\mathbf{n} = \mathbf{g} - \mathbf{b}$, described by $\mathrm{pr}_{\mathbf{n}}(\mathbf{g} - \mathbf{b} \,|\, \mathbf{b})$. The likelihood of the data under T_1 is then found by averaging over the ensemble of possible backgrounds:

$$\mathrm{pr}(\mathbf{g} | T_1) = \int_{\infty} d^M b \, \mathrm{pr}_{\mathbf{n}}(\mathbf{g} - \mathbf{b} \,|\, \mathbf{b}) \mathrm{pr}_{\mathbf{b}}(\mathbf{b}). \qquad (9.39)$$

For the signal-present condition, T_2, the noise is just $\mathbf{n} = \mathbf{g} - \mathbf{b} - \mathbf{s}$ for a known signal $\mathbf{s}$ and a particular realization of the random background. The likelihood on the data under this hypothesis is then

$$\mathrm{pr}(\mathbf{g} | T_2) = \int_{\infty} d^M b \, \mathrm{pr}_{\mathbf{n}}(\mathbf{g} - \mathbf{b} - \mathbf{s} \,|\, \mathbf{b}) \mathrm{pr}_{\mathbf{b}}(\mathbf{b}). \qquad (9.40)$$

Forming the ratio of Eq. (9.40) to Eq. (9.39) yields the likelihood ratio.

As a simple example, consider a multivariate normal background with mean $\overline{\mathbf{b}}$ and covariance matrix $\mathbf{K_b}$. With uncorrelated, additive Gaussian noise, the overall covariance matrix of the data is now $\mathbf{K_g} = \sigma^2 \mathbf{I} + \mathbf{K_b}$, where $\mathbf{I}$ is the identity matrix. The signal-absent likelihood is then

$$\text{pr}(\mathbf{g}|T_1) \propto \exp\left[-\frac{1}{2}(\mathbf{g} - \overline{\mathbf{b}})^t \mathbf{K_g}(\mathbf{g} - \overline{\mathbf{b}}) \right], \tag{9.41}$$

and the signal-present density is given by

$$\text{pr}(\mathbf{g}|T_2) \propto \exp\left[-\frac{1}{2}(\mathbf{g} - \overline{\mathbf{b}} - \mathbf{s})^t \mathbf{K_g}(\mathbf{g} - \overline{\mathbf{b}} - \mathbf{s}) \right]. \tag{9.42}$$

Now the log-likelihood ratio can be found:

$$\lambda = \mathbf{s}^t \mathbf{K_g^{-1}}(\mathbf{g} - \overline{\mathbf{b}} - \mathbf{s}). \tag{9.43}$$

The ideal strategy is to subtract the known signal and mean background from the data, multiply by the inverse of the data covariance matrix, and then correlate with the expected signal. We call the filtering with the inverse of $\mathbf{K_g}$ a generalized prewhitening operation because it looks like the prewhitening operation of Eq. (9.29). In Eq. (9.43) the ideal observer compensates for the correlations in the data that result from measurement noise plus object variability, which are both contained in $\mathbf{K_g}$.

Note that Eq. (9.43) represents a linear strategy; the data appear just once in the expression. The special case of a flat but varying background can be found asymptotically by appropriately modifying the covariance matrix $\mathbf{K_b}$, which captures the correlation length of $\mathbf{b}$.

The use of other types of random backgrounds, either theoretical, simulated, or those from actual clinical images, is the subject of current research (see later chapters in this volume).

9.3.2.3 Signal parameter uncertainty

Another form of object randomness is the case where the form of the signal is specified, but there is randomness in P of its defining parameters [24]. For example, the signal to be detected might have known shape, but unknown amplitude or location. Another example is a sinusoidal signal of random frequency. We can arrange these random parameters into a vector $\boldsymbol{\alpha}_j$ with probability density $\text{pr}_{\alpha}(\boldsymbol{\alpha}_j)$ under hypothesis T_j. We assume that the statistics of $\boldsymbol{\alpha}_j$ and $\mathbf{b}$ are independent.

The data under T_j can now be represented by $\mathbf{g} = \mathbf{s}(\boldsymbol{\alpha}_j) + \mathbf{b} + \mathbf{n}$. The likelihood of the data is determined by performing a double average, first over the possible backgrounds for each particular signal form, and then over the ensemble of signals:

$$\text{pr}(\mathbf{g}|T_j) = \int_{\infty} d^P\alpha \int_{\infty} d^M b\, \text{pr}_{\mathbf{n}}(\mathbf{g} - \mathbf{b} - \mathbf{s}(\boldsymbol{\alpha}_j)|\mathbf{b})\text{pr}_{\mathbf{b}}(\mathbf{b})\text{pr}_{\alpha}(\boldsymbol{\alpha}_j). \tag{9.44}$$

Consider the problem of detecting a signal with random location on a known background **b**. For additive white noise, the likelihood on the data in the signal-absent state is given by Eq. (9.22) with $\overline{g}_{m1} = b_m =$ the value of the known background at detector m. The signal-present hypothesis is characterized by the random location parameter $\mathbf{r}_0$ which has density function $\mathrm{pr}_{\mathbf{r}}(\mathbf{r}_0)$. The signal contribution at the mth channel is $s_m(\mathbf{r} - \mathbf{r}_0)$, which means the signal is shifted to position $\mathbf{r}_0$ and sampled at position m. The probability density function under this hypothesis is then given by

$$\mathrm{pr}(\mathbf{g}|T_2) \propto \int_\infty d^2\mathbf{r}_0 \exp\left[-\frac{1}{2\sigma^2} \sum_{m=1}^{M} \left(g_m - b_m - s_m(\mathbf{r} - \mathbf{r}_0)\right)^2 \right] \mathrm{pr}_{\mathbf{r}}(\mathbf{r}_0). \quad (9.45)$$

The likelihood ratio for this problem can be found to be

$$\Lambda \propto \int_\infty d^2\mathbf{r}_0 \, \mathrm{pr}_{\mathbf{r}}(\mathbf{r}_0) \exp\left[\frac{1}{\sigma^2} \sum_{m=1}^{2} (g_m - b_m) s_m(\mathbf{r} - \mathbf{r}_0) \right]. \quad (9.46)$$

The ideal observer subtracts the background, correlates with the signal for shift $\mathbf{r}_0$, divides by the noise variance, and exponentiates. This is done for each possible signal shift and the results are averaged with respect to the prior density on the shift variable. The behavior of the ideal observer for the location-uncertain problem was explored by Nolte and Jaarsma [26] and more recently by Brown *et al.* [27].

The ideal strategy in the random-location problem with a Gaussian random background is in essence a combination of Eqs. (9.43) and (9.46). In that case the *mean* background is subtracted from the data, the result is prewhitened by the overall data covariance, and then the correlation with the possible signal alternatives occurs.

Other forms of signal-parameter uncertainty can be modeled by appropriate choice of the parameter vector $\boldsymbol{\alpha}_j$ and its prior. The likelihood ratio has been computed by Clarkson and Barrett [28] for Bayesian detection with amplitude, scale, orientation and position uncertainty.

9.3.2.4 *The effect of limited data sets*

When an imaging system has a very nonlocal point response function (PRF), such as a tomographic imaging system with a limited number of views, the image of a point source is very noncompact. The PRF for a limited-view tomography system will have streak artifacts that are deterministic, but object dependent. Given the problem of detection of a known object, say a compact disk, when the measurement system is a limited-view tomography system, an ideal observer that knew the disk location would account for the noncompact PRF as part of its procedure for detecting a disk in that particular location. For this SKE/BKE task, the ideal observer suffers a performance penalty compared to its performance on the same detection task on an image generated by an imaging system with a compact PRF. The penalty arises because the ideal observer's strategy, given in Eq. (9.27), is to match filter using the expected streaky image of the disk, thereby collecting more noise than when it uses a compact template.

The real problem with limited data sets comes when the task is also complicated by object variability. When a disk to be detected has a random location, the artifacts in the image will vary depending on the location of the disk [29]. Even worse, object variability in the form of a random background results in an image that has nonlocal contributions from all of the nonsignal components in the object. Thus it is all the more important that the evaluation of systems in which the data are limited involves tasks that incorporate some form of object variability for accurate assessment of system performance.

Hanson and collaborators have presented a task-based framework for the evaluation of tomographic imaging geometries and reconstruction algorithms [30–32]. In the early phase of this work, machine observers inspired by Bayesian decision theory were utilized for comparison of reconstruction algorithms. A true ideal-observer performance calculation was not done, because the statistics of the images were not well understood, particularly in the case of nonlinear reconstruction algorithms. Later the reconstruction algorithms were evaluated using neural networks to approximate ideal performance [33–35].

A number of investigators in the field today are working toward improved understanding of the statistics of reconstructed images. The full multivariate probability density function for the expectation-maximization algorithm has been determined theoretically by Barrett *et al.* [36] and verified through Monte Carlo simulation by Wilson *et al.* [37]. For other algorithms the statistics of the reconstructions have been determined through second order [38–42]. Second-order statistics are sufficient to determine the optimal linear discriminant for tasks using the reconstructions. (See subsequent chapters in this volume.) Further work is needed to improve our understanding of the higher-order image statistics that result from the variety of reconstruction algorithms being developed for tomography to assess their utility in a Bayesian framework.

Theoretically, the ideal observer can make optimal use of the raw data and has no need of post-processing. In the projection data the statistics of the noise are known to be Poisson, and perhaps approximately Gaussian. The form of the likelihood of the data conditioned on a particular object is then of the form found in Section 9.3.1. However, the object variability is sometimes more easily understood at least intuitively in the reconstruction space. Thus, the overall likelihood might be computed based on either the projection data or the reconstructions, depending on mathematical convenience. If the likelihood is computed based on the reconstructions, the statistics of the noise following post-processing by the reconstruction algorithm must be determined, and the considerations of the preceding paragraph come into play.

Unlike the ideal observer, the human observer has a real need for a reconstruction in order to make sense of the detected data. Few human observers are able to make diagnoses on the basis of projection data. Ideal-observer performance is germane for the assessment of the quality of the raw detected data, giving an upper bound on the performance of any observer who uses the data to perform some prescribed task [43]. Human performance studies are especially relevant for the assessment of reconstruction algorithms and displayed data. Assessment of reconstructed images requires a much broader range of considerations, including the null functions of the imaging system, the reconstruction artifacts that result, and the need for reconstruction constraints and object class models to reduce these effects. Subsequent chapters in this volume are devoted to models for predicting human performance on reconstructions.

9.4 Comparison with human performance

In publications dating back 50 years, Rose suggested the use of an absolute scale for evaluating human performance on visual tasks [44]. While Rose's work was based on a statistical approach, it preceded the development of the Bayesian theory of signal detection. 1958, Tanner and Birdsall introduced figures of merit relating human performance to ideal-observer performance [45]. Human efficiency as we shall use it is defined as the squared ratio of the measured d_A of the human observer to the computed d_A of the ideal observer [46].

In this section we review the results of investigations of human performance for tasks in which performance of the ideal observer has been calculated, to show how well (or not!) human performance is predicted by SNR_I.

9.4.1 Noise-limited tasks

For tasks in which the signal and background are known and the ideal observer is limited by uncorrelated quantum or thermal fluctuations in the data, we have seen that the optimal strategy is to perform a linear template-matching operation on the image to calculate the ideal decision variable. For such tasks, the ideal observer of Bayesian decision theory has been found to be a good predictor of human performance. Human efficiency has been found to be 30–50% for a range of detection and discrimination tasks [47, 48].

For an SKE/BKE task in correlated noise, the ideal strategy is to first perform a prewhitening operation on the data before cross-correlating it with the expected difference signal. A number of investigators have measured human performance in images degraded by colored noise. Human efficiency for images with low pass noise is not significantly degraded relative to performance in white noise [48–50]. When the noise is high pass, such as when it is characterized by a ramp-shaped noise power spectrum as in the case of a computed-tomography (CT) imaging system, human efficiency relative to the ideal observer falls to about 20%. Noise characterized by power-law behavior at low frequency, that is, with a power spectrum of the form ν^n (where ν is spatial frequency and the exponent $n = 1, 2, 3, 4$) has been shown to cause dramatic degradation in human detection performance relative to the ideal observer as n increases. This inability to perform the prewhitening operation has been shown to be consistent with the requirement that human observers process visual information through frequency-selective channels [51]. The investigation of channelized observers that predict human performance over a wider range of tasks is an area of active research, as described by subsequent chapters in this volume.

9.4.2 Effect of signal spatial extent

An ideal observer is assumed to make perfect use of all available signal information, which naturally includes signal size and shape. These elements are incorporated into the description of the signal embodied in $f(\mathbf{r})$ in object space ($\mathbf{s}$ in data space). For compact signals (signals with limited spatial extent) in white noise, human performance can be predicted by an ideal observer that is known to position a template over the location of the expected signal and perform a linear filtering operation. However, human efficiency relative to the ideal observer degrades when the signal extent evidently becomes sufficiently large that some limitation in the integration area of the human is reached [52]. Interestingly, signals that are large in spatial extent without needing a large integration area for detection are still detected quite effectively by the human observer. An example is the detection of a known grid of bright lattice points in a noisy background [53]. Another example is the detection of mirror symmetry patterns of dots [54, 55]. It has been postulated that the human achieves high efficiency for such tasks possibly by utilizing a series of local template matching operations [56].

9.4.3 Statistically-defined signals and backgrounds

We now consider tasks represented by the distributions in Figure 9.2 labeled "quantum noise and object variability." When the task is the detection of 1 of N orthogonal signals of limited spatial extent, human performance has been shown to be again roughly 50% efficient compared to the ideal observer performing the same task [57–60]. That is, the performance penalty experienced by the human observer is no greater than the performance penalty paid by the ideal observer for the same object variability. Nolte and Jaarsma [26] showed that the very complicated (and highly nonlinear) form of the ideal observer's test statistic given in Eq. (9.46) could be almost matched in performance by an observer that simply performs a sequence of linear filtering operations, one for each of the N signals, and chooses in favor of whichever signal alternative gives the maximum filter output. It is therefore possible that the human performs this nonlinear task through the simple mechanics of applying a sequence of linear templates to the image, one for each signal alternative.

More recently, studies of signal detection with background variability in a Bayesian framework have been performed by Burgess [61–63], following the work of Rolland [64], Yao [65], and Barrett [66]. When the object variability is such that the signal is a known Gaussian object on a statistically defined background, Rolland and Yao showed that the detection performance of humans was predicted quite well by a channelized Hotelling observer, the subject of a subsequent chapter in this volume. However, the form of background variability they studied did not lend itself to calculations of the full ideal-observer detectability.

Burgess investigated human performance for objects with statistically defined backgrounds similar to those of Rolland [64] and Yao [65]. By generating the random, spatially nonuniform background structure through the use of a filtered Gaussian field, he was able to use an expression like Eq. (9.43) to calculate SNR_I. He found human efficiency to be again around 50% for backgrounds with long-range structure relative to the signal, but dropping to as low as 15% when the background correlation distance approaches the size of the signal. The ideal observer must be handicapped by frequency-selective channels to predict human performance across the full range of experimental parameters, a result that is consistent with the findings of Rolland and Yao.

For non-compact signals with uncertainty, human efficiency can be extremely low. This has been shown to be true in a number of studies, for example, the detection of a "jittery" grid—analogous to the SKE/BKE experiment mentioned in the previous section in which a grid of bright lattice points is to be detected, but where now the locations of the bright points are jittered, or individually randomized, about their means [53], the detection of random dot patterns as the number of dots grows large [67, 68], and the detection of diffuse liver disease [69]. These results may be driven by the complexity of the calculation required to derive the ideal decision variable—the human may not have the ability to use all the numbers the ideal observer can, perhaps because of memory or time limitations.

9.4.4 Tasks limited by artifacts

One might guess from the nonlocal SKE/BKE task performance described in Section 9.4.2 that human efficiency would be quite low for tasks involving images in which significant artifacts are present, because the human might not be able to compensate for the long-range nature of artifact structures. We have investigated human performance for two discrimination tasks on images reconstructed from a limited number of tomographic views. The first was the detection of low-contrast disks at known locations in scenes also containing many randomly located high-contrast disks [70]. The second was the discrimination of exactly specified single and binary objects (the "Rayleigh" task) in an image of many such objects placed randomly to generate artifacts in the reconstructions [71]. To approximate the ideal observer's performance, neural network decision performance was determined on the same tasks [33, 34]. We found human performance to be remarkably well modeled by a machine observer that performed only simple linear operations on the images. Human efficiency relative to the neural network observer was substantially lower. Other authors in this volume report similar experience, in that human performance is much more accurately predicted by linear observers for many tasks.

Long-tailed PRFs also arise in imaging systems where septal penetration in collimators occurs, when veiling glare is present as in image intensifier systems, or because of scattered radiation in the body. Human performance on images from such systems has been shown to improve following deconvolution filtering of such images, which has the effect of narrowing the overall system PRF [72]. The ideal observer's performance is unchanged by an invertible filter acting on a raw data set. So here again we find that human efficiency is low for a system with a noncompact PRF, and post-processing can improve human performance.

When considering artifacts, their impact on human performance, and the concomitant implications for system design, a few more points should be made. First, even though it is often possible to post-process images to reduce artifacts, there is always an attendant noise penalty. Also, while an observer might be able to learn that certain objects generate artifacts of a known general structure, artifacts can lessen clinicians' confidence by putting the burden on them to know what is an artifact and what is biology. And finally, an imaging system is rarely used for a single task. While certain detection or discrimination tasks might be performed reasonably well in the presence of artifacts, those same artifacts can also make performance of estimation tasks on the same image inaccurate. As always, the system design should be for a range of tasks, where all these factors are considered.

9.5 Estimation of ideal observer performance from finite samples

The closed-form solutions and numerical methods for determining SNR_I suggested in Section 9.3. assume that the noise PDF is known and therefore ensemble statistics can be employed. Recently Gagne and Wagner have investigated the characteristics of SNR_I when it is determined from experimental measurements [73]. The problem they address is one in which a finite number of sample images from a radiographic system viewing a simple (phantom) object are obtained, and in some of these a nonrandom signal is present. Thus each image represents a noise or signal-plus-noise realization in an SKE/BKE paradigm. This work has applicability for quality-assurance applications in which sample images are used to determine the imaging performance of a particular imaging device in a clinic. Current practice involves having a human reader evaluate a small number of test images, but this process is fraught with variability and imprecision. Tapiovaara and Chakraborty have proposed experimental methods for estimating suboptimal observer performance for mammographic and fluoroscopic applications, among others [74–76]. The contribution of Gagne and Wagner is the characterization of the statistical properties (bias and variance) of the estimated SNR_I. Wear has performed a similar investigation into estimates of ideal-observer detectability in ultrasound [77].

9.6 Estimation tasks

We have concentrated in this chapter on classification tasks, yet we know that increasingly in medical imaging the task is one of quantitation or estimation of one or more parameters from a data set. We have ignored this task primarily because this volume is concerned with image perception, and humans are often left out of the loop when quantitation tasks are performed on images. Computer algorithms simply tend to be more accurate and precise for such tasks.

For those readers interested in the design, optimization, and evaluation of imaging systems for estimation tasks, the same statistical decision theoretic framework is applicable. Several investigators have utilized estimation tasks in the assessment of medical images [79]. Kijewski evaluated imaging systems for a detection task with size and location uncertainty by determining the performance of an estimator of the uncertain parameters [80, 81]. Barrett has derived figures of merit for both classification and estimation tasks and shown their relationship [82]. Although this analysis is limited to linear observers, it nevertheless shows the connectedness of the two types of tasks and illustrates how one can determine the effect of changes in the imaging system or post-processing on each task. With this framework one can see how to avoid optimizing a system for a detection task while degrading it for an estimation task.

More recently, Barrett *et al.* have shown how a simple type of object variability—random location—relates the design of a system for a classification task intimately with the design of a system that is optimized for estimation [83]. This powerful approach is not restricted to shift-invariant systems, yet it describes an imaging system's performance in terms of its ability to recover Fourier components of the object. The Fourier domain is as useful as ever for image evaluation, even for nonstationary, shift variant imaging systems.

9.7 Closing remarks

We have known for some time that assessment of linear, shift-invariant systems using simple tasks leads to the NEQ approach of Eq. (9.31). A consensus in the community has developed on how to make the measurements necessary to characterize the measurement noise and the system transfer characteristics in order to determine this performance metric [84]. Recently, we have seen much progress in the development of analytical and numerical methods for the computation of ideal-observer task performance for more complex tasks and more realistic models of the imaging system.

For ideal-observer performance measures to be meaningful, the imaging system must be modeled accurately, including both its deterministic and stochastic properties. The imaging matrix can be measured for some modalities and used to determine the sensitivity function [85]. If it is simulated, it is important that the continuous-to-discrete nature of the imaging process be modeled appropriately. A hybrid model of the data statistics can often be formulated, with theory guiding the noise model and simulation or measurements determining the object statistics [86]. The object statistics can frequently be assumed to be independent of the noise. Even nonlinear imaging systems can be modeled as having additive noise. In all cases, a thorough understanding of the physics of the imaging process is key to image assessment.

We have described studies of progressively more complicated tasks that have been investigated to determine how well ideal-observer models can be used to predict human performance. These investigations have resulted in a better understanding of how to balance the emission imaging design trade-off between resolution and noise in the presence of a lumpy background, for example, and what choice of post-processing options best serves the observer for a visual task based on tomographic data. For tasks in which the optimal strategy can be approximated by one or more linear operations using compact filters, the human has been shown to be fairly efficient. This is true with the caveat that there appear to be limits to the integration area and contrast sensitivity of the human observer. Both these limitations can often be handled by changing the system magnification, in the first case, or by post-processing that alters local or global contrast, in the second case. For more complicated tasks that require either much more number crunching or a large amount of memory, the human often falls off severely in performance compared to the ideal observer.

The beauty of the statistical-decision-theory approach to image assessment is that once we have a measure of ideal-observer performance, we have a basis of comparison from which we can state in absolute terms when human performance is particularly high or low. When the human observer is found to be grossly inefficient at some task, the message is clear—the system designer should consider revisiting the design to enable the human to more readily extract the information required to perform the given task, or the human might be augmented by a machine reader.

The progress being made in our ability to calculate ideal-observer performance for more clinically realistic tasks is being matched by advancements in methodologies for determining human performance for the same tasks. Assessment of raw data by ideal observer performance, displayed data by human observer performance, and the ultimate determination of human efficiency for complex tasks inevitably requires collaboration among imaging physicists, perceptual scientists, radiologists, and statisticians. We look forward to continued interaction between investigators from these varied areas of expertise as we strive to expand our toolbox of image assessment models and methods in the future.

Acknowledgments

I want to thank Hal Kundel for the invitation to write this brief summary of the contributions of many innovative investigators in the field of image perception and image assessment. I want to especially thank Harry Barrett, David Brown, Art Burgess, Bob Gagne, Ken Hanson, Charles Metz, Markku Tapiovaara, and Bob Wagner for the many enlightening communications and collaborations over the years that have influenced this write-up.

References

[1] ICRU Report 54. "Medical Imaging—The Assessment of Image Quality." Bethesda, MD: International Commission on Radiation Units and Measurements, 1996.

[2] Barrett HH, Myers KJ. *Foundations of Image Science*. New York: Wiley, 2001.

[3] Barret HH, Denny JL, Wagner RF, Myers KJ. "Objective Assessment of Image Quality. II. Fisher Information, Fourier Crosstalk, and Figures of Merit for Task Performance." J Opt Soc A 12:834–852, 1995.

[4] Van Trees HL. *Detection, Estimation, and Modulation Theory*, Vol. I. New York: Wiley, 1968.

[5] Melsa JL, Cohn DL. *Decision and Estimation Theory*. New York: McGraw-Hill, 1978.

[6] Fukunaga K. *Introduction to Statistical Pattern Recognition*, 2nd Edition. New York: Academic, 1990.

[7] Metz CE. "Fundamental ROC Analysis." In Van Metter R, Beutel J, Kundel H (Eds.) *Handbook of Medical Imaging: Volume 1, Progress in Medical Physics and Psychophysics*. Bellingham, WA: SPIE, 1999.

[8] Barrett HH, Abbey CK, Clarkson E. "Objective Assessment of Image Quality. III. ROC Metrics, Ideal Observers, and Likelihood-Generating Functions." J Opt Soc Am A15:1520–1535, 1998.

[9] Swensson RM, Green DM. "On the Relations between Random Walk Models for Two-Choice Response Times." J Math Psychol 15:282–291, 1977.

[10] Papoulis A. *Probability, Random Variables and Stochastic Processes*. McGraw-Hill, 1965.

[11] Shapiro JH. "Bounds on the Area under the ROC Curve." J Opt Soc Am 16:53–57, 1999.

[12] Clarkson E, Barrett HH. "Approximations to Ideal-Observer Performance on Signal Detection Tasks." Appl Opt, to be published in Apr 2000 edition.

[13] Wagner RF, Brown DG. "Unified SNR Analysis of Medical Imaging Systems." Phys Med Biol 30:489–518, 1985.

[14] Shaw R. "The Equivalent Quantum Efficiency of the Photographic Process." J Photog Sci 11:199–204, 1963.

[15] Wagner RF, Brown DG, Metz CE. "On the Multiplex Advantage of Coded Source/Aperture Photon Imaging." Proc SPIE 314, 1981, pp. 72–76.

[16] Barrett HH, Swindell W. *Radiological Imaging: The Theory of Image Formation, Detection, and Processing*, revised Edition. San Diego: Academic Press, 1996.

[17] Burgess AE. "The Rose Model, Revisited." J Opt Soc Am A16:633–646, 1999.

[18] Tsui BMW, Metz CE, Atkins FB, Starr SJ, Beck RN. "A Comparison of Optimum Spatial Resolution in Nuclear Imaging Based on Statistical Theory and on Observer Performance." Phys Med Biol 23:654–676, 1978.

[19] Myers, KJ, Wagner RF, Brown DG, Barrett HH. "Efficient Utilization of Aperture and Detector by Optimal Coding." Proc SPIE 1090:164-175, 1989.

[20] Barrett HH, Rolland JP, Wagner RF, Myers KJ. "Detection and Discrimination of Known Signals in Inhomogeneous, Random Backgrounds." Proc SPIE 1090, 1989, pp. 176–182.

[21] Myers KJ, Rolland JP, Barrett HH, Wagner RF. "Aperture Optimization for Emission Imaging: Effect of a Spatially Varying Background." J Opt Soc Am A7:1279–1293, 1990.

[22] Myers KJ, Wagner RF. "Detection and Estimation: Human vs. Ideal as a Function of Information." Proc SPIE 914, 1988, pp. 291–297.

[23] Barrett HH, Myers KJ, Wagner RF. "Beyond Signal-Detection Theory." Proc SPIE 626, 1986, pp. 231–239.

[24] Wagner RF, Barrett HH. "Quadratic Tasks and the Ideal Observer." Proc SPIE 767, 1987, pp. 306–309.

[25] Barrett HH, Abbey CK. "Bayesian Detection of Random Signals on Random Backgrounds." In Duncan J, Gindi G (Eds.) *Information Processing in Medical Imaging, Proceedings of the 15th International Conference, IPMI 97*, Poultney, VT, 1997. Lecture Notes in Computer Science. Berlin: Springer-Verlag, 1997.

[26] Nolte LW, Jaarsma D. "More on the Detection of one of M Orthogonal Signals." J Acoust Soc Am 41:497–505, 1967.

[27] Brown DG, Insana MF, Tapiovaara M. "Detection Performance of the Ideal Decision Function and Its McLaurin Expansion: Signal Position Unknown." J Acoust Soc Am 97:379–398, 1995.

[28] Clarkson E, Barrett HH. "Bayesian Detection with Amplitude, Scale, Orientation and Position Uncertainty." In Duncan J, Gindi G (Eds.) *Information Processing in Medical Imaging, Proceedings of the 15th International Conference, IPMI 97*. Poultney, VT, 1997. Lecture Notes in Computer Science. Berlin: Springer-Verlag, 1997.

[29] Myers KJ, Wagner RF, Hanson KM, Barrett HH, Rolland JP. "Human and Quasi-Bayesian Observers of Images Limited by Quantum Noise, Object Variability, and Artifacts." Proc SPIE 2166, 1994, pp. 180–190.

[30] Hanson KM. "Method of Evaluating Image-Recovery Algorithms Based on Task Performance." J Opt Soc Am A7:1294–1304, 1990.

[31] Myers KJ, Hanson KM. "Comparison of the Constrained Algebraic Reconstruction Technique with the Maximum Entropy Technique for a Variety of Tasks." Proc SPIE 1232, 1990, pp. 176–187.

[32] Myers KJ, Hanson KM, Wagner RF. "Task Performance Based on the Posterior Probability of Maximum-Entropy Reconstructions Obtained with MEMSYS 3." Proc SPIE 1443, 1991, pp. 172–182.

[33] Brown DG, Anderson MP, Myers KJ, Wagner RF. "Comparison of Neural Network, Human, and Sub-Optimal Bayesian Performance on a Constrained Reconstruction Detection Task." Proc SPIE 2167, 1994, pp. 614–622.

[34] Myers KJ, Anderson MP, Brown DG, Wagner RF, Hanson KM. "Neural Network Performance for Binary Discrimination Tasks. Part II: Effect of Task, Training, and Feature Pre-Selection." Proc SPIE 2434, 1995, pp. 828–837.

[35] Ruck DW, Rogers SK, Kabrisky M, Oxley ME, Suter BW. "The Multilayer Perceptron as an Approximation to a Bayes Optimal Discriminant Function." IEEE Trans. on Neural Networks 1:296–298, 1990.

[36] Barrett HH, Wilson DW, Tsui BMW. "Noise Properties of the EM Algorithm: I. Theory." Phys Med Biol 39:833–846, 1994.

[37] Wilson DW, Tsui BMW, Barrett HH. "Noise Properties of the EM Algorithm: II. Monte Carlo Simulations." Phys Med Biol 39:847–872, 1994.

[38] Fessler JA. "Mean and Variance of Implicitly Defined Biased Estimators (Such as Penalized Maximum Likelihood): Applications to Tomography." IEEE Trans Med Imag 5:493–506, 1996.

[39] Wang W, Gindi G. "Noise Analysis of Regularized EM for SPECT Reconstruction." IEEE Nuclear Science Symposium Conference Record 3:1933–1937, 1996.

[40] Wang W, Gindi G. "Noise Analysis of MAP-EM Algorithms for Emission Tomography." Phys Med Biol 42:2215–2232, 1997.

[41] Soares EJ, Byrne CL, Pan TS, Glick SJ. "Modeling the Population Covariance Matrices of Block-Iterative Expectation-Maximization Reconstructed Images." Proc SPIE 3034, 1997, pp. 415–425.

[42] Qi J, Leahy RM. "A Theoretical Study of the Contrast Recovery and Variance of MAP Reconstructions with Applications to the Selection of Smoothing Parameters." In *IEEE Nuclear Science Symposium Conference Record*, 1998.

[43] Wagner RF, Brown DG, Pastel MS. "Application of Information Theory to the Assessment of Computed Tomography." Med Phys 6:83–94, 1979.

[44] Rose A. "The Sensitivity Performance of the Human Eye on an Absolute Scale." J Opt Soc Am 38:196–208, 1948.

[45] Tanner Jr WP, Birdsall TG. "Definitions of d' and η as Psychophysical Measures." J Acoust Soc Am 30:922–928, 1958.

[46] Barlow HB. "The Absolute Efficiency of Perceptual Decisions." Philos Trans R Soc Lond Ser B290:71–82, 1980.

[47] Burgess AE, Wagner RF, Jennings RJ, Barlow HB. "Efficiency of Human Visual Signal Discrimination." Science 214:93, 1981.

[48] Burgess AE. "Statistical Efficiency of Perceptual Decisions." Proc SPIE 454, (1985), pp. 18–26.

[49] Judy PF, Swensson RG. "Lesion Detection and Signal-to-Noise Ratio in CT Images." Med Phys 8:13–23, 1981.

[50] Myers KJ, Barrett HH, Borgstrom MC, Patton DD, Seeley GW. "Effect of Noise Correlation on Detectability of Disk Signals in Medical Imaging." J Opt Soc Am A2:1752–1759, 1985.

[51] Myers KJ, Barrett HH. "Addition of a Channel Mechanism to the Ideal-Observer Model." J Opt Soc Am A4:2447–2457, 1987.

[52] Burgess AE, Humphrey K, Wagner RF. "Detection of Bars and Discs in Quantum Noise." Proc SPIE 173, 1979, pp. 34–40.

[53] Wagner RF, Insana MF, Brown DG, Garra BS, Jennings RJ. "Texture Discrimination: Radiologist, Machine, and Man." In Blakemore C (Ed.) *Vision: Coding and Efficiency*. Cambridge: University Press, 1990, pp. 310–318.

[54] Barlow HB. "The Efficiency of Detecting Changes in Density in Random Dot Patterns." Vision Res 18:637–650, 1978.

[55] Barlow HB, Reeves BC. "The Versatility and Absolute Efficiency of Detecting Mirror Symmetry in Random Dot Displays." Vision Res 19:783–793, 1979.

[56] Wagner RF, Myers KJ, Brown DG, Tapiovaara MJ, Burgess AE. "Higher-Order Tasks: Human vs. Machine Performance." Proc SPIE 1090, 1989, pp. 183–194.

[57] Starr SJ, Metz CE, Lusted LB, Goodenough DJ. "Visual Detection and Localization of Radiographic Images." Radiology 116:533–538, 1975.

[58] Swensson RG, Judy PF. "Detection of Noisy Visual Targets: Models for the Effects of Spatial Uncertainty and Signal-to-Noise Ratio." Percept and Psychophys 29:521–534, 1981.

[59] Burgess AE, Ghandeharian H. "Visual Signal Detection. II. Signal-Location Identification." J Opt Soc Am A1:906–910, 1984.

[60] Burgess AE. "Visual Signal Detection. III. On Bayesian Use of Prior Knowledge and Cross Correlation." J Opt Soc Am A2:1498–1506, 1985.

[61] Burgess AE. "Statistically Defined Backgrounds: Performance of a Modified Non-Prewhitening Observer Model." J Opt Soc Am A11:1237–1242, 1994.

[62] Burgess AE, Li X, Abbey CK. "Visual Signal Detectability with Two Noise Components: Anomalous Masking Effects." J Opt Soc Am A14:2420–2442, 1997.

[63] Burgess AE. "Visual Signal Detection with Two-Component Noise: Low-Pass Spectrum Effects." J Opt Soc Am A16:694–704, 1999.

[64] Rolland JP, Barrett HH. "Effect of Random Background Inhomogeneity on Observer Detection Performance." J Opt Soc Am A9:649–658, 1992.

[65] Yao J, Barrett HH. "Predicting Human Performance by a Channelized Hotelling Observer Model." Proc SPIE 1768, 1992, pp. 161–168.

[66] Barrett HH, Yao J, Rolland JP, Myers KJ, "Model Observers for Assessment of Image Quality." Proc Natl Acad Sci USA 90:9758–9765, 1993.

[67] Maloney RK, Mitchison GJ, Barlow HB. "Limit to the Detection of Glass Patterns in the Presence of Noise." J Opt Soc Am A4:2336–2341, 1987.

[68] Tapiovaara M. "Ideal Observer and Absolute Efficiency of Detecting Mirror Symmetry in Random Images." J Opt Soc Am A7:2245–2253, 1990.

[69] Garra BS, Insana MF, Shawker TH, Wagner RF, Bradford M, Russell MA. "Quantitative Ultrasonic Detection and Classification of Liver Disease: Comparison with Human Observer Performance." Invest Radiol 24:196–203, 1989.

[70] Wagner RF, Myers KJ, Hanson KM. "Task Performance on Constrained Reconstructions: Human Observer Performance Compared with Sub-Optimal Bayesian Performance." Proc SPIE 1652, 1992, pp. 352–362.

[71] Myers KJ, Wagner RF, Hanson KM. "Rayleigh Task Performance in Tomographic Reconstructions: Comparison of Human and Machine Performance." Proc SPIE 1898, 1993, pp. 628–637.

[72] Rolland JP, Barrett HH, Seeley GW. "Quantitative Study of Deconvolution and Display Mappings for Long-Tailed Point-Spread Functions." Proc SPIE 1092, 1989, pp. 17–21.

[73] Gagne RM, Wagner RF. "Prewhitening Matched Filter: Practical Implementation, SNR Estimation and Bias Reduction." Proc SPIE 3336, 1998, pp. 231–242.

[74] Tapiovaara MJ, Wagner RF. "SNR and Noise Measurements for Medical Imaging: I. A Practical Approach Based on Statistical Decision Theory." Phys Med Biol 38:71–92, 1993.

[75] Tapiovaara MJ. "SNR and Noise Measurements for Medical Imaging: II. Application to Fluoroscopic Equipment." Phys Med Biol 38:1761–1788, 1993.

[76] Chakraborty DP. "Physical Measures of Image Quality in Mammography." Proc SPIE 2708, 1996, pp. 179–193.

[77] Wear KA, Gagne RM, Wagner RF. "Uncertainties in Estimates of Lesion Detectability in Diagnostic Ultrasound." J Acoust Soc Am 106: 1999.

[78] Hanson KM. "Optimal Object and Edge Localization in the Presence of Correlated Noise." Proc SPIE 454:9–17, 1984.

[79] Mueller SP, Kijewski MF, Moore SC, Holman BL. "Maximum-Likelihood Estimation—A Model for Optimal Quantitation in Nuclear Medicine." J Nucl Med 31:1693–1701, 1990.

[80] Kijewski MF, Mueller SP, Moore SC, Rybicki FJ. "Generalized Ideal Observer Models for Design and Evaluation of Medical Imaging Systems." Presented at the *77th Assembly of the Radiological Society of North America*, Chicago, 1991.

[81] Kijewski MF. "The Barankin Bound: A Model of Detection with Location Uncertainty." Proc SPIE 1768, 1992, pp. 153–160.

[82] Barrett HH. "Objective Assessment of Image Quality: Effect of Quantum Noise and Object Variability." J Opt Soc Am A7:1266–1278, 1990.

[83] Barrett HH, Denny JL, Wagner RF, Myers KJ. "Objective Assessment of Image Quality. II. Fisher Information, Fourier Crosstalk, and Figures of Merit for Task Performance." J Opt Soc Am A12:834–852, 1995.

[84] Cunningham I, Shaw R. "Signal-to-Noise Optimization of Medical Imaging Systems." J Opt Soc Am A43:621–632, 1999.

[85] Rowe RK, Aarsvold JN, Barrett HH, Chen J-C, Klein WP, Moore BA, Pang IW, Patton DD, White TA. "A Stationary Hemispherical SPECT Imager for Three-Dimensional Brain Imaging." J Nucl Med 34:474–480, 1993.

[86] Fiete RD, Barrett HH, Smith WE, Myers KJ. "The Hotelling Trace Criterion and Its Correlation with Human Observer Performance." J Opt Soc Am A4:945–953, 1987.

CHAPTER 10
A Practical Guide to Model Observers for Visual Detection in Synthetic and Natural Noisy Images

Miguel P. Eckstein, Craig K. Abbey and François O. Bochud
Cedars Sinai Medical Center, UCLA School of Medicine

CONTENTS

10.1 Introduction

When an investigator is developing a new image-processing technique or manipulating an image-acquisition technique they are confronted with the question of whether the new technique will improve clinical diagnosis. A first approach is to look at individual physical properties of the image such as image contrast and resolution. Although these properties might be useful, it has long been known that the noise characteristics of the image system need to be taken into consideration to appropriately evaluate the quality of an image whether it will be used to detect, classify, and/or estimate a signal (Cunningham and Shaw, 1999). One useful measure of the noise characteristics is the noise-equivalent quanta (NEQ) that expresses the image noise in terms of the number of Poisson-distributed input photons per unit area at each spatial frequency (Wagner and Brown, 1985). The NEQ can be thought of as a measure inversely related to the amount of noise as a function of spatial frequency.

However, when the diagnostic decision involves a human observer, medical image quality can be defined in terms of human performance in visual tasks that are relevant to clinical diagnosis (Barrett, 1993). In this context, receiver operating characteristics (ROC) studies are the standard method of evaluating the impact of a particular image manipulation on clinical diagnosis. In these studies, the physicians scrutinize a set of medical images (under the different image-acquisition or processing conditions) and rate their confidence about the presence of the lesion. The investigator infers from these ratings a measure of performance known as the area under the ROC curve.

Often, the number of possible conditions is large and ROC studies become time consuming and costly because they require a large number of human observations. Other times, the investigator might want to optimize a parameter or a set of parameters. In such cases, the number of conditions suffers a combinatorial explosion, and therefore ROC studies become unfeasible. Thus it is desirable to develop a metric of image quality that could be used for fast evaluation and optimization of image quality but also would have the predictive power of ROC studies.

Computer-model observers are algorithms that attempt to predict human visual performance in noisy images and might represent the desired metric of image quality when the diagnostic decision involves a human observer and a visual task. Development of models to predict human visual signal detection in noise goes back to work by Rose (1948) who studied the detectability of a flat-topped disk embedded in white noise (see Burgess, 1999a, for a review). In the last two decades, many studies have concentrated on finding a model observer that can predict human performance across many types of synthetic backgrounds. More recently, model observers have been applied to real medical-image backgrounds. The hope is that eventually model observers will become common metrics of task-based image quality for evaluation of medical-image quality as well as optimization of imaging systems. Presently, the variety of model observers and methodologies to calculate

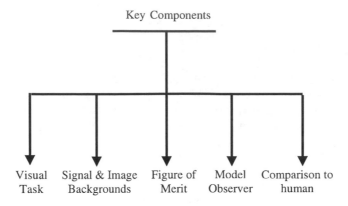

Figure 10.1:   Key components required for the use of model observers for medical-image-quality evaluation/optimization.

their performance make some of the choices of model observers for image quality evaluation/optimization difficult. What type of task and images to use? Which of the available model observers should be chosen to evaluate human performance for a given background type? How to calculate model-observer performance (figure of merit)? How to compare model-observer and human performance?

The vast number of psychophysical experiments, background types, and even author notation style can be overwhelming for an investigator unfamiliar with the field. The purpose of the present chapter is to survey past work on development and application of model observers to synthetic and real backgrounds. The hope is that the chapter can serve as a sort of starting point or "road map" for researchers unfamiliar with the field yet interested in applying model observers to a given task or image modality.

10.2 Key components for the use of model observers

In order to use model observers, a number of key components must be defined (Figure 10.1). First, the investigator needs to choose the visual task where the model observer will be evaluated or optimized. Second, a background type and a signal must be chosen for the visual task. Third, a model observer or a set of model observers to perform the visual task must be chosen from the large variety of available models. Fourth, a method to calculate model observer performance in the selected visual task must be determined. Finally, if human performance in the same task has been measured then a method for comparing model and human performance is required. The following five sections discuss in detail issues related to these key components.

10.3 Visual tasks for model observers

In most medical-image tasks, the physician searches over the regions of interest within the image with multiple eye movements fixating at points of interest. The

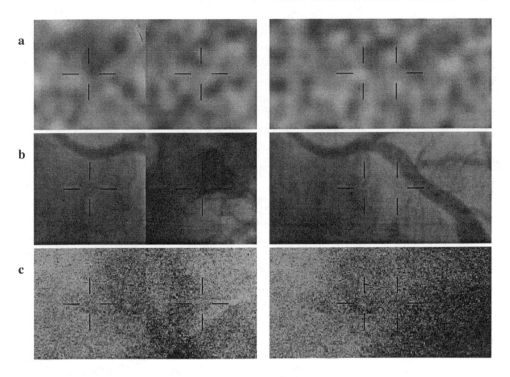

Figure 10.2: Acoss-image 2-AFC task (left) vs within-image 2-AFC task (right). The black lines are cues indicating to the observer the exact possible signal locations. From top to bottom: (a) low-pass comupter-generated noise; (b) x-ray coronary angiographic background; (c) x-ray mammographic background.

physician then decides whether a particular lesion is present or absent (yes/no). In other cases (e.g., x-ray angiography), the physician must classify an anatomic feature in one of N categories (e.g., mild, medium, severe stenosis). These tasks are theoretically complex and computationally time consuming and there are currently, for the most part, no image-based model observers to predict human performance in these tasks. Instead model observers are developed for tasks that are a simplification of the real-world physician's tasks but are theoretically more tractable. A commonly used task is the multiple-alternative forced-choice task (MAFC) where the lesion might appear in one of M-specified locations. The task of the observer is to indicate which of the M locations contains the target. Other tasks, such as a yes/no task with no location uncertainty, can also be used for the model observer. In this task the signal always appears on a specified location with some probability and the task is to decide whether it is present or absent on a given image. In some cases, performance in these simpler tasks can be mathematically mapped to performance in the more complex realistic tasks where the signal can appear at any location within an image (Hermann *et al.*, 1993). In other instances, no mapping is available, but performances in both types of tasks are positively correlated. For example, an image-processing technique that improves performance in the simple

MAFC detection task will improve performance in the more complex realistic task (Eigler *et al.*, 1994).

The present chapter will only address model observers in the context of MAFC tasks (for a yes/no task or a rating task see Chapter 11). When using MAFC tasks, an important issue is whether each of the possible signal locations will be located within independent samples of backgrounds or within one sample background. Figure 10.2 shows an across-image 2-AFC task (left column) versus a within-image 2-AFC task (right column) for three different background types (from to top to bottom: low-pass noise, x-ray coronary angiograms, and x-ray mammograms). Although the difference might seem trivial at first, the calculation of model-observer performance for these two tasks (across-image vs. within-image MAFC tasks) will require different methods. Most studies in the literature use an across-image MAFC task that makes calculation of model-observer performance simpler. The less used within-image MAFC task (Eckstein *et al.*, 1999a, 1999b) has the advantage of being similar to the physicians' task of scrutinizing a number of locations within a medical image but may require more complex methods for calculation of model performance.

10.4 Signals and backgrounds

The investigator is also confronted by the question of what backgrounds and signals to use to evaluate a particular imaging modality and imaged anatomy. One approach is to use computer-simulated backgrounds that visually appear similar to the real image backgrounds for the particular imaging modality with the hope that the model observer results with the synthetic backgrounds will generalize to the real backgrounds.

For example, computer-generated white noise (spatially uncorrelated) has been used because it mimics the image-noise of quantum origin. However, image receptor blur present in many imaging modalities introduces background correlations. When the background is correlated, the random variations in luminance at different spatial positions in the image background co-vary. A positive correlation between neighboring regions of a background implies that if the random variation is an increase (rather than a decrease) in luminance at one point in the image the random variation at a neighboring point in the image will also tend to be an increase in luminance. In these circumstances low-pass filtered white noise seem to be a better representation of the image backgrounds. In other imaging modalities such as computed tomography (CT), the reconstruction algorithms produce a noise with increasing power with spatial frequency. Ramp noise power spectrum is therefore often used to simulate CT noise (Hanson, 1980). Furthermore, medical images also contain spatial variations in luminance attributable to anatomical structures that are irrelevant to the signal to be detected (Revesz *et al.*, 1974; Ohara *et al.*, 1989). In order to generate images that include such structures Rolland and Barrett (1992) developed a method known as lumpy background that involves creating Gaussian blobs at different random positions of the image. These "blobs" give the image a structured look similar to nuclear-medicine images. Recently Bochud *et al.* (1999a) have extended this technique to create elongated structures with a common orientation grouped into clusters (clustered lumpy background). This technique mimics the local structures such as fibers in mammograms.

A different approach altogether is to use real anatomic backgrounds from patient data rather than computer-simulated backgrounds. This latter method requires a large database of patient images so that the model-observer results can be generalized to the population of patient images.

The advantage of the computer-simulated backgrounds is that the statistical properties of the backgrounds are known and satisfy many statistical properties that make calculation of model performance simpler (see section on figures of merit). The crucial statistical property is that the mean and variance (across many samples or realizations of a background) is the same at every pixel and the covariance between two pixels only depends on their relative position (not their absolute position in the image). When a set of images satisfies these properties, it is said to be stationary (see Bochud *et al.*, 1999b for a treatment on stationarity in image backgrounds). The stationarity assumption greatly simplifies the calculation of model-observer performance and allows calculation of model performance within the Fourier-spectrum framework (Wagner and Brown, 1985).

The advantage of real anatomic backgrounds is clearly their realism. The disadvantage is that often real anatomic backgrounds do not obey the stationarity property and therefore some of the standard techniques for calculating model performance in stationary backgrounds do not always generalize to these real background scenarios.

An important issue is that the investigator needs to generate (for synthetic backgrounds) or gather (for patient backgrounds) a large number of sample backgrounds so that the model-observer performance in the samples used in the visual task generalize to the population of synthetic/real backgrounds.

Table 10.1 shows a sample of a variety of different backgrounds used in the literature, a mathematical equation and a graph describing the noise power spectrum (power versus spatial frequency), their main application to medical imaging, and relevant references.

The next step is to select a signal to be detected in the visual task. Signals almost always are computer generated and often are designed to mimic a realistic feature of interest in the medical images: lumps or microcalcifications for x-ray mammograms (Burgess, 1999b; Bochud *et al.*, 1999b), nodules in chest images (Judy and Swensson, 1985; Seltzer *et al.*, 1994; Samei *et al.*, 1997), filling defects or arterial stenosis in coronary angiography (Ohara *et al.*, 1989; Eckstein and Whiting, 1996).

Finally, a method to combine the signal with the backgrounds must be selected. Again, one approach is to attempt to model the combination of the signal and background so that it mimics the image-generation process of the imaging modality of interest. Sometimes these realistic methods make model-observer performance calculations more complex and therefore investigators choose to simply add the signal to the background, which leads to simpler expressions for model-observer performance calculations (Bochud *et al.*, 1999b).

Table 10.1: Table summarizes many of the backgrounds (synthetic or real) used in visual detection experiments, the mathematical description in terms of the noise power spectra, their main application to medical imaging, models successfully used to predict human performance and sample references

Noise Type	Sample Image	Mathematical Description of Noise Power Spectra	Graph of Noise Power Spectra	Stationary?
White noise		$N(u) = k$, u is the spatial frequency in the radial direction and k is a constant		Yes
Low-pass (Gaussian filtered white noise)		$N(u) = |e^{-2\pi^2 s_b^2 u^2}|^2$, where s_b is the standard deviation of the Gaussian		Yes
Band-pass		$N(u) = |(|u - \Delta u|^{n/2})$ $\times e^{-B_f^2 u^2}|^2$		Yes
Ramp noise		$N(u) = |u|$		Yes
Power law		$N(u) = \dfrac{k \cos(\pi u)}{(u_0^\beta + u^\beta)}$, where u_0 is the lowest frequency supported by the image and β is in the range of 0 and 4		Yes
Lumpy background II		$N(u) = \dfrac{\overline{K}}{A} b_0^2$ $\times \exp(-2\pi^2 r_b^2 |u|^2)$, where K/A is mean number of lumps per detector area and b_0^2 is the strength of the blob		Yes
Clustered lumpy Background		$N(u) = \dfrac{\overline{Kn}}{A}(N_b(u)$ $+ n N_s(u))$, K and n are mean number of clusters and blobs respectively; A is the area of a single image; $W_b(u)$ power spectrum component from the blob; $W_s(u)$ power spectra from the interaction of blob and cluster shape		Yes
x-ray mammogram		$N(u) = 1/u^{3.7}$ for $u_0 < u < u_f$, where $u_0 > 0$ is the lowest frequency supported by the image and u_f is the highest frequency determined by the Nyquist limit		No
x-ray angiograms		$N(u) = 1/u^{3.4}$ for $u_0 < u < u_f$		No

Table 10.1:   (Continued)

Gaussian Model Responses?	Main Application	Signals Used in Experiments	Successful Model Observers	Reference
Yes	Photon noise	Blurred disk, sinewaves, Gabor signals	Suboptimal non-prewhitening matched filter model, Hotelling (internal noise, porportional noise, sampling efficiency, uncertainty)	Burgess *et al.*, 1981; Burgess and Ghandeharian, 1984; Swensson and Judy, 1981; Eckstein *et al.*, 1997
Yes	Photon noise Focal spot blur-nuclear imaging	Sharp edge disk Gaussian profile	Channelized Hotelling	Burgess *et al.*, 1997; Rolland and Barrett, 1992
Yes	Gamma-ray-imaging	Disk with ramp edge	Non-prewhitening matched filter model with an eye filter (NPWE)	Myers *et al.*, 1985
Yes	Computed tomography	Disks	Region of interest (ROI)	Hanson, 1980
Yes	General patient anatomy	Gaussian, simulated nodules	Hotelling	Burgess *et al.*, 1997; Burgess, 1999b
Unknown	Nuclear medicine	Gaussian profile	NPWE Channelized Hotelling-Hotelling	Myers *et al.*, 1990; Roland and Barrett, 1994
Yes	X-ray mammography	Simulated masses and microcalcifications	Unknown	Bochud *et al.*, 1999a
Approximately	X-ray mammography	Simulated masses and microcalcifications	Unknown	Bochud *et al.*, 1999b
Approximately	X-ray angiography	Projected hemispheres (blurred disks)	Channelized Hotelling-NPWE	Eckstein *et al.*, 1998a, 1999b

10.5 Model observers

Given that the task, signal, and background have been defined, the investigator needs to choose an appropriate model observer among a large variety of models. The purpose of the this section is to classify the existing models into categories to create a taxonomy of model observers that allows readers to have a broader and clearer understanding of the differences and relationships across model observers.

10.5.1 Image discrimination models

In general, there are two traditions of models in human visual detection. The first types of models were developed to predict human visual detection of a single or a compound of sinusoidal signals superimposed on uniform backgrounds or another sinusoidal grating (masking models). These models typically included a set of spatial-frequency-tuned filters and a nonlinear combination of information across the filters. Some of these nonlinear decision rules have been shown to perform at a lower performance level than human observer when random variations in the backgrounds are introduced (Eckstein *et al.*, 1998b).

More recently this tradition of models has concentrated on predicting visual detection of a signal superimposed on one of two identical copies of more complex backgrounds such as an airport runway or a natural image (Ahumada *et al.*, 1995; Daly, 1993). These models are often referred to as image-discrimination models and attempt to predict the detectability of a target or artifact superimposed on one of two copies of a particular background. The images in these tasks are typically displayed for brief durations (60–500 ms).

The models predict the reduction in the visibility of the target atributable to a nonlinear compressive transducer and/or divisive inhibition across channels (Foley, 1994, Watson and Solomon, 1997). Image-discrimination models have not been extensively applied to medical images. Recent work has applied these models to predict the presence of a lesion in one of two identical coronary angiographic backgrounds (Eckstein *et al.*, 1997b) and to evaluate the effect of image compression on mammograms (Johnson *et al.*, 1999). Their application is somewhat limited by the fact that they have been designed to predict performance detecting a signal superimposed on one of two identical backgrounds. However, this task is different from the physicians' task, which is to compare different locations within a medical image that contains backgrounds that have different random variations.

10.5.2 Models for detection in noise

A second family of models has been designed to predict human performance detecting signals embedded in visual noise. These models typically include linear decision strategies that make use of knowledge about the signal and background statistics. These types of models are based on statistical decision theory (Peterson *et al.*, 1954) that was first applied to detection problems in radar.

Most of the model observers currently used for visual detection in noisy images are linear models. Linear model observers compare a template with the data by computing the correlation at each of the possible signal locations. For an M-alternative forced-choice (MAFC) task where the signal appears in one of M possible locations, the model observer is assumed to obtain the template output at each location and select the location that elicits the highest response. The general form for linear models is

$$\lambda_i = \sum_{x=1}^{N} \sum_{y=1}^{N} w(x, y) g_i(x, y), \tag{10.1}$$

where the scalar λ_i is scalar response of the model to ith location, $w(x, y)$ is the two-dimensional template, and $g_i(x, y)$ is the data at a given ith location.

A convenient and often used framework for a model observer is the use of a matrix formulation (Barrett et al., 1993; Myers et al., 1985). We can adopt the matrix formulation by ordering the elements of the $N \times N$ template into and $N^2 \times 1$ column vector and doing the same with the data (see Appendix A for details). In the matrix/vector formulation the correlation is given by (Barrett et al., 1993):

$$\lambda_i = \sum_{n=1}^{N^2} w_n g_n = \mathbf{w}^t \mathbf{g}_i, \tag{10.2}$$

where $\mathbf{w}$ and $\mathbf{g}$ are vectors and the superscript t refers to the transpose.

The variety of current model observers can be classified based on different properties. First, models can be classified based on the prior knowledge they use to derive the template. Figure 10.3 shows all the models to be presented classified based on the amount of knowledge they use about the signal and background. As the different models are presented, the reader is encouraged to refer back to Figure 10.3 to see how the models compare in the amount of knowledge used to derive the template.

For example, some models use information about the signal; others use information about the signal and the background statistics. Second, given that these models are attempting to predict human performance, many of them include information-processing constraints intended to reflect properties of the human visual system derived from psychophysical or physiological findings. Therefore, models differ in the components they include to reflect constraints imposed by the human visual system. These components could include differential sensitivity of the human visual system to different spatial frequencies (Robson et al., 1966), neural noise (Tolhurst et al., 1983) modeled as a constant additive internal noise (Burgess et al., 1981) or an internal noise component proportional to the external noise (Burgess and Colborne, 1988), intrinsic uncertainty about the spatial position or spatial properties of the signal (Tanner, 1961; Pelli, 1985). Table 10.2 describes a number of these possible components that can be included in the model.

A fundamental component that distinguishes two groups of noise models is processing by a set of channels that are spatial-frequency and sometimes orientation tuned (Sachs et al., 1971). These channels are intended to reflect the response

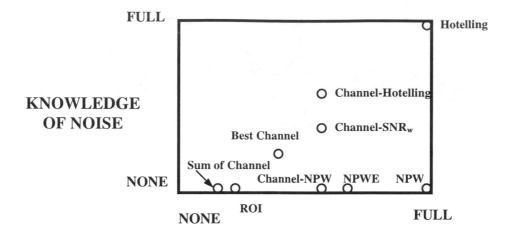

KNOWLEDGE
OF SIGNAL

Figure 10.3: A quantitative plot of model observers based on the knowledge they use about the signal and background statistics to build the template. Particular signals might favor one model over another. The diagram ranks the models on their use of knowledge to derive templates averaged over all possible signals.

properties of receptive fields of cells in the visual cortex area V1 which selectively respond to signals with a given spatial frequency and orientation (Movshon *et al.*, 1978). We therefore present models in two categories: (a) Non-channelized models; (b) Channelized models.

In the following we discuss the general concepts behind each of the models. For the relationship of these models with the best-possible observer, the ideal observer, see Chapter 12. In addition, for each model, Table 10.3 shows the mathematical representation of the templates used by each of the models as well as relevant references in the literature. Tables 10.4a and 10.4b also show the definition of all symbols used in this chapter.

10.5.2.1 Non-channelized models

10.5.2.1.1 Region of interest (ROI).   One of the most basic models is the region-of-interest model (ROI). The ROI model uses knowledge about the possible location of the signal but not about its profile. It uses a uniform template that simply integrates the pixel values over a given region. The equal weighting of each pixel is done irrespective of the profile of the signal (Hanson, 1980).

10.5.2.1.2 Non-prewhitening matched filter (NPW).   The NPW model has a long history with extensive application in medical imaging (see for review Wagner and Weaver, 1972; Burgess *et al.*, 1981; Judy and Swensson, 1987). The NPW

Table 10.2: Components that can be included in model observers to reflect constraints in processing by the human visual system

Human Visual System Component	Description	Reference
Optics and receptor sampling	Reduction in sensitivity to high spatial frequencies due to the optical properties of the pupil and receptor lattice on the retina	Geisler and Davila, 1985
Contrast sensitivity function (CSF)	Reduction in sensitivity to high and low spatial frequencies including optical factors as well as neural factors	After visual adaptation to a uniform background (Robson, 1966); after adaptation to natural, noisy and fractal images (Webster and Myahara, 1997)
Spatial frequency channels	Reflects the response properties of cells in the visual cortex that preferentially respond to visual stimuli with a specific spatial frequency and orientation	Gabor (Watson, 1983); difference of Gaussians (Wilson and Bergen, 1979); difference of Mesa (Daly, 1993); square (Myers et al., 1985)
Constant internal noise	Additive noise to the observers internal response due to variation in the firing of cells as well as fluctuations in decision criteria	Pelli (1985); Burgess and Colborne (1988); Eckstein et al. (1997a)
Induced internal noise	Additional internal noise induced within the observer due to the presence of a high-contrast background or external noise in the image	Burgess and Colborne (1988); Eckstein et al. (1997a)
Intrinsic uncertainty	Inherent uncertainty within the observer about the spatial position, spatial frequency or other parameter of the signal	Pelli (1985); Eckstein et al. (1997a)
Nonlinear transducer	A non-linear relationship between the image contrast and the observer's internal response	Legge and Foley (1980); Lu and Dosher (1999)

consists of a template that exactly matches the signal profile (Table 10.3). This approach is optimal in white noise but becomes suboptimal in correlated noise where the optimal strategy is to use a template that takes into account the correlations in the backgrounds. The term non-prewhitening refers to the NPW's inability to take into account noise correlations (an operation known as prewhitening). The NPW model has been successful at predicting human performance in white noise but fails to predict it in low-pass filtered noise and real anatomic backgrounds (Rolland and Barrett, 1992; Eckstein *et al.*, 1998a).

10.5.2.1.3 Non-prewhitening matched filter with eye filter (NPWE). One extension of the NPW model that takes into account properties of the human visual system is the non-prewhitening matched filter with an eye filter (NPWE; also known as the modified non-prewhitening matched filter). This model uses information about the signal but takes into account the differential human visual sensitivity to different spatial frequencies. The contrast sensitivity function (CSF) is derived from experiments where the contrast threshold for human visual detection of sinusoidal patterns is measured as a function of the spatial frequency of the pattern superimposed on uniform fields. The NPWE model therefore uses a template that matches the signal filtered by the CSF function (Table 10.3; Ishida *et al.*, 1984; Giger and Doi, 1985; Burgess, 1994).

More recent versions of the NPWE model (Eckstein *et al.*, 1998a, 1999b) use contrast sensitivity functions measured after visual adaptation to white and $1/f$ noise (Webster and Myahara, 1997) rather than after adaptation to uniform luminance fields. The NPWE model has been able to predict many results including white noise, lumpy backgrounds (Burgess, 1994), and real anatomic backgrounds. However, recent work by Burgess has shown that when the signal frequency amplitude is broadband with respect to the noise, then the NPWE model is not a good predictor of human performance (Burgess *et al.*, 1997; Burgess, 1999b).

10.5.2.1.4 Hotelling observer. The Hotelling observer was proposed as a model observer by Barrett and colleagues (Myers *et al.*, 1985; Fiete *et al.*, 1987; Barrett *et al.*, 1993; Rolland and Barrett, 1992). It is the ideal observer when image statistics are Gaussian and is also known as the prewhitening matched filter when the image statistics are stationary (North, 1963; Wagner and Brown, 1983). Unlike the NPW model, the Hotelling observer derives a template that takes into account knowledge about not only the signal profile but also the background statistics. In white noise, no compensation for background statistics is needed and the Hotelling observer uses a template identical to that of the matched filter. However, in correlated noise, the Hotelling observer derives a template that decorrelates the noise prior to matched filtering.

The template for the Hotelling observer is derived from the inverse of the covariance matrix of the background (Table 10.3). The covariance matrix for a background describes the variance at each pixel in the image and the covariance between pairs of pixels. When the noise is computer generated, then the covariance matrix is known a priori and can be related mathematically to the background noise power spectra (Bochud *et al.*, 1999b). On the other hand, when the backgrounds

Table 10.3: Templates for different linear observers for detection in noise

Noise Models	Templates: Discrete Matrix Notation (spatial domain)	Templates: Fourier Continuous Notation	Sample Reference
Non-prewhitening matched filter	$\mathbf{w} = [\langle \mathbf{g_s} \rangle - \langle \mathbf{g_n} \rangle]$, where $\langle \mathbf{g_s} \rangle$ is the mean signal-present image and $\langle \mathbf{g_n} \rangle$ is the mean noise-only image and $\mathbf{w}$ is the template vector	$\widetilde{w}(u, v) = \widetilde{s}(u, v)$, where $\widetilde{w}(u, v)$ is the template in the Fourier domain and $\widetilde{s}(u, v)$ is the Fourier transform of the signal	Wagner and Weaver, 1972; Burgess et al., 1981
Non-prewhitening matched filter with eye filter	$\mathbf{w} = \mathbf{E}^{\mathrm{T}}[\langle \mathbf{g_s} \rangle - \langle \mathbf{g_n} \rangle]\mathbf{E}$. where $\mathbf{E}$ is a matrix containing the eye filter	$\widetilde{w}(u, v) = \widetilde{s}(u, v)\,\widetilde{E}(u, v)$, where $\widetilde{E}(u, v)$ is the eye filter in the Fourier domain	Ishida et al., 1974; Burgess, 1994
Hotelling	$\mathbf{w} = \mathbf{K_p}^{-1}[\langle \mathbf{g_s} \rangle - \langle \mathbf{g_n} \rangle]$, $\mathbf{K_p}^{-1}$ is the variance covariance matrix of the image	$\widetilde{w}(u, v) = \widetilde{s}(u, v)/N(u, v)$, where $N(\mathrm{u}, v)$ is the noise power spectrum	Myers et al., 1985; Barrett et al., 1993; Burgess, 1999b
Sum across channels	$\mathbf{w} = \mathbf{V1}$, where $\mathbf{V}$ is a matrix consisting of columns representing each channel profile and $\mathbf{1}$ is the column vector of 1's	$\widetilde{w}(u, v) = \sum \widetilde{v}_j(u, v)$, where $\widetilde{v}_j(u, v)$ is the jth channel in the Fourier domain	Graham, 1989
Most sensitive channel	$\mathbf{w} = \mathbf{V}\mathbf{max}[[\mathbf{Diag}(\mathbf{K_v})]^{-1}[\langle \mathbf{g_{v/s}} \rangle - \langle \mathbf{g_{v/n}} \rangle]]$, where $\mathbf{V}$ is defined as above, $\langle \mathbf{g_{v/s}} \rangle$ is the mean signal present image as seen through the channels, $\langle \mathbf{g_{v/n}} \rangle$ is the mean noise only image as seen through the channels, $\mathbf{K_v}$ is the covariance of the channel responses given by $\mathbf{K_v} = \mathbf{V}^{\mathrm{T}}\mathbf{K_p}\mathbf{V}$, the $\mathbf{Diag}$ operation zeroes all off diagonal elements (covariance terms) and the $\mathbf{max}$ function takes the maximum element from the matrix	$\widetilde{w}(u, v) = \mathbf{max}(\widetilde{K}_v^{-1}\widetilde{s}_v(u, v))$, where $\widetilde{s}_v(u, v)$ is the signal as seen through the channels in the Fourier domain and $\widetilde{K}_v$ is the covariance of channels in the Fourier domain	Graham, 1989

Table 10.3: (Continued)

Noise Models	Templates: Discrete Matrix Notation (spatial domain)	Templates: Fourier Continuous Notation	Sample Reference
Channelized matched filter to the signal as seen through the channels	$\mathbf{w} = \mathbf{V}[\langle \mathbf{g}_{v/s}\rangle - \langle \mathbf{g}_{v/n}\rangle]$	$\tilde{w}(u,v) = \tilde{s}_v(u,v)$, where $[\tilde{s}_v(u,v)]_j$ $= \int \overline{\tilde{v}_j(u,v)}\tilde{s}(u,v)\,du\,dv$	Eckstein *et al.*, 1998b
Channelized matched filter to the spatial domain signal	$\mathbf{w} = \mathbf{V}\mathbf{K}_v^{-1}[\langle \mathbf{g}_{v/s}\rangle - \langle \mathbf{g}_{v/n}\rangle]$, where $K_v = \mathbf{V}^T\mathbf{I}\mathbf{V}$ and $\mathbf{I}$, the identity matrix is the covariance for white noise	$\tilde{w}(u,v) = \tilde{\mathbf{K}}_v^{-1}\tilde{\mathbf{s}}_v(u,v)$, $[\tilde{\mathbf{K}}_v]_{i,j}$ $= \int \overline{\tilde{v}_i(u,v)}\,\tilde{v}_j(u,v)\,du\,dv$	Eckstein and Whiting, 1995
Channelized Hotelling	$\mathbf{w} = \mathbf{V} = \mathbf{K}_v^{-1}[\langle \mathbf{g}_{v/s}\rangle - \langle \mathbf{g}_{v/n}\rangle]$, where $\mathbf{K}_v = \mathbf{V}^T\mathbf{K}_p\mathbf{V}$	$\tilde{w}(u,v) = \tilde{\mathbf{K}}_v^{-1}\tilde{\mathbf{s}}_v(u,v)$, where $[\tilde{\mathbf{K}}_v]_{i,j}$ $= \int \overline{\tilde{v}_i(u,v)}\,N(u,v)\tilde{v}_j(u,v)\,du\,dv$	Myers *et al.*, 1987; Yao *et al.*, 1994; Barrett *et al.*,1993
Channelized SNR-weighted	$\mathbf{w} = \mathbf{V}[\mathbf{Diag}(\mathbf{K}_v)]^{-1}[\langle \mathbf{g}_{v/s}\rangle - \langle \mathbf{g}_{v/n}\rangle]$, where the **Diag** operation zeroes all off diagonal elements (covariance terms) of the variance-covariance matrix	$\tilde{w}(u,v) = \mathbf{Diag}(\tilde{\mathbf{K}}_v^{-1})\tilde{\mathbf{s}}_v(u,v)$, $[\tilde{\mathbf{K}}_v]_{i,j}$ $= \int \overline{\tilde{v}_i(u,v)}\,N(u,v)\tilde{v}_j(u,v)\,du\,dv$	Eckstein, *et al.*, 1998b

Table 10.4a: Definition of symbols for model observer templates

Symbol	Definition
$\mathbf{g}_s$	Vector corresponding to the data at the signal-present location.
$\mathbf{g}_n$	Vector corresponding to the data at the noise-only location.
$\mathbf{g}_{v/s}$	Vector containing the data at the signal-present location as seen through the channels.
$\mathbf{g}_{v/n}$	Vector containing the data at the noise-only location as seen through the channels.
$\langle\ \rangle$	Expectation value.
$\mathbf{w}$	Column vector containing the values of the model template.
$\mathbf{E}$	Matrix containing the eye filter.
$\mathbf{K}$	Covariance matrix describing the variance and covariance of image-pixel values.
$\mathbf{V}$	Matrix where each column contains the spatial weights of each channel profile.
$\mathbf{K_v}$	Covariance matrix describing variance and covariance of channel responses.
$\eta_{i,j}$	Response of jth channel at the ith location.
c_j	Scalar weight applied to the jth channel response.
$\mathbf{I}$	Identity matrix.
$\widetilde{w}(u, v)$	2-dimensional function containing the Fourier amplitude of the template.
$\overline{\widetilde{w}(u, v)}$	Complex conjugate of template
$N(u, v)$	Noise power spectra of the background.
$\widetilde{E}(u, v)$	Eye filter expressed in the Fourier domain.
$\widetilde{s}(u, v)$	Fourier amplitude of the signal.
$\widetilde{s}_v(\mathbf{u}, \mathbf{v})$	Fourier amplitude of the signal as seen through the channels.
$\widetilde{\mathbf{K}}_v$	Covariance describing the covariance of channels in the Fourier domain.
$\widetilde{\mathbf{v}}_j(u, v)$	Fourier amplitude of jth channel.
$\mathbf{Diag}$	Operation that zeroes all off diagonal elements of the matrix.
$\mathbf{Max}$	Operation that takes the maximum value of a vector or matrix.

Table 10.4b: Definition of symbols for figures of merit for model observers

Symbol	Definition
Pc	Percent correct of trials in which the model correctly identifies the signal location.
M	Number of possible signal locations in the task.
H	Total number of images or trials to which the model is applied.
$\phi(x)$	Gaussian probability density function.
$\Phi(x)$	Cumulative Gaussian probability
d'	Index of detectability, a figure of merit for model performance in MAFC tasks when the model responses are statistically independent and Gaussian.
λ_s	Response of model-template to data at the signal location.
λ_n	Response of model-template to data at the noise only location.
σ_λ	Standard deviation of the response of the model-template. Assumed to be the same for signal-present locations and noise-only locations.
d'_r	Index of detectability for correlated model responses.
$r_{p,q}$	Correlation between the model responses at two different locations.
$\mathbf{K}_{p,q}$	Covariance matrix describing the correlation between pixels at two different locations at which the signal might appear.

are real then the covariance matrix is not known and must be estimated from the samples. One potential problem in these cases is that the number of samples needed to obtain a stable estimate of the covariance matrix might be as high as 10 to 100 times the size of the covariance matrix (Barrett *et al.*, 1998). Therefore if one estimates a covariance matrix for a 200×200 image, then one will obtain a covariance of $200^2 \times 200^2$ and will require at least 400,000 to 4,000,000 sample images for stable estimations. Clearly gathering of such a large number of sample images is difficult.

A first possible solution to reduce the dimensionality problem of the covariance estimation is to constrain the data to $b \times b$ square pixel regions or windows around the possible signal locations. If the signal is 6 to 8 pixels wide, then typical values for the square window (b) are 12×12 pixels (Eckstein *et al.*, 1998b; 1999a, 1999b). The limitation of this approach is that the Hotelling template is then constrained spatially to the dimensions of the spatial square window used to calculate the covariance matrix. This spatial constraint of the template may introduce systematic degradation in the Hotelling-model performance.

A second solution proposed by Barrett *et al.* (1998) is to use a set of linear pre-processing filters that capture the main features of the Hotelling template. The

Hotelling model does not act on the pixels itself but rather on the set of values resulting from the dot product of the feature filters and the data. The model then derives the best linear combination of the feature filters that maximally discriminates the mean response (across all images) of the model to the signal location from the mean response of the model to the nonsignal locations. The appropriate choice of the functions might depend on the type of signal used in the experiment. Barrett *et al.* (1998) used the first six terms of Laguerre–Gauss polynomials. Note that these functions are not meant to model channels in the human visual system but rather to introduce some smoothness assumptions to the estimation of the Hotelling-observer template to reduce the dimensionality problem. However, if the signal is not rotationally symmetric, use of the Laguerre–Gauss functions will present constraints in the estimation of the Hotelling template.

10.5.2.2 Channelized models

A second family of model observers includes preprocessing of the image by a set of channels that are tuned to a given spatial frequency and sometimes orientation. All channelized models have the same general framework in that the model computes the correlation between each channel and the data at the possible signal locations obtaining one scalar output per channel[1]:

$$\eta_{ij} = \mathbf{v}_j^t \mathbf{g}_i, \tag{10.3}$$

where η_{ij} is the response of the jth channel to the ith location, $\mathbf{v}_j$ is a vector containing the spatial weights of the jth channel, and g_i is the data as previously defined.

The responses of all channels to a given location are then linearly combined with a given set of weightings resulting in a single scalar response per location:

$$\lambda_i = \sum_j^J c_j \eta_{ij}, \tag{10.4}$$

where λ_i is the model response to the ith location and c_j is the weight applied to the response of the jth channel. For an MAFC task, the models then choose the location resulting in the highest response (λ_i).

The decision rule of channelized models can also be restated in a mathematically equivalent (and conceptually useful) way by substituting Eq. (10.3) into Eq. (10.4)

$$\lambda_i = \left[\sum_j^J c_j [\mathbf{v}_j^t \mathbf{g}_i] = [\mathbf{Vc}]^t \mathbf{g}_i = \mathbf{w}^t \mathbf{g}_i \right], \tag{10.5}$$

---

[1] Note that the channelized models for detection in noise do not typically use channels positioned at every spatial position in the image. Therefore there is a reduction of information when going from the pixel representation of the image to the channel representation.

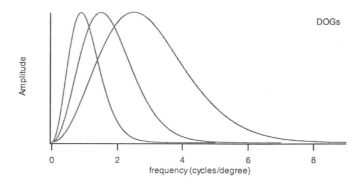

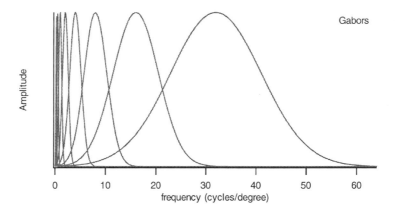

Figure 10.4: Spatial frequency amplitude of two different sets of channel profiles: (a) Top: Difference of Gaussians; (b) Bottom: Gabor channel mechanism.

where **c** is a column vector with the weights applied to each channel and **V** is a matrix consisting of columns with each of the different J channels. In Eq. (10.5), the channelized model can be thought as applying a single template **w** to the different locations but where this template is built from and constrained by the set of channels.

There are number of different channel profiles in the literature including square channels (Myers *et al.*, 1987; Yao and Barrett, 1992), difference of Gaussians (Wilson and Bergen, 1979; Abbey and Barrett, 1995), difference of Mesa filters (Daly, 1993; Burgess *et al.*, 1997), and Gabor channels (Eckstein *et al.*, 1998a, 1999b). The latter three have the advantage of being closer to the response properties of cells measured by physiological studies. For example, Marcelja (1980) used Gabor mathematical functions to model the response of cells in area V1 of the cat (Movshon *et al.*, 1978). Watson (1983) subsequently used these functions for his model of spatial form. Figure 10.4 shows spatial frequency weighting function of the DOG channel profiles and the Gabor channel profiles.

In addition, channelized models can also be classified based on the way they combine each of the channel responses into a single scalar response (the selection of the weights applied to each channel, c). Depending on how they are defined, channelized models differ in the amount of knowledge used about the signal and background statistics in order to combine information across channels. In the following, we briefly describe some of these models. Table 10.3 also summarizes the equations to obtain the templates for the different models.

10.5.2.2.1 Sum of channel responses.   One of the most basic rules to combine information across channels is to perform a straight summation across the responses of the different channels. This decision rule has been previously used as a possible combination rule to predict performance detecting sinusoidal gratings in the absence of noise (Graham, 1989). It can also be thought of in essence as a channelized ROI because it does not use information about the signal or background to combine the channel responses.

10.5.2.2.2 Most sensitive channel.   Another possible decision rule used is that the observer monitors the single most sensitive channel among the all the channels (Graham, 1989). In our context "most sensitive" is defined as the single channel that achieves the best performance detecting the signal (under Gaussian assumptions). In other words, this model does not have the ability to combine information across channels and is constrained to using the one best channel. When the signal exactly matches one of the channel's spatial functions (such as in many basic visual psychophysics experiments) then the most sensitive channel is identical to the NPW model.

10.5.2.2.3 Non-prewhitening channelized matched filter I (matched to the signal as seen through the channels).   This is a NPW model constrained to the information encoded by the channels. There are two different versions of this model. In this first version, the weights applied to each channel match the expected output of the channel to the signal. That is, the model matches the signal as seen through the channel mechanism. This strategy would be optimal combination rule if there was no external noise on the image, and performance is limited by internal noise which is independent from channel to channel. However, it becomes suboptimal when there is external noise in the image.

10.5.2.2.4 Non-prewhitening channelized matched filter II (matched to the signal on the image).   In the second version of the non-prewhitening channelized matched-filter model, the weights applied by the model to combine responses across models are adjusted so that the linear combination of the channels match as close as possible the spatial signal on the images (Eckstein and Whiting, 1995). It is the optimal linear combination of channel responses when the external noise is white but becomes suboptimal in correlated noise. Interestingly, the two types of non-prewhitening channelized matched-filter models are identical when the channels are orthogonal and, therefore, the channel responses to external white noise are uncorrelated.

10.5.2.2.5 Channelized Hotelling. The channelized Hotelling observer is similar to the Hotelling but is constrained by a reduction in information content by the processing through the channels (Myers *et al.*, 1987; Yao *et al.*, 1994; Abbey and Barrett, 1995; Burgess *et al.*, 1997; Eckstein *et al.*, 1998a; 1999b). Like the Hotelling model, it takes into consideration signal information transmitted by each channel and in addition it weighs the variance of the channel responses as well as the covariance between the different channel responses. The channelized Hotelling template is the best template (under Gaussian noise assumptions) that can be derived from a linear combination of the channel profiles. The channelized Hotelling template is calculated from the inverse of the covariance matrix of the channel responses (Table 10.3). When the external noise is white the channelized Hotelling model is identical to the non-prewhitening channelized matched filter II.

10.5.2.2.6 Channelized SNR weighted. The channelized SNR (the word SNR is used in a broad sense an refers to the channels' d' defined as the mean response of the channel to the signal location minus the mean response of the channel to the nonsignal response divided by the standard deviation of the channel response) weighted model weights each channel by the amount of signal information encoded by the channel and inversely to the standard deviation of the response (Eckstein *et al.*, 1998b). However, this strategy is not the optimal linear strategy for combining channel responses because, it does not take into account the correlation between the channels. For example, if two channels have a high SNR but are highly correlated, the SNR weighted model would assign large weights to both these channels while the Hotelling model would realize that the channels are highly correlated, encode similar information, and therefore reduce the weights to them. When the channels are orthogonal, the channelized SNR weighted model is equivalent to the channelized Hotelling model.

10.5.3 Which model to choose?

Given the vast number of model observers, one might wonder what criteria to use in order to choose one model observer or another. If the investigator is using image backgrounds and signal profiles that have been previously studied, then one approach would be to use model observers that have been good predictors of human performance in that background. The second to last column of Table 10.1 shows a list of successful models for each of the given backgrounds based on previous studies.

10.6 Calculation of figures of merit

Having chosen the task, the backgrounds, the signal to be used, and the model observers to be tested, the investigator must decide how to measure performance of the model observer in the visual task.

10.6.1 Percent correct from template application

The most basic way to measure performance in an MAFC task is to compute the probability of a correct outcome in each trial. A correct outcome occurs when the

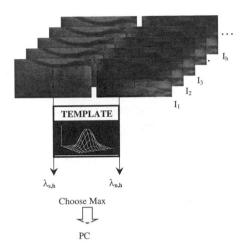

Figure 10.5: Direct application of template to images for a 2-alternative forced choice (2-AFC). For each trial (I_h), the template is applied to the possible signal tocations (indicated with the fudiciary marks) resulting in two scalar responses (λ). The model then chooses the location eliciting the highest response. Performance of the model is measured by the percent of trials (Pc) where the model identified the correct location for the signal.

response to the signal location exceeds the maximum response to the background-only locations, $\text{Prob}(\lambda_s > \max(\lambda_n))$. One obtains an estimate of this probability from samples by applying the template to the different locations in the image and tallying the percent of trials where the model correctly identifies the signal location (Figure 10.5). This can be mathematically expressed as

$$\widehat{Pc} = \frac{1}{H} \sum_{h=0}^{H} \text{step}(\lambda_{s,h} - \max(\lambda_{n,i,h})), \tag{10.6}$$

where $\lambda_{s,h}$ is the response of the template to the signal plus background in the hth trial, $\lambda_{n,i,h}$ is the output correlation to background-only location at the ith location in the hth trial, and H is the total number of trials. The **max** function takes the maximum among the template responses to the $M-1$ non-signal locations. The **step** function is 1 when the argument is larger than 0 and is 0 when the argument is less than 0.

An advantage of Pc is that it makes no assumptions about the statistical properties of the model responses (e.g., Gaussian, independent). One disadvantage is that it requires application of the template to every image sample, which makes the calculation computationally costly. In addition, performance as measured by Pc for a given MAFC task cannot be related easily to Pc in a different MAFC task or a yes/no task unless properties about the model responses are assumed or known.

10.6.2 *Index of detectability,* d′: *Detection across independent backgrounds*

In most tasks, the signal appears in one of M locations where each location is within an independent background sample (Figure 10.2). If the backgrounds are synthetic then each independent sample corresponds to a different realization of the background. If the backgrounds are real then a different sample generally refers to backgrounds coming from different patients. In these cases the pixel value variations in each of the possible signal locations are typically independent, which will result in template responses that are statistically independent from one location to another. A common assumption is that the template responses obey Gaussian distributions. When the backgrounds are computer generated, they are often created to meet this property by design under assumptions of a linear model. When the backgrounds are samples from real medical images, the assumption needs to be verified. However, the Gaussian-model response seems to be in many cases (x-ray coronary angiograms and mammograms, Bochud *et al.*, 1999d) a good approximation.

With these two assumptions, one can represent the model-observer responses to the signal location and to the noise-only locations as being sampled from two univariate Gaussian distributions. The distribution of model responses to the signal location has often a larger mean than that to the noise location. Performance can then be defined in terms of the distance in standard-deviation units between the signal-plus-noise and the noise-only distribution. This metric is known as the index of detectability, d' (Greeen and Swets, 1966):

$$d' = \frac{\langle \lambda_s \rangle - \langle \lambda_n \rangle}{\sigma_\lambda}, \tag{10.7}$$

where $\langle \lambda_s \rangle$ is the mean model response to the signal plus background, $\langle \lambda_n \rangle$ is the mean model response to the background only, and σ_λ are the standard deviation of the model responses assumed to be the same for the signal-present background and background-only locations respectively.

The advantages of the d' index of detectability are: (1) It does not depend on the number of possible locations in the task; (2) It can be calculated without actually applying the template to the images and is therefore computationally easier.

When the response of the model is Gaussian distributed and the responses to each location are statistically independent, then d' can be used to calculate Pc for any alternative forced-choice experiment by calculating the probability of the signal response taking a larger value than all the non-signal locations (Green and Swets, 1966):

$$Pc(d', M) = \int_{-\infty}^{+\infty} \phi(x - d') \left[\Phi(x) \right]^{M-1} dx, \tag{10.8}$$

where

$$\phi(x) = \frac{1}{\sqrt{2\pi}} e^{-x^2/2}.$$

Also, $\Phi(x)$ is the cumulative Gaussian distribution function, $\Phi(x) = \int_{-\infty}^{x} \phi(y)\,dy$ and M is the number of possible signal locations in the experiment.

10.6.2.1 Calculating d' from image statistics: stationary versus non-stationary backgrounds

One advantage of the index of detectability is that it can be calculated directly from image statistics without having to apply the template directly to every image sample (Figure 10.6; Table 10.5). The mean response of the template to the signal location, $\langle \lambda_s \rangle$, can be calculated from the response of the template to the mean image containing the signal (and similarly for the mean response to the noise-only location). The variance of the template response is calculated from the template and the covariance of the image background (see Appendix A).

Furthermore, when the images obey the stationarity assumption, then the Fourier transform domain is often used to represent the signal and the noise, and d' is calculated from the Fourier representation of the template and signal Fourier amplitudes and the noise power spectrum (Table 10.5). Note that the expression are valid for an additive signal only. Similar expressions for a multiplicative signal can be found elsewhere (Bochud *et al.*, 1999b).

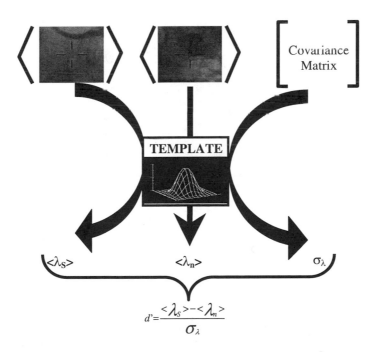

Figure 10.6: Index of detectability d' calculated directly from image statistics. Instead of applying the template to the images on each trial, performance is measured by applying the template to the mean data at the signal present location, the mean data at the noise only location, and calculating the variance of the model-template response from the covariance matrix (see Appendix A for details).

Table 10.5: Calculating the index of detectability and the index of detectability for correlated responses. Symbols defined in Tables 10.4a and 10.4b

	Index of Detectability	Index of Detectability for Response Correlation
General definition	$$d' = \frac{\langle \lambda_s \rangle - \langle \lambda_n \rangle}{\sigma_\lambda}$$	$$d'_r = \frac{d'}{\sqrt{1-r}}$$
Non-stationary backgrounds	$$d' = \frac{\mathbf{w}^t(\langle \mathbf{g}_s \rangle - \langle \mathbf{g}_n \rangle)}{\sqrt{\mathbf{w}^t \mathbf{K} \mathbf{w}}}$$	$$d'_r = \frac{\mathbf{w}^t(\langle \mathbf{g}_s \rangle - \langle \mathbf{g}_n \rangle)}{\sqrt{\mathbf{w}^t \mathbf{K} \mathbf{w} - \mathbf{w}^t \mathbf{K}_{p,q} \mathbf{w}}}$$
Stationary backgrounds	$$d' = \frac{\int_{-\infty}^{+\infty}\int_{-\infty}^{+\infty} \overline{\tilde{w}(\mathbf{u},\mathbf{v})}\, \tilde{s}(\mathbf{u},\mathbf{v})\, d\mathbf{u}\, d\mathbf{v}}{\left[\int_{-\infty}^{+\infty}\int_{-\infty}^{+\infty} |\tilde{w}(\mathbf{u},\mathbf{v})|^2 \mathbf{N}(\mathbf{u},\mathbf{v})\, d\mathbf{u}\, d\mathbf{v}\right]^{1/2}}$$	$$d'_r = \frac{\int_{-\infty}^{+\infty}\int_{-\infty}^{+\infty} \overline{\tilde{w}(\mathbf{u},\mathbf{v})}\, \tilde{s}(\mathbf{u},\mathbf{v})\, d\mathbf{u}\, d\mathbf{v}}{\left[\int_{-\infty}^{+\infty}\int_{-\infty}^{+\infty} |\tilde{w}(\mathbf{u},\mathbf{v})|^2 \mathbf{N}(\mathbf{u},\mathbf{v})[1 - e^{-2\pi i(\Delta x u + \Delta y v)}]\, d\mathbf{u}\, d\mathbf{v}\right]^{1/2}}$$

10.6.3 Index of detectability for correlated responses d_r': Within-image detection tasks

Sometimes the investigator chooses a task where the signal can appear in two locations within an image rather than in two independent images (see Figure 10.2). One potential problem is that for backgrounds with spatially slow-varying luminance changes (e.g., low-pass noise or $1/f^\beta$ power spectra images such as natural and medical images) the pixel values at the different possible signal locations might be correlated. Correlations between the pixels might lead to correlations between the template response to the different possible signal locations. In this case, use of Eq. (10.8) to calculate Pc in a task with M locations from an estimated d' (calculated from Eq. (10.7)) will result in an erroneous Pc. This is because Eq. (10.8), treats the responses as statistically independent even if they are not. For these tasks, the investigator should not use d' as a figure of merit and instead should use Pc by directly applying the template to the images to quantify model performance. Another possibility is to use a modified index of detectability d_r' that takes into account response correlations (Eckstein *et al.*, 1999a):

$$d_r' = \frac{d'}{\sqrt{1-r}},\tag{10.9}$$

where r is the correlation coefficient between the responses to two different locations defined as:

$$r_{p,q} = \frac{\langle(\lambda_{p,i} - \langle\lambda_p\rangle)(\lambda_{q,i} - \langle\lambda_q\rangle)\rangle}{\sqrt{\langle(\lambda_{p,i} - \langle\lambda_p\rangle)^2\rangle}\sqrt{\langle(\lambda_{q,i} - \langle\lambda_q\rangle)^2\rangle}},\tag{10.10}$$

where $\lambda_{p,i}$ is the model response at location p in the ith trial and $\lambda_{q,i}$ is the model response at location q in the ith trial.

This new metric, d_r', is in essence a correction on d' that takes into account the correlation across responses and allows the investigator to preserve the Pc versus d' relationship in the case of statistically independent responses (Eq. (10.5)). As with d', d_r' has the advantages of being independent of the number of possible signal locations in the MAFC task and can also be computed directly without applying the template (Table 10.5).

Equation (10.9) holds when the pairwise correlations among the responses to the different locations in the MAFC task are constant. This might not be the case in many cases and then d_r' should be used with caution. On the other hand, recent results have shown robustness of d_r' to small departures from the constant correlation assumption for a 4-AFC task in x-ray coronary angiograms (Eckstein *et al.*, 1999a).

10.6.4 What figure of merit to use?

Based on whether the visual task is an across-image MAFC or a within-image MAFC, on whether the backgrounds are stationary or non-stationary, and whether

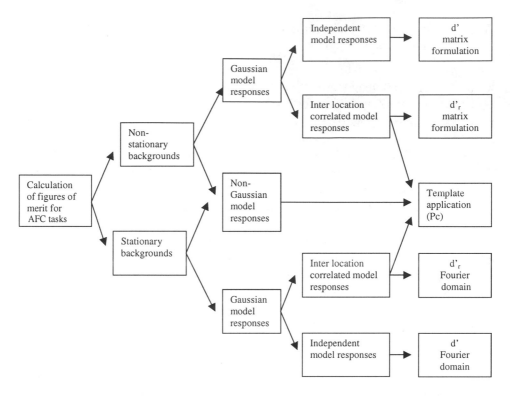

Figure 10.7: Decision tree to choose an appropriate figure of merit for a given visual task and background.

there is reason to believe that the model responses are or are not Gaussian, the investigator should choose a figure of merit appropriate to the circumstances. Figure 10.7 is a decision tree that might assist the investigator making the decision on the figure of merit to be used for the given conditions.

10.7 Comparing model to human performance

Given that there are many model observers one might use, often times a preliminary human psychophysics study is conducted in order to determine which one of a number of model observers best predicts observer performance. In these instances, the investigator obtains human and model performance in the visual task. The first step in trying to compare human and model-observer performance is to have performance measured by the same metric (Pc or d'). If model performance is measured with a d' metric, then one must obtain a similar metric for human observers. However, the investigator does not have direct access to the human templates response for each image and therefore cannot directly calculate a d' metric from Eq. (10.7). Instead the investigator simply has access to the location that the human observer chose on for each image. Therefore human performance is first quantified by computing the percent of trials in which they correctly identified the signal location

(Pc; Eq. (10.1)). Next, a d' metric for the human observer is inferred from the measured Pc using Eq. (10.8), assuming that the responses of the human observer are Gaussian distributed and statistically independent. The Gaussian assumption has been shown to be a good approximation to the internal response of human observers for visual detection in white noise (Swensson and Judy, 1981; Burgess and Ghandeharian, 1984), x-ray coronary angiograms (Eckstein and Whiting, 1996), and x-ray mammograms (Bochud *et al.*, 1999d).

A typical problem is that performance of the model observers is typically better than that of human performance so comparison between the two is nontrivial. There are two commonly used methods to make comparisons: (1) The constant efficiency method; (2) Degradation of model-observer performance.

10.7.1 The constant efficiency method

If the index of detectability has been used to quantify model and human performance then one method to compare whether a model performance is a good predictor of human performance is to compute the efficiency of human performance with respect to the model observers defined as the square ratio of d's: $(d'_{human}/d'_{model})^2$. The investigator looks at how the efficiency with respect to a given model varies across conditions. If the model is a good predictor of human performance then the efficiency should be approximately constant across the different conditions (Myers *et al.*, 1985).

10.7.2 Degrading model observer performance

A second method to compare model and human performance is to add additional sources of degradation to the model observer so that the model observer performs at human levels. There are different methods of degrading model performance. The most common is to include internal noise in the model. Experimental work has shown that there are two components to human internal noise. A first component is additive and generally dependent on the mean luminance of the images (Burgess and Colborne, 1988). A second component that is generally a more significant source of performance degradation is proportional to the variance produced by the external noise (Burgess and Colborne, 1988).

10.7.2.1 Proportional internal noise and scaling d'

In some special cases the effect of adding an internal noise component to a model that is proportional to the external noise is equivalent to multiplying d' across conditions by a scaling factor (Burgess *et al.*, 1997; Burgess, 1999b). The scaling factor can be adjusted to match performance between human and model performance in one condition or could be fit in order to minimize the overall discrepancy between model and human observer across all conditions studied. The scaling procedure should not be used indiscriminately because it is only valid when the use of d' is warranted (Gaussian, independent responses).

10.7.2.2 Injecting internal noise as a random variable

The more general and robust procedure to degrade model performance involves directly injecting internal noise into the template application procedure (Eckstein *et al.*, 1998a, 1999b). In this approach, a random variable (with zero mean) is added to the model template response to each of the locations for each image. If the internal noise is proportional then it is related through a proportionality constant to the variance in the template response produced by the external noise. The amount of injected internal noise is iteratively adjusted so that model and human Pc in a given condition are matched or to minimize the discrepancy between human and model performance across all conditions been studied. The advantage of this latter method is that it does not make any inherent assumptions about the Gaussian statistical independence of the template responses nor about the constancy of the mean response of the model to the signal across conditions. The disadvantage is that it is computationally more costly than the scaling method.

10.7.2.3 Other methods to degrade human performance

Although the internal noise method is the most commonly used method to degrade human performance other possibilities are available. Intrinsic uncertainty (Pelli, 1985) in the human observer about signal parameters is another source of inefficiency. The observer is assumed to be uncertain about the spatial position, temporal position, spatial frequency, or orientation of the signal. The observer therefore monitors on each trial not only the response of a single template but the response of many templates, each of which are at different spatial locations, temporal positions, spatial frequencies, or orientations. In most versions of the simplified uncertainty model (Pelli, 1985; Eckstein *et al.*, 1997a) the responses of the additional "uncertain templates" are assumed to encode no signal information and be statistically independent from the signal relevant template.

Additional methods to degrade performance of models for detection in noise that have not been extensively investigated are a nonlinear transducer (Lu and Dosher, 1999; Foley and Legge, 1981) and divisive inhibition across channels (Heeger, 1992; Geisler and Albrecht, 1992; Watson and Solomon, 1997).

10.8 Concluding remarks

Metrics based on arbitrary properties of an image are poor predictors of human visual detection in clinically relevant tasks. However, a vast number of studies have shown that model observers can be successfully used to predict human performance in visual tasks in synthetic noisy images and more recently in real anatomic backgrounds. With the increase of digital archival of medical images it is becoming easier to perform model-observer-based evaluation and optimization of medical-image quality. The purpose of the present chapter was to make some of the tools and methodologies needed to use model observers more accessible to new investigators with the hope that model observers will become common metrics of medical-image quality.

Acknowledgements

This was work was supported by National Institute of Health (NIH) grant RO1 HL53455 and NASA grant 50827. The work is a result of many lively discussions over the years with Al Ahumada, Harry Barrett, Art Burgess, Dick Swensson, Beau Watson, and other outspoken researchers in the image perception and vision communities to which I am thankful for sharing their knowledge with me. The authors thank Jay Bartroff for his help with many of the figures.

References

Abbey CK, Barrett HH. "Linear Iterative Reconstruction Algorithms: Study of Observer Performance." In Bizais Y, Barillot C, Di Paola R (Eds.) *Proc 14th Int Conf On Information Processing in Medical Imaging.* Dordrecht: Kluwer Academic, 1995, pp. 65–76.

Ahumada Jr AJ, Watson AB, Rohally AM. "Models of Human Image Discrimination Predict Object Detection in Natural Backgrounds." In Rogowitz B, Allebach J (Eds.) *Human Vision, Visual Proc and Digital Display VI.* Proc SPIE 2411, 1995, pp. 355–362.

Barrett HH, Abbey CK, Gallas B, Eckstein MP. "Stabilized Estimates of Hotelling-Observer Detection Performance in Patient Structured Noise." Proc SPIE 3340, 1998.

Barrett HH, Yao J, Rolland JP, Myers KJ. "Model Observers for Assessment of Image Quality." Proc Natl Acad Sci USA 90:9758–9765, 1993.

Bochud FO, Abbey CK, Eckstein, MP. "Statistical Texture Synthesis of Mammographic Images with Clustered Lumpy Backgrounds." Optics Express 4:33–43, 1999a.

Bochud FO, Abbey, CA, Eckstein MP. "Visual Signal Detection in structured backgrounds IV, Calculation of Figures of Merit for Model Observers in Non Stationary Backgrounds." J of the Opt Soc of Am A 1999b (in press).

Bochud FO, Abbey CK, Eckstein MP. "Further Investigation of the Effect of Phase Spectrum on Visual Detection in Structured Backgrounds." Proc SPIE 3663, 1999c.

Bochud FO, Abbey CK, Bartroff JL, Vodopich DJ, Eckstein MP. "Effect of the Number of Locations in MAFC Experiments Performed with Mammograms." In *Far West Image Perception Conference*, Nakoda Lodge, AB, Canada, 1999d.

Burgess AE. "The Rose Model, Revisited." J Opt Soc Am A16:633–646, 1999a.

Burgess AE. "Visual Signal Detection with Two-Component Noise: Low-Pass Spectrum Effect." J Opt Soc Am A16:694–704, 1999b.

Burgess AE, Li X, Abbey CK. "Visual Signal Detectability with Two Noise Components: Anomalous Masking Effects." J Opt Soc Am A14:2420–2442, 1997.

Burgess AE. "Statistically Defined Backgrounds: Performance of a Modified Non-Prewhitening Observer Model." J Opt Soc Am A11:1237–1242, 1994.

Burgess AE and Colborne B. "Visual Signal Detection IV: Observer Inconsistency." J Opt Soc Am A5:617–627, 1988.

Burgess AE, Ghandeharian H. "Visual Signal Detection. II. Signal Location Identification." J Opt Soc Am A1:900–905, 1984.

Burgess AE, Wagner RB, Jennings RJ, Barlow HB. "Efficiency of Human Visual Signal Discrimination." Science 214:93–94, 1981.

Cunningham IA, Shaw R. "Signal-to-Noise Optimization of Medical Imaging Systems." J Opt Soc Am A16:621–632, 1999.

Daly S. "The Visual Differences Predictor: An Algorithm for the Assessment of Image Fidelity." In Watson AB (Ed.) *Digital Images and Human Vision.* Cambridge, Mass: MIT Press, 1993, pp. 179–206.

Eckstein MP, Abbey CK, Bochud FO. "Visual Signal Detection in Structured Backgrounds. III. Figure of Merit for Model Performance in Multiple-Alternative Forced-Choice Detection Task with Correlation Response." J Opt Soc Am A, 1999a (in press).

Eckstein MP, Abbey CK, Bochud FO, Whiting JS. "The Effect of Image Compression in Model and Human Observers." In *Proceedings SPIE Image Perception* 3663, 1999b, pp. 243–252.

Eckstein MP, Abbey CK, Whiting JS. "Human Vs Model Observers in Anatomic Backgrounds." Proc SPIE 3340, 1998a, pp. 15–26.

Eckstein MP, Abbey CK, Bochud FO. "Models for Visual Detection in Complex Backgrounds II: Applications." In *Annual Meeting of the Optical Society of America*, Baltimore, MD, 1998b.

Eckstein MP, Ahumada AJ, Watson AB. "Visual Signal Detection in Structured Backgrounds II. Effect of Contrast Gain Control, Background Variations and White Noise." J Opt Soc of Am (Special issue on Visual Contrast Sensitivity) A14:2406–2419, 1997a.

Eckstein MP, Ahumada AJ, Watson AB. "Image Discrimination Models Predict Visual Detection in Natural Image Backgrounds." In *Proceedings to SPIE Electronic Imaging, Hum Vis & App* 3016, 1997b, pp. 44–56.

Eckstein MP, Whiting JS. "Visual Signal Detection in Structured Backgrounds I: Effect of Number of Possible Spatial Locations and Signal Contrast." J Opt Soc Am A13:1777–1787, 1996.

Eckstein MP, Whiting JS. "Lesion Detection in Structured Noise." Academic Radiology 2:249–253, 1995.

Eigler NL, Eckstein MP, Mahrer K, Honig D, Whiting JS. "Effect of a Stenosis Stablilized Display on Morphological Features." Circ 96:1157–1164, 1994.

Fiete RD, Barrett HH, Smith WE, Myers KJ. "The Hotelling Trace Criterion and Its Correlation with Human Observer Performance." J Opt Soc Am A4:945–953, 1987.

Foley JM. "Human Luminance Pattern-Vision Mechanisms: Masking Experiments Require a New Model." Opt Soc Am A11:1710–1719, 1994.

Foley JM, Legge GE. "Contrast Detection and Near Threshold Discrimination in Human Vision." Vision Res 21:1041–1053, 1981.

Geisler WS, Albrecht DG. "Cortical Neurons: Isolation of Contrast Gain Control." Vision Res 32:1409–1410, 1992.

Geisler WS, Davila KD. "Ideal Discriminators in Spatial Vision: Two-Point Stimuli." J Opt Soc Am A2:1483–1497, 1985.

Giger ML, Doi K. "Investigation of Basic Imaging Properties in Digital Radiography. 3. Effect of Pixel Size on SNR and Threshold Contrast." Med Phys 12:201–208, 1985.

Graham NVS. *Visual Pattern Analyzers.* New York: Oxford University Press, 1989.

Green DM, Swets JA. *Signal Detection Theory and Psychophysics.* New York: Wiley, 1966.

Hanson K. "Detectability in Computed Tomographic Images." Med Phys 6:441–451, 1980.

Heeger DJ. "Nonlinear Model of Neural Responses in Cat Visual Cortex." Vis Neurosci 181–197, 1992.

Hermann C, Buhr E, Hoeschen D, Fan SY. "Comparison of ROC and AFC Methods in a Visual Detection Task." Medical Physics 20:805–812, 1993.

Ishida M, Doi K, Loo L, Metz CE, Lehr JL. "Digital Image Processing: Effect on Detectability of Simulated Low-Contrast Radiographic Patterns." Radiology 150:569–575, 1984.

Johnson JP, Lubin J, Krupinski EA, Peterson HA, Roehrig H, Baysinger A. "Visual Discrimination Model for Digital Mammography." *Proceedings SPIE Image Perception* 3663, 1999, pp. 253–263.

Judy PF, Swensson RG. "Detection of Small Focal Lesions in CT Images: Effects of Reconstruction Filters and Visual Display Windows." Br J Radiol 58:137–145, 1985.

Judy PF, Swensson RG. "Display Thresholding of Images and Observer Detection Performance." J Opt Soc Am A4:954–965, 1987.

Marcelja S. "Mathematical Desription of the Responses of Simple Cortical Cells." J Opt Soc Am A70: 1297–1300, 1980.

Lu ZL, Dosher BA. "Characterizing Human Perceptual Inefficiencies with Equivalent Internal Noise." J Opt Soc Am A16:764–78, 1999.

Movshon JA, Thompson ID, Tolhurst DJ. "Spatial Summation in the Receptive Fields of Simple Cells in the Cat's Striate Cortex." J Physiol London 283:53–77, 1978.

Myers K, Barrett HH. "Addition of a Channel Mechanism to the Ideal Observer Model." J Opt Soc Am A4:2447–2457, 1987.

Myers KJ, Barrett HH, Borgstrom MC, Patton DD, Seeley GW. "Effect of Noise Correlation on Detectability of Disk Signals in Medical Imaging." J Opt Soc Am A2:1752–1759, 1985.

North DO. "Analysis of the Factors Which Determine Signal-Noise Discrimination in Pulsed Carrier Systems." RCA Tech Rep PTR6C, 1943; reprinted in Proc IRE 51:1016-1-28, 1963.

Ohara K, Doi K, Metz CE, Giger ML. "Investigation of Basic Imaging Properties in Digital Radiography. 13. Effect of Simple Structured Noise on the Detectability of Simulated Stenotic Lesions." Med Phys 16:14–21, 1989.

Pelli DG. "Uncertainty Explains Many Aspects of Visual Contrast Detection and Discrimination." J Opt Soc Am A2:1508–1530, 1985.

Peterson WW, Birdsall TG, Fox WC. "The Theory of Signal Detectability." Trans of the IRE PGIT 4:171–212, 1954.

Revesz G, Kundel HL, Graber MA. "The Influence of Structured Noise on the Detection of Radiologic Abnormalities." Invest Radiol 9:479–486, 1974.

Robson JG. "Spatial and Temporal Contrast-Sensitivity Functions of the Visual System." J Opt Soc Am 56:1141–1142, 1966.

Rolland JP, Barrett HH. "Effect of Random Inhomogeneity on Observer Detection Performance." J Opt Soc Am A9:649–658, 1992.

Rose A. "The Sensitivity Performance of the Human Eye on an Absolute Scale." J Opt Soc Am A38:196–208, 1948.

Sachs M, Nachmias J, Robson J. "Spatial Frequency Channels in Human Vision." J Opt Soc Am A61:1176–1186, 1971.

Samei E, Flynn MJ, Eyler WR. "Simulation of Subtle Lung Nodules in Projection Chest Radiography." Radiology 202:117–124, 1997.

Seltzer SE, Judy PF, Swensson RG, Nawfel R, Chan KH. "Flattening of Contrast-Detail Curves for Liver CT." Med Phys 21:1547–1555, 1994.

Swesson RG, Judy PF. "Detection of Noisy Visual Targets: Model for the Effects of Spatial Uncertainty and Signal to Noise Ratio." Percept Psychophys 29:521–534, 1981.

Tanner WP. "Physiological Implications of Psychophysical Data." Annals of the New York Academy of Sciences 166:172, 1961.

Tolhurst DJ, Movshon JA, Dean AF. "The Statistical Reliability of Signals in Single Neurons in Cat and Monkey Visual Cortex." Vision Research 23:775–785, 1983.

Wagner RF, Brown DG. "Unified SNR Analysis of Medical Imaging Systems." Phys Med Biol 30:489–518, 1985.

Wagner RF, Weaver KE. "An Assortment of Image Quality Indices for Radiographic Film-Screen Combinations—Can they be Resolved?" In Carson PL, Hendee WH, Zarnstorff WC (Eds.) Application of Optical Instrumentation in Medicine I. Proc SPIE 35, 1972, pp. 83–94.

Watson AB, Solomon, JA. "A Model of Contrast Gain Control in Human Vision." J Opt Soc Am A14:2379–2391, 1997.

Watson AB. "Detection and Recognition of Simple Spatial Forms." In Bradick OJ, Sleigh AC (Eds.), Physical and Biological Processing of Images. New York: Springer-Verlag, 1983.

Webster MA, Myahara E. "Contrast Adaptation and the Spatial Structure of Natural Images." J Opt Soc Am A9:2355–2366, 1997.

Wilson H, Bergen J. "A Four-Mechanism Model for Threshold Spatial Vision." Vision Research 19:19–32, 1979.

Yao J, Barrett HH. "Predicting Human Performance by a Channelized Hotelling Observer Model." SPIE Math Methods Med Imaging 1768, 1992, pp. 161–168.

Appendix A: Definitions of matrix-formulation components for model observers non-channelized models

Image Vectorized image

$$g(x, y) = \begin{bmatrix} g_{0,0} & g_{0,1} & \cdots & g_{0,m} \\ g_{1,0} & g_{1,1} & \cdots & g_{1,m} \\ \vdots & \vdots & \ddots & \vdots \\ g_{n,0} & g_{n,1} & \cdots & g_{n,m} \end{bmatrix} \longrightarrow \quad \mathbf{g} = \begin{bmatrix} g_{0,0} \\ g_{0,1} \\ g_{0,m} \\ g_{1,0} \\ g_{1,1} \\ \vdots \\ g_{n,m} \end{bmatrix},$$

where $g_{n,m}$ is the digital value of the image in the nth and mth pixel position of the image

Template Vectorized template

$$w(x, y) = \begin{bmatrix} w_{0,0} & w_{0,1} & \cdots & w_{0,m} \\ w_{1,0} & w_{1,1} & \cdots & w_{1,m} \\ \vdots & \vdots & \ddots & \vdots \\ w_{n,0} & w_{n,1} & \cdots & w_{n,m} \end{bmatrix} \longrightarrow \quad \mathbf{w} = \begin{bmatrix} w_{0,0} \\ w_{0,1} \\ w_{0,m} \\ w_{1,0} \\ w_{1,1} \\ \vdots \\ w_{n,m} \end{bmatrix}.$$

Mean signal present/signal absent vectors:

$$\langle \mathbf{g}_s \rangle = (1/N) \Sigma \mathbf{g}_s,$$
$$\langle \mathbf{g}_n \rangle = (1/N) \Sigma \mathbf{g}_n.$$

Noise covariance matrix:

$$\mathbf{K} = \langle [\mathbf{g} - \langle \mathbf{g} \rangle]^{\mathrm{T}} [\mathbf{g} - \langle \mathbf{g} \rangle] \rangle =$$

$$\mathbf{K} = \begin{bmatrix} \langle (g_{0,0} - \langle g_{0,0}\rangle)^2 \rangle & \langle (g_{0,0} - \langle g_{0,0}\rangle)(g_{0,1} - \langle g_{0,1}\rangle) \rangle & \cdots & \langle (g_{0,0} - \langle g_{0,0}\rangle)(g_{n,m} - \langle g_{n,m}\rangle) \rangle \\ \langle (g_{0,1} - \langle g_{0,1}\rangle)(g_{0,0} - \langle g_{0,0}\rangle) \rangle & \langle (g_{0,1} - \langle g_{0,1}\rangle)^2 \rangle & \cdots & \langle (g_{0,1} - \langle g_{0,1}\rangle)(g_{n,m} - \langle g_{n,m}\rangle) \rangle \\ \vdots & \vdots & \ddots & \vdots \\ \langle (g_{n,m} - \langle g_{n,m}\rangle)(g_{0,0} - \langle g_{0,0}\rangle) \rangle & \langle (g_{n,m} - \langle g_{n,m}\rangle)(g_{0,1} - \langle g_{0,1}\rangle) \rangle & \cdots & \langle (g_{n,m} - \langle g_{n,m}\rangle)^2 \rangle \end{bmatrix},$$

where $\langle \mathbf{g} \rangle$ is the expectation value of the image $\mathbf{g}$ and ^{T} is the transpose matrix. Note that the covariance matrix is assumed to be equal for the signal present and signal absent images.

Mean response of model template:

$$\langle \lambda_s \rangle = \mathbf{w}^{\mathrm{T}} \langle \mathbf{g}_s \rangle,$$
$$\langle \lambda_n \rangle = \mathbf{w}^{\mathrm{T}} \langle \mathbf{g}_n \rangle.$$

Variance of response of model template:

$$\sigma_\lambda^2 = \mathbf{w}^{\mathrm{T}} \mathbf{K} \mathbf{w}.$$

The basic methodology to compute performance for channelized model observers is essentially the same except that instead of starting with the values of the pixels the models operate on the responses of the channels to the signal present and signal absent images.

CHAPTER 11
Modeling Visual Detection Tasks in Correlated Image Noise with Linear Model Observers

Craig K. Abbey, François O. Bochud
UCLA School of Medicine

CONTENTS

11.1 Introduction

A perceptual phenomena that has received considerable attention in the medical imaging community is the influence of image variability on signal-detection tasks. This subject is relevant to medical imaging because detection tasks are a common use of diagnostic images, and these images have two well known sources of variability [1–10]. The first source of variability results from system noise obtained during image acquisition. System noise is usually defined by the physical processes that govern the imaging device such as counting statistics, film-grain noise, or amplifier noise. The other source of variability in medical images has to do with the variable nature of the objects being imaged. Patient-to-patient variability—sometimes referred to as "anatomical" noise—is more difficult to characterize than system noise but can be an important factor that limits detection performance.

For detection tasks in the presence of image variability, a general approach to modeling human observers has been to use signal detection theory to define mathematical algorithms that perform the same detection task as the human observer. These sorts of models are often referred to as "model observers" because they mimic the role (as well as, it is hoped, the performance) of a human observer. Linear observers are an important class of model observers because they have been widely studied for simple detection tasks in noise, where there is no signal uncertainty [11] (see Chapter 9).

In medical imaging, predictive models of task performance have an important application as an aid to optimizing diagnostic-imaging systems. The basic precept of objective assessment of image quality is that the best system will result in images that allow an observer (usually a clinician) to best perform a diagnostic task of interest [3]. In principle then, the process of optimizing imaging systems involves numerous evaluations of human-observer performance in the task of interest. However, human-observer studies are costly and time consuming. Predictive models for detection performance would greatly reduce the need for these studies and allow for tuning more parameters in the diagnostic-imaging chain [11].

This chapter considers the most basic detection task, signal-known-exactly (SKE) detection. The SKE task epitomizes the notion of controlled stimuli. The signal-present images of an SKE task have a fixed (nonrandom) signal profile that is fixed at a given location, orientation, and size. In principle, the signal contrast is also presumed to be fixed, although some experimental methodologies adjust the signal contrast to achieve a predetermined level of performance [12]. SKE tasks are certainly simpler than clinical detection tasks which contain varying degrees of uncertainty in the signal parameters. However, this simplicity can be an advantage in basic studies of perceptual performance because it removes possible confounds from the resulting observed data. For example, consider the detection of a signal at an unknown location in an image and in the presence of image noise. This is not an SKE detection task because of uncertainty in the signal location. Poor performance in this task by human observers could be explained by some combination of image-noise effects and an inefficient visual search strategy. Fixing the signal at a particular location isolates the image-noise effects, and can provide a point of reference for further studies exploring interactions between noise and search effects.

The goal of this chapter is to present a review of linear model observers for SKE detection in the presence of image variability. We shall focus on linear observers because they constitute the majority of models used in the medical-imaging literature for SKE detection in noise, and they have some attractive mathematical properties as well. A central premise of model observers is that they can perform the same task as the human observer, and hence we shall see how a model observer can be used to generate results in various detection experiments. We shall also investigate how statistical properties of images influence these models and their performance. Performance in each of these experiments is then tied to a common figure of merit, the observer detectability index d'. Some particular observers are then described to illustrate how the image statistics influence the definition of these observers as well.

11.2 Mathematical preliminaries

Before commencing with the main topics, we will review some of the basic notation and statistical quantities used throughout this chapter.

11.2.1 Continuous and discrete image representations

One common representation of an image is as a function of spatial position. For a two-dimensional image, we can equate a location on the image with a two-dimensional column vector $\mathbf{r}$ that contains the horizontal and vertical coordinates of the location. The intensity of the image at the location is given by the function $g(\mathbf{r})$. The image is presumed to exhibit some form of random variability, and hence $g(\mathbf{r})$ can be considered a random variable for every $\mathbf{r}$, or equivalently, the function g can be considered a random function. Descriptions of random functions and numerous mathematical results about them can be found in the large and well developed field of stochastic processes [13].

For digital images, it may be more convenient to use a discrete representation because these images consist of a finite set of pixel values. In this case, the image can be considered an M-dimensional vector $\mathbf{g}$, where M is the number of pixels in the image. The mth element of the image vector, $[\mathbf{g}]_m$, is the intensity of the mth pixel. A common convention is for m to index image pixels starting in the upper left corner of the image ($m = 0$) and proceeding row by row to the lower right corner ($m = M - 1$). This sort of index is referred to as a lexicographical index [14]. Figure 11.1 shows how a lexicographical index works diagrammatically. Image variability leads to the interpretation of $\mathbf{g}$ as a random vector governed by a multivariate probability-density function (pdf).

A connection between continuous and discrete representations of images can be made by the operation of sampling. Intuitively, the role of sampling is to evaluate a function at a specified list of points and, hence, this operation converts a continuously defined function into a discrete vector. A more general definition of sampling uses a sampling function that, for imaging purposes, can also be called

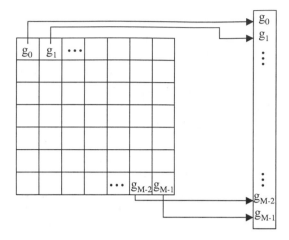

Figure 11.1: Lexicographical index. This diagram shows how pixel intensities are remapped from a two-dimensional image to a one-dimensional column vector by a lexicographical index.

a "pixel" function. The pixel function is the luminance profile of a single pixel. Ideally, this two-dimensional function is a small rectangle of constant intensity. An element of the vector $\mathbf{g}$ is defined by integrating $g(\mathbf{r})$ against the pixel function, denoted by ϕ, to obtain

$$[\mathbf{g}]_m = \int d\mathbf{r} g(\mathbf{r}) \phi(\mathbf{r} - \mathbf{r}_m), \qquad (11.1)$$

where $\mathbf{r}_m$ specifies the location of the mth pixel and $[\mathbf{g}]_m$ is the mth element of the vector $\mathbf{g}$. The integral used here (with a boldface differential, $d\mathbf{r}$) indicates an integration over all components of $\mathbf{r}$. For $\mathbf{r} = (x, y)^t$ where the superscript t indicates the transpose, the integral $\int d\mathbf{r}$, is equivalent to $\int\int dx \, dy$.

Both the continuous and discrete image representations just described have situations in which they are advantageous. However, for the present purpose we find the discrete representation somewhat easier to use. Hence, the rest of the chapter will present developments for the discrete image representation.

11.2.2 Signal-present and signal-absent images in detection tasks

The signal-detection task categorizes images into one of two possible classes. Signal-present images are those that contain a signal of interest, regardless of whether the signal profile can be readily visualized in the image. A signal-absent image does not contain the signal. In medical imaging, a signal-present image is defined as an image of a patient with disease while a signal-absent image comes from a patient that does not have disease. Hence the definitions of signal-present and signal-absent images are associated with the state of the patient being imaged and not necessarily with the content of the image. A patient with disease is identified with the signal-present hypothesis (referred to as h_2), and a patient without disease is identified with the signal-absent hypothesis (h_1). The notions of signal-present or signal-absent classes of images can thus be thought of as images that are conditional on one of these two hypotheses.

For the purposes of modeling signal detection, it is necessary to associate the signal-present and signal-absent hypotheses with sets of images. We refer to equations that describe the combination of image components in an image under each hypothesis as the image-generating equations. Image components are such quantities as the signal profile, anatomical background, and system noise. If an additive combination of components is assumed, the generating equations for a image-vector $\mathbf{g}$ are

$$
\begin{aligned}
&\text{Signal-present images } (h_2)\text{: } \quad \mathbf{g} = \mathbf{b} + \mathbf{n} + \mathbf{s} \\
&\text{Signal-absent images } (h_1)\text{: } \quad \mathbf{g} = \mathbf{b} + \mathbf{n},
\end{aligned}
\tag{11.2}
$$

where $\mathbf{s}$ is the signal profile, $\mathbf{b}$ is the background (or nonsignal-related anatomical features), and $\mathbf{n}$ is the image fluctuations attributable to system noise.

11.2.3 Image statistics

Image statistics are used to characterize the variability in a set of images and play two important roles in modeling detection tasks. The first is that variability in the images propagates through the model and influences the performance of the model. Hence the performance of a given model is largely determined by the statistical properties of the images on which it is used. The other role played by statistical properties lies in defining the models themselves. As seen in Section 11.4 on linear-model observers (and elsewhere in this handbook), most models of detection use specific statistical properties as components of the model.

Two statistical properties will be of interest in this chapter, the image mean and covariance. The image mean is itself an image (although in the case of an image vector, it may not be quantized to a finite number of bits on a grey scale). The image covariance is somewhat more complicated and depends on pairs of points in the image.

11.2.3.1 Image mean

The image mean is defined as the expected value of the image at each point. For an image vector, $\mathbf{g}$, the image mean is defined as another vector, $\bar{\mathbf{g}}$, where each element is defined by the vector-valued expectation

$$
\bar{\mathbf{g}} = \langle \mathbf{g} \rangle.
\tag{11.3}
$$

The angular brackets indicate the expected value over an ensemble of possible image vectors represented by $\mathbf{g}$.

The image generating equations given in Eq. (11.2) can be used to relate the image mean to the effects of the signal and background under each of the detection hypotheses. Because the system noise is generally assumed to have a mean value of zero at all locations, it does not affect the image mean in any way (i.e., $\langle \mathbf{n} \rangle = 0$). With this assumption, the image mean under each of the signal-detection hypotheses is

$$\text{Signal-present images } (h_2): \quad \overline{\mathbf{g}} = \mathbf{s} + \overline{\mathbf{b}}$$
$$\text{Signal-absent images } (h_1): \quad \overline{\mathbf{g}} = \overline{\mathbf{b}}. \tag{11.4}$$

11.2.3.2 Image covariance

The image covariance characterizes departures from the mean value at any two points in the image. For an image with M pixels, the image covariance is an $M \times M$ matrix defined by the matrix valued expectation

$$\mathbf{K_g} = \langle (\mathbf{g} - \overline{\mathbf{g}})(\mathbf{g} - \overline{\mathbf{g}})^t \rangle,$$

where $(\mathbf{g} - \overline{\mathbf{g}})(\mathbf{g} - \overline{\mathbf{g}})^t$ is the outer product of the vector $(\mathbf{g} - \overline{\mathbf{g}})$ with itself.

As with the image mean, the image covariance can be related to the components of the image-generating equations to illustrate the role played by the signal, background, and system noise. Under the assumption that the background and system noise are uncorrelated with each other, and not influenced by the presence of the signal, the image covariance is identical under both of the signal-detection hypotheses, and given by

$$\mathbf{K_g} = \mathbf{K_b} + \mathbf{K_n}, \tag{11.5}$$

where $\mathbf{K_b}$ and $\mathbf{K_n}$ are the covariance matrices associated with the background and system noise respectively.

11.2.4 Scalar products with an image

Linear observers utilize a scalar product with the image as a fundamental part of the detection process. The scalar product serves to reduce the image to a scalar-valued decision variable (sometimes referred to as a test statistic or an internal response variable). A decision on the presence or absence of a signal is based on the value of this variable. For a given model, the statistical properties of the images influence the perceptual process to the extent that they propagate through the scalar product to the decision variable.

For a linear observer, the decision variable utilizes a weighted sum of the image intensity at all points in an image where the weights are independent of the image intensity. For discrete image vectors, the weights can be thought of as an

M-dimensional vector, like the image. The decision variable, denoted by λ, is computed from the sum

$$\lambda = \sum_{m=0}^{M-1} [\mathbf{w}]_m [\mathbf{g}]_m = \mathbf{w}^t \mathbf{g}. \tag{11.6}$$

The second equality of Eq. (11.6) serves to introduce the more compact vector notation for a scalar product between the vectors $\mathbf{w}$ and $\mathbf{g}$. Because $\mathbf{w}^t$ is a $1 \times M$ dimensional array and $\mathbf{g}$ is an $M \times 1$ dimensional array, their product is 1×1: a scalar. Vector notation will be used to avoid numerous summation symbols in the remaining formulas. The weighting vector, $\mathbf{w}$, is often referred to as an observer "template" because it is used in a pointwise multiplication of the image before summing to get λ.

The mean and variance of λ in Eq. (11.6) are completely determined by the image mean and covariance matrix. The mean value of λ, denoted $\bar{\lambda}$, is defined by the action of $\mathbf{w}$ on the image mean as

$$\bar{\lambda} = \mathbf{w}^t \bar{\mathbf{g}}. \tag{11.7}$$

The definition of $\bar{\lambda}$ can be specified to the signal-present or signal-absent hypotheses by substituting the appropriate expression from Eq. (11.4) for $\bar{\mathbf{g}}$. The variance of λ, denoted σ_λ^2, is determined from $\mathbf{w}$ and the image covariance $\mathbf{K_g}$ by the quadratic form

$$\sigma_\lambda^2 = \mathbf{w}^t \mathbf{K_g} \mathbf{w}. \tag{11.8}$$

11.3 Modeling signal-detection tasks

The preliminaries developed in the last section will now be used to describe an approach to modeling SKE detection. We begin with the formation of a decision variable as a function of an image. This step is common to any model of the signal-detection process. The discussion then turns to how the decision variable is used to make decisions regarding the presence or absence of the signal in a number of different kinds of detection experiments. This connection is motivated by the conviction that a model observer must be able to perform the same task as a human observer. Finally, the relationship of the detectability index to performance in each of the experimental paradigms is described. This relation is the basis for using the detectability index as a common figure of merit for detection performance.

11.3.1 Generation of a decision variable

Any method for performing a detection task can be cast as the formation of a scalar decision variable followed by a decision based on it. As in Section 11.2.4, the decision variable is denoted by λ. A general decision variable can be defined by the transformation

$$\lambda = w(\mathbf{g}) + n_{\text{int}}, \tag{11.9}$$

where $w(\mathbf{g})$ is a scalar-valued function (not necessarily a linear function) of the image vector $\mathbf{g}$, and n_{int} incorporates the effects of internal noise in the decision maker. Internal noise is a known component of human performance in detection tasks, and hence, important to include in models of perceptual performance [15, 16]. Internal noise is used to explain why human observers will make different decisions on the same set of images in repeated trials. Internal noise also accounts for one source of suboptimal performance in human observers.

The term "model" observer is used to describe a mathematical model that generates a decision variable. In other words, a particular functional form for w in Eq. (11.9) defines the deterministic component of a model observer. The model is not fully described until the distribution of the stochastic internal-noise component has been specified as well.

Linear-model observers, the subject of this chapter, generate a decision variable that is a linear function of the image with an added internal noise component. Hence the decision variable used by this class of observers can be written according to Eq. (11.6) using a scalar product between the image and a vector of weights. Linear observers specialize Eq. (11.9) to

$$\lambda = \mathbf{w}^t \mathbf{g} + n_{\text{int}}, \tag{11.10}$$

where $\mathbf{w}$ is the weighting vector, often referred to as the observer template. The weights determine how each point in the image is used to perform the task.

11.3.2 Making a decision

The way that a decision variable is used to actually make a decision depends on the type of detection task being performed. The decision process is described here for three different detection tasks. The goal is to show how a model observer test statistic, as defined in Eq. (11.10) can be used to generate the output of a detection experiment. For practical advantages and disadvantages of the experimental methods described here, see Burgess[17]. A thorough treatment of experimental methods in detection tasks can be found in Green and Swets [18].

11.3.2.1 The yes-no detection task

In a yes-no detection task, the observer is shown a single image and asked to indicate whether a signal is present or not in the image. For a model observer, the decision in a yes-no detection task is implemented by comparing the decision variable, λ defined in either Eq. (11.10) (or more generally in Eq. (11.9)), to a

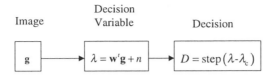

Image   Decision
               Variable   Decision

g → $\lambda = \mathbf{w}'\mathbf{g} + n$ → $D = \text{step}(\lambda - \lambda_c)$

Figure 11.2: Yes-no detection task. A schematic diagram of the model for deriving a decision for an input image stimuli.

threshold t. Let the decision be denoted by the variable D which is

$$D = \begin{cases} \text{Signal-present,} & \text{if } \lambda > t \\ \text{Signal-absent,} & \text{if } \lambda < t. \end{cases}$$

Note that a continuous distribution of λ has been assumed, and hence the probability of an equivocal decision in which $\lambda = t$ is negligible.

For a binary decision, it is common to associate the number 0 with a signal-absent decision, and 1 with a signal-present decision (regardless of whether these decisions are correct). Using this convention, D can be more compactly written as

$$D = \text{step}(\lambda - t),$$

where the step function is a binary-valued function that has a value of 1 for arguments greater than 0 and a value of 0 for arguments less than 0. Figure 11.2 illustrates the formation of a decision in a yes-no detection task.

11.3.2.2 The rating-scale detection task

In a rating-scale task, the observer is asked to give a score for each image indicating their confidence that a signal is present or absent. The score is presumed to have a monotonic relationship with the decision variable. The score can be obtained on an ordinal scale by recording decisions on a 6- or 10-point rating scale. In the lower limit of a two-point rating scale, this task is identical to yes-no detection. Ratings can also be recorded on an effectively continuous scale using a graphical device such as a slide-bar.

For an N-point rating scale, the decision, D, is commonly described by an integer from 1 to N. Conventions differ in the labelling of rating scales. For the purposes here, we will say values of D near N imply a high confidence that the signal is actually present in the image while values near 1 imply a high confidence that the signal is not present. Values of D in the middle of the rating scale indicate less confidence. The decision can be thought of as a quantized version of λ using

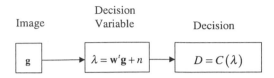

Figure 11.3: Rating-scale detection task. The diagram for deriving a decision in a rating-scale task for an input image stimuli.

multiple thresholds, t_1 to t_{N-1} according to

$$D = \begin{cases} 1 & \text{for } -\infty < \lambda < t_1 \\ \vdots & \vdots \\ i & \text{for } t_{i+1} < \lambda < t_i \\ \vdots & \vdots \\ N & \text{for } t_{N-1} < \lambda < \infty. \end{cases}$$

For a continuous score, there is no need to quantize the decision variable into a fixed number of categories. In this case the recorded decision can be thought of as a transformation of the decision variable to a confidence rating,

$$D = C(\lambda),$$

where C is presumed to be a monotonic function of the decision variable. Note that the decision in an N-point rating scale task can be thought of in terms of a "stair-step" function for $C(\lambda)$ with $N - 1$ steps occurring at t_1 to t_{N-1}. Figure 11.3 illustrates the formation of a decision in a rating-scale detection task.

11.3.2.3 Forced-choice detection

In forced choice detection, the observer is presented with M_A (where $M_A \geqslant 2$) images and asked (forced) to identify the image that contains the signal. Alternatively, a single image may be presented with multiple possible signal locations. Note that the number of alternatives in a forced-choice detection experiment is often referred to by the variable M. We use M_A to avoid confusion with the prior use of M as the number of pixels in the image (and hence the number of elements in the vector $\mathbf{g}$). The decision made in each trial identifies the image or a location within the image that is the most likely to contain the signal. Hence the decision is an index from 1 to M_A. A model observer for forced-choice detection tasks is be implemented by indexing the response to each image so that the M_A alternatives result in responses λ_j, $j = 1, \ldots, M_A$. The decision is then defined as the index of the maximum response.

While the actual decision made in each trial is the choice of an image, it is often more convenient to analyze the trial outcome—a binary variable that is 1 if the observer chooses the correct image in the trial and 0 otherwise. A model observer

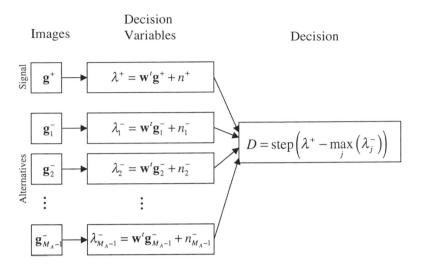

Figure 11.4: Multiple-alternative forced-choice detection task. The diagram for deriving a decision in a forced-choice task for M_A input image stimuli.

for forced-choice detection tasks can be implemented by presuming that the observer chooses the image with the largest response variable. Hence the outcome of the trial is 1 if the response to the signal-present image is larger than the response to any of the signal-absent images. If we denote the response to the signal-present image as λ^+, and to each of the signal-absent images as λ_j^-, where j runs from 1 to $M-1$, the resulting "decision" is given as

$$D = \text{step}\left(\lambda^+ - \max_{j=1,M_A-1}(\lambda_j^-)\right).$$

In the simplest case of a two-alternative forced-choice experiment, there is only one signal-absent image and hence the max is unnecessary, as is the subscript j. In this case the decision is defined as

$$D = \text{step}\left(\lambda^+ - \lambda^-\right).$$

Figure 11.4 illustrates the formation of a decision in a forced-choice detection task.

11.3.3 The detectability index as a figure of merit for detection performance

The detectability index, d', is a figure of merit that can be derived from all three of the detection experiments just described. Because d' has been used at times for various quantities that are equivalent only under assumptions, we will briefly describe the usage followed here. We begin by defining the observer signal-to-noise ratio for a detection task as

$$\text{SNR} = \frac{\bar{\lambda}^+ - \bar{\lambda}^-}{\sqrt{\frac{1}{2}\sigma_{\lambda^+}^2 + \frac{1}{2}\sigma_{\lambda^-}^2}}, \tag{11.11}$$

where $\bar{\lambda}^+$ and $\bar{\lambda}^-$ are the mean signal-present and signal-absent response, and $\sigma^2_{\lambda+}$ and $\sigma^2_{\lambda-}$ are their respective variances. Statisticians define a signal-to-noise ratio as the mean of a random variable divided by its standard deviation. As such, it is the inverse of the coefficient of variation. The random variable whose SNR is given in Eq. (11.11) is $\sqrt{2}(\lambda^+ - \lambda^-)$, where λ^+ is presumed to be independent of λ^-. For a modification to accommodate correlation between λ^+ and λ^-, see Eckstein *et al.* [19], Chapter 10.

We will follow the guidelines of Green and Swets [18] and define d' as a special case of the observer SNR in which λ^+ and λ^- are presumed to be independent Gaussians distributed with equal variance. In this case, $\sigma^2_{\lambda+} = \sigma^2_{\lambda-} = \sigma^2_{\lambda}$ and the expression in Eq. (11.11) reduces to

$$d' = \frac{\bar{\lambda}^+ - \bar{\lambda}^-}{\sigma_{\lambda}}. \tag{11.12}$$

For a linear observer, the detectability index can be expressed directly in terms of the image mean and covariance in the two signal-detection hypotheses, the observer template, and the variance of the internal noise component. Using the definitions of signal-present and signal-absent images in Eq. (11.2), it is straightforward to obtain the mean and variance of λ^+ and λ^-. These, combined with σ^2_{int}, the variance of the internal noise component, result in

$$d' = \frac{\mathbf{w}^t \mathbf{s}}{\sqrt{\mathbf{w}^t \mathbf{K_g} \mathbf{w} + \sigma^2_{\text{int}}}}. \tag{11.13}$$

Yes-no, rating-scale, and forced-choice detection experiments can all be used to obtain detectability indices that are equivalent to d' under some attendant assumptions. Because of these assumptions, it is important to make clear the distinction between d' given in Eq. (11.13) and detectability indices derived from the various detection tasks. The detectability indices defined below have a subscript indicating the task from which each was derived. Formulas for the detectability in each experiment are given along with the conditions necessary for equivalence to d'.

11.3.3.1 Yes-no detection

The yes-no detection task described above in Section 11.3.2.1 is performed by comparing the decision variable, λ, to a threshold, t. There are four possible outcomes of this comparison in any given trial. When the signal is actually present and the observer correctly identifies it as so, the decision is called a true positive (TP). Alternatively, the observer may incorrectly identify the image as signal absent, in which case the decision is called a false negative (FN). When a signal is not actually present in the image and the observer incorrectly decides that it is, the decision is called a false positive (FP). Finally, if the observer correctly decides that the signal is absent, the decision is called a true negative (TN).

The true-positive fraction (TPF) is the probability that $D = 1$ (a signal-present decision is made) given that the signal is truly present in the image. The TPF is defined in terms of the observer response variable and the threshold as $\Pr(\lambda^+ > t)$ (recall that λ^+ is the observer response variable given that the image is present and λ^- is the response given that the signal is absent). The false-negative fraction (FNF) is defined as the probability that $D = 0$ (a signal-absent decision is made) given that a signal is truly present in the image. This probability is given by $\Pr(\lambda^+ < t)$, and is therefore determined by $1-$ TPF. The false-positive fraction (FPF) is the probability that $D = 1$, given that the signal is not actually present in the image. The FPF is given by $\Pr(\lambda^- > t)$. Finally, the true-negative fraction (TNF) is defined as the probability that $D = 0$ given that the signal is absent. Like the TPF and FNF, the TNF (given by $\Pr(\lambda^- < t)$) is completely determined by $1 -$ FPF.

Because of the close relation between the TPF and FNF, and between the FPF and TNF, the detection performance in a yes-no task is conventionally summarized by the TPF and FPF observed in an experiment. A detectability index for yes-no detection tasks can be defined from the TPF and FPF as

$$d_{\text{YN}} = \Phi^{-1}(\text{TPF}) - \Phi^{-1}(\text{FPF}), \qquad (11.14)$$

where Φ^{-1} is the inverse of the cumulative normal distribution function. Under the assumption that λ^+ and λ^- both obey Gaussian distributions that have equal variances ($\sigma_{\lambda^+}^2 = \sigma_{\lambda^-}^2$), $d_{\text{YN}} = d'$ within measurement error.

11.3.3.2 Rating-scale detection

The yes-no detection task is often thought of as producing a single point on the receiver-operating-characteristic (ROC) curve whereas rating-scale detection experiments can generate the entire ROC curve. An ROC curve plots the TPF as a function of the FPF as the detection threshold, t, goes from ∞ to $-\infty$. Hence, progressing from left to right on the ROC curve implies moving t from right to left. The curve starts at the point $(0, 0)$ and increases monotonically to the point $(1, 1)$. The point $(0, 0)$ corresponds to setting the yes-no detection threshold higher than any possible observer response (for example $t = \infty$). This point is the equivalent of a yes-no experiment in which the observer always decides "signal absent" regardless of the image data. Such an observer would never make a false-positive decision because a positive (signal-present) decision is never made. As a result, the FPF is zero for this threshold setting. The TPF is zero for the same reason. At the other extreme, the point $(1, 1)$ corresponds to setting t lower than any possible observer response. In this case, the detection strategy decides "signal present" regardless of the image. The monotonic increase in the curve results from the increase in the TPF and FPF as t is decreased. A description of the process by which the ROC curve is estimated from rating-scale data is beyond the scope of this chapter. However, thorough treatments of this subject can be found in the work of Dorfman *et al.* [20–22], Green and Swets [18], Swets and Pickett [23], and Metz [24–26]. There is also a chapter of this volume dedicated to ROC methodology (Chapter 15).

The ROC curve provides a flexible and complete description of detection performance by an observer. However, the ROC curve itself is not a scalar figure of merit, and hence one has to know how to say one ROC curve is better than another in order to say that one system is better than another. Typically, the area under the ROC curve (AUC) is used to summarize an entire ROC curve in a single scalar figure of merit that can be used for optimizing diagnostic imaging. In principle, the AUC ranges from 0 to 1, but generally it should be above the chance level of 0.5; a detection strategy that results in an AUC that is less than the chance level probably indicates a misspecification of the task to the observer. The opposite detection strategy, one that chooses signal present whenever the original detector chooses signal absent and vice versa, results in higher performance than the original. The detectability index derived from a rating-scale experiment is defined as

$$d_A = \sqrt{2}\Phi^{-1}(\text{AUC}). \tag{11.15}$$

If the internal decision variable is normally distributed under each hypothesis with equal variance, then d_A is equivalent to d'. If the decision variable is Gaussian but with different variances, d_A is still equivalent to the observer SNR of Eq. (11.11). Hence, this equivalence is slightly more general than the equivalence in yes-no detection tasks because it holds even when the internal response variables have different variances under the two signal-detection hypotheses.

11.3.3.3 Forced-choice detection

The result of a forced-choice detection experiment is usually an estimate of proportion correct (PC), the fraction of trials that are answered correctly on average. Because PC is scalar valued and can be readily related to detection performance (better performance implies increased PC), it is often reported as a figure of merit.

The detectability is defined implicitly from PC by the formula

$$\text{PC} = \int d\lambda\, \phi(\lambda - d_{\text{MAFC}})\Phi(\lambda)^{M_A - 1}, \tag{11.16}$$

where $\phi(\cdots)$ is the standard normal probability density function. The detectability index is determined by finding the value of d_{MAFC} such that equality holds. The implicit equation for d_{MAFC} can be solved using tabulated values [27], or by standard root finding methods from numerical analysis [28]. In the special case of two-alternative forced choice (2AFC), the integral for PC can be determined analytically as

$$\text{PC} = \int d\lambda\, \phi(\lambda - d_{\text{2AFC}})\Phi(\lambda)$$
$$= \Phi\left(\frac{d_{\text{2AFC}}}{\sqrt{2}}\right).$$

This leads to an explicit formula for $d_{2\text{AFC}}$ as

$$d_{2\text{AFC}} = \sqrt{2}\Phi^{-1}(\text{PC}). \tag{11.17}$$

The close resemblance of $d_{2\text{AFC}}$ in Eq. (11.17) to d_{AUC} in Eq. (11.15) reflects that fact that AUC and PC from 2AFC are identical quantities as long as the definition of the internal response variable remains consistent between the two experiments [18]. With human observers, differences between $d_{2\text{AFC}}$ and d_{AUC} have been observed [29] with detectability determined from forced-choice experiments generally slightly larger than the detectability determined from rating-scale experiments. This disparity may result from inefficient use of the rating scale by the observers in the form of additional "rating-scale noise" in the internal noise of the observer.

11.4 Linear model observers

In this section we describe a few specific observers as examples of how observer templates are defined. A more extensive treatment of various model observers is given in Chapter 10. A review of attempts to match human-observer performance with these models (and others) can also be found in Chapter 10 and in a recent report from the International Commission on Radiation Units and Measurements [4]. The treatment given here is derived from Abbey [30].

11.4.1 The Hotelling observer

The Hotelling observer was introduced to medical imaging from the pattern recognition literature [31] by Barrett and coworkers [32–34] by means of the Hotelling trace criterion (HTC). This figure of merit, in turn, had been brought to pattern recognition from the work of Harold Hotelling in the mathematical-statistics literature beginning the early 1930s [35].

The HTC is a figure of merit for task performance that applies to general classification tasks. In the special case of detection tasks (a classification task with only two classes), the HTC reduces to the observer SNR defined in Eq. (11.11).

The Hotelling observer is the observer template used for the HTC in a detection task. For an SKE detection tasks in the presence of Gaussian-distributed image variability, the Hotelling observer is equivalent to the ideal observer as described in Chapter 9. The detectability of the Hotelling observer given below is identical to that given in Eq. (9.30) of that chapter.

The Hotelling observer is computed from the image mean and covariance, and can be shown to maximize d' in Eq. (11.13) in the absence of internal noise ($\sigma_\varepsilon^2 = 0$). Furthermore, if the images in a SKE detection task are Gaussian distributed with equal covariance matrices for both the signal-present and signal-absent classes then the Hotelling observer is equivalent to the ideal observer. These two properties make the Hotelling observer an attractive observer to consider in place of the ideal observer when the image distributions are unknown or difficult to evaluate.

In the absence of internal noise and assuming an invertible image covariance matrix, the Hotelling-observer template is given by

$$\mathbf{w}_{\text{Hot}} = \mathbf{K_g}^{-1}\mathbf{s}, \tag{11.18}$$

where $\mathbf{K_g}$ is the image covariance matrix and $\mathbf{s}$ is the mean signal. The functional form of $\mathbf{w}_{\text{Hot}}$ can be shown to maximize d'. Under the given conditions, the detectability of the signal by the Hotelling observer simplifies to

$$d'_{\text{Hot}} = \sqrt{\mathbf{s}^t \mathbf{K_g}^{-1} \mathbf{s}}. \tag{11.19}$$

When $\mathbf{K_g}$ is singular, the definition of the Hotelling observer given in Eq. (11.18) and the Hotelling-observer detectability in Eq. (11.19) can be modified by using the Moore-Penrose pseudoinverse provided that $\mathbf{s}$ does not contain any null vectors of $\mathbf{K_g}$.

Because the Hotelling observer is defined in terms of the inverse (or pseudoinverse) of the image covariance, some care must be used in its evaluation. Direct inversion of the image covariance may be a prohibitive operation because of the large size of the matrix. Fiete [36] suggests a viable alternative to direct inversion of $\mathbf{K_g}$ by casting the Hotelling-observer template as the solution of the linear system of equations

$$\mathbf{K_g}\mathbf{w}_{\text{Hot}} = \mathbf{s}.$$

This linear system can be solved iteratively using any of a number of algorithms for large linear systems [37].

Including internal noise in the Hotelling observer response requires some care. If the variance of the internal-noise component is simply fixed at a constant value, then it is clearly advantageous in Eq. (11.13) to let the magnitude of the template get large enough that σ_ε^2 is negligible when compared to $\mathbf{w}^t \mathbf{K}\mathbf{w}$. To avoid this sort of magnitude effect, the internal-noise variance can be made proportional to the amplitude of the template. One way to do this is to define the internal noise variance as

$$\sigma_\varepsilon^2 = \mathbf{w}^t \mathbf{K}_{\text{Int.}}\mathbf{w}.$$

This approach is derived from the work of Ahumada [38] who describes it as putting the internal noise into the image. Note that with σ_ε^2 defined in this way, d' is invariant to a change in the amplitude of the template. For the internal noise covariance $\mathbf{K}_{\text{Int.}}$, the Hotelling observer template is given by

$$\mathbf{w}_{\text{Hot}} = (\mathbf{K_g} + \mathbf{K}_{\text{Int.}})^{-1}\mathbf{s},$$

and the Hotelling observer detectability is

$$d'_{\text{Hot}} = \sqrt{\mathbf{s}^t (\mathbf{K_g} + \mathbf{K}_{\text{Int.}})^{-1} \mathbf{s}}.$$

Particular care must be taken when estimating the mean and covariance used in the Hotelling observer from samples. It is tempting to estimate $\mathbf{w}_{\text{Hot}}$ by simply replacing the image mean and covariance by their sample estimates. The resulting estimate of detectability may be highly inaccurate because the inverse of a sample covariance is generally a poor estimate of the inverse covariance unless an enormous number of sample images are available. Better estimates of the inverse covariance are possible when constraints apply. Examples of constraints that have been used to this end are stationarity [39] and limitations in spatial extent [40]. Another approach that uses feature responses is described below in Section 11.4.3.

11.4.2 Nonprewhitening observer

The nonprewhitening (NPW) observer is defined as the output of a template that is tuned (or adapted) to the mean value of the signal. The observer does not incorporate knowledge of the image covariance matrix into the into the observer template, and hence, when strong pixel-to-pixel correlations exist in the images, the NPW observer can be highly suboptimal. In a number of earlier works [41–46], and a few more recent ones [47], the suboptimal performance of the NPW observer was found to match the performance of human observers. However, other recent works [6, 10] have shown that this is not always the case. In particular, Burgess *et al.* [10] presented human-observer data in which the correlation structure of the noise was manipulated so that an observer which did not adapt to the correlation structure of the noise would achieve a slope of unity on a particular log-log plot. They found that human-observer performance did not have a slope of unity indicating that human observers can incorporate knowledge of the image covariance (in some form) into their detection strategy. Nonetheless, the NPW observer is easy to evaluate and remains an interesting model observer because of the number of cases in which it has been predictive of human performance.

The NPW observer presented in Eq. (11.20) is equivalent to the Hotelling observer when the image covariance is proportional to the identity matrix (i.e., $\mathbf{K_g} = \sigma^2 \mathbf{I}$). Hence the NPW is equivalent to the ideal observer when the image variability is Gaussian-distributed white noise.

The observer template associated with the NPW observer is defined by

$$\mathbf{w}_{\text{NPW}} = \mathbf{s}. \tag{11.20}$$

It is evident from the form of Eq. (11.20) that the image covariance does not explicitly enter into the form of the observer template, and hence the observer template does not depend on pixel-to-pixel correlations in the image. Even though the image covariance does not affect the observer template, the covariance will still be a factor determining the observer detectability.

The NPW observer is often modified to incorporate a contrast sensitivity function meant to model the contrast sensitivity of the human visual system [41, 47]. There is no general consensus on the form of this contrast-sensitivity function, other than it is bandpass with a peak frequency in the range of the optimal visual contrast-sensitivity human near four cycles per degree visual angle. This eye-filtered NPW observer, abbreviated NPWE, is defined by

$$\mathbf{w}_{\mathrm{NPWE}} = \mathbf{E}\mathbf{s},$$

where the matrix $\mathbf{E}$ represents the linear process of filtering by the visual contrast-sensitivity function. Incorporation of an eye filter generally improves the agreement with human observers.

11.4.3 Channelized-Hotelling observers

The channelized-Hotelling observer was introduced by Myers [48], and Myers and Barrett [49] as a way to incorporate elements from human visual system into models of signal detection for medical imaging. The notion of spatial-frequency-selective channels (or receptive fields) in the human visual system has long been part of the field of vision science [50–52], and has often been incorporated into models of visual detection in this field [53, 54]. The inclusion of channel mechanisms gave a visual "front end" to model observers in medical imaging. The addition of channels to the Hotelling detection strategy led to agreement with human observers in a number of detection experiments that included correlated noise with both highpass and lowpass power spectra [11].

In the first implementations of the channelized-Hotelling observer just described, the channel responses were formed by integrating distinct (nonoverlapping) octave-wide bands of radial frequencies. This particular form for the channel profiles had attractive orthogonality properties for signals embedded in stationary noise. The lack of orientation channels was justified on the grounds that rotationally symmetric signals embedded in noise with an isotropic noise-power spectrum do not result in any preferential orientations.

More recent implementations of the channelized-Hotelling observer have used nonorthogonal, overlapping channel profiles [55–57]. In a few cases, orientation-tuned channels have been used as well [10, 58]. The channelized Hotelling observer has generally resulted in good agreement with human-observer data. However, it is important to note that the various implementations of this observer used different choices of the channel parameters (such as the channel profiles, or total number of channels), and hence it is not yet clear whether one choice of model parameters will simultaneously fit all the human data.

A somewhat different use of the channelized-Hotelling observer has been as an approximation to the Hotelling observer. The channelized-Hotelling observer is equivalent to the Hotelling observer when the observer template of the latter can be expressed as a linear combination of the channel profiles. In this case the channels are not chosen to represent components of the human visual system, but rather as a limited set of basis vectors for representing the Hotelling-observer template. As will be seen below, the resulting expression for the observer template does not require the inversion of the full image covariance. Barrett *et al.* [59] have successfully applied this strategy using Laguerre–Gauss functions for the channel profiles.

The channelized-Hotelling observer performs a detection task after first reducing the image to a set of channel-response variables. The channels of the channelized-Hotelling observer provide a mechanism for partial adaptation to image statistics and suboptimal performance. The role of the channels is to reduce the input image to a set of channel responses by inner products between the image $\mathbf{g}$ and the filter associated with each channel. A diagram of the formation of a decision variable is given in Figure 11.5. For a channel model with a total of N_C channels, the channel responses are the elements of an N_C-dimensional vector $\mathbf{u}$, defined as

$$\mathbf{u} = \mathbf{T}^t \mathbf{g} + \boldsymbol{\varepsilon}, \tag{11.21}$$

where $\mathbf{T}$ is an $M \times N_C$ matrix whose columns are of the various channel filters, and $\boldsymbol{\varepsilon}$ is a random vector representing the internal noise present (if any) in each channel response. In most practical implementations of channelized observers, N_C/M is in the range of 10^{-2} to 10^{-5}, and hence the transformation from $\mathbf{g}$ to $\mathbf{u}$ represents a large dimensionality reduction. These dimensions make $\mathbf{T}$ a highly rectangular matrix.

The internal noise in the channels is presumed to be zero mean with a covariance matrix $\mathbf{K}_{\boldsymbol{\varepsilon}}$. The internal noise in each channel response is usually assumed to be independent from channel to channel, and hence $\mathbf{K}_{\boldsymbol{\varepsilon}}$ is an $N_C \times N_C$ diagonal matrix with each diagonal element representing the variance of the internal-noise component in the corresponding channel.

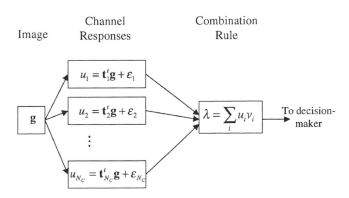

Figure 11.5: Diagram of the formation of a decision variable by a channelized-Hotelling observer. Each of the channel filters, $\mathbf{t}_1, \ldots, \mathbf{t}_{N_C}$, is a column of the channel matrix $\mathbf{T}$. The channel weights are given in $v_1 \ldots v_{N_C}$.

In order to produce a scalar test statistic, the observer must compute a scalar function from the vector $\mathbf{u}$. The act of reducing the channel-response vector to a scalar defines a channel-combination rule. We will consider linear-combination rules in this work although nonlinear-combination rules are often used to explain detection performance in classical masking experiments from vision science. A linear-combination rule is defined by an inner product between the channel responses in $\mathbf{u}$ and a fixed vector, $\mathbf{v}$, of channel weights. The resulting observer response is given by

$$\lambda = \mathbf{v}^t \mathbf{u}$$
$$= \mathbf{v}^t \left(\mathbf{T}^t \mathbf{g} + \boldsymbol{\varepsilon} \right). \tag{11.22}$$

If we equate the deterministic components of Eq. (11.22) to the deterministic components of the linear-observer template of Eq. (11.10), we see that the channelized-observer template is given by

$$\mathbf{w}_{\text{Chan}} = \mathbf{T}\mathbf{v}. \tag{11.23}$$

Similarly, the random components of Eq. (11.22) and Eq. (11.10) can be equated yielding an internal noise component defined by

$$n_{\text{int}} = \mathbf{v}^t \boldsymbol{\varepsilon}.$$

The variance of the internal noise term used in formulas for the SNR is then given by

$$\sigma_{\text{int}}^2 = \mathbf{v}^t \mathbf{K}_\varepsilon \mathbf{v}. \tag{11.24}$$

The channelized-Hotelling observer can be thought of as the Hotelling-observer strategy applied to the channel responses, $\mathbf{u}$, rather than the image vector, $\mathbf{g}$. In order to apply the Hotelling strategy, we need to know the first- and second-order moments of $\mathbf{u}$ under each of the task hypotheses. Because the operations involved in forming the channel responses are linear, the moments of $\mathbf{u}$ can be obtained by straightforward transformations of the moments of $\mathbf{g}$. The mean value of $\mathbf{u}$ under the two task hypothesis are given by

$$\text{Signal-present images } (h_2): \quad \bar{\mathbf{u}} = \mathbf{T}^t (\mathbf{s} + \bar{\mathbf{b}})$$
$$\text{Signal-absent images } (h_1): \quad \bar{\mathbf{u}} = \mathbf{T}^t \bar{\mathbf{b}}. \tag{11.25}$$

The covariance matrix for $\mathbf{u}$ is the same under the two task hypotheses and is given by

$$\mathbf{K_u} = \mathbf{T}^t \mathbf{K_g} \mathbf{T} + \mathbf{K}_\varepsilon. \tag{11.26}$$

For the two mean channel-response vectors given in Eq. (11.25), and channel co-variance given in Eq. (11.26), the combination rule corresponding to the Hotelling strategy is given by

$$\mathbf{v}_{\text{Hot}} = \mathbf{K_u}^{-1}\mathbf{T}^t\mathbf{s}. \tag{11.27}$$

The detectability associated with these channel weights is derived from Eq. (11.19) to be

$$d'_{\text{CH}} = \sqrt{\mathbf{v}_{\text{Hot}}^t\mathbf{K_u}^{-1}\mathbf{v}_{\text{Hot}}}. \tag{11.28}$$

The channelized-Hotelling observer template can be obtained by substituting Eq. (11.27) into Eq. (11.23) to get

$$\begin{aligned}\mathbf{w}_{\text{CH}} &= \mathbf{T}\mathbf{v}_{\text{Hot}} \\ &= \mathbf{T}\mathbf{K_u}^{-1}\mathbf{T}^t\mathbf{s}.\end{aligned}$$

We can further tie definition of the channelized-Hotelling observer to the image domain by replacing $\mathbf{K_u}$ by its definition in Eq. (11.26) to obtain

$$\mathbf{w}_{\text{CH}} = \mathbf{T}(\mathbf{T}^t\mathbf{K_g}\mathbf{T} + \mathbf{K_\varepsilon})^{-1}\mathbf{T}^t\mathbf{s}. \tag{11.29}$$

The internal noise variance in the channelized-Hotelling decision variable caused by noise in the channels is derived from Eq. (11.24) to be

$$\begin{aligned}\sigma_{\text{int}}^2 &= \mathbf{v}_{\text{Hot}}^t\mathbf{K_\varepsilon}\mathbf{v}_{\text{Hot}} \\ &= \mathbf{s}\mathbf{T}(\mathbf{T}^t\mathbf{K_g}\mathbf{T} + \mathbf{K_\varepsilon})^{-1}\mathbf{K_\varepsilon}(\mathbf{T}^t\mathbf{K_g}\mathbf{T} + \mathbf{K_\varepsilon})^{-1}\mathbf{T}^t\mathbf{s}.\end{aligned} \tag{11.30}$$

Equations (11.29) and (11.30) demonstrate that the channelized-Hotelling observer can be implemented as a single spatial template with an internal noise component, and hence, this observer fits the definition of a linear observer in Eq. (11.10). The observer template and the internal noise variance of the channelized-Hotelling observer can be used to obtain the performance of the channelized-Hotelling observer in terms of the mean signal and image covariance (as well as $\mathbf{T}$ and $\mathbf{K_\varepsilon}$). The detectability of the channelized-Hotelling observer is found by using the template and internal noise variance from Eq. (11.29) and Eq. (11.30) in Eq. (11.13). The resulting expression simplifies to

$$d'_{\text{CH}} = \sqrt{\mathbf{s}^t\mathbf{T}(\mathbf{T}^t\mathbf{K_g}\mathbf{T} + \mathbf{K_\varepsilon})^{-1}\mathbf{T}^t\mathbf{s}}. \tag{11.31}$$

A very important practical point is that the channelized-Hotelling observer avoids some computational difficulties of the Hotelling observer. Because of the transformation by $\mathbf{T}$, the dimension of the necessary inverse has been reduced to the dimension of the channel responses. This reduction in dimension is generally great enough that the inverse of the channel covariance matrix, $\mathbf{T}^t \mathbf{K_g T} + \mathbf{K}_\varepsilon$, can be obtained directly even when the large dimension of $\mathbf{g}$ makes inversion of $\mathbf{K_g}$ infeasible. The reduction in dimension also allows reasonable estimates of the inverse matrix from samples.

11.5 Summary

In this chapter we have described an approach to modeling human-observer performance in noise-limited signal-detection tasks. The central premise of the approach has been that the human observer adopts a linear-detection strategy in which the pixel intensities of the image are weighted and then summed to form a decision variable. The distribution of the decision variable can be used to obtain various quantities that describe how well the observer performs the task such as the ROC curve, the detectability index d', proportion correct PC, and sensitivity and specificity. Under Gaussian assumptions on the decision variable, these figures of merit for detection performance are all directly related to each other and determined by the mean and variance of the internal response. The fact that we can obtain these quantities from the model observers and compare them to estimates of the same quantities for human observers forms the basis for using these models as way to both understand how human observers perform this kind of detection task and to predict performance levels without time-consuming observer-performance studies.

A few particular model observers have been described in detail (many more are described in Chapter 10) to illustrate some of the variety of models that have been investigated in this context. The differences between the various models illustrate how statistical properties of the images influence the form of these models. Examples included the nonprewhitening observer that is only sensitive to the mean spatial profile of the signal and the Hotelling observer that uses perfect knowledge of both the signal profile and the covariance of the noise. Other models, such as the nonprewhitening eye-filter observer and channelized Hotelling observer, mediate knowledge of the image statistics by known components of the human visual system such as contrast sensitivity, visual channels, and internal noise.

The ultimate goal of finding a single model observer that will predict human-observer performance in all relevant situations is still an area of active research. In the meantime, model observers are increasing being used to augment, or even replace, human-observer studies. For evaluating areas such as lossy image compression, image reconstruction, and novel imaging geometries, model observers are increasingly being used to fine-tune imaging parameters for better observer performance.

Acknowledgments

The authors have benefitted from discussions and input from Harrison Barrett, Arthur Burgess, Miguel Eckstein, Harold Kundel, and Kyle Myers. The first author would like to thank in particular Miguel Eckstein, for a careful reading of the manuscript, and Harrison Barrett, for introducing him to the subject matter and teaching him the approach presented here. CKA was supported by NIH R01 HL54011 and FOB was supported by NIH R01 HL53455.

References

[1] Revesz G, Kundel HL, Graber MA. "The Influence of Structured Noise on the Detection of Radiologic Abnormalities." Invest Radiol 9:479–486, 1974.

[2] Ruttiman UE, Webber RL. "A Simple Model Combining Quantum Noise and Anatomical Variation in Radiographs." Med Phys 11:50–60, 1984.

[3] Barrett HH. "Objective Assessment of Image Quality: Effects of Quantum Noise and Object Variability." J Opt Soc Am A 7:1266–1278, 1990.

[4] ICRU Report 54, "Medical Imaging—the Assessment of Image Quality." International Commission on Radiation Units and Measurements, 1995.

[5] Myers KJ, Rolland JP, Barrett HH, Wagner RM. "Aperture Optimization for Emission Imaging: Effect of a Spatially Varying Background." J Opt Soc Am A 7:1279–1293, 1990.

[6] Rolland JP, Barrett HH. "Effect of Random Background Inhomogeneity on Observer Detection Performance." J Opt Soc Am A 9:649–658, 1992.

[7] Eckstein MP, Whiting JS. "Visual Signal Detection in Structured Backgrounds I. Effect of Number of Possible Locations and Signal Contrast." J Opt Soc Am A 14:2406–2419, 1996.

[8] Samei E, Flynn MJ, Beue GH, Peterson E. "Comparison of Observer Performance for Real and Simulated Nodules in Chest Radiography." Proc SPIE 2712:60–70, 1996.

[9] Eckstein MP, Ahumada AJ, Watson AB. "Visual Signal Detection in Structured Backgrounds. II. Effects of Contrast Gain Control, Background Variations, and White Noise." J Opt Soc Am A 13:1777–1787, 1997.

[10] Burgess AE, Li X , Abbey CK. "Visual Signal Detectability with Two Noise Components: Anomalous Masking Effects." J Opt Soc Am A 14:2420–2442, 1997.

[11] Barrett HH, Yao J, Rolland JP, Myers KJ. "Model Observers for the Assessment of Image Quality." Proc Natl Acad Sci 90:9758–9765, 1993.

[12] Watson AB, Pelli DG. "QUEST: a Bayesian Adaptive Psychometric Method." Perceptual Psychophysics 33:113–120, 1983.

[13] Hoel PG, Port SC, Stone CJ. *Introduction to Stochastic Processes*. Illinois: Waveland Press, 1972.

[14] Smith WE, Barrett HH. "Hotelling Trace Criterion as a Figure of Merit for the Optimization of Imaging Systems." J Opt Soc Am A 11:1237–1242, 1994.

[15] Burgess AE, Colborne B. "Visual Signal Detection. IV. Observer Inconsistency." J Opt Soc Am A 5:617–627, 1988.

[16] Pelli D. Effects of Visual Noise, Ph.D. Dissertation, University of Cambridge, Cambridge, 1981.

[17] Burgess AE. "Comparison of Receiver Operating Characteristic and Forced Choice Observer Performance Measurement Methods." Med Phys 22(5):643–655, 1995.

[18] Green DM, Swets JA. *Signal Detection Theory and Psychophysics.* New York: John Wiley and Sons, 1966.

[19] Eckstein MP, Abbey CK, Bochud FO. "Visual Signal Detection in Structured Backgrounds IV. Figures of Merit for Model Performance in Multiple Alternative Forced Choice Detection Tasks with Correlated Responses." Accepted for publication in J Opt Soc Am A.

[20] Dorfman DD, Alf E. "Maximum Likelihood Estimation of Parameters of Signal Detection Theory and Determination of Confidence Intervals-Rating Method Data." Journal of Mathematical Psychology 6:487–496, 1969.

[21] Dorfman DD. "RSCORE 11." In Swets JA, Pickett MR (Eds.) *Evaluation of Diagnostic Systems: Methods from Signal Detection Theory.* New York: Academic Press, 1982.

[22] Dorfman DD, Berbaum KS. "RSCORE-J: Pooled Rating-Method Data: A Computer Program for Analyzing Pooled ROC Curves." Behavior Research Methods, Instruments, & Computers 18:452–462, 1986.

[23] Swets JA, Pickett RM. *Evaluation of Diagnostic Systems.* New York: Academic Press, 1982.

[24] Metz CE. "Basic Principles of ROC Anaysis." Seminars in Nucl Med 8:283–298, 1978.

[25] Metz CE. "ROC Methodology in Radiological Imaging." Invest Radiol 21:720–733, 1986.

[26] Metz CE. "Some Practical Issues of Experimental Design and Data Analysis in Radiological ROC Studies." Invest Radiol 24:234–245, 1989.

[27] Elliot P. "Forced Choice Tables," Appendix I. In Swets JA (Ed.) *Signal Detection and Recognition by Human Observers: Contemporary Readings.* New York: Wiley and Sons, Inc., 1964.

[28] Dahlquist G, Björck A. *Numerical Methods.* New Jersey: Prentice-Hall, Inc., 1974.

[29] Herrmann C, Buhr E, Hoeschen D, Fan SY. "Comparison of ROC and AFC Methods in a Visual Detection Task." Phys Med Biol 20:805–811, 1993.

[30] Abbey CK. Assessment of Reconstructed Images, Ph.D. Dissertation, University of Arizona, Tucson, 1998.

[31] Fukunaga K. *Introduction to Statistical Pattern Recognition.* New York: Academic, 1972.

[32] Barrett HH, Myers KJ, Wagner RF. "Beyond Signal-Detection Theory." Proc SPIE 626:231–239, 1986.

[33] Fiete RD, Barrett HH, Smith WE, Myers KJ. "The Hotelling Trace Criterion and Its Correlation with Human Observer Performance." J Opt Soc Am A 3:717–725, 1987.

[34] Fiete RD, Barrett HH. "Using the Hotelling Trace Criterion for Feature Enhancement in Image Processing." Optics Letters 12:643–645, 1987.

[35] Hotelling H. "The Generalization of Student's Ratio." Ann of Math Statist 2:360–378, 1931.

[36] Fiete RD. The Hotelling Trace Criterion Used for System Optimization and Feature Enhancement in Nuclear Medicine, Ph.D. Dissertation, University of Arizona, Tucson, 1987.

[37] Golub GH, Van Loan CF. *Matrix Computations*, Second Edition. Baltimore: Johns Hopkins University Press, 1989.

[38] Ahumada AJ. "Putting the Noise of the Visual System Back in the Picture." J Opt Soc Am A 4:2372–2378, 1987.

[39] Wagner RF, Brown DG. "Unified SNR Analysis of Medical Imaging Systems." Phys Med Biol 30:489–518, 1985.

[40] Eckstein MP, Whiting JS. "Lesion Detection in Structured Noise." Acad Radiol 2:249–253, 1995.

[41] Loo L-N, Doi K, Metz CE. "A Comparison of Physical Image Quality Indices and Observer Performance in the Radiographic Detection of Nylon Beads." Phys Med Biol 29:837–856, 1984.

[42] Ishida M, Doi K, Loo L-N, Metz CE, Lehr JL. "Digital Image Processing: Effect on Detectability of Simulated Low-Contrast Radiographic Patterns." Radiology 150:569–575, 1984.

[43] Loo L-N, Doi K, Metz CE. "Investigation of Basic Imaging Properties in Digital Radiography. 4. Effect of Unsharp Masking on the Detectability of Simple Patterns." Med Phys 29:209–214, 1985.

[44] Myers KJ, Barrett HH, Borgstrom MC, Patton DD, Seeley GW. "Effect of Noise Correlation on the Detectability of Disk Signals in Medical Imaging." J Opt Soc Am A 2:1752–1759, 1985.

[45] Judy PF, Swensson RG. "Detectability of Lesions of Various Sizes on CT Images." Proc SPIE 535:38–42, 1985.

[46] Judy PF, Swensson RG. "Size Discrimination of Features on CT Images." Proc SPIE 626:225–230, 1986.

[47] Burgess AE. "Statistically Defined Backgrounds: Performance of a Modified Nonprewhitening Matched Filter Model." J Opt Soc Am A 11:1237–1242, 1994.

[48] Myers KJ. Visual Perception in Correlated Noise, Ph.D. Dissertation, University of Arizona, Tucson, 1985.

[49] Myers KJ, Barrett HH. "The Addition of a Channel Mechanism to the Ideal-Observer Model." J Opt Soc Am A 4:2447–2457, 1987.

[50] Campbell FW, Robson JG. "Application of Fourier Analysis to the Visibility of Gratings." J Physiol Lond 197:551–556, 1968.

[51] Sachs M, Nachmias J, Robson JG. "Spatial-Frequency Channels in Human Vision." J Opt Soc Am 61:1176–1186, 1971.

[52] Graham N, Nachmias J. "Detection of Grating Patterns Containing Two Spatial Frequencies: A Comparison of Single-Channel and Multiple-Channels Models." Vis Res 11:251–259, 1971.

[53] Watson AB. "Detection and Recognition of Simple Spatial Forms." In Sander OJ, Sleigh AJ (Eds.) *Physical and Biological Processing of Images*. Berlin: Springer-Verlag, 1983.

[54] Daly S. "The Visible Differences Predictor: An Algorithm for the Assessment of Image Fidelity." In Watson AB (Ed.) *Digital Images and Human Vision*. Cambridge, Mass: MIT Press, 1993.

[55] Abbey CK, Barrett HH. "Linear Iterative Reconstruction Algorithms: Study of Observer Performance." In Bizais Y, Barillot C, Di Paola R (Eds.) *Proc 14th Int Conf on Information Processing in Medical Imaging*. Dordrecht: Kluwer Academic, pp. 65–76, 1995.

[56] Abbey CK, Barrett HH, Wilson DW. "Observer Signal-to-Noise Ratios for the ML-EM Algorithm." Proc SPIE 2712:47–58, 1996.

[57] King MA, de Vries DJ , Soares EJ. "Comparison of the Channelized Hotelling and Human Observers for Lesion Detection in Hepatic SPECT Imaging." Proc SPIE 3036:14–20, 1997.

[58] Eckstein MP, Whiting JS. "Lesion Detection in Structured Noise." Acad Radiol 2:249–253, 1995.

[59] Barrett HH, Abbey CK, Gallas B, Eckstein MP. "Stabilized Estimates of Hotelling Observer Performance in Patient-Structured Noise." Proc SPIE 3340:27–43, 1998.

CHAPTER 12
Effects of Anatomical Structure on Signal Detection

Ehsan Samei
Duke University

William Eyler
Henry Ford Hospital

Lisa Baron
Medical University of South Carolina

CONTENTS

12.1 Introduction

Many factors influence the detection of abnormalities in medical images. Poor acquisition technique, improper processing and presentation of the image data, and sub-optimal viewing of the images are among these factors. However, even when from a technical standpoint such processes are optimal, subtle abnormalities in the image can go unrecognized. For example, subtle lesions in chest radiographs and in mammograms, and subtle fractures in muscloskeletal images are frequently missed (Muhm, 1983; Bird, 1992; Wallis, 1991; Hu, 1994). The difficulty in the detection of subtle abnormalities can be attributed to the statistical nature of decision-making in conjunction with psychophysical elements, both perceptual and cognitive, affecting the detection process. An attribute of medical images that greatly influences the psychophysics of detection is the anatomical structure within which the abnormalities are to be detected.

Anatomical structure within medical radiological images is created by the normal anatomy of the patient. In cross-sectional imaging, such as Computed Tomography (CT) and Magnetic Resonance Imaging (MRI), the structure results from the anatomy present in the cross-sectional slab of the image. In projection imaging, such as radiography and mammography, the anatomical structure is more complex, as the projection of the three-dimensional anatomy creates overlays in the two-dimensional image plane. The anatomical structure in either type of image influences the detection of abnormalities in the image, elevating the contrast threshold for detection, complicating the localization of the signals, and creating false signals.

The perceptual effects of anatomical structure on detection, though well recognized, have not been well-understood (Greening, 1954; Boynton, 1956; Smith, 1967; Neitzel, 1998). This chapter focuses on these effects from a visual/perceptual standpoint. First, the noise characteristics of anatomical structure are discussed. An attempt is then made to delineate some of the mechanisms through which anatomical structure affects detection. Finally, the influence of anatomical structure on signal detection is demonstrated in a few specific clinical examples. The chapter ends by outlining some methods for reducing the influence of anatomical structure.

12.2 Anatomical structure as noise

The detection of an abnormality (i.e., signal) in medical images is generally understood to be limited by the amount of *noise* in the image.[1] In a radiological image, there are usually two major sources of noise: (1) quantum noise (mottle) or background fluctuations within the image attributable to the finite number of quanta forming the image; and (2) anatomical structure or background fluctuations formed by the surrounding or overlying anatomy apart from the signal (Figure 12.1).

The relative influence of quantum noise and anatomical structure has been investigated for a variety of detection tasks including those in chest radiography,

---

[1] In this chapter, noise is defined as the ensemble of all the features present in the two-dimensional image apart from the "true" signal. Thus signal and noise are relative terms and are dependent on the particular diagnostic task that is being performed.

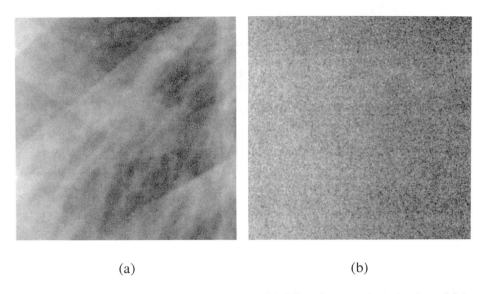

(a)   (b)

Figure 12.1: Examples of quantum noise (mottle) (a) and anatomical structure (b) in a chest radiograph. The quantum pattern is created by the fluctuations in the number of x-ray photons forming the image. The anatomical pattern is created by the projection of anatomical features in the thorax such as ribs, pulmonary vessels, and lung tissue.

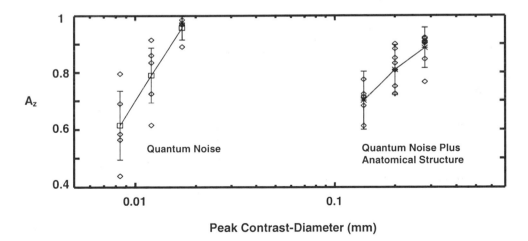

Peak Contrast-Diameter (mm)

Figure 12.2: Relative influence of quantum noise and anatomical structure in the detection of lung nodules in chest radiographs (from Samei, 1999). The data illustrate the detectability of nodules in quantum noise and in quantum noise plus anatomical structure backgrounds as a function of contrast-diameter product of the nodules.

dental radiography, mammography, and angiography (Samei, 1999; Kundel, 1985; Ruttimann, 1984; Whiting, 1996; Bochud, 1997). One outcome of such comparative studies has been the recognition of two zones associated with the detection process: a quantum-limited zone in which the detection of abnormalities is substantially influenced by the level of quantum noise in the image, and a quantum-saturated zone in which the anatomical structure plays a more substantial role (Ruttimann, 1984; Barrett, 1990). With the current state of medical-imaging technology and the radiology standards in place, most medical images are acquired with a low level of quantum noise, and thus many, if not most, of the signal-detection tasks in medical imaging today are in the quantum-saturated zone. For example, in chest radiography, the anatomical structure of the thorax plays a much more prominent role in the detection of subtle lung nodules than quantum noise; the presence of anatomical structure increases the contrast threshold in terms of the diameter of the nodule by a factor of four (Figure 12.2) (Samei, 1999). Furthermore, a nodule that is completely visible against the quantum-noise background of the chest radiograph (A_z approaching a value of 1.0)[2] is fully masked when the fluctuations of the anatomical structure are added.

The influence of quantum noise on visual perception has been well substantiated (Burgess, 1982; Rose, 1948). The detection of single circular objects in quantum noise may be described by the classical model of Albert Rose (Rose, 1948). In this model, contrast threshold is linearly proportional to the signal-to-noise ratio calculated on the basis of the variance or the root-mean-square of the fluctuations. This model has been found applicable in the detection of disk-shaped objects as well as objects with a Gaussian contrast profile in uncorrelated noise (Rose, 1948; Dobbins, 1992; Marshall, 1994; Launders, 1995; Judy, 1995a; Judy, 1995b). Thus, first-order statistics (e.g., variance) are usually sufficient to describe the influence of quantum noise on the detection of simple targets.

There has been a natural tendency to study the influence of anatomical structure using first-order statistics, in a manner similar to the approach taken for quantum noise (Seeley, 1984; Ruttimann, 1984). Such studies show good agreement with observer results in dental radiography and in nephrography. However, the findings may not be generalized to other detection tasks in medical imaging, as quantum noise and anatomical structure have substantially different statistical and spatial characteristics. While quantum noise is a poorly-correlated[3] stationary pattern that can be modeled with a Poisson distribution and described by its variance, anatomical structure is highly correlated and non-stationary.[4] In the presence of anatomical structure, variance is not a good indicator of perceptual performance, as the observer results depend not only on the *magnitude* of the noise power spectrum[5] but also its *shape* (Burgess, 1982). The treatment of anatomical structure with only its first-order statistics neglects the spatial characteristics of the structure and its

---

[2] A_z is the area under the receiver-operating-characteristic, ROC, curve, and is commonly used as an index of visibility/performance in detection tasks. It commonly varies between 0.5 (50% detection probability, pure chance) and 1.0 (100% detection with no false positives).

[3] Correlation here refers to the spatial correlation of the signal-intensity fluctuations (quantum or anatomical) in the adjacent areas of a two-dimensional image.

[4] Stationarity is a condition in which the noise characteristics of an image are independent of the location in the image.

[5] The noise-power spectrum or Wiener spectrum is a measure of second-order statistics of noise in the image that describes not only the magnitude of the noise but its spatial characteristics in terms of spatial frequencies.

possible local correlation with the signal, a situation that is commonly encountered in projection radiography.

To what extent anatomical structure can be considered "noise" in a perceptual sense (i.e., to what extent it hinders the detection of signals) is a subject of debate. The highly correlated nature of anatomical structure creates a dichotomy in the detection of signals: in some detection tasks, the correlation degrades the observer performance beyond that predicted by its first-order statistics. This situation has been demonstrated by Myers *et al.* in the detection of simple disk objects against a correlated background typical of those created by filtering operations in nuclear-medicine imaging (Myers, 1985). In some other detection tasks, however, the observer is able to distinguish a "fixed pattern" associated with the anatomy and "remove" (or nullify) the pattern during the detection process, thus performing better than would be expected based on noise variance. In the image-perception literature, this "removal" process is known as "prewhitening." In the detection of two-dimensional Gaussian signals against a certain kind of nonhomogeneous (so-called "lumpy") background, Rolland and Barrett found that observers are able to prewhiten the noise (Rolland, 1992), a finding that has not been reproduced in another similar study (Judy, 1996). Although few such studies have been performed on real anatomical backgrounds, it can be hypothesized that most detection tasks fall somewhere between the two extremes of total prewhitening and none.

Therefore, not all the fluctuations in the image associated with anatomical structure act as noise. In the context of signal detection, anatomical structure exhibits a dual nature: a component of the fluctuations acts as noise and directly deteriorates the visual detection, while the observer is able to recognize and prewhiten the other component during the detection process. To what extent the human observer is able to prewhiten the correlation of anatomical structure, or will be negatively influenced by it, depends on the modality and the task at hand. For example, a recent study demonstrates that human observers are able to partially prewhiten the anatomical structures in the detection of nodules in mammography (Bochud, 1999). For the detection of microcalcifications, however, the results were highly image dependent, varying from total prewhitening to none.

The prewhitening ability of human perception is an active area of research. Most of the effort in this line of research is to model the human visual and cognitive mechanisms underlying signal detection in medical images, thus enabling the performance-based optimization of diagnosis and the attributes of the imaging systems without costly observer-performance experiments. In order to achieve this objective, it is important to derive a single model that accurately predicts the varying prewhitening ability of human observers.

Two classes of observer models have been particularly successful in describing human perceptual performance in the presence of correlated noise. The non-prewhitening matched-filter model (NPW), which matches a template with the image data to "detect" a signal, and which accounts for noise correlation in the image, has been successful in modeling signal detection in correlated backgrounds created by filtering operations (Myers, 1985). However, the model has failed in lumpy backgrounds. In such backgrounds, the Hotelling model, which prewhitens the background correlation before the matched filtering, has been particularly successful. However, this model has failed in the filtered backgrounds of the former type (Rolland, 1992).

Burgess has recently suggested a modified version of the NPW model, which includes the spatial-frequency response of the human visual system (Burgess, 1994). The new model has been able to predict signal detection in both types of backgrounds described above. Similar prediction ability has been achieved by modifying the Hotelling model to include a finite number of visual channels of various spatial frequencies (Myers, 1990; Yao, 1992; Burgess, 1995), based on the belief that the human visual system employs such channels (Sachs, 1971). These observer models have been described in detail in other chapters. At present, the prewhitening ability of human observers in perceiving correlated noise and anatomical structure remains unclear and awaits further research.

One of the limitations of prior investigations in modeling the perceptual process has been the utilization of images of synthetic nonuniform background patterns with simple superimposed signals. Synthetic backgrounds with known statistical characteristics keep the mathematical model tractable. However, these backgrounds fall short of simulating the complex anatomical structure of real images. Some new developments in synthesizing more realistic yet mathematically tractable synthetic backgrounds are described in another chapter of this book. It is evident that if the perceptual performance of humans and the influence of anatomical structure on signal detection are to be better understood, more realistic signals and backgrounds should be utilized.

12.3 Perceptual effects of anatomical structure

The perceptual mechanisms through which anatomical structure influences the detection of signals in medical images are complicated. The mechanisms cannot be cleanly compartmentalized into independent categories. Furthermore, there are multitudes of psychophysical processes in human vision that we are just beginning to understand. However, three types of effects may be identified, that describe, at least in part, the way in which anatomical structure influences detection. They include the visual search effect, the global effect, and the local effect of anatomical structure.

12.3.1 Visual search effect

The first step in detecting a signal is to localize it by visually searching the image. There have been many studies on visual search processes (Krupinski, 1997), a topic that is covered in another chapter of this book in detail. In general, the need for visual search arises from the limited angular coverage of the high-acuity foveal vision of the eye. The fovea subtends an angle of only about 2 degrees, and the visual acuity sharply drops beyond the "foveal cone" (i.e., the solid angle that is covered by the fovea) (Sharp, 1997). At a typical viewing distance of 30–60 cm

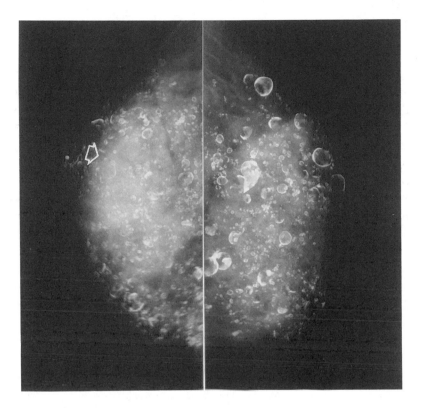

Figure 12.3: Left and right mediolateral mammograms in a 66-year-old patient presenting a left breast mass. The patient had bilateral silicone injections in her twenties. It is difficult to appreciate the 5-cm breast cancer in the left breast through the dense tissue and the globally complex mammographic pattern created by diffuse calcifications (calcified silicone granulomas).

(1–2 ft) from the image, the foveal vision of the eye only covers an area of about 1–2 cm diameter. Therefore, it is necessary to search the image for potential targets.

The search process usually starts with a rapid sub-second global view of the whole image during which suspect areas of the image are identified (Kundel, 1987; Nodine, 1987; Krupinski, 1996). During this stage, peripheral vision is believed to play a major role. Subsequently, the observer proceeds to scan the areas of interest by moving the foveal cone across the image in rapid jumping movements, between which the target areas are examined in short fixations. The fixations usually form clusters that define areas of interest. If no suspicious region is identified during the so-called global impression phase, the observer usually scans the image with the aid of the anatomy. The anatomical structure in the image plays a role both in the global-impression phase and in the subsequent scanning phase of the search process.

In the global-impression phase, all the complexities of the anatomy directly influence the way the observer comprehends the image. Figure 12.3 shows an example of a mammogram in which complexity associated with the presence of multiple calcifications in the breast may dominate the global impression of the image. Consequently, the observer may not identify the presence of a nodule. Because the global impression is an important stage of the detection process in which broad suspect areas and even potential targets are first identified, and because the impression loosely "guides" the subsequent scanning phase, the layout of anatomical structure can substantially affect the outcome.

Anatomical structure also affects the scanning phase of the search process, not only indirectly through the global impression, but also directly in the way the observers scan the image. The effects of variations in scanning pattern on detection have not been fully quantified, neither is it clear how anatomical structure directs the scanning pattern. However, studies have shown that some abnormalities are missed because the observer has failed to fixate close to the abnormality (Hu, 1994; Kundel, 1978). The scanning pattern of an image is highly dependent on the observers, especially on their experience in reading similar kinds of images. Other factors, such as clinical history and the tendency of the observer to search for certain types of abnormalities in the image, also affect the scanning pattern (Carmody, 1984; Kundel, 1969).

12.3.2 Global effect

There are cases in which a suspect area is identified during the search process, but the perception does not lead to a positive finding by the radiologist. In such cases, the anatomical structure of the image hinders the detection by two kinds of interference: (1) "global" interference, where the influence can be characterized by the global statistical characteristics of the background in relation to the signal associated with the abnormality, and (2) "local" interference, where the background pattern immediately surrounding the nodule alters the presentation of the abnormality.

Global statistical characteristics of anatomical structure tend to create false signals. False signals are either parts of the normal anatomy (e.g., end-on vessels in the detection of lung nodules in chest radiographs) or are created by constructive overlaying of projected anatomy. At the global level, the detectability of a true signal is determined by the degree of its identification or *distinctiveness* from these false signals. In the cases in which signal and background have substantially different characteristics (e.g., different spatial-frequency spectra), the global interference of the background is minimal. However, in many situations, false signals and true signals have very similar visual characteristics (Figure 12.4(a–b)). Kundel has demonstrated how this limits the minimum size of a pulmonary lesion that can be reliably detected in chest radiographs; the study shows that nodules smaller than 0.8 to 1 cm cannot be clearly distinguished from the "false" nodules created by anatomical structure (Kundel, 1981). The global effect of anatomical structure can be approached (though not fully modeled) by the statistical decision theory (Burgess, 1997) and quantified by analyzing the false-positive results of observer studies (Revesz, 1985).

The global characteristics of the image may also influence detection through the satisfaction-of-search (SOS) effect. SOS refers to a situation in which an observer, after finding an abnormality in the image, tends to overlook additional abnormalities and thus stop the search prematurely. It has been shown that the presence of simulated nodules in chest radiographs, for example, affects the detection of native lesions (Berbaum, 1990). The detection of false signals created by the global characteristics of anatomical structure can influence the detection of true signals through the same process.

12.3.3 Local effect

Considering only the global influence of anatomical structure and ignoring the complications associated with the search process, we would expect detection to be independent of the signal location. However, there have been indications that slight changes in the location of a signal significantly affect its detectability (Samei, 1996), suggesting that the local characteristics of anatomical structure play an important role in the detection process. This influence takes place when anatomic overlays or immediate surroundings partially or fully obscure the abnormality, or

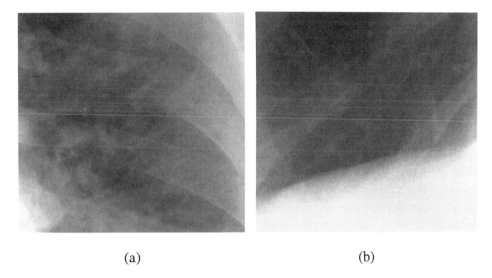

(a)   (b)

Figure 12.4: Simulated tissue-equivalent pulmonary nodule, with 6.3% contrast and 6.4 mm diameter, superimposed at the center of five lung areas from chest radiographs (a–e). The global influence can be appreciated in (a) and (b) in which the presence of similar-looking structures created by the overlay of normal anatomical features may confuse the observer in identifying the true lesion. The significant variation in the presentation of the nodule in c–e illustrates the local influence of anatomical structure. For comparison, (f) shows a 1.3% contrast, 1.3-mm-diameter centrally located simulated nodule against a background that contains only the quantum noise mottle from a typical chest radiograph. The detectability of this nodule is the same as the average detectability of those in the other five anatomical images (Samei 1999).

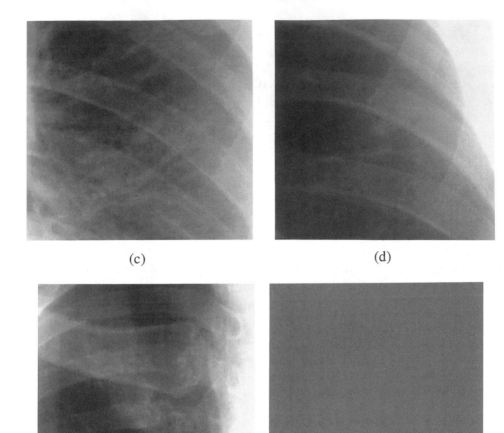

(c)

(d)

(e)

(f)

Figure 12.4: (Continued).

significantly alter its presentation and/or its contrast (Kundel 1976; Kundel 1989) (Figure 12.4(c–e)). The abnormality is thus "camouflaged." The phenomenon is obviously less pronounced in cross-sectional imaging, but it is not absent either.

In an effort to quantify the local influence of anatomical structure on the detection of lung nodules, in the 1970s, Kundel and Revesz adapted Engel's concept of conspicuity (Engel, 1971; Engel, 1974) to define a conspicuity index (Revesz, 1974). The index, defined as the ratio of the mean density change normal to the contour of a lesion to that tangential to the contour, showed a linear correlation with the results of a number of observer studies (Revesz, 1974; Revesz, 1977; Kundel, 1976; Kundel, 1979). However, the correlation was less favorable in some later studies (Hallberg, 1978; Brogdon, 1978). The discrepancy was most likely

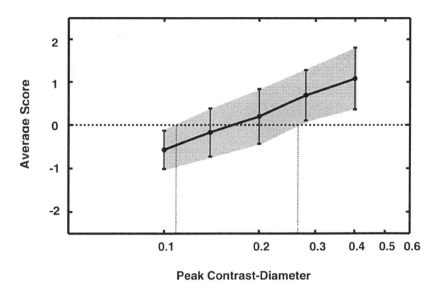

Figure 12.5: The average observer score for visibility as a function of nodule contrast-diameter product in chest anatomical backgrounds. The error bars show ±1 standard deviation of changes due to the nodule location.

attributable to the dependence of the measurement method on the characteristics of the signal and the image (e.g., the influence of the edge definition of the nodule on the index), in addition to the fact that it did not account for complications arising from the search and localization of the signal or those from the global influence of anatomical structure (Revesz, 1985).

In order to be able to quantify the local influence of anatomical structure, we performed an experiment in which the locations of simulated nodules were varied slightly against anatomical backgrounds of chest radiographs (Samei, 1998). The variation in location allowed different local background patterns to overlay the nodules while the global background remained the same. Considering only ±1 standard-deviation variations, the results indicated that the variation in detectability of a nodule due to the influence of its local background surroundings is equivalent to that caused by changing the size of the nodule by fifty percent (Figure 12.5). That corresponds to a significant change of about 0.2 in A_z based on signal-known-exactly (SKE)[6] experiments (Samei, 1999).

In summary, anatomical structure within an image influences the detection of abnormalities through a combination of at least three perceptual effects: search, global effects, and local effects. These mechanisms are often interrelated during the interpretation of medical images, and it is their overall effect in conjunction with psychological elements of visual perception that determines the outcome.

---

[6]SKE refers to the studies in which the observer has the full knowledge of what and where the potential targets are.

12.4 Effects of anatomical structure in selected clinical applications

This section presents a few examples of the influence of anatomical structure on detection in selected radiologic imaging applications. The illustrations are pictorial so that readers might develop a visual appreciation for this influence.

In chest radiography, the large dynamic range presents at once a challenge to represent all of the anatomical structures and the opportunity to detect small lesions, especially in the air-containing portions of the lung. The normal vasculature may hide a nodule (Figure 12.6) but a second projection may reveal the lesion. Mediastinal and skeletal structures often project over a lesion making recognition difficult. Ribs alone cover approximately two-thirds of the lung regions in postero-anterior/antero-posterior chest radiographs (Waring, 1926) affecting the presentation of most abnormalities in the thoracic cavity. Examples of such overlay are shown in Figures 12.7 and 12.8. The anatomical background of the lung also often changes as a result of diffuse pulmonary disease such as sarcoidosis (Figure 12.8), idiopathic fibrosis, or chronic obstructive pulmonary disease. Cellular and fibrotic thickening of interstitial tissues in the lung may at first produce a fine reticular pattern, reducing contrast, but as the process becomes more granular and nodular, identification of new disease of other etiology may become more difficult. CT and MRI increase the sensitivity of the diagnostic process.

The muscloskeletal system, like other solid organs, offers a less favorable anatomical background than the lung. The cortical and trabecular parts of the skeletal system present a variety of anatomical backgrounds that must be *learned* in order to detect early disease. The radiographic imaging of the muscloskeletal system usually shows the bones to advantage while providing a less-rewarding display of the soft tissues. Ultrasound, MRI, CT, and nuclear medicine images usually provide additional information on changes in the anatomical background of fat, water, and calcified opacities (Figure 12.9). The cortical and trabecular bony structures provide a high contrast and varied background, which is specific to given regions and must also be learned.

In abdominal imaging, both solid and hollow viscera, provide anatomical backgrounds less favorable for the detection of early lesions than the chest. The detection of lesions in the solid organs (e.g., liver, spleen, pancreas, adrenals and kidneys) depends in great measure on the use of contrast materials and cross-sectional imaging, as anatomical structure significantly obscures the abnormality in standard radiographic applications. The use of CT, MRI, and angiographic approaches is often mandatory; oral and intravenous contrast media play a large role.

In mammography, complex mammographic patterns often diminish the perception of mammographic lesions that could indicate cancer including masses, microcalcifications, skin thickening, tissue asymmetry (focal or diffuse), architectural distortion, and the appearance of new densities or calcifications. Anatomical characteristics of a difficult mammographic background include dense glandular tissue, diffuse nodularity, or abundant calcifications. Local interference in mammography occurs when a malignant process is interspersed within an area of similar structures in the anatomical background. When viewing a mammogram, the observer

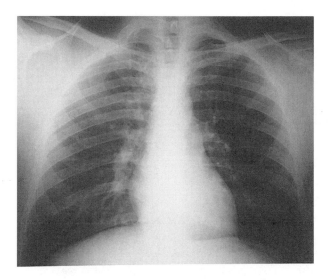

(a)

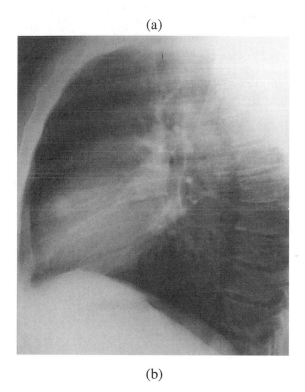

(b)

Figure 12.6: Right middle lobe nodule. (a) The postero-anterior radiograph shows a 19-mm nodule largely obscured by the lower portion of the right lung root and the posterior portion of the right 10th rib. (b) A left lateral projection shows the nodule well. (c) An enlargement of the medial right lower thorax provides better detail. (d) A postero-anterior view of the medial right lower thorax 4 years later, at which time the slowly growing nodule of carcinoma is 30 mm in diameter.

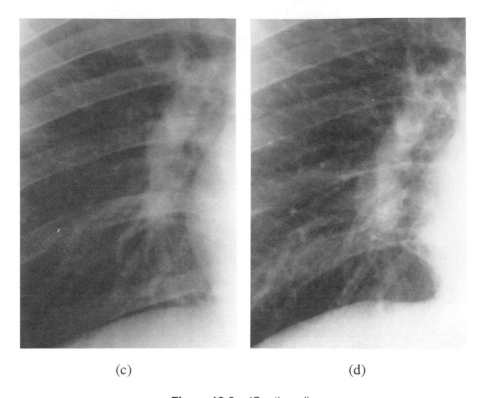

(c)   (d)

Figure 12.6: (Continued).

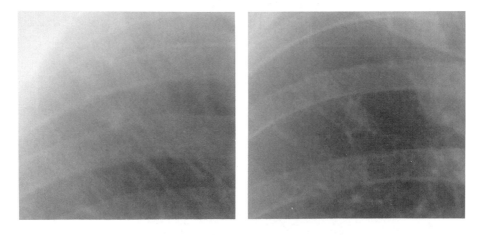

Figure 12.7: Similar small right upper lobe carcinomas from two patients. (left) The lesion is projected free of bone just lateral to the anterior portion of the second rib. (right) A similar lesion overlies the anterior second rib and vessels and is more difficult to see.

needs to mentally subtract, or prewhiten, the overlying structure away from a potential cancer. This task can be especially difficult in dense breasts. Figure 12.10 demonstrates a dense breast pattern with a 3-cm palpable mass in the upper outer

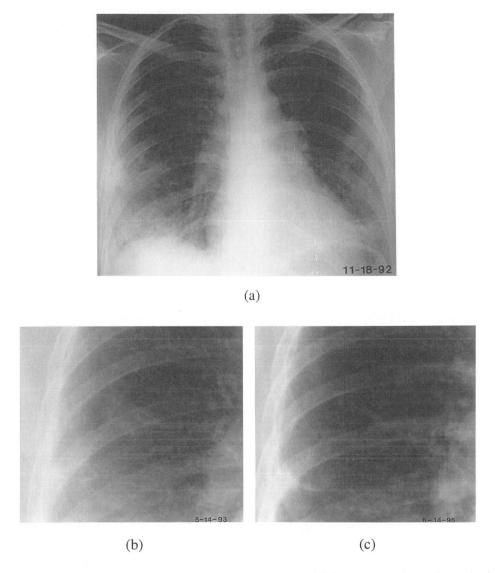

(a)

(b)   (c)

Figure 12.8: Sarcoidosis of the lungs and lymph nodes. (a) Postero-anterior radiograph of 11-18-92 shows a reticular nodular pattern in the lungs, most marked at the bases. There are a few small strands of scar or atelectasis laterally in right midchest. The lung roots and the azygous area display enlarged nodes. (b) Right midthorax of 5-14-93 shows no change from the preceding study. (c) Right midthorax of 6-14-95 shows no change from the previous studies except for interval occurrence of fracture of the 6th rib, healed at time of the examination. (d) Right midthorax of 12-12-95 at full inspiration. Diffuse parenchymal reticular-nodular pattern, small band of atelectasis, scar or fissure, and healed rib fracture are shown again. There is now an irregular opacity, approximately 1 cm in diameter overlying the posterior portion of the 7th rib (arrow). (e) Right midthorax of 12-12-95 with incomplete inspiration. While less complete inspiration results in increased diffuse changes, the irregular nodule is now projected over the thin anterior 3rd rib, but free of the heavier posterior 7th rib. While a better display of a nodule would be expected with full inspiration, the more favorable relation to the ribs has resulted in better depiction of the small carcinoma.

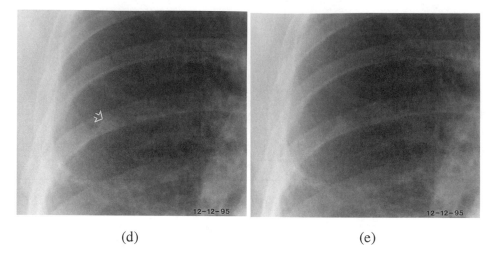

(d)   (e)

Figure 12.8: (Continued).

quadrant of the breast. The mammogram illustrates how the tumor almost completely blends into the surrounding breast tissue; only the superior and anterior margins are clearly visualized.

Dense breast tissue can also hinder the detection of calcifications by obscuring the calcifications within the glandular tissue. Calcifications are an important abnormality to perceive because some cancers only present as nonpalpable calcium deposits. The dense glandular tissue in Figure 12.11 obscures the suspicious calcifications in the outer breast. The magnified view further illustrates the impact of the dense tissue in the detection of the subtle malignant calcifications. Focal nodular densities, in an otherwise fatty breast, can also complicate the perception of a cancer. This is partially related to the necessity of prewhitening; the observer must subtract the normal nodular breast tissue away from a potential breast cancer. Figure 12.12 demonstrates mainly fat-replaced breast tissue with a scattering of parenchymal densities. Hidden within the center of this benign pattern is an 8-mm cancerous lesion. A heightened awareness of subtle differences in nodularity may alert the observer to the presence of the tumor.

Architectural distortion is perhaps one of the most difficult abnormalities to appreciate on the mammogram. Distortion occurs when a process within the breast (cancerous or noncancerous) disrupts the normal flowing pattern of arcing curvilinear lines. This occurs as a result of the desmoplastic reaction caused by the growing tumor. Disturbance of this normal symmetric flow, especially when the normal lines are directed away from the nipple, should be regarded with a high degree of suspicion. These subtle changes are especially challenging to detect in a globally dense breast. The surrounding dense tissue in Figure 12.13 hinders the perception of the mild retraction of the stroma by the cancer. The ability to perceive this cancer is markedly reduced because of the surrounding noise from the normal glandular tissue.

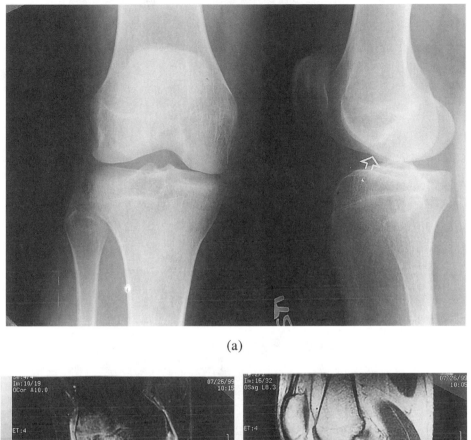

(a)

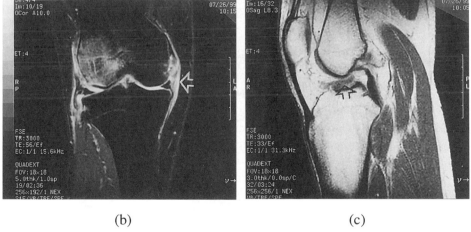

(b)   (c)

Figure 12.9: Trauma to the knee with both soft tissue and bone injuries. (a) Antero-posterior and lateral projections of the right knee. Joint effusion and a small indentation on the lateral femoral condylar joint surface (arrow). The anatomic background does not permit the recognition of the bruise by radiograph. (b) Fast spin echo T2 weighted fat suppressed (TR 3000, TE 56 eff.) antero-posterior MR study shows damage to the medial collateral ligament (arrow) and extensive bone bruising in the lateral condyle. (c) Fast spin echo proton density weighted (TR 3000, TE 33 eff.) lateral projection shows joint effusion and tear of the anterior cruciate ligament (arrow).

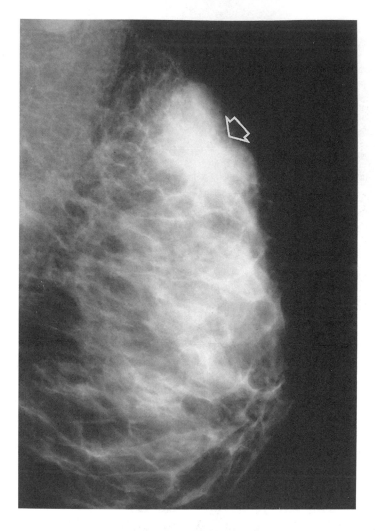

Figure 12.10: Mediolateral oblique film screen mammogram of a 50-year-old patient with a palpable upper-quadrant breast lesion. The mammogram demonstrates moderately dense breast tissue. The 3.0-cm breast cancer located in the upper portion of the breast is partially obscured by the dense glandular tissue.

Global interference from surrounding breast parenchyma can also interfere with the perception of breast cancer. In the example of Figure 12.14, the breast parenchyma is predominantly fat-replaced and relatively easy to interpret. There is a focal region of benign-appearing calcifications in the lower portion of the breast. However, closer inspection reveals that although most of these calcifications are benign in appearance, several have a more suspicious morphology. A biopsy demonstrated extensive cancer throughout the interior portion of the breast. Interestingly, a majority of the cancer was located in the mammographically normal-appearing breast tissue.

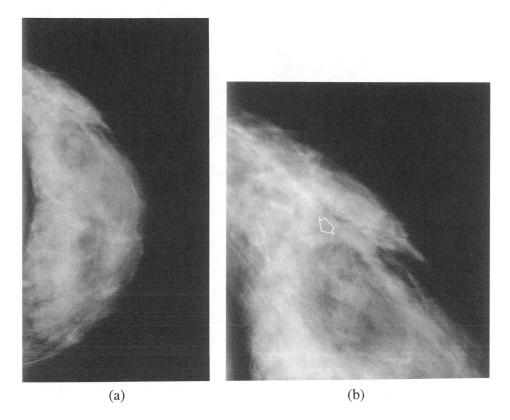

(a)   (b)

Figure 12.11: Mammograms of a 38-year-old asymptomatic patient presenting for a screening mammogram. (a) Full view of the craniocaudal mammogram demonstrates extremely faint calcifications in the outer portion of the breast. (b) Magnified image demonstrates faint pleomorphic calcifications. Biopsy revealed cancer.

12.5 Methods for reducing the effects of anatomical structure

Through the years, imaging methods have been developed that suppress anatomical fluctuations and reduce the overall influence of anatomy on detection. Now, it is possible to image the body using different imaging modalities that present the anatomy differently and can provide different prospectives on the same body part.

In projection imaging, the acquisition of multiple views (e.g., lateral, oblique, postero-anterior, etc.) has been a low-cost and simple method to reduce the influence of anatomical structure. Views from different angles can provide the observer with an opportunity to find abnormalities that might have been camouflaged in a single view (Figure 12.6). The angular separation between the views is most commonly 90 degrees. It should be noted that using large angular separations, it is sometimes difficult to use the three-dimensional spatial information (i.e., correlation of the anatomical features) in identifying the abnormalities from the back-

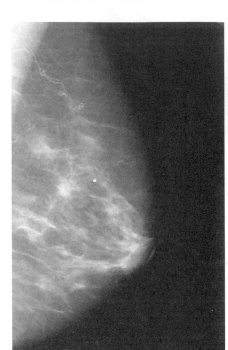
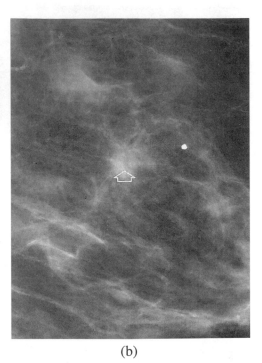

(a)   (b)

Figure 12.12: Mediolateral oblique film-screen mammogram of a 77-year-old asymptomatic patient presenting for a screening mammogram. (a) The mammogram demonstrates a primarily fat-replaced breast parenchymal pattern with scattered nodular densities. (b) Magnified view demonstrates the subtle spiculated cancer in the midbreast.

ground, and thus the benefit of this approach in reducing the effects of anatomical structure is limited.

Cross-sectional imaging is the most effective method to reduce the influence of anatomical structure. MRI, CT, Single Photon Emission Computed Tomography (SPECT), Positron Emission Tomography (PET), and ultrasound all are able to provide clinical images with practically no overlay of the anatomy. It should be noted, however, that the influence of anatomical structure is not completely eliminated, as the complexity of the anatomy in the two-dimensional plane of the image still influences visual perception. In addition, cross-sectional modalities create more data per case compared to projection imaging, making the evaluation of the data more time-consuming. Widespread utilization of these imaging methods is also limited by cost considerations.

In the case of thoracic imaging, as mentioned above, ribs have a role in masking abnormalities, especially lung nodules (Austin, 1992; Kundel, 1981). The bony anatomical structure from a chest radiograph can be eliminated by utilizing the difference in the spectral absorption characteristics of bone and soft tissue in a technique known as dual-energy digital radiography (Stewart, 1990; Lehmann, 1981;

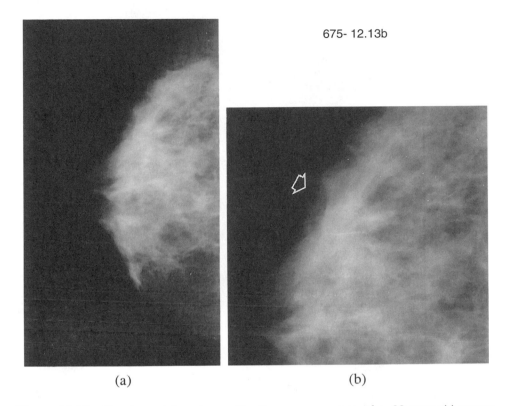

675- 12.13b

(a)   (b)

Figure 12.13: Craniocaudal and magnification mammograms of a 62-year-old asymptomatic patient who presented for a screening mammogram. (a) Note the dense breast tissue. There is a subtle area of architectural distortion in the outer breast. The degree of distortion is difficult to appreciate due to the surrounding dense tissue. (b) Magnified view illustrating the area of architectural distortion (arrow). A biopsy of this lesion documented cancer.

Kamimura, 1995). In the most common approach to dual-energy imaging, the detector is made of two sensitive layers with a metal filter in between which preferentially blocks lower-energy photons in the x-ray spectrum that are unabsorbed in the first detector layer from reaching the second layer. "Soft-tissue" and "bone" images are then constructed by subtraction of the low-energy and high-energy images acquired from the two detector layers. The image-quality characteristics of these systems, and particularly their noise characteristics, have not been fully evaluated. Some studies have reported improved detection of lung nodules using this technique (Kelcz, 1994; Ergun, 1990; Kido, 1995). A relatively new technology with only one system commercially available, dual-energy imaging is currently under clinical evaluation.

Stereoscopic imaging is another method that can diminish the influence of anatomical structure. In contrast to multi-view imaging, the method can provide positive reinforcement of the signal and thereby improve detection. Two images

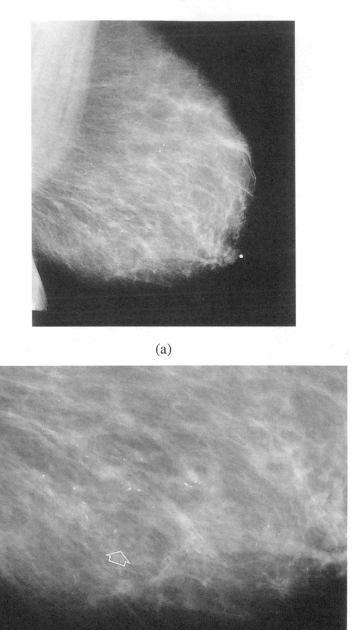

(a)

(b)

Figure 12.14: Mediolateral oblique and magnified views in a 65-year-old asymptomatic patient. (a) The breast tissue is primarily fat-replaced. There are no nodules, masses or areas of distortion. However, calcifications are apparent in the lower portion of the breast. (b) Magnified view depicts the calcifications. Although a majority of the calcifications appear relatively benign there are some worrisome ones scattered within the population. A biopsy demonstrated cancer throughout the entire lower portion of the breast.

of the body part are acquired at two different projections with a small angular separation. The images are then viewed either side by side or stereoscopically. Stereoscopic imaging was extensively used in the past, especially for chest imaging (Levitin, 1943; Bowie, 1944). However, it lost its popularity by the middle of the century, and was gradually replaced by two-view, postero-anterior/lateral chest radiography (Lewis, 1946). There were a variety of reasons for discontinuation of the practice (Daves, 1962; Batson, 1944; McGrigor, 1942; Meservey, 1938). More relatively recent studies, however, have suggested that stereoscopic imaging might be effective in the detection of nodules in chest radiographs (Brogdon, 1978; Kelsey, 1982) and in mammograms (Getty, 1999). Currently, the method is rarely used clinically.

Digital tomosynthesis is a multi-projection modality under current investigation that is effective in reducing the detrimental effects of anatomical structure. The method is similar to conventional tomography in which images of a single plane within the body part are acquired by linear movement of the x-ray source and the receptor in opposite directions during the acquisition (Johns, 1983). The linear movement blurs the objects outside of the image plane, but the blurred signal remains within the image and degrades its quality and its contrast. In digital tomosynthesis, multiple projection images of the body part are acquired by a moving x-ray source and a digital detector with a fast read-out response (Zwicker, 1997). Acquired images are then processed for either three-dimensional reconstruction or cine presentations. The method reduces the influence of overlays on detection. Preliminary evaluations of this technique have shown improved detection of lesions in breast imaging and in chest imaging (Niklason, 1997; Dobbins, 1998).

Like tomosynthesis, image processing is a method that became possible with the advent of digital imaging in radiology. Image processing has the potential to reduce the influence of anatomical structure on detection. Currently, various image-processing algorithms for enhanced image display such as gray scaling, spatial-frequency processing, and gray-scale equalization are utilized in clinical applications. An ideal processing method should enhance the features of the abnormality while suppressing the anatomical background. Because in many situations, abnormalities and the anatomical structures have similar characteristics (e.g., similar contrast and power in the spatial-frequency space), the apparent enhancement of image quality might adversely increase the number of false positives. The characteristics of the human visual system in conjunction with those of the abnormality and anatomical background should be taken into account in design and implementation of image-processing algorithms for specific detection tasks. More advanced task-dependent image-processing algorithms currently await clinical evaluation (Laine, 1994; Laine, 1995; Vuylsteke, 1994).

12.6 Conclusions

Anatomical structure plays a major role in the detection of abnormalities in radiological images. Although this influence has been well recognized, it has not been well understood. Three effects have been identified through which anatomical structure influences detection, namely, the effects on the search process, the global or "false-signal" effect, and the local or "camouflaging" effect. Better characterization of the signals associated with abnormalities, anatomical structure, and human perceptual and decision-making processes is the underlying knowledge by which we may better understand the mechanisms of this influence. In the last few years, there has been major progress in modeling human performance for simple detection tasks. Slowly but surely, investigators are making their way toward modeling the more complex tasks associated with real backgrounds and real signals. However, modeling human performance with complex anatomical structures cannot by itself improve the outcome. New acquisition modalities and image-processing methods that can suppress anatomical textures and thus improve diagnostic performance are being developed. In the design and optimization of both new and existing methods, accurate modeling of perceptual performance is a significant element, and therefore remains an important area of research.

References

Austin JHM, Romney BM, Goldsmith LS. "Missed Bronchogenic Carcinoma: Radiographic Findings in 27 Patients with a Potentially Resectable Lesion Evident in Retrospect." Radiology 182:115–122, 1992.

Barrett HH, Swindell W. *Radiological Imaging: The Theory of Image Formation, Detection, and Processing*. New York, NY: Academic Press, 1981.

Barrett HH. "Objective Assessment of Image Quality: Effects of Quantum Noise and Object Variability." JOSA 7:1266–1278, 1990.

Batson OV, Carpentier VE. "Stereoscopic Depth Perception." AJR 51:202–204, 1944.

Berbaum KS, Franken Jr EA, Dorfmann DD *et al.* "Satisfaction of Search in Diagnostic Radiology." Invest Rad 25:133–140, 1990.

Bird RE, Wallace TW, Yankaskas BC. "Analysis of Cancers Missed at Screening Mammography." Radiology 184:613–617, 1992.

Bochud FO, Verdun FR, Valley JF, Hessler C, Moeckli R. "Importance of Anatomical Noise in Mammography." Proc SPIE 3036, 1997, pp. 74–80.

Bochud FO, Valley JF, Verdun FR, Hessier C, Schnyder P, Abbey CK. "Measurement of Human-Observer Responses with a 2-AFC Experiment." Med Phys 26:1365–1370, 1999.

Boynton RM, Bush WR. "Recognition of Forms Against a Complex Background." JOSA 46:758–764, 1956.

Bowie ER, Jacobson GG. "Routine Chest Roentgenography on Negro Inductees at Fort Benning, Georgia." AJR 52:500–504, 1944.

Brogdon BG, Moseley RD, Kelsey CA, Hallberg JR. "Perception of Simulated Lung Lesions." Invest Radio 13:12–15, 1978.

Burgess AE, Wagner RF, Jennings RJ. "Human Signal Detection Performance in Medical Images." In *IEEE Computer Society International Workshop on Medical Imaging*, 1982, pp. 99–105.

Burgess AE. "Statistically Defined Backgrounds: Performance of a Modified Non-Prewhitening Observer Model." JOSA 11: 1237–1242, 1994.

Burgess AE. "Comparison of Non-Prewhitening and Hotelling Observer Models." Proc SPIE 2436, 1995, pp. 2–9.

Burgess AE, Li X, Abbey CK. "Nodule Detection in Two Component Noise: Toward Patient Structure." Proc SPIE 3036, 1997, pp. 2–13.

Carmody DP, Kundel HL, Nodine CF. "Comparison Scans while Reading Chest Images: Taught but Not Practiced." Invest Radiol 19:462–466, 1984.

Daves ML, Dalrymple GV. "Objective stereoscopy." Radiology 48:801–805, 1962.

Dobbins JT, Ergun DL, Blume H, Rutz LJ. "Detective Quantum Efficiency of Three Generations of Computed Radiography Acquisition Systems." Radiology 185(P):159, 1992.

Dobbins JT, Webber RL, Hames SM, "Tomosynthesis for Improved Pulmonary Nodule Detection." Radiology 209(P):280, 1998 (abstract).

Engel FL. "Visual Conspicuity and Directed Attention and Retinal Locus." Vision Research 11:563–576, 1971.

Engel FL. "Visual Conspicuity and Selective Background Interference in Eccentric Vision." Vision Research 14:459–471, 1974.

Ergun DL, Mistretta CA, Brown DE, Bystrianyk RT, Sze WK, Kelcs F, Naidich DP. "Single-Exposure Dual-Energy Computed Radiography: Improved Detection and Processing." Radiology 174:242–249, 1990.

Getty GJ, Pickett RM, D'Orsi CJ, Karellas A. "Stereoscopic Digital Mammography: What Can You See in a Stereo View of the Breast that You Can't See in Two Standard Orthogonal 2D Films." In *Proceedings of the 8th Far West Image Perception Conference*, Alberta, Canada (abstract), 1999.

Greening RG, Pendegrass EP. "Postmortem Roentgenography with Particular Emphasis upon the Lung." Radiology 62:720–724, 1954.

Hallberg JR, Kelsey CA, Briscoe D. "Some Effects of Method on the Measured Conspicuity of Chest Lesions." Invest Radiol 13:439–443, 1978.

Hu CH, Kundel HL, Nodine CF, Krupinski EA, Toto LC. "Searching for Bone Fractures: A Comparison with Pulmonary Nodule Search." Acad Radiol 1:25–32, 1994.

Johns HE, Cunningham JR. *The Physics of Radiology*. Springfield, IL: Charles C Thomas Publisher, 1983.

Judy PF, Kijewski MF, Fu X, Swensson RG. "Observer Detection Efficiency with Target Size Uncertainty." Proc SPIE 2436, 1995a, pp. 10–17.

Judy PF, Swensson RG, Kijewski MF. "Observer Detection Efficiency of Disk and Gaussian Targets." Radiology 197:356, 1995b.

Judy PF. "Detection of Clusters of Simulated Calcifications in Lumpy Noise Backgrounds." Proc SPIE 2712, 39–46, 1996.

Kamimura R, Takashima T. "Clinical Application of Single Dual-Energy Subtraction Technique with Digital Storage Phosphor Radiography." J Digital Imaging 8S:21–24, 1995.

Kelcz F, Zink FE, Peppler WW, Kruger DG, Ergun DI, Istretta CAM. "Conventional Chest Radiography Versus Dual-Energy Computed Radiography in the Detection and Characterization of Pulmonary Nodules." AJR 162:271–278, 1994.

Kesley CA, Moseley RD, Mettler FA, Briscoe DE. "Cost-Effectiveness of Stereoscopic Radiographs in Detection of Lung Nodules." Radiology 142:611–613, 1982.

Kido S, Ikezoe J, Naito H, Arisawa J, Tamura S, Kozuka T, Ito W, Kato H. "Clinical Evaluation of Pulmonary Nodules with Single-Exposure Dual-Energy Subtraction Chest Radiography with an Interactive Noise-Reduction Algorithm." Radiology 194: 407–412, 1995.

Krupinski EA. "Visual Scanning Patterns of Radiologists Searching Mammograms." Acad Radiol 3:137–144, 1996.

Krupinski E. "Visual Search: Mechanisms and Issues in Radiology." In *Workshop, SPIE Medical Imaging Conference*, Newport Beach, CA, 1997.

Kundel E. "Perception Errors in Chest Radiography." Seminars in Resp Med 10:203–210, 1989.

Kundel HL, Nodine CF, Thickman D, Toto L. "Searching for Lung Nodules: A Comparison of Human Performance with Random and Systematic Scanning Models." Invest Radiol 22:417–422, 1987.

Kundel HL, Nodine CF, Carmody D. "Visual Scanning, Pattern Recognition and Decision-Making in Pulmonary Nodule Detection." Invest Radiol 13:175–181, 1978.

Kundel HL, Wright DJ. "The Influence of Prior Knowledge on Visual Search Strategies During the Viewing of Chest Radiographs." Radiology 93:315–320, 1969.

Kundel HL, LaFollette PS. "Visual Search Patterns and Experience with Radiological Images." Radiology 81:288–292, 1981.

Kundel HL. "Predictive Value and Threshold Detectability of Lung Tumors." Radiology 139:25–29, 1981.

Kundel HL, Revesz G. "Lesion Conspicuity, Structural Noise, and Film Reader Error." AJR 126:1233–1238, 1976.

Kundel HL *et al.* "Contrast Gradient and the Detection of Lung Nodules." Invest Radiol 14:18–22, 1979.

Kundel HL *et al.* "Nodule Detection with and without a Chest Image." Invest Radiol 20:94–99, 1985.

Laine A, Fan J, Yang W. "Wavelets for Contrast Enhancement of Digital Mammography." In *IEEE Engineering in Medicine and Biology*, 1995, pp. 536–550.

Laine AF, Schuler S, Fan J, Huda W. "Mammographic Feature Enhancement bu Multiscale Analysis." IEEE Trans Med Imaging 13:725–752, 1994.

Launders JH, Cowen AR. "A Comparison of the Threshold Detail Detectability of a Screen-Film Combination and Computed Radiology under Conditions Relevant to High-kVp Chest Radiography." Physics in Medicine and Biology 40:1393–1398, 1995.

Lehmann LA, Alvarez RE, Mocovski A, Brody WR, Pelc NJ, Riederer SJ, Hall AL. "Generalized Image Combination in Dual kVp Digital Radiography." Med Phys 8:659–667, 1981.

Levitin J. "Ten Thousand Chest Examinations with the Stereoscopic Roentgen Unit." AJR 49:469–475, 1943.

Lewis I, Morgan RH. "The Value of Stereoscopy in Mass Radiography of the Chest." Radiology 46I:171–172, 1946.

Marshall NW, Faulkner K, Busch HP, Lehmann KJ. "The Contrast-Detail Behaviour of a Photostimulable Phosphor Based Computed Radiography System." Physics in Medicine and Biology 39:2289–2303, 1994.

McGrigor DB. "Radiographic Stereoscopy." British J Radiology 15:273–281, 1942.

Meservey AB. "Depth Effects in Roentgenograms." AJR 39:439–449, 1938.

Muhm JR, Miller WE, Fontana RS, Sanderson DR, Uhlenhopp MA. "Lung Cancer Detected During a Screening Program Using Four-Month Chest Radiographs." Radiology 148:561–565, 1983.

Myers KJ, Barrett HH, Bergstrom MC, Patton DD, Seeley GW. "Effect of Noise Correlation on Detectability of Disk Signals in Medical Imaging." JOSA 2:1752–1759, 1985.

Myers KJ, Rolland JP, Barrett HH, Wagner RF. "Aperture Optimization for Emission Imaging. Effect of a Spatially Varying Backgrounds." JOSA 7:1279–1293, 1990.

Neitzel U, Pralow T, Schaefer-Prokop C, Prokop M. "Influence of Scatter Reduction on Lesion Signal-to-Noise Ratio and Lesion Detection in Digital Chest Radiography." Proc SPIE 3336, 1998, pp. 337–347.

Niklason LT, Christian BT, Niklason LE, Kopans DB, Castleberry DE et al. "Digital Tomosynthesis in Breast Imaging." Radiology 205:399–406, 1997.

Nodine CF, Kundel HL. "The Cognitive Side of Visual Search in Radiology." In O'Regan JK, Levy-Schoen A (Eds.) Eye Movements: From Physiology to Cognition. New York: Elsevier Science, 1987, pp. 573–582.

Revesz G, Kundel HL, Graber MA. "The Influence of Structured Noise on the Detection of Radiologic Abnormalities." Invest Radio 9:479–486, 1974.

Revesz G, Kundel HL. "Psychophysical Studies of Detection Errors in Chest Radiology." Radiology 123:559–562, 1977.

Revesz G. "Conspicuity and Uncertainty in the Radiographic Detection of Lesions." Radiology 154:625–628, 1985.

Rolland JP, Barrettt HH. "Effect of Random Background Inhomogeneity on Observer Detection Performance." JOSA 9:649–658, 1992.

Rose A. "The Sensitivity Performance of the Human Eye on an Absolute Scale." JOSA 38:296–208, 1948.

Ruttimann UE, Webber RL. "A Simple Model Combining Quantum Noise and Anatomical Variation in Radiographs." Medical Physicss 11:50–60, 1984.

Sachs M, Nachmisa J, Robson J. "Spatial-Frequency Channels in Human Vision." JOSA 61:1176–1186, 1971.

Samei E, Flynn MJ, Beute GH, Peterson E. "Comparison of Observer Performance for Real and Simulated Nodules in Chest Radiography." Proc SPIE 2712, 1996, pp. 60–70.

Samei E, Flynn MJ, Eyler WR, Peterson E. "The Effect of Local Background Anatomical Patterns on the Detection of Subtle Lung Nodules in Chest Radiographs." Proc SPIE 3340, 1998, pp. 44–54.

Samei E, Flynn MJ, Eyler WR. "Relative Influence of Quantum and Anatomical Noise on the Detection of Subtle Lung Nodules in Chest Radiographs." Radiology 1999 (accepted, in print).

Seeley GW, Roehrig H, Hillman BJ. "A Computerized Method for Measurement of Conspicuity: Comparison of Film and Digital Nephrograms." Invest Radio 19: 583–586, 1984.

Sharp PF, Philips R. "Physiological Optics." In Hendee WR, Wells PNT (Eds.) *The Perception of Visual Information.* New York, NY: Springer-Verlag, 1997.

Smith MJ. *Error and Variations Diagnostic Radiology.* Springfield, IL: Charles C. Thomas, 1967.

Stewart BK, Huang HK. "Single-Exposure Dual-Energy Computed Radiography." Medical Physics 17:866–875, 1990.

Vuylsteke P, Schoeters E. "Multiscale Image Contrast Manipulation (MUSICA)." Proc SPIE 2167, 1994, pp. 551–560.

Wallis RE, Walsh MT, Lee JR. "A Review of False Negative Mammography in a Symptomatic Population." Clin Radiol 44:13–15, 1991.

Waring JJ, Wasson WW. "The Imperfections of the Stereoscopic Maneuver in Radiography of the Chest." Radiology 6:298–203, 1926.

Whiting SW, Eckstein MP, Morioka CA, Eigler NL. "Effect of Additive Noise, Signal Contrast and Feature Motion on Visual Detection Structured Noise." Proc SPIE 2712, 1996, pp. 26–38.

Yao J, Barrett HH. "Predicting Human Performance by a Channelized Hotelling Observer Model." Proc SPIE 1768, 1992, pp. 161–168.

Zwicker RD, Atari NA. "Transverse Tomosynthesis on a Digital Simulator." Med Phys 24:867–971, 1997.

CHAPTER 13
Synthesizing Anatomical Images for Image Understanding

Jannick P. Rolland
School of Optics/CREOL, the University of Florida

CONTENTS

13.1 Introduction

The main goals of research in medical and biomedical imaging are to create "better" imaging systems, more accurate reconstructions, and develop methods of image processing that utilize the most important information present in an image or set of images, for accurate, timely, and cost-effective diagnosis and treatment of disease. How well desired information can be extracted best serves to define image quality and consequently the performance of imaging systems. Furthermore, as we deepen our understanding of medical images, new systems and new methods of image processing and image display may help optimize performance and assist radiologists in their challenge for accurate diagnostics.

Image quality is thus best measured by the performance of an observer on specific tasks [1]. The observer may be human such as a physician making a diagnosis, or a mathematical model such as an ideal observer [2], or a computer algorithm. Specific tasks may be the detection of a lesion in a chest x ray [3], the estimation of the percent stenosis of a detected aneurysm [4], or the registration of images such as the superimposition of anatomical atlases on patient data [5]. Regardless of the task considered, however, methods to assess image quality based on task performance are most important.

Traditionally, the conception of improved imaging systems in medical imaging has been accomplished by designing and constructing proposed systems and characterizing them from an engineering point of view, by reporting parameters such as resolution, modulation transfer function, and pixel signal-to-noise ratio. Naturally, such evaluation is not sufficient to predict the performance that the system will have in the clinic, given that it does not take into account either information about the types of objects being imaged or the tasks being carried out.

To fully assess the system, clinical trials based on specific tasks must be conducted. While clinical trials are required for final system assessment, the reliance on clinical trials for system design and optimization has severe limitations. First, the construction of proposed systems is costly and time consuming. In addition, if the system requires further optimization, it may take multiple trials and errors to find the best set of parameters and tradeoff to satisfy required task-based image-quality criteria. Finally, it is nearly impossible to know the anatomical underlying structures of the acquired clinical images unless the diagnosis is verified by physical examination. Instead, disease states are most often estimated by interpreting the images and looking for correlation with previous cases established statistically as well. The approach of building systems and conducting trial-and-error changes based on clinical images thus constitutes a highly impractical means of optimizing imaging systems.

For quantitative image-quality assessment, ensembles of images with equivalent statistics are required. When anatomical structures are imaged, it is important to note that the statistical properties are not only unknown, but are widely varying from patient to patient. It can therefore be elusive in several cases to attempt to classify clinical images in order to form statistical ensembles for image-quality assessment. For example, breast tissues vary on a quasi-continuum in terms of fibrosity and fat amount, and establishing classes of images with equivalent statistical properties is not always possible with clinical images.

Another approach to improving imaging systems in medical imaging is to employ images acquired from mechanical phantoms. While mechanical phantoms are well specified, the main limitation is typically the lack in flexibility to vary parameters in the phantom to account for either natural variations in the data, or the presence of different types of abnormality.

In this chapter, we shall describe how synthetic images of anatomical images obtained either from a mathematical or a procedural model provide a useful tool to enhance our understanding of images. We shall also discuss how they enable quantifying image quality without the limitations of other methods previously mentioned. Employing synthetic images also has the benefit to yield cost-effective investigations.

In order to ensure a realistic level of complexity, synthetic images that model the statistics of anatomical images are desired to ensure transfer of findings to image-quality assessment of clinical images. If we cannot demonstrate the validity of a predictive task-based model in mathematically specified images relevant to medical imaging, we foresee that such a model will most likely fail to predict performance in clinical images.

In this chapter, we provide methods for synthesizing several types of synthetic images: angiograms, lumpy backgrounds, nuclear-medicine liver scans, ultrasound B scans, and generally speaking textured images with application to simulation of x-ray mammograms. The statistical properties of statistically defined images or image components are detailed.

13.2 Computer-simulated angiograms

Angiography is a radiological imaging modality that allows visualization of the normally radioluscent vascular anatomy. High radiographic attenuation is achieved in the vessels of interest by the injection, prior to exposure with diagnostic radiation, of a radio dense contrast agent. One of the many tasks performed with this modality is to detect or measure the extent of aneurysms or stenoses in blood vessels. The presence of such blood-vessel abnormality may be indicative of vascular disease, and accurate diagnosis is essential in prevention of catastrophic vascular malfunction resulting from the rupture of an aneurysm or constricted blood flow in a major vessel.

The motivation for employing computer-simulated angiograms comes from the need to precisely control the stimuli in performance experiments employing either the human observer or a mathematical observer. We shall show that aspects of the vessel generation in three dimensions can be parameterized in order to enable acquisition of tightly specified, but realistic stimuli. Moreover, statistically defined curvature and torsion, as well as irregular edges further allow for realistic, yet mathematically specified, blood vessels.

Tasks that have been considered using these simulated images are the detection and the estimation of aneurysms and stenoses for image understanding and medical-image interpretation. Specifically, computer-generated angiograms were employed in testing by means of psychophyscial experiments whether the curvature of the blood vessel at the location of a lesion had any impact on the detectability of the lesion in both a location known exactly and in a search task.

In a location known-exactly task, the detectability of lesions was measured. We found that the detection thresholds increased with curvature [6]. This experiment was then followed by an investigation of lesion detectability in a search experiment, referred to as lesion saliency. The more salient a lesion, the faster it was found. In this location-unknown task, the percent narrowing or bulging of the blood vessel was adjusted for all lesions to be equally detectable in a location known-exactly task. We then found that curvature had no impact on the saliency of the lesions. They were all equally salient once equally detectable in a location known-exactly task [7]. This experiment led to deeper understanding of lesion detection in angiograms, and allowed us to investigate independently detectability in a location known-exactly task versus detectability in a search task, where location was unknown.

The computer-generated angiograms were also used in some estimation task experiments. Under controlled conditions, the ability of human observers to estimate a change in the shape of a blood vessel corresponding to either some aneurysm or a stenosis embedded in a tree of similar shaped objects (i.e., blood vessels) was measured. In these experiments, the control of the stimuli allowed to investigate the accuracy of estimation as a function of the location of the lesion with respect to other underlying structures close to the blood vessels [8].

Another task that may be considered with computer-simulated angiograms is the assessment of 3D reconstruction algorithms. In this case, branching blood vessel trees would be required. An algorithm for simulating individual three-dimensional (3D) blood vessels with lesions in user-specified regions of interest is now described. The methods may be extended to simulation of branching blood vessel trees.

13.2.1 Overall approach for angiogram simulations

The simplest simulation of an angiogram with realistic geometry of individual blood vessels may be achieved by simulating individual three-dimensional blood vessels that curve and twist in a predefined volume, followed by the summation of several of their projections [9]. While clinical angiograms clearly possess many branching blood vessels, the simple approach to angiogram simulation described here leads to images that have been mistaken to be real angiograms by radiologists. Moreover, the simulation of 3D individual blood vessels described here constitutes the foundation for developing a method for branching blood vessels.

The approach to blood vessels simulation consists in viewing 3D blood vessels as general cylinders defined by a medial axis, and a corresponding diameter function coupled with a curvature and torsion associated with each point along the axis. The simulation of an individual blood vessel consists then of the following steps: (1) generating a space curve that bends and twists in space, which mathematically represents the medial axis of the blood vessel, (2) defining a region of interest on the two-dimensional (2D) projection of the space curve to locate potential lesions, (3) generating the 3D blood vessel from a space curve and the parameters that characterize the blood vessel; for example, diameter, type of lesion if any, lesion parameters such as the size of the lesion, and (4) generating one or several 2D projections of the 3D blood vessel. Each step of the simulation is now described.

13.2.2 Space curve generation

Initially, a curve is generated which specifies the path of the vessel in three-dimensional space as shown in Figure 13.1. The curve is specified by the Frenet formulas that mathematically specify the curvature and the torsion of a space curve as the curve traces a path in space. The Frenet description given by O'Neill Barrett (1966) can be summarized as follows [10].

The velocity vector of a curve β at position s is $\beta'(s)$, and the speed of the curve at s is the length of the velocity vector, or $\|\beta'(s)\|$, where the double-side bar denotes the norm of a vector. Let β be a unit speed curve, such that along β, $\|\beta'(s)\| = 1$. Then $T = \beta'$ is called the unit *tangent vector* field on β. The derivative of T denoted T' equal β'' and measures the way in which the curve is turning in space. T' is called the *curvature vector* field of β. The length of T' gives a numerical measurement of the turning of β. The function $\kappa(s)$ equal $\|T'(s)\|$ is called the *curvature function* of β. κ is positive and the larger κ, the sharper is the turning of β. T' is always normal to β. If we impose the restriction that κ is strictly positive, then the unit vector field N equal T'/κ on β indicates the *direction* in which β is turning at each point, and is called the *principal normal vector* field of β. Then the vector field B equal T cross product N on β is called the *binormal vector* field of β.

The three vector fields T, N, and B are unit vectors that are mutually orthogonal at each point along the curve. The set of these three vectors (T, N, B) is called the Frenet frame field of β. The key to the successful study of the geometry of a curve β is to use its Frenet frame field, for it contains all descriptive information about β.

The Frenet formulas then express the change or derivatives (T', N', B') of the Frenet frame field (T, N, B). If β is a unit-speed curve with curvature $\kappa(s)$ and torsion $\tau(s)$ then

$$
\begin{aligned}
T' &= \kappa N, \\
N' &= -\kappa T + \tau B, \\
B' &= -\tau N.
\end{aligned}
\tag{13.1}
$$

Given the curvature and torsion functions along the curve or values at each point along the arc length of the space curve, the Frenet formulas can be used to compute the new Frenet frame field at a point $s + \delta s$ as a function of κ, τ, and (T, N, B) at s. In the simulation, a curvature κ and torsion τ are chosen at each point along the space curve according to specified statistical distributions about previous values as we shall describe. The next location in space (x, y, z) of the

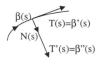

Figure 13.1: Definition of the normal and tangent to a space curve.

space curve is then computed given a small increment in arclength δs and the coordinates T_x, T_y, and T_z of the tangent vector along x, y, and z at s.

13.2.3 Curvature and torsion specification

The values of curvature and torsion along the space curve are defined statistically to allow for realistic simulations. Because 3D angiograms are not readily or even typically available, and realistic simulations may only be obtained if the blood vessels are first simulated in 3D before being projected, we have selected a range of variation based on theoretical ground (i.e., positivity constraint) as well as empirical investigations.

The curvature may be specified to take on values greater than 0 and less than or equal to 0.3. These values correspond to an infinite radius of curvature (i.e., a straight curve) and a radius of curvature equal to about 3 pixels, respectively. Smaller radii of curvature were disallowed.

Following the requirement that the curvature κ be positive, a Poisson distribution for small values of the curvature or an approximation to a Poisson distribution for larger values is a natural choice. Another possible choice would be a Gaussian with positivity constraint. A Poisson distribution was chosen in the simulation demonstrated, and the values of κ were thus first scaled by a factor of 1000 in order to work with integer values.

For such a range, if the scaled previous curvature value is less than 10 or greater than 290, the next value is chosen according to a Poisson distribution about the scaled previous value. If the previous curvature value is within those two values, the next value is chosen from a Gaussian distribution whose mean value equals the scaled previous curvature value, and whose standard deviation equals the mean.

In the same way that curvature values greater than 0.3 were disallowed, torsion values τ were restricted to the range -0.3 to 0.3. New values of τ are sampled from a Gaussian distribution of standard deviation small with respect to the range to ensure a smooth change in torsion as the curve is generated. A Gaussian, whose mean value was the previous torsion value, and the standard deviation was 0.02, was chosen.

Finally, if the newly selected curvature or torsion values were outside their range of variation (0.0 to 0.3 for κ, and -0.3 to 0.3 for τ), or the percent change in the curvature or torsion was greater than 30%, the current curvature or torsion was assigned to the previous value. A mechanism for preventing extensive or continuous high curvature or torsion "loops" that would lead to "pig tails" was also put into place. A count of consecutive curvature and torsion values greater than 0.29

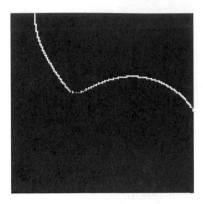

Figure 13.2: An example of a 2D projected space curve.

was kept. When the count exceeded a value as a function of δs, a new curvature or torsion value was assigned, which was in the case presented here the previous curvature or torsion divided by a factor of three.

From the space curve, a projected space curve denoted $\kappa_{2D}(s)$ is generated as shown in Figure 13.2. A file however maintains values of s, κ, and τ for each position along the curve, as well as the 2D curvature values of the projected space curve (O'Neill, 1966) [10]. The validation of the range of values selected for the curvature and the torsion of the 3D blood vessels, while not conducted in the work referenced here, would consist in comparing the values of $\kappa_{2D}(s)$ obtained in the simulated blood vessels to that of clinical 2D angiograms.

13.2.4 Blood vessels and possible lesions simulation

The positions at which lesions (i.e., aneurysms or stenoses) may form in the vessel can be specified along the projected space curve, where user-defined regions of interest (ROIs) may be specified as shown in Figure 13.3. While specified along the projected, thus 2D, space curve, the ROIs location and dimensions subsequently serves in the generation of the 3D blood vessels.

Starting with the generation of a single blood-vessel angiogram, at each position along the space curve defining the location of the blood vessel, a solid sphere of specified diameter is placed. The simulation of the 3D blood vessel is equivalent to rolling the sphere along the 3D space curve. Possible lesions are then automatically generated in 3D by allowing the sphere to vary in diameter within the specified ROIs.

The shape of lesions may be specified by some function. We shall demonstrate the case of a Gaussian function of given height and width, where the height represents the percent fraction of the blood-vessel diameter, and the width represents the length of the lesion expressed in units of pixel. Specifically, the sum of a constant and a Gaussian function centered at the location of a lesion, for example, describes the diameter of the rolling sphere as it passes through the lesion region.

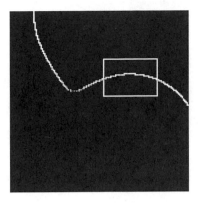

Figure 13.3: A region of interest has been drawn on the projected curve.

13.2.5 Example of simulated angiograms

To simulate 2D angiograms, 3D blood vessels, with or without lesions, are generated individually and projected in a 2D plane. An example of a segment of a blood vessel with an aneurysm is shown in Figure 13.4. Additional examples are shown in Figures 13.5 and 13.6. In Figure 13.5, the vessel has a diameter of 10 pixels, and a 50% aneurysm of length 20 pixels located in the lower right corner. In Figure 13.6, the vessel has an initial diameter of 15 pixels which tapers by a factor of −0.001 from its starting position, and a 50% stenosis of length 10 pixels positioned roughly halfway along the path of the vessel, near the center of the image. The images shown here were cropped from 256 × 256 images.

Individual 2D blood vessels can then be added. Examples are shown in Figure 13.7. In the case of the simulation shown, all blood vessels had the same diameter, except at the location of lesions, as required for a controlled psychophysical experiment where we did not want the diameter of the blood vessels to create a confounding factor for studying the effect of curvature on detection [7]. Simulations may include blood vessels of different, as well as spatially varying, diameter.

13.2.6 Simulation of edge noise

The diameter of the blood vessel may be varied randomly as well in order to simulate natural variations in the diameter of the vessel walls. In a healthy patient, vessel walls are indeed smooth. However, in older patients or patients with vascular disease such as artherosclerosis, small plaques form on the interior wall of the vessel, causing the vessel imaged with contrast agent to have a lumpy or non-smooth boundary. We shall refer to such variations as edge noise.

Edge noise can be generated by employing grayscale morphology methods to randomly erode or dilate the level contours in the image [9]. The lumpy appearance of the boundary of the vessel is a form of texture. The generation of noise is done iteratively. The number of iterations dictates, along with the correlation of

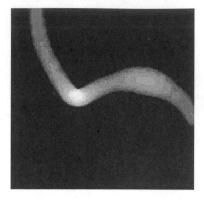

Figure 13.4:   A blood vessel was generated with an aneurysm in the specified region of interest in 3D. The 2D projection is shown.

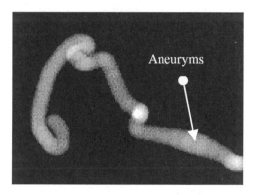

Figure 13.5:   A blood vessel with an aneurysm is shown.

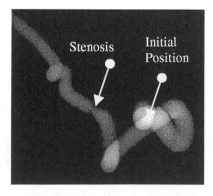

Figure 13.6:   A blood vessel with an stenosis is shown.

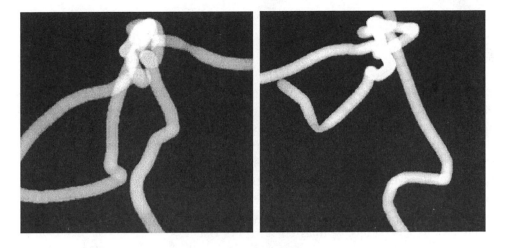

Figure 13.7: Examples of computer-simulated angiograms.

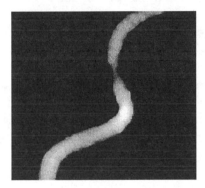

Figure 13.8: Edge noise was added to the blood-vessel simulation.

the noise, the extent of the effect. An example of edge noise simulation is shown in Figure 13.8.

13.2.7 Statistical ensembles

As stated in Section 13.1, quantitative image-quality assessment requires ensembles of images with equivalent statistics. The ability to mathematically synthesize blood vessels importantly allows us to define classes of images with equivalent statistical descriptions regarding the geometry of the blood vessels such as their distributions of curvature, torsion, and blood-vessel diameters, as well as the types of lesions and their locations. For example, in the studies reported by Rolland *et al.* (1996) [7], ensembles of computer-simulated angiograms with lesions at either low, medium, or high curvature values were generated to investigate the effect of curvature on lesion detection.

13.3 Synthesizing lumpy backgrounds

The need for spatially varying backgrounds was generated by an unsolved problem in planar emission imaging systems. Such a system generally consists of an x ray or gamma-ray source, an aperture element, and a detector. The challenge was how to specify the optimal photon-collecting aperture. Large apertures yield high photon counts but with positional uncertainty or poor resolution, while small apertures yield low photon counts and high resolution.

Finding the optimal trade-off between collection efficiency and resolution is important in the design and utilization of these systems, and requires quantitative specification of the imaging system from object space to the detector. The most challenging is typically the specification of the object to be imaged, which may be thought of as the combination of a lesion embedded in an anatomical background, or as an anatomical image that may or may not present abnormal changes in its texture. Examples of such objects are lesions and architectural distortions in mammographic images, respectively.

Cases of backgrounds where the performance of statistical observer models could be easily calculated were given in Chapter 9. The case of a known-exactly lesion (i.e., characteristics and location are exactly specified) embedded in an infinite uniform background of known strength led to an aperture which is infinite in extent. The generalization of this problem to include a background of unknown strength combined with a finite detector size led to the contrary to a finite optimal aperture size which better reflects clinical experience [11].

Another problem, presented by Wagner *et al.* (1981) consisted of a high-contrast Rayleigh task in which the ideal observer was computed to determine whether a noisy image was that of a single or double Gaussian two-dimensional signal [12]. Harris (1964) suggested that this discrimination task as a function of the object width and separation is a useful test of imaging system performance [13]. What was referred to as the signal in the Wagner paper, is the equivalent of a lesion in medical imaging. The signal was superimposed in this case on a uniform background of known and constant strength. The only randomness in the image resulted from Poisson statistics. Wagner *et al.* chose to image this object through different apertures including a pinhole and a large open aperture twenty times the size of the pinhole. They found that, for the ideal observer, the large aperture outperformed the small pinhole for all source widths and separations. This finding did not agree with experimental practices in emission imaging. For example, in nuclear medicine, spatial resolution of 1 cm, measured as the width of the point spread function, seems to give the best subjective image quality. The detection and Rayleigh tasks that found superior performance for large apertures have two common features: one is the complete specification of the background and signal, the other is the infinite size of the detector area.

To investigate the paradox brought by the Tsui and Wagner studies, Myers *et al.* (1990) increased the complexity of the task by relaxing the property of an exactly specified background while keeping the object size and similarly the detector size infinite [14]. Specifically, researchers simulated spatially varying backgrounds that are known as lumpy backgrounds [15, 16]. Detectability of several mathematical observers was computed and it was found that the Hotelling observer predicted an optimal aperture size for detectability, also found for the human observer.

The intent behind the lumpy-backgrounds simulation was not to replicate mathematically specific types of images. Rather it was intended to simply allow for the spatially varying property often encountered in medical images, while ensuring that the gray-level statistical properties were fully determined and known so that the performance of mathematical observers could be computed and hypotheses tested. Lumpy backgrounds have since been employed in various image-quality assessment tasks for medical imaging [17–21]. It is implicitly assumed in such approaches to simulating quasi-anatomical images that a system optimized for a model observer and a specified task would also be optimal not only for the human observer but also for more realistic tasks.

13.3.1 Assumptions for the simulation of lumpy backgrounds

In the simulation of lumpy backgrounds, the ability to create a spatially inhomogeneous background while knowing its first and second-order statistical properties are of primary importance. The variability in the background can be achieved in many different ways, but only certain models lead to descriptions that are mathematically tractable [16].

We make several assumptions to simplify the mathematics. First, we assume that the background is a wide-sense stationary process, where the autocorrelation function is a function of only the distance $\mathbf{r}$ between two observation points. Second, we assume that the background autocorrelation function is a Gaussian function of the form

$$R_f(\mathbf{r}) = \frac{W_f(0)}{2\pi r_b^2} \exp(-|\mathbf{r}|^2/2r_b^2), \qquad (13.2)$$

where r_b is the correlation length of the autocorrelation function and $W_f(0)$ is the value of the power spectrum at zero frequency. The subscript f here emphasizes the fact that the autocorrelation function refers to the object $f(\mathbf{r})$ rather than the image $g(\mathbf{r})$. The notation $W_f(0)$ comes from the notations used for the power spectrum because, for stationary statistics, the power spectrum $W_f(\boldsymbol{\Delta})$ can be defined as the Fourier transform of the autocorrelation function, so that

$$W_f(\boldsymbol{\Delta}) = W_f(0) \exp(-2\pi^2 r_b^2 |\boldsymbol{\Delta}|^2), \qquad (13.3)$$

where $\boldsymbol{\Delta}$ is the 2D frequency variable in the Fourier domain conjugate to $\mathbf{r}$. $W_f(0)$ is chosen as a measure of lumpiness. We shall now proceed to a description of two simulation schemes that yield stationary statistics and Gaussian autocorrelation functions.

13.3.2 Type-I lumpy backgrounds

The first approach to lumpy backgrounds is to simulate uncertainty in the image by randomly superimposing Gaussian functions upon a constant background of strength B_0 over the object space [15]. We refer to these Gaussian functions as Gaussian blobs or simply blobs. To keep the mathematics simple, we assume that the Gaussian blobs are of constant amplitude $b_0/\pi r_b^2$ and constant half-width r_b. An object formed with these blobs can be described mathematically as the sum of two terms: a constant term and a lumpy component term. The lumpy component term is the convolution of a set of delta functions of equal amplitude randomly located in object space, with a Gaussian function of constant strength and width. The lumpy component of the background, denoted $b(\mathbf{r})$, is then given by

$$
b(\mathbf{r}) = \left[\sum_{j=1}^{K} \delta(\mathbf{r} - \mathbf{r}_j) \right] * \left[\frac{b_0}{\pi r_b^2} \exp\left(-\frac{|\mathbf{r}|^2}{r_b^2} \right) \right]
$$

$$
= \sum_{j=1}^{K} \frac{b_0}{\pi r_b^2} \exp\left(-\frac{|\mathbf{r} - \mathbf{r}_j|^2}{r_b^2} \right), \tag{13.4}
$$

where $\mathbf{r}_j$ is a uniformly distributed random variable over the object area that describes the location of the jth blob, and K is the number of blobs in the background. Note that r_b is the $1/e$ width of the blobs as well as the correlation length (defined as a standard deviation) of R_f.

The description of a nonuniform background given by Eq. (13.4) is not sufficient to yield a Gaussian autocorrelation function. The calculation of the autocorrelation function presented in Section 13.3.3 shows that the number of blobs K must itself be a random variable with the mean of K equal to its variance. A Poisson distribution is chosen for K as it will satisfy this condition. The expression for $R_f(\mathbf{r})$ reduces to

$$
R_f(\mathbf{r}) = \frac{\overline{K}}{A_f} \frac{b_0^2}{2\pi r_b^2} \exp\left(-\frac{|\mathbf{r}|^2}{2r_b^2} \right), \tag{13.5}
$$

where A_f is the area of the object. The expression for R_f, or equivalently W_f given by

$$
W_f(\mathbf{\Delta}) = \frac{\overline{K}}{A_f} b_0^2 \exp\left(-2\pi^2 r_b^2 |\mathbf{\Delta}|^2 \right) \tag{13.6}
$$

describes the complete second-order statistics of the lumpy background thus generated. By comparing Eq. (13.3) to Eq. (13.6), we find that the lumpiness, measured in units of counts^2/(s^2 mm^2) is given by

$$
W_f(0) = \frac{\overline{K}}{A_f} b_0^2. \tag{13.7}
$$

We note that lumpiness as defined is a function of only the mean number of blobs per unit area and the strength of the blobs, not their actual size and shape. The size and shape of the blobs may be an important factor, however, in relation to the task to be performed. For example, in a lesion-detection task, the shape and size of the blobs are important in relation to the size and shape of the lesion to be detected.

13.3.3 Computation of first and second-order statistics for type-I lumpy backgrounds

The random variable used to describe the lumpiness in the background given by Eq. (13.4) can be written as

$$b(\mathbf{r}) = \left[\sum_{j=1}^{K} \delta(\mathbf{r} - \mathbf{r}_j)\right] * y(\mathbf{r}), \tag{13.8}$$

where the asterisk denotes 2D convolution, and

$$y(\mathbf{r}) = \frac{b_0}{\pi r_b^2} \exp\left(-\frac{|\mathbf{r}|^2}{r_b^2}\right). \tag{13.9}$$

The first-order statistics can be expressed most generally as the gray-level histogram averaged over the ensemble of objects. In the case of lumpy backgrounds, the histogram is Gaussian by construction. The mean of the histogram, which is also the expected value $\overline{B}$ of the background over the ensemble of objects, can be derived analytically and its expression will be required in the computation of second-order statistics. The expression for the mean level $\overline{B}$ is given by

$$
\begin{aligned}
\overline{B} &= B_0 + \langle b(\mathbf{r})\rangle_{f,K} \\
&= B_0 + \left\langle \sum_{j=1}^{K} \frac{1}{A_f} \int d^2\mathbf{r}_j \, y(\mathbf{r} - \mathbf{r}_j)\right\rangle_K \\
&= B_0 + \frac{\overline{K}}{A_f} b_0,
\end{aligned}
\tag{13.10}
$$

where we assumed that A_f tends to infinity, and $\langle b(\mathbf{r})\rangle_{f,K}$ is the expectation value of $b(\mathbf{r})$ averaged over two random variables, the random positions r_j for a fixed number of blobs (i.e., average over f), and the various values of K. Note that B_0 is in units of counts/(s mm^2), $\overline{K}/A_f$ is in units of counts/mm^2, and b_0 is in units of counts/s. The mean background $\overline{B}$ is then expressed as the number of counts/(s mm^2).

For a Gaussian random process, the second-order statistics is fully described by the autocorrelation function. Similarly, to compute the autocorrelation of this random process, we shall average over f and K. The autocorrelation of the lumpy background $b(\mathbf{r})$ is given by

$$
\begin{aligned}
R_f(\mathbf{r}) &= \langle R_{f|K}(\mathbf{r}' - \mathbf{r}'')\rangle_K \\
&= \langle\langle[b(\mathbf{r}') - \langle b(\mathbf{r}')\rangle_{f|K}][b(\mathbf{r}'') - \langle b(\mathbf{r}'')\rangle_{f|K}]\rangle_{f|K}\rangle_K,
\end{aligned} \tag{13.11}
$$

where $\mathbf{r}''$ and $\mathbf{r}'$ are 2D position vectors and $\langle b(\mathbf{r}')\rangle_{f|K}$ is the expectation value of $b(\mathbf{r}')$ averaged over the random positions of blobs that constitute the lumpy backgrounds. The expression for $R_{f|K}$ given in Eq. (13.11) can be shown to reduce to the difference of two terms [16]

$$
R_{f|K}(\mathbf{r}) = \langle b(\mathbf{r}')b(\mathbf{r}'')\rangle_{f|K} - \langle b(\mathbf{r}')\rangle_{f|K}\langle b(\mathbf{r}'')\rangle_{f|K}. \tag{13.12}
$$

The second term of Eq. (13.12) is given by

$$
\langle b(\mathbf{r}')\rangle_{f|K}\langle b(\mathbf{r}'')\rangle_{f|K} = \left\langle\sum_{j=1}^{K}y(\mathbf{r}' - \mathbf{r}_j)\right\rangle_{f|K}\left\langle\sum_{j=1}^{K}y(\mathbf{r}'' - \mathbf{r}_j)\right\rangle_{f|K} = K^2\frac{b_0^2}{A_f^2}. \tag{13.13}
$$

The first term of Eq. (13.12) can be written

$$
\begin{aligned}
\langle b(\mathbf{r}')b(\mathbf{r}'')\rangle_{f|K} &= \left\langle\sum_{i=1}^{K}y(\mathbf{r}' - \mathbf{r}_i)\sum_{j=1}^{K}y(\mathbf{r}'' - \mathbf{r}_j)\right\rangle_{f|K} \\
&= \int d^2r_1\,\mathrm{pr}(\mathbf{r}_1)\ldots\int d^2r_K\,\mathrm{pr}(\mathbf{r}_K) \\
&\quad\times\sum_{i=1}^{K}y(\mathbf{r}' - \mathbf{r}_i)\sum_{j=1}^{K}y(\mathbf{r}'' - \mathbf{r}_j),
\end{aligned} \tag{13.14}
$$

where $\mathrm{pr}(\mathbf{r}_i)$ is the probability associated with the random variable $\mathbf{r}_i$. If $i = j$, each term of the sum over i and j contributes in the same fashion to term 1. Since there are K terms such that $i = j$, the first term of Eq. (13.12) becomes for $i = j$,

$$
\langle b(\mathbf{r}')b(\mathbf{r}'')\rangle_{f|K}(i = j) = \frac{K}{A_f}\frac{b_0^2}{2\pi r_b^2}\exp\left(-\frac{|\mathbf{r}|^2}{2r_b^2}\right). \tag{13.15}
$$

Similarly, since they are $(K^2 - K)$ terms with $i \neq j$, the contribution of the terms $i \neq j$ to the first term of Eq. (13.12) is given by

$$
\langle b(\mathbf{r}')b(\mathbf{r}'')\rangle_{f|K}(i \neq j) = (K^2 - K)\frac{b_0^2}{A_f^2}. \tag{13.16}
$$

Thus the autocorrelation function R_f is given by

$$R_f(\mathbf{r}) = \frac{\overline{K}}{A_f}\frac{b_0^2}{2\pi r_b^2}\exp\left(-\frac{|\mathbf{r}|^2}{2r_b^2}\right) + \overline{(K^2 - K)}\frac{b_0^2}{A_f^2} - \overline{K}^2\frac{b_0^2}{A_f^2}, \tag{13.17}$$

which is Gaussian only if K satisfies $\overline{(K^2 - K)} = \overline{K}^2$ or $\overline{(K^2 - \overline{K}^2)} = \overline{K}$. If K is a Poisson random variable, such relationship will be satisfied and the autocorrelation reduces to a Gaussian given by

$$R_f(\mathbf{r}) = \frac{\overline{K}}{A_f}\frac{b_0^2}{2\pi r_b^2}\exp\left(-\frac{|\mathbf{r}|^2}{2r_b^2}\right). \tag{13.18}$$

The power spectrum, which is defined as the Fourier transform of the autocorrelation function is given by

$$W_f(\mathbf{\Delta}) = \frac{\overline{K}}{A_f}b_0^2\exp\left(-2\pi^2 r_b^2|\mathbf{\Delta}|^2\right) \quad \text{thus} \quad W_f(0) = \frac{\overline{K}}{A_f}b_0^2. \tag{13.19}$$

13.3.4 Type-II lumpy backgrounds

A second approach to lumpy backgrounds with a Gaussian autocorrelation function is to filter uncorrelated Gaussian noise. If the filter function is chosen to be a Gaussian function of correlation length r_b, a mathematical description of the background generated from filtered uncorrelated Gaussian noise is best given in the discrete form

$$b(\mathbf{r}_j) = \sum_i a(\mathbf{r}_i)\frac{H(0)}{\pi r_b^2}\exp\left(-|\mathbf{r}_j - \mathbf{r}_i|^2/r_b^2\right), \tag{13.20}$$

where $a(\mathbf{r}_i)$ is a random variable normally distributed with mean value A_0 and standard deviation σ, with i specifying the ith blob located at the ith pixel, and r_j is the location of the jth pixel in the background. In this model, the randomness resides in the amplitude of the Gaussian blobs instead of in their position.

13.3.5 Computation of first and second-order statistics for type-II lumpy backgrounds

The mean background $\overline{B}$ of the random process $b(\mathbf{r}_j)$ can be evaluated by taking the ensemble average over the random variable, which in this case, is the amplitude of the noise impulses at each pixel location j in the image. $\overline{B}$ is given in counts/(s pixel) by

$$\begin{aligned}
\overline{B} &= \langle b(\mathbf{r})\rangle_a \\
&= \left\langle \frac{H(0)}{\pi r_b^2}\sum_i a(\mathbf{r}_i)\exp\left(-|\mathbf{r}_j - \mathbf{r}_i|^2/r_b^2\right)\right\rangle_a \\
&= \frac{1}{\varepsilon^2}H(0)A_0,
\end{aligned} \tag{13.21}$$

where A_0 in units of counts/(s pixel) is defined as $\langle a(\mathbf{r}_i)\rangle_a$, and ε^2 is the pixel area.

By definition, the power spectrum of uncorrelated noise $W(\boldsymbol{\Delta})$ is constant, and if we denote by $H(\boldsymbol{\Delta})$ the Gaussian filter used to filter Gaussian noise, the resulting power spectrum is given by

$$W_f(\boldsymbol{\Delta}) = W(\boldsymbol{\Delta})\big|H(\boldsymbol{\Delta})\big|^2. \tag{13.22}$$

To generate lumpy backgrounds of type II with the same autocorrelation function as lumpy backgrounds of type I, we define $H(\boldsymbol{\Delta})$ as

$$H(\boldsymbol{\Delta}) = H(0)\exp\!\left(-\pi^2 r_b^2|\boldsymbol{\Delta}|^2\right), \tag{13.23}$$

where $H(0)$ is the amplitude of the filter and r_b is the correlation length of the resulting autocorrelation function. The filtered power spectrum is then given by

$$W_f(\boldsymbol{\Delta}) = W(0)\big[H(0)\big]^2\exp\!\left(-2\pi^2 r_b^2|\boldsymbol{\Delta}|^2\right). \tag{13.24}$$

The expression for the autocorrelation function is then given by the inverse Fourier transform of the power spectrum as

$$R_f(\mathbf{r}) = \frac{W(0)[H(0)]^2}{2\pi r_b^2}\,\exp\!\left(-\frac{|\mathbf{r}|^2}{2r_b^2}\right). \tag{13.25}$$

The measure of lumpiness is now given by

$$W_f(0) = W(0)\big[H(0)\big]^2, \tag{13.26}$$

where $H(0)$ is simply a number and $W(0)$ is in units of counts per unit time and per unit area. Therefore, $W_f(0)$ is again in units of $\text{counts}^2/(\text{s}^2\,\text{mm}^2)$ for example. In the case of discretization of all quantities for digital simulations, $W_f(0)$ will be expressed in units of $\text{counts}^2/(\text{s}^2\,\text{pixel})$.

13.3.6 Examples of lumpy backgrounds type I and II

Examples of lumpy backgrounds of types I and II are shown in Figure 13.9(a) and (b), respectively. In Figure 13.9(a), the mean background $\overline{B}$ increases from left to right with values of 384, 1664, and 3200 counts/(s pixel), and the lumpiness increases from top to bottom with $W_f(0)$ equals 10^4, 10^5, and 10^6 $\text{counts}^2/(\text{s}^2\,\text{pixel})$. As the lumpiness increases, the strength of the blobs b_0 increased from 1280, 4047, and 12,800 counts/s, while the mean number of blobs is 100. In Figure 13.9(b), the value of $\overline{B}$ and $W_f(0)$ are the same as in Figure 13.9(a). As the lumpiness increases, the variance of the noise increases with σ equal 33.33, 105.41, and 333.33 pixels, respectively. As $\overline{B}$ increases, the strength of the filter takes the values 3, 13, and 25, respectively.

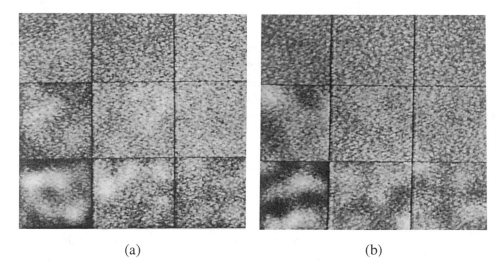

(a)   (b)

Figure 13.9: (a) Lumpy backgrounds of type I. (b) Lumpy backgrounds of type II.

13.4 Modeling liver scans

Cargill (1989) proposed a computer-generated 3D model of liver with the possibility to include various disease states [22]. Such a model, when combined with a model of imaging in nuclear medicine, was applied to imaging-system design optimization. Specifically, Cargill investigated the correlation of the Hotelling observer (presented in Chapter 11 of this book in the context of lumpy backgrounds) with human performance for nine different systems. This study was one of the milestones in showing that the Hotelling observer can be used to predict human performance.

Cargill also investigated how changes in texture correlated with disease states. In such investigation, the aim was to establish quantitative measures of the power spectrum of livers independently of the imaging system. Cargill estimated the contribution of the imaging system to real scans, and used the mathematical liver model to validate the approach. This investigation was one step forward in the development of imaging systems designed to optimize the amount of information related to, in this case, the texture associated with the liver being imaged. The methods may apply equally well to other organs [23].

Modeling the liver includes defining its three-dimensional shape and filling its volume. Object classes of normal livers were constructed by randomly perturbing the surface of the normal liver.

Liver diseases may be classified as focal or diffuse. Focal lesions correspond to reduced uptake of tracer in the liver. Focal lesions are typically liver tumors, metastatic lesions, and inflammatory disease such as amebic abscesses. In the case of diffuse disease, the entire liver structure is altered. Liver diseases were modeled to represent tumors, metastatic disease, and forms of inflammatory and diffuse diseases that we shall summarize here [22].

13.4.1 Modeling the shape of the liver

In modeling the shape of the liver, it was assumed that the surface of the liver could be expressed as an analytic function of vectors drawn from the origin of a coordinate system to points on the surface of the liver. This function was obtained from a set of measurements of points on the surface of a normal liver. The sampled function was then expanded in a set of orthogonal basis functions which spanned its vector space [24]. The three-dimensional fitted liver is then constructed by placing it at the center of a 3D grid attached to a coordinate system. The space is then divided into equal volume elements, or voxels. If a voxel is established to be inside the liver volume, the voxel is assigned a constant value that represents in nuclear medicine the uniform uptake of tracer throughout normal liver tissue.

In mapping the surface of the liver, because the liver appeared to possess approximate symmetry relative to spherical coordinates, the measurement data set acquired was mapped in a spherical polar coordinate system. The data set will be denoted $f(\theta, \phi)$. Spherical harmonics, denoted $Y_{lm}(\theta, \phi)$ are given by

$$Y_{lm}(\theta, \phi) = (-1)^m \sqrt{\frac{2n+1}{4\pi} \frac{(n-m)!}{(n+m)!}} P_{lm}(\cos\theta) e^{im\phi}, \qquad (13.27)$$

where l and m are integers to keep the functions single valued, $-l \leqslant m \leqslant l$, and $P_{lm}(\cos\theta)$ are the associated Legendre polynomials given by

$$P_{nm}(x) = \frac{1}{2^n n!} (1 - x^2)^{m/2} \frac{d^{m+n}}{dx^{m+n}} (x^2 - 1)^n. \qquad (13.28)$$

Because the spherical harmonics are orthonormal and complete, any single-valued function of θ and ϕ evaluated over the surface can be expanded in a uniformly convergent double series of spherical harmonics, a Laplace series,

$$f(\theta, \phi) = \sum_{l=0}^{\infty} \sum_{m=-l}^{l} a_{lm} Y_{lm}(\theta, \phi). \qquad (13.29)$$

If $f(\theta, \phi)$ is known, the expansion coefficients a_{lm} are determined by evaluating the product of the function to be fitted with the corresponding spherical harmonic over the unit sphere

$$a_{lm} = \int_0^{2\pi} \int_0^{\pi} Y_{lm}^*(\theta, \phi) f(\theta, \phi) \sin\theta \, d\theta \, d\phi, \qquad (13.30)$$

where the asterisk denotes the complex conjugate. Once the expansion coefficients have been determined, the function $f(\theta, \phi)$ can be reconstructed using the spherical harmonics.

In practice, the function $f(\theta, \phi)$ is sampled at discrete values of θ and ϕ, denoted θ_k and ϕ_n, given by

$$\theta_k = \frac{k\pi}{K}, \qquad \phi_n = \frac{2n\pi}{N}. \tag{13.31}$$

The sampled spherical harmonics $Y_{lm}(\theta_k, \phi_n)$ are not in general orthogonal and therefore

$$\sum_{k=1}^{K} \sum_{n=1}^{N} Y_{l'm'}^*(\theta_k, \phi_n) Y_{lm}(\theta_k, \phi_n) = \varepsilon_{l'm'lm}, \tag{13.32}$$

where $\varepsilon_{l'm'lm}$ can be considered a nonzero residue. The residue does not allow the double sum over l and m to be eliminated, and the calculation of one expansion coefficient cannot be isolated from the others. As the values of K and N become large, the residue becomes negligible, and the contribution of the coefficients where $l' = l$ and $m' = m$ are acceptably small.

There are useful recursion relations that relate adjacent values of l and m in the associated Legendre polynomials contained in the spherical harmonics [25]. These recursion relations facilitate calculating the spherical harmonics up to any desired value of l, once the few lowest-order terms have been computed, without having to perform the multiple differentiations that occur in the definition of the associated Legendre polynomials. The recurrence formula relating adjacent values of l is given by

$$P_{l+1,m}(x) = \frac{2l+1}{l-m+1} x P_{lm}(x) - \frac{l+m}{l-m+1} P_{l-1,m}(x). \tag{13.33}$$

The expression relating adjacent values of m is given by

$$P_{l,m+1}(x) = \frac{-2mx}{(1-x^2)^{1/2}} P_{lm}(x) - (l+m)(l-m+1) P_{l,m-1}(x). \tag{13.34}$$

There is also an expression relating spherical harmonics with index $-m$ to those with index m given by

$$Y_{l,-m}(\theta, \phi) = (-1)^m Y_{lm}^*(\theta, \phi). \tag{13.35}$$

Each expansion coefficient can then be calculated directly once the corresponding spherical harmonic term has been established. The surface of the liver can then be reconstructed from typically a truncated set of the spherical harmonics.

An ensemble of normal livers can be generated efficiently by perturbing randomly the spherical harmonics coefficients, from which new livers may be reconstructed. In doing so, the basic shape of the liver remains unchanged but the changes introduced represent normal size and shape variations.

13.4.2 Examples of mathematically fitted liver

For the case of the liver modeled by Cargill, the function $f(\theta, \phi)$ was typically sampled over 24 values of azimuthal angle ϕ (every 15°) and 36 values of polar angle θ (every 5°), giving a total of 840 values. For an expansion up to $l = 7$, the largest residue was 0.001, considered negligible. In the case of coarser sampling, where the residue cannot be ignored, a Schmidt orthogonalization procedure on the spherical harmonics allows creation of a new set of functions composed of

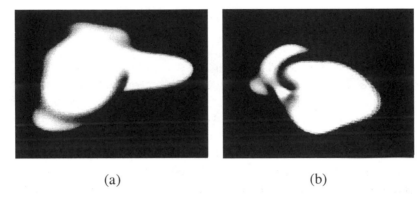

(a)   (b)

Figure 13.10: Simulation of a mathematically fitted liver scan (a) anterior view and (b) right lateral view (courtesy of Ellen Cargill, 1989).

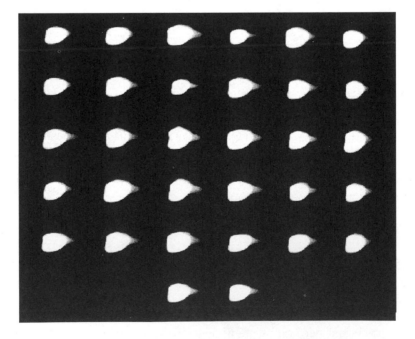

Figure 13.11: In this figure, 32 normal livers obtained from perturbing randomly the spherical harmonics coefficients are displayed (courtesy of Ellen Cargill, 1989).

weighted sums of the spherical harmonics that will be closer to being orthogonal over the sample space [25]. Figure 13.10 depicts shaded representations of an anterior view and a right lateral view of the mathematically fitted liver. Figure 13.11 shows two-dimensional projections of 32 normal livers created by perturbing randomly the spherical harmonics coefficients.

13.4.3 Modeling focal liver disease

Disease that is local in nature is referred to as focal disease. The most common primary focal liver tumor is hepatoma. Such lesions were modeled as ellipsoids within the liver parenchyma having uptake equal to 10% of normal liver tissue. Simulated lesions were located randomly within the liver volume.

13.4.4 Modeling metastatic disease

A major function of the liver is to process blood coming from the digestive system. Thus the liver is likely to track metastatic cells originating from the digestive system because of its proximity and the fact that it is the first extensive capillary network the cells encounter. If the liver fails to destroy these cancer cells, they may further metastasize. Consequently, the liver has a high rate of involvement in metastatic disease. Metastatic lesions can be modeled as multiple cold ellipsoids randomly located and oriented to represent lesions of various sizes randomly located within the liver volume.

Hepatomegaly, which is the enlargement of the liver, often accompanies the development of metastatic disease and is modeled by scaling the liver uniformly by multiplying the spherical harmonic coefficients by a constant.

13.4.5 Modeling inflammatory disease

Inflammation of the liver may be a response to infection. If the infection is focal in nature, such as an abscess, then the inflammation is likely to be focal in nature. In this case, cold ellipsoids randomly localized in the volume of the liver may be used to model abscesses. However, inflammation may also be associated with viral hepatitis, in which case the inflammation will be generalized and be modeled as diffuse disease.

13.4.6 Modeling of diffuse disease

Diseases that affect the overall parenchyma of the liver are referred as diffuse disease. Hepatitis and cirrhosis are common examples. The development of cirrhosis follows the self-similar structure of the liver. Rappaport *et al.* (1983) identified three basic types of lesions based on the degree of involvement of the higher orders of parenchyma organization [26]. They suggested to classify nodules based on their state of vascularization, which lead to defining triadal, paratriadal, and atriadal nodules. In addition, changes that may occur in the liver include hepatomegaly, left-lobe hypertrophy, righ-lobe blunting, heterogenous uptake, and low overall uptake. Other features related to the spleen and the vertebral bone marrow may also be present to some degree.

Changes in morphology of the liver may manifest as hepatomegaly or atrophy, or local enlargement. Atrophy can be modeled by altering the original data set representing the surface and refitting the deformed surface by a set of new coefficients. This perturbation involves varying the points on the modeled surface over some angular range. Most importantly, the data set must be perturbed in a smooth fashion to ensure a good fit of spherical harmonics to the perturbed data set [22]. Given a deformed liver, an ensemble may be simulated by varying the spherical harmonics coefficients.

Heterogenous uptake in the liver occurs frequently in cirrhosis of the liver. Such uptake manifests as a patchy appearance of the liver or texture. This is the result of portions of the liver parenchyma being replaced by scar tissue, and consequently not taking up any of the tracer. Patchy uptake was simulated by using a 3D texture in the volume of the liver. A 3D texture was obtained by filtering white noise in the Fourier domain with a $1/f^n$ spectrum. We shall further address more advanced methods for texture synthesis in Section 13.6.

13.5 Synthesizing ultrasound B-scan images

Pioneer work in texture synthesis for image-quality assessment in medical imaging can be found in ultrasound imaging. The need for synthetic images in ultrasound imaging first arose from the need to test novel methods for processing ultrasound signals [27]. Fink (1983) investigated the use of short-time Fourier analysis to provide an estimation of the echographic spectral composition as a function of time. Simulated echographic data from a one-dimensional tissue model was used to test this new method.

Insana *et al.* (1986) investigated how tissue signatures may be obtained from first and second-order statistics of ultrasonic B-scan textures [28]. In order to isolate second-order statistics, they identified nonstochastic stuctures in Rician noise fields such as blood vessels. The identification was established by thresholding a correlation image obtained from using a matched-filter technique in which a one-dimensional function is cross-correlated with the ultrasound image. Correlation thresholds were established by studying simulated images with known statistics. In another related investigation, Wagner *et al.* (1986) simulated images with Rician statistics and presented an algorithm for automatically ranking the images based on their statistical properties [29].

Momenan *et al.* (1988) employed simulated ultrasound B-scan-like images to establish which statistical parameters were most useful in discriminating tissue types. The main use of synthetic images was in the validation of image-processing techniques [30].

Finally, Valckx and Thijssen (1997) investigated the potentials of co-occurrence matrix analysis for the characterization of echographic image textures [31]. They simulated one-dimensional data sets with different number densities of the randomly distributed scatterers, and with different levels of structural scattering strength.

13.5.1 Modeling ultrasound B-scan images

The scattering of a radio-frequency (rf) wave from a random medium such as soft tissue involves a random walk in two dimensions corresponding to the real and imaginary components of the rf signal [32, 33]. Ultrasonic backscattered or echo pulses from soft tissues, when displayed as a clinical B-scan image, form a texture pattern that is characteristic of both the imaging system and the tissue being imaged [34]. The resulting images have the granular structure described as texture or speckle, which results from interactions (i.e., absorption, reflection, scattering) between the coherent ultrasonic pulses transmitted into the body and the microscopic (0.008 mm to 2 mm) structures of the tissue [35]. Scattering, responsible for the random character of the images, occurs at multiple sites randomly distributed within the resolution cell of the ultrasonic transducer.

Histological studies have shown that tissue scatterers vary in size and shape and that the different structures have varying degrees of spatial order. The organization of scattering stuctures for most biological media falls somewhere between blood, which is completely disordered and consists of randomly distributed scatterers, and skeletal muscle tissue, which is highly ordered with nearly periodic scatterers that repeat over a long range [36].

In the synthesis of ultrasonic B-scan texture images, soft tissues may be repre-sented as an acoustically uniform medium that comprises two different classes of scatterers [29]. In this modeling approach, the first class of scatterers consists in randomly positioned scatterers according to a uniform distribution. This scatterer class corresponds to diffuse scatterers within tissue. The process of interference for the diffuse component can be geometrically described as a random walk of component phasors and the received complex signal such as the rf voltage output V_d of the ultrasound transducer can be modeled as the sum of N complex signals from individual identical discrete scatterers

$$V_d = \sum_{j=1}^{N} a_j = \sum_{j=1}^{N} |a_j| \exp(i\phi_j) = a_{dr} + i a_{di}, \tag{13.36}$$

where the index d denotes the diffuse component, the index r and i denote the real and imaginary parts, respectively, and N represents the number of scatterers per resolution cell.

The second class of scatterers consists in nonrandomly distributed scatterers with long-range order. This can be modeled by adding a complex signal to the random sum, represented most generally as a phasor of real component a_{sr} and imaginary component a_{si}. The quantity $I_s = (a_{sr}^2 + a_{si}^2)$ is referred to as the specular intensity. Because this specular contribution is distributed over a region of the tissue or source of scattering, it is referred to as distributed specularity. The output voltage V is in this case given by

$$V = (a_{sr} + i a_{si}) + (a_{dr} + i a_{di}). \tag{13.37}$$

Examples of specular scatterers in tissues with resolvable long-range order are the portal triads and lobules in liver parenchyma and the collagenous sheaths that surround muscle bundles. Structures such as blood vessels and organ surfaces are not considered part of the texture, and are thus not included in this ultrasound texture model.

13.5.2 First and second-order statistics of ultrasound images

The first-order statistics are determined by the gray-level histogram of the B-scan or magnitude image. Considering first the diffuse scatter component, when the number of scatterers within a resolution cell is large and the phases of the scattered waves are independent and distributed uniformly between 0 and 2π, the complex amplitude V_d resulting from the random walk has real and imaginary components a_{dr} and a_{di} whose joint probability density function (pdf) is a circular Gaussian given by

$$p(a_{dr}, a_{di}) = \frac{1}{2\pi\sigma} \exp\left[-\left(a_{dr}^2 + a_{di}^2\right)/2\sigma^2\right]. \tag{13.38}$$

This is simply the product of two independent Gaussian density functions with zero mean and variance that can be shown to depend on the mean-square scattering amplitude of the particles in the scattering medium [37]. The average incoherent backscattered intensity component represented as the mean square of the complex amplitude averaged over all particles in the scattering medium is given by

$$\langle V_d V_d^* \rangle = \langle a_{dr}^2 + a_{di}^2 \rangle = 2\sigma^2 = I_d, \tag{13.39}$$

and will be referred to as the mean diffuse intensity I_d. The pdf associated with $|V_d| = \sqrt{I_d}$ can be shown to follow a Rayleigh pdf, while the pdf associated with $|V_d|^2 = I_d$ is an exponential pdf. The magnitude $\sqrt{I_d}$ is the quantity of interest, as ultrasound B-scan displays the envelope of the echo of the received signals, and the envelope is the instantaneous value of the magnitude of the phasor when the signal is sufficiently narrowband [33].

When the distributed specular component is also considered, the joint pdf of the real and imaginary components a_{dr} and a_{di} then becomes

$$p(a_{dr}, a_{di}) = \frac{1}{2\pi\sigma^2} \exp\left[-\left((a_{dr} - a_{sr})^2 + (a_{di} - a_{si})^2\right)/2\sigma^2\right], \tag{13.40}$$

where Eq. (13.37) was considered. The pdf associated with $|V|$ when both diffuse and specular reflections are considered, can be shown to follow a Rician probability density function generalized to include a spatially structured specular signal [32].

Wagner *et al.* (1983) found that the most fruitful second-order measure for analyzing ultrasound textures was the autocorrelation function and its Fourier transform, the texture power spectrum [38]. They have derived them, using the analytical apparatus of Middleton (1960), for the cases of the signal amplitude and signal intensity. They found that the straightforward study of the intensity signal led to the same results that follow from the more complicated envelope analysis [39]. The results for intensity are thus reported in this chapter.

The average correlation between one intensity measurement I at position x, and another measurement, I' at position $x' = x + \Delta x$, where the second measurement is obtained by translating the transducer a fixed distance Δx, can be shown to reduce to

$$
\begin{aligned}
\langle I I' \rangle &= I_d^2\left(1 + |\rho|^2\right) + I_d(I_s + I_s') + \langle(I_s \otimes I_s')\rangle + 2I_d\rho\langle(a_{sr} \otimes a_{sr}' + a_{si} \otimes a_{si}')\rangle \\
&= I_d^2\left(1 + |\rho|^2\right) + 2I_d\langle\overline{I_s}\rangle + \langle(I_s \otimes I_s')\rangle \\
&\quad + 2I_d\rho\langle(a_{sr} \otimes a_{sr}' + a_{si} \otimes a_{si}')\rangle,
\end{aligned} \tag{13.41}
$$

where the angle brackets denote expectation value, the symbol $\otimes$ indicates the conventional correlation operation, and $\langle\otimes\rangle$ further denotes the correlation operation averaged over the record length X of the position variable x. Also, the parameter ρ is the complex coherence factor (i.e., normalized autocovariance of the complex field) defined as

$$
\rho = \langle V V'^* \rangle / \sqrt{\langle |V|^2 \rangle \langle |V'|^2 \rangle}. \tag{13.42}
$$

The Fourier transform of the autocorrelation function yields the expression for the power spectrum detailed in Wagner *et al.* (1987) [39].

13.5.3 *Examples of simulated ultrasound B-scan images*

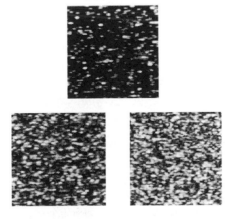

Figure 13.12: Sample images of ultrasound Bscans generated by computer simulation. The top images corresponds to fewer than 1 scatterer per resolution volume. The lower left and right images correspond to 2 and 6 scatterers per resolution volume, respectively. (Courtesy of Robert Wagner, FDA, Maryland.) (Copyright 1997, American Institute of Physics [62].)

13.6 Texture synthesis

In the same way that patchy uptake in the liver may be represented as a texture [22, 28], other medical images such as parenchyma in breast tissue and the inner structure of bones, may also be modeled as textures [40, 41]. Abnormality in the breast tissue parenchyma may manifest itself as architectural distortions in mammography for example. Loss in bone strength, generally with aging, is known as osteoporosis. Osteoporosis can be diagnosed from loss in bone density, yet the change in structure itself, while harder to measure is also thought to be important to establishing the state of disease and the effectiveness of drugs, for example, to rebuild bone strength [42].

Texture synthesis is the ability to create, from one acquired texture sample, an ensemble of images that look visually similar in structure, yet differ pixel to pixel from the acquired sample. As pointed to earlier in this chapter, the importance of synthesized textures in the assessment of image quality in medical imaging lies in the ability to be able to generate large ensembles of statistically equivalent images [43]. These images may serve as background images into which one may or may not insert objects of interest (i.e., lesions), or may serve as the object of interest itself [44]. Such statistically equivalent ensembles provide an effective means to assess image quality in medical systems such that findings will more easily transfer to clinical images.

13.6.1 General method of texture synthesis

Various natural textures have been effectively synthesized using a multi-layer pyramid transform that allows decomposition of a sample image at different scales and orientations [45]. After decomposition of a sample image, the histograms of the subimages thus obtained were employed to modify the histogram of a uniformly distributed white noise image that had been submitted to the same decomposition. The reconstruction, or synthesis, of the modified noise subimages yields a synthesized texture. Each new synthesis requires a new realization of the noise image.

13.6.2 Pyramid transform and image decomposition

An n-layer steerable pyramid transform constitutes the basis for the texture synthesis algorithm. One layer of the pyramid is depicted in Figure 13.13. Layers are connected by a factor of two *decimation*, of the image [46]. Decimation is a downsampling operation that consists in retaining every other pixel in an image. It is applied after low-pass filtering of the image, represented as "blur filter" on the left-hand side of the pyramid. Within each layer, the image is then filtered by a set of bandpass filters and followed by a set of orientation filters that form a quadrature mirror filter bank [47–50]. Four scales and four orientations 17 × 17 size filters, corresponding to 0-degree, 45-degree, 90-degree, and 135-degree orientations, were adopted in the simulation shown here.

During the decomposition synthesis, the sample texture image is processed through the left-hand side of the pyramid. It is represented in Figure 13.13 as an

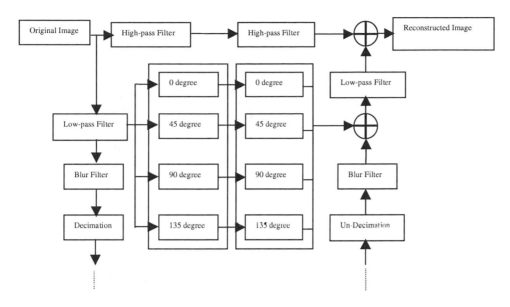

Figure 13.13: A layer of the steerable pyramid transform employed in the texture synthesis algorithm is shown. The image in the upper-right corner is either a texture sample or a realization of a white noise. The left hand of the pyramid is used for decomposing the two images. The right-hand side of the pyramid is used for image reconstruction or synthesis.

input to the pyramid in the upper left corner. In parallel, a realization of uniformly distributed white noise is processed through the same pyramid. The role of the white noise image is to provide a starting point for the synthesis.

13.6.3 Histogram matching and synthesis

The method of texture synthesis employs a technique known as histogram matching of two images. Histogram matching, sometimes referred to as histogram specification, is an image processing technique, specifically a point operation, which modifies a candidate image so that its histogram matches that of a model image [51]. While histogram matching is not widely employed in image processing, it is a generalization of histogram equalization, an image processing technique commonly employed to enhance low-contrast images [52–54].

The histograms of the subband noise images at multiple scales and multiple orientations are then matched to the corresponding histograms of the subband sample images. Fast algorithms for histogram matching have been proposed and investigated for enhancing the efficiency of the synthesis process [55]. Efficiency of the histogram matching operations is important in texture synthesis because the operations of decomposition and histogram matching are performed recursively, where the first synthesized image serves as the input noise image in the second iteration of the algorithm. While a quantification of the optimal number of iterations is subject to current investigation, five to seven iterations are typically performed.

The modified subband noise images are then recombined according to the right-hand side of the steerable pyramid transform shown in Figure 13.13. Starting from the lowest layer, images are undecimated from layer to layer. Undecimation is an upsampling operation that consists in inserting zero values in between pixels of the image. Such operation is followed by a blurring of the image represented as "blur filter" on the right-hand side of the pyramid. Moreover, at each upsampling operation, the intensity values are multiplied by four to compensate for the loss in image brightness that resulted during the downscaling of the images during the decomposition phase [43].

13.6.4 A two-component decomposition approach

The approach to texture synthesis described was extended to synthesize medical images such as mammograms [41]. The key to the successful synthesis of such images was an additional decomposition of the sample texture image into two components: the larger spatial variations in the image and a smaller relative scale underlying texture, shown in the upper-right and lower-left corners of Figure 13.14,

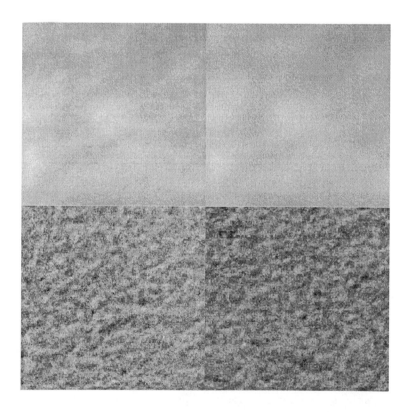

Figure 13.14: A segment of a mammographic image is shown in the upper-left corner. The extracted larger scale component is shown in the upper-right corner. The relatively smaller-scale component is shown in the lower-left corner. Finally a synthetic realization of the smaller-scale component is shown in the lower-left corner.

respectively. The larger scale images are reminiscent of lumpy images described earlier. One realization of the synthesized smaller scale texture is also shown in the lower right corner of the figure.

13.6.5 A breast-tissue mathematical phantom

The synthesis of an ensemble of images $M_i(x, y)$ can be established using an adaptive linear combination of realizations from the two model components: a realization of a broadly spatially varying texture, such as a lumpy image, denoted as $L_i(x, y)$, and a realization of the synthesized underlying texture component denoted as $T_i(x, y)$. The resulting synthesized image is then given by

$$M_i(x, y) = \alpha L_i(x, y) + (1 - \alpha)T_i(x, y), \qquad (13.43)$$

where α ranges from 0 to 1. Such a combination allows spanning of a wide range of tissue types with relative amounts of the broadly spatially varying component and the smaller-scale texture component. Such an approach to the synthesis of medical images may naturally find application to other types of images beside mammographic tissue.

13.6.6 Computation of first- and second-order statistics of synthetic textures

The first-order statistics of synthetic textures is the gray-level histogram of the sample texture employed in the synthesis given that histogram matching is part of the synthesis process, and it is also performed as a last step of the synthesis.

For Gaussian random processes, such as the lumpy backgrounds described earlier, the autocorrelation function or equivalently the power spectrum fully characterizes the second-order statistics. Knowledge of the first-order statistics and the autocorrelation function are in fact sufficient to compute the statistical properties of the random process to any order.

For non-Gaussian random processes, the complete second-order statistics are defined as the two-point probability density function (2P-PDF) also known as the co-occurrence matrix, especially in the literature on image processing. Julez first used gray-tone spatial dependence co-occurrence statistics in texture discrimination experiments [56].

A component of the complete 2P-PDF is computed as the frequency of simultaneous occurrence of two gray levels from two pixels separated by a directional distance $\mathbf{d}$ [60]. As $\mathbf{d}$ varies in size and orientation, the complete 2P-PDF is formed. A few components of the complete 2P-PDF for the small-scale mammographic texture are shown in Figure 13.15. Both components of the 2P-PDF of the original texture (i.e., left image) and a synthetic realization of the same texture (i.e., right image) are shown. Specifically, components of the 2P-PDF for values of $\mathbf{d}$ equal $(-5, -5)$, $(-3, -5)$, $(3, -5)$, and $(5, -5)$ from upper left to right, and $(-5, -5)$, $(-5, -3)$, $(-5, 3)$, and $(-5, 5)$ from top left to bottom left are presented. For each component shown, the co-occurrence of two gray levels varying between 0–255 is coded as intensity values.

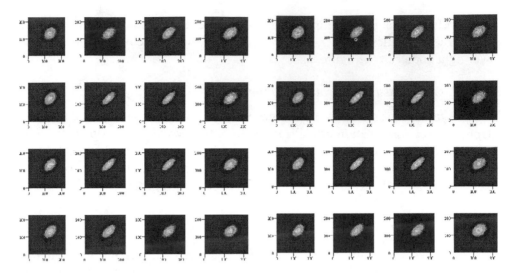

Figure 13.15: On the left, components of the 2P-PDF of the small-scale mammographic texture image are shown for values of **d** equal $(-5, -5)$, $(-3, -5)$, $(3, -5)$, and $(5, -5)$ from upper left to right, and $(-5, -5)$, $(-5, -3)$, $(-5, 3)$, and $(-5, 5)$ from top left to bottom left. On the right, the same components for a synthetic realization of the texture are shown. On each component, the co-occurrence of two gray levels varying between 0–255 is coded as intensity values.

Given that computing the complete 2P-PDF is quite demanding, various statistical measures have been extracted from the 2P-PDF for use in automatic texture discrimination [57]. The autocorrelation function or equivalently the power spectrum, for example, have been some of the measures most widely employed in analyzing statistical images like natural scenes. While the fact that the power spectra of natural images such as textures follow some power law may be found to be significant, it is important to note that power spectra do not provide complete descriptors of second-order statistics if the process is non-Gaussian. The power spectrum can be computed from the 2P-PDF but the reverse is not true.

Importantly, specifically two studies demonstrate that two sets of images with equal power spectra, yet having Fourier spectra that differ in phase, yield different detectability performance for human observers [58, 59]. In both investigations, ensembles of images with their natural noise, and ensembles of images with their natural-phase spectra replaced with random-phase spectra were considered in the study. Furthermore in Bochud (1995), ensembles of images with equal power spectra but with Fourier spectra of different phases were obtained by filtering various realizations of white noise with the desired power spectrum. Bochud considered a location know-exactly detection task, where human subjects were asked in a two-alternative forced choice experiment which image contained a small object. The object to be detected was six pixels in size in a 256×256 image, and aimed at simulating microcalcifications in mammography. Thomson (1997) looked at the ability to visually discriminate between two textures presented in a temporal-sequential paradigm. These investigations pointing to the importance of the phase spectra of texture images document the importance of looking at the complete second-order statistics, not simply the power spectra, to characterize texture images and quantify task performance in textured images.

It must be noted that the first-order statistics have a significant impact on the form of the 2P-PDF. In the limit of large **d** values, the 2P-PDF becomes the product of the 1P-PDFs, that is the first-order statistics or histograms. Thus, if textures are compared based on their second-order statistics, they must be first equaled in first-order statistics. Harris (1999) investigated histogram matching to either a uniformly distributed random process, which is equivalent to histogram equalization, or a Gaussian distribution [61]. After equalization of first-order statistics, a simple distance measure was computed between two 2P-PDFs as

$$D(p^a, p^b) = \frac{1}{N_\mathbf{d}} \sum_\mathbf{d} \left(\sum_{ij} \left[p^a(\mathrm{GL}_i, \mathrm{GL}_j; \mathbf{d}) - p^b(\mathrm{GL}_i, \mathrm{GL}_j; \mathbf{d}) \right]^2 \right)^{1/2}, \quad (13.44)$$

where ij is a pair of gray levels, p^a and p^b are the 2P-PDFs for texture a and b, respectively, and $N_\mathbf{d}$ is the number of directional distances considered. Other distance measures that may provide enhanced classification are currently subject to investigation.

Based on the distribution of distance values within ensembles of texture images, and the mean distance values across different ensembles of texture images, Harris found higher performance for texture discrimination in the case of matching to a Gaussian distribution. Optimization of the Gaussian parameters for specific medical data sets may provide improved means of texture classification based on the complete 2P-PDF.

For the problem of texture classification, a crucial part of the classification algorithm is the estimation of the 2P-PDF for a given texture realization. While the simplest way to estimate a 2P-PDF is the relative-frequency method, it generally yields noisy estimates. A question is how many sample points should be considered to estimate a probability density function with known accuracy using the relative-frequency method? An estimate based on the maximum-entropy (ME) method, where moments of the random process are used to constrain the estimate, yields smoother estimates. Similarly, one must ask in this case how many moments should be considered? The problem of 2P-PDF estimation was investigated an reported in Goon and Rolland (1999) [60]. Results show that the maximum-entropy method yields accurate estimates, however efficient computational methods must be investigated.

13.7 Conclusion and future work

Mathematically synthesized images have played and will continue to play an important role in deepening our understanding of images and in quantifying image quality in medical imaging. Computer-simulated angiograms, lumpy backgrounds, and the synthesis of 3D livers, ultrasound B-scans, and mammographic textures were reviewed.

The ability to simulate angiograms allowed researchers to investigate the role of blood-vessel curvature in the detection of lesions, as well as the impact of structural context near lesions. Furthermore, it allowed controlled experiments where detectability in a search experiment could be investigated, given that the detectability in the location-known-exactly task could be measured and set equal across the conditions investigated for the search experiment. The simulations thus allowed for designing experiments that would not be realizable using clinical images.

The ability to simulate images with spatially varying components, yet well defined statistics, as found in the lumpy backgrounds, allowed us to model detection of lesions in spatially varying backgrounds often encountered in medical images. The use of spatially varying backgrounds, rather than previously chosen constant backgrounds, allowed researchers to resolve the long existing paradox between predictive models of detection and clinical experience. It also allowed further test of the validity of observer models, reported in another chapter of this book, to predict human performance in various classification tasks.

A method for the simulation of organs was presented. The application to modeling liver scans was shown as well as the ability to model various liver diseases. Such mathematical phantoms played an important role in demonstrating the ability of the Hotteling observer to predict human performance in a classification task.

Finally, methods for synthesizing texture images were presented including the synthesis of ultrasound B-scan images, and the synthesis of mammographic textures. The goal of texture synthesis is to render an ensemble of images with statistical properties that are equivalent to those encountered in clinical images. The complete 2P-PDF is considered a meaningful measure of second-order statistics of texture images for non-Gaussian random processes.

Lumpy backgrounds, ultrasound B-scan modeling, and mammographic-tissue synthesis constitute pioneer work in the modeling of texture images. Extensive work is yet to come to investigate and compare various approaches to texture synthesis for medical imaging, establishing efficient methods to estimate 2P-PDFs for effective texture characterization, and further validating the ability to effectively classify medical textures based on second-order statistics as well as possibly higher-order statistics. Moreover, statistical models of medical textures may be employed in establishing priors for image reconstruction.

Finally, in the same manner that we simulated lumpy backgrounds based on wanting to render texture images with a given autocorrelation function, methods to synthesize textures that satisfy specific predefined statistics may provide a useful tool to the field of image understanding and quality assessment in medical imaging.

Acknowledgments

I thank Kyle Myers for her inputs in presenting this material and for her kind review of the manuscript and suggestions. I am thankful to Harry Barrett for providing original pictures regarding the synthesis of liver scans, but most importantly for providing me with a vision and continued encouragement that inspires me always. Finally, I thank Keith Wear and Robert Wagner for their inputs on the section on synthesizing ultrasound B-scans and providing an illustration as well.

References

[1] Swets JA. "Measuring the Accuracy of Diagnosis Systems." Science 240:1285–1293, 1988.

[2] Barrett HH, Yao J, Rolland JP, Myers KJ. "Model Observers for Assessment of Image Quality." Proc Natl Acad Sci 90:9758–9765, 1993.

[3] Revesz G, Kundel HL, Graber MA. "The Influence of Structured Noise on Detection of Radiologic Abnormalities." Invest Radiol 9:479–486, 1974.

[4] Tobis J, Nalcioglu O, Iseeri L *et al.* "Detection and Quantitation of Coronary Artery Stenoses from Digital Substraction Angiograms Compared with 35 Millimeter Film Cineangiograms." Am J Cardiol 54:489–496, 1984.

[5] Davatzikos C. "Spatial Transformation and Registration of Brain Images Using Elastically Deformable Models." Comp Vis and Image Understanding, Special Issue on Medical Imaging 66(2):207–222, 1997.

[6] Rolland JP, Muller K, Helvig CS. "Visual Search in Medical Images: A New Methodology to Quantify Saliency." Proc SPIE 2436, 1995, pp. 40–48.

[7] Rolland JP, Helvig CS. "Visual Search in Angiograms: Does Geometry Play a Role in Saliency?" Proc SPIE 2712, 1996, pp. 78–88.

[8] Puff D. "Human Vs. Vision Model Performance for Two Medical Image Estimation Tasks." Ph.D Dissertation, University of North Carolina at Chapel Hill, 1995.

[9] Rolland JP, Puff D. "Angiogram Simulation Software Documentation." Technical Report TR93-018, University of North Carolina at Chapel Hill, 1993.

[10] O'Neill Barrett. *Elementary Differential Geometry.* Orlando: Academic Press, 1966, p. 75.

[11] Tsui BMW, Metz CE, Atkins FB, Starr SJ, Beck RN. "A Comparison of Optimum Spatial Resolution in Nuclear Imaging Based on Statistical Theory and Observer Performance." Phys Med Biol 23:654–676, 1978.

[12] Wagner RF, Brown DG, Metz CE. "On the Multiplex Advantage of Coded Source/Aperture Photon Imaging." In Brody W (Ed.) *Digital Radiography, Proc. Soc. Photo-Opt. Instrum. Eng.* 314, 1981, pp. 72–76.

[13] Harris JL. "Resolving Power and Decision Theory." J Opt Soc Am A54:606–611, 1964.

[14] Myers KJ, Rolland JP, Barrett HH, Wagner RF. "Aperture Optimization for Emission Imaging: Effect of a Spatially Varying Backgrounds." J Opt Soc Am A7:1279–1293, 1990.

[15] Rolland JP. "Factors Influencing Lesion Detection in Medical Imaging." Ph.D Dissertation, University of Arizona, 1990.

[16] Rolland JP, Barrett HH. "Effect of Random Background Inhomogeneity on Observer Detection Performance." J Opt Soc Am A9:649–658, 1992.

[17] Burgess AE. "Statistically-Defined Backgrounds: Performance of a Modified Nonprewhitening Observer Model." J Opt Soc Am A11:1237–1242, 1994.

[18] Eckstein MP, Whiting JS. "Lesion Detection in Structured Noise." Acad Radiol 2:249–253, 1995.

[19] Judy PF. "Detection of Clusters of Simulated Calcifications in Lumpy Noise Backgrounds." Proc SPIE 2712, 1996, pp. 39–46.

[20] Whitting JS, Eckstein MP, Moriaka CA, Eigler NL. "Effect of Additive Signal Contrast and Feature Motion on Visual Detection in Structured Noise." Proc SPIE 2712, 1996, pp. 26–38.

[21] Gallas BD, Barrett HH. "Detectability for a Lumpy Background Model as a Function of Background Parameters." OSA Annual Meeting (abstract) 1997.

[22] Cargill EB. "A Mathematical Liver Model and Its Application to System Optimization and Texture Analysis." Ph.D Dissertation, University of Arizona, 1989.

[23] West BJ, Goldberger AL. "Physiology in Fractal Dimensions." American Scientist 75:354–365, 1987.

[24] Harper C. *Introduction to Mathematical Physics*. Englewood Cliffs: Prentice Hall, 1976, pp. 217–218.

[25] Park D. *Introduction to the Quantum Theory*. New York: McGraw-Hill, 1974, pp. 631–646.

[26] Rappaport AM, McPhee PJ, Fisher MM, Phillips MJ. "The Scarring of the Liver Acini (Cirrhosis)." Virchows Archive A402:107–137, 1983.

[27] Fink M, Hottier F, Cardoso JF. "Ultrasonic Signal Processing for In-Vivo Attenuation Measurement: Short Time Fourier Analysis." Ultrasonic Imaging 5:117–135, 1983.

[28] Insana MF, Wagner RF, Garra BS, Brown DG, Shawker TH. "Analysis of Ultrasonic Image Texture Via Generalized Rician Statistics." Optical Engineering 25(6):743–748, 1986.

[29] Wagner RF, Insana MF, Brown DG. "Unified Approach to the Detection and Classification of Speckle Texture in Diagnostic Ultrasound." Opt Eng 25(6):738–742, 1986.

[30] Momenan R, Wagner RF, Loew MH, Insana MF, Garra BS. "Characterization of Tissue from Ultrasound Images." IEEE Control Systems Magazine 49–53, 1988.

[31] Valckx FMJ, Thijssen JM. "Characterization of Echographic Image Texture by Cooccurence Matrix Parameters." Ultrasound in Med and Biol 23(4):559–571, 1997.

[32] Goodman JW. *Statistical Optics*. New York: John Wiley and Sons, 1985.

[33] Middleton D. *An Introduction to Statistical Communication Theory*. New York: McGraw-Hill, 1960.

[34] Fellingham-Joynt L. "A Stochastic Approach to Ultrasonic Tissue Characterization." Ph.D thesis, Stanford University, also published as Tech. Report No G 557-4, 1979.

[35] Wear KA, Wagner RF, Brown DG. "Statistical Properties of Estimates of Signal-to-Noise Ratio and Number of Scatterers per Resolution Cell." J Acoust Soc Am 102(1):635–641, 1997.

[36] Shung KK, Sigelmann RA, Reid JM. "Scattering of Ultrasound by Blood." IEEE Trans Biomed Eng BME-23:460–467, 1976.

[37] Goodman JW. "Statistical Properties of Laser Speckle Patterns." In Dainty JC (Ed.) *Laser Speckle and Related Phenomena*. Berlin: Springer-Verlag, 1975, pp. 9–75.

[38] Wagner RF, Smith SW, Sandrik JM, Lopez H. "Statistics of Speckle in Ultrasound B-Scans." IEEE Trans Sonics Ultrason SU-30:156–163, 1983.

[39] Wagner RF, Insana MF, Brown DG. "Statistical Properties of Radio-Frequency and Envelope-Detected Signals with Applications to Medical Ultrasound." J Opt Soc Am A4:910–922, 1987.

[40] Strickland RN. "Wavelet Transforms for Detecting Microcalcifications in Mammograms." IEEE Transactions on Medical Imaging 15(2):218–229, 1996.

[41] Rolland JP, Strickland R. "An Approach to the Synthesis of Biological Tissue." Optics Express 1(13) 1997.

[42] Nicholson PHF, Mueller R, Lowet G, Cheng XG, Hildebrand T, Ruegsegger P, Van der Perre G, Dequeker J, Boonen S. "Do Quantitative Ultrasound Measurements Reflect Structure Independently of Density in Human Vertebral Cancellous Bone?" Bone 23:425–431, 1998.

[43] Rolland JP, Goon A, Yu L. "Synthesis of Textured Complex Backgrounds." Opt Eng 37(7):2055–2063, 1998.

[44] Harris C. "Normalized Second-Order Statistics for Texture Characterization." Master Dissertation, University of Central Florida, Orlando FL, 1999.

[45] Heeger DJ, Bergen JR. "Pyramid-Based Texture Analysis/Synthesis." Computer Graphics Proceedings 229–238, 1995.

[46] Vaidyanathan PP. *Multivariate Systems and Filter Banks*. Englewood Cliffs, NJ: Prentice Hall, 1993.

[47] Woods JW. *Subband Image Coding*. Norwell MA: Kluwer Academic Publishers, 1991, pp. 43–192.

[48] Simoncelli EP, Freeman WT, Adelson EH, Heeger DJ. "Shiftable Multi-Scale Transforms." IEEE Transactions on Information Theory, Special Issue on Wavelets 38:587–607, 1992.

[49] Perona P. "Deformable Kernels for Early Vision." IEEE Transactions on Pattern Analysis and Machine Intelligence 7(5):488–489, 1995.

[50] Simoncelli EP, Freeman WT. "The Steerable Pyramid: A Flexible Architecture for Multi-Scale Derivative Computation." In *Proc IEEE Int Conf Image Processing*, Washington, DC, 1995.

[51] Castleman KR. *Digital Image Processing*. Upper Saddle River NJ: Prentice Hall, 1996.

[52] Hall EH. "Almost Uniform Distributions for Computer Image Enhancement." IEEE Trans Comput C-23(2):207–208, 1974.

[53] Pizer SM, Amburn EP, Austin JD, Cromartie R, Geselowitz A, Greer T, Romeny BTH, Zimmerman J, Zuiderveld K. "Adaptive Histogram Equalization and Its Variations." Computer Vision, Graphics, and Image Processing 39:355–368, 1987.

[54] Paranjape RB, Morrow WM, Rangayyan RM. "Adaptive-Neighborhood Histogram Equalization for Image Enhancement." Graphical Models and Image Processing 54(3):259–267, 1992.

[55] Rolland JP, Vo V, Abbey CK, Yu L, Bloss B. "Fast Algorithms for Histogram Matching: Application to Texture Synthesis." Journal of Electronic Imaging 9(1), 2000.

[56] Julez B. "Visual Pattern Discrimination." IRE Trans Inform Theory 8(2):84–92, 1962.

[57] Haralick RM. "Statistical and Structural Approaches to Texture." Proc IEEE 67(5):786–804, 1979.

[58] Bochud FO, Verdun FR, Hessler C, Valley JF. "Detectability on Radiological Images: The Influence of Radiological Noise." Proc SPIE 2436, 1995, pp. 156–164.

[59] Thomson MGA, Foster DH. "Role of Second- and Third-Order Statistics in the Discriminability of Natural Images." J Opt Soc Am A14(9):2081–2090, 1997.

[60] Goon A, Rolland JP. "Texture Classification Based on Comparison of Second-Order Statistics I: 2P-PDF Estimation and Distance Measure." J Opt Soc Am A16(7):1566–1574, 1999.

[61] Harris C. "Normalized Second-Order Statistics for Texture Characterization." Master Thesis, University of Central Florida, 1999.

[62] Weir KA, Wagner RF, Brown DG, Insana MF. "Statistical Properties of Estimates of Signal-to-noise Ratio and Number of Scatterers per Resolution Cell." J Acoust Soc Am 102(1):635–641, 1999.

CHAPTER 14
Quantitative Image Quality Studies and the Design of X-Ray Fluoroscopy Systems

David L. Wilson
Case Western Reserve University and University Hospitals of Cleveland

Kadri N. Jabri, Ravindra M. Manjeshwar
Case Western Reserve University

CONTENTS

14.1 Introduction

14.1.1 X-ray dose and image quality

X-ray fluoroscopy is a medical-imaging technique whereby low-dose high-acquisition-rate x-ray images are obtained [1, 2]. Fluoroscopy provides quantum-limited high-definition digital-television viewing of structures inside the body. It makes possible many minimally invasive treatments such as balloon angioplasty, neuroembolizations, and transjugular intrahepatic portosystemic shunts (TIPS). Despite many recent developments in MR and CT imaging, x-ray fluoroscopy remains the principal imaging method for image-guided therapy.

Although the x-ray dose per acquisition is low, very long sessions of fluoroscopy are required during complex interventional procedures giving relatively large doses to patients and operators [3]. Procedures lasting 4 hours with fluoroscopy times over 100 minutes are documented [4, 5], and some interventional neuroangiography procedures last 8 to 12 hours with fluoroscopy times exceeding 75 min [6]. The FDA has documented reports of severe skin injury [7, 8]. In a public health advisory, the FDA warns of "... occasional, but sometimes severe radiation-induced skin injuries to patients resulting from prolonged, fluoroscopically-guided, invasive procedures." The advisory points out that injury can occur after less than one hour of fluoroscopy at normal exposure rates of 2 to 5 rad/min [9]. Such exposures are easily reached in complex procedures. Hence, on average fluoroscopy accounts for one half of the population diagnostic x-ray dose [10] and for exceptionally large doses to those patients getting the most intricate procedures.

Simply reducing x-ray exposure produces images with a reduced signal-to-noise ratio and with an unacceptable image quality for intricate interventions. Interventional angiography procedures require the visualization of arteries and embolic materials as well as small, pixel-size devices such as guide wires, coils, and stents. In neuroangiography, catheters are sometimes 2.5 F (0.82 mm) and guide wires are 0.4 mm in diameter and smaller [6]. This is nearly as small as a pixel! Fluoroscopy image quality is also an issue in cardiac interventional angiography, where guide wires are commonly 0.3 mm to 0.5 mm [11]. Perhaps even smaller interventional devices would be developed if imaging techniques were improved. Some stents used in cardiology are virtually invisible under fluoroscopy. Although fluoroscopy at special high exposure levels is discouraged, interventionalists continue to use it for improved visualization [11].

Thus, on the one hand, there is a public health interest to lower x-ray dose to patients and staff. On the other, enhanced image quality will improve current procedures and possibly help create new ones. X-ray fluoroscopy images are quantum-limited noisy images, and the need to lower x-ray dose conflicts with the need to maintain, or improve, image quality. Engineering methods for reducing dose while maintaining or even improving image quality are varied. Such methods include the x-ray fovea [12] and the similar region-of-interest fluoroscopy technique [13], low-acquisition-rate pulsed fluoroscopy [14, 15], time-varying acquisition rate pulsed fluoroscopy [16], and digital noise-reduction filtering of fluoroscopy sequences [17–23].

The goal of our laboratory is to minimize x-ray dose and maximize image quality by optimizing the acquisition and processing of x-ray fluoroscopy images. To achieve this, we quantitatively study how engineering choices in the imaging chain affect human perception. In most studies, we use a very objective measure of image quality, the detection of low-contrast objects in noisy image sequences. We use both experiments and computer models of human detection.

Our experiments are all aimed at practical issues in x-ray fluoroscopy system design. These include studies on low-acquisition-rate fluoroscopy, continuous x ray versus pulsed x-ray acquisitions with reduced motion blurring, last-image-hold, digital temporal filtering, and digital spatial filtering. We have performed experiments with and without target motion. There is a new important impetus for our work. New large-area, semiconductor-based, flat-panel x-ray detectors are being developed. Unlike conventional systems that use an image intensifier and video camera, these systems have minimal temporal and spatial blurring. This allows for a variety of new and potentially more effective processing techniques to enhance image quality. In order to evaluate and optimize these techniques, perception studies are needed to reliably determine quantitative image quality for clinically relevant tasks.

14.1.2 Image sequences and visual perception

In addition to x-ray fluoroscopy, many important medical-imaging methods such as ultrasound, cardiac cine MRI, ultrafast CT, x-ray angiography, and MRI fluoroscopy consist of sequences of medical images. Relatively little quantitative image-quality work has been done on such sequences requiring aspects of time and motion.

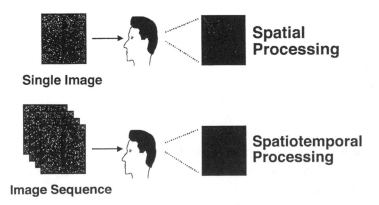

Figure 14.1: When one views a sequence of noisy fluoroscopy images, there is spatio-temporal processing in the visual system that results in a clearly seen target (bottom). If the display is frozen at a single frame, there is no temporal processing and only spatial visual processing is done. The target is seen less well and can disappear in the noise (top).

As shown in Figure 14.1, there is a simple demonstration of the fundamental difference between the perception of a single image and an image sequence. When a human examines a sequence of noisy fluoroscopy images, there is spatio-temporal processing in the visual system and objects are easily recognized because of temporal processing that acts to reduce the effective noise. If the display is stopped at a single frame, there is no temporal processing and only spatial visual processing occurs. The display becomes perceptually noisier; objects become more difficult to see; and some disappear altogether. This experiment demonstrates that special considerations are required for last-image-hold displays in fluoroscopy.

The added temporal dimension of the display involves additional visual processing, and image quality results from single images cannot be simply extrapolated to image sequences. Our laboratory has led the work on perception in fluoroscopy image sequences [14, 15, 24–34], and highlights of this research will be reviewed in this chapter.

14.2 Modeling

Using variations on a so-called *modified non-prewhitening matched-filter* model, we have successfully modeled a variety of experimental results. Models incorporate a psychophysically determined, spatio-temporal contrast-sensitivity function (Figure 14.2). We use models having at most one free parameter consisting of a single scaling factor to match absolute values of detection. Nevertheless,

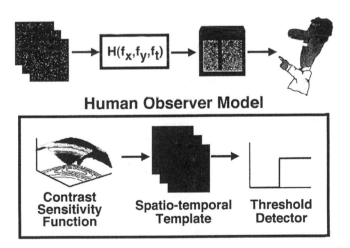

Figure 14.2: Block diagram of the observer model, a modified non-prewhitening matched filter that includes a spatio-temporal visual-system contrast-sensitivity response function. A noisy image sequence is acquired and undergoes processing by a transfer function, H, that depends upon image-acquisition rate and optional digital filtering. The output image sequence is observed on a monitor. The human-observer model consists of a spatio-temporal filter (contrast sensitivity function), a non-prewhitening matched filter (template), and a threshold detector.

many interesting aspects of human detection are described. The success comes from the spatio-temporal contrast-sensitivity function measured several years ago by Kelly [35] and described more fully later. Despite being measured under very different experimental conditions, this measurement contains truths for human detection in noise-limited image sequences. We next describe our basic models and implementation issues.

14.2.1 Spatio-temporal modified non-prewhitening matched filter

In many cases, we apply a full spatio-temporal template for detection [29, 30]. Below is the result for the case of an infinite cylinder vertically aligned along the y axis. Calculations are performed in the Fourier domain along two dimensions, f_x and f_t:

$$\text{SNR} = \frac{A_y \int_{f_x} \int_{f_t} \{ S(f_x, f_t) V_{st}(f_x, f_t) \} \{ [S(f_x, f_t)^* * W_t(f_t)] V_{st}(f_x, f_t)^* \} \, df_t \, df_x}{\sqrt{\int_{f_x} \int_{f_t} \{ |[S(f_x, f_t) * W_t(f_t)]|^2 |V_{st}(f_x, f_t)|^2 \} \{ |V_{st}(f_x, f_t)|^2 P_n(f_x, f_t) \} \, df_t \, df_x}}, \qquad (14.1)$$

where, A_y is a constant resulting from integration along f_y; $S(f_x, f_t)$ is the spatio-temporal template; $V_{st}(f_x, f_t)$ is the spatio-temporal contrast sensitivity function, and $P_n(f_x, f_t)$ is the power spectrum of the noise. Humans have a limited capacity to use information in a sequence of images [27]. To model this, we include a temporal window function, $W_t(f_t)$, that exponentially attenuates the temporal response from past inputs. Details are given in previous publications [29, 30].

For the case of continuous infinite motion, we can simplify Eq. (14.1) [29]. We assume white noise in the image display with a constant noise-power density, $P_n(f_x, f_t) = \sigma_e^2$. With the cylinder moving at a constant velocity, v, the signal becomes $s(x, t) = s(x - vt)$, and we get

$$\text{SNR} = \frac{A_y \int |S(f_x) V(f_x, v)|^2 \, df_x}{\sqrt{\int |S(f_x) V(f_x, v)|^2 |V(f_x, v)|^2 \sigma_e^2 \, df_x}}. \qquad (14.2)$$

A variation on the full spatio-temporal model was developed by Aufrichtig et al. for detection of a stationary object at a known location [24]. In this case, we apply a two-dimensional template for detection in sequences. The SNR of this model is given by

$$\text{SNR} = \frac{\int_{f_x} \int_{f_y} |S(f_x, f_y) V_{st}(f_x, f_y, 0)|^2 \, df_y \, df_x}{\sqrt{\int_{f_x} \int_{f_y} \{ |S(f_x, f_y) V_{st}(f_x, f_y, 0)|^2 \} \{ \int_{f_t} |V_{st}(f_x, f_y, f_t)|^2 P_n(f_x, f_y, f_t) \, df_t \} \, df_y \, df_x}}. \qquad (14.3)$$

If the visual response function, $V_{st}(f_x, f_y, f_t)$, is separable in space and time $(V_{st}(f_x, f_y, f_t) \stackrel{\text{def}}{=} V_s(f_x, f_y) V_t(f_t))$, we get

$$\text{SNR} = \frac{V_t(0) \int_{f_x} \int_{f_y} |S(f_x, f_y) V_s(f_x, f_y)|^2 \, df_y \, df_x}{\sqrt{\int_{f_x} \int_{f_y} \{ |S(f_x, f_y) V_s^2(f_x, f_y)|^2 \} \{ \int_{f_t} |V_t(f_t)|^2 P_n(f_x, f_y, f_t) \, df_t \} \, df_y \, df_x}}. \qquad (14.4)$$

If examined very carefully, one finds that Eqs. (14.3) and (14.4) are not exactly special cases of Eqs. (14.1) and (14.2). This is described in detail in another publication [36] where a more complex model structure is introduced that roughly describes an extraordinarily large number of experiments. Although more general, this latter model less accurately describes some specific experiments reviewed here. Hence, we compare results to Eqs. (14.1) through (14.4). Rather than attempting to fine tune a single complex human-observer model, we find it beneficial to develop multiple relatively simple models where each one accurately predicts fluoroscopy image quality over a range of experiments. Because a particular acquisition or processing technique is accurately described, we can use a model to effectively guide x-ray system design.

14.2.2 Visual response function

The visual-system spatio-temporal contrast sensitivity is measured from flicker experiments using either stationary [37–39] or traveling [35, 40] sinewave stimuli. In traveling sinewave experiments, Kelly measured a contrast-sensitivity function with a stabilized visual field and reported the result in terms of a function:

$$V(f_x, v) = [6.1 + 7.3 \, |\log(v/3)|^3] \times v f_x^2 \exp[-2 f_x (v+2)/45.9], \qquad (14.5)$$

where v is the velocity of the traveling sinewave [35]. We can substitute f_t/f_x for v to get a function $V(f_x, f_t)$. Kelly also measured unstabilized contrast sensitivities with eye motion. The unstabilized response for stationary sinewaves was very close to the stabilized response at $v = 0.15$ deg/s [35]. For $v > 0.15$ deg/s, the unstabilized and stabilized responses were both described by Eq. (14.5). In our experiments, we conduct unstabilized perception experiments with both moving and stationary projected cylinders. For $v > 0.15$ deg/s, we use Eq. (14.5) and for $0 \leqslant v \leqslant 0.15$ deg/s, we substitute $V(f_x, 0.15)$ from Eq. (14.5).

14.2.3 Computations

The computations should mimic the experiments as closely as possible. Various acquisition rates are possible; the display occurs at discrete time instances; pixels are discrete; and the cylinder moves as many as 16 pixels between frames when we simulate low-acquisition-rate imaging. These features imply that we should use a discrete formulation and digital signal processing concepts. In discrete calculations, we replace integrations and differentials with summations and sampling intervals. In low-acquisition-rate simulations, there are periodic repetitions in the frequency domain. Better fits to the data are obtained when S in the signal template is replaced with the signal expected for the continuous case [29]. This effectively limits the impact of the periodic repetitions and perhaps mimics the natural situation where views of the external world are continuous rather than discretely sampled images.

14.2.4 Temporal and spatial filtering

In temporal filtering experiments, we apply a digital temporal filter to each pixel as a function of time. It is a low-pass first-order recursive filter that is implemented on x-ray systems for fluoroscopy noise reduction [1]. In the time domain, the output of the filter, $y(t)$, is given by

$$y(t) = y(t-1) + \frac{1}{k}\big[x(t) - y(t-1)\big], \quad \text{for } k \geqslant 1, \tag{14.6}$$

where $x(t)$ is the input value at the current time instant, and k is the filter gain. When $k = 1$, there is no filtering ($y(t) = x(t)$); when k approaches infinity, the current sample is ignored ($y(t) \approx y(t-1)$); and in general for $k > 1$, the filtered noise variance is $1/(2k-1)$ of the input noise variance [41]. The frequency response is given by

$$H_k(f) = \frac{1/k}{1 - \dfrac{k-1}{k}\exp(-j2\pi f \Delta t)}. \tag{14.7}$$

For spatial filtering experiments, we investigate three different spatial filters that are independently applied to each frame in an image sequence. The filters are 3×3 center-weighted averagers with different weight assignments. The output of the center-weighted averager, $y(m,n)$, is given by

$$y(m,n) = \frac{\sum_{i=-1}^{+1}\sum_{j=-1}^{+1} a_{ij}x(m+i, n+j)}{K+8},$$

$$\text{where } a_{ij} = \begin{cases} K & \text{if } i = j = 0, \\ 1 & \text{otherwise,} \end{cases} \tag{14.8}$$

where m and n are the discrete spatial coordinates in image space and K is the center weight. When $K = 1$, the filter becomes a simple 3×3 averager that reduces noise variance by a factor of $1/9$. As K increases, less filtering is achieved. We use three levels of filtering that reduce pixel-noise variance by factors of 0.75, 0.50, and 0.25. In experiments, we simulate ideal edge-preserving spatial filters by first filtering background noise only and then adding the signal for detection. As a result, no edge blurring is introduced by the digital filters, and the filters are "ideal" in that sense. This construction is deliberately chosen so as to mimic the large variety of edge-preserving filters described later (Section 14.5.2).

14.3 Methods

In our laboratory, we have evaluated image quality in some medical applications other than x-ray fluoroscopy. Other techniques are sometimes more suitable than the forced-choice detection paradigm. For optimization of digital subtraction angiography, we used a quality rating of specific features [42]. For optimization of fast MRI methods, we used quantitative comparisons to gold standard images using a perceptual-difference model [43]. In x-ray fluoroscopy, we used paired-comparison experiments [14] and found results quite similar to forced-choice experiments. Nevertheless, the forced-choice detection experimental paradigm is the most objective measure of image quality, and we use it almost exclusively in this chapter. Some years ago, we began to use an adaptive forced-choice technique [15, 34, 44]. Some advantages of this technique are described below, and many more are reviewed in detail elsewhere [15, 34].

14.3.1 Experimental paradigm

Our basic experiment is an M-alternative forced choice (M-AFC) where a target is placed randomly in the center of one of M panels. Targets are typically disks or projected cylinders (Figure 14.3). The subject rightly or wrongly chooses the position where she, or he, thinks the object resides.

The method is adaptive [45–47]. That is, based upon all previous responses, detectability is estimated and the next contrast or dose is adjusted so as to maintain a constant probability correct, typically 80% in our experiments. In standard forced choice, fixed contrast values are used, and preliminary experiments are necessary to avoid contrasts where subjects approach perfect performance (always detect target) or chance performance (pure guessing). These extremes are referred to as the ceiling and floor, respectively [48], and they must be avoided because no graded information is obtained. In our adaptive method, no preliminary experiments are needed and subjects quickly converge to a fixed performance level. By fixing the performance level, we can design efficient experiments that minimize measurement uncertainty [34].

In experiments, we always compare detection under two conditions, for example, fluoroscopy at 15 acq/s and conventional fluoroscopy at 30 acq/s. We alternate such reference and test presentations. By interspersing presentations, we ensure that the condition of the subject is the same for both. This controls for undesirable variables such as subject attention level, fatigue, and possible physiologic variability.

For data analysis, we use a signal-detection model that hypothesizes a continuous decision variable internal to the observer with Gaussian probability density functions for the cases of *target present* and *no-target present*. Between the means of the two overlapping distributions, there is a distance d' that is normalized by the standard deviation. The variable d' is a detectability index that can be interpreted as a decision variable signal-to-noise ratio [49]. For our adaptive technique, we require a simplified model relating d' to variables of interest. We assume that d' is proportional to the *image* contrast-to-noise ratio, C/σ_n, where C is contrast and σ_n is the standard deviation of the image-display noise. The Rose model for a disk [50] and the ideal observer model for a given object both have this form [51]. In an x-ray system that maintains a constant gray level, σ_n^2 is inversely related to the number of x-ray quanta and hence x-ray dose, D, and we have

$$d' = uCD^{1/2}, \tag{14.9}$$

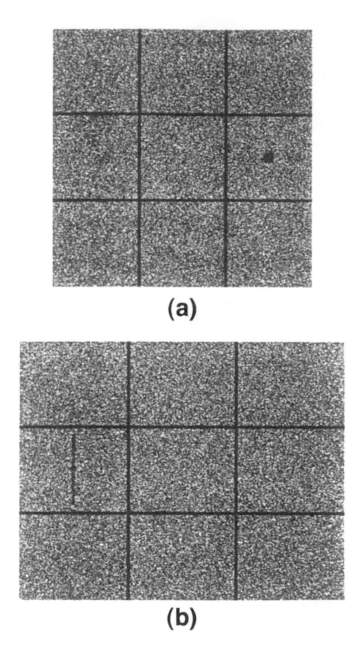

(a)

(b)

Figure 14.3: In this 9-AFC display, a low-contrast target, either a disk (a) or projected cylinder (b) is randomly placed in the center of one of the panels. The target can be moving or stationary. Images are viewed in a noisy image sequence typically consisting of 64 unique image frames. The noise obscures the target, and the subject correctly or incorrectly chooses the panel containing the target. Noise or contrast levels are adapted in subsequent presentations. Noise is reduced in this figure for clarity.

where u is the detectability parameter to be determined. Because we use an adaptive method that clamps the probability correct, this model must be applicable over a limited operating range. For fixed object contrast and dose, it becomes easier to discriminate between target and no-target as u increases. In experiments, the value of u depends upon independent variables such as the number of frames, pulsed acquisition rate, and filter transfer function.

As a function of d', one can calculate the probability of a correct choice in an M-AFC experiment using the equation below where $g(t)$ and $G(t)$ are probability-density and cumulative-probability functions for a Gaussian, respectively [34, 52]:

$$\text{prob}(correct) = p(d') = \int_{t=-\infty}^{\infty} [G(t)]^{M-1} g(t - d') \, dt. \qquad (14.10)$$

For a 9-AFC, a probability correct of 80% uniquely defines a constant, $d'_{80\%} = 2.405$.

Eqs. (14.9) and (14.10) relate u to the probability of a correct response. We use a maximum-likelihood technique to estimate u from all responses. In an adaptive contrast measurement, we use a constant standard dose, estimate u, and compute a new contrast, $C = d'_{80\%}/(u D^{1/2})$, for the next trial. In an adaptive-dose measurement, we use a constant contrast and compute $D = [d'_{80\%}/(uC)]^2$ for the next trial.

We have used two basic experimental designs. First, we adapt contrast and then use identical contrasts for reference and test presentations. Dose (and noise) is adapted to make the comparison between reference and test presentations. Estimates of u are reported for comparison of measurements. Because we are interested in dose utilization, we sometimes present results in the form of an equivalent-perception dose ratio, or EPDR. Second, contrasts for reference and test presentations are adapted independently of each other while dose (and noise) remained fixed. In these experiments, we compare contrast thresholds for 80% probability correct in terms of a contrast sensitivity, $1/C$. This quantity is easy to interpret and has a linear relationship with u, as seen in Eq. (14.9).

The output of a typical interspersed reference/test experiment is shown in Figure 14.4. The reference/test method starts with 25 or 50 reference (e.g., 30 acq/s pulsed fluoroscopy) trials in which a maximum-likelihood estimate of u is obtained; a fixed dose (and noise) is used; and a new contrast is determined for each new trial. Next, there are 25 or 50 test (e.g., 15 acq/s pulsed fluoroscopy) trials. In this case, we use a constant contrast from the reference trials and adapt the dose so that the response is on average 80% correct. Finally, we alternate reference and test trials and adapt contrast and dose, respectively. The contrast for the test (pulsed-15) presentation is always the same as that for the last reference (pulsed-30) presentation. Between 200 and 400 total trials are applied. Outputs are u, contrast, and dose values as a function of trial number. The final dose value for test is the EPDR. Standard deviations of all parameters are computed assuming binomial statistics, and other details are described elsewhere [34].

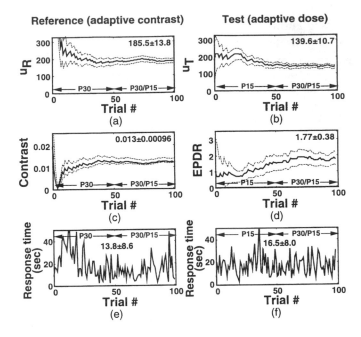

Figure 14.4: Plots are from a pulsed-30/pulsed-15 experiment with a disk diameter of 16 pixels. As a function of trial number, maximum-likelihood estimates and standard deviations of u are shown for pulsed-30 (a) and pulsed-15 (b). The adapted contrast for both the reference and test displays is shown in (c). The dose for the test method is adapted during the experiments (d), and the final value is EPDR $= 1.77 \pm 0.38$. Response times for pulsed-30 and pulsed-15 are shown in (e) and (f), respectively. Mean values for the last 50 response times are given in the figure. In the regions of the curves identified by $\langle P30 \rangle$ or $\langle P15 \rangle$, only pulsed-30 or pulsed-15 trials, respectively, are given. In the case of $\langle P30/P15 \rangle$, pulsed-30 and pulsed-15 trials are alternated. There are 100 pulsed-30 and 100 pulsed-15 trials giving a total of 200 presentations in this session. We often use 400 or more trials in an experiment.

14.3.2 Display and images

We use a display system consisting of software running on a conventional PowerMac personal computer. We typically display 60 to 100 frames in a repeating cine-loop. The 8-bit display has a carefully linearized luminance versus gray-level response. Display rates are accurately obtained using the vertical synch pulse on the PowerMac as a time standard. The display runs at 66 frame/s, non-interlaced. Each frame is repeated twice to mimic 33 acq/s fluoroscopy, a rate close to a conventional acquisition at 30 acq/s. For simplicity, we shall refer to pulsed and continuous acquisitions at 33 acq/s as *pulsed-30* and *continuous-30*, respectively. Repeating each frame four times simulates an acquisition rate of 16.5 acq/s, and we call this *pulsed-15*. Randomized noisy image sequences are constructed between trials from noise arrays stored in random-access memory (RAM) or are read from a very fast hard drive. Relatively complex calculations are required to estimate detectability, and the code is optimized for speed. A new noise sequence presentation is created within 3 to 7 s. Details of software and validation are described elsewhere [34].

The 9-AFC images are typically 384×384 pixels for stationary targets and 480×384 pixels for moving targets. Images are separated into 9 fields (Figure 14.3) and a low-contrast target, which is either a disk or cylinder (stationary or moving), is placed randomly in one of the field centers. The contrast, C, is

$$C = \frac{|\mu_b - \mu_d|}{\mu_b + \mu_d},$$ (14.11)

where μ_b is the mean gray-scale value of the background, and μ_d is a minimum gray-scale value from the noise-free target. This definition of contrast ranges between 0 and 1. At the low contrasts found in detection experiments, C is proportional to the gray-level difference $|\mu_b - \mu_d|$. A Poisson distribution of x-ray quanta that mimics fluoroscopy is used, and parameters are chosen to approximate an x-ray system [1, 15]. For cylinder targets, x-ray system blur is introduced in each frame by convolving the cylinder profile with a one-dimensional kernel representing the line spread function (LSF).

14.3.3 Experimental sessions

Experiments are conducted in a darkened room. Typically, we use 3 to 5 experienced subjects, and some are naive to hypotheses. Subjects have normal, or corrected-to-normal vision and are adequately trained in each experiment before data collection begins. Subjects are urged to give accurate responses and are rewarded with a computer beep when they successfully select the target. The presentation is terminated on a mouse-press response. Subjects are aware that the time for a response is recorded. A typical experimental session lasts one hour and consists of 100 reference and 100 test trials. Such an experiment uses 20,000 unique noisy image frames.

14.4 Results and discussion

14.4.1 X-ray acquisition

14.4.1.1 Low-acquisition-rate pulsed fluoroscopy

Low-frame-rate pulsed acquisition is commonly advertised as a dose-saving technique for x-ray fluoroscopy systems. In pulsed fluoroscopy, short x-ray pulses are produced and images are obtained with minimal motion blurring. At reduced acquisition rates, gap filling is done to produce images suitable for standard display systems; for example, at 15 acq/s, each image is repeated once to create a 30 frame/s display. Prior to our experiments, there were two common arguments regarding x-ray exposure calibration. One idea was to fix the exposure per acquisition giving dose savings of 50% for an acquisition at 15 acq/s as compared to 30 acq/s. Second, some argued that because humans temporally averaged over a

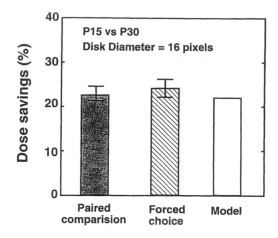

Figure 14.5:   Dose savings for pulsed-15 as compared to pulsed-30 acquisitions are shown. Predictions of the human-observer model are compared to forced-choice [15, 34] and paired-comparison [14] experiments for a disk of diameter 16 pixels. The average dose savings are 22%, 24% and 22% for paired-comparison, forced-choice experiments and model predictions respectively. Model Eq. (14.3) is used, and data are averages across three subjects. Similar dose savings were measured for pulsed-15 with disk targets of diameters ranging from 8 to 32 pixels [14].

few frames, at 15 acq/s one must double the exposure per acquisition to get equivalent perception. This latter calibration would result in no dose savings.

Using our quantitative methods, we determined appropriate exposure values for equivalent perception [14, 15, 24]. We used two experimental paradigms: paired-comparison and forced-choice, and compared the measured dose savings to predictions from a human observer model (Figure 14.5). Targets were stationary disks of diameter 16 pixels. Average dose savings of 22% and 24% were measured with the paired-comparison and forced-choice methods, respectively. The predictions of the human-observer model (22%) compared very favorably with measurements. These experiments convincingly demonstrated dose savings with pulsed-15 for threshold contrast target detection (forced-choice experiments) as well as supra-threshold object visibility (paired comparison experiments). Even larger dose savings are obtained at 10 and 7.5 acq/s [14].

For pulsed-15 and pulsed-30, the detection of moving objects is examined as a function of velocity and object size in Figure 14.6. Targets are projected cylinders simulating arteries, catheters, and guide wires in x-ray fluoroscopy, and diameters are 1, 5, and 21 pixels. To facilitate the comparison of experiments to theory, we introduce a single normalization factor. Theoretical curves are normalized signal-to-noise ratios, $SNR/SNR_{1,0}$, where $SNR_{1,0}$ is the prediction for a stationary 1-pixel-diameter cylinder and a pulsed-30 acquisition. Similarly, measurements are given in terms of $u/u_{1,0}$, where $u_{1,0}$ is measured under the aforementioned conditions. Several important results stand out. First, comparing all curves, detection at pulsed-30 is better than detection at pulsed-15. Second, from ratios of u values,

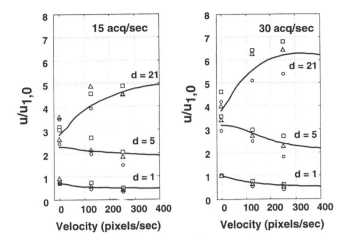

Figure 14.6: Effect of velocity and cylinder size on detectability for pulsed-15 and pulsed-30 acq/s are shown in (a) and (b), respectively. Normalized experiment data (symbols) and model predictions (curves) are plotted. Normalized data are $u/u_{1,0}$ where $u_{1,0}$ is the detectability parameter for a stationary 1-pixel-diameter cylinder at 30 acq/s. Model predictions are also normalized to give $SNR/SNR_{1,0}$ where $SNR_{1,0}$ is the model prediction for the stationary 1-pixel-diameter cylinder. A discrete version of model Eq. (14.1) is used [29], and data are from three subjects.

the dose savings of pulsed-15 relative to pulsed-30 are practically unaffected by motion and are similar to values reported in Figure 14.5. Third, in the case of the thin 1-pixel-diameter cylinder, detection decreases by as much as 50% as velocity increases from 0 to 256 pixels/s. Fourth, detection of the thick 21-pixel-diameter cylinder clearly improves with increasing velocity. Hence, large objects become easier to see when they are moving and small objects become harder to see. The human-observer model quantitatively predicts all of these results.

14.4.1.2 Continuous versus pulsed acquisition

Continuous x-ray exposure blurs moving objects, and x-ray system motion blur can be reduced with a pulsed acquisition whereby short x-ray exposures are used to acquire images. For both acquisition types, moving objects are potentially "blurred" by temporal processing in the human visual system. In the elegant experiments described below, we selectively investigated effects of x-ray system and visual system motion blurring [30].

In Figure 14.7, we examine detection with continuous and pulsed acquisition of stationary and moving targets. In the case of a continuous acquisition, there is x-ray-system and visual-system motion blur. In the case of a pulsed acquisition, there is visual-system blur only. The normalized detectability parameter, $u/u_{1,0}$, for 1-pixel-diameter moving cylinders is plotted. Again, the human-observer model quantitatively predicts human detection-performance for both pulsed-30 (solid curve) and continuous-30 (dashed curve) over the range of velocities. Importantly,

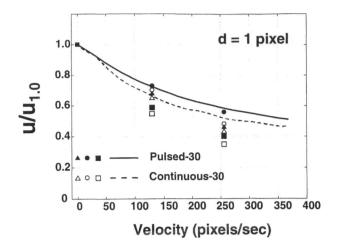

Figure 14.7: Pulsed-30 and continuous-30 detectability measurements are compared to model predictions for a moving 1-pixel-diameter cylinder. For each subject, $u/u_{1,0}$ is plotted as a function of velocity for pulsed-30 (filled symbols) and continuous-30 (unfilled symbols) acquisitions. SNR predictions from the human-observer model, $SNR/SNR_{1,0}$ are also plotted for pulsed-30 (solid curve) and continuous-30 (dashed curve) acquisitions. The discrete form of model Eq. (14.2) is used [30], and data are from three subjects.

the measured difference between pulsed-30 and continuous-30 is less than the effect of velocity. This indicates that the effect of visual-system blur dominates the effect of x-ray system motion blur. This result is not surprising if one considers the low-pass temporal filtering in the human visual system. Elsewhere, results of intermediate calculations show this conclusively [29].

To isolate the effect of x-ray motion blur from visual-system motion blur, we motion-blurred cylinders but presented them at fixed locations. Cylinders were blurred identically to the moving cylinders in Figure 14.7 using an effective "blurring velocity." In Figure 14.8, the ratio of detectability parameters, ($u_{continuous}/u_{pulsed}$) are plotted for (a) blurring without motion and (b) blurring with motion. In the case of a static target, motion blurring significantly degrades detection. However, when the targets are moving, motion blurring has relatively little effect. Hence, blurring of a stationary target greatly degrades detection performance, and this has profound implications for last-image-hold, as described in the next section.

14.4.1.3 Last-image hold

In fluoroscopy last-image-hold (LIH), an image is maintained on the monitor after terminating the x-ray exposure. LIH is a dose-savings feature, as it allows physicians to contemplate the last image and plan the next move in an interventional procedure. The image quality in an LIH frame should be at least as good as in the preceding sequence of images. As described previously with regard to Figure 14.1, visualization of an LIH frame is degraded because there is no longer tem-

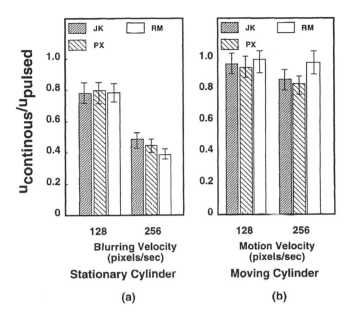

Figure 14.8: The ratio of the detectability parameters for continuous and pulsed acquisitions are shown at blurring velocities of 128 and 256 pixels/s. Note that for a static target, there is no difference between a continuous and pulsed acquisition, giving a ratio of unity. (a) The cylinder target of diameter 1 pixel is stationary and is blurred by a motion blur kernel with an "effective blur velocity." The ratio, $u_{continuous}/u_{pulsed}$, decreases to an average of $\approx$40% at a blurring velocity of 256 pixels/s. (b) The 1-pixel-diameter cylinder target is moving and blurred by the "motion velocity." The ratio, $u_{continuous}/u_{pulsed}$, degrades by only 7%.

poral processing to effectively reduce the noise. We next use quantitative image-quality techniques to investigate noise and exposure requirements for LIH [15, 25].

We investigated detection in single image frames that simulate LIH and in a sequence of N unique frames displayed in a continuous cine loop (Figure 14.9). We plotted the ratio of the detectability parameter, u_N, for N frames, to the detectability parameter, u_1, of a single frame. The x-ray dose per acquisition was equal for the image sequences and the single images. In the figure, detection improves significantly as the number of frames increases from 1 to 30 while there is no significant difference beyond 30 frames. We are interested in the asymptotic value that approximates the case for a very long fluoroscopy acquisition. For disk targets, the average ratios of detectability parameters, u_N/u_1, is 2.6 for N greater than 30. This implies that the noise variance in the single image should be reduced by a factor of $\approx$6 ($= u_N^2/u_1^2$) for equivalent perception as compared to a long image sequence. To put it another way, processing by the human visual system effectively reduces the noise variance by a factor of $\approx$6 for image sequences. Effectively, this corresponds to an averaging of about 6 image frames. (An analogy to averaging is given for simplicity. The effective temporal frequency response differs from a simple averager [27].)

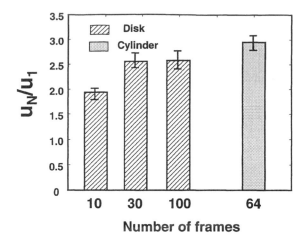

Figure 14.9: This shows the effect on detection of the number of unique noise frames in a repeating loop. The target is either a disk or cylinder, and pulsed-30 is used. Data are plotted as a ratio, u/u_1, where u_1 is the detectability parameter for a single frame. The ratio u/u_1 increases as the number of frames increases from 1 to 30. There is no significant improvement in this ratio beyond 30 frames. The average ratio, beyond 30 frames, for a disk target of diameter 16 pixels is 2.6. The average ratio is 3.0 for a cylinder target of diameter of 5 pixels.

Although experiments in Figure 14.8 on x-ray-system motion blurring were performed with image sequences, we anticipate that similar effects will be found on experiments using single images. There is a large degradation in detection of stationary blurred targets, and this has important ramifications for fluoroscopy last-image-hold. If one images a moving guide wire with continuous fluoroscopy and displays it as a last-image hold, detection can be degraded by as much as 40% as compared to a pulsed-30 acquisition without blurring. Assuming Eq. (14.9), such a change in d' can correspond to a decrease in the probability correct from 80% to 35%, less than 25% above the chance value of 11% in a 9-AFC experiment. This dramatic effect on static targets is the most significant difference between pulsed-30 and continuous-30. It also demonstrates that simply averaging the last 6 frames for LIH might give unacceptable image blurring.

14.4.2 Digital noise reduction filtering

As reviewed later in Section 14.5.2, there are many potential techniques for digitally filtering x-ray-fluoroscopy images. Digital filtering is a potential dose-reduction technique because one can acquire images at reduced exposure and restore images to original image quality. A commonly used metric for image quality improvement is the reduction in display noise variance. (Signal blurring is also assessed, but we neglect that for now.) Noise variance is a naive assessment of image quality, as it does not consider the interaction with the human observer. Hence, we again use our quantitative image-quality methods to study the ability of filtering to

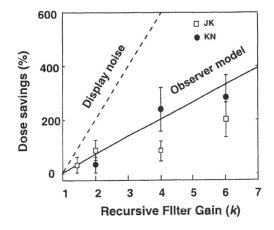

Figure 14.10: Dose savings with temporally filtered sequences are plotted as a function of filter gain k. Measurements compare favorably to the human-observer model while display noise pixel variance greatly overestimates the effect of filtering. Model Eq. (14.4) is used [27]. Data are plotted for two subjects.

restore image quality of acquisitions at reduced exposure. We assess both spatial and temporal digital filtering. In order to mimic existing image-filtering techniques that reduce spatial and temporal blurring of signals, we investigate some idealized cases. We consider temporal filtering without target motion, and we investigate spatial filtering of noise only without target blurring. Our results should therefore provide an upper limit on realistic image-filtering techniques.

14.4.2.1 Temporal filtering

A first-order recursive, low-pass temporal filter (Eq. (14.6)), commonly implemented on commercial x-ray fluoroscopy systems [1, 27], is evaluated. Because the temporal filter is applied at each pixel location as a function of time, the spatial noise in each frame remains white, but the noise across time is correlated. We measure dose savings as a function of the temporal filter gain, k (Figure 14.10). The human-observer model compares very favorably with the data. However, the predictions from the ratio of pixel-noise variances greatly overestimate filter effectiveness.

14.4.2.2 Spatial filtering

There are many reports concerning the effect of spatially correlated noise [53–55], and statistically defined structured backgrounds [56, 57] on detection in single images. These studies show that for equal noise variances, human detection performance can be degraded in the presence of spatial noise correlation. Surprisingly, there have been only scattered, sometimes anecdotal, comments in the literature about the effects of noise-reduction filtering with small kernels. Such filters either slightly improve detection [53] or potentially degrade detection [54].

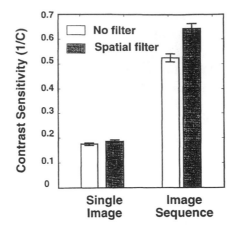

Figure 14.11: Contrast-sensitivity $(1/C)$ measurements for unfiltered and spatially filtered single images and image sequences are plotted. The variance reduction ratio for the center-weighted averaging filter is 0.25. There is a significant improvement ($p < 0.05$) in detection with filtering for image sequence. The effect of filtering on single images is not significant ($p > 0.05$). Plotted data are averages across three subjects. In this figure, we do not normalize contrast; instead $C = |\mu_b - \mu_d|$.

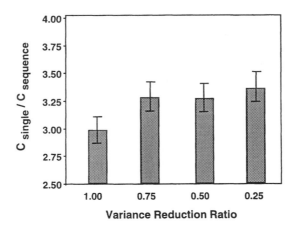

Figure 14.12: The ratio of contrast thresholds in image sequences to single images is plotted as a function of the variance reduction ratio of the noise. Average measurements from three subjects are plotted along with standard error bars. At all filtering levels there is a significant effect ($p < 0.05$) of filtering on this ratio. In this figure, we do not normalize contrast; instead $C = |\mu_b - \mu_d|$.

Our principal interest is spatial filtering in image sequences. We filter each image independently of the others. Hence, each image contains spatially correlated noise, but each frame is independent of the rest, and across time, noise is white. To examine mechanisms in detail, we quantitatively evaluated human detection in spatially filtered image sequences and single image frames [32].

For single images and image sequences, contrast thresholds, $1/C$, are plotted for both unfiltered and spatially filtered images in Figure 14.11. The target is a projected cylinder with a diameter of 5 pixels, and the noise variance is reduced by 0.25 after filtering. While there is no statistically significant effect on single images, filtering significantly improves detection in image sequences. Thus, while spatial filtering might not be particularly useful for single images, it is quite effective on image sequences. To compare effects on image sequence versus single images, we plot the ratio of the contrast thresholds as a function of filtering level (Figure 14.12). The average ratio is significantly increased when noise is filtered. Hence, the temporal processing by the human visual system becomes more efficient as image sequences are increasingly spatially processed.

We propose an explanation. When one spatially low-pass filters a single image, the reduction in pixel noise variance acts to improve detection, but the spatial noise correlation acts to degrade it. As a result, we see little or no net improvement in detection. When viewing a spatially filtered image sequence, the negative effect of spatial noise correlation in single images is reduced as the spatial correlation in one frame is independent of that in the next. In this case, detection is significantly improved.

14.5 Implications for x-ray system design

Several results are applicable to the design of x-ray fluoroscopy systems. There are important implications for both image acquisition and digital processing.

14.5.1 Image acquisition

We have extensively studied pulsed-fluoroscopy acquisitions at reduced acquisition rates (pulsed-15, pulsed-10, etc.) and compared them to conventional 30 acq/s pulsed fluoroscopy (Figures 14.5 and 14.6, and several publications [14, 15, 24, 29, 36]). Comparing pulsed-15 to pulsed-30, we find that one can calibrate the x-ray system with a dose savings of 20–25% and get equal detection. Similar results are obtained with and without motion (Figures 14.5 and 14.6). Alternatively, one can elect to double the exposure per pulse and keep a constant temporal exposure rate when pulsed-30 is dropped to pulsed-15. In this case, we estimate that detectability will increase by $\approx 12\%$. This will correspond to more easily visualized interventional devices. As reviewed elsewhere [14], dose savings for pulsed-10 and pulsed-7.5 are even greater. Our experiments represent the first objective image quality measures of dose savings with such acquisitions. Although as discussed later, low-acquisition-rate fluoroscopy can result in a choppy display, it is acceptable to many. Regardless, we believe that the detection criterion provides an excellent way to objectively estimate a proper dose-savings calibration.

Pulsed x-ray fluoroscopy acquisitions demand fast on and off switching of x-ray production. This capability requires special x-ray system modifications, and extra cost, to remove the effect of cable capacitance. Hence, in a separate study, we compared pulsed-30 to continuous x-ray acquisitions, giving acquisitions without and with x-ray system motion blurring, respectively. In the case of moving targets, there is very little difference in detectability between pulsed-30 and continuous acquisitions (Figure 14.7). We surmise that this is because visual-system motion blurring dominates x-ray-system blurring in these experiments without eye pursuit [30]. Importantly, when targets are blurred with simulated x-ray-system motion blur and then viewed in a static fashion, there is a very significant degradation of detection as compared to a pulsed acquisition. Hence, pulsed fluoroscopy does indeed improve visualization. Surprisingly, the effect is much more prevalent in a last-image-hold image than when a target is rapidly in motion.

Some additional experiments reported elsewhere should be considered with regard to x-ray-system motion blurring. In Figure 14.7, experiments are conducted without eye pursuit, and motion degrades and enhances detection of small and large objects, respectively. In other experiments, we use a marker near the moving target that enables eye pursuit [33]. In this case, both the degradation and enhancement with motion are quantitatively reduced in a manner consistent with a reduced velocity on the retina. In the case of clinical fluoroscopy, objects are above the contrast threshold and eye pursuit is possible. In this event, retinal velocity is reduced and the effect of x-ray-system motion blur will be more prominent. X-ray-systems can be designed with various pulse durations. It will be important to reexamine this issue with a variety of pulse durations under conditions of eye pursuit.

In x-ray fluoroscopy, there are emerging techniques to which quantitative perception methods can be applied. One interesting idea is to vary the image-acquisition rate during a clinical study. Abdel-Malek *et al.* have proposed an adaptive gating approach for x-ray dose reduction in cardiac interventional imaging [16]. In their method, image-acquisition rate is adjusted to match the motion during the cardiac cycle, with decreased rates during periods of reduced motion. The highest acquisition rates are reserved for periods of greatest motion (ventricular ejection) to eliminate choppiness in the display. In periods of less motion (isovolumetric contraction and relaxation) acquisition rate is reduced to 10 or 15 acq/s, where one can reduce the dose per unit time. Although we have not conducted experiments with a time-varying acquisition rate, our studies suggest that for equivalent perception at the reduced acquisition rate of 10 to 15 acq/s, the x-ray dose savings should be 20–38%. Additional experiments using a time-varying acquisition rate are warranted.

As described with regard to Figure 14.1, when a fluoroscopy sequence is fixed at a single frame, visualization of low-contrast objects significantly degrades because there is no longer temporal processing in the visual system to decrease the effect of noise. We examined image-quality requirements for such a last-image-hold visualization (Section 14.4.1.3) and found that the noise variance in a last-image-hold display must be reduced by a factor of 6 to give detection equivalent to that in the sequence. This corresponds to a summation of 6 fluoroscopy frames, a value even larger than previously determined with paired comparison experiments [25]. An additional important design issue for last-image-hold is that motion blurring of small interventional targets greatly degrades perception (Figure 14.8) [30].

There are several potential engineering solutions for last-image-hold. One is to simply increase the exposure on the detector by a factor of six for last-image-hold.

Raising the kVp unacceptably affects image contrast, and increasing the tube current normally takes time. Hence, the most appropriate way to increase exposure is to prolong the x-ray pulse duration by a factor of six. Because this will normally be the last pulse for some seconds, tube loading should not be a significant issue. Detection and display gains must be appropriately adjusted. Motion blurring can be a problem, but normally physicians will not stop x-ray production when an interventional device is rapidly moving. A second approach is to average six image frames together. One possibility is to create a running average of the last six frames and produce this on demand. Another is to create an average of the next six frames following a command, but this is probably inadvisable in situations where a test contrast injection is being viewed. Averaging of six image frames can lead to considerable motion blurring, a very undesirable effect. With the ability to calculate motion detection on the fly, one could maintain a running average and terminate the acquisition when motion is less prevalent. As reviewed later, image filtering techniques that effectively reduce motion blurring are also applicable. Finally, because many x-ray fluoroscopy systems include recursive digital filtering, one could simply display the output of a recursive digital filter that reduces noise variance by a factor of six. Of these possibilities, increasing the x-ray pulse duration might be preferred. Note that last-image-hold following a contrast injection for road-mapping has other design requirements [58–60].

14.5.2 Digital filtering

Owing to the increasing use of digital video, there has been significant work in digital filtering of dynamic image sequences (see Brailean et al. [61] for an excellent review). In general, whenever one filters a sequence of images, there can be spatial or temporal motion blurring, and methods are developed to decrease these effects. To reduce motion blur, many x-ray fluoroscopy systems include temporal filtering with motion detection whereby recursive temporal filtering is reduced whenever motion is "detected" from pixel changes above a threshold [1]. More advanced methods of motion compensation are possible with filtering along motion trajectories [22]. We can categorize filtering methods in terms of temporal filters, temporal filters with motion detection, temporal filters with motion compensation, spatial contrast-enhancement filters, spatio-temporal filters with motion and/or object motion detection, and spatio-temporal filters with motion compensation. A special class of filters consist of nonlinear order statistic filters. In our laboratory, we have developed a motion-detection filter that uses Kalman filtering [62–65], a temporal-filtering method that responds to motion of objects of interest such as vessels and interventional devices [23], and an order-statistic spatio-temporal filter that preserves edges [66].

Not only have we developed practical filters for x-ray fluoroscopy, we have applied quantitative image-quality methods to determine how filtering interacts with the human visual system [27, 28, 32]. In Figure 14.10, we quantified the effect of a temporal recursive filter on human perception. We found that detection was much less improved than predicted from noise-variance measurements. The reason is that the human visual system temporally filters an image sequence, and digital filtering is only effective when it attenuates noise at temporal frequencies not dominated by visual-system filtering. This is very clearly demonstrated in other experiments where high- and low-pass digital filters having equal noise reduction are compared [27]. We have considerable confidence in the ability of the model to predict the effect of temporal filtering.

Spatial noise-reduction filtering can also be an effective image-enhancement method for image sequences (Figure 14.11) [32]. Although small-kernel spatial-noise-reduction filters do not statistically improve detection in single images, image sequences are significantly enhanced (Figures 14.11 and 14.12). The effect of spatial noise-correlation that acts to degrade detection in a single frame is reduced whenever images are shown in a sequence.

To date, our emphasis with quantitative evaluation of filters has been to understand the interaction with the human visual system. As described above, there are a very large number of potential image-filtering methods. Recently, we have examined a spatio-temporal order-statistic filter that acts to reduce both spatial and motion blurring. With filtering, we find significant improvement in detection, as well as discrimination experiments where the task is to choose the target having a contrast higher than other targets [66]. The methods and models that we have created can help us understand and optimize fluoroscopy image filtering. They will enable us to proceed with optimization in a systematic fashion.

14.5.3 Potential limitations

Although we refer to our image sequences as x-ray fluoroscopy, this is a simplification. We do not consider factors in conventional fluoroscopy such as electronic noise, camera-lag temporal blurring, and image intensifier spatial blurring. However, our purpose is to selectively study the effect of a specific type of acquisition or processing, and this is best done in a simplified controlled setting. In addition, new flat-panel detectors virtually eliminate spatial and temporal blurring.

It is also understood that detectability measurements do not encompass all image-quality issues. For example, a reduced-rate acquisition can result in a choppy display [67–69]. One does not perceive a choppy display with the low-contrast phantoms used in our experiments. However, with high contrast, small cylinders moving at the highest velocity, pulsed-15, can appear choppy. These observations are consistent with those of Watson et al. [70]. Sampled motion gives periodic spectral replications in the frequency domain. Watson et al. report that sampled displays look continuous whenever the periodic replications are below the contrast threshold. Because we use low-contrast objects, the periodic repetitions are always below threshold; a choppy display is not observed; and there is no confound in our experiments. Even if a display is perceived to be choppy, the dose requirements from detection experiments are probably valid.

In the case of cardiac angiography, some believe that the quality of fluoroscopy at 15 acq/s is quite sufficient and use it routinely. One problem is that 15 acq/s appears choppy when the x-ray system is panned, but this can obviously be solved with appropriate x-ray system design. In the case of noncardiac applications, motion is more isolated, and very-low-acquisition-rate pulsed fluoroscopy (3 acq/s) is accepted by some European radiologists [71].

14.6 Conclusions

We described a large number of experimental and theoretical results. Many were unexpected. For example, spatial filtering enhanced the image quality of image sequences but had little effect on single images. Large targets were easier to see when they were moving, but small targets were harder to see. Although we obtained such basic information about human perception, experiments were directly related to practical aspects of fluoroscopy acquisition and processing. The success of this endeavor shows that one can use image-perception studies to help engineer imaging systems. Many studies remain, but we believe that quantitative image-quality experiments will eventually lead to acquisition and processing strategies for x-ray fluoroscopy that are optimized for the human observer.

Acknowledgments

This work was supported by National Institutes of Health grant R01-HL48918. We recognize the significant efforts of Richard Aufrichtig and Ping Xue in much of this work.

References

[1] Krestel E (Ed.). *Imaging Systems for Medical Diagnostics*. Berlin, Germany: Siemens AG, 1991.

[2] Bushberg JT, Seibert AJ, EML Jr, Boone JM. *The Essential Physics of Medical-Imaging*. Williams and Wilkins, 1994.

[3] National Council on Radiation Protection and Measurement, Bethesda, MD, Report 107, *Implementation of the Principle of as Low as Reasonably Achievable (ALARA) for Medical and Dental Personnel*, 1990.

[4] Berthelsen B, Cederblad Å. "Radiation Dose to Patients and Personnel Involved in Embolization of Intercerebral Arteriovenous Malformations," Acta Radiol 32:492–497, 1991.

[5] Lindsey BD, Eichling JO, Ambos D, Cain ME. "Radiation Exposure to Patients and Medical Personnel During Radiofrequency Catheter Ablation for Supraventricular Tachycardia," Am J Cardiol 70:218–223, 1992.

[6] Smith TP. "Diagnostic and Interventional Radiology," In Balter S, Shope TB (Eds.) *Syllabus: A Categorial Course in Physics, Physical and Technical Aspects of Angiography and Interventional Angiography*. Oak Brook, IL: RSNA Publications, 1995, pp. 31–36.

[7] Presentation by Shope TB, Center for Devices and Radiological Health, FDA, In Workshop sponsored by the Mid-Atlantic Chapter of the AAPM; titled "Fluoroscopy: Exposure, Injuries, and Interventional Procedures." September 22–23, 1995.

[8] Shope TB. "Radiation-Induced Skin Injuries from Fluoroscopy." Radiology 197(P):209, 1995 (abstract).

[9] FDA Public Health Advisory. Avoidance of Serious X-Ray Induced Skin Injuries to Patients During Fluoroscopically-Guided Procedures. September 30, 1994.

[10] National Council on Radiation Protection and Measurement, Bethesda, MD, Report 100. Exposure of the U.S. Population from Diagnostic Medical Radiation, 1989.

[11] Smith TP. "Cardiac Diagnostic and Interventional Procedures." In Balter S, Shope TB (Eds.) *Syllabus: A Categorial Course in Physics, Physical and Technical Aspects of Angiography and Interventional Angiography* Oak Brook, IL: RSNA Publications, 1995, pp. 45–48.

[12] Labbe VS, Chiu M-Y, Rzeszotarski MS, Wilson DL. "The X-Ray Fovea, a Device for Reducing X-Ray Dose in Fluoroscopy." Med Phys 21:471–481, 1994.

[13] Rudin S, Bednarek DR. "Region of Interest Fluoroscopy." Med Phys 19:1183–1189, 1992.

[14] Aufrichtig R, Xue P, Thomas CW, Gilmore GC, Wilson DL. "Perceptual Comparison of Pulsed and Continuous Fluoroscopy." Med Phys 21:245–256, 1994.

[15] Xue P, Wilson DL. "Pulsed Fluoroscopy Detectability From Interspersed Adaptive Forced Choice Measurements." Med Phys 23:1833–1843, 1996.

[16] Abdel-Malek A, Yassa F, Bloomer J. "An Adaptive Gating Approach for X-Ray Dose Reduction During Interventional Procedures." IEEE Trans Med Imag 13:2–12, 1994.

[17] Dubois E, Sabri S. "Noise Reduction in Image Sequences Using Motion-Compensated Temporal Filtering." IEEE Trans Commun COM-32:826–831, 1984.

[18] Huang TS, Hsu YP. "Image Sequence Enhancement." In Huang TS (Ed.) *Image Sequence Analysis*. Berlin, Germany: Springer Verlag, 1981, pp. 290–310.

[19] Kuan DT, Sawchuk AA, Strand TC, Chavel P. "Adaptive Noise Smoothing Filter for Images with Signal-Dependent Noise." IEEE Trans Pattern Anal Mach Intell PAMI-7:165–177, 1985.

[20] Jiang S-S, Sawchuk AA. "Noise Updating Repeated Wiener Filter and Other Adaptive Noise Smoothing Filters Using Local Image Statistics." Applied Optics 25:2326–2337, 1986.

[21] Chan CL, Katsaggelos AK, Sahakian AV. "Image Sequences Filtering in Quantum-Limited Noise with Applications to Low-Dose Fluoroscopy." IEEE Trans Med Imag 12:610–621, 1993.

[22] Singh A. *Optic Flow Computation: A Unified Perspective*. Los Alamitos, CA: IEEE Computer Society Press, 1992.

[23] Aufrichtig R, Wilson DL. "X-Ray Fluoroscopy Spatio-Temporal Filtering with Object Detection." IEEE Trans Med Imag 14:733–746, 1995.

[24] Aufrichtig R, Thomas C, Xue P, Wilson DL. "A Model for Perception of Pulsed Fluoroscopy Image Sequences." J Opt Soc Am A 11:3167–3176, 1994.

[25] Wilson DL, Xue P, Aufrichtig P. "Perception of Fluoroscopy Last-Image-Hold." Med Phys 21:1875–1883, 1994.

[26] Wilson DL, Xue P, Aufrichtig R. "Perception in X-Ray Fluoroscopy." In Kundel HL (Ed.) *Proceedings of SPIE Medical Imaging 1994: Image Perception*, Vol. 2166. Bellingham, Washington: SPIE, 1994, pp. 20–23.

[27] Wilson DL, Jabri KN, Aufrichtig R. "Perception of Temporally Filtered X-Ray Fluoroscopy Images." IEEE Trans Med Imag 18:22–31, 1999.

[28] Wilson DL, Jabri KN, Xue P, Aufrichtig R. "Perceived Noise Versus Display Noise in Temporally Filtered Image Sequences." Journal of Electronic Imaging 5:490–495, 1996.

[29] Xue P, Wilson DL. "Detection of Moving Objects in Pulsed X-Ray Fluoroscopy." J Opt Soc Am A 15:375–388, 1998.

[30] Xue P, Wilson DL. "Effects of Motion Blurring in X-Ray Fluoroscopy." Med Phys 25:587–599, 1998.

[31] Jabri KN, Srinivas Y, Wilson DL. "Quantitative Image Quality of Spatially Filtered X-Ray Fluoroscopy." In *Proceedings of SPIE Medical Imaging 1999: Image Perception*, Vol. 3663. Bellingham, Washington: SPIE, 1999, pp. 296–303.

[32] Jabri KN, Wilson DL. "Detection Improvement in Spatially Filtered X-Ray Fluoroscopy Image Sequences." J Opt Soc Am A 16:742–749, 1999.

[33] Wilson DL, Manjeshwar RM. "Role of Phase Information and Eye Pursuit in the Detection of Moving Objects in Noise." J Opt Soc Am A 16:669–678, 1999.

[34] Xue P, Thomas CW, Gilmore GC, Wilson DL. "An Adaptive Reference/Test Paradigm: Application to Pulsed Fluoroscopy Perception." Behavior Research Methods, Instruments, & Computers 30:332–348, 1998.

[35] Kelly DH. "Motion and Vision, II: Stabilized Spatio-temporal Threshold Surface." J Opt Soc Am 69:1340–1349, 1979.

[36] Wilson DL, Jabri KN, Xue P. "Modeling Human Visual Detection of Low-contrast Objects in Fluoroscopy Image Sequences." In Kundel HL (Ed.) *Proceedings of SPIE Medical Imaging 1997: Image Perception*, Vol. 3036. Bellingham, Washington: SPIE, 1997, pp. 21–30.

[37] Robson JG, "Spatial and Temporal Contrast-Sensitivity Functions of the Human Visual System." J Opt Soc Am 56:1141–1142, 1966.

[38] Kelly DH. "Frequency Doubling in Visual Responses." J Opt Soc Am A 56:1628–1633, 1966.

[39] Kelly DH, "Retinal Inhomogeneity. I. Spatiotemporal Contrast Sensitivity." J Opt Soc Am 1:107–113, 1984.

[40] van Nes F, Koenderink JJ, Nas H, Bouman MA, "Spatiotemporal Modulation Transfer in the Human Eye." J Opt Soc Am 57:1082–1088, 1967.

[41] Candy JW, *Signal Processing. The Modern Approach.* New York, NY: McGraw-Hill, 1988.

[42] Talukdar AS, Wilson DL. "Optimization of Image Quality for DSA Warping Registration." In *Proceedings of SPIE Medical Imaging 1999: Image Processing*, Vol. 3661. Bellingham, Washington: SPIE, 1999, pp. 819–827.

[43] Salem KA, Duerk JL, Wendt M, Wilson DL. "Evaluation of Keyhole MR Imaging with a Human Visual Response Model." In *Proceedings of SPIE Medical Imaging 1999: Image Perception*, Vol. 3663. Bellingham, Washington: SPIE, 1999, pp. 232–242.

[44] Xue P, Jabri KN, Wilson DL. "The Adaptive Reference/Test Forced-Choice Method with Application to Fluoroscopy Perception," In Kundel HL (Ed.) *Proceedings of SPIE Medical Imaging 1997: Image Perception*, Vol. 3036. Bellingham, Washington: SPIE, 1997, pp. 298–307.

[45] Pentland, A. "Maximum Likelihood Estimation: The Best PEST." Percep Psychophys 28:377–379, 1980.

[46] Watson AB, Pelli DG. "QUEST: A Bayesian Adaptive Psychometric Method." Percep Psychophys 33:113–120, 1983.

[47] King-Smith PE, Grigsby SS, Vingrys AL, Benes SC, Supowit A. "Efficient and Unbiased Modifications of the QUEST Threshold Method: Theory, Simulations, Experimental Evaluation and Practical Implementation." Vision Research 34:885–912, 1994.

[48] Green D, Swets JA. *Signal Detection Theory And Psychophysics.* New York: Krieger, 1974.

[49] Burgess AE. "Comparison of Receiver Operating Characteristic and Forced Choice Observer Performance Measurement Methods." Med Phys 22: 643–655, 1995.

[50] Rose A. *Vision: Human And Electronic.* New York: Plenum, 1973.

[51] Wagner RF, Brown DG. "Unified SNR Analysis of Medical Imaging Systems." Phys Med Biol 30:489–518, 1985.

[52] Ohara K, Doi K, Metz CE, Giger ML. "Investigation of Basic Imaging Properties in Digital Radiography. 13. Effect of Simple Structured Noise on the Detectability of Simulated Stenotic Lesions." Med Phys 16:14–21, 1989.

[53] Guignard PA, "A Comparative Method Based on ROC Analysis for the Quantitation of Observer Performance in Scintigraphy." Phys Med Biol 27:1163–1176, 1982.

[54] Myers KJ, Barrett HH, Borgstrom MC, Patton DD, Seeley GW. "Effect of Noise Correlation on Detectability of Disk Signals in Medical Imaging." J Opt Soc Am A 2:1752–1759, 1985.

[55] Blackwell KT. "The Effect of White and Filtered Noise on Contrast Detection Thresholds." Vision Research 38:267–280, 1998.

[56] Rolland JP, Barrett HH. "Effect of Random Background Inhomogeneity on Observer Detection Performance." J Opt Soc Am A 9:649–658, 1992.

[57] Burgess AE, Li X, Abbey CK. "Visual Signal Detectability with Two Noise Components: Anomalous Masking Effects." J Opt Soc Am A 14:2420–2442, 1997.

[58] Kump KS, Sachs P, Wilson DL. "The X-Ray Angiography Short-Bolus Technique." In *Proceedings of the Conference of the IEEE Engineering in Medicine Biology Society*, Vol. 16. Piscataway, NJ: IEEE, 1994, pp. 506–507.

[59] Kump K, Wilson D. "Optimization of Image Stacking as Applied to X-Ray Angiographic Sequences." In *Proceedings of SPIE Medical Imaging 1996: Physiology and Function from Multidimensional Images*, Vol. 2709. Bellingham, Washington: SPIE, 1996, pp. 76–81.

[60] Wilson DL, Chen C-H, Sahin M, Bao L, Tarr RW. "Image Stacking for Visualization of Low-Contrast Arteries." Radiology 189(p): 277, 1993 (abstract).

[61] Brailean JC, Kleihorst RP, Efstratiadis SN, Katsaggelos AK, Lagendijk RL. "Noise Reduction Filters for Dynamic Image Sequences: A Review." Proc IEEE 83:1272–1292, 1995.

[62] Aufrichtig R, Singh A, Wilson DL. "Kalman Filtering with Motion Compensation of Fluoroscopic Image Sequences." Radiology 189(p):249, 1993 (abstract).

[63] Aufrichtig R, Geiger D, Singh A, Wilson DL. "Spatio-Temporal X-Ray Fluoroscopy Filtering Using Object Detection." In *Computers in Cardiology*. Washington, DC: IEEE Computer Society Press, 1993, pp. 587–590.

[64] Singh A, Wilson D, Aufrichtig R. "Enhancement of X-Ray Fluoroscopy Images." In *Proceedings of SPIE Medical Imaging*, Vol. 1898. Bellingham, Washington: SPIE, 1993, pp. 304–310.

[65] R. Aufrichtig, Perception and Filtering of Interventional X-Ray Fluoroscopy Image Sequences. PhD Thesis, Case Western Reserve University, May, 1994.

[66] Sanchez F, Srinivas Y, Jabri KN, Wilson DL. "Quantitative Image Quality Analysis of a Non-Linear Spatio-Temporal Filter." IEEE Trans on Image Processing (submitted).

[67] Grollman JJH, Klosterman H, Herman MW, Moler CL, Eber LM, MacAlpin RN. "Dose Reduction Low Pulse-Rate Fluoroscopy." Radiology 105:293–298, 1972.

[68] Grollman JJH. "Radiation Reduction by Means of Low Pulse-Rate Fluoroscopy During Cardiac Catheterization and Coronary Arteriography." Am J Roentgenol 121:636–641, 1974.

[69] Fritz SL, Mirvis SE, Pais SO, Roys S. "Phantom Evaluation of Angiographer Performance Using Low Frame Rate Acquisition Fluoroscopy." Med Phys 15:600–603, 1988.

[70] Watson AB, Albert J, Ahumada J, Farrell JE. "Window of Visibility: A Pschophysical Theory of Fidelity in Time-Sampled Visual Motion Displays." J Opt Soc Am A 3:300–307, 1986.

[71] Ammann E, Wiede G. "Generators and Tubes in Interventional Radiology." In Balter S, Shope TB (Eds.) *Syllabus: A Categorical Course in Physics, Physical and Technical Aspects of Angiography and Interventional Angiography.* Oak Brook, IL: RSNA Publications, 1995, pp. 59–74.

CHAPTER 15
Fundamental ROC Analysis

Charles E. Metz
The University of Chicago

CONTENTS

15.1 Introduction

Receiver operating characteristic (ROC) analysis is accepted widely as the most complete way of quantifying and reporting accuracy in two-group classification tasks. Based in statistical decision theory [1], ROC methodology was developed initially for evaluation of detectability in radar [2, 3] but soon was extended to applications in psychology and psychophysics [4–8] and in other fields [9–11]. The use of ROC analysis in medical decision making, medical diagnosis and medical imaging was first proposed by Lusted [12–15], who pointed out that a diagnostician or radiologist can achieve different combinations of sensitivity and specificity by consciously or unconsciously changing the "threshold of abnormality" or "critical confidence level" which is used to distinguish nominally positive test results (or images) from nominally negative outcomes, and that ROC analysis is ideally suited to the task of separating such "decision threshold" effects from inherent differences in diagnostic accuracy. Subsequently, ROC techniques have been employed in the evaluation of a broad variety of diagnostic procedures [16–21], especially in medical imaging [22–30]. The medical applications of ROC analysis have fostered a number of methodological innovations, particularly in ROC curve fitting, in elucidating distinctions among several sources of variation in ROC estimates, and in testing the statistical significance of differences between such estimates.

This chapter surveys conventional ROC methodology from a broad perspective, both to acquaint the reader with the current state of the art and to guide the reader to other literature that provides greater conceptual and/or methodological detail. Variants of ROC analysis that take localization into account [31–38] are described in a subsequent chapter, whereas relationships between ROC analysis and cost/benefit analysis [22, 39–43] as well as the use of ROC analysis in predicting and quantifying the gains in accuracy obtained from multiple readings of each image [44, 45] are discussed elsewhere.

15.2 The ROC curve as a description of diagnostic accuracy

Use of ROC analysis in medical imaging acknowledges that the practical value of an imaging system in diagnostic medicine generally depends not only upon the physical characteristics of the system and of the disease and nondisease states of interest, but also upon the perceptual characteristics of the human and/or automated observers who will interpret the images and upon the "critical confidence level" that a particular observer employs to distinguish nominally "positive" images from nominally "negative" images. Changing the setting of this critical confidence level changes both an imaging procedure's sensitivity (i.e., the probability that an actually-positive image will be classified correctly as "positive" with respect to a given disease) and the procedure's specificity (the probability that an actually-negative image will be classified correctly as "negative"). Therefore, one cannot completely assess an imaging-system/observer combination's ability to classify images as "positive" or "negative" with respect to a given disease simply in terms of a single pair of numbers that represents sensitivity and specificity; instead, one must estimate and report all of the tradeoffs between sensitivity and specificity that the imaging-system/observer combination can achieve. In effect, an ROC curve is a graph of these tradeoffs. However, for historical reasons, ROC curves usually plot sensitivity (also called "true positive fraction," or "TPF") not as a function of specificity, but rather as a function of [1.0 − specificity] ("false positive fraction," or "FPF"). The conceptual basis for ROC analysis and the limitations of alternative methodologies for evaluation of diagnostic techniques have been described elsewhere in much greater detail [5, 7, 8, 13, 20, 22–26, 29, 30].

In terms of a six-tiered hierarchical model of diagnostic efficacy [27, 28], ROC analysis describes diagnostic performance at Level 2: the extent to which diagnostic decisions agree with actual states of health and disease. However, in some situations ROC curves can be combined with data on disease prevalence and judgments of decision utilities to predict efficacy at higher levels [22, 39–43].

15.3 Independent variables and sources of bias

Decision accuracy in medical imaging depends upon the difficulty of the cases that must be classified and the skill of image readers, so ROC curves depend upon these factors as well. Therefore, the cases and readers employed in an ROC study must be chosen to represent fairly the populations of cases and readers about which conclusions are to be drawn.

Case factors that may influence decision accuracy include disease stage, lesion size, the extent to which actually-negative cases are potentially confusing or distracting, the kind of prior information (if any) that is available to the image reader, and the inclusion or exclusion of cases for which diagnostic "truth" is difficult to establish. Reader factors, on the other hand, include training and experience with a particular imaging modality, familiarity with morphological manifestations of the disease in question and with potentially confusing normal variants, and motivation in a study setting.

Each of these factors can be considered an independent variable worthy of scientific investigation to the extent that it may be identified and either controlled or represented by an appropriate spectrum of examples; however, each factor is also a potential source of bias that can undermine a study's scientific validity. Bias issues and their remedies in evaluations of diagnostic techniques have been discussed elsewhere [46–50]. Sometimes it is helpful to distinguish between evaluation studies that strive to determine diagnostic accuracy in absolute terms and those that seek only to rank diagnostic techniques, because some potential sources of bias in the former situation may have little or no effect in the latter [50].

15.4 ROC indices

Although knowledge of the entire ROC curve is required in order to describe the performance of a diagnostic test completely for a defined disease, group of patients, readers, etc., often one would like to summarize the curve by a single number, particularly when one wishes to draw a conclusion concerning which of two ROC curves is "better." Evidence from a broad variety of fields indicates that specification of a complete ROC curve almost always requires at least two parameters [51], so summarizing the curve by a single univariate index generally discards information that the full ROC provides. However, summary indices can be meaningful if they are chosen with a clear appreciation of a particular comparison's practical goal and an understanding of the ways in which such indices can be misleading.

The most commonly employed univariate summary of a conventional ROC curve is the area under the entire curve when it is plotted in a unit square. This index (denoted by A_z when it has been estimated by fitting a conventional "binormal" ROC curve) has the advantage of several intuitive interpretations [25, 26, 52, 53], and it provides a meaningful basis for ranking ROC curves if the curves in question do not cross. However, the "total area" index is a global measure of decision performance that implicitly considers all of the points on an ROC curve to be of equal importance, and this may not be the case in clinical applications of a diagnostic test, because a particular "operating point" (i.e., combination of TPF and FPF) always is most efficacious in a cost-benefit sense for any given disease prevalence and set of utility judgments [22]. Therefore other, more sharply-focused summary indices should be employed in comparisons of diagnostic performance when a particular region of the TPF vs. FPF graph is of primary interest and/or when ROC curve estimates cross. Three basic classes of such indices have been proposed: those that compare the TPF (or FPF) values of two ROC curves at a particular FPF (or TPF) [54, 55]; those that compare the average TPF (or FPF) values of two ROC curves in a particular range of FPF (or TPF) [56–58]; and those that compare the maximum values of a measure of efficacy on two ROC curves [22, 43]. Parametric ROC curves can be compared also in terms of a vector difference in curve-parameter space [55, 59, 60], but this approach does not allow the curves to be ranked in any intuitive way.

15.5 Confidence-rating scales

Because ROC analysis seeks to determine all of the combinations of sensitivity and specificity that can be achieved by use of different decision-threshold settings, it requires that test-result data be collected on a graded (rather than binary) ordinal scale. For many years, ROC curves that described the accuracies of human judgments were estimated from confidence ratings collected on a discrete ordinal scale with 4 to 7 (often 5) categories. This limited number of categories was found empirically to provide ROC curve estimates with sufficient precision if each observer employed the scale so that its category boundaries were distributed across the range of possible stimuli in a fashion that provided a more-or-less uniform of spread of "operating" points along the ROC curve. However, the way in which a human observer employs a discrete ordinal scale cannot be controlled directly by the investigator, so such scales sometimes were found to provide poorly-distributed sets of points on the ROC, thereby reducing the precision with which the curve could be determined and sometimes—especially with small data sets—yielding "degenerate" data sets with characteristics that could not be analyzed by conventional curve-fitting methods [50].

Recently, in an attempt to overcome such problems, several investigators have proposed the use of continuous (or fine-grained—e.g., 100-point) reporting scales in ROC studies that involve human judgments [61, 62]. The important potential advantage of such scales is that they do not impose an artificial "front-end quantization" of the data, but instead allow each observer to report seemingly meaningful distinctions that would be lost if use of a small number of reporting categories were imposed. Although this approach has been criticized on the grounds that human variability causes judgment data to be less reproducible when it is collected on a fine-grained or continuous scale, these objections overlook the fact that ROC curve estimates depend only upon the rank-order statistics of the confidence ratings obtained from actually-positive and actually-negative cases, and not upon the confidence ratings themselves. Experience to date with 100-point reporting scales (which observers can interpret intuitively as subjective-probability scales) in ROC experiments has been encouraging. Statistical methods for fitting ROC curves to human judgment data collected on fine-grained reporting scales (or quantitative test-result data collected on inherently continuous scales) are discussed in Section 15.8, below.

15.6 Other issues in experimental design

15.6.1 The need to establish truth

Both the ease with which observer performance experiments are conducted and the results that those experiments provide depend upon the objects about which decisions must be made and upon the images that are used as a basis for those decisions. Therefore, careful attention must be devoted to the selection of objects and images if the results of an observer performance experiment are to provide meaningful indicators of image quality.

Questions of image quality in diagnostic medicine ultimately concern the ability of radiologists or other trained observers to correctly decide patients' states of health and disease from images made under clinical conditions. Therefore, observer performance experiments that employ clinical images can provide direct assessments of image quality, and such studies should be conducted whenever they are feasible and scientifically valid. Several practical considerations often make the use of clinical images difficult, however.

In any objective evaluation of a diagnostic system, the true state of the object (e.g., patient) from which each image is made must be known by the data analyst, so that observers' responses can be compared with truth. Unfortunately, the establishment of diagnostic truth in clinical images is sometimes difficult, both in principle (because "truth" is ultimately a philosophical matter) and in practice (because great effort may be required to determine the actual state of health or disease of a particular patient at a particular point in time "beyond a reasonable doubt"). Important issues that must be confronted in establishing truth in clinical evaluation studies have been reviewed elsewhere [24, 25, 46, 49]. In particular, attention must be focused on biases that may be caused by the omission of clinical cases for which truth is particularly difficult to establish [47–49]. Carefully designed clinical image-evaluation studies can be done and useful conclusions can be drawn from them [24, 25], but studies that employ nonclinical images—though subject to other limitations, as noted below—often are less demanding and may be adequate.

Some of the practical difficulties of clinical images in observer performance experiments are overcome by employing specially-designed inanimate objects ("phantoms") instead of human patients. "Truth" is defined by the phantom's construction in this situation, and the features to be detected or distinguished by the observers are readily controlled. Images of carefully designed phantoms can accurately represent virtually all of the physical aspects of the clinical image-forming process. The task of selecting object features and/or images with an appropriate level of difficulty has been discussed elsewhere [50], but the detectability (e.g., average area under two ROC curves to be compared) that yields optimal statistical power has not yet been determined precisely. The chief limitation of phantom images in observer performance experiments usually is the problem of designing and manufacturing phantoms that represent clinical object structures with realism sufficient to ensure that the experiment's results are similar to those that would be obtained in clinical practice. Accurate representation of complex anatomical background is often difficult or impossible, particularly because that background must vary from image to image if it is to represent the normal anatomical variation among patients which typically complicates clinical image interpretation. Also, generation of large numbers of phantom images sometimes can be laborious, especially when the positioning and/or background of the phantom is varied in a controlled way to simulate clinical conditions. Phantom images are most useful in observer performance studies when the determination of truth in clinical cases is difficult and an absence of realistic, variable background structure is considered unlikely to affect the results sought from the study.

Alternatively, large numbers of images for use in an observer performance study can be generated quickly and inexpensively by digital computer and subsequently displayed on film or a video monitor. Knowledge of the physical processes associated with a particular imaging modality often can be used to produce images that closely approximate those that could be obtained more laboriously with phantoms. The object features to be detected and/or image background structures can be varied stochastically with relative ease. A unique advantage of computer-generated images in research is their ability to simulate the images that would be produced by hypothetical imaging modalities or combinations of imaging parameters in existing modalities. The chief disadvantage of computer-generated images is that the accuracy with which they represent real images is sometimes limited or unknown, either because inclusion of the full complexity of the physical image-forming process may be difficult or because computer-modeled object features and background structures may be oversimplified.

In an attempt to combine the advantages of clinical and computer-simulated images in observer performance experiments that involve lesion detection, actually-normal clinical images can be modified by computer to represent the inclusion of abnormal object features. Hybrid images of this kind reduce the difficulty of determining clinical truth, allow a detection experiment to include lesions with any desired size, shape, and contrast, and automatically include realistic—indeed, real—variations in normal anatomical background. The task of determining truth is reduced to one of ensuring that lesions of the class to be detected are truly absent from the clinical images. Often this can be accomplished on the basis of clinical follow-up alone, particularly with modalities such as chest radiography and mammography that are used for periodic screening of large and predominantly normal populations. Hybrid images are produced most easily with modalities such as computed tomography and scintigraphy, in which clinical images are readily available in digital form and the imaging process is essentially linear, but they can be generated also in other modalities such as screen/film radiography by digitization of analog images and appropriate attention to sensitometric effects. Simulated lesions superimposed upon actually normal clinical images must take into account the contrast rendition and spatial resolution of the imaging system, and they must include the effects of any (significant) perturbations which the presence of a lesion would impose on the detected radiation field. Production of realistic hybrid images may be difficult in ultrasonography, for example, due to complex effects of reflections between normal and abnormal structures, and in radionuclide imaging when the abnormality constitutes a reduced concentration of activity, because Poisson-statistical variation in the image due to normal local activity cannot be removed exactly.

15.6.2 Disease prevalence

Empirically, the case-sample components of variance in ROC curve estimates and their indices are roughly proportional to $[(1/M_{pos}) + (1/M_{neg})]$, where M_{pos} and M_{neg} represent the numbers of actually-positive and actually-negative cases, respectively, upon which the estimate is based. If M_{neg} is much larger than M_{pos}, this proportionality indicates that a large fraction of each observer's time is devoted to reading cases that do not contribute substantially to increased precision in the ROC study's result. ROC curves do not depend upon the prevalence of actually-positive cases in a study if an observer's decision-making strategy does not change with prevalence., so most ROC studies are designed to include roughly equal numbers of actually-positive and actually-negative cases. On the other hand, important diseases can be rather rare in populations of practical interest in medical imaging (only about one-half percent of women screened by mammography have incident breast cancer, for example), and one may conjecture that image-reading and/or decision-making strategy does, in fact, change at such low prevalences. Therefore, a question may arise as to whether the prevalence of actually-positive cases in an ROC study should be chosen to approximate the disease prevalence in a clinically-relevant population, despite the greater resources and effort that such an approach would require. No clear-cut answer to this question is available at present, but several points seem worthy of note.

First, if the total number of cases employed in an experiment is held fixed, then small departures from a 50:50 case mix have little effect on the precision with which ROC curves and their indices can be estimated. On the other hand, large departures cause precision to degrade rapidly. For example, with a fixed total number of cases, the expression provided in the previous paragraph indicates that case-sample components of variance increase by only about 50% when prevalence changes from 0.50 to 0.20, but then increase by an additional 50% as prevalence changes from 0.20 to 0.15. Also, the use of realistic prevalences in ROC studies may impose an enormous burden in terms of the total number of images—and, therefore, observer time—that is needed to obtain a desired standard error in estimates of decision accuracy. For example, when reader variation is ignored and only 1 out of 200 cases is actually positive (i.e., with prevalence equal to 0.005), a total of 5000 images would be needed to obtain the same precision that could be obtained with 100 images if half of those were actually positive. Taken together, these observations provide strong practical justification for use of prevalences in the range of 0.20 to 0.80 if decision accuracy does not depend strongly on disease prevalence.

Unfortunately, due to the logistical difficulty of quantifying prevalence effects with high precision, no data obtained to date indicate clearly the extent to which image-reading and/or decision-making strategy may change at prevalences as low as those often encountered in clinical settings. Additional investigation is sorely needed.

15.6.3 Reading-order effects

The sequence in which images are read by human observers can influence their interpretation and, thus, the result of an ROC study. Therefore, an important issue in experimental design is the need to ensure that the image-reading order used in an experiment does not bias the result of the study toward or against any of the imaging conditions under comparison.

Perhaps the most important reading-order bias can occur when images of a single case sample are read in two or more imaging and/or display modalities and all of the images from one modality are read before all of those from another. If cases are recognized during their second reading in this situation and any diagnostically relevant information is recalled from the first reading, then the ROC curve achieved from the second reading reflects the diagnostic value not of the second imaging modality alone, but instead the value of a combination of the two modalities, which may be complementary. Therefore, the result of the ROC experiment may be biased in favor of the second modality in this situation.

Two approaches can be used to reduce or eliminate such reading-order effects; the common theme is to vary the order in which the modalities' images are read in a way such that reading-order effects tend to cancel out. With either method, readings of images of a given patient by the same observer should be separated by as much time as possible.

The simpler approach (which we consider here for two modalities) is to have half of the observers read the images from modality A first and those from modality B second, whereas the other observers read the two modalities in the opposite order. This technique addresses the problem by attempting to make reading-order effects cancel across observers. It may often be adequate, but its results remain vulnerable to second-order effects, such as the possibility that one of the groups will be skewed toward observers who "remember cases" better, thereby biasing the study's results in favor of the modality read second by that group.

A more complex approach seeks to cancel reading-order effects within each observer's results. Here, the patient sample is broken into several subsets, and the various modality-subset combinations are sequenced so that each observer sees half the patients first in each modality. Sequences of modality-subset combinations should be chosen to separate readings of different modalities' images of the same patient by as much time as possible, and ideally a different (but always internally balanced) sequence of modality-subset combinations should be used for each observer, with the different sequences chosen to balance all potential modality/reading-order interactions across observers as much as possible. An example of this latter approach is described elsewhere [50].

Perhaps the only situation in which reading-order effects are appropriate occurs when both of two conditions are satisfied: (i) a stand-alone imaging modality is to be compared with the combination of that imaging modality and a supplementary modality; and (ii) the stand-alone modality is always read before the combination in clinical practice. In this situation, which occurs in assessing some computer-aided diagnostic (CAD) techniques, for example [63], if the experimental design provides an amount of time between the first and second readings of each image similar to that which would occur in clinical practice, the potential benefit of the first reading to interpretations made from the second reading becomes not a bias, but instead a factor of realistic experimental design.

15.7 Comments on forced-choice methodology

ROC analysis provides a more complete description of observer performance than other currently available evaluation methodologies, and in principle it can be applied to any two-state classification task. However, ROC studies often require substantial time and effort from their observers, because each image reading must be reported on a confidence scale that the observer must attempt to hold constant throughout his/her participation in the experiment. In situations where only a summary index is sought and the full ROC is not required, "forced choice" methodology provides an alternative and sometimes more efficient approach.

As noted in Section 15.4, the total area under an ROC curve provides a useful summary of discrimination performance. Perhaps surprisingly, this area can be measured directly in a "two-alternative forced-choice" (2-AFC) experiment [5, 52, 53] without measurement of—or explicit reference to—the ROC curve.

The observer in a 2-AFC experiment views independent pairs of images together. One image in each pair is always actually positive, whereas the other is always actually negative, and the observer is required to state which image is which. If the actually-positive image is varied randomly in each pair (between left and right, say, with equal probability), then the percentage of correct decisions in this task can range from 0.5 (indicating chance performance) to 1.0 (indicating perfect performance). With this paradigm, the observer does not need to adopt any confidence threshold; instead, his impressions of the two images are compared with each other. It can be shown, under very general assumptions, that the expected fraction of correct decisions in this 2-AFC experiment equals the expected area under the ROC curve that would be measured with the same images viewed one at a time in a conventional ROC experiment [5, 52, 53]. Thus, if only the total ROC area is of interest, it can be measured directly by the 2-AFC paradigm, with some apparent saving in experimental effort.

The chief disadvantage of the 2-AFC approach lies in the fact that the trading relationship between sensitivity and specificity (i.e., the ROC curve) is never determined. Therefore, the result of a 2-AFC experiment cannot be used in higher-order efficacy analyses involving costs and benefits [22, 39–43], where a particular compromise between sensitivity and specificity must be considered. Also, the 2-AFC paradigm can be more efficient than the ROC approach in terms of observer time, but it is less efficient in terms of the number of images required for an experiment, because greater statistical precision in the ROC-area index can be gained with a given number of images if confidence-rating data, which determine the ROC, are obtained from the observer [53]. Hence, the 2-AFC technique should be considered for use primarily in situations where the conventional ROC-area index provides an adequate summary of performance and where observer time— rather than the number of images available with truth—is the scarce experimental resource.

A generalization of the 2-AFC paradigm involves a task in which exactly one of $M > 2$ simultaneously-presented images (or locations in a single image) is actually positive, and the observer is required to identify the actually positive image (or location). The level of performance achieved by the observer is represented by the fraction of such trials in which his/her decision is correct [30, 64]. For a given level of image quality, the difficulty of this "multiple-alternative forced-choice" (M-AFC) task increases with M, the number of images (or candidate locations) presented to the observer in each trial. An advantage of the M-AFC paradigm is that statistical power can be optimized, for any given level of image quality (signal-to-noise ratio), by use of an appropriate value of M. The M-AFC technique also provides substantially better sampling statistics than 2-AFC experiments for a given number of decision trials and allows the investigation of observer performance at higher signal-to-noise ratios [64]. However, a disadvantage of the approach is that the theoretical relationship between performance in a M-AFC experiment and in an ROC experiment becomes more strongly dependent upon the shape of the ROC curve as M increases [30].

15.8 ROC curve fitting

An "empirical ROC curve" is swept out if one plots the set of all possible (FPF, TPF) pairs that can be calculated from the test results (e.g., confidence ratings) by adopting various settings of the critical test-result value which distinguishes nominally positive results from nominally negative results. Aside from the $(0, 0)$ and $(1, 1)$ points that terminate every conventional ROC curve, all such empirical ROCs are comprised of $(K - 1)$ points if the test-result data include K distinct values. For example, an empirical ROC can involve no more than 4 off-corner points if its data are collected on a 5-category discrete scale, whereas it will be represented by $(M_{pos} + M_{neg} - 1)$ points if test results from M_{pos} actually-positive cases and M_{neg} actually-negative cases are collected without tied values on a continuous scale. In the latter hypothetical situation, all line segments drawn between neighboring points are either vertical or horizontal; neighboring points are separated by $1/M_{pos}$ in the vertical direction or by $1/M_{neg}$ in the horizontal direction; and vertical or horizontal "runs" of points on the ROC graph correspond to "truth-state runs" in the rank-ordered test-result data. Each such run tends to become shorter if M_{pos} and M_{neg} are increased in proportion, thereby causing the empirical ROC to converge toward a smooth curve in the limit of an infinitely large case sample. Hence, to estimate a population ROC curve, which must be continuous if the test-result scale is not inherently discrete, many investigators prefer to fit a smooth ROC curve to data collected on either kind of scale.

All widely-used curve-fitting approaches require that one adopt some functional form with adjustable parameters for the ROC curve and then select the values of these parameters to fit the data best in some sense. For reasons described elsewhere [60], ROC curves are fit more appropriately by maximum-likelihood estimation than by least-squares methods. An important aspect of the maximum-likelihood approach is that it does not require a strict assumption concerning the underlying decision-variable distributions, but instead requires only that a form be assumed for a latent (i.e., effective) pair of decision-variable distributions. In practice, this means that one must assume the form of the underlying distributions only to within a monotonic transformation of the decision variable (which need not be known), because ROC curves are invariant under such transformations.

The conventional "binormal" model, which assumes that real-world ROC curves have the same form as those produced by an underlying pair of normal distributions, is employed most widely [65–67] and has been shown to provide good fits to ROC data collected in a very broad variety of situations [51, 68]. In order to ensure that appropriately-shaped fits are obtained with small data sets, some attention has focused recently on alternative "proper" ROC curve-fitting models [69–71], which ensure that all fitted ROCs are convex. However, to date no reliable methods have been developed for testing the statistical significance of differences between ROC curve estimates obtained from these new "proper" models.

Maximum-likelihood estimation of ROC curves requires extensive calculations and careful attention to numerical methods. Fortunately, computer programs developed specifically for this purpose and refined on the basis of experience with many data sets are available at no cost from several sources [72].

15.9 Statistical tests for differences between ROC estimates

Usually one would like an ROC curve to describe the performance of a particular diagnostic test when it is applied to a defined population of cases (i.e., patients), but in practice only an estimate of the curve can be obtained by applying the test to a finite sample of cases that has been drawn from the population of interest. Moreover, when the test must be interpreted by human observers, as in medical imaging, one usually would like the ROC curve to represent the typical performance of the test when it is interpreted by a defined population of readers (e.g., radiologists with a particular amount of experience in mammography), even though the curve must be estimated from a finite sample of readers who will, in general, have varying degrees of skill. The often complicated statistical methodologies that have been developed for ROC curve fitting and statistical significance testing reflect this wish to use data obtained from samples of cases and readers to draw conclusions about the performance of diagnostic tests in populations of cases and/or readers.

The extent to which the result of an experiment can be generalized to a population of cases and/or readers depends upon the kinds of variation that have been taken into account in determining the statistical significance of the result. Recall that a "p-value" represents the probability that a difference at least as large as that found in the experiment would occur by chance if the experiment were repeated many times and no difference exists, in fact, between the conditions being compared. Therefore, the calculated p-value should depend upon the way in which one imagines the experiment to be repeated. For example, suppose that, on one hand, an ROC experiment is repeated many times with independently-sampled cases but always with the same readers or, on the other hand, with independently-sampled cases and with independently-sampled readers. Clearly, one should expect the result of the experiment to vary more in the latter situation than in the former, because variation in reader skill then would be added to variation in the difficulty of the case sample [24, 73]. If both of these sources of variation were taken into account in calculating a p-value for a particular result of the experiment, then one could conclude that a statistically significant difference applies to the populations of both cases and readers that were sampled in the experiment. However, if only case-sample variation were taken into account in calculating the p-value and reader variation were ignored, then the conclusion could be generalized to a population of cases but would be restricted to the particular sample of readers that was employed in the experiment. Conversely, if only reader variation were taken into account in calculating the p-value and case-sample variation were ignored, then the conclusion could be generalized to a population of readers but would be restricted to the particular sample of cases that was employed.

This perspective suggests two fundamentally different ways of contrasting the statistical tests that have been developed for analyses of ROC studies: either in terms of the source(s) of variation [73] taken into account or in terms of the particular ROC index for which values are to be compared [50, 72]. Other, more technical, distinctions among statistical tests include questions of whether the case samples for the two diagnostic modalities to be compared are independent or paired, whether the statistical test employs parametric or nonparametric methods, and whether covariate factors (such as lesion size, for example) are taken into account [72].

Student's t test takes only reader variation into account when it is applied to differences between ROC index estimates [50], whereas most other current statistical tests for the significance of differences between ROC estimates take only case-sample variation into account [43, 53–55, 57–60, 74–78]. However, several approaches are now available with which to account for both reader variation and case-sample variation in statistical testing, thereby allowing the conclusions of a study to be generalized to both a population of readers and a population of cases [24, 79–86].

Free software for testing differences between ROC estimates has been listed elsewhere [72].

15.10 Ordinal regression techniques

As mentioned earlier in this chapter, ROC curves in medical imaging depend upon the difficulty of cases and the skill of image readers. Therefore, one would expect ROC curves to rise in a smooth way if one were to perform experiments with increasingly larger lesions or with readers who have an increasingly larger number of years of training, for example.

Most ROC studies conducted to date either have employed lesions with a particular size and/or readers with a particular amount of training, in order to draw conclusions about specific situations, or have included diverse spectra of lesion size and/or reader experience in order to draw conclusions that apply to heterogeneous populations. However, suppose that one wishes to quantify the dependence of an ROC curve upon both lesion diameter and years of reader training, for example. One approach would be to: (i) conduct numerous experiments, with lesion size and training period held fixed at different pairs of values in each experiment; (ii) fit an ROC curve to the ordinal response data obtained from each combination of lesion size and training period; and then (iii) fit a two-dimensional surface (e.g., by least-squares techniques) to the results of the ROC curve fitting in order describe the functional dependence of some ROC index (e.g., total area under the curve) upon lesion diameter and training period.

A more powerful and much more elegant technique would be to combine steps (i) through (iii) above in order to estimate simultaneously the ROC curves and their dependence on "covariates" such as lesion diameter and training period. This approach to ROC analysis, called "ordinal regression," was first proposed by Tosteson and Begg [87] and has been developed subsequently by Toledano and Gatsonis [84–86]. However, several theoretical and technical issues (such as a current inability to analyze continuously-distributed data and lack of readily-available software) must be resolved before this potentially powerful approach can be employed widely.

15.11 An overview

Conventional ROC analysis provides an objective and meaningful approach for assessment of decision-performance in two-group classification tasks. Much methodological progress—particularly in experimental design and data analysis— has been made during the past two decades in developing ROC techniques for medical-imaging applications, but several important practical issues remain unresolved, thereby providing opportunities for future research.

Acknowledgments

Several sections of this chapter are based upon the author's written contributions to an ICRU committee chaired by Professor Peter Sharp of the University of Aberdeen. Professor Sharp's skill in guiding the efforts of that committee and in editing its report [30] is acknowledged with gratitude. Also gratefully acknowledged are the contributions of Dr. Heber MacMahon of The University of Chicago, who pointed out the appropriateness of reading-order effects in some CAD-evaluation studies, as described at the end of Section 15.6.3.

The manuscript for this chapter was supported by grant R01-GM57622 from the National Institutes of Health (C.E. Metz, principal investigator). Much of the work described here was supported by the same grant, by a University of Chicago contract with the University of Iowa under grant R01-CA62362 from the National Institutes of Health (D.D. Dorfman, principal investigator), or by grant DE FG02–94ER6186 from the U.S. Department of Energy (C.E. Metz, principal investigator). The content of this chapter is solely the responsibility of the author and does not necessarily represent the official views of the sponsoring organizations.

References

[1] Wald A. *Statistical Decision Functions*. New York: Wiley, 1950.

[2] Van Meter D, Middleton D. "Modern Statistical Approaches to Reception in Communication Theory." IRE Trans PGIT-4:119, 1954.

[3] Peterson WW, Birdsall TG, Fox WC. "The Theory of Signal Detectability." IRE Trans PGIT-4:171, 1954.

[4] Swets JA, Tanner Jr WP, Birdsall TG. "Decision Processes in Perception." Psych Rev 68:301, 1961.

[5] Green DM, Swets JA. *Signal Detection Theory and Psychophysics*. New York: Wiley, 1966; (reprint with corrections: Huntington, NY: Krieger, 1974).

[6] Swets JA. "The Relative Operating Characteristic in Psychology." Science 182:990, 1973.

[7] Egan JP. *Signal Detection Theory and ROC Analysis*. New York: Academic Press, 1975.

[8] Swets JA. *Signal Detection Theory and ROC Analysis in Psychology and Diagnostics: Collected Papers*. Mahwah, NJ: Lawrence Erlbaum Associates, 1996.

[9] Swets JA. "Effectiveness of Information Retrieval Methods." American Documentation 20:72, 1969.

[10] Swets JA, Green DM. "Applications of Signal Detection Theory." In Pick HA, Liebowitz HL, Singer A *et al.* (Eds.) *Psychology: From Research to Practice.* New York: Plenum, 1978, p. 311.

[11] Swets JA. "Assessment of NDT Systems (Parts I and II)." Materials Evaluation 41:1294, 1983.

[12] Lusted LB. "Logical Analysis in Roentgen Diagnosis." Radiology 74:178, 1960.

[13] Lusted LB. *Introduction to Medical Decision Making*. Springfield, IL: Thomas, 1968.

[14] Lusted LB. "Decision-Making Studies in Patient Management." New Engl J Med 284:416, 1971.

[15] Lusted LB. "Signal Detectability and Medical Decision-Making." Science 171:1217, 1971.

[16] McNeil BJ, Keeler E, Adelstein SJ. "Primer on Certain Elements of Medical Decision Making." New Engl J Med 293:211, 1975.

[17] McNeil BJ, Adelstein SJ. "Determining the Value of Diagnostic and Screening Tests." J Nucl Med 17:439, 1976.

[18] Griner PF, Mayewski RJ, Mushlin AI, Greenland P. "Selection and Interpretation of Diagnostic Tests and Procedures: Principles and Applications." Annals Int Med 94:553, 1981.

[19] Robertson EA, Zweig MH, Van Steirtghem AC. "Evaluating the Clinical Efficacy of Laboratory Tests." Am J Clin Path 79:78, 1983.

[20] Swets JA. "Measuring the Accuracy of Diagnostic Systems." Science 240:1285, 1988.

[21] Zweig MH, Campbell G. "Receiver-Operating Characteristic (ROC) Plots: A Fundamental Evaluation Tool in Clinical Medicine." Clinical Chemistry 39:561, 1993. [Erratum published in Clinical Chemistry 39:1589, 1993.]

[22] Metz CE. "Basic Principles of ROC Analysis." Seminars in Nucl Med 8:283–298, 1978.

[23] Swets JA. "ROC Analysis Applied to the Evaluation of Medical Imaging Techniques." Invest Radiol 13:109, 1979.

[24] Swets JA, Pickett RM. *Evaluation of Diagnostic Systems: Methods from Signal Detection Theory*. New York: Academic Press, 1982.

[25] Metz CE. "ROC Methodology in Radiologic Imaging." Invest Radiol 21:720, 1986.

[26] Hanley JA. "Receiver Operating Characteristic (ROC) Methodology: The State of the Art." Critical Reviews in Diagnostic Imaging 29:307, 1989.

[27] Fryback DG, Thornbury JR. "The Efficacy of Diagnostic Imaging." Med Decis Making 11:88, 1991.

[28] National Council On Radiation Protection and Measurements. *An Introduction to Efficacy in Diagnostic Radiology and Nuclear Medicine* (NCRP Commentary 13). Bethesda, MD: NCRP, 1995.

[29] Metz CE, Wagner RF, Doi K, Brown DG, Nishikawa RN, Myers KJ. "Toward Consensus on Quantitative Assessment of Medical Imaging Systems." Med Phys 22:1057, 1995.

[30] International Commission On Radiation Units and Measurements. *Medical Imaging: The Assessment of Image Quality* (ICRU Report 54). Bethesda, MD: ICRU, 1996.

[31] Egan JP, Greenberg GZ, Schulman AI. "Operating Characteristics, Signal Detection, and the Method of Free Response." J Acoust Soc Am 33:993, 1961.

[32] Starr SJ, Metz CE, Lusted LB, Goodenough DJ. "Visual Detection and Localization of Radiographic Images." Radiology 116:533, 1975.

[33] Metz CE, Starr SJ, Lusted LB. "Observer Performance in Detecting Multiple Radiographic Signals: Prediction and Analysis Using a Generalized ROC Approach." Radiology 121:337, 1976.

[34] International Atomic Energy Agency. "IAEA Co-Ordinated Research Programme on the Intercomparison of Computer-Assisted Scintigraphic Techniques: Third Progress Report." In *Medical Radionuclide Imaging, Vol. 1.* Vienna: International Atomic Energy Agency, 1977, p. 585.

[35] Bunch PC, Hamilton JF, Sanderson GK, Simmons AH. "A Free Response Approach to the Measurement and Characterization of Radiographic Observer Performance." Proc SPIE 127:124, 1977.

[36] Chakraborty DP. "Maximum Likelihood Analysis of Free-Response Receiver Operating Characteristic (FROC) Data." Med Phys 16:561, 1989.

[37] Chakraborty DP, Winter LHL. "Free-Response Methodology: Alternate Analysis and a New Observer-Performance Experiment." Radiology 174:873, 1990.

[38] Swensson RG. "Unified Measurement of Observer Performance in Detecting and Localizing Target Objects on Images." Med Phys 23:1709, 1996.

[39] Metz CE, Starr SJ, Lusted LB, Rossmann K. "Progress in Evaluation of Human Observer Visual Detection Performance Using the ROC Curve Approach." In Raynaud C, Todd-Pokropek AE (Eds.) *Information Processing in Scintigraphy.* Orsay, France: Commissariat à l'Energie Atomique, Département de Biologie, Service Hospitalier Frédéric Joliot, 1975, p. 420.

[40] Swets JA, Swets JB. "ROC Approach to Cost/Benefit Analysis." In Ripley KL, Murray A (Eds.) *Proceedings of The Sixth IEEE Conference on Computer Applications in Radiology.* New York: IEEE Computer Society Press, 1979, p. 203. Reprinted in *Introduction to Automated Arrhythmia Detection* New York: IEEE Computer Society Press, 1980, p. 57.

[41] Phelps CE, Mushlin AI. "Focusing Technology Assessment." Med Decis Making 8:279, 1988.

[42] Sainfort F. "Evaluation of Medical Technologies: A Generalized ROC Analysis." Med Decis Making 11:208, 1991.

[43] Halpern EJ, Alpert M, Krieger AM, Metz CE, Maidment AD. "Comparisons of ROC Curves on the Basis of Optimal Operating Points." Academic Radiol 3:245, 1996.

[44] Metz CE, Shen J-H. "Gains in Accuracy from Replicated Readings of Diagnostic Images: Prediction and Assessment in Terms of ROC Analysis." Med Decis Making 12:60, 1992.

[45] Swensson RG. "Gains in Accuracy from Averaging Ratings of Abnormality." Proc SPIE 663:100, 1999.

[46] Ransohoff DF, Feinstein AR. "Problems of Spectrum and Bias in Evaluating the Efficacy of Diagnostic Tests." New Engl J Med 299:926, 1978.

[47] Begg CB, Greenes RA. "Assessment of Diagnostic Tests when Disease Verification is Subject to Selection Bias." Biometrics 39:207, 1983.

[48] Gray R, Begg CB, Greenes RA. "Construction of Receiver Operating Characteristic Curves when Disease Verification is Subject to Selection Bias." Med Decis Making 4:151, 1984.

[49] Begg CB, McNeil BJ. "Assessment of Radiologic Tests: Control of Bias and other Design Considerations." Radiology 167:565, 1988.

[50] Metz CE. "Some Practical Issues of Experimental Design and Data Analysis in Radiological ROC Studies." Invest Radiol 24:234, 1989.

[51] Swets JA. "Form of Empirical ROCs in Discrimination and Diagnostic Tasks: Implications for Theory and Measurement of Performance." Psychol Bull 99:181, 1986.

[52] Bamber D. "The Area Above the Ordinal Dominance Graph and the Area Below the Receiver Operating Graph." J Math Psych 12:387, 1975.

[53] Hanley JA, McNeil BJ. "The Meaning and Use of the Area under a Receiver Operating Characteristic (ROC) Curve." Radiology 133:29, 1982.

[54] McNeil BJ, Hanley JA. "Statistical Approaches to the Analysis of Receiver Operating Characteristic (ROC) Curves." Med Decis Making 4:137, 1984.

[55] Metz CE, Wang P-L, Kronman HB. "A New Approach for Testing the Significance of Differences between ROC Curves Measured from Correlated Data." In Deconinck F (Ed.) *Information Processing in Medical Imaging*. The Hague: Nijhoff, 1984, p. 432.

[56] McClish DK. "Analyzing a Portion of the ROC Curve." Med Decis Making 9:190, 1989.

[57] Thompson ML, Zucchini W. "On the Statistical Analysis of ROC Curves." Stat Med 8:1277, 1989.

[58] Jiang Y, Metz CE, Nishikawa RM. "A Receiver Operating Characteristic Partial Area Index for Highly Sensitive Diagnostic Tests." Radiology 201:745, 1996.

[59] Metz CE, Kronman HB. "Statistical Significance Tests for Binormal ROC Curves." J Math Psych 22:218, 1980.

[60] Metz CE. "Statistical Analysis of ROC Data in Evaluating Diagnostic Performance." In Herbert D, Myers R (Eds.) *Multiple Regression Analysis: Applications in the Health Sciences*. New York: American Institute of Physics, 1986, p. 365.

[61] Rockette HE, Gur D, Metz CE. "The Use of Continuous and Discrete Confidence Judgments in Receiver Operating Characteristic Studies of Diagnostic Imaging Techniques." Invest Radiol 27:169, 1992.

[62] King JL, Britton CA, Gur D, Rockette HE, Davis PL. "On the Validity of the Continuous and Discrete Confidence Rating Scales in Receiver Operating Characteristic Studies." Invest Radiol 28:962, 1993.

[63] Kobayashi T, Xu X-W, MacMahon H, Metz CE, Doi K. "Effect of a Computer-Aided Diagnosis Scheme on Radiologists' Performance in Detection of Lung Nodules on Chest Radiographs." Radiology 199:843, 1996.

[64] Burgess AE. "Comparison of Receiver Operating Characteristic and Forced Choice Observer Performance Measurement Methods." Med Phys 22:643, 1995.

[65] Dorfman DD, Alf E. "Maximum Likelihood Estimation of Parameters of Signal Detection Theory and Determination of Confidence Intervals—Rating Method Data." J Math Psych 6:487, 1969.

[66] Grey Dr, Morgan BJT. "Some Aspects of ROC Curve-Fitting: Normal and Logistic Models." J Math Psych 9:128, 1972.

[67] Metz CE, Herman BA, Shen J-H. "Maximum-Likelihood Estimation of ROC Curves from Continuously-Distributed Data." Stat Med 17:1033, 1998.

[68] Hanley JA. "The Robustness of the "Binormal" Assumptions Used in Fitting ROC Curves." Med Decis Making 8:197, 1988.

[69] Dorfman DD, Berbaum KS, Metz CE, Lenth RV, Hanley JA, Dagga HA. "Proper ROC Analysis: The Bigamma Model." Academic Radiol 4:138, 1997.

[70] Pan X, Metz CE. "The "Proper" Binormal Model: Parametric ROC Curve Estimation with Degenerate Data." Academic Radiol 4:380, 1997.

[71] Metz CE, Pan X. " 'Proper' Binormal ROC Curves: Theory and Maximum-Likelihood Estimation." J Math Psych 43:1, 1999.

[72] Metz CE. "Evaluation of CAD." In Doi K, MacMahon H, Giger ML, Hoffmann KR (Eds.) *Computer-Aided Diagnosis in Medical Imaging*. Amsterdam: Elsevier Science (Excerpta Medica International Congress Series, Vol. 1182), 1999, p. 543.

[73] Roe CA, Metz CE. "Variance-Component Modeling in the Analysis of Receiver Operating Characteristic Index Estimates." Academic Radiol 4:587, 1997.

[74] Hanley JA, McNeil BJ. "A Method of Comparing the Areas under Receiver Operating Characteristic Curves Derived from the Same Cases." Radiology 138:839, 1983.

[75] DeLong Er, DeLong DM, Clarke-Pearson DL. "Comparing the Areas under Two or More Correlated Receiver Operating Characteristic Curves: A Nonparametric Approach." Biometrics 44:837, 1988.

[76] Wieand S, Gail MH, James BR, James KL. "A Family of Nonparametric Statistics for Comparing Diagnostic Markers with Paired or Unpaired Data." Biometrika 76:585, 1989.

[77] Zhou XH, Gatsonis CA. "A Simple Method for Comparing Correlated ROC Curves Using Incomplete Data." Stat Med 15:1687, 1996.

[78] Metz CE, Herman BA, Roe CA. "Statistical Comparison of Two ROC Curve Estimates Obtained from Partially-Paired Datasets." Med Decis Making 18:110, 1998.

[79] Dorfman DD, Berbaum KS, Metz CE. "ROC Rating Analysis: Generalization to the Population of Readers and Cases with the Jackknife Method." Invest Radiol 27:723, 1992.

[80] Dorfman DD, Metz CE. "Multi-Reader Multi-Case ROC Analysis: Comments on Begg's Commentary." Academic Radiol 2(supplement 1):S76, 1995.

[81] Roe CA, Metz CE. "The Dorfman–Berbaum–Metz Method for Statistical Analysis of Multi-reader, Multi-Modality ROC Data: Validation by Computer Simulation." Academic Radiol 4: 298, 1997.

[82] Dorfman DD, Berbaum KS, Lenth RV. "Multireader, Multicase Receiver Operating Characteristic Methodology: A Bootstrap Analysis." Academic Radiol 2:626, 1995.

[83] Dorfman DD, Berbaum KS, Lenth RV, Chen Y-F, Donaghy BA. "Monte Carlo Validation of a Multireader Method for Receiver Operating Characteristic Discrete Rating Data: Factorial Experimental Design." Academic Radiol 5:591, 1998.

[84] Toledano AY, Gatsonis C. "Regression Analysis of Correlated Receiver Operating Characteristic Data." Academic Radiol 2(supplement 1):S30, 1995.

[85] Toledano AY, Gatsonis C. "Ordinal Regression Methodology for ROC Curves Derived from Correlated Data." Stat Med 15:1807, 1996.

[86] Toledano AY, Gatsonis C. "GEEs for Ordinal Categorical Data: Arbitrary Patterns of Missing Responses and Missingness in a Key Covariate." Biometrics 22:488, 1999.

[87] Tosteson A, Begg C. "A General Regression Methodology for ROC Curve Estimation." Med Decis Making 8:204, 1988.

CHAPTER 16
The FROC, AFROC and DROC Variants
of the ROC Analysis

Dev P. Chakraborty
University of Pennsylvania

CONTENTS

771

16.1 FROC methodology

16.1.1 Introduction

Receiver operating characteristic (ROC) methodology [1–5] is widely used in diagnostic radiology to measure imaging task performance. A ROC experiment yields a measure A_z, the area under the ROC curve, which is independent of disease prevalence and the criteria used by the observer in reporting decisions. The ROC method is strictly applicable only to tasks that call for a binary decision on the part of the observer: is the image normal or abnormal, and most diagnostic tasks do not satisfy this requirement. For example, in nodule detection in chest radiography, the clinical task requires specification of location(s) of the perceived nodule(s). This information is of clinical relevance as it may guide subsequent surgical intervention, yet this information must be ignored in ROC studies, resulting in an imprecise or fuzzy scoring method. In particular, if the observer's decision was abnormal for an actually positive image but he indicated an incorrect location, the ROC paradigm would not penalize this reader. This event would be scored as a true positive even though the reader committed *two* errors on this image: missing the actual lesion (local false negative) and selecting a location that was nodule free (local false positive). Another issue is that when multiple lesions may present on the same image, ROC analysis ignores additional information (more than 1 perceived lesion) that the reader is prepared to provide. For an image with two nodules, one reader may detect only one of the nodules while the other detects both nodules. Both readings would be scored identically in the ROC method. However, the clinical consequences of missing one of the nodules could be very significant.

Neglect of lesion location information must compromise the power (i.e., the probability of detecting a true difference between two modalities) of the ROC experiment. To recover the lost power one could use large numbers of matched cases and readers [1], but this increases the overall cost and duration of the study. ROC experiments already have a reputation for being costly and time consuming. Another option is to use sophisticated statistical models that allow multi-reader and multi-modality ROC studies to be more accurately analyzed [6–8]. These models attempt to maximize the statistical precision of the estimates resulting from ROC studies. However, none of these approaches addresses the basic problem that information is being lost at the front-end of the ROC experiment.

Some attempts have been made at addressing the basic problem by devising other observer performance experiments [9, 10]. Reference [9] describes a method where 0 or 1 lesion is present in each image, and the observer is required to localize the lesion to one of several adjacent congruent subregions. An LROC (localization ROC) plot was described in Ref. [9] to describe the observer's performance under these conditions. Reference [10] describes an experiment in which multiple lesions could be present in an image. The observer was asked to detect them but localization was not required. These methods have rarely been used as they lacked procedures for statistical analyses and curve fitting the experimental data points. More recently Swensson [11] has developed a maximum likelihood solution to the LROC experiment and applied it to several experiments. The LROC approach is promising, but it is limited to tasks where there can be zero or one lesions per image, and the observer is forced to make a localization decision *even if he believes that the image is normal.*

We have studied free-response observer performance experiments that use the lesion location information. This section reviews these methodologies and gives guidelines for their use. We describe the free-response receiver operating characteristic (FROC) experiment, the available analytical tools and variants on the free-response experiment: alternative free-response receiver operating characteristic (AFROC) scoring, and the free-response forced error (FFE) experiment. Next we discuss the validity of the assumptions made in FROC analysis and the power of the FROC experiment. We describe how correlated AFROC data should be analyzed and discuss the localization accuracy needed. We discuss an application of FROC analysis to computer-aided diagnosis (CAD) and make a number of suggestions on how future studies ought to be conducted. We also respond to some criticism of the FROC method that has appeared in the literature.

16.1.2 The FROC experiment

Egan [12] was the first to introduce the term "free-response" in the context of detection of auditory signals occurring at arbitrary times in a given time interval. The time uncertainty in auditory detection experiments and the spatial location uncertainty in medical images have obvious parallels. Bunch *et al.* [13, 14] adapted this approach to the medical imaging situation. They described an observer performance experiment that accommodated both location uncertainty, multiple lesions per image and free-response. They introduced the FROC plot, see Figure 16.1, which is a plot of lesion localized fraction versus mean number of false positives per image or sample-area (see below for clarification of the image versus sample-area distinction). Finally, they deduced the mathematical connection between FROC and ROC curves under certain simplifying assumptions. However,

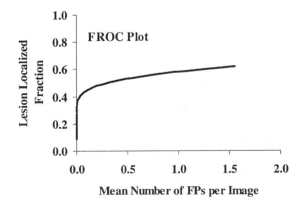

Figure 16.1: The FROC curve is defined as a plot of TP fraction versus mean number of FPs per image.

they did not solve the problems of statistical fitting of the FROC data points and identification of a summary index of performance. The FROC plot they proposed is unbounded in the positive x direction and does not, by itself, lead to a summary performance index. Sorenson *et al.* [15] described a method involving transformation of the FROC data to ROC coordinates and application of a least-squares fitting procedure. The analogous procedure in ROC methodology has been largely supplanted by the maximum likelihood Dorfmam and Alf procedure [16]. Chakraborty *et al.* [17] applied the FROC methods to a clinical evaluation problem, conventional chest radiography versus an experimental digital device. They used the interpolated y value corresponding to a specified x value on the FROC plot, as the summary index of performance. This suffered from difficulties with interpolating the data if "straddling" points were unavailable and the fact that not all FROC ratings data were used in these estimates. Still lacking was a way to fit all the FROC ratings data and assessment of statistical significance. Chakraborty [18] subsequently introduced a binormal FROC model and its maximum likelihood solution. This resulted in theoretical fits to FROC data points, a summary performance index and error estimates. In a later publication [19] Chakraborty and Winter suggested another way of analyzing FROC data, called AFROC (for alternative FROC) analysis. They showed how the widely available ROCFIT program could be applied to analyze AFROC scored data, yielding estimates of summary performance and errors. In this paper they also introduced the free-response forced error (FFE) experiment, which yields a nonparametric estimate of summary performance.

FROC methodology requires an image set where the experimenter knows the truth, that is, whether the images are normal or abnormal and the location of each lesion. Each image can contain zero or more localized lesions. The reader is asked to search each image for lesions and to *indicate and rate according to confidence level* the suspicious locations. A high rating could mean high confidence that the location in question is actually a lesion. Typically 4 response categories are used with 4 = very likely to be a lesion, 3 = likely to be a lesion, 2 = possibly a lesion and 1 = probably not a lesion. Some investigators prefer to use the 1 rating for the most confident lesion, but this is a trivial point as far the FROC method is concerned. Multiple responses are allowed for each image, including no responses. If an indicated location is within a *clinically relevant acceptance region* of an actual lesion centroid, the event is scored as a true positive (TP) and otherwise it is scored as a false positive (FP). These are the only two unambiguous events, namely TP and FP in an FROC experiment and terms like true negative and false negative can be confusing. (TN events could refer to when a reader does not indicate any locations on a normal image, or it could refer to non-indicated non-lesion locations on an abnormal image. Likewise, FN events could refer to when the reader does not indicate any location on an abnormal image or it could refer to non-indicated lesion locations.) A plot of TP fraction versus mean number of FPs per image, denoted by λ, is defined as the FROC curve, see Figure 16.1. Near the origin the observer is adopting a strict criterion for reporting lesions, ensuring few TPs and few FPs. As the criterion is relaxed, the observer attains higher values of TP fraction, and the mean number of FPs per image grows. Note that when the abnormalities are relatively difficult the FROC curve does not reach TP fraction $= 1$, except at very large values of mean number of false positives per image.

16.1.3 The FROC model

Unlike the single decision variable per image of the ROC model, the FROC model proposes a plurality of position-dependent decision variables per image. For example, for a numerical observer, the decision variables could be the outputs of cross-correlation calculations performed at independent (non-overlapping) locations on the image. Locations that match the expected target template would yield larger cross-correlation values than locations that did not match. The higher the cross-correlation value the more suspicious is the corresponding location for presence of lesion, and the higher the confidence level of the numerical observer. For a human observer a similar search procedure is assumed, with the cross-correlation calculation modified by the observer's perceptual filtering. It is not necessary to assume that the human observer samples every location on the image as this affects the maximum number of lesions detected, which will be reflected in the FROC summary measure. The FROC model assumes that the observer (numerical or human) sets up internal threshold levels that are held constant over the duration of the experiment. The number of thresholds depends on the rating scale employed. A 4-rating FROC experiment requires 4 such threshold levels. The observer is assumed to mark as level-4 lesions the independent locations where the local decision variable exceeds the level-4 threshold. There could be more than one location that satisfies these criteria on an image, and if so, the observer is assumed to mark each of them. Based on clinical knowledge the observer is assumed to arbitrate neighboring suspicious locations as either 2 distinct lesions or as a single lesion. Similarly, the observer marks as level-3 lesions all independent locations on an image where the decision variable exceeds his level-3 threshold but is smaller than his level-4 threshold, etc. In this model it is assumed that unmarked images did not produce values of the decision variable greater than the level-1 threshold.

Signal distribution: With reference to Figure 16.2, the distribution of decision variable values at actual signal locations, the *signal* distribution, is assumed to be $\varphi(x, \mu_1, \sigma_1)$, i.e., a Gaussian with mean μ_1 and standard deviation σ_1. Let the area under the Gaussian that is intercepted above the observer's chosen threshold (T_λ) be defined as $\nu(T_\lambda)$, see Eq. (16.1):

$$\nu(T_\lambda) = \int_{T_\lambda}^{\infty} \varphi(x, \mu_1, \sigma_1)\, dx. \tag{16.1}$$

This is identified as the *expected* fraction of lesions that are detected and localized at threshold T_λ. For example, $\nu(T_4)$ is the area under the signal distribution intercepted above the level-4 threshold denoted by T_4. The observed cumulative FROC lesion detected fraction is denoted by the symbol v, which is an estimate of ν. The quantities v_4, v_3, v_2, v_1 satisfy the inequalities $1 \geqslant v_1 \geqslant v_2 \geqslant v_3 \geqslant v_4 \geqslant 0$. Also,

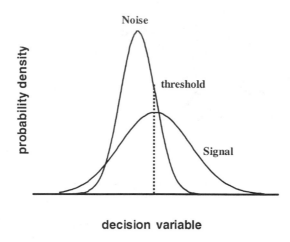

decision variable

Figure 16.2: Illustrating the FROC binormal model. The two distributions are each assumed to be Gaussian. The curve labeled "Noise" is the distribution of the highest confidence-level noise-event. The curve labeled "Signal" is the distribution for lesion locations. The dotted line is the threshold adopted by the observer. The area above the threshold and under the noise distribution is the FPI fraction, and the area above the threshold and under the signal distribution is the corresponding TP fraction.

$v_3 - v_4$ is an estimate of the area under the signal curve above the 3 level but below the 4 level, and so on.

Noise distribution: The total number of possible false positive locations per image is potentially large and unknown. For a given TP fraction, the *exact* number of false positive events generated on any image cannot be predicted but, provided one makes an assumption, the *average* number can. The average number of false positives per image is denoted by the symbol λ. If one assumes that the false positives are Poisson distributed with mean λ, then the probability of generating N false positives on an image is given by the Poisson distribution $P(N, \lambda)$, see Eq. (16.2),

$$P(N, \lambda) = \frac{\exp(-\lambda)\lambda^N}{N!}. \tag{16.2}$$

Because $P(0, \lambda)$ is the probability of generating *no* false positives, then $1 - P(0, \lambda)$ must be the probability of generating one or more false positives on an image. The event "one or more false positives" has special significance in FROC theory: it is called a false positive image (FPI) event. The probability of generating a FPI at λ FPs per image is denoted by *PFPI* (λ), see Eq. (16.3),

$$PFPI(\lambda) = 1 - P(0, \lambda) = 1 - \exp(-\lambda). \tag{16.3}$$

The distribution of FPI events is assumed to be a Gaussian with mean μ_2 and standard deviation σ_2. A FPI is generated every time a sample from this distribution exceeds the observer's threshold, see Eq. (16.4)

$$PFPI(\lambda) = \int_{T_\lambda}^{\infty} \varphi(x, \mu_2, \sigma_2)\, \mathrm{d}x. \tag{16.4}$$

The FPI distribution is identical to that of the decision variable at the highest noise location, or most suspicious signal-free location. For a specific image, if the observer selects a cutoff below the highest noise value, he will generate one or more false positives, that is, an FPI event. For example, $PFPI$ (4) is the probability of generating FPI's at the 4-level. If $PFPI(4) = 0.20$, 20% of the images generated one or more false positives at the 4-level. Some of these images may have additional 4 - and lower-level level false positives: these do not count as additional FPIs. Each image can produce at most one FPI and this characterizes the noise properties of the image. For a given reader, a FPI at a low level (e.g., 0 or 1) is characteristic of an image that is unlikely to generate FPs, making it easier to visualize possible lesions. Likewise an image that generates a FPI at the 4-level is more likely to generate FPs, making it harder to visualize possible lesions. Continuing with the example, $PFPI$ (3) is the probability of generating FPI's at the 3-level. $PFPI$ (3) $- PFPI$ (4) is an estimate of the area under the FPI distribution above the 3-level but below the 4-level, and so on. Note that

$$1 \geqslant PFPI(1) \geqslant PFPI(2) \geqslant PFPI(3) \geqslant PFPI(4) \geqslant 0. \tag{16.5}$$

To summarize, in FROC theory one assumes two distributions labeled *signal* and *noise*. For a chosen threshold T_λ, the area under the signal distribution intercepted above the threshold T_λ is the expected value of the lesion localized fraction, $v(T_\lambda)$. The corresponding area under the noise distribution is the expected probability $PFPI$ (λ) of generating a FPI. To convert from $PFPI$ to the FROC x-axis coordinate, namely λ, one uses Eq. (16.3). The connection between T_λ and λ is implicit in Eqs. (16.3) and (16.4), with large values of T_λ leading to small values of λ, and conversely.

As the observer's threshold criterion is lowered, $v(T_\lambda)$ rises and tends to 1 in the limit $\lambda = \infty$. Also, $PFPI$ (λ) rises, tending to 1 in the same limit. To achieve $PFPI = 1$ with certainty, the observer must mark *every* location (noise and signal) on *every* image. This guarantees the detection of all signals at the price of generating an FPI on every image. This fact assures the correct normalization of the two Gaussians to unit areas. The total number of signals eventually detected must equal the total number of actual lesions, and the total number of FPIs generated must equal the total number of images.

This was the approach taken by Chakraborty [18], which describes the maximum likelihood solution of the above model. The FROCFIT program described in that paper implements the maximum likelihood algorithm to estimate the parameters of the FROC binormal model from FROC data points (i.e., v_i, λ_i, $i = 1, 2, \ldots, N$, for a N-rating FROC experiment). Note that a plot of v (T_λ) versus $PFPI$ (T_λ) is a ROC-like curve that follows from the model. It is "ROC-like"

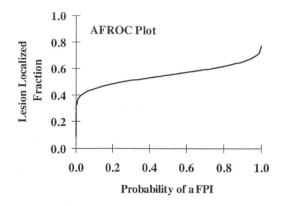

Figure 16.3:   The AFROC curve: the area under this curve is the FROC performance metric, denoted by A_1.

in the sense that it is generated by two latent gaussian distributions. This curve is called the alternative free-response receiver operating characteristic (AFROC), see Figure 16.3. The area under the AFROC curve was proposed as the performance measure in the FROC task. To avoid confusion with A_z of ROC methodology, the area under the AFROC is denoted by the symbol A_1. The FROCFIT program produces an estimate of A_1 and its sampling error (due to the finite number of cases). Unlike A_z, which ranges from 0.5 to 1, A_1 ranges from 0 to 1. A randomly guessing observer will produce $A_1 = 0$ if the lesion size is small compared to the image area, and a perfect observer will produce $A_1 = 1$.

Image size effects: In their paper Bunch *et al.* [13] defined the x-axis of the FROC plot as "number of FPs per *image area*." The images they experimented with had a size of 50×50 mm^2. They also conducted experiments with these images regarded as subdivided into 25×25 mm^2 and 12.5×12.5 mm^2 regions. They showed that the mean number of false positives per image area (the parameter λ in Eq. (16.2) was *proportional* to the image area. This lended support to their view that, for the type of targets they studied (each less than 2.2 mm^2 in area), FP generation was a point process and obeyed Poisson statistics.

Based on this result one can qualitatively predict the dependence of A_1 on image area, for tasks that obey Poisson statistics. Consider first the case where the number of lesions per unit image area is unchanged. As there are proportionately more lesions in a larger image area, then at constant threshold the lesion-detected fraction will be unchanged. This is the plotted quantity along the y-axis of the AFROC plot in Figure 16.3. As the image area increases one expects λ to increase proportionately and from Eq. (16.3) one expects *PFPI* to increase. According to Figure 16.3 this will "pull" each point on the AFROC curve towards the right, i.e., to higher values of *PFPI* causing the A_1 value to drop, i.e., performance will be degraded. If the total number of lesions in the image set is unchanged, there is a further drop in A_1. This is because it is more likely that a given target will be missed in a larger area, i.e., the points on the AFROC curve will also be pulled down. The combined effect is expected to lead to a greater drop in performance than in the first case.

It is clear that different investigators can obtain different A_1 values simply due to variations in image size. A model of the size dependence, which would allow such data to be reconciled, is presently not available.

Lesion number effects: If the FROC events are independent (see discussion of asumptions below), then as the number of lesions increases, one expects A_1 to be unchanged—with more lesions the number of TPs will increase in proportion, but the lesion-localized fraction will be unchanged. By the independence assumption, the FP events are unaffected and hence A_1 will be constant. Note however, that the independence assumption may break down as the number of lesions increases. Likewise, adding a number of images with no lesions (normals) should not change the AFROC data points—the x-axis data points will simply become statistically more precise while the y-data points will be unchanged. Thus, one expects A_1 to be unchanged.

16.1.4 AFROC analysis

A second approach, termed AFROC scoring [19], is to directly obtain estimates of PFPI from the images by counting the observed FPI events. Let FPI_i and V_i ($i = 0, 1, 2, 3, 4$) denote the observed *uncumulated counts* of FPIs and lesion-detection events in an FROC experiment at threshold T_i. Specifically, FPI_4 is the number of FPIs when only level 4 responses are considered and FPI_3 is the number of FPIs when only level 3 responses are considered, and so on, and similarly for the V_i. The zero response symbolizes *non-events*, where the observer does not provide explicit events. In FROC theory the non-events are analyzed on an equal footing with actual events. FPI_0 is the number of images on which no FPIs (and hence no FPs) were generated and V_0 is the number of lesions that were undetected. Initially all FPI_i and V_i ($i = 0, 1, 2, 3, 4$) are initialized to zeroes. Figure 16.4 illustrates AFROC scoring: observer indicated locations and confidence levels are shown as the open circles with an accompanying numerical rating. Figure 16.4(a) shows an image with two nodules, both of which were detected and localized at the 4-level. An additional 4-response was a false positive. This image would be scored as two hits at the 4-level and one FPI at the 4-level and we increment V_4 by 2 and FPI_4 by 1. Two other false positives at levels 1 and 2 are also shown but do not enter the analysis because they may *not* be independent events. Because the observers decision threshold T_4 was smaller than the highest-noise value on this image, one expects to see additional false positives at lower confidence levels. Figure 16.4(b) shows a solitary nodule that was missed, as the observer made no responses on this image. This image is scored as a hit at the 0-level and a FPI at the 0-level and we increment V_0 by 1 and FPI_0 by 1. Figure 16.4(c) is scored as one hit at the 1-level and one FPI at the 2-level. Finally, Figure 16.4(d) is scored as one hit at the 4-level, one at the 1-level and a FPI at the 2-level.

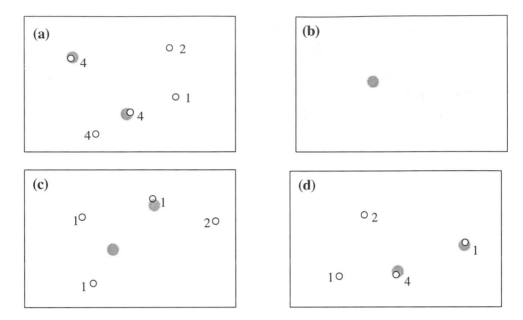

Figure 16.4: The sub-panels illustrate AFROC scoring. Figure 16.4(a) is scored as a 2 TPs at the 4-level, and one FPI at the 4-level. Figure 16.4(b) is scored as both a TP and a FPI at the 0-level. Figure 16.4(c) is scored as one hit at the 1-level and one FPI at the 2-level. Figure 16.4(d) is scored as one hit at the 4-level, one at the 1-level and a FPI at the 2-level.

Note that V_i and FPI$_i$ are uncumulated quantities. The relationship of these to v and *PFPI* are shown in Eq. (16.6),

$$\overline{v_\lambda} = \sum_{i \geqslant \lambda} V_i \bigg/ N_L,$$
$$\overline{PFPI_\lambda} = \sum_{i \geqslant \lambda} FPI_i \bigg/ N_I, \qquad 0 < \lambda < N, \qquad (16.6)$$

where the bar denotes an expectation value and N is number of ratings employed. The set of numbers (V_i, FPI$_i$, where $i = 0, 1, 2, \ldots, N$) can be analyzed using ROCFIT. One enters the total number of lesions for the number of positive cases, the total number of images for the number of negative cases and $N + 1$ for the total number of categories. The FROC i-response formally corresponds to the ROC $i + 1$ response, and the 4-level FROC experiment formally corresponds to the 5-level ROC experiment. The area parameter value produced by ROCFIT produced A_z value is interpreted as A_1. The advantage of AFROC analysis is that it does not make the Poisson distribution assumption. To perform AFROC scoring one needs an image by image record of all responses on all images, where each record must include the confidence level and whether it was a TP or a FP.

16.1.5 FFE experiment

It is also possible to measure A_1 directly without performing a rating experiment. This involves a procedure, called the free-response forced error (FFE) experiment [19], where the observer enumerates all suspicious locations on an image in *decreasing* order of confidence level, until he makes a false positive decision. The number of lesions detected before the first error is counted. Summing this over the entire image set and dividing by the total number of lesions one gets an estimate of A_1. This method of counting implies equal weighting to the lesions. Another way [19] is to do the calculation of A_1 on an image-by-image basis, and subsequently average over all images, which is equivalent to assigning equal weighting to the images. Note that FROCFIT calculates A_1 on the basis of equal weighting of lesions. It is desirable to have a version of FROCFIT that equally weights images, and similarly for AFROC analysis. The advantage of FFE analysis is that it is nonparametric and independent of the Gaussian distribution assumption. Like the 2AFC experiment it is expected to be less efficient than the corresponding AFROC or FROCFIT analyses. It does have the advantage of simplicity and could be used as a robust performance measure. Few would argue against the proposition that detecting and localizing more lesions without making any errors is desirable. The FFE experiment could be done retrospectively after the FROC data has been collected. One asks the reader to resolve "ties" by rank ordering all indicated locations on an image that share the same confidence level. For example, if an image has two 4-level responses, then he indicates which is most suspicious (4-a) and which is least suspicious (4-b).

16.1.6 The validity of the FROC assumptions

The assumptions of the FROCFIT analysis model are as follows. (1) The occurrences of lesions in an image are independent events. (2) The observer maintains constant confidence levels for the duration of the experiment. (3) The false-positives are independent Poisson distributed events. (4) The events (FPs and TPs) are mutually independent, as are the FPIs and TPs. (5) The FPIs and TPs are Gaussian distributed events. In AFROC analysis all assumptions involving FPs are unnecessary, as the method is not concerned with individual FP events. We note at the outset that the FROC scoring must be performed so that the observer can generate *only single events that are classifiable either as TPs or as FPs*. If this requirement is violated the experimenter will have introduced additional dependencies between TPs and FPs that may not be present at the perceptual level. This is discussed later in the context of applications of CAD to microcalcification detection.

Assumption 1: The occurrences of lesions in an image are independent events. The presence of a lesion should not affect the probability of more lesions being present. The validity of this assumption is expected to depend on the clinical task. In a patient with a metastatic tumor of the lung, several regions of the lung may be simultaneously abnormal. A similar issue may affect the occurrence of clustered specks in mammography. The validity of this assumption can best be judged with clinical input. In phantom studies, on the other hand, this is never an issue as it is completely under the experimenter's control.

Assumption 2:   The confidence levels (CLs) are maintained at constant values by the observer. This requires constancy of CLs between different image presentations over the course of the study, and between different responses made on the same image. The latter constancy assumption has been criticized in the literature [11]. Because the limitation of the observer's memory, maintaining constant CLs between different images is obviously more difficult than maintaining them on the same image—the images could be viewed over a long time interval (typically weeks). Therefore, the limiting assumption could be constancy of CLs between different images. This assumption is identical to that used in ROC analysis. It is true that for some detection tasks (such as metastatic lung cancer) detecting a high category lesion increases the a-priori odds of other lesions being present, which could cause the reader to apply a lower criterion to other pereceived lesions on the same image. Clearly work is needed to show if this effect can be distinguished from the image-to-image fluctuations of the confidence level.

Assumption 3:   The false positives on an image are independent Poisson distributed events. This assumption allows the transformation of the FROC abscissa to FPI, see Eq. (16.3) and follows from the view advocated by Bunch *et al.* [14] of regarding FP generation as a "point" process. Metz has questioned the Poisson assumption [20], but definitive experimental data to prove or disprove this assumption are lacking. To assess the validity of the Poisson Assumption one needs to compare the actual number of FPs to the predicted number and calculate the chi-squared statistic. If the total area occupied by the target objects is much smaller than the image area, then the reader has many opportunities for false positives on the same image. It seems reasonable that a Poisson process can approximate the occurrence of false positives under this condition. To the extent that Assumption 1 (lesion independence) is not true, it could affect the validity of the Poisson assumption. For example, the radiologist may consider multiple regions as suspicious for the same disease process and tend to mark all of them. When he does make FP errors, they would tend to be clustered together on certain images, thereby violating the Poisson and the FP independence assumptions. When the conditions of the Poisson and FP independence assumption are not met, it is advisable to use AFROC scoring and analyze the data using ROCFIT. The disadvantage is that AFROC scoring does not use all the FP information provided by the reader. For example, multiple FP events on a single image can produce at most one FPI event. This is expected to lead to some loss of statistical power.

Assumption 4:   The observer events (FPs and TPs or FPIs and TPs) are all mutually independent. Independence of FPs and TPs on the same image may be a problem because of the failure of Assumption 1. Also, as opportunities for further events become depleted by existing events, this assumption will fail. For example, site depletion will affect the occurrence of subsequent FPs and TPs making them less likely. A relevant variable is the ratio, per image, of the total number of actual events to the number of potential independent sites. If this ratio is small, additional events are unlikely to deplete the number of potential FP sites significantly. Under this condition, the independence assumption is expected to be reasonably valid. To ensure validity of this assumption it is recommended that the ratio be smaller than about 0.05 (this number is based on our past nodule detection study [19], where reasonable fits to the theory were obtained, but further studies are needed to define it more precisely). In support of non-independence is the "satisfaction-of-search" (SOS) effect: the presence of a distracter nodule on an image may make it less likely that a native nodule will be reported [21]. Similar remarks apply to the independence of FPIs and TPs.

Assumption 5:   The FPIs and TPs are Gaussian distributed events. This assumption is justified from the central limit theorem and the precedent that a similar assumption is widely used in ROC analysis. Also, as has been shown in simulation studies, the consequences of departures from Gaussian are difficult to observe under practical conditions of limited numbers of cases [22].

Assumptions 1, 3, and 4 are probably the three most limiting ones in FROC theory and research to circumvent them is needed. However their lack of validity may be less relevant to imaging system *comparison* studies. Most investigators are interested in differences between modalities when using matched cases and readers. The lack of validity of the assumptions will affect the absolute A_1 values. However, differences in A_1 values are less likely to be affected. In our opinion, the lack of independence concerns should not deter investigators from using FROC in imaging system comparison studies. Conversely, the consequence of applying ROC methodology inappropriately, to detection tasks that it was not designed to handle, could be worse. True differences between modalities could be missed or the wrong methodology could be selected as superior, see below.

16.1.7 Power of a FROC study

The power of the AFROC method is expected to be superior to that of a ROC experiment using the same cases. This is because every image will contribute a FPI event (including the "zero" level) but only normal cases contribute FPs in the ROC case. In other words a better estimate of the noise properties will result in the FROC study. Also, each positive image will contribute at least one TP event in AFROC scoring but will contribute only one TP in a ROC study, leading to a better estimate of the signal properties. Moreover, the TP events in AFROC are *precise*. In ROC analysis an image such as Figure 16.5(a) where two errors have occurred (a FP and a FN) would be scored as a high confidence level TP. In fact it would be scored *identically* as Figure 16.5(b), where the lesion was correctly localized at the 4-level. Consider that Figure 16.5(a) is the first-modality image and Figure 16.5(b) is the second-modality image of the same patient. It is obvious that although the B modality is superior to the A modality for this patient, ROC scoring does not distinguish between them. In AFROC scoring Figure 16.5(a) would count as a low ("0") confidence level hit and a high confidence level FPI and Figure 16.5(b) would be scored as a high confidence level hit and a low ("0") confidence level FPI. For this patient, on both detection and avoidance of false positive criteria, modality B would be correctly judged superior by the AFROC method. The extent of this power improvement would depend on the relative frequency of errors such as that shown in Figure 16.5 in ROC experiments. This issue is now receiving attention from Swensson [11] who has shown that error estimates obtained by his LROCFIT program are substantially smaller than those estimated by ROCFIT on the same data sets. Smaller error will lead to enhanced power. The difference between the LROC method and ROC method is the neglect, in the latter, of events with detection but incorrect localization.

The above example illustrates the superiority of FROC over ROC for the case when there is *only* one lesion per image. We stress this as there is a misconception that FROC is only useful in phantom-based work when there can be multiple lesions per image, allowing good statistics to be built up rapidly while using only a few images (using few images is undesirable, see below). While the advantage of FROC for multiple lesions per image is certainly true, that does not negate the advantage of FROC even in the case where there is only 0 or 1 lesion possible in

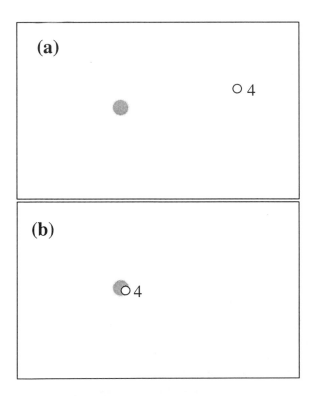

Figure 16.5: On the fuzzy scoring in the ROC study and why this must lead to loss of statistical power as compared to an AFROC study. In ROC analysis both cases (a) and (b) would be scored as TP events, which would show no difference between the modalities. Modality B would be judged superior by the AFROC method on both detection and avoidance of false positive criteria.

every image. The only situation where we expect equivalent powers in FROC and ROC experiments is when localization of lesions is not an issue.

16.1.8 The application of CORROC2 to AFROC rating data

When the same observer reads a set of images under two conditions (or modalities), a correlated analysis using CORROC2 is possible [23]. One regards the image set as N_I "normal" images and N_L "abnormal" images, where N_I = number of images and N_L = number of lesions. The procedure is to first perform AFROC scoring on an image in the first reading condition: the FPI confidence level and the confidence levels of the lesions (including the 0 ratings for images with no FPs and undetected lesions) are noted. This is repeated for the corresponding image in the second reading condition. All FROC ratings are increased by unity before entry into the CORROC2 input file, so that the 0 to 4 scale becomes a 1-5 scale. The FPI ratings for the two imaging conditions are entered as the responses for the first patient regarded as a normal patient. The ratings for the first lesion (assuming that at least one lesion is present) are entered in pairs as the responses for the first image regarded as an abnormal patient. The procedure is continued until all lesions in the first patient are used up. There will be as many abnormal patient entries for this image as there are lesions in the image. It is important to pair the lesion responses correctly so that they apply to the same physical lesions. The process is repeated for each image in the case set. The CORROC2 input data will consist of N_I pairs of ratings for the normal images and N_L pairs of ratings for the abnormal images. All ratings submitted to CORROC2 will range from 1 to 5, and the program needs to be told that 5 is the most confident rating level. The CORROC2 output allows the determination whether the difference observed for the reader was significant.

16.1.9 The localization accuracy needed for a TP event

In FROC analysis, if an indicated location is within a *clinically relevant acceptance region* of an actual lesion centroid, the event is to be scored as a true positive (TP) and otherwise it is to be scored as a false positive (FP). For simple target shapes the acceptance region is frequently chosen to be the size of the target, that is, the indicated location of a nodule should be within a nodule radius of the real nodule. For very small objects this requirement should be relaxed so that normal human pointing uncertainty (say hand jitter) does not become the determining factor. For clinical detection tasks, the acceptance region should be determined by what radiologists consider acceptable uncertainty in communicating their findings to other radiologists, surgeons, and clinicians. In such studies it is desirable to consult with radiologists to ascertain the scoring of questionable indicated locations. To the extent that the scoring criteria are still arbitrary after following these rules, it will limit the ability to report a measure of performance that is independent of the acceptance region [20]. This is not a serious problem for modality comparison studies, where the same lesions are present in both modalities and the same scoring rules are applied. We believe that criticism of FROC on this account applies especially to ROC methodology, which neglects the localization altogether. We recommend that all FROC experimenters report the details of the scoring criteria actually adopted.

16.1.10 Evaluating segmentation algorithms

Most work in evaluating segmentation algorithms has involved developing similarity measures between the region indicated by the algorithm and the actual lesion region. Such approaches do not distinguish between FP and FN errors, do not allow for the dependence of sensitivity and specificity on the confidence level of the segmentation algorithm and lack a threshold independent assessment of the classifier performance. A ROC-like approach has been proposed [24] to deal with this problem. It involves characterizing the region D indicated by the classifier with two fractional numbers, FPLE (false positive localization error) and FNLE (false negative localization error), which depend on the degree of overlap between the region D and the true lesion region L and can be calculated for each image. This has the advantage that a false positive region that is located far from a true lesion yields a higher FPLE than a region that is closer to an actual lesion. Similarly, a FN region that is farther from the indicated region D counts as a larger FNLE error that one closer to D. A plot of 1-FNLE versus FPLE is defined as the DL-ROC (distance-based localization ROC) curve. The DL-ROC curve is transformed to z-deviate axes and the data points are least squares fitted to obtain the parameters of the underlying binormal ROC model. The least-squares fitting procedure is known to be non-optimal because it assumes that the data points are independent. In fact, it corresponds to the way in which ROC curves were analyzed before the maximum likelihood procedure of Dorfman and Alf became widely available. In spite of this drawback it is our opinion the basic idea of penalizing distant FPs more than near FPs is desirable to include in a FROC model.

16.1.11 Applications of FROC analysis to computer aided diagnosis (CAD)

While the FROC method has not been as widely used as ROC, nonCAD applications of FROC have been steadily rising [25–32]. In computer aided diagnosis (CAD) however, FROC has met with limited acceptance. Some researchers have simply compared FROC curves without fitting them [33]. In one application to microcalcification detection the FROC approach was apparently not successful. We discuss this influential CAD microcalcification study [34] as it sheds light on how the scoring employed can affect the validity of the FROC method. The details of the CAD algorithm are not relevant to this discussion, but we note that before the CAD algorithm could report a suspected microcalcification site, that site had to meet a clustering requirement, namely it had to be close to at least 3 other sites. The 4 or more adjacent specks were termed a cluster. The clustering criterion was chosen because of the need to improve CAD performance. While the CAD reporting criterion was *cluster* based, the FROC scoring criterion was *speck* based. A suspicious location was scored as a TP if it fell within 10 pixels of a true speck and otherwise it was counted as a FP. The *cluster* based reporting and the *speck* based scoring implied that *CAD was unable to report single events that are either TP or FP.*

Disallowing this ability violated the assumptions of the FROC analytical model. In particular it invalidated the likelihood function given in Chakraborty [18]. The authors attributed the failure of FROC analysis to the dependence of FP events. Actually the dependence problem applies to both TP and FP events. The tools needed to analyze the experiment reported by Chan *et al.* [34] presently do not exist. One solution is to use a cluster-based approach for both reporting and scoring the specks, as some investigators have done. This discussion also explains why FROC methods have been more successfully applied to nodule-detection CAD studies [35, 36]. The CAD nodule algorithm produces an overall coordinate that is compared to a true nodule location to score it as a TP or a FP. Note that all events are single events that are either a TP or a FP.

16.1.12 Discussion

The need for a sufficient number of cases and case and reader matching is just as true for FROC as it is for ROC. A sufficient number of cases are needed for reliable estimation of both signal and noise properties. Cases with no lesions should be included, as they allow the noise properties to be better estimated and because they are typically the majority of cases viewed by the clinician. The cases should be subtle, that is, not too easy or too difficult. In the former case the observer may be able to detect all the lesions without generating any false positives and such data cannot be analyzed by FROC methods. Typical values of the A_1 parameter in the literature range from 0.4 to 0.9. Phantom-based work lends itself easily to FROC methodology, as the lesion locations are precisely known, but the number of lesions per image should be kept low in our opinion: typically no more than 1 or 2, depending on the task. The intent of experimenters (including the author) who have used larger numbers in FROC studies was to augment the statistics. However, this can lead to violation of assumptions and poor fits. As stated earlier, the power gain of the FROC experiment also applies to cases with only one lesion per image.

Training of observers is very important in FROC studies. The observer must become familiar with the appearance of TPs and FPs and learn how to distribute his confidence levels. It is important that the subjects provide adequate sampling of the FROC curve, and not be too conservative or too lax. An excessively conservative observer will only sample the sharply rising part of the FROC curve and may not provide any data point on the level part of the curve. Conversely, a lax observer will make too many false-positive errors and inadequately sample the sharply rising part of the curve. The confidence level training is often not given sufficient attention in FROC studies. As a rule-of-thumb the observer should generate less than about 2 FPs on each image at the lowest confidence level. Screening mammography FP rates are much lower, but performing FROC experiments under similar conditions would be expensive. The experimenter can use FROC curves generated from preliminary readings to appropriately instruct the reader. The scoring must ensure that only single events (TP or FP) are possible. The acceptance region for TP events should be consistently used and reported. The search area of the image and the lesion area should be reported.

In some applications of FROC to CAD we have noticed that the FROC curve is presented as a finely sampled curve. This is made possible by varying the threshold against which CAD output is compared. The finely sampled curve implies precise knowledge of the FROC curve. This may be misleading as the errors in the curve increases with fewer entries in the categories, and moreover the errors at higher FPs increase because of the cumulation. Sampling errors of FROC data points are discussed by Chakraborty *et al.* [17]. The number of events in the individual ratings categories analyzed by FROCFIT should not be allowed to fall below 5, and ideally should be larger than 10. This will require binning the data before analysis by FROCFIT. A fair comparison of the quality of fits produced by FROCFIT would be to quote the chi-squared statistic calculated by the program. If there are less than 5 entries in any category, FROCFIT tries to merge adjacent categories to achieve this requirement. The experimenter who pays attention to the binning can avoid this automatic merging. An attempt should also be made to show that the binning does not sensitively influence the results.

Which FROC method should the experimenter use: FROCFIT, AFROC, or FFE? FROCFIT should be used to start as it is expected to yield the best statistics. The quality of the fits produced by FROCFIT should be assessed using the chi-squared statistic (each category must have at least 5 responses in order to get a meaningful value). If the fits are unsatisfactory, then AFROC analysis should be tried and the quality of the fits reassessed. AFROC analysis will yield less power than FROCFIT, but because it does not make the Poisson assumption or assume independent FPs, the fitting may be improved. If the quality of the fits is still unsatisfactory, or if the experimenter is conservative, we recommend the FFE experiment. As noted above, this can be performed retrospectively on the original data set. FFE is expected to yield the least power of all three methods. Simply comparing FROC or AFROC curves (without calculating A_1) is indefensible practice, in our opinion, as it unnecessarily sacrifices power.

Present FROC theory represents a small step in removing the binary-decision limitation of ROC methodology. In addition to location uncertainty there are other dimensions to the radiologist's reporting process that need to be considered. For example, in mammography the task involves detecting the lesion, localizing it, and finally characterizing the lesion as benign or malignant. Accommodation of such higher/order tasks is crucial if observer performance methodology is to be more useful to radiologists. The importance of research in this area can hardly be over emphasized [37].

In conclusion, we have described what we believe is the current state-of-the-art in FROC methodology. While ROC methodology is widely accepted, the FROC approach is the more natural experiment from a clinician's viewpoint. We have made specific recommendations on how FROC experiments should be conducted. Several areas where FROC methodology could be improved are also indicated.

16.2 DROC methodology

16.2.1 Introduction

The second variant of ROC methodology to be described is the differential receiver operating characteristic (DROC) [38] method. The problem being addressed here is the efficiency and cost of the ROC experiment. In the ROC method one first determines the *absolute* performance (A_z) for each modality and then differences these values to determine which modality is superior. Frequently, the experimenter's primary interest is in the *difference* between two modalities, not in the *absolute* values. For such problems an alternative method that is more sensitive to image-quality differences is desirable. The increased sensitivity could be used to detect smaller differences in A_z values, or to detect a specified difference with fewer images and readers.

16.2.2 Theory

The DROC method involves viewing pairs of images of the same patient, one from each modality denoted by A and B. The patient can be normal or abnormal but this information is not known to the observer. For example, a normal (abnormal) A modality image is displayed paired with a normal (abnormal) B modality image. The following information is elicited for each image pair:

(a) The diagnosis (D1): D1 = 0 for normal or D1 = 1 for abnormal.

(b) The confidence level (D2) for the diagnosis D1: low, medium, or high, or on a 100-point scale.

(c) The preferred image (D3) that yields greater confidence in the diagnosis D1: D3 = 0 for the left image or D3 − 1 for the right image.

(d) The confidence level (D4) for the preference D3: low, medium, or high, or on a 100-point scale.

The well-known ROC model uses the concept of a *decision variable* (x) to analyze the ratings data. It is assumed that each presentation of an image to the reader is accompanied by an occurrence of a value x of the decision variable (DV). High values of x are associated with high confidence that the image is positive and low values with high confidence level that the image is negative. The DROC analysis model is based on the concept of the *differential decision variable* (z), which measures preference for a modality for a particular diagnosis when case matched images are presented simultaneously. A high value of z (say $z \to +\infty$) corresponds to high preference for the B modality for a positive finding. Similarly, a very small value of z (say $z \to -\infty$) corresponds to a high preference for the B modality for a negative finding. If the observer has no bias for a modality then

$z = x_B - x_A$. A binormal model is assumed for the two distributions of z, corresponding to actually positive and negative cases. As the threshold is varied, these distributions generate a ROC-like curve known as the DROC curve. The latter is defined as a plot of B-preferred positive pair fraction versus B-preferred negative pair fraction. The DROC curve is binormal and can be determined using available ROC software. The area under the DROC curve is termed A_d. If the area under the DROC is greater than 0.5, then B modality is predicted to be superior for the stated detection task.

16.2.3 Analysis

The left versus right order is coded by the logical variable ARHS (read "A modality on the right-hand-side") as follows: ARHS = 0 if the A modality was on the left-hand-side, and ARHS = 1 otherwise. One defines the variable B_A (read "B minus A") as follows:

$$B\_A = (2 \bullet ARHS - 1) \bullet (1 - 2 \bullet D3). \tag{16.7}$$

Note that B_A has the following properties: B_A = 1 if the B modality was preferred, that is, if Pref(B) > Pref(A) and B_A = −1 if the A modality was preferred, that is, if Pref(B) < Pref(A). Assume that a 100-point pseudo-continuous rating scheme is adopted, with 0 corresponding to least confidence and 100 to highest confidence. The diagnosis index D1 determines the direction of D3. For example, for D1 = 0 (normal image pair) we interpret D3 = 0 as meaning that the left image was *preferred for normal*. Likewise, for D1 = 1, D3 = 0 means that the left image was preferred for abnormal. Similarly, for D3 = 1 the right image is preferred for normal (if D1 = 0) or for abnormal (if D1 = 1). Eq. (16.7) allows conversion of the left–right information to the preferred modality. The indicated confidence level D4 is converted to the differential confidence level z as follows:

$$z = (2 \bullet D1 - 1) \bullet D4 \bullet B\_A. \tag{16.8}$$

Note that if B_A = 1, z varies for −100 (B is strongly preferred to A for negative diagnosis) to +100 (B is strongly preferred to A for positive diagnosis). The variable z is the differential rating expressed on a continuous scale. The z data for positive and negative images can be analyzed using LABROC to determine the separation of the underlying Gaussian distributions and the DROC curve. The critical ratio is calculated from Eq. (16.9),

$$CR_{DROC} = \frac{A_d - 0.5}{\sigma(A_d)}, \tag{16.9}$$

where the denominator, the standard deviation of A_d, is available from the LABROC output.

The procedure described above was used to test the basic ideas of DROC analysis [38]. In this experiment the confidence level D2 was not acquired. Interleaved

ROC and DROC experiments were performed on a common phantom-generated image set. Abnormal images were simulated using speck-containing ROIs extracted from ACR phantom images. Normal images were simulated by extracting background regions that did not contain any specks. The unprocessed images formed the B modality (or baseline modality). A noise addition processing was used to simulate the A modality. Six readers interpreted these images under ROC and DROC conditions. Discrete confidence levels were used in this study: low, medium, and high. It was found that DROC and ROC indicated the same direction of change (i.e., the unprocessed images were superior to the noise added images) but the DROC critical ratio was larger than the corresponding ROC critical ratio. The ROC critical ratio was obtained from CORROC2 analysis of the ROC ratings-data.

As noted above, the procedure outlined above assumes a bias-free obscrver. Initial claims that DROC is bias free are incorrect. The presence of bias can distort the observed A_d value: a reader who always picks the B modality as superior will elevate A_d as he will shift the positive z distribution to the right and the negative z distribution to the left, thereby increasing their separation. To solve this problem we are now collecting the D2 information, the confidence level for the detection task. This allows a correlated analysis of performance in the two tasks represented by $y = x_B + x_A$ and $z = x_B - x_A$. Note that the z is the differential DV defined previously. The quantity y is thc DV for the paired-image detection task. In our model the detection DV is the sum of the individual detection DVs of the two modalities, and the differential DV is the difference of these values. The indicated confidence level D2, which varied from 0 to 100, is converted to y using Eq. (16.10),

$$y = (2 \bullet D1 - 1) \bullet D2. \tag{16.10}$$

One can regard y and z as two correlatcd decision variables, along the lines of the CLABROC bivariate model. These values are supplied to the CLABROC program as different modalities. CLABROC will yield A_z values corresponding to the tasks y and z, denoted by $A_z(y)$ and $A_z(z)$, respectively, and their correlation ρ_A. The quantity $A_z(z)$ is identified as the uncorrected area under the DROC curve A_d, and $A_z(y)$ is the corresponding ROC area for the paired image detection task. If the observer introduces no bias, it can be shown that $A_z(y)$ and $A_z(z)$ will be uncorrelated. If he does introduce bias, modeled as a diagnosis-independent value, then the measures become correlated. The method of bias removal that suggests itself is to insert a negative bias into the analysis program, and adjust its magnitude until cancellation occurs, that is, when ρ_A is minimized. At this point the observed $A_z(z)$ value will the desired bias–free A_d value.

16.2.4 Results

The bias-reduction procedure was tested with simulation experiments in the IDL (Interactive Data Language, Research Systems, Boulder, Colorado) programming language. The Gaussian random-number generator RANDOMN was used to simulate the decision variables. A routine CRANDOMN was written to generate correlated random numbers with a specified correlation ρ and shift Δ. For example, CRANDOMN $(\rho, N, \Delta, \mu, \sigma)$ produced two arrays of size N (1/4 the total number of images, divided equally between negative and positive and between A and B modalities) representing N samples of x_A and x_B. Here x_A and x_B were drawn from two correlated Gaussian distributions with common standard deviation σ. In other words, x_A was drawn from a Gaussian of mean μ, and x_B was drawn from a Gaussian of mean $\mu + \Delta$, and the two samples had the desired correlation ρ. In this way we simulated the two modalities A and B. We set $\rho = 0.9$ for the positive cases and $\rho = 0.5$ for the negative cases. We also set $N = 900$ corresponding to 3600 total number of cases. We set the standard deviation of the two negative ROC distributions at 1.0 and those of the two positive ROC distributions at 1.4. The d' parameter for the A modality was set at 1.50 (corresponding to an A_z (A) of 0.856). A zero shift was assumed for the negative distribution, and it was assumed that the positive B modality distribution was positive-shifted by 0.5 d' units relative to the positive A modality. This corresponds to an expected A_z (B) of 0.921 for the B modality. With no bias effects the expected A_d is 0.664. Bias was introduced into the model by adding a term $B_0 \bullet (2 \bullet D1 - 1)$ to the differential confidence level D4. This corresponds to an observer who adds (or subtracts) B_0 to the true difference ratings, and increases the differential rating of images he believes to be positive while decreasing the differential rating of images believed to be negative. Bias correction consisted of subtracting a similar term $B \bullet (2 \bullet D1 - 1)$ from the observed D4, where B is a guess at the bias. When the guess is correct, the two biases cancel each other and the corresponding $A_z(z)$ value will the desired bias–free A_d value.

The bias correction procedure appears to work in this simulation study. For $N = 900$ and $B_0 = 20$, the magnitude of the area correlation was minimized at close to B = 20, see Figure 16.6. The corrected value of A_d obtained at this point was 0.672 versus the predicted 0.664. For the smaller case sample ($N = 90$) the agreement was actually better ($A_d = 0.662$) even though the minimum was at B = 16, rather than 20, but this could be a sampling artifact. The correction procedure is promising but needs further study under different conditions. For the method to be useful, it should apply to $N = 90$ images or less.

16.2.5 Discussion

The DROC method attempts, paradoxically, to get diagnostic accuracy from preference data. It represents an attempt to put conventional preference testing on firmer ground. In commonly performed preference studies a reader *with no diagnostic ability* can mislead the experimenter simply by choosing the preferred modality for all image pairs. It is important to note that the DROC study is free from this type of bias as such a reader will pick the preferred modality equally for positive and negative pairs. DROC methodology has the potential of substantially decreasing the time and expense of observer performance evaluation studies. The reason is that observers are ex-

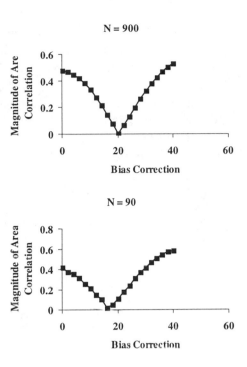

Figure 16.6: Illustrating the proposed bias reduction procedure for DROC experiments. When the bias correction value equals the actual bias (assumed to be 20 in this case) the area correlation value is minimized.

pected to detect small inter-modality differences in image quality when they are shown the images in pairs. Detecting the small differences may not be possible when the images are presented sequentially, often after a large time interval.

In conclusion, the DROC method has the potential of significantly increasing the power of imaging system comparison studies. However, the DROC method is comparatively new and there is a specific issue with bias that needs to be further resolved. While the bias-correction method we have proposed appears to be promising, it needs more testing before we can recommend it for general use.

Acknowledgments

This work was partially supported by a grant from the Department of Health and Human Services, National Institutes of Health, National Cancer Institute, RO1-CA75145.

References

[1] Green DM, Swets JA. *Signal Detection Theory and Psychophysics*. Huntington, NY: RE Krieger, 1974.

[2] Swets JA, Pickett RM. *Evaluation of Diagnostic Systems: Methods from Signal Detection Theory*. New York: Academic Press, 1982.

[3] Metz CE. "ROC Methodology in Radiologic Imaging." Investigative Radiology 21:720–733, 1986.

[4] Metz C. "Some Practical Issues of Experimental Design and Data Analysis in Radiological ROC studies." Investigative Radiology 24:234–245, 1989.

[5] Chesters MS. Human Visual-Perception and ROC Methodology in Medical Imaging. Phys Med Biol 37(7): 1433–1476, 1992.

[6] Dorfman DD, Berbaum KS. "Degeneracy and Discrete Receiver Operating Characteristic Rating Data." Academic Radiology 2:907–915, 1995.

[7] Obuchowski NA. "Multireader, Multimodality Receiver Operating Characteristic Curve Studies: Hypothesis Testing and Sample Size Estimation Using an Analysis of Variance Approach with Dependent Observations." Academic Radiology 2(Suppl 1):S22-9; discussion S57-64, S70-1 pas, 1995.

[8] Obuchowski NA. "Multireader Receiver Operating Characteristic Studies: A Comparison of Study Designs." Academic Radiology 2(8):709–716, 1995.

[9] Starr SJ, Metz CE, Lusted LB, Goodenough DJ. "Visual Detection and Localization of Radiographic Images." Radiology 116:533–538, 1975.

[10] Metz CE, Starr SJ, Lusted LB. "Observer Performance in Detecting Multiple Radiographic Signals. Prediction and Analysis Using a Generalized ROC Approach." Radiology 121:337–347, 1976.

[11] Swensson RG. "Unified Measurement of Observer Performance in Detecting and Localizing Target Objects on Images." Medical Physics 23(10):1709–1725, 1996.

[12] Egan JP, Greenburg GZ, Schulman AI. "Operating Characteristics, Signal Detectability and the Method of Free Response." J Acoust Soc Am 33:993–1007, 1961.

[13] Bunch PC, Hamilton JF, Sanderson GK, Simmons AH. "A Free-Response Approach to the Measurement and Characterization of Radiographic Observer Performance." SPIE Proceedings, Optical Instrumentation in Medicine VI 4, 1977, pp. 124–135.

[14] Bunch PC, Hamilton JF, Sanderson GK, Simmons AH. "A Free-Response Approach to the Measurement and Characterization of Radiographic Observer Performance." Journal of Applied Photographic Engineering 4:166–171, 1978.

[15] Sorenson JA, Mitchell CR, Armstrong 2d JD, Mann H, Bragg DG, Mann FA, Tocino IB, Wojtowycz MM. "Effects of Improved Contrast on Lung-Nodule Detection. A Clinical ROC Study." Invest Radiol 22(10):772–780, 1987.

[16] Dorfman DD, Alf Jr. E. "Maximum-Likelihood Estimation of Parameters of Signal-Detection Theory and Determination of Confidence Intervals-Rating-Method Data." Journal of Mathematical Psychology 6:487–496, 1969.

[17] Chakraborty DevP *et al.* "Digital Vs. Conventional Imaging of the Chest: A Modified ROC Study Using Simulated Nodules." Radiology 158:35–39, 1986.

[18] Chakraborty DevP. "Maximum Likelihood Analysis of Free-Response Receiver Operating Characteristic (FROC) Data." Medical Physics 16:561–568, 1989.

[19] Chakraborty DevP, Loek Winter HL. "Free-Response Methodology: Alternative Analysis and a New Observer Performance Experiment." Radiology 174:873–881, 1990.

[20] Metz C. "Evaluation of Digital Mammography by ROC Analysis." In Doi K, Giger ML, Nishikawa RM, Schmidt RA (Eds.) *Digital Mammography '96, Proceedings of the 3rd International Workshop on Digital Mammography.* Elsevier, 1996, pp. 61–68.

[21] Berbaum KS, Franken EA, Dorfman DD *et al.* "Satisfaction of Search in Diagnostic Radiology." Inv Rad 26:133–140, 1990.

[22] Hanley JA. "The Robustness of the 'Binormal' Assumptions Used in Fitting ROC Curves." Medical Decision Making 8:197–203, 1988.

[23] This is available from Professor Charles Metz at the University of Chicago. Available on the web at http://www-radiology.uchicago.edu/sections/.

[24] Lirio RB, Garcia LG, Sosa PV *et al.* "Localization Error in Biomedical Imaging." Comput Biol Med 22(4):277–286, 1992.

[25] Mansson LG, Kheddache S, Schlossman D *et al.* "Digital Chest Radiography with a Large Image Intensifier—Evaluation of Diagnostic Performance and Patient Exposure." Acta Radiol 30:337–342, 1989.

[26] Burl MC, Asker L, Smyth P *et al.* "Learning to Recognize Volcanoes on Venus." Mach Learn 30:165–194, 1998.

[27] Fearon T, Vucich J, McSweeney WJ, Potter BM, Brallier DR, McIlhenny J, Tepper J, Markle BM. "A Comparative Evaluation of Rare Earth Screen-Film Systems. Free-Response Operating Characteristic Analysis and Anatomic Criteria Analysis." Investigative Radiology 21:734–742, 1986.

[28] Anastasio MA, Kupinski MA, Nishikawa RM. "Optimization and FROC Analysis of Rule-Based Detection Schemes Using a Multiobjective Approach." IEEE Trans Med Imaging 17:1089–1093, 1998.

[29] Tourassi GD, Floyd CE. "Artificial Neural Networks for Single-Photon Emission Computed-Tomography—A Study of Cold Lesion Detection and Localization." Invest Radiol 28(8):671–677, 1993.

[30] Miettunen R, Korhola O, Bondestam S, Standertskjold-Nordenstam CG, Lamminen A, Somer K, Soiva M. "Combination of Multiple Pencil-Beam Imaging to Computed Storage Phosphor Radiography: A New Method." European Journal of Radiology 12:161–166, 1991.

[31] Schultze Kool LJ, Busscher DLT, Vlasbloem H *et al.* "Advanced Multiple Beam Equalization Radiography in Chest Radiology: A Simulated Nodule Detection Study." Radiology 169:35–39, 1988.

[32] Kido S, Ikezoe J, Naito H *et al.* "Clinical-Evaluation of Pulmonary Nodules with Single-Exposure Dual-Energy Subtraction Chest Radiography with an Iterative Noise-Reduction Algorithm." Radiology 194(2):407–412, 1995.

[33] Xu XW, Doi K, Kobayashi T *et al.* "Development of an Improved CAD Scheme for Automated Detection of Lung Nodules in Digital Chest Images." Med Phys 24(9):1395–1403, 1997.

[34] Chan HP, Niklason LT, Ikeda DM *et al.* "Digitization Requirements in Mammography—Effects on Computer-Aided Detection of Microcalcifications." Med Phys 21(7):1203–1211, 1994.

[35] Mendez AJ, Tahoces PG, Lado MJ *et al.* "Computer-Aided Diagnosis: Automatic Detection of Malignant Masses in Digitized Mammograms." Med Phys 25(6):957–964, 1998.

[36] Petrick N, Chan HP, Wei DT *et al.* "Automated Detection of Breast Masses on Mammograms Using Adaptive Contrast Enhancement and Texture Classification." Med Phys 23:1685–1696, 1996.

[37] Krupinski EA, Kundel HK. "Update on Long-term Goals for Medical Image Perception Research." Acad Rad 5:629–633, 1998.

[38] Chakraborty DP, Kundel HL, Nodine C, Narayan TK, Devaraju V. The Differential Receiver Operating Characteristic Method. SPIE Vol. 3338, 1998, pp. 234–240.

CHAPTER 17
Agreement and Accuracy Mixture Distribution Analysis

Marcia Polansky
MCP-Hahnamann University, School of Public Health

CONTENTS

17.1 Introduction

Correctly diagnosing the disease from which the patient suffers is the first step in developing an appropriate treatment plan. Therefore, it is essential to assess the accuracy of diagnostic tests, that is, the likelihood that a reader is correct with respect to an established standard. There are difficulties involved in determining the accuracy of a diagnostic imaging test. It may not be possible to definitively diagnose all cases because of variation in the presentation of the disease, the inaccessibility of the disease within the body and the concomitant invasiveness of the definitive diagnostic procedure, and the difficulty with making a differential diagnosis from other conditions with similar presentations. The diagnostic test under study may itself be the gold standard. There are also potential biases when a panel of experts is used to obtain a definitive diagnosis. Typically, the panel reviews the clinical data as well as the results of the diagnostic procedures to arrive at a consensus diagnosis. The effectiveness of the panel depends on the quality, completeness, and unambiguity of the information which is available to them (which may be quite limited for reasons discussed above) for making their decision. When there is a lack of consensus, an influential member of the panel can sway other members of the group to his/her view so that the panel becomes equivalent to a single reader with strong convictions (Revesz et al. [1], Greenes and Begg [2], Kundel and Polansky [3], and Hillman et al. [4]). The difficult cases require a large investment of time of the panel and in the end the diagnosis of the patient is not always resolved. One approach for insuring that the diagnoses of the study cases are accurate is to exclude cases for which the diagnosis is uncertain. However this limits the generalizability of the results of the accuracy study to general practice. It is also considered desirable to include cases which are difficult to assess radiologically but which have definitive diagnoses (based on clinical follow-up or pathological tests). These difficult-to-assess cases ("stress" cases) are believed to more likely detect differences among diagnostic tests because presumably easy cases could be correctly diagnosed by even a fairly insensitive test. As a result, initial studies of the accuracy of diagnostic tests are generally done using carefully selected subsets of all cases.

Additional issues arise when one is interested in evaluating the performance of a diagnostic test when it is used for diagnosis of disease in a real clinical population. In a naturalistic study, unlike in a laboratory study, it is important that the sample be representative of the population. Ideally then the cases should be a random sample of cases from the clinical population for which the test is intended to be used. A definitive diagnosis is required for every case to insure generalizability of the results to the clinical population. Also, a large number of cases needs to be included in the study to insure that there were adequate numbers of hard cases ('stress' cases) in the sample. Verification of large numbers of cases and particularly the difficult to diagnose cases is expensive and as discussed above is not always an option.

Another approach to evaluating the performance of a diagnostic test in its natural setting (either after its initial evaluation in the well controlled but artificial laboratory setting or when it is not possible to study accuracy) is to conduct an agreement study rather than an accuracy study. In an agreement study, multiple readers independently read and give a diagnosis for each case. The diagnosis of the majority of the readers is used in lieu of obtaining a diagnosis using case verification. A limitation of a study of agreement among readers is that the readers could all be wrong because of some misleading feature of the image. However, although the diagnosis of the majority of readers is not necessarily the true diagnosis, it is the most accurate diagnosis that is possible using the particular diagnostic method (and the accepted radiological standard). That is, any error remaining is the result of inherent limitations in the diagnostic method and not human error. Knowledge of the agreement of one reader and more generally the agreement of several readers with a "majority of readers" is directly clinically relevant in that it determines how many readers would be required to review an image in order to obtain a diagnosis which is as accurate as is possible with the particular diagnostic method. The notion of multiple readings is fundamental to diagnostic medicine in terms of the use of second opinions. Because in studies of agreement it is not necessary to do case verification, the time involved in evaluating each case is considerably reduced.

An earlier approach to conceptualizing agreement was to focus on the agreement of one reader with another reader (rather than the agreement of one reader with the majority). Cohen's Kappa [5] and Aickin's Alpha [6] are measures of agreement of one reader with another reader (i.e., pair wise agreement), which we will discuss. In terms of medical decision making, this framework has limitations because it is of limited direct interest whether two readers agree with each other. Of greater interest is how likely it is that one reader's diagnosis will agree with that of the majority of readers. Hence our approach is to consider the probability that a reader (or an initial reading and a second opinion reading) would agree with the diagnosis of an infinite majority of potential readers if they were to diagnose that case. Also of interest, would be to determine the proportion of all readers who would be expected to give the same diagnosis, (e.g., whether almost all the readers would give the same diagnosis for the case or whether say only 75% of all readers would give the same diagnosis). If readers have similar training and skill, the probability that a typical reader agrees with the majority is equal to the average agreement for the cases,

The probability that a typical reader agrees with the majority is equal to the average agreement for the cases even if the agreement rate differs among cases. For example, suppose there is a subgroup of images with high agreement, say 90%, and another subgroup of images with lower agreement, say 70%, and that 80% of the images are in the high-agreement subgroup and 20% are in the low-agreement subgroup. The probability that one reader would agree with the majority is $0.8*0.90+0.2*0.70=0.86$. Also of interest is whether second opinions can be used to confirm a diagnosis in the sense that if the second opinion (second reading) agrees with the first reading, then these readings would agree with the majority. In this case though, the probability that a pair of consistent readings agree with the majority depends on whether the agreement is the same for all images or whether there are subgroups of images with high and low agreement (the latter corresponding more closely to reality). It becomes clearer why the agreement among several readings increases the probability that their common diagnosis will agrees with the greater majority diagnosis, if we consider a more extreme case when there are, say, five readings done. If there are five readings and all five readings are disease positive, then we would be confident that the majority of all readers would give a disease-positive reading. If the cases were not homogenous in terms of agreement, the high observed agreement rate of five out of five instead of, say, three out of five would also suggest that this case belonged to the high-agreement subgroup rather than the low-agreement subgroup, thus further increasing our confidence in the reading agreeing with the majority. If all the cases are homogenous (i.e., same agreement rate when there are an infinite number of readers), the high observed agreement rate of five out of five instead of three out of five would increase our confidence that the observed readings agree with the (infinite unobserved) majority, but not as much so as if the cases were heterogeneous in terms of agreement (because there is no high-agreement subgroup). The belief of many radiologists that if two readers agree then we should have very high confidence in the truth of the readings while if two readers disagree we should be concerned that this is a hard case to read and one will never be sure of the diagnosis no matter how many readers are brought in (because they will also disagree) supports the notion that there is one subgroup of images that are very easy to read and another group of images that is indeterminate.

The existence of variation in image difficulty induces a statistical dependence among readings in that the results of preceding images provide information as to the likely results of subsequent readings (e.g., if the first two readers agree, the case is likely to be easy and all subsequent readings will agree, while if the first two readers disagree, it is likely to be an indeterminate case and there is likely to be disagreement among other radiologists as well). In summary, if the images differ in their "readability" it is not enough to know the overall agreement rate when it is of interest to determine the agreement of several readings with the majority reading. Rather, the multivariate distribution of the ratings must be determined (and then using the laws of probability, the probability of more than one reading agreeing with the majority can be determined). The multivariate distribution of ratings are the probabilities for each possible set of multiple reading outcomes. For example, if there are two readings, then there are four possible multiple or paired reading outcomes: two positive readings, two negative readings, first reading is positive and second reading is negative, and vice versa.

Knowledge of the distribution of images in terms of agreement is of interest in and of itself. However it also has implications in designing agreement studies and in generalizing the results of agreement studies. If agreement is homogenous among images then a smaller sample of images can be used to study agreement. If there is a subgroup of high-agreement images and a small subgroup of low-agreement images, then a larger study would be needed to insure the inclusion of the rare low-agreement images. Alternatively, it might be of interest to focus on the low-agreement images because these are the hard images in that different diagnosticians come to different conclusions ("stress set" in terms of agreement) and it might be for these low-agreement images that a new diagnostic test or improvement would be more sensitive than the original test. In terms of generalizing the results of an agreement study to other populations, one would be more cautious if there were subgroups of images differing in their degree of agreement. Caution would be advisable because different populations might have more or less images from each subgroup. For example, in a general population that is being screened for disease, there will be a higher proportion of low-agreement disease-positive images (i.e., "subtle" cases in the early stages of disease) than there will be for a group of symptomatic patients, some of whom will have advanced disease. There may also be significant differences among readers in how often they agree with the consensus. Some readers may agree less often with the majority of readers because they are less accurate. Others may agree with the majority of readers less often because they are more accurate and they are detecting disease others are missing or are not misled by atypically appearing normal cases. The latter is less likely, because these more skilled readers would make fewer errors on the easy cases so overall they would agree more often than other readers with the majority reading (because they would be correct for the easy cases). Differences among readers, however, is less of an issue when it is of interest to determine the agreement of several readings with the majority readings because the readers will average each other out.

The observation that images vary in difficulty and that there is variation among readers has led to the development of models for agreement which explicitly include terms for these sources of differences. Models of agreement including those developed by Hui and Walter [7], Espeland and Handelman [8], Qu *et al.* [9]. Agresti and Lang [10], and Kundel and Polansky [3] will be discussed after we review the classic measures of agreement.

17.2 Kappa coefficient and Aicken's Alpha

An early measure of agreement, which is still in widespread use at the present time, is Cohen's Kappa [5]. Kappa is referred to as 'chance corrected agreement' but this is a misnomer and can be misleading to the unwary. Kappa is the relative increase in agreement over agreement resulting from pure guessing with the rates of guessing disease-positive readings set equal to the observed disease-positive rates of each reader. The rationale often given for comparing observed agreement to agreement by guessing is that two readers can artificially increase their agreement by altering the proportion of cases which they give a disease-positive rating. However, as will be shown below, the agreement that can be obtained by guessing also depends on disease prevalence. The dependence of Kappa on disease prevalence makes it difficult to interpret and invalidates its use in comparing the agreement of diagnostic tests that are studied in populations with different prevalences. These drawbacks of Kappa may offset its desirable property of adjusting for differences among readers in how conservative they are in diagnosing disease, which can be minimal and decrease the usefulness of Kappa as a general measure of agreement in diagnostic medicine.

Kappa values lie on a scale of +1 to −1. A Kappa value of 1 corresponds to perfect agreement and a value of 0 corresponds to pure guessing. A Kappa of less then 0 indicates that the readers are systematically disagreeing, that is, they are doing worse than would be expected if they guessed. This could occur if one reader is using positive and negative that are different from the other reader or if the reader has a reversed notion of disease prevalence.

It is easiest to define Kappa when the agreement data are presented as a two-way table. We consider the most basic case of agreement data in radiology that consisting of two readers who classify cases as either disease positive (D+) or disease negative (D−). A 2 × 2 (as the only possible reading outcomes are present or absent) two-way table is obtained with the row dimension defined to correspond to reader 1 and the column dimension to reader 2 as shown in Table 17.1.

The formula for Kappa (κ) is then as follows:

$$\kappa = \frac{p_o - p_e}{1 - p_e}, \tag{17.1}$$

where p_o, observed agreement (i.e., the sum of the proportions on the diagonal of the table, $\Sigma p_{ii} = p_{11} + p_{22} + \cdots$); p_e, expected agreement for guessing based on observed rates of diagnosing the presence of disease for each reader (i.e., the sum of the expected proportions for the diagonal cells for this type of guessing). The expected proportions are obtained by multiplying the marginal row and column percents for the cell so that (total) expected agreement, $p_e = \Sigma p_{i+} p_{+i}$ where p_{i+}, the proportion of objects with a rating of i for rater 1 and p_{+i}, the proportion of objects with a rating of i for rater 2.

For example, consider the hypothetical Table 17.2 with the ratings of two readers who give either a positive or a negative reading for each image.

In order to compute Kappa, we begin by computing the observed agreement (p_o) and the expected agreement by guessing (p_e). The observed agreement is obtained by adding the proportion of cases with two positive readings and the proportion of cases with two negative readings (i.e., summing the cell proportions on the diagonal of Table 17.2) and is $p_o = 0.3 + 0.5 = 0.8$. The overall expected agreement by guessing based on the reader's rates of disease-positive readings, is

Table 17.1: Agreement data

| | | Reader 1 | | |
		D+	D−	Row totals
Reader 2	D+	p_{11}	p_{12}	p_{1+}
	D−	p_{21}	p_{22}	p_{2+}
Column totals		p_{+1}	p_{+2}	1.00

obtained by summing the expected proportions of two positive readings and two negative readings. Expected proportions for reading outcomes for a pair of readers can be obtained by multiplying the row and column proportions corresponding to the cell for that outcome in the table of agreement (as indicated in Eq. (17.1)). For example, the expected proportion of cases with positive readings (i.e., the cell in the first row and column) by both readers is $p_{11} = p_{1+} * p_{+1} = 0.35 * 0.45 = 0.16$. The expected proportions for the other possible reading outcomes are computed by multiplying the appropriate marginal totals in an analogous manner and are shown in Table 17.3.

The expected agreement by guessing is the sum of the diagonal of the table and is $p_c = 0.16 + 0.36 = 0.52$. Kappa is then:

$$\kappa = \frac{0.8 - 0.52}{1 - 0.52} = 0.58.$$

Agreement when guessing when the disease prevalence is known (and the readers set their disease-positive rates to be equal to the true prevalence), is greater when the proportion of cases in each diagnostic category is unbalanced. In diagnostic medicine, diagnostic categories are generally unbalanced because most people who are tested do not have the disease. In order to show that agreement increases with prevalence, we will begin by determining the expected proportion of paired readings with each of the four possible joint outcomes (i.e., both readings are positive, first reading is positive and second reading is negative, etc.). Note that the guessing we are considering here is slightly different then the guessing which is assumed when computing Kappa. Here we assume that the true prevalence is known and the probability of guessing disease positive is set to the true prevalence

Table 17.2: Observed proportions

		Reader 1		
		D+	D−	Row totals
Reader 2	D+	0.30	0.05	0.35
	D−	0.15	0.50	0.65
Column totals		0.45	0.55	1.00

Table 17.3: Expected proportions

		Reader 1		
		D+	D−	Row totals
Reader 2	D+	0.16	0.19	0.35
	D−	0.29	0.36	0.65
Column totals		0.45	0.55	1.00

while for Kappa each reader is assumed to have their own rate of diagnosing disease. Readers might have different rates of diagnosing disease if they differed in how conservative they are. One reader might over-diagnose disease so as not to miss any disease-positive people while the other might not (or do this to a lesser extent), so that one or both of the reader's personal prevalences might differ from the true disease prevalence. Nevertheless one would expect that readers' personal prevalences would not be overly different from the true prevalences.

The formulas for the expected values for guessing based on true prevalence can be derived from the formulas given for computing Kappa, except that we use the prevalence instead of the observed disease-positive rates. First, we consider the probability of two positive readings when guessing based on prevalence. The probability of two positive readings is the probability that the first reading is positive multiplied by the probability that the second reading is positive. Because the probability of a positive reading is equal to the prevalence for each reader, the probability of a pair of positive readings is

$$P(\text{two positive readings when optimally guessing}) = \text{prev} * \text{prev} = \text{prev}^2.$$

The probabilities for the other possible outcomes for paired readings are obtained similarly and are shown below:

P (first reading positive and second reading negative when optimally guessing)
$= \text{prev} * (1 - \text{prev})$,
P (first reading negative and second reading positive when optimally guessing)
$= (1 - \text{prev}) * \text{prev}$,

and,

$$P(\text{two negative readings when optimally guessing}) = (1 - \text{prev})^2.$$

Note that the probability of the first reading being positive and the second reading being negative is the same as the first reading being negative and the second reading being positive. Also, as can be seen, the probability of two positive readings and two negative readings when guessing based on prevalence depends exclusively on the disease prevalence. In order to quantitatively assess the effect of prevalence on the probabilities, and thereby agreement, we computed these probabilities first for a disease prevalence of 0.05 (a rare disease) and then for a disease prevalence of 0.5 (a common medical problem). The probabilities for paired reading outcomes when the prevalence is 0.05 are shown below.

P (two positive readings when prev $= 0.05) = 0.05 * 0.05 = 0.0025$,
P (one positive reading and one negative reading in a specified order
when prev $= 0.05) = 0.05 * 0.95 = 0.0475$,

and

$$P(\text{two negative readings when prev} = 0.05) = 0.95 * 0.95 = 0.90.$$

When the prevalence is 0.5, the joint probabilities for paired readings are as follows:

$P(\text{two positive readings when prev} = 0.5) = 0.5 * 0.5 = 0.25,$
$P(\text{one positive reading and one negative reading in a specified order}$
   $\text{when prev} = 0.5) = 0.5 * 0.5 = 0.25,$

and

$$P(\text{two negative readings when prev} = 0.5) = 0.5 * 0.5 = 0.25.$$

The probabilities of outcome pairs for two ratings under guessing are shown below in Table 17.4.

The diagnosis by guessing for the low-prevalence population results in a very high agreement rate between the two readers (agreement rate $= 0.904 + 0.0025 = 0.91$), while for the evenly divided population the observed agreement rate was very low (agreement rate $= 0.25 + 0.25 = 0.50$). Kappa is the same and zero in both cases, because Kappa describes the fractional increase in agreement over that achieved by prevalence-based guessing and prevalence-based guessing was in fact used (i.e., the numerator of Eq. (17.1) is 0 because $p_o = p_e$, so Kappa is 0).

We now consider the effect of prevalence on agreement and Kappa for a diagnostic test with diagnostic value (instead of for prevalence-based guessing as

Table 17.4: Expected probabilities when guessing based on prevalence

| | | Prevalence $= 0.05$ Reader 2 | | |
		D−	D+	Row totals
Reader 1	D−	0.904	0.0475	0.95
	D+	0.0475	0.0025	0.05
Column totals		0.95	0.05	1.00
		Prevalence $= 0.5$ Reader 2		
		D+	D−	Row totals
Reader 1	D−	0.25	0.25	0.50
	D+	0.25	0.25	0.50
Column totals		0.50	0.50	1.00

in the previous illustration). We will use as an example, a diagnostic test which has sensitivity $= 0.9$ and specifity $= 0.9$. We will compare the agreement when the diagnostic test is used for a population with 50% prevalence of disease and for a population with a disease prevalence of only 5% (the same prevalences were used above for determining the effect of prevalence on agreement when guessing). First we construct a table of paired reading outcomes that would arise for such a diagnostic test. The expected proportion (probability) of cases with two positive readings is obtained by summing the expected proportion of cases with two positive ratings when disease is present and the expected proportion of cases with two positive ratings when the disease is absent after weighting by prevalence (prev) for a diagnostic test with 90% sensitivity and specificity as shown below:

$$
\begin{aligned}
P\,&(\text{two positive ratings}) \\
&= P\,(\text{two positive readings if true disease positive}) * \text{prev} \\
&\quad + P\,(\text{two positive readings if true disease-negative}) * (1 - \text{prev}).
\end{aligned}
$$

Because the cases are assumed to be read independently by the two readers, the probability of two positive readings, given the disease status of the case, is obtained by multiplying the probabilities of a positive reading given the disease status of the case for each reader so that

$$
\begin{aligned}
P\,&(\text{two positive readings if true disease positive}) \\
&= P\,(\text{reading 1 is disease positive if true disease positive}) \\
&\quad * P\,(\text{reading 2 is disease positive if true disease positive}) \\
&= \text{sensitivity} * \text{sensitivity} = \text{sensitivity}^2,
\end{aligned}
$$

and similarly,

$$
\begin{aligned}
P\,&(\text{two positive readings if true disease negative}) \\
&= P\,(\text{reading 1 is disease positive if true disease negative}) \\
&\quad * P\,(\text{reading 2 is disease positive if true disease negative}) \\
&= (1 - \text{specificity})^2,
\end{aligned}
$$

so that,

$$
\begin{aligned}
P\,&(\text{two positive readings}) \\
&= P\,(\text{two positive readings if true disease positive}) \\
&\quad + P\,(\text{two positive readings if true disease negative}) \\
&= \text{sensitivity}^2 * \text{prev} + (1 - \text{specificity})^2 * (1 - \text{prev}).
\end{aligned}
$$

The probability of two negative readings can be obtained in a similar manner and is as follows:

$$
\begin{aligned}
P\,&(\text{two negative readings}) \\
&= (1 - \text{sensitivity})^2 * \text{prev} + \text{specificity}^2 * (1 - \text{prev}).
\end{aligned}
$$

The probability of the first reading being positive and the second reading being negative is the same as the probability of the first reading being negative and the second reading being positive and is

$$
\begin{aligned}
P(\text{1st reading positive and 2nd reading negative}) \\
= P(\text{1st reading positive and 2nd reading negative}) \\
= \text{sensitivity} * (1 - \text{sensitivity}) * \text{prev} \\
+ (1 - \text{specificity}) * \text{specificity} * (1 - \text{prev}).
\end{aligned}
$$

The above equations can also be used to compute the joint distribution of a pair of ratings when the prevalence is 0.5 as shown below:

$$
\begin{aligned}
P(\text{two positive readings}) &= (0.9 * 0.9) * 0.5 + (0.1 * 0.1) * 0.5 - 0.41 \\
P(\text{first reading positive and second reading negative}) \\
&= (0.9 * 0.1) * 0.5 + (0.1 * 0.9) * 0.5 = 0.09 \\
P(\text{first reading negative and second reading positive}) \\
&= (0.1 * 0.9) * 0.5 + (0.9 * 0.1) * 0.5 = 0.09, \text{ and} \\
P(\text{two negative readings}) &= (0.1 * 0.1) * 0.5 + (0.9 * 0.9) * 0.5 = 0.41.
\end{aligned}
$$

The joint probability distribution for paired readings when the prevalence is 0.05 is as follows:

$$
\begin{aligned}
\text{Prop(two positive readings)} &= (0.9 * 0.9) * 0.05 + (0.1 * 0.1) * 0.95 = 0.77. \\
\text{Prop(first reading positive and second reading negative)} \\
&= (0.9 * 0.1) * 0.05 + (0.1 * 0.9) * 0.95 = 0.09 \\
\text{Prop(first reading negative and second reading positive)} \\
&= (0.1 * 0.9) * 0.05 + (0.9 * 0.1) * 0.95 = 0.09 \\
\text{Prop(two negative readings)} &= (0.1 * 0.1) * 0.05 + (0.9 * 0.9) * 0.95 = 0.05.
\end{aligned}
$$

The expected proportions for this diagnostic test with 90% sensitivity and specificity are shown in Table 17.5(a, b).

We see that the agreement rates are identical for the population with a prevalence of 0.05 and the population with a prevalence of 0.5 because the sum of the diagonal is the same for both Tables 17.5(a) and 17.5(b) ($p_0 = 0.77 + 0.05 = 0.82$ when the prevalence is 0.05 and $p_0 = 0.41 + 0.41 = 0.82$ when the prevalence is 0.5). The equality of the agreement rates is intuitively appealing because we had set the sensitivity equal to the specificity so that the prevalence would not be expected to have an effect on the agreement rate.

We now compute Kappa for the diagnostic test with 90% sensitivity and specificity when the prevalence is 0.05 and when the prevalence is 0.5. For both prevalences, we have just shown that the agreement rate is $p_0 = 0.82$. To compute Kappa we must construct the expected table when guessing using the marginal totals of Table 17.5. For example, to obtain the probability of two positive readings, we multiply the proportion of cases with the first reading being positive by the proportion of cases with the second reading ($p_{1+} * p_{+1} = 0.86 * 0.86 = 0.73$ for a

Table 17.5(a): Proportions expected for a diagnostic test with 90% sensitivity and specificity

| | | Prevalence = 0.05 Reader 2 | | Column total |
		D−	D+	
Reader 1	D−	0.77	0.09	0.86
	D+	0.09	0.05	0.14
Row total		0.86	0.14	1.00

| | | Prevalence = 0.5 Reader 2 | | Column total |
		D−	D+	
Reader 1	D−	0.41	0.09	0.50
	D+	0.09	0.41	0.50
Row total		0.50	0.50	1.00

Table 17.5(b): Expected proportions when Guessing is based on prevalence

| | | Prevalence = 0.05 Reader 2 | | Column total |
		D−	D+	
Reader 1	D−	0.73	0.13	0.86
	D+	0.13	0.01	0.14
Row total		0.86	0.14	1.00

| | | Prevalence = 0.5 Reader 2 | | Column total |
		D−	D+	
Reader 1	D−	0.25	0.25	0.50
	D+	0.25	0.25	0.50
Row total		0.50	0.50	1.00

prevalence of 0.05 and ($p_{1+} * p_{+1} = 0.5 * 0.5 = 0.25$ for a prevalence of 0.5. The complete tables of expected proportions assuming chance assignment are shown in Table 17.5(b).

Referring to Table 17.5(b), we find that the expected agreement by guessing is $p_e = 0.73 + 0.01 = 0.74$ for a prevalence of 0.05 and the expected agreement by guessing is $p_e = 0.25 + 0.25 = 0.5$ for a prevalence of 0.5.

Now substituting into Eq. (17.1) we obtain the Kappas as follows:

$$Kappa_{prev=0.05} = (0.82 - 0.74)/(1 - 0.74) = 0.31$$
$$Kappa_{prev=0.5} = (0.82 - 0.50)/(1 - 0.5) = 0.64.$$

As can be seen, Kappa, which compares observed agreement to prevalence-based guessing, is low when the prevalence is 0.5 (Kappa $= 0.64$) and even lower when the prevalence is 0.05 (Kappa $= 0.31$) despite the high sensitivity and specificity of the test (90%). The low values of Kappa for a test with high diagnostic value indicates that Kappa should not be subjectively interpreted as having been measured on the same scale as raw agreement and that Kappa values for highly diagnostic tests are typically less than 0.75. Also of interest is that the large difference in the Kappa's is attributable to differences in disease prevalence and not to any difference in the accuracy of the diagnostic test, because by the construction of the example, the same diagnostic test was used in the populations with different prevalences.

Figure 17.1 below shows the strong relationship between prevalence and Kappa for a range of prevalences for a diagnostic test with 90% accuracy.

The above examples and Figure 17.1 highlight the characteristic of Kappa, which is often overlooked, that Kappa does not assess solely or even primarily the characteristics of the test but also reflects the prevalence of disease in the population for which it is used. The limitation of Kappa is that it cannot distinguish between the effect of prevalence on agreement and the effect of the stringency of the cut point used to classify cases as disease positive and disease negative.

Feinstein and Cicchetti [11] have studied the properties of Kappa and have expressed similar views as this author. Swets [12] has also studied the properties of

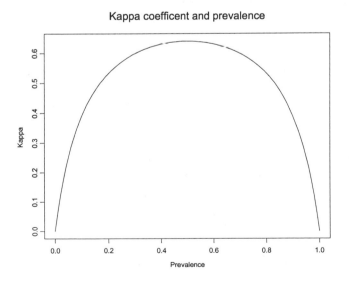

Figure 17.1: Kappa coefficient and prevalence.

Kappa in the context of ROC analysis. He concluded that Kappa should not be used as a measure of accuracy (i.e., agreement of a reading with the truth) because the study of empirical ROC curves has shown that the assumptions underlying Kappa are not consistent with the shapes of ROC curves which are naturally found in many fields including diagnostic imaging. Generalizations of Kappa which exist include the weighted Kappa which allows for partial credit for close scores (Cohen [13], 1968) and a Kappa for agreement with majority (Landis and Koch [14]).

Aickin [6] developed a modified Kappa-like statistic, which is based on an explicit model of agreement between two raters. Aicken assumed there were two types of objects, objects for which the disease category to which they belonged was obvious to any appropriately trained person viewing the image, so that readers would always agree for these objects and another group of objects which were impossibly difficult to classify so that all agreement was attributable chance alone. This joint probability distribution of a paired ratings based on the assumptions above is

$$
\begin{aligned}
p(i, j) &= (1 - \alpha) * p_r(i) p_c(j) + \alpha \quad \text{if } i = j \\
&= (1 - \alpha) * p_r(i) p_c(j) \qquad \text{if } i \neq j,
\end{aligned} \tag{17.2}
$$

where $p(i, j)$, the probability that rater 1 gives rating i and rater 2 gives rating j; α, the proportion of objects with complete agreement; $(1 - \alpha)$, the proportion of objects for which all agreement can be explained by chance; $p_r(i)$, the probability of rater r giving a rating of i, and $p_c(i)$, the probability of rater c giving a rating of i.

The proportion of objects with perfect agreement is alpha (α). Aickin showed that α follows the pattern of a Kappa-like statistic. The only difference between Aickin's Alpha and Cohen's Kappa is that the marginal probabilities of the sub-population of hard-to-classify objects are used instead of the full marginal probabilities.

The difficulty with using this model in agreement studies in diagnostic radiology is that the objects are assumed to be so easy that there is always perfect agreement or so hard that all agreement is by chance. However this is generally not so in medical diagnosis. For example, suppose there is a subgroup of cases for which the accuracy is 90%. The agreement between two readers of 0.81 ($0.9 * 0.9$) is not mainly by chance, it is because they each agree with the truth. The agreement is really more "by cause," because each reader is highly accurate (although not perfectly accurate). It follows that Aiken's Alpha, like Cohen's Kappa, reflects the disease prevalence as well as the accuracy of the test, although Aicken's Alpha will be somewhat less sensitive to prevalence than Cohen's Kappa because the improvement in agreement for the diagnostic test is expressed as a percent of only the subgroup of hard cases.

The value of Aickin's approach is that he explicitly models agreement and introduces the notion of agreement by cause and that he uses a mixture distribution to model agreement. A mixture distribution is a general class of distributions that are used for data that are assumed to come from more than one population. A mixture distribution would then include the distributions for each of the populations contributing to the sample and the mixing probabilities which corresponds to the proportion of observations from each population. Aicken's model is a two-component mixture distribution because there are two subgroups of objects, those with perfect agreement and those that agree only "by chance." When there are only two readers (i.e., raters in Aicken's terminology), the number of parameters that can be included in the mixture model is limited to three parameters (so that the solution is unique). Because Aicken's model allows the marginal probabilities for the hard images to differ, his model already has three parameters, and no additional subgroups (e.g., intermediate difficulty images) can be added to his assumed mixture distribution. A more detailed discussion of mixture distributions is included in Section 17.3 in which we discuss the mixture of binomial models suggested by Kundel and Polansky for three and more readers.

17.3 Other models for agreement

Hiu and Walter [7] were among the first statisticians to use a mixture model for estimating the sensitivity and specificity of diagnostic tests when there was no gold standard. Their focus was to compare two different diagnostic tests when there was a single reading done using each diagnostic test. In order to make the link from agreement to accuracy, they assumed that the majority diagnosis was the true diagnosis. Recognizing the limited number of parameters, which can be included when there are only two readings, they proposed to use samples from two populations with different prevalences of disease. They also made the assumption that the sensitivity of the test would be the same for both populations. Similarly, the specificity of the test was assumed to be the same for both populations. However the sensitivity and the specificity of the test were allowed to differ from each other. The mixture distribution that follows from these assumptions when there are two populations each with diseased (D+) and nondiseased (D−) cases is a mixture of four multinomial distributions, each corresponding to one of the four subgroups of images (the disease positive images from population 1, the disease negative images from population 1, the disease positive images from population 2, and the disease negative images from population 2). The model has six parameters: the sensitivity of each test, the specificity of each test, and the disease prevalence in each population. This model can be expressed in terms of the joint probabilities of paired readings from diagnostic test r and diagnostic test c as follows:

$$p(i, j) = p_r(i \mid D-)p_c(j \mid D-)p_1(D-)s_1$$
$$+ p_r(i \mid D+)p_c(j \mid D+)p_1(D+)s_1$$
$$+ p_r(i \mid D-)p_c(j \mid D-)p_2(D-)(1 - s_1)$$
$$+ p_r(i \mid D+)p_c(j \mid D+)p_2(D+)(1 - s_1)$$

for $i = 0, 1$ and $j = 0, 1$,   where $0 = D-$ reading and $1 = D+$ reading,   (17.3) and where s_1, proportion of the total cases from population 1 and $(1 - s_1)$, proportion from population 2; $p_i(D+)$, the prevalence of disease in population i; $p_r(i \mid D+)$, the probability that diagnostic test r gives a reading of i if disease is present so that the sensitivity of diagnostic test r is $p_r(i = 1 \mid D+)$; $p_r(i \mid D-)$, the probability that diagnostic test r gives a reading of i if disease is not present so that the specificity of diagnostic test r is $p_r(i = 0 \mid D-)$; $p_c(i \mid D+)$, the probability that diagnostic test c gives a reading of i if disease is present so that the sensitivity of diagnostic test c is $p_c(i = 1 \mid D+)$; $p_c(i \mid D-)$, the probability that diagnostic test c gives reading of i if disease is not present so that the specificity of diagnostic test c is $p_c(i = 0 \mid D-)$.

As discussed, the implicit assumption underlying their interpretation of the parameters of the model is that the majority rating is the true diagnosis. If we don't make this assumption, we can view $p_r(i = 0 \mid D-)$ as the percent of time a reader will agree with the majority reading of no disease or the specificity of the diagnostic test relative to the majority diagnosis (relative specificity). Similarly, $p_r(i = 1 \mid D+)$ is the agreement for the disease-positive cases (i.e., the relative sensitivity). Using Aickin's terminology, agreement with the majority could be viewed as agreement by cause, and may be an improvement over his original definition because agreement either all by chance or all by cause is not required. For example, if a reader agrees with the majority for 90% of cases, then the agreement by cause would be 90%. Also note that Hui and Walter's model untangles prevalence from agreement as a consequence of a clearer notion of agreement by cause. This paves the way for determining agreement for a population with a different disease prevalence. For example if Hui and Walter's model is fit to agreement data and the relative sensitivity and specificity for one of the tests are estimated to be 0.90 and 0.80, respectively, and the prevalence is estimated to be 0.05, then a reader will agree with the majority for 81% cases (i.e., $0.9 * 0.05 + 0.8 * 0.95 = 0.81$). If this diagnostic test is used in a population with a higher prevalence, say, of 0.40, then a reader will agree with the majority for 0.84 ($9 * 0.40 + 0.8 * 0.60 = 0.84$) of the cases.

The model proposed by Hui and Walter has the disadvantage that all images in the same diagnostic category are assumed to be equally difficult to read. However, there are likely to be differences in agreement rates within diagnostic groups because images undoubtedly vary in difficulty within diagnostic groups. Two approaches have been used to take into account this variability. One approach is to consider there to be discrete subgroups of images within each diagnostic category, perhaps a very high agreement group, a moderate agreement group, and an indeterminate group. An alternate approach is to assume that there is only one group but that there is some variation in agreement around a common mean (i.e., a unimodal distribution for agreement). Qu et al. [9] used the latter approach. He assumed that the variation in agreement about the common mean has a normal distribution. His model also includes an effect of rater, so that differences among raters can be assessed.

Qu *et al.*'s approach can be used if the variation in agreement rates has an approximately normal or symmetric distribution. However, in many of the agreement studies in radiology which Kundel and Polansky have conducted, agreement rates were highly skewed or bimodal. They found that in a naturalistic study (a cross-sectional study of a clinical population) there is a typically a large subgroup of images that have very high agreement, another group of images with moderate agreement, and a very small group with no agreement. In one such study, a random sample of 95 hard-copy chest images were taken in an intensive care unit and were read independently by four radiologists. The true diagnosis was known for each case based on a review of clinical records including information on the subsequent course of the disease. The expected number of positive readings among the four radiologists was obtained separately for the disease-positive and the disease-negative images assuming a one-group model (all cases of equal difficulty) and then a two-subgroup model (i.e., hard and easy cases). They assumed the same agreement rate for all images within the group (for the one-group model) and for each of the two subgroups (in the two-subgroup model) to keep the number of parameters in the model sufficiently small. Our meaning by the statement that the agreement rate within groups (subgroups) was assumed to be constant requires some clarification. A constant agreement rate within a group (subgroup) does not mean that if each image is read by a small number of readers, say four readers, that exactly three out of four readings will be disease positive for all the cases. Rather, what we mean by a constant rate in a group is that if there were an infinite number of readings done for each image, the agreement rate for each image would equal the agreement rate of all the other images. For example if a group has a constant agreement rate of 75%, and a very large number of readings are done for each image, then all the images will have agreement very close to 75%. Our interpretation for why there were not always exactly three of only four is that unknown factors or circumstances when the reading took place influenced the readings in a nonsystematic (i.e., random) way. All of the radiologists were chest specialists, so we can assume that they interpret images in a similar way.

If we assume that the disease-positive images have the same agreement rate and readers are interchangeable, then the number of positive readings for multiple readings has a binomial distribution (constant-rate model). When the two-homogenous-subgroup model holds, the probability distribution for the number of positive readings is a mixture distribution for two binomials. The above two models were fit separately for the disease-positive images and the disease-negative images. We discuss mixture-of-binomial distributions in greater depth and a method for estimating the parameters of the mixture distribution in Section 17.4.

As can be seen in Table 17.6, the two-subgroup model (i.e., mixture of two binomials) appears to fit considerably better than the constant-rate model (Table 17.1) for both the disease-positive and the disease-negative groups. For the disease-negative images, there appear to be two subgroups, a large very accurate subgroup (99% accuracy which comprises about two thirds of the images) and a second group with moderate accuracy (67% accuracy which comprises one third of the images). The lack of fit of the one group model is attributable to the over estimation of the number of images with all but one reader agreeing and the under-estimation of the number of images with fair accuracy.

There also may be a small group of images that provide no diagnostic or mis-leading information (5% to 10% of the data) but there were not sufficient images to fit a three-binomial mixture to determine if this was the case. The disease-positive images also appear to have two subgroups but there were only 30 images, so it is more difficult to determine whether there are two subgroups of disease-positive images. One could also raise the possibility that there are not really two distinct groups of images (within each diagnostic category) but one group with a highly skewed distribution. However, it is very difficult to model asymmetric distribu-tions, because of the complicated functional form and the parameters of the model would not have straightforward interpretations. Therefore, we are satisfied with making the simplifying assumption that there are two homogenous subgroups of images rather than one heterogeneous group with a highly skewed distribution for agreement.

It is of interest that only three of the thirty-six true disease-negative images had a majority diagnosis of disease positive (and none had unanimous readings). However, there were 7 of 30 disease-positive images with a false disease-negative majority diagnosis. It is striking that the frequencies of images with all but one agreeing is almost the same as the number of images with complete agreement for the disease-positive images (11 vs 8) while for the disease-negative images there is a preponderance of images with complete agreement (43 vs 12). This suggests that there is more disagreement among radiologists for the disease-positive cases. That is, perfect agreement does not occur as often for disease-positive cases as for disease-negative cases. Also of interest are the estimates of the proportions of images in each of the subgroups and the accuracy rates for images in each sub-group. We see that for the disease-negative images, the accuracy (i.e., specificity because these are true disease-negative cases) for one subgroup of images is 0.99 (Table 17.7), so we can think of this subgroup as being an easy subgroup of cases. This subgroup includes slightly more than half the images (62% approximately). The other subgroup has much lower accuracy (66%). Because of the smaller num-ber of disease-positive images, it is difficult to make definitive interpretations of the estimates of the parameters for the disease-positive images. With this caution in mind, it appears that the accuracy (i.e., sensitivity because these are true disease-positive cases) may be less for the easy disease-positive cases (0.87 compared to 0.99 and the approximately equivalent numbers of images with all but one agreeing and images with complete agreement discussed above). Also of interest is that for the hard subgroup, a minority of the readers detect the disease (0.32), that is, the majority diagnosis is not the correct diagnosis. Table 17.7 also includes the overall estimate of the accuracy of the diagnostic test for each disease group. The overall accuracy for each disease group is obtained by computing the weighted average of the accuracies of the easy and hard subgroups as shown below:

$$ACC = ACC_{easy} * p_{easy} + ACC_{hard} * (1 - p_{hard}).$$

Table 17.6: Expected number of positive readings for the one-group model and for the two-subgroup model

Disease negative images ($n = 65$)					
Number of D+ readings	0	1	2	3	4
Observed number of cases	43	12	7	3	0
Expected for one-group model	37	22	5	1	0
Expected for two-group model	44	11	7	2	1

Disease positive images ($n = 30$)					
Number of D+ readings	0	1	2	3	4
Observed number of cases	2	5	4	8	11
Expected for one-group model	0	3	9	12	6
Expected for two-group model	2	4	5	8	11

Table 17.7: Estimates of the parameters of mixtures of two binomials separately for the disease-positive group of images and for the disease-negative group

Disease Group	Accuracy Rate		Proportion of Easy Images	Accuracy for Disease Group
	Easy Subgroup	Hard Subgroup		
Disease $-$	0.99	0.66	61.8%	86.5%
Disease $+$	0.87	0.32	64.9%	80.2%

The accuracy as defined here corresponds to the specificity for disease-negative images and the sensitivity for disease-positive images.

A number of investigators have used the subgroup approach to modeling agreement including Espeland and Handelman [8], Agresti and Lang [10], and Kundel and Polansky [3]. Aickin's model is an extreme version of this approach in which he defines a group of perfect agreement images and a group of impossibly hard to diagnose images. Agresti and Lang's [10] model for agreement belongs to the class of mixture models referred to as a qualitative latent-factor model. A qualitative latent-factor model is a model used for qualitative data when the data come from several populations, and the population, from which each observation originated from is not known. In Agresti and Lang's model, each class of the qualitative latent factor represents a subgroup of the images with a unique pattern of ratings. For example there may be a class that includes the images with a high proportion of positive readings, another class with images with mainly negative readings, and a third class with images with mixed readings. The first class could be considered the high-agreement positive images, the second class the high-agreement negative images, and the third class the low-agreement images. Agresti and Lang's model allows for differences among readers. A restriction to the nature of these differences is that if a reader gives a higher proportion of positive readings in one class than the model assumes that the reader gives a higher proportion of positive readings in all the other classes. However, a highly accurate reader would not give more positive readings for all classes of images. For the class with high-agreement positive images this reader would have a very high rate of positive readings, but for the high agreement negative images this skilled reader would have a high rate of negative readings. Therefore this model cannot be used to study differences in the reliability of readers.

Espeland and Handelman [8] also used a qualitative latent-factor analysis to model agreement. They modeled agreement among dentists who read radiographs for diagnosing dental caries. The most general model they considered assumed five subgroups of images. They assumed that there was a group of radiographs with all readers agreeing that the tooth had caries, a group of radiographs with perfect agreement that the tooth was normal, an equivocal positive-caries group, and an equivocal caries-negative group. For the equivocal groups, it was assumed that a certain unknown percent of the time, greater than 50% the readers would correctly classify the image as carious if it were truly carious and not carious if it were truly not carious. The fifth group was assumed to be the indeterminate images for which there was exactly a 50% chance that the image would receive a caries-positive or a caries-negative judgment.

Differences in agreement rates among readers were assumed to be possible for the equivocal images. For example, one dentist could correctly detect caries in 80% of the true disease-positive cases while another dentist might only detect disease for 70% of the disease-positive cases. Unlike the model proposed by Agresti and Lang, their model did not have a restriction as to the functional form of the reader differences. That is, a reader could give a high proportion of caries-positive judgments for the equivocal positive images and a high proportion of caries-negative judgments for the equivocal negative images and could therefore be viewed as a better-than-average reader. Espeland and Handelman's model can be thought of as being comprised of a series of log-linear models, one for each subgroup of images. They also introduced the notion of relative sensitivity and specificity. The relative sensitivity was the rate of positive-carie judgments when the image belonged to a positive latent class (i.e., the perfect-agreement positive-caries subgroup or the equivocal positive-caries subgroup). The relative specificity was defined analogously for the readings of the negative-caries images). The prevalence of each level of the latent factor could also be estimated from the parameters of their models. They also formulated the idea that the levels of the latent factors could be thought of as the consensus diagnosis for subgroups of images.

17.4 Mixture distributions of binomials

Kundel and Polansky [3] used a mixture of binomials model to assess agreement. Each binomial distribution corresponds to a subgroup of images with its own rate of agreement. Typically four or five subgroups would be required to encompass the full variation in differences in the interpretability of images. The five subgroups would typically be a high-agreement disease-positive subgroup, a moderate-agreement disease positive, a very-low-agreement disease positive, a moderate-agreement disease negative, and a high-agreement disease negative. The readers are assumed to have the same agreement rates, so that the number of disease-positive readings has a binomial distribution with a rate of positive readings specific to the subgroup to which the image belongs.

The equation for the binomial distribution for the number of positive readings for a subgroup of images (subgroup i) with the same agreement rate of m_i, is shown below:

$$\text{Bin}(x, m_i; r) = \left(\frac{r!}{(r-x)!x!} \right) m_i^x (1 - m_i)^{r-x}, \qquad (17.4)$$

where x, the number of positive readings; r, the number of readers; m_i, rate of positive readings for the ith subgroup.

For example, if there are seven readers and an images is an easy disease-positive image (i.e., is a member of the fourth subgroup so $i = 4$) then the probability of 6 positive readings out of the 7 readings is.

Figure 17.2 shows a hypothetical mixture of four binomials for radiologic images. The bar height-represent the proportion of cases in each of the image subgroups. The most prevalent subgroup is the easy normals and the next most prevalent group is the easy disease-positives. Also note that the disease-positive cases are shown to have less agreement than the disease-negatives (the bars are closer to the center than for the negative cases), which is also commonly found in practice (and in the ER example above).

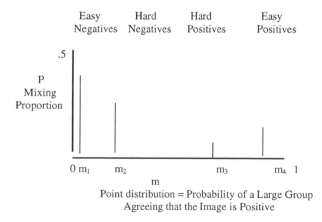

Figure 17.2: An example of a mixture distribution showing four point distributions for easy and hard positive and negative cases.

The general equation for a mixture of binomials with the number of subgroups denoted as 'I' (i.e., if $I = 5$ then there are five subgroups of cases) is shown below:

$$f(x; m_i, \ldots, m_I, p_i, \ldots, p_I, r) = \sum_{i=1}^{I} p_i \text{bin}(x; m_i, r), \qquad (17.5)$$

where x, the number of positive readings; r, then number of readers; m_i, parameter of ith binomial and p_i, mixing probability for the ith binomial and $p_I = 1 - (p_1 + p_1 + \cdots + p_{i-1})$.

The proportion of images (prevalence) belonging to the ith subgroup corresponds to the mixing parameter for the ith binomial (p_i). The expected proportion of positive readings for an image from the ith subgroup is p_i. The rate of agreement between a reader and the majority reading (relative agreement) is also m_i when m_i is greater than 0.5. (The majority diagnosis is disease positive since the binomial parameter is greater than 0.5 and the probability of a positive reading equals m_i for the binomial. Hence the probability of a reader agreeing with the majority is m_i.) If m_i is less then 0.5, then the majority reading is disease negative so that the agreement is: $1 - m_i$, since $1 - m_i$ is the probability of a disease negative reading. For example, if $m_1 = 0.2$ then only 20% of all readers would give a positive reading for images in subgroup i, while 80% (1–20%) would give a negative reading so that the majority reading is negative. The rate of agreement of one reader with the majority would also be 80% by the binomial assumption.

An estimate of the overall agreement rate (i.e., the percent agreement among a large number of radiologists for all subgroups of cases combined) can be obtained by taking a weighted average of the agreement rates of each subgroup as follows:

$$RPA = \sum_{i=1}^{I} p_i m_i^*, \qquad (17.6)$$

where

$$m_i^* = m_i \text{ if } m_i > 0.5; \quad m_i^* = 1 - m_i \text{ if } m_i \leqslant 0.5.$$

For example, we can consider the following hypothetical image set, which has four subgroups of images with the following estimated parameters for the mixing probabilities and the rates of positive readings (Table 17.8).

Then the overall percent agreement relative to the consensus (relative percent agreement or RPA) is

$$RPA = 0.40 * 0.99 + 0.15 * 0.75 + 0.10 * 0.65 + 0.35 * 0.94 = 0.90.$$

The number of readers limits the number of subgroups or binomial distributions which can be included in a mixture model. In general, if the number of parameters

Table 17.8: Hypothetical example of a four-component mixture distribution of binomials for agreement data

	Proportion (p_i)	Rate of Positive Readings (m_i)	Agreement Rate $(m_i^* = 1 - m_i)$
Easy disease negatives	0.40	0.01	0.99
Hard disease negative	0.15	0.25	0.75
Hard disease positives	0.10	0.65	0.65
Easy disease positives	0.35	0.94	0.06

in a model equal the number of data points, the model is saturated and the predicted values from the model will equal the observed data. If there are more parameters than data points, the estimates are not unique in that different sets of estimates of the parameters will give the same predicted values (which will also equal the observed values). The data for estimating mixtures of binomials is the frequency distribution of the number of positive readings. If there are r readers then there are $r + 1$ values for the number of positive readings (i.e., $0, 1, \ldots, r$). Each binomial, except the last binomial, which is included in the mixture distribution, has two parameters, the mixing proportion (p_i) and the binomial rate (m_i). Because the mixing proportions by definition always add to 1, the last binomial does not require a mixing proportion parameter, as the value of its mixing proportion is the others subtracted from 1 (Eq. (17.5)). Therefore the number of parameters in a mixture-of-binomials model is $I * 2 - 1$, where I is the number of binomials. It follows that the number of parameters, $I * 2 - 1$, must be less than or equal to $r + 1$ for the estimates to be unique. For example, if there are four readers ($r = 4$) than $r + 1 = 5$. For a three-component binomial mixture ($I = 3$), there are $I * 2 - 1 = 5$ parameters, so three binomials is the maximum number of parameters which can be included in the mixture distribution when there are four readers.

17.4.1 Emergency room study

This first example of the-use-of mixture distribution methodology (MDA) which we will present is for a study of agreement of a cross section of radiographs read in an emergency room to diagnose trauma or an acute disease process. One hundred patients were sequentially enrolled in the study to provide a representative sample of patients presenting to an emergency room in an academic medical center. Eight radiologists independently and in random order reviewed all the exams for the patient and then made a diagnosis as to the presence or absence of disease present, or whether it was equivocal. For the purposes of the analysis shown here, we combined the equivocal diagnoses with disease-positive images. The distribution of agreement is shown in Table 17.9.

Mixture distributions with varying numbers of component binomials were fit to the data and estimates for the parameters of the mixture distributions were obtained and are shown in Table 17.10.

Table 17.9: Distribution of ER images

	Number of Positive Readings									
	0	1	2	3	4	5	6	7	8	Total
Number of Images	35	17	8	7	3	6	4	6	14	100

Table 17.10: Mixture distribution for ER agreement study

Number of Binomials in Mixture	m_1	p_1	m_2	p_2	m_3	p_3	m_4	p_4	m_5	p_5	RPA
2	0.11	67.8	0.84	32.2							87.6
3	0.06	56.7	0.49	22.4	0.95	20.9					84.5
4	0.04	45.4	0.25	22.2	0.67	15.2	0.97	17.2			87.1
5 (saturated)	0.04	45.4	0.25	17.9	0.26	4.6	0.67	15.2	0.97	17.2	87.1

Table 17.11: Observed and expected percent of positive images

Number of Binomials in Mixture Distribution	Number of Positive Readings								
	0	1	2	3	4	5	6	7	8
(Observed)	35	17	8	7	3	6	4	6	14
2	28	26	11	3	1	3	8	12	8
3	34	19	7	6	6	5	3	7	14
4	35	17	9	6	4	5	5	6	14

Inspection of the parameters of the four-component mixture distribution shows that there is a large group of disease-negative images that have very high agreement (agreement rate of $1 - 0.04 = 0.96$ and which comprise approximately 70% of the disease-negative images) and the remaining disease-negative images having moderate agreement (a 75% agreement rate). There was less agreement for the disease-positive images. Approximately half of the disease-positive images had an agreement rate of only 67%. As can be seen, the two-component binomial mixture distribution did not provide a good fit for the observed readings (Table 17.11). The lack of fit was attributable to the predicted number of cases with all but one reader agreeing exceeding the observed number of cases with all but one reader agreeing. For example, there were only 17 cases with all but one negative reading while the estimated number from the two-component model was much larger (26). The three- and four-component-mixture models fit the data considerably better than the two-component-mixture model. The expected numbers of images with all but one agreeing (for disease positive and disease negative) were less for these models so that they were closer to the observed values. It is of interest that when the five component-binomial mixture was fit to the data, two of the binomials had almost identical rates (0.74 and 0.75 for the binomial rates respectively), which suggests that there are only four subgroups of distinct images.

The models, which we fit, all assumed discrete subgroups of homogenous images (within a disease category). The alternative model of Qu *et al.* assumes that the images in a disease category (i.e., the disease-positive category and the disease-negative category respectively) belong to one group with variation within the group. The variation in observed agreement rates is assumed to follow a normal distribution. This model would not fit this ER data because of the skewed (and therefore non-normal) distribution of reading rates. More specifically, the abrupt drop off in the number of images with all but one reader agreeing from all readers agreeing is a specific type of non-normality of the rates, which suggests bimodality (i.e., two distinct subgroups). However whether there are two distinct subgroups within each disease group or whether the distribution of agreement rates is just very highly skewed cannot be determine with certainty with the limited number of readings per image. However the four-subgroup model is consistent with subjective clinical experience that there is a large subgroup of disease-positive (disease-negative) images that is very easy to interpret and another group of disease-positive (disease-negative) images that is difficult to interpret. The empirical support for using the four-subgroup model is that it fits the data well. It also has the advantage of its ease of interpretation.

17.4.2 Musculoskeletal abnormalities

This second example is a comparison of analog film radiography and computed radiography. The cases consisted of 140 radiographs made for a variety of musculoskeletal abnormalities such as fractures, joint dislocations, bone neoplasms, arthritis, foreign bodies, and discrete soft-tissue tumors (courtesy of Larry T. Cook and Glendon G. Cox at the University of Kansas Medical Center). The images were rated on a 5-point scale with 5 = definitely abnormal. Because there were seven readers, it is possible to fit a mixture of four point distributions. We also explored the effect of varying the cut point used for classifying a reading as a positive reading. We used three different cutoffs for classifying an image as abnormal: $\geqslant 3$, $\geqslant 4$, and $\geqslant 5$. The distribution of the number of readers who classify each image as abnormal using each of these cutoffs is shown in Table 17.12.

We also computed 95% confidence intervals using the bootstrap method (Efron and Tibshirani [15]). The estimates and 95% confidence intervals for the parameters of the mixture distributions are shown in Table 7.13.

As can be seen, the estimated proportions of images with abnormal reports $(p_1 + p_2)$ decreases as the cutpoint is made more stringent (increased) and the proportion of normal reports increases. The RPA also increases as the cutoff is increased. Also of interest is that for the cut point of 2, m_3 and m_4 have approximately the same value (0.73 and 0.74 respectively), suggesting that only a three-binomial mixture distribution is needed to model agreement (for this cut point).

Table 17.12: Distribution of number of positive reports for musculoskeletal abnormalities

Cut point	Number (proportion) of Positive Reports							
	0	1	2	3	4	5	6	7
2	8 (0.06)	13 (0.09)	21 (0.15)	8 (0.06)	10 (0.07)	15 (0.11)	10 (0.07)	55 (0.39)
3	40 (0.29)	14 (0.10)	15 (0.11)	5 (0.04)	14 (0.10)	8 (0.06)	8 (0.06)	36 (0.26)
4	70 (0.50)	12 (0.09)	12 (0.09)	6 (0.04)	7 (0.05)	8 (0.06)	13 (0.09)	12 (0.09)

Table 17.13: Estimates and 95% CIs for parameters of a four component mixture distribution for readings of images of musculoskeletal abnormalities

a) Estimated Probabilities of Positive Readings for each Sub-population

Cut point	m_4	m_3	m_2	m_1
2	0.999(0.98–0.99)	0.73(0.62–0.81)	0.72(0.23–0.73)	0.24(6.4e–07–0.28)
3	0.99 (0.94–0.99)	0.64(0.41–0.72)	0.21(0.19–0.67)	0.007(1.23e–10–0.11)
4	0.86 (0.80–0.99)	0.41(0.21–0.79)	0.25(0.16–0.43)	0.009(1.58e–06–0.04)

b) Estimated Mixing Proportions

Cut point	p_4	p_3	p_2	p_1	Relative percent agreement (RPA)
2	0.36(0.27–0.46)	0.20(0.15–0.32)	0.08(0.04–0.36)	0.36(0.06–0.39)	0.84(0.30–0.87)
3	0.26(0.18–0.37)	0.23(0.12–0.31)	0.26(0.10–0.36)	0.25(0.20–0.51)	0.86(0.79–0.88)
4	0.25(0.05–0.29)	0.08(0.05–0.28)	0.17(0.08–0.31)	0.50(0.38–0.64)	0.88(0.85–0.92)

17.4.3 Application of the EM algorithm to compute the maximum likelihood estimates of the parameters of a binomial mixture

The EM algorithm [16] can be used to estimate the maximum likelihood estimates of the parameters of the mixture distribution. Agresti and Lang [10] (1993) discuss the use of the EM algorithm for the more general quasi-symmetric latent-class model of which the binomial mixture is a special case. We briefly describe the EM algorithm and provide the equations for estimating the parameters of a mixture of binomials.

To apply the EM algorithm, the observed data are viewed as being a part of a more complete data set, which has a more tractable likelihood than that of the observed data (and is the likelihood of the complete data, which is maximized). The EM algorithm has two steps, an expectation step and a maximization step. In the expectation step, the expected value of the missing data, given the observed data, is used in place of the missing data in the likelihood equation for the complete data. In the maximization step, the likelihood of the complete data is maximized.

Data from mixture distributions can be viewed as incomplete because we do not know which component distribution generated the data. If there are only a limited number of readers, say 4, and 3 out of 4 of these readers agree a case is disease positive, this could be a case from an easy subgroup or a hard subgroup. We could only determine with certainty which subgroup a case belongs to if there are many readers. The complete data are then the group membership of each object (which is unknown) and the multiple rating of each object (which is known). We can write the formula for the complete data most simply in terms of the number of positive ratings for the kth object (x_k) and by using the indicator variables z_{ik} where $z_{ik} = 1$ if the kth object is from the ith distribution. The likelihood is then as follows:

$$L(x_1, \ldots, x_K, z_{11}, \ldots, z_{1,K}, z_{I1}, \ldots, z_{I,K}) = \prod_{k=1}^{K} \prod_{i=1}^{I} (p_i \operatorname{Bin}(x_k; m_i, r))^{z_{ik}}.$$

$$(17.7)$$

Taking the log of the likelihood we find that each term includes only one parameter. Separate maximizations of the terms involving each parameter, give the following simple expressions for the parameters:

$$p_i = \Sigma z_{ik}/K \quad \text{and}$$
$$m_i = (\Sigma z_{ik} * x_k)/(r \Sigma z_{ik}) \quad \text{for } i = 1 \text{ to } I.$$

The expected value of the missing data given the observed data for the E step of the algorithm can be obtained in a straightforward manner using Bayes Theorem and is

$$E(z_{ik} = 1 \mid x = x_k, m_i; r)$$
$$= \operatorname{prob}(x = x_k, z_{ik} = 1; m_i, r)/\Sigma \operatorname{prob}(x = x_k, z_{ik} = 1; m_i, r),$$

$$(17.8)$$

where $\operatorname{prob}(x = x_k, z_{ik} = 1; m_i, r) = p_i * \operatorname{bin}(x = x_k; m_{i,}, r)$

The probability that an image is from subgroup i given it has a specified number of positive images is assumed to be the same for all images (i.e., prob($z_{i1} = 1$) = prob($z_{i2} = 1$) = $\cdots$ = prob($z_{iK} = 1$) so that the expression can also be written as:

$$E(z_{ik} = 1 \mid x = x_k, m_i; r) = E(z_i = 1 \mid x, m_i; r) = \frac{\text{prob}(x, z_i = 1; m_i, r)}{\Sigma \text{prob}(x, z_i = 1; m_i, r)},$$

where $x = x_k$.

The advantage of this latter equation is that it highlights that the expected values do not need to be computed individually for every image since all images with the same number of disease positive readings will have the same conditional expectations.

Because z_{ik} takes on the value of one if the case is from the ith subgroup and is 0 otherwise, the above conditional expected value of z_{ik} is the expected proportion of images which would come from subgroup i among images with the same number of positive readings (as the kth image). (This is analogous to the mean equalling the proportion of ones, when the data include only the values of zero and one.) Stated concisely, the above conditional expectation is the conditional probability of an image belonging to subgroup i given the observed number of positive readings for that image.

The EM algorithm then involves selecting starting values for the parameters of the mixture distribution, computing the $E(z_i = 1 \mid x, m_i; r)$'s and then computing new estimates of the parameters of the mixture distribution. In the next iteration of the EM algorithm, the expected values of the missing data are recomputed using the estimates of the parameters from the previous iteration and then the parameters of the mixture distribution are re-estimated. Subsequently, in each iteration of the EM algorithm, the estimates of the parameters from the previous iteration are used in computing new expected values of the missing data and new estimates of the parameters. We will refer to the present iteration as the $p + 1$ iteration and the previous iteration (from which the estimates of the parameters are obtained) as the pth iteration. The steps of the EM algorithm are shown below:

Step 1 of the $p + 1$ iteration: Computing expected values of missing data (i.e., expected proportions in each subgroup):

Compute the estimates of the probabilities that an image belongs to subgroups $1, 2, \ldots, I$ given the number of positive readings are $0, 1, \ldots, r$ respectively using the values for the parameters of the mixture distribution from the previous iteration. In the first iteration, the starting values for the parameters are used instead of estimates from the previous iteration. The equation for the expected values of the missing data in the $p + 1$ iteration based on the estimates of the parameters from the previous iteration (pth iteration) of the algorithm is shown below:

$$\widehat{E}^{p+1}(z_i = 1 \mid x; \widehat{m}_i^p, r)$$
$$= \hat{p}_i^p \text{bin}(x; \widehat{m}_i^p, r) / \sum_i \hat{p}_i^p \text{bin}(x; \widehat{m}_i^p, r) \quad \text{for } i = 1 \text{ to } I \quad \text{and } x = 0 \text{ to } r.$$

Step 2 of the $(p + 1)$th iteration: Computing new estimates of the binomial parameters and mixing probabilities:

Compute the $(p+1)$th iteration estimates of the parameters of the binomial mixture distribution after substituting in the estimated conditional expected values for the unknown z_i's as follows:

$$\hat{p}_i^{p+1} = \sum_l n_l \widehat{E}^{p+1}(z_i \mid l; m_i^p, r)/K$$

$$\widehat{m}_i^{p+1} = \sum_l l n_l \widehat{E}^{p+1}(z_i \mid l; m_i^p, r)/r\hat{p}_i^{p+1} K \quad \text{for } i = 1 \text{ to } I, \qquad (17.9)$$

where n_l, number of images with l positive readings.

The above two steps are repeated until the algorithm converges.

Because the EM algorithm does not always converge to the global maximum (i.e., the MLE), it is necessary to try different starting values. Our experience using the algorithm has shown that if any values of $\widehat{m}_i$ are 0 or 1 then the algorithm has likely not converged to the MLE. Also if the $\widehat{m}_i$ switch order (in terms of magnitude) from their order as starting values, the algorithm is likely to have converged to a local maximum. Different starting values should then be tried.

We illustrate the use of the EM algorithm for the agreement study with eight readers done in an emergency room (Table 17.9). Specifically, we sketch the use of the EM algorithm to estimate the parameters of the four component binomial mixture distribution given in Table 17.10. We start with starting values for the parameters which reflect our prior knowledge that one of the four groups typically is a high-agreement group of disease negative images and another group is a high-agreement disease positives (hence $m_1 = 0.01$ and $m_4 = 0.99$). Also we set one of the two middle binomial parameters to be less than 0.5 and one to be greater than 0.5 because we anticipate that there might be a group of low-agreement disease-positive cases and a group of low-agreement disease-negatives cases (Table 17.14).

We will illustrate the use of EM algorithm to compute the MLE estimates of p_1 and m_1, which are the rate of disease-positive readings, and the proportion of cases in the high-agreement disease-negative group. In the course of showing the computations, we will also provide an intuitive basis for the various formulas

Table 17.14: Starting values for EM algorithm

Binomial(i)	p_i	m_i
1	0.4	0.01
2	0.1	0.4
3	0.3	0.84
4	0.2	0.99

that are used. In the first step of the EM algorithm, the expected values of the missing data (i.e., the probability or expected proportion of cases belonging to each subgroup based on the number of positive readings for the case) are computed. These expected proportions are computed for no positive readings, two positive readings, and up to all r readers agreeing. We will illustrate this computation for the expected proportion of cases belonging to subgroup 1 for those cases with no positive readings. Obtaining this expectation (which is a conditional expectation because it is the expected proportion belonging to subgroup 1 given the observed number of positive readings), involves using Bayes Theorem (Eq. (17.8)). Bayes Theorem enables one to obtain a conditional probability (which is unknown) using the reverse conditional probability (which is assumed to be known). In this case, we know the probability that a case has no positive readings given the case belongs to subgroup 1 but we do not know the probability that a case belongs to subgroup 1 given it has no positive readings (until we apply Bayes Theorom). In order to use Bayes Theorem, the (joint) probability that a case belongs to subgroup i and had no agreement is computed for all the i subgroups (using the multiplication rule of probability and multiplying the probability that a case belongs to subgroup i by the probability these is no agreement given it belongs to subgroup i). These joint probabilities can be most easily obtained by making a table with the $\hat{p}_i^0$'s and $\widehat{m}_i^0$'s, computing the probabilities of no positive readings ($x = 0$) for the binomial distributions corresponding to each subgroup of images (i.e., for each i) and then multiplying each binomial probability by the proportion of cases in the subgroup as shown (Table 17.15).

Bayes Theorom is then used to computed the desired expected (conditional) proportion (which for the sake of this example is the expected proportion of cases belonging to subgroup 1 given there were no positive readings). The numerator of Bayes equation is the expected proportion of cases with no positive readings and who are from subgroup 1 and the denominator is the sum of the expected proportions for all the subgroups so we can obtain the expected proportion of cases belonging to subgroup 1 if there are no positive readings as follows:

$$\widehat{E}^{p+1}(z_1 = 1 \mid x; \widehat{m}_1^0, 8) = \frac{\hat{p}_1^0 \text{bin}(x; \widehat{m}_1^0, 8)}{\sum_i \hat{p}_1^0 \text{bin}(x; \widehat{m}_1^0, 8)} = 0.369/0.371 = 0.995.$$

Table 17.15: Computations to obtain expected values

i	$\hat{p}_i^0$	$\widehat{m}_i^0$	$\text{bin}(x = 0; \widehat{m}_i^0, 8)$	$\text{bin}(x = 0; \widehat{m}_i^0, 8)\hat{p}_i^0$
1	0.4	0.01	0.923	0.369
2	0.1	0.4	0.017	0.0016
3	0.2	0.84	0	0
4	0.3	0.99	0	0
sum				3708

As can be seen, the expected value for the 1st mixture is 0.995, that is, if 8 of the 8 readings were disease negative for a case then the probability that the case would have come from the mixture distribution with the disease positive reading rate of 0.01 (i.e., the high-agreement disease-negative group) is almost a certainty (0.995).

The expected conditional probabilities of a case belonging to the first binomial for each possible number of positive readings are needed for the second step of the EM algorithm and can be obtained similarly as was done for $x = 0$. These expectations are shown in the first column below (Table 17.16) and are used in the second step of the EM algorithm.

In the second step of the EM algorithm we compute the estimates of $\hat{p}_1^1$'s and $\widehat{m}_1^1$ (Eq. (17.8)) so that

$$\hat{p}_1^1 = \sum_l n_l \widehat{E}^1(z_i \mid l; m_i^0, 8)/100 = 48.285/100 = 0.48,$$

and

$$\widehat{m}_1^1 = \sum_l ln_l \widehat{E}^1(z_i \mid l; m_i^0, r)/r\hat{p}_1^1 K = 13.85/(8 \cdot 0.48 \cdot 100) = 0.36.$$

The computation of the estimates for all four binomial distributions (in the mixture distribution) would complete the first iteration of EM algorithm. These estimates are used in the second iteration to obtain new expected values for the missing data and in turn new estimates of the binomial parameters. Further iterations would then be done until the algorithm converged.

17.4.4 The number of images and readers that are required for the MDA method

We simulated a reading study to determine the means and standard errors of the estimates of RPA for different numbers of images and readings. Our interest in determining the mean of the estimates of the RPA was to determine if the estimated RPA was unbiased. The standard errors can be used to determine how much sampling error there is in the estimated RPA. For simplicity we used a three-binomial mixture distribution. The outer two groups were assumed to be images for which there was agreement beyond chance and they were assumed to have the same agreement rate and in equal proportions. The middle group was assumed to be an indeterminate group so that the agreement rate (with the consensus) was set to 0.5 (i.e., guessing). The proportion of images in the indeterminate group was set at proportions ranging from 0 to 30%. The values of m and p which corresponded to a specified RPA (which are unique under the above assumptions) and were determined using an equation which was derived for this purpose. RPAs ranging from 70% to 90% were simulated.

As can be seen in Table 17.14, the mean estimated values of RPA was relatively close to the true RPA value for most values of RPA of interest (generally

Table 17.16: Computations to obtain parameter estimates for the 1st binomial (in mixture distribution)

j	$\widehat{E}^{p+1}(z_1=1 \mid x=j; \widehat{m}_1^0, 8)$	n_j	$n_j \widehat{E}^{p+1}(z_1=1 \mid x=j; \widehat{m}_1^0, 8)$	$n_j j \widehat{E}^{p+1}(z_1=1 \mid x=j; \widehat{m}_1^0, 8)$
0	0.995	35	34.825	0
1	0.769	17	13.073	13.073
2	0.0478	8	0.3824	0.7648
3	0.0007	7	0.0049	0.0147
4	0	3	0	
5	0	6	0	
6	0	4	0	
7	0	6	0	
8	0	14	0	
sum			48.2853	13.8525

within 1). As be seen in Table 17.14, increasing from four to six readers greatly decreased the variance of the RPA. For example, with six readers and 200 images, an RPA of 0.90, and 10% indeterminate images, the standard error of the RPA is 1.25. When there were only four readers, then between 400 and 500 images will provide the same standard error as 200 images. Thus a reading study with 6 readers and 200 to 300 images (each read using both modalities) would be sufficient to compare two diagnostic modalities with high agreement rates (i.e., about 90% (e.g., a difference in RPA of about 5 would be detectable) and would be preferable to a four-reader study (because the total number of readings needed would be less for the former). If the agreement rate is low (80%), 400 to 500 images with six readers would be needed to detect a difference of 5 percentage points. When there are more that four subgroups, more readers will be needed to insure that there is a unique solution for the MLE. We have found there to be five subgroups on occasion (the very-high-agreement disease-positive and disease-negative cases, the equivocal disease-positive and disease-negative cases and the indeterminate group). In this case the minimum number of readers required would be nine. More readers are also advantageous because this allows for greater generalizability of the results of the study to other readers. We have not yet determined how many readings and images are needed to statistically compare individual parameters (m's and p's) of the mixture distribution between two modalities.

17.4.5 Bootstrap confidence intervals

As discussed, bootstrap confidence intervals can be computed for the RPA. The bootstrap is a resampling method that can be used to standardize errors and construct confidence intervals for estimates of parameters. Briefly, the bootstrap method involves repeatedly taking samples from the data with replacement. The same size samples are taken as the original sample. The RPA is computed for each of these samples and the 95th percentile and the 5th percentile are the upper and lower ends of the 95% confidence interval (Efron [17] and Efron and Tibshirani [15]).

17.4.6 Using MDA to determine the relative percent agreement of a diagnostic test for a different population (adjusted RPA)

The agreement rate (with the consensus) is typically greater for disease negative images than it is for disease positive images. Therefore the overall agreement rate will generally depend on the prevalence of disease. It may be of interest to estimate the (overall) agreement rate for a population with a different disease prevalence. This can easily be done using the MDA because the model is parameterized in terms of subgroups of images. The subgroups with consensus of disease positive are collectively the disease positive images so that the sum of their prevalences (as estimated in the MDA) is the prevalence of disease. The only further assumption that is needed in order to estimate the RPA for the new prevalence (adjusted RPA) is that the relative proportions in each disease positive subgroup in the new population is the same as that in the original population (the analogous assumption must

Table 17.17: Expected values and standard errors of RPA for four and six readings

Four Readings

N	Fixed RPC = 0.90		Fixed RPC = 0.80		
	p_2		p_2		
	0%	10%	0%	10%	20%
100	89.4 (2.0)[1,2]	90.0 (3.0)	78.1 (3.6)	79.1 (3.7)	81.0 (3.7)
200	89.6 (1.3)	89.9 (1.8)	78.4 (2.7)	79.3 (2.8)	80.9 (2.9)
300	89.7 (1.1)	89.9 (1.4)	78.6 (2.3)	79.4 (2.5)	80.9 (2.5)
400	89.7 (1.0)	89.9 (1.3)	78.8 (2.1)	79.5 (2.2)	80.9 (2.2)
500	89.7 (0.8)	89.8 (1.1)	79.9 (1.9)	79.6 (2.0)	80.9 (2.0)

Fixed RPC = 0.70

	p_2				
N	0%	10%	20%	30%	40%
100	67.0 (4.5)	67.9 (4.4)	69.3 (4.2)	70.9 (4.3)	71.7 (4.4)
200	67.1 (3.4)	67.9 (3.5)	69.2 (3.6)	70.6 (3.8)	71.2 (3.9)
300	67.2 (3.1)	67.9 (3.3)	69.2 (3.3)	70.6 (3.4)	70.9 (3.5)
400	67.2 (3.0)	67.9 (3.0)	69.2 (3.1)	70.6 (3.3)	70.8 (3.3)
500	67.2 (2.8)	67.9 (2.9)	69.2 (3.0)	70.6 (3.1)	70.7 (3.1)

Six Readings

N	Fixed RPC = 0.90		Fixed RPC = 0.80		
	p_2		p_2		
	0%	10%	0%	10%	20%
100	89.9 (1.57)	90.5 (1.87)	79.4 (2.13)	80.3 (2.12)	82.0 (2.37)
200	89.9 (1.08)	90.3 (1.25)	79.5 (1.55)	80.3 (1.85)	81.9 (1.74)
300	89.9 (1.00)	90.3 (1.02)	79.6 (1.37)	80.3 (1.57)	81.7 (1.52)
400	89.9 (0.69)	90.2 (1.04)	79.6 (1.13)	80.3 (1.31)	81.6 (1.50)
500	89.9 (0.60)	90.2 (0.86)	79.6 (0.93)	80.3 (1.30)	81.5 (1.28)

Fixed RPC = 0.70

	p_2				
N	0%	10%	20%	30%	40%
100	68.2 (3.19)	69.1 (3.19)	70.5 (3.07)	72.0 (3.21)	72.4 (3.38)
200	68.3 (2.50)	69.1 (2.45)	70.5 (2.49)	71.9 (2.53)	72.1 (2.74)
300	68.4 (2.13)	69.2 (2.24)	70.5 (2.16)	71.8 (2.26)	71.9 (2.31)
400	68.4 (1.98)	69.2 (1.90)	70.4 (2.02)	71.7 (2.05)	71.8 (2.19)
500	68.5 (1.92)	69.2 (1.86)	70.4 (1.94)	71.7 (1.90)	71.7 (2.01)

[1] Mean(SD).
[2] The means and standard deviations are based on 40,000 simulations.

be made for the disease negative subgroups). The formula for this 'prevalence-adjusted rate' (RPA_{adj}) for a four-binomial mixture is shown in Eq. (17.10):

$$RPA_{adj} = \frac{m_1 * (1 - prev) * p_1}{(p_1 + p_2)} + \frac{m_2 * (1 - prev) * p_2}{(p_1 + p_2)}$$
$$+ \frac{m_3 * prev * p_3}{(p_3 + p_4)} + \frac{m_4 * prev * p_4}{(p_3 + p_4)}, \quad (17.10)$$

where prev, disease prevalence in the new population.

Returning to the earlier hypothetical example, (Table 17.8) of a four-component mixture distribution, we can compute the RPA if the disease prevalence is 20% (prev $= 0.20$) rather than the original prevalence 45% (the prevalence was obtained from adding the proportion of hard disease-positive and easy disease-positive images which were 0.10 and 0.35 from Table 17.8)

$$RPA_{adj} = \frac{0.99 * (1 - 0.2) * 0.4}{(0.4 + 0.15)} + \frac{75 * (1 - 0.2) * 0.15}{(0.4 + 0.15)}$$
$$+ \frac{0.65 * 0.2 * 0.10}{(0.10 + 0.35)} + \frac{0.94 * 0.2 * 0.35}{(0.10 + 0.35)} = 0.92.$$

Note that the new relative percent agreement is slightly greater than the original RPA (0.92 vs 0.90) because the prevalence of the disease was reduced and the agreement was higher disease-positive cases than for disease-negative cases.

A caution with this approach is that the relative proportions of high- and low-agreement cases within disease categories (disease positive and disease negative) may also differ in the new population relative to the original population. Depending on how great this difference waserror could be introduced into the adjusted RPA.

These adjusted RPA are similar in concept to adjusted rates in epidemiological studies. For example, in an epidemiological study of skin cancer it may be of interest to determine the increase in rates resulting from sun exposure. For this purpose it would be of interest to compare the rates of a disease (e.g., skin cancer) in a northern and southern populations (e.g., residents of Florida vs residents of Pennsylvania). However if the age distribution is different in the two populations, there will be a difference in rates caused by age as well as sun exposure (the risk factor of interest). Age-adjusted disease rates can be computed for each population by assuming the same age distribution for both populations and using (age) strata-specific disease rates (this is referred to as the direct method of adjustment). In this case instead of adjusting for age, we are adjusting for disease prevalence, but otherwise the method is identical.

17.5 Summary

Agreement studies can provide useful information about the diagnostic value of tests including how many readings will reliably provide a diagnosis that would be consistent with the diagnosis of the majority of similarly trained individuals.

An early measure of agreement, Kappa, although it has the advantage that it can be calculated when there are only two readers, cannot distinguish between (relative) sensitivity and specificity and is confounded by prevalence. As discussed, because of this confounding, it is not meaningful to compare Kappas when Kappas are computed for populations with different prevalences. Although Kappa is commonly referred to as chance-corrected agreement, this is a misnomer. Kappa is a measure of the relative improvement in agreement over a certain type of guessing, and consequently Kappa values will be smaller than agreement values. As we have shown, a diagnostic test with very high accuracy could have only a modest Kappa when the disease prevalence is low.

Modeling agreement can increase our understanding of agreement. Most models of agreement can be used to assess the agreement of a reader(s) with a hypothetical majority of readers with similar training and experience. The agreement of one reader with the 'consensus of the diagnostic community' is more relevant to diagnostic medicine than whether two readers agree with each other. However, modeling agreement requires multiple readers because a realistic model for agreement will be more complex. One complexity is that the agreement rate may differ among subgroups of images. The MDA methodology provides a way to identify subgroups of images that differ in ease of interpretation as well as providing an overall measure of agreement.

References

[1] Revesz G, Kundel HL, Bonitatibus M. "The Effect of Verification on the Assessment of Imaging Techniques." Investigative Radiology 18(2):194–197, 1983.

[2] Greenes RA, Begg CB. "Assessment of Diagnostic Technologies: Methodology for Unbiased Estimation from Samples of Selectively Verified Patients." Academic Radiology 751–756, 1985.

[3] Kundel HL, Polansky M. "Mixture Distribution and Operating Characteristic Analysis of Portable Chest Imaging Using Screen-Film and Computed Radiography." Academic Radiology 4:1–7, 1997.

[4] Hillman BJ, Hessel SJ, Swenson RG, Herman PG. "Improving Diagnostic Accuracy: A Comparative Study of Interactive and Delphi Consultations." Investigative Radiology 12:112–115, 1977.

[5] Cohen J. "A Coefficient of Agreement for Nominal Scales." Educational and Psych Meas 20:37–46, 1960.

[6] Aickin M. "Maximum Likelihood Estimation of Agreement in the Constant Predictive Probability Model and Its Relation to Cohen's Kappa." Biometrics 46:293–302, 1990.

[7] Hui S, Walters SD. "Estimating the Error Rates of Diagnostic Tests." Biometrics 36:167–171, 1980.

[8] Espeland MA, Handelman SL. "Using Latent Class Models to Characterize and Assess Relative Error in Discrete Measurements." Biometrics 45:587–599, 1989.

[9] Qu Y, Tan M, Kutner MH. "Random Effects Models in Latent Class Analysis for Evaluating Accuracy of Diagnostic Tests. Biometrics 52:797–810, 1996.

[10] Agresti A, Lang JB. "Quasi-Symmetric Latent Class Models with Application to Rater Agreement." Biometrics 49:131–139, 1993.

[11] Feinstein AR, Cicchetti DV. "High Agreement but Low Kappa: I. The Problems of Two Paradoxes." J Clin Epidemiol 43:543–549, 1990.

[12] Swets J. "Form of Empirical ROCs in Discrimination and Diagnostic Tasks: Implications for Theory and Measurement of Performance." Psychological Bulletin 88:181–198, 1986.

[13] Cohen J. "Weighted Kappa: Nominal Scale Agreement with Provision for scaled Disagreement or Partial Credit." Psychol Bull 70:213–220, 1968.

[14] Landis JR, Koch G. "An Application of Hierachical Kappa-Type Statistics in the Assessment of Majority Agreement Among Multiple Observers." Biometrics 33:363–374, 1977.

[15] Efron B, Tibshirani RJ. *An Introduction to the Bootstrap.* Chapman Hall, 1993, Chapter 14, pp. 185–186.

[16] Dempster A, Laird N, Rubin D. "Maximum Likelihood from Incomplete Data Via the EM Algorithm." J Royal Stat Soc B39:1–38, 1977.

[17] Efron B. "Better Bootstrap Confidence Intervals." JASA 82:171–185, 1987.

[18] Begg CB, Metz. "CE Consensus Diagnoses and 'Gold Standards' (Commentary on Henkelman)." Medical Decision Making 10:129–31, 1990.

[19] Epstein DM, Dalinkas MK, Kaplan FS, Aronchick JM, Marinelli DL, Kundel HL. "Observer Variation in the Detection of Osteopenia." Skeletal Radiol 15:347–349, 1986.

[20] Henkelman RM, Kay I, Bronskill MJ. "Receiver Operator Characterisic (ROC) Analysis with Truth." Medical Decision Making 10(1):24–29, 1996.

[21] Fletcher EWL, Griffiths GJ, Williams LA, McLachlan MSF. "Observer Variation in Assessing Renal Scarring." BJ Radiol 53:428–431, 1980.

[22] Gilchrist J. "QROC Curves and Kappa Functions: New Methods for Evaluating the Quality of Clinical Decisions." Opthal Physiol 12:350–360, 1992.

[23] Herman PG, Khan A, Kallman CE, Rojas KA, Carmody DP, Bodenheimer MM. "Limited Correlation of Left Ventricular End-Diastolic Pressure with Radiographic Assessment of Pulminary Hemodynamics." Radiology 174:721–724, 1990.

[24] Jannarone RJ, Macera CA, Garrison CZ. "Evaluating Inter-Rater Agreement Through 'Case-Control' Sampling." Biometrics 43:433–437, 1987.

[25] Kerr M. "Issues in the Use of Kappa." Invest Radiol 26:78–83, 1991.

[26] Kraemer H. "Assessment of 2 × 2 Associations: Generalization of Signal Detection Methodology." The American Statistician 42:37–49, 1988.

[27] Markus JB, Somers S, Franic SE, Moola C, Stevenson GW. "Inter-Observer Variation in the Interpretation of Abdominal Radiographs." Radiology 171:69–71, 1989.

[28] Musch DC, Landis JR, Higgins ITT, Gilson JC, Jones RN. "An Application of Kappa-Type Analyses to Inter-Observer Variation in Classifying Chest Radiographs for Pneumoconiosis." Stats in Med 3:73–83, 1984.

[29] Oden N.L. "Estimating Kappa from Binocular Data." Stats in Med 10:1303–1311, 1991.

[30] Titterington DM, Smith AFM, Makov UE. *Statistical Analysis of Finite Mixture Distributions*. Wiley, 1995.

[31] Ubersax JS, Grove, WM. "Statistical Modeling of Expert Ratings on Medical Treatment Appropriateness." JASA 88:421–427, (1993).

[32] Wackerly DD, McClave JT, Rao PV. "Measuring Nominal Scale Agreement Between a Judge and a Known Standard." Psychometrika 43(2):213–223, 1978.

CHAPTER 18
Visual Search in Medical Images

Harold L. Kundel
University of Pennsylvania School of Medicine

CONTENTS

18.1 Introduction

18.1.1 Definition of search tasks

Searching is a common human activity. We search for a book in the library by looking systematically along the shelves; we search for a friend in a crowd by looking for a familiar face; we search for a pin on the floor by crawling around and feeling for the pin. The common elements in search tasks are a known object that is the purpose of the search, some knowledge about how and where the object is hidden, and a deliberate concentration on the performance of search. In technical terms, search involves a target, prior-knowledge about the target-background relationship, and selective attention. Visual search implies that the visual perceptual system is being used to conduct the search.

18.1.2 Searching for targets in medical images

This chapter will focus on searching for small targets in medical images. Tumors are commonly used as targets in studies of visual search because they rank highly among the abnormalities that are overlooked by radiologists in everyday practice [1]. An investigator who wishes to study tumor detection can find many examples of tumors that are small and inconspicuous. (The terms "nodule" and "mass" are frequently used when referring to tumors and will be used interchangeably in this chapter without any specific nuance of meaning implied. They are all solid lumps of tissue. Nodule is frequently used for lung and liver tumors whereas mass is used for to breast tumors.) However, images with naturally occurring tumors may not be entirely suitable for use as stimuli because the tumors may either occur in combination with other distracting abnormalities or may vary too much in physical characteristics. To overcome these disadvantages, tumors are frequently simulated on carefully chosen background images. Simulation makes available large numbers of tumors with well defined physical characteristics that can be placed anywhere on selected backgrounds. Pulmonary nodules have been simulated on chest images optically [2, 3] and digitally [4, 5]. Microcalcifications and masses have been simulated on mammograms [6] and tumors have been simulated in computed tomograms of the liver [7]. Some critics have argued that simulated lesions are not sufficiently authentic because subtle characteristics might not be included [8]. As a response to such criticism and using the power of computer-illustration programs, investigators have cut lesions out of abnormal images and transplanted them into normal images to produce "hybrids" that come closer to reality than directly synthesized lesions [6].

18.1.3 Imaging tasks

Search is an important part of many of the more general tasks carried out by diagnostic radiologists. Diagnostic imaging tasks can be divided roughly into the five categories shown in Table 18.1: detection, comparison, location, classification, and estimation. Detection and location certainly involve search, and the other tasks might involve search as well.

Table 18.1:   Common diagnostic imaging tasks

Detection	Presence or absence of an abnormality; Yes-No or Rating Scale.
Comparison	Change in appearance; Same-Different, Greater Than or Less Than.
Location (Staging)	Determine the anatomical extent of a known abnormality.
Classification	Assign an abnormality to a predefined class of objects.
Estimation	Quantify the size, shape, or intensity of an object.

18.1.4 The nature of visual search

If you look straight ahead, objects in the center of the field are seen with greater clarity. Although you are aware of objects extending in a broad ellipse about the center of the field of view, they are not distinct. In order to see something in the peripheral part of the visual field more distinctly you can either move your eyes, your head, or, more commonly, both. When searching an image, the visual system is involved in two activities, examining the retinal image for the target and scanning the eyes over the image. These activities are necessary because the retinal field of view, although very broad, is not uniformly sensitive to stimuli. An understanding of the anatomical and physiological organization of the visual system can be helpful for understanding the complex interplay of examining the retinal image and shifting the axis of the gaze. The next section will briefly review some of the salient features of visual system organization.

18.2 The organization of the visual system

18.2.1 The retinal sensory array

The retina consists of a roughly hexagonal mosaic of two types of sensory cells called rods and cones. The rods are sensitive to low levels of light intensity but not to color. They are used primarily for night (scotopic) vision. The cones are used for daylight (photopic) and color vision. There are three types of cone with spectral sensitivity in the long (red), middle (green), and short (blue) wavelength part of the visible spectrum. The 10^6 cones and 10^8 rods of the primate retina are non-uniformly distributed over the surface. A small area on the axis of the gaze in the center of the retina called the fovea centralis, or simply the fovea, contains only densely packed cones. The packing density decreases toward the peripheral retina and is correlated with spatial resolution, which is greatest in the fovea and decreases steeply toward the periphery. The foveal cones are spaced at about 2 to 2.5 μm, and human beings can resolve two points that are about 5.5 μm apart on the fovea. This amounts to about 1 minute of arc or 0.15 mm at 60 cm. At this distance, the fovea subtends about 2 deg of visual angle, which is about equivalent to the size of a quarter held at arms length. The bottom illustrations in Figure 18.1. indicate the approximate size of the foveal field when a chest image is viewed at about 60 cm.

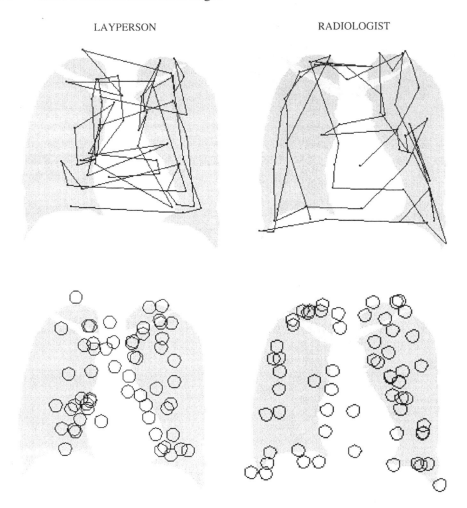

Figure 18.1: Scanpaths (top) and foveal fixation distributions (bottom) of a layperson and a radiologist looking at a normal chest radiograph for about 20 s.

The rods and cones make multiple synapses with other cells in the retina. Although there are many lateral connections, the main pathway from the sensory cells to the interior of the brain is by way of bipolar cells which, in turn, connect with the ganglion cells whose axons form the optic nerves that course from the retinas to the lateral geniculate bodies in the brain. The stimulus from the roughly 10^8 sensory cells is conducted to the lateral geniculate bodies by about 10^6 ganglion cells. The convergence of the neural pathways is explained by the organization of the sensory mosaic into roughly circular receptive fields that feed into the ganglion cells. The response from a stimulus applied to cells in the center of the field is modified by the stimulus applied to the surrounding field and the combined response is transmitted to a single ganglion cell. Neurophysiologists have identified two types of ganglion cell (large and small) that perform different functions and that project to different layers of the six-layered lateral geniculate nucleus. The magnocellular system (large cells) is color blind, has high contrast sensitivity, fast temporal resolution, and low spatial resolution; while the parvocellular system (small cells) is color selective, has low contrast sensitivity, slow temporal resolution, and high spatial resolution [9]. The major point to be made here is that the retina is not a passive array of sensors that passes information to other centers in the brain for processing but rather is an active neural network that achieves considerable functional differentiation at an early stage of visual processing.

18.2.2 The retinal image and the perceived field of view

Although the entire visual field of view is perceived to be of equal clarity, the center of the field has the greatest resolving power and there is a gradual decrease in the visibility of objects by the peripheral vision. This results partly from the physical structure of the retinal sensory array and partly from the neural connections to the visual cortex that favor the foveal cones. The dominance of the central vision for the visibility of details can be demonstrated easily by looking at the words in the center of a printed page and trying to read words at the edges of the page without moving the eyes. This phenomenon is expressed as a decrease in spatial resolving power from the center to the edge of the retina. There is also a decrease in the perception of low-contrast objects by the peripheral retina. The detectability of low-contrast objects is a smoothly varying function of visual eccentricity [10]. This is illustrated for pulmonary nodules in Figure 18.2(a). Even though the sensitivity of the retina decreases smoothly, albeit nonlinearly, with retinal eccentricity, for convenience many investigators divide the visual field into the central (or foveal) and the peripheral vision and attribute different functions to each. Using this model, the scanning component of visual search is conceptualized as a spotlight that is moved over the scene. An immediate question that arises is how large to make the spotlight. That is, how large a field size should be used in order to be sure that all of the targets are detected? This has led to the concept of a functional or useful visual field [11] that is moved over the scene by eye and head movement. The spotlight model is useful for explaining some scanning behavior especially with tasks that require rectilinear scanning such as reading. It is less useful when trying to explain search tasks involving more complicated images because it neglects the activity of the peripheral vision. In addition, there is no anatomical or neurophysiological support for such a model. The retina is not divided into two zones and there is no neurophysiological data to support a functional differentiation into central and peripheral retina. Kundel and Nodine [12, 13] have conceptualized search in terms of a global-focal search model that combines a preliminary analysis of the total retinal image with specific analysis of selected locations by the fovea. The global-focal model considers perception as an hypothesis-testing, decision-oriented process as proposed by Gregory and Rock [14, 15]. This will be discussed in more detail in Section 18.2.4.

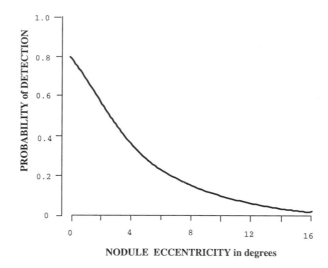

Figure 18.2a: The probability of detecting a pulmonary nodule as a function of nodule displacement (eccentricity) from the fixation point. The data are averaged over two readers. The nodules were about 1 cm in diameter and had a contrast of about 5%. Their probability of detection was 80% when viewed for 360 ms. Taken from Carmody *et al.* [10].

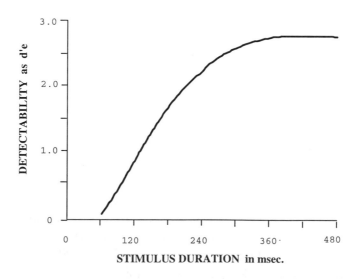

Figure 18.2b: The detectability of a 1 cm, 5% contrast pulmonary nodule as a function of the duration of the exposure to the stimulus within a single fixation. The detectability is expressed as the index of detectability d'e. The data are taken from Carmody *et al.* [10].

18.2.3 The fixation as the fundamental unit of visual processing

Moving the head and eyes largely compensates for the limitations of contrast sensitivity and resolving power resulting from the anatomy of the retinal sensory array and the functional differentiation of the neural network of the retina. The six muscles that control each eye are capable of producing very intricate movements. Most of the movements can be divided into three broad categories called fine saccades, coarse saccades, and smooth pursuit movements [16, 17]. The coarse saccades are the high-velocity ballistic movements that rapidly jump the axis of the gaze from place to place. The saccades are interspersed with fixations that average between 200 to 300 ms in duration. The fixation is the fundamental unit of visual information processing. The image projected onto the retina is processed during each fixation. Although perception seems instantaneous, the brain actually requires time to process visual information both within fixations and over a number of fixations. The processing within a single fixation can be demonstrated by using an exposure to a display that is only a fraction of the duration of a fixation [12, 18, 19] or by suddenly modifying a display of text in the middle of a fixation [20]. Experiments using a brief exposure utilize a device called a tachistoscope and show that when the duration of the exposure is very short, less than 30 ms, only simple or very familiar objects can be recognized. As the exposure duration is increased, more complicated objects and more details can be identified. The experiments are done by having the viewer push a button while looking at a small dot in the center of a uniformly illuminated display. When the button is pushed, the test image flashes on for a short time and is followed immediately by a masking stimulus consisting of a random pattern that acts to erase the previous stimulus from the visual short-term memory. An experiment was done to determine how much a radiologist can identify in a chest image in one fixation [12]. Three radiologists and 7 radiology residents were shown 22 PA chest images, 5 with abnormal lungs, 5 with abnormally shaped hearts, and 12 with no abnormalities. In a 200-ms exposure, radiologists can make cardiac diagnoses that require shape recognition and pulmonary diagnoses that require mass recognition with accuracy significantly better than chance. The area under the receiver operating characteristic (ROC) curve for pooled data was 0.75 for a 200-ms look and 0.96 for free viewing. Small objects such as lung nodules have to be close to the axis of the gaze to be seen in a single fixation, and during a single fixation detectability depends on both the stimulus duration and the displacement from the center of the gaze axis [10] (see Figure 18.2(a) and 18.2(b)). Many small objects can be detected in one 200-ms fixation, but some of them may require multiple fixations. Nodules that are reported are typically viewed by a cluster of fixations that can have a total duration of 0.5 to 2.0 s. During a 15- to 20-s viewing period, a nodule that is reported is typically fixated repeatedly for a total gaze duration of 1 to 3 s [21]. This type of scanning behavior is illustrated in Figure 18.3.

The time spent examining the nodules should not be confused with the time spent scanning the image before the nodule is discovered. The detection of most subtle pulmonary nodules occurs very rapidly, typically requiring 10 to 20 s or 30

TRUE POSITIVE RESPONSE   **FALSE NEGATIVE RESPONSE**

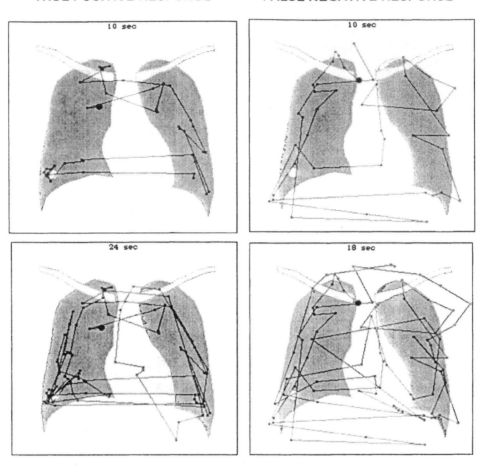

Figure 18.3: The top row shows the scanpaths of a radiologist for the first 10 s of viewing a chest image that contained a subtle pulmonary nodule in the right lower lobe. The white dot shows the location of the nodule. The bottom row shows the scanpath for 20 s of viewing. The radiologist reported the nodule on the left but did not report the nodule on the right.

to 60 fixations [13, 22]. Occasionally nodules are discovered late in the scanning process. When a nodule is discovered, the perception of the image is modified to include the new finding. Sometimes, a nodule is fixated for a few seconds and is not perceived or reported. The resulting false negative response can be classified as a decision error [23] and indicates the importance of covert decision making to basic visual perception.

18.2.4 Perception as a decision process: the Gregory–Rock model

Gregory and Rock [14, 15] have proposed decision-centered models for visual perception. Perception starts with a rapid process occurring in a few hundreds of ms (see Figure 18.4). This produces what Rock called the "literal" perception [15].

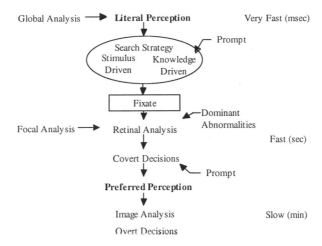

Figure 18.4: A flow diagram of the development the perception.

This is also called the "bottom-up" process in which the retinal signal is broken down into visual primitives that express form, color, movement, depth, and texture [9]. A slower phase, the so called "top-down" process, uses knowledge about the organization of the external world to create a "preferred" perception composed of definable objects. Gregory [14] called this applying the "object hypothesis." This phenomenon is familiar to most radiologists who have had abnormalities pointed out that they did not see initially. Usually the abnormalities are small and inconspicuous, such as lung nodules and fractures, although occasionally they are quite conspicuous and may involve completely reorganizing the perception of the image. Usually the perception is changed in response to information about the implied meaning of the image [24]. In radiology, this information is frequently supplied by the clinical history.

The detection of inconspicuous lung nodules on chest radiographs is an example of modification of the literal perception. When the radiologist first views the chest image, conspicuous abnormalities are recognized rapidly. Inconspicuous nodules, by definition, must be viewed by the central visual field to be detected with any level of reliability. The optimal visual field size for detecting low-contrast lung nodules of about one cm diameter is about five degrees in diameter, which is equivalent to a 5-cm circle on a chest image at 60-cm viewing distance [13]. During visual search, potential nodule sites have to be identified and inspected. At each site, the perceptual system must decide if any image features at the site are sufficiently characteristic to be considered as a nodule in the preferred perception. The decision to perceive or not to perceive is covert; it is made at a preconscious level. The decision not to perceive leaves the perception of the image unchanged. The decision to perceive results in the addition of the nodule features to the perception. Once nodule features are perceived, an overt or conscious decision can be made about whether the features constitute a real tumor or just normal structures masquerading as a tumor.

18.2.5 Visual search: the global-focal model

The global-focal perception hypothesis follows directly from the Gregory–Rock model and hypothesizes that two different types of scene analysis, global and focal, are performed sequentially, sometimes within a single fixation and sometimes in a cluster of fixations centered on a particular location in the image. Global analysis uses the sensory data from the entire retina and produces a general interpretation of the visual scene. The retinal network extracts low-spatial-frequency boundary information at the onset of each fixation, and establishes the spatial relationship of major objects in the scene. It also identifies perturbations, which are novel or unexpected features, and maps the location for closer scrutiny. Focal analysis concentrates on the information collected by the central retinal fields and provides a detailed interpretation of the part of the visual scene that is centered on the axis of the gaze. Although there is no direct neurophysiological evidence, it is easy to imagine that these functions represent the operation of the magnocellular

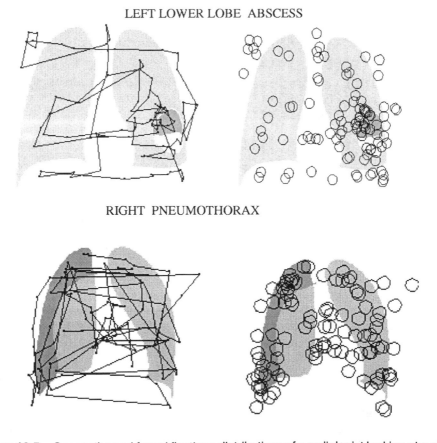

Figure 18.5: Scanpaths and foveal fixations distributions of a radiologist looking at a chest radiograph with a focal lung abscess in the left lower lobe (top) and with a pneumothorax on the right side. Notice how the fixations concentrate on the abnormal areas.

and parvocellular systems respectively. The size of the visual field that is being analyzed during focal fixations is variable, ranging from 2 to 6 deg, and it is often called the useful visual field. The image features within this field have been selected for analysis either as a result of peripheral attraction by a perturbation noted during the global analysis or as a result of cognitive guidance. No matter how the eyes are directed, eye-position recordings invariably show that coverage of a scene by the central vision is selective and not exhaustive. Figure 18.5 shows the scanpaths and the coverage of two abnormal chest images by a 2-deg-diameter field representing the fovea. Note that there are large lung regions that are not viewed by the fovea. This is commonly observed even when radiologists are specifically instructed to search for lung nodules or fractures [25]. This does not necessarily mean that search is inefficient but it does illustrate the importance of the parafoveal retina in the analysis of images.

There is a great deal of anecdotal and experimental evidence showing that the visual system has a limited capacity for processing information. The title of Miller's often-quoted review, "The magic number seven, plus or minus two: some limits on our capacity for processing information" almost gives away the whole story [26]. The visual system deals with the richness of detail in the visual world by excluding or filtering unwanted information and focusing on the objects that are important for current behavior. The subject of selective visual attention will not be discussed here. The interested reader is referred to a recent review by Desimone and Duncan [27].

18.3 Visual scanning as a method for studying visual search

18.3.1 Studying visual search

Search can be studied in two basic ways, either by determining the time required for finding and locating a target or by observing the visual scanning pattern. Search time studies are easy to perform and allow the accumulation of enough data to test statistical hypothesis with reasonable power. However, the search time includes both the time required to find the target and the time spent fixating the target to determine whether or not it should be added to the preferred perception. Visual scanning studies are difficult to perform because they require special apparatus to record head and eye position [28]. The apparatus may be intrusive and usually requires calibration before and after viewing. However, in addition to the time required to find a target, visual scanning studies also provide data about when and where visual attention was allocated in the image including on those targets that were not reported as well as those targets that were reported.

18.3.2 Studies of visual scanning in radiology

Tuddenham and Calvert [29] were the first investigators to record the scanning patterns of radiologists. They presented four radiologists with "a series of paper roentgenograms of normal and abnormal chests" in a dimly lighted room. The radiologists scanned the image with a movable spotlight while a motion picture camera recorded the location of the spot on the image. Each radiologist was asked to set the size of the spot to the smallest comfortable circle before beginning the experiment. The scanning pattern was reconstructed by playing back the motion pictures. They made a number of important observations based of an analysis of 43 scanning patterns

First, they found that observers selected a scanning circle that was much larger than the field of view subtended by the fovea. Unfortunately, they did not report the size of the spot. Subsequent research has suggested that the optimal scanning field size for low contrast targets is about 5 deg in diameter [13] which is about 5 cm on a chest film viewed from a distance of 55 cm. The 5-degree estimate is drawn mainly from studies of lung nodule detection. The calculation was based on a model in which the viewer was required to maximize the detection of lung nodules on a chest image in a fixed viewing time. The optimal size results from the tension between visual field size and scanning time. Clearly, given a large amount of time, the entire 2-degree fovea could be scanned over the image systematically. This just does not happen. In fact the higher the level of expertise as measured by task performance, the shorter the time required to perform the task [30, 31].

Second, Tuddenham and Calvert [29] found that coverage of the images by the scanning circle was non-uniform. They speculated that non-uniform coverage could account for reader error. A number of subsequent studies have confirmed that coverage is, indeed, non-uniform but the relationship of non-uniform coverage by the central vision to errors of omission is far from clear. Most missed lung nodules [23], linear fractures [25], and masses on mammograms [32] are fixated by the central visual field. The data in Table 18.2 are taken from a study of lung-nodule detection [23] in which the fixation dwell time by a field of 5.6 deg diameter (6 cm on the chest image) was calculated. Seventy percent (14/20) of the missed nodules were fixated for intervals ranging from 0.2 to 2.1 s. Some of the nodules received a cluster of fixations while others were fixated once and then re-fixated later. The nodules were divided into three categories on the basis of the total fixation dwell time. Scanning errors were scored when the nodule was not located within 2.8 deg (3 cm) of the center of a fixation. Recognition errors were scored when the total fixation dwell time was less than 1 s. Decision errors were scored when the total

Table 18.2: Dwell times in seconds for high-confidence false-negative responses to 1-cm simulated lung nodules (from Kundel *et al.* [23])

Number Of Images	Pct.	Initial Dwell		Total Dwell		Error Designation
		Mean	Range	Mean	Range	
8	30	0	0	0	0	Scanning
5	25	0.24	0.2–0.3	0.50	0.2–0.6	Recognition
9	45	0.46	0.15–0.8	1.23	0.8–2.1	Decision

fixation dwell time was more than 1 s. It should be made clear that the readers in the study did not report anything unusual at the locations of the missed nodules. The readers made covert decisions not to perceive a nodule and the nodule features were not added to the preferred perception.

Third, Tuddenham and Calvert [29] observed that there was great variability in the patterns. One reader showed a systematic pattern and one reader showed an initial circumferential pattern followed by a more complex pattern. The other two readers had complex unclassifiable patterns. Investigators who record eye movements have always been fascinated by eye search patterns or scanpaths [33]. Yarbus [16] showed qualitative changes in the scanpaths and the distribution of fixations in response to questions that were asked about a picture that was being viewed. Yet the analysis of scanpath patterns has not contributed much to the understanding of visual search. The patterns of the scanpaths shown in Figure 18.6 are different but the fixation distributions are almost identical. It is not clear if the sequence in which visual information is collected by the visual system is important for performance. Experts seem to make more efficient use of information from the peripheral retina and fixate abnormal locations in the image more quickly and efficiently than non-experts. Llewellyn-Thomas and Lansdown [34] were the first investigators to record the eye-position of radiology trainees during the viewing of chest radiographs. They found that the trainees concentrated their fixations on the strong borders in the image. Kundel and Lafollette [35] recorded the eye-position of people at various stages of medical training ranging from none, through medical

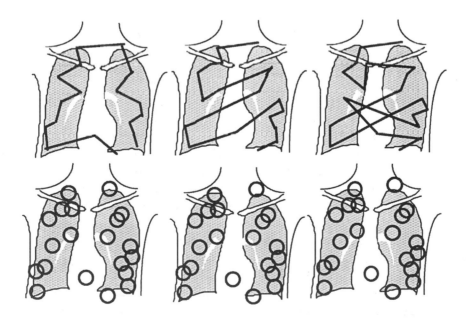

Figure 18.6: The three scanpaths in the upper part of the figure are qualitatively very different. They represent a circumferential, a zigzag, and a complex pattern. Each scanpath resulted in an identical distribution of fixations.

school and radiology residency, and on to staff radiologists. Qualitative evaluation of the patterns on a normal chest image (see Figure 18.1) shows an evolution of the scanpath pattern from one that concentrates on the edges of the heart to an apparently deliberate circumferential sweep of the chest centered on the lungs. Similarly, qualitative evaluation of the patterns on an abnormal chest image shows that the most experienced people immediately view the abnormalities sometimes to the exclusion of the rest of the chest. Nodine and Kundel [36] have proposed that the observed scanpath is the result of three activities that determine the location of fixations, checking, discovery and idling. Checking fixations sample the areas identified by the global analysis of the image. Discovery fixations sample areas that are identified by the cognitive component of the search mechanism. They sample areas where there is a high probability of finding a target based upon prior knowledge. Finally, when the visual system is occupied with decision making based upon evidence already accumulated, the preferred perception is periodically refreshed and the fixations just continue to sample the major features already identified and entered into the preferred perception. The expert using the peripheral vision in a global response quickly identifies potential abnormalities and checks them. Discovery, search, and decision making are efficient and, consequently there are only a few discovery fixations and very little idling. Consequently, the expert is fast and shows an orderly scanpath (see Figures 18.3, 18.5, and 18.7).

18.3.3 Visual dwell time and decision errors

Table 18.2 shows that many false-negative decisions are associated with prolonged visual fixation times. Dwell times are measured by defining a region or zone on an image and measuring the total fixation time within that zone. The zone usually is defined in relation to a small target object. For a lung nodule, fractures, or a mass on a mammogram, it is defined as a circular or elliptical zone usually with a radius between 2 and 3 deg. The dwell time is measured for each of the four basic decision outcomes: true positive, true negative, false positive, and false negative. The zone is placed over the lesion location for measurement of true-positive and false-negative dwell times and it is placed over appropriately defined control locations for true-negative decisions. It is placed over the location indicated by the observer for false-positive decisions. A mean or median dwell time over trials and readers can be calculated, but statistical comparisons are difficult because the dwell times are not normally distributed. The technique of survival analysis has provided useful statistical tools [37]. Figure 18.7 is a plot of the survival of fixation dwell times on a 4-degree-diameter circular location in an image. In the test condition, the location contained a simulated nodule about 1 cm in diameter (approximately 1 degree at 60 cm viewing distance) and of low contrast so that it was just visible when the location was known exactly. In the control condition, there was no nodule in exactly the same location on the image. The total fixation dwell times for the first 15 s of viewing pooled over readers and trials were grouped according to decision outcome. The survival curve can be described as follows. At time 0, all of the fixations are represented and all of the curves start at 100%. About 90%

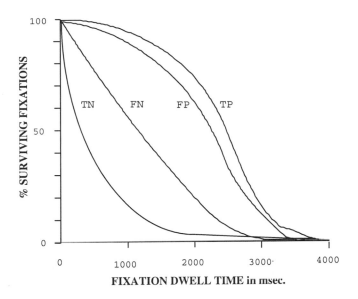

Figure 18.7: Survival curves for the fixations landing within a 5-deg-diameter circle on a test chest image that contained a nodule or a control image that was nodule free. The first 15 s of viewing was included. The data are pooled from 6 radiology residents viewing 20 test and 20 control images [47].

of the fixations that were classified as true negatives were shorter than 1000 ms and at 1000 ms, only the 10% that are longer than 1000 ms remain. The situation is different for the true-positive decisions. Only 10% of the fixations on correctly identified nodules were shorter than 1000 ms and at the 1000 ms time mark about 90% remain. The important point about these curves is that false-negative decisions have dwell times between the positives (true and false) and the true negatives. This is interpreted to mean that the nodule sites were fixated long enough for nodule features to be detected but that a decision was made not to perceive the features.

18.3.4 Satisfaction of search

Tuddenham [38] suggested that lesions were missed in the presence of other abnormalities because the viewer, having looked at the image long enough, was satisfied with the current perception. This phenomenon, which many radiologists report anecdotally has been called either "satisfaction of search" (SOS) or "satisfaction of meaning." Berbaum *et al.* [39] were the first investigators to actually demonstrate the phenomenon in a controlled experiment. They found that simulated nodules added to images with subtle native abnormalities decreased the number of the native abnormalities that were reported. Samuel *et al.* [40] did a similar experiment but reversed the stimuli. They added subtle lung nodules to chest images with obvious native abnormalities and found that the detection of the lung nodules was decreased in the presence of the obvious native abnormalities. The effect can be demonstrated reproducibly in the laboratory but there is not a satisfactory, perceptually sound, explanation for the cause. The simple explanation that search is terminated before all of the abnormalities can be found is not supported by the laboratory evidence. Eye-position analysis shows that the most missed abnormalities are not neglected by the central vision, they are fixated and then ignored [41, 42]. This observation suggests that the explanation for satisfaction of search must be sought in the decision mechanisms that determine how attention is allocated rather than in the scanning and data-acquisition mechanisms that characterize visual search.

18.4 Current problems in visual search

18.4.1 Prompts and cues

Prompts are hints about the image that cannot be derived from the actual pictorial content. Most prompts are verbal statements that suggest either where to look in the image or what kind of disease to expect in the image. In radiology, the clinical history or the indication for the imaging exam provides a strong prompt. There has been controversy about whether a radiologist should look at the images without knowledge of the clinical history and provide a supposedly objective assessment, unbiased by the clinical information or whether the clinical history should be provided so as to get the best possible consultation about that particular patient.

Cues are hints about the image that are part of the pictorial content. Internal cues are image findings that suggest other findings. For example, if a breast is missing on a chest image suggesting that the patient has had surgery for breast cancer, the radiologist might look more carefully at the lungs and bones for evidence of metastases. External cues are arrows and circles that are placed on the image to call attention to a particular place. External cues are used by some radiologists to indicate the location or type of abnormalities on images. External cues such as arrows and circles are also used by the emerging technologies of computer-aided diagnosis (CAD), and computer-aided perception (CAP) for marking the sites of potential abnormalities on images [43, 44]. Prompts and cues will be discussed separately.

18.4.2 Prompts from clinical history

Berbaum *et al.* [45] reviewed the studies of the effect of clinical history on diagnostic accuracy and noted that they could be divided into two categories, those that used subtle clinical cases of all sorts and those that used simulated nodules. The studies using clinical cases all showed that the prompt provided by the clinical history improved performance whereas the studies using simulated nodules showed either no effect or a shift in diagnostic criteria without a change in performance. Berbaum *et al.* [45] performed a study in which 6 experienced radiologists diagnosed 43 cases, 25 with subtle abnormalities including 5 with nodules and 18 normals. They showed (see Table 18.3) that the prompt improved diagnostic accuracy when decisions on all of the cases were considered but that there was either no effect or a minimal effect on the detection of nodules.

Table 18.3: The area under the ROC curve for prompted and unprompted clinical radiographs

	unprompted	prompted
All cases (25 abn. 18 normal)	0.79	0.88
Nodules (5 abn. 11 normal)	0.83	0.85

Prompts may work by changing the allocation of attention to various parts of the image. Eye-position studies [46] have shown that the effect of clinical history is to change the coverage of normal images by visual fixations. When the history was specific for nodules, 65% of the fixations were on the lungs and 5% were on the peripheral part of the chest, whereas when the history was a general one, 43% of the fixations were on the lungs and 18% were on the peripheral part of the chest.

18.4.3 External pictorial cues

As part of a study of computer-assisted perception of lung nodules on chest images, external cues in the form of circles were placed on the image [47]. The test condition, a second look at the image with circles about the nodules, was compared with the control condition, a second look at the image without circles about the nodules. The images with the circles resulted in a 26% improvement in the detection of lung nodules. Krupinski [48] then studied the effect of external cues as an independent phenomenon and showed that a complete circle composed of solid concentric white and black lines increased the detectability of nodules located inside the circle and decreased the detectability of nodules located immediately outside the circle. A partial circle composed of a dotted or dashed concentric line increased detectability but not as much as the solid circle. Increased detectability with a circle was also shown for simulated masses on mammographic backgrounds [49]. The perceptual process that is responsible for the improved detection is unknown. In studies of CAD it may be necessary to control for the effect of having the computer add a cue to the image.

18.4.4 Static and dynamic displays

Llewellyn-Thomas [50] pointed out that people search three types of display: static, dynamic and intermittent. Searching a static display consisting of either a single image or an array of images is the most common form of viewing images in radiology. Despite some early interest [51], dynamic displays such as those seen on fluoroscopes and cine images have received almost no attention in radiology. Intermittent displays are common in surveillance tasks such as radar where an observer must watch a display for a rare event. This is a problem of vigilance and has little application in radiology except possibly screening situations where targets such as tumors might be rare. The development of digital displays and the attempt to use only a few monitors for very large cross-sectional studies has raised the issue of using serial instead of parallel displays. There have been no comparative studies of eye position during the viewing of parallel and serial displays. This is a fertile area for perceptual research that could have important implications for the practice of radiology.

18.4.5 Teaching radiology

Those of us engaged in perceptual research are frequently asked how to search images or what to tell students about searching images. Llewellyn-Thomas [50] reviewed search behavior and made some common sense observations about searching images but they were based on very scanty hard information about visual search in radiology. Carmody [52] surveyed a number of textbooks and found that when advice about searching images was given, it included making comparisons and scanning the image systematically. Studies of eye scanpaths have shown that this advice is not followed by the experts. Kundel and Wright [46] reported that only 2 of 25 scanpaths of the chest showed symmetrical comparison movements. Carmody [52] using more liberal criteria for comparison and found that board certified radiologists and radiology residents used comparison scans less than 4% of the time. The comparisons were not specific to anatomy or pathology. These results show that comparison does not occur at the sampling level, however, it may go on at higher levels of the perceptual process [53].

Carmody [52] in a survey of radiology residents and radiologists, found that most of them advocated some sort of systematic search and claimed that they used a systematic approach to searching images. However, eye-position studies on the same people showed that systematic search was very rare. Fifty-eight percent (29/50) of the scans of radiologists were too complex to classify, 34% (17/50) were circumferential and 8% (4/50) were zigzag, confirming prior observations [29, 46]. Modeling has shown that although complicated, the scans of radiologists searching chest images for lung nodules are not random [13].

I believe that it is not possible to prescribe a search strategy because search is a component of the mechanism of attention. The reader who tries to use a deliberate search strategy is paying attention to search and not to the task of image interpretation. Mechanical search aids may be able to direct search, but their value in radiology has never been tested and they do not reinforce what experts do naturally.

I advise students to use a three-step attention-directing strategy. First, view the image without any clinical information and come to a conclusion. Second, briefly divert the attention away from the image by reading the clinical information, even if it is limited to the patient's age and then look at the image again. Finally, look at the image while dictating a report that mentions all of the pertinent organ systems. In this way there are three opportunities to view the image, and at the end there is a systems review that may uncover abnormalities that were not previously perceived.

References

[1] Berlin L, Berlin JW. "Malpractice and Radiologists in Cook County, IL: Trends in 20 Years of Litigation." American Journal of Roentgenology 165:781–788, 1995.

[2] Kundel HL, Revesz G, Stauffer HM. "Evaluation of a Television Image Processing System." Investigative Radiology 3:44–50, 1968.

[3] Kundel HL, Revesz G, Toto L. "Contrast Gradient and the Detection of Lung Nodules." Investigative Radiology 14:18–22, 1979.

[4] Kundel HL, Nodine CF, Thickman DI, Carmody DP, Toto LC. "Nodule Detection with and without a Chest Image." Investigative Radiology 20:94–99, 1985.

[5] Sherrier RH, Johnson GA, Suddarth S, Chiles C, Hulka C, Ravin CE. "Digital Synthesis of Lung Nodules." Investigative Radiology 20:933–937, 1985.

[6] Burgess AE, Chakraborty S. "Producing Lesions for Hybrid Mammograms: Extracted Tumors and Simulated Microcalcifications." In Krupinski EA (Ed.) *Medical Imaging 99: Image Perception and Performance.* Proc SPIE 3663, 1999, pp. 316–322.

[7] Wester C, Judy PF, Polger M, Swensson RG, Feldman U, Seltzer SE. "Influence of Visual Distractors on Detectability of Liver Nodules on Contrast-Enhanced Spiral Computed Tomography Scans." Acad Radiol 4:335–342, 1997.

[8] Sorenson JA, Nelson JA, Niklason LA, Klauber MR. "Simulation of Lung Nodules for Nodule Detection Studies." Investigative Radiology 15:490–495, 1980.

[9] Livingstone M, Hubel D. "Segregation of Form, Color, Movement, and Depth: Anatomy, Physiology, and Perception." Science 240:740–749, 1988.

[10] Carmody DP, Nodine CF, Kundel HL "An Analysis of Perceptual and Cognitive Factors in Radiographic Interpretation." Perception 9:339–344, 1980.

[11] Nelson WW, Loftus GR. "The Functional Visual Field During Picture Viewing." Journal of Experimental Psychology: Human Learning and Memory 6:391–399, 1980.

[12] Kundel HL, Nodine CF. "Interpreting Chest Radiographs without Visual Search." Radiology 116:527–532, 1975.

[13] Kundel HL, Nodine CF, Thickman DI, Toto LC. "Searching for Lung Nodules a Comparison of Human Performance with Random and Systematic Scanning Models." Investigative Radiology 22:417–422, 1987.

[14] Gregory RL. *The Intelligent Eye.* New York: McGraw-Hill, 1970.

[15] Rock I. *The Logic of Perception.* Cambridge, MA: The MIT Press, 1983.

[16] Yarbus AL. *Eye Movements and Vision.* New York: Plenum Press, 1967.

[17] Carpenter R. *Movements of the Eyes.* London: Pion Limited, 1977.

[18] Sperling G. "The information available in brief visual presentations." Psychological Monographs: General & Applied 74:1–29, 1960.

[19] Loftus GR. "Tachistoscopic Simulations of Eye Fixations on Pictures." Journal of Experimental Psychology: Human Learning and Memory 7:369–376, 1981.

[20] McConkie GW, Underwood NR, Zola D, Wolverton GS. "Some Temporal Characteristics of Processing During Reading." Journal of Experimental Psychology: Human Perception and Performance 11:168–182, 1985.

[21] Kundel HL, Nodine CF, Krupinski EA. "Searching for Lung Nodules: Visual Dwell Indicates Locations of False-Positive and False-Negative Decisions." Investigative Radiology 24:472–478, 1989.

[22] Oestmann JW, Greene R, Kushner DC, Bourgouin PM, Linetsky L, Llewellyn HJ. "Lung Lesions: Correlation Between Viewing Time and Detection." Radiology 166:451–453, 1988.

[23] Kundel HL, Nodine CF, Carmody DP. "Visual Scanning, Pattern Recognition, and Decision Making in Pulmonary Nodule Detection." Investigative Radiology 13:175–181, 1978.

[24] Kundel HL, Nodine FC. "A Visual Concept Shapes Image Perception." Radiology 146:363–368, 1983.

[25] Hu CH, Kundel HL, Nodine CF, Krupinski EA, Toto LC. "Searching for Bone Fractures: A Comparison with Pulmonary Nodule Search." Academic Radiology 1:25–32, 1994.

[26] Miller G. "The Magic Number Seven, Plus or Minus Two: Some Limits on Our Capacity for Processing Information." Psychol Rev 63:81–97, 1956.

[27] Desimone R, Duncan J. "Neural Mechanisms of Selective Visual Attention." Annual Rev Neuroscience 18:193–222, 1995.

[28] Nodine CF, Kundel HL, Toto LC, Krupinski EA. "Recording and Analyzing Eye-Position Data Using a Microcomputer Workstation." Beh Res Meth Inst & Comp 24:475–485, 1992.

[29] Tuddenham WJ, Calvert WP. "Visual Search Patterns in Roentgen Diagnosis." Radiology 76:255–256, 1961.

[30] Christensen EE, Murry RC, Holland K, Reynolds J, Landay MJ, Moore JG. "The Effect of Search Time on Perception." Radiology 138:361–365, 1981.

[31] Nodine CF, Kundel HL, Lauver SC, Toto LC. "Nature of Expertise in Searching Mammograms for Breast Masses." Academic Radiology 3:1000–1006, 1996.

[32] Krupinski EA, Nodine FC. "Gaze Duration Predicts the Locations of Missed Lesions in Mammography." In Gale AG, Astley SM, Dance DR, Cairns AY, (Eds.) Digital Mammography. Amsterdam: Elsevier, 1994, pp. 399–403.

[33] Stark L, Ellis SR. "Scanpaths Revisted: Cognitive Models Direct Active Looking." In Fisher M, Senders (Ed.) Eye Movements; Cognition and Visual Perception, 1981, pp. 193–226.

[34] Llewellyn-Thomas E, Lansdown EL. "Visual Search Patterns of Radiologists in Training." Radiology 81:288–291, 1963.

[35] Kundel HL, LaFollette PS. "Visual Search Patterns and Experience with Radiological Images." Radiology 103:523–528, 1972.

[36] Nodine CF, Kundel HL. "The Cognitive Side of Visual Search in Radiology." In O'Regan JK, Levy-Schoen A (Eds.) *Eye Movements: From Physiology to Cognition*. North Holland: Elsevier Science Publishers, 1987, pp. 573–582.

[37] Anderson S, Auquier A, Hauck WW, Oakes D, Vandaele W, Weisberg HI. *Statistical Methods for Comparative Studies*. New York: John Wiley & Sons, NY, 1980.

[38] Tuddenham WJ. "Roentgen Image Perception—A Personal Survey of the Problem." Radiological Clinics of North America 3:499–501, 1969.

[39] Berbaum KS, Franken JEA, Dorfman DD, Rooholamini SA, Kathol MH, *et al.* "Satisfaction of Search in Diagnostic Radiology." Investigative Radiology 25:133–140, 1990.

[40] Samuel S, Kundel HL, Nodine CF, Toto LC. "Mechanism of Satisfaction of Search: Eye Position Recordings in the Reading of Chest Radiographs." Radiology 194:895–902, 1995.

[41] Berbaum KS, Franken JEA, Dorfman DD, Miller EM, Caldwell RT, Kuehn DM, Berbaum ML. "Role of Faulty Visual Search in the Satisfaction of Search Effect in Chest Radiography." Academic Radiology 5:9–19, 1998.

[42] Kundel HL, Nodine CF, Toto L. "An Eye-Position Study of the Effects of a Verbal Prompt and Pictorial Backgrounds on the Search for Lung Nodules in Chest Radiographs." In Krupinski EA (Ed.) *Medical Imaging 99: Image Perception and Performance*. Proc SPIE 3663, 1999, pp. 122–128.

[43] Nishikawa RM, Giger ML, Doi K, Vyborny CJ, Schmidt RA, Metz CE, Wu Y, Yin FF, Jiang Y, Huo Z, Lu P, Zhang W, Ema T, Bick U, Papaioannou J, Nagel RH. "Computer-Aided Detection and Diagnosis of Masses and Clustered Microcalcifications from Digital Mammograms." Proceedings SPIE: Biomedical Image Processing and Biomedical Visualization 1905, 1993, pp. 422–432.

[44] Krupinski EA, Nodine CF, Kundel HL. "Enhancing Recognition of Lesions in Radiographic Images Using Perceptual Feedback." Optical Engineering 37:813–818, 1998.

[45] Berbaum KS, Franken JEA, Dorfman DD, Barloon TJ, Ell SR, Lu CH, Smith W, Abu-Yousef MM. "Tentative Diagnoses Facilitate the Detection of Diverse Lesions in Chest Radiographs." Investigative Radiology 21:532–539, 1986.

[46] Kundel HL, Wright DJ. "The Influence of Prior Knowledge on Visual Search Strategies During the Viewing of Chest Radiographs." Radiology 93:315–320, 1969.

[47] Kundel HL, Nodine CF, Krupinski EA. "Computer Displayed Eye Position as a Visual Aid to Pulmonary Nodule Interpretation." Investigative Radiology 25:890–896, 1990.

[48] Krupinski EA, Nodine CF, Kundel HL. "Perceptual Enhancement of Tumor Targets in Chest X-Ray Images." Perception and Psychophysics 53:519–526, 1993.

[49] Kundel HL, Nodine CF, Lauver SC, Toto LC. "A Circle Cue Enhances Detection of Simulated Masses on a Mammographic Background." Presented at *Medical Imaging 1997: Image Perception*, 1997.

[50] Llewellyn-Thomas E. "Search Behavior." Radiol Clinics of N America 7:403–417, 1969.

[51] Potsaid MJ. "Cine and TV Methods of Analyzing Search in Roentgen Diagnosis." Journal of the SMPTE 74:731–736, 1965.

[52] Carmody DP, Kundel HL, Toto LC. "Comparison Scans While Reading Chest Images: Taught, but not Practiced." Investigative Radiology 19:462–466, 1984.

[53] Locher PJ, Nodine CF. "The Perceptual Value of Symmetry." Comp Math Appl 17:475–484, 1989.

CHAPTER 19
The Nature of Expertise in Radiology

Calvin F. Nodine, Claudia Mello-Thoms
University of Pennsylvania Medical Center

CONTENTS

19.1 Introduction

This chapter is about expertise in radiology. In the domain of radiology, expertise is largely acquired through massive amounts of case-reading experience. But just as everyone who is taught how to read is not an expert reader, so too everyone who is taught how to read medical images is not an expert image interpreter. The criterion that defines an expert medical-image interpreter is consistent and reliably accurate diagnostic performance. Nothing less will do. For example, despite intensive study and training, it has been shown that radiology residents at the end of residency training are significantly below the average of a large national sample of U.S. radiologists in overall accuracy of screening mammograms for breast cancer (Nodine, Kundel, Mello-Thoms *et al.*, 1999). This finding is not surprising when considered within the framework of research on expertise, which stresses that expert performance in many domains is, statistically speaking, rare, and usually accomplished only after extensive training and practice (Chi, Glasser, Farr, 1988; Ericsson and Charness, 1994).

We view expertise as the ability to acquire and use contextual knowledge that differentiates one from one's peers in a particular field. In this sense, expertise is a contextual concept, because the knowledge-structured skills that make an expert in one domain do not transfer to other domains (Nodine and Krupinski, 1998; Patel and Groen, 1991). Moreover, expertise is composed of a sum of different parts, each having a unique influence on the total. For example, in the context of medical image interpretation, an expert is someone that has had more experience, meaning diagnosed more cases, thus providing a broader range of variations of normalcy against which to differentiate abnormal findings. An expert is also someone who has a natural talent to perform within a chosen domain. Again, from a radiological perspective, different radiologists may have seen a similar number of medical images, but some will stand out in their ability to diagnose abnormalities, and perform the task faster. This component of expertise is called by us talent, but there is no doubt that motivational factors may be coloring what is termed talent (Ericsson, 1996, p. 27; Ericsson and Charness, 1994, pp. 728–729).

Although expertise has been extensively studied in many domains, the concept is still very elusive. If at this point one was able to pinpoint what makes an expert in any given field, one could certainly go out and create an artificial expert in that field simply by teaching a machine the skills that make one an expert. This has been tried many times, and some success has been achieved. Expert systems have been developed to find calcifications in mammograms (Nishikawa, Jiang, Giger *et al.*, 1994), to detect signs of lung cancers in chest radiographs (Lo, Lin, Freeman *et al.*, 1998), to differentiate benign from malignant lesions in mammograms (Zheng, Greenleaf, Gisvold, 1997). However, we are still very far from having an intelligent system that can actually read and interpret a medical image as reliably, accurately, and efficiently as a human expert.

The reason for this may be in the nature of expertise itself. As previously mentioned, medical expertise is formed by two parts, one that is computable, which responds to training by learning, and one that is uncomputable, which is independent of training, referred to as talent. We can design models that approximate the logical reasoning of experts when they are examining an image and making a decision, but there has been little success modeling internal processes that are responsible for the talent part (see Ericsson and Charness, 1994). Furthermore, these processes do not seem to arise from a structured thinking hierarchy, but rather seem to evolve spontaneously.

Thus, one is forced to consider the possibility that machine expertise will be restricted to the acquired part that makes up human expertise, which is related to training, to structured knowledge, to rule-based thinking. This is not to say that the performance of expert systems should not be compared with human experts, but rather, that expert systems possess a different kind of expertise. This by no means invalidates the need for intelligent systems in medical diagnosis. As shown elsewhere (Nodine, Kundel, Mello-Thoms *et al.*, 1999) it takes a great number of cases for one to become an expert mammogram reader, and it is here that intelligent systems will find their niche, by either providing a second, informed diagnosis, or by working as tutors, helping less experienced radiologists or radiology residents make as many correct decisions as possible, while keeping errors to a minimum. It is our belief that in contexts where both parts of expertise are operating, expert systems will surpass human performance in the computable part, but remain void when it comes to the talent component of expertise.

19.2 Plan of the chapter

Radiology is largely a visual discipline. This means that rather than relying on direct observation of patients, radiologists rely on interpreting image representations (usually generated by x-ray imaging) to gather diagnostic information about the medical status of patients. They may also read the patient's clinical history either to guide or to clarify image interpretation.

The interpretation of medical images depends on both image perception and cognitive processes. Often-cited perceptual skills include visual search, visual information processing, and visual discrimination and differentiation which are part of perceptual learning. In addition to perceptual skills, the interpretation of medical images depends on cognitive skills primarily related to diagnostic reasoning and decision making. Expertise represents a honing of these perceptual and cognitive skills. But, how much of expertise in radiology is learning to understand what one is looking at anatomically (basic science) and how much is what one sees within a clinical context as signaling pathology (clinical problem solving) is difficult to estimate.

In this chapter we shall summarize some of the findings on expertise in radiology. The theme is to show how image perception interacts with decision making to produce skilled diagnostic interpretation of medical images. The basic information-processing flow to achieve this is: VISUAL SEARCH—OBJECT RECOGNITION— DECISION MAKING. This is our "brand" of expertise theory (Nodine and Kundel, 1987). It is biased toward the perceptual side, whereas many radiology expertise studies are biased toward the cognitive side. Our perceptual bias is reflected in our choice of theory and methodology. This is true of the cognitive camp as well. Thus, we look at radiology expertise as primarily visual problem solving. Our methods depend heavily on generating theoretical inferences from eye-position data, whereas many studies using the cognitive approach depend on generating theoretical inferences from verbal-protocol data (e.g., Lesgold, Feltovitch, Glaser *et al.*, 1981; 1988). Note that a third approach exists, namely, the connectionist approach (Dawson, 1998), which models information processing in artificial intelligence (AI) using artificial neural networks (or ANNs). This approach will be discussed later in this chapter.

We will use a recent study of mammography expertise to illustrate some basic points: First, how experience influences the acquisition of expertise, and a discussion of the imperfect translation of experience as an error-correction feedback mechanism for training radiology residents. Second, how the three components of information processing, search, recognition and decision making, combine to produce diagnostic-decision outcomes. Third, how the information-processing model works across radiology subdomains by comparing research findings in chest and breast radiology, and pointing out some important differences in the two subdomains that may result in negative transfer.

19.3 Expertise roots

Expertise research has its roots in the intersection of cognitive psychology and computer science, now known as artificial intelligence, or AI. The cognitive psychology side of this research was concerned with identifying human information-processing skills associated with solving intellectual problems (e.g., playing chess, solving physics problems, diagnosing disease), and the computer-science side was interested in modeling cognitive processes by developing programmable algorithms that would generate performance outcomes with the ultimate goal of creating expert systems. The overarching framework for research on expert systems was learning theory generally and problem solving specifically. Man was conceived of as a processor of information, and the process of seeking information was analyzable in terms of contingencies of reinforcement, that is, feedback, that corrected erroneous behavior and thus guided the course of learning.

A lot of water has passed over that dam since AI began the study of expertise. The late Alan Newell, one of the founding fathers of AI predicted in 1973 that "... when we arrive in 1992 (Newell's retirement date from Carnegie-Mellon University) we will have homed in on the essential structure of mind" (Newell, 1973, p. 306). Needless to say, that prediction was a bit optimistic, but it does reflect the enthusiasm and hopes that one of its founders had for AI. Some would say the defining moment for the beginning of AI was George Miller's article on the limits of human information-processing capacity (Miller, 1956). Cognitive psychology was thought, at the time of its inception in the 50's, as reflecting a shift away from behaviorist learning theory toward finding mental structures (rules for learning and problem solving). Looking back today, almost 50 years later, it is somewhat amusing to see how stubbornly reinforcement (albeit redefined), the cornerstone of behavioristic theory, continues to survive within mainstream learning theory in spite of the cognitive revolution which spured cognitive theory, cognitive science, and artificial neural networks.

As already indicated, research on expertise has been wide ranging and it is not the purpose of this chapter to review it all. Rather, the goal is to provide a glimpse of expertise research by focusing on radiology. When it comes to studying expertise, the domain of radiology is broad. In today's era of specialization in medicine, we have experts in subdomains of radiology, as for example, breast imaging (mammography), thoracic imaging, angiography, etc., and an expert in mammography is unlikely to also be an expert in another subdomain.

The hierarchial ordering from general to specific domains is important to recognize in studying expertise in radiology because, although radiology resident training provides mentoring experiences in a number of subdomains of radiology, the ultimate goal of such training is to make a radiologist who is Master of one subdomain, rather than Jack of all subdomains. The result is that radiology expertise is subdomain specific. This emphasis on subdomain-specific training and experience fine tunes the radiologists such that performance of an experienced mammographer may suffer if asked to interpret a chest radiograph, or performance of an experienced chest radiologist may falter if asked to interpret a mammogram. From the standpoint of a learning theory framework, expertise skills are specific to a given subdomain and do not effectively transfer to other subdomains within radiology. This is true of medical expertise in general (Patel and Groen, 1991).

19.4 Expertise, acquired or innate?

Most expert performance is acquired, not innate (Ericsson and Charness, 1994). This is not to say that native talent plays no role, but its role is limited, particularly in medicine. Perceptual tests to identify visual skills of prospective radiologists have not generally been successful (Bass and Chiles, 1990; Smoker, Berbaum, Luebke et al., 1984). This is because what the test purports to measure (e.g., spatial relations) is either too abstract or too far removed from the radiology task. Thus there is little or no transfer of test skills to radiology reading skills. A good example is finding NINA in Al Hirschfeld's drawings of theater scenes. Hirschfeld's task calls on visual-search skills for locating NINA targets within the theater scene, and object-recognition skills for disembedding letters from features of theatrical scenery in order to recognize NINA's name. These search and recognition skills seem to be very close to what is required of the radiologist searching a chest image for a lung nodule, but we have found that radiologists are no better than laypersons at finding NINAs (Nodine and Krupinski, 1998). This result seems to argue that expertise in radiology is very narrow and subdomaine specific. In the following section we will examine expertise in different domains, and see how expertise in chess and in the medical field compare to expertise in radiology.

19.4.1 Chess-playing expertise

Parallels have been made between the chess master and the radiology expert performing their tasks (Wood, 1999). Both have built extensive, organized, and searchable mental arrays containing task-specific information such as configurations of chess pieces mapped to feasible game-playing moves, or radiographic patterns of anatomy mapped to pathological signs that are used in solving their respective problems. These mental arrays are often referred to as schemas.

Expertise research starting with de Groot's (1965) and Chase and Simons' (1973) seminal studies and generalizing across a number of expertise domains has found practice to be the major independent variable in chess skill. For example, Charness, Krampe and Mayr (1996) have shown that "deliberate practice" is critical for acquiring skill in chess playing. What is meant by deliberate practice is self-motivated effortful study. We believe that this definition, broadly stated, describes the type of study medical residents go through during residency training. Their study is closely supervised by mentors who motivate learning and guide training by drawing on a vast data base of clinical experience. In chess, for example, Charness *et al.* estimate that 32,000 hours of deliberate practice over 9 to 10 years are necessary on average to achieve grandmaster levels (2500 Elo points; Elo was the name of the man who developed the scale). It is important to note the Charness *et al.* distinction between deliberate practice, and casual practice which involves playing games with others. Deliberate practice correlates higher with chess skill ($r = 0.60$) than does casual practice ($r = 0.35$), which lead them to conclude that deliberate practice is the primary change agent influencing chess skill. One reason this conclusion is so important to our discussion of radiology expertise is because acquiring radiology skill depends on highly motivated and supervised learning, and Charness *et al.* have shown that this type of learning produces more effective cognitive-skill outcomes than casual learning and book reading. This realization has important implications for training radiology residents where supervised learning takes the form of mentor-guided experiences.

Another reason to look carefully at chess expertise is because chess skill has a perceptual component of search that draws on schematic representations of chess-move patterns leading to "best" game moves (Gobet and Simon, 1996) in much the same way as radiology skill has a perceptual component of search that draws on schematic representations of normal anatomic patterns against which to compare new image input for signs of abnormality. Studies of expertise in both chess and radiology have been modeled as problem-solving tasks of the general form: SEARCH & DETECT—EVALUATE—DECIDE. Both chess and radiology have a strong visual-spatial component.

19.4.2 Medical expertise

The study of medical expertise draws heavily on linguistic analysis of the semantic content of propositional statements of physicians recorded as verbal protocols, or thinking out loud. The verbal protocols are scored for the recall of medical-knowledge representations and reasoning processes used to generate either data-driven inferences or hypothesis-driven facts leading to diagnostic explanations (Patel and Groen, 1991). In contrast, the study of radiology expertise, because the focus is shifted from observations of a live patient to medical images, focuses on perceptual analysis of image features, or statements about the interpretation of image features (see Raufaste, Eyrolle, Marine, 1998).

19.4.3 Radiology expertise

The study of expertise in radiology has been limited to the subdomains of chest radiology and mammography. The radiologist's task in both cases has been modeled within a visual problem-solving framework. However, different experimental methods have been used to gain insights into the nature of perceptual-cognitive skills underlying medical-image interpretation. The cognitive approach as exemplified by Lesgold (1984) and Lesgold, Feltovitch, Glaser *et al.* (1981, 1988) uses a form of verbal-protocol analysis involving analyses of observers' diagnostic reports and sketches of abnormal regions to identify cognitive structures that presumably interact recursively between hypotheses and image features to generate diagnostic outcomes.

The perceptual approach as exemplified by our research (e.g., Nodine, Kundel, Mello-Thoms *et al.*, 1999; Kundel and Nodine, 1975) has used a combination of measures derived primarily from eye-position data to characterize schema-driven search strategies leading (or following) focal analyses of perceptual features from which diagnostic decisions are inferred. The eye-position data include percent coverage of the image by a fixed circular field approximating the size of the fovea plus error tolerance, time spent dwelling on selected image location (target or nontarget) referred to as cumulative gaze duration or visual dwell, and time to detect a target referred to as search time to a hit. In our most recent work in mammography, we compared speed-accuracy performance as a function of level of expertise using a chronometric analysis of decision time. Decision time is similar to reaction time used by Posner (1986). We used decision time to measure how training influenced information-processing skills in screening mammograms for breast cancer.

Expertise in radiology, and in medicine more generally, refers to reliably accurate diagnostic problem solving. This does not mean that radiologists are infallible. They make errors, and much of our research and that of others has focused on the error side of the coin rather than the accuracy side (e.g., Kundel, Nodine, Krupinski, 1990; Parasuraman, 1986).

19.4.4 Mammography expertise

To illustrate the importance of training and experience (practice) on the acquisition of medical-image interpretive skills, we recently concluded a study of mammography expertise in which we compared performance of experienced breast imagers (mammographers) with radiology residents undergoing mammography training and mammography technologists. Our study was designed to compare observers having differing degrees of interpretive skill reading mammograms in an effort to shed light on how such skill is acquired and reflected in performance. As part of this study, in order to provide a clearer picture of how the three groups differ in experience interpreting mammograms, we obtained data about the number of mammographic reports generated by residents and mammographers. This was done as a way of quantifying the amount of mentor-guided image-reading experience residents received. The 19 radiology residents who were part of the study represented mainly third-year ($n = 7$) and fourth-year ($n = 8$) residents, plus 4 fellows, with mammography reading experience varying from 10 to 2465 cases over a 3-year interval. The average reading experience at the end of resident training was 650 cases for our resident sample. Over the same period, each of the 3 mammographers read 9459 to 12,145 cases.

Figure 19.1 shows the relationship between log (base 10) cumulative number of mammogram cases read over a 3-year interval and A1, the area under the AFROC (alternative free operating characteristic) curve, which is a measure of overall diagnostic accuracy.

This figure shows a significant linear-regression fit of the data ($R^2 = 0.667$) with a positive slope suggesting that interpretive-skill competence as reflected by A1 performance (area under the AFROC) increases directly with log case-reading experience. This finding is strikingly similar to that found by Charness et al. (1996) between log cumulative practice alone (deliberate practice) and current Elo rating (chess-skill rating measure) for chess players under 40 year of age. A log scale was used to represent the effects of case reading experience because several investigators have suggested that the relationship between practice and learning is best expressed by a power function and this has been referred to as the Power Law of learning (e.g., Newell and Rosenbloom, 1981; Anderson, 1995).

The range of case-reading experience in Figure 19.1 was from about 1 log case readings to 4.1 log case readings, or about 10 to 12,000 cases. This range includes two residents at the beginning of mammography training with very little case reading experience (<1 log case) who performed at an A1 of about 0.500, where 0.000 is chance performance under the AFROC curve, and 3 mammographers with from 10,000 to 12,000 case reading experience (>4.1 log cases) who performed at A1 $= 0.840$. The training level of the observers is indicated by numbers or letters associated with the data points. Overall performance increases directly with experience, and in an orderly progression with training level. The fact that the beginning residents' performance is above chance at the start of mammography rotation can probably be attributed to reading experience from other specialities encountered during residency rotations as well as book reading and didactic sessions on mammography. Talent is also a factor that plays a role in the relationship shown in Figure 19.1, and shows the greatest variability in the third- and fourth-year residents who are nearing the end of their training experience.

The main point of Figure 19.1 is that logarithmic increases in mentor-guided mammography reading experiences are required to produce skilled mammography reading performance, and even at the end of mammography training, residents' interpretive skills are significantly below that of their mentors and will, according

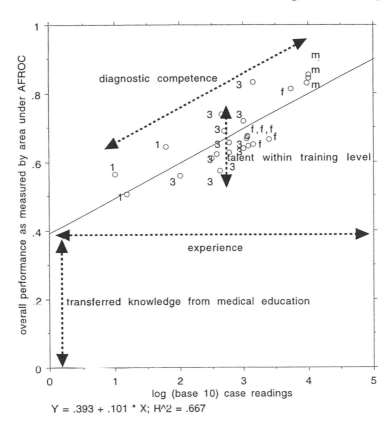

Figure 19.1: A regression analysis of overall performance measured as A1 as a function of log (base 10) number of cases read over a 3-year period by 3 experienced mammographers and 19 radiology residents undergoing clinical mammography rotation. When case readings is zero, the regression line intercepts the y-axis at 0.393 A1. With mentor-guided case-reading training and experience, A1 performance increases. The numbers next to the data points indicate the level of training and experience of the observers: 1 = first- and second-year residents; 3 = third- and fourth-year residents; f = fellows; and, m = mammographers. As indicated by the diagram below the data, competence increases with experience. Differences within levels are assumed to be due either to talent or random variation.

to this plot, require massive further amounts of reading experience. The interesting question is whether other forms of training more closely aligned to the notion of deliberate practice, which might be achievable by providing computer-assisted feedback as part of the training, would produce more effective learning. This makes the computer the mentor, but as such the computer can only be programmed to provide "plausible" feedback to student inquiries since image "truth" is unknown.

19.5 What is learned from reading medical images?

The usual answer to what is learned is knowledge, which is translated into various forms of cognitive skills and decision strategies. The knowledge skills that are learned provide a perceptual basis for recognizing disease states in medical images and a cognitive basis for translating image perceptions into diagnostic disease categories. The details of these cognitive skills and strategies are elusive because the experimental means of getting at them is indirect and usually couched in cognitive theory. This is why expert systems have not generally led to practical results. If these skills and strategies cannot be identified, they cannot be taught. The simplest solution is to override the perceptual-cognitive analyses that attempt to identify the skills and strategies and instead resort to performing massed practice on the task that best represents the domain of expertise. It is agreed by many researchers from both perceptual and cognitive camps that massed practice is the main change agent in achieving expertise. Thus, if the goal is to be a radiologist, then the prescription for gaining expertise is to learn about radiology by practicing reading radiographs. Practicing reading radiographs has to be supplemented by feedback about whether the readings match reality in terms of diagnostic truth, and making appropriate adjustments (error-correction feedback). This means that training in medicine, particularly anatomy and pathology, as well as in radiology, which depends on 3D spatial abilities, is a necessary prerequisite. So the sequence for gaining expertise in radiology is: TRAIN & READ RADIOGRAPHS—SEEK FEEDBACK—ADJUST READING TO FIT DIAGNOSTIC FACTS.

We will use examples from the research literature on radiology expertise to compare the perceptual and cognitive approaches designed to answer the question, what is learned? The general framework for problem solving in the radiology domain for both approaches can be summarized as:
SEARCH & DETECT—RECOGNIZE—DECIDE.

In other words, three different aspects benefit from learning: developing a heuristic search and detection strategy, fine-tuning visual recognition of targets through practice, and balancing the likelihood of being correct against the possibility, and cost, of error in decision making. A recent version of the perceptual model is shown in Figure 19.2.

This figure shows that a global percept can be extracted from the image. This corresponds to obtaining an overall impression of what is being displayed. From this global percept, objects are separated and representations of disease-free areas are segregated from representations of possible-lesion areas. The lesion candidates are then scanned for feature extraction, which is the initial step in hypothesis formation by the observer. These features will work as guides to the expert, by suggesting the possible diagnostic outcomes. Once this diagnostic list is generated, it is confirmed against the features observed, which gives the expert a probabilistic distribution of the possible diseases. The possible disease list is checked with the objects perceived in the image, and a new search activated. In this way expert reasoning works in two directions, bottom-up, by carrying out object segmentation and feature extraction, and top-down, by checking the image elements against the diagnostic list.

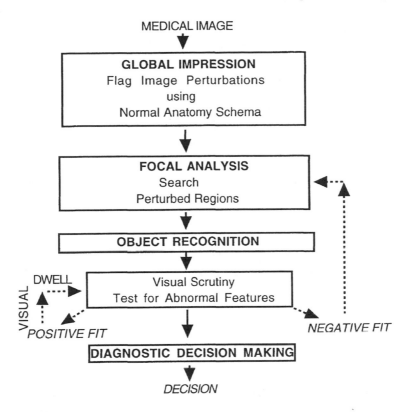

Figure 19.2: A perceptual model of the radiology task. The model shows the information-processing flow from the presentation of the image to diagnostic decision. Initially, a medical image elicits a global impression that flags perturbations setting up focal analysis in which perturbed regions of the image are searched. This results in recognition of objects that are tested for abnormality. The outcome of each test is either a positive or negative fit to the abnormality being tested. In either case, the testing is recursive. If a positive fit is found, the object is scrutinized by multiple eye fixations resulting in a build up of visual dwell in the region of interest. If a negative fit is found, attention shifts back to the medical image for a new global impression flagging another perturbed region, focal analysis searches it, a new object may be recognized and recursive testing for abnormalities continues until the observer is satisfied that enough evidence has accumulatied to make a diagnostic decision. Under this model, true abnormalities may be detected and receive fixation dwell but fail to be reported.

19.5.1 Search

A key question that drives both the perceptual and cognitive approaches is: How is search guided by knowledge (Newell and Simon, 1972), whether searching the visual display or searching the problem space for a diagnostic solution? The perceptual approach attempts to derive answers by analysis of eye-position data that search and test image features for diagnostic information leading to a decision outcome. The cognitive approach attempts to derive answers from analysis of verbal protocol data that reveal cognitive structures embedded in propositional-statement logic referring to image findings used to generate diagnostic solutions.

19.5.1.1 Eye movements and searching the visual-image space

Searching with the Eyes—One of the earliest attempts to study the role of search in radiology expertise was carried out by Kundel and La Follette (1972). They were interested in the evolution of expert search patterns. Kundel and Wright (1969) had already provided evidence that radiologists frequently use a circumferential search pattern when searching for lung nodules in chest radiographs. The circumferential pattern reflects a heuristic search strategy for selectively sampling information on the radiograph based on prior knowledge about the type of target abnormality (e.g., lung nodule), or expectations about disease type (e.g., clearly recognizable multiple abnormalities). The evolution of a heuristic search was clearly demonstrated in a follow-up study which compared eye-fixation patterns of untrained laymen, medical students, radiology residents, and staff radiologists viewing normal and abnormal chest radiographs without prior knowledge about type of target abnormality. According to the authors, this heuristic search strategy evolved mainly as a result of "... knowledge of radiographic anatomy, pathology, and clinical medicine rather than upon formal radiologic training as given in residency programs." A specific form of the knowledge that guides search is "... clear and unambiguous definitions of 'normal' and 'abnormal'" (Kundel and La Follette, p. 528). This knowledge comes from years of experience reading chest radiographs to gain familiarity with features that distinguish targets of search from their anatomic backgrounds.

These early studies represent the beginnings of the perceptual approach to the study of expertise. They are important because they point out that radiology expertise is characterized by heuristic, not random, search. The term heuristic is popular in AI research, and books have been written arguing about its meaning and significance in AI (e.g., Groner, Groner, Bischof, 1983). We refer to heuristic search here meaning that experts choose an approach in searching a radiograph which draws on prior knowledge and experience to form an initial hypothesis that guides search rather than searching in a trial and error manner without preconceptual guidance. This strategizing is an interesting trade off that human observers choose in solving problems, in contrast to machines that typically use an exhaustive sampling of the problem space until the target of search is detected. A good example of this can be found in world champion-level chess programs which are capable of a 14-ply full-width search, where ply refers to one move and countermove. Contrast this brute-force search with skilled human chess players who typically look only one or two plies deep, even though they could look 8–10 plies deep (Charness, 1981). Humans are unwilling to expend the energy required to carry out an exhaustive search for the small amount of gain that it yields. Applied to searching radiographs, this translates into a search strategy in which the observer attempts to use the smallest effective visual field to sample the most informative image areas in a minimum amount of time (Kundel, Nodine, Thickman, *et al.*, 1987). An expert uses structured knowledge to adjust the visual field size, determine the informative areas of the image, and keep track of the information yield over the time course of search.

Evidence that structured knowledge guides the search of experts comes from comparing random versus systematic-scanning (exhaustive) models based on human eye-fixation parameters. This comparison shows that radiologists confine their scanning to the lungs, in a chest radiograph, with a visual field between 2 and 3 deg (radius), searching for lung nodules. We speculate that gobal-image properties define the boundaries of the target-containing area. By 10 sec the radiologists have covered 85 percent of the lungs and detected most of the lung nodules. In the same time, the exhaustive model has covered more of the chest area, but not more lung area. The search pattern of the radiologists has been shown to exhibit more consistency with a circumferential pattern most common when searching for lung nodules, but for more general search tasks consistency gives way to idiosyncratic patterns that are too complex to categorize (Kundel and Wright, 1969). These findings suggest that scanning patterns of radiologists are not random but rather dependent on what the radiologist perceives to be the task, and what is seen during the course of scanning the image.

19.5.1.2 Verbal protocols, thinking out loud and searching the cognitive-problem space

Searching with the Mind—The cognitive approach has downplayed the visual component of radiology expertise and focused on the observer's cognitive evaluation of the radiographic display. The approach is similar to that used by Chase and Simon for studying chess in that a perceptual phase and a cognitive phase are separately tested. As an example, we use the experimental protocol of Lesgold, Feltovitch, Glaser *et al.* (1981, 1988). First the observer is given a brief view of the radiograph (2 sec), and asked what was seen with experimenter prompts to test the limits of the initial perceptual phase. Second, a verbal protocol is elicited by having the observer read the radiograph while "thinking out loud." This is followed by a formal dictated diagnostic report. Finally, the observer is given the patient history, re-examines the radiograph, and if necessary makes modifications in the diagnostic report. The goal of the perceptual phase is to identify how the stimulus is initially represented and schematically encoded within the problem space and to get at tentative hypotheses. The goal of the verbal protocol phase is to identify reasoning paths to a diagnostic solution. The reasoning step was modified in the experimental protocol by dropping the initial perceptual phase and expanding the verbal protocol phase to include having observers circle key areas on the radiograph that were considered critical in the reasoning path to diagnosis.

Lesgold, Feltovitch, Glaser *et al.* studied expertise in chest radiology by comparing verbal protocols of radiology residents at various levels with those of experienced radiologists. Analyses of verbal protocols led to a two-stage model of the diagnostic process. In the first stage a perceptual decision is generated. This yields a probabilistically-weighted set of perceptual features that diagnostically characterizes the radiographic image leading to a single outcome. The initial stage is followed by a decision-making analysis of the perceptual features within a cognitive framework of diagnostic problem solving (see Selfridge, 1959). The first stage depends heavily on the observer's schematic knowledge in the form of an anatomic representation—a map of chest features. The second stage depends on cognitive testing of perceptual features that are translated into radiologic findings used to feed diagnostic reasoning chains. Radiology expertise was reflected by a richly structured anatomic schema mapping x-ray features to normal anatomy. This rich schema provides the basis for detecting "left over" features signaling and localizing possible abnormalities on new chest x-ray image instances. A schema is called up faster in experts than trainees giving experts a faster start in searching the radiograph and a more accurate roadmap of abnormal features likely to trigger a decision-making rule leading to a diagnostic solution.

The skill component of expertise was demonstrated by the fact that experts exceeded trainees on all quantitative measures derived from protocol analysis (e.g., more findings, more and bigger clusters of findings, more relationships among findings, and more inferential thinking using findings). Experts were also better than trainees at recognizing and localizing perturbations in normal anatomic structures that signaled pathology. Analysis of protocol statements emphasized the problem-solving flexibility of experts in generating schemata to fit specific cases, holding them tentative and accepting or rejecting them only after rigorous testing. The experts seemed to be able to generalize the x-ray findings from specific cases to idealized patterns of disease by drawing on mental models of patients' anatomy and medical history. Trainees showed less flexibility, generating schema so tightly bound to perceived x-ray findings that they often led to false solutions. For Lesgold, Feltovitch, Glaser *et al.*, the schema is the key to successful problem solving and "... acquisition of expertise consists in ever more refined versions of schemata developing through a cognitively deep form of generalization and discrimination." (p. 340). For most radiographic diagnoses, a shallow level of cognitive processing will suffice, and may even be more accurate than deeper reasoning (Proctor and Dutta, 1995). It is only with complex diagnoses that the advantage of deep cognitive processing becomes apparent. This deep form of cognitive processing comes about as a result of extended practice that makes expertise in radiology possible. Raufaste, Eyrolle, Marine (1998) expand on this conclusion by testing what they call a "pertinence generation" model of radiology diagnosis. Protocol analysis of 22 radiologists' interpretations of two "very difficult" cases revealed two qualitatively different kinds of expertise, basic and super. The super experts were distinguished by increased pertinence in the interpretation of diagnostic findings. Pertinence generation refers to linking visual signs (radiologic findings) to diagnostic inferences which increases with level of expertise. The cognitive processing behind pertinence generation is schema driven but the reasoning chain is more deliberate and reflective in super experts than basic experts or radiology residents. Super expertise is not simply acquired through more and more experience. Rather, at least for Raufaste, Eyrolle, Marine (1998), super expertise is the integration of reading experience with teaching and research experiences. These provide a basis for integrating understanding about how radiologic findings are translated into plausible (pertinent) diagnostic hypotheses and logically tested for pathologic process leading to a diagnosis in much the same deliberate manner as deductive reasoning is carried out in a scientific experiment.

19.5.2 Visual recognition—features vs patterns vs objects

We have talked a lot about the importance of schemata in radiologic problem solving. Neisser (1976) built his theory of cognition around the concept of anticipatory schemata. According to his view, perception is a constructive process of discovering what the visual world (or image) is like and adapting to it. This discovery and adaptation process is, in the most general sense, the goal of visual information processing. It is possible to view radiographic diagnosis as a constructive process. For Neisser, the perceptual cycle is elicited by a schema that directs visual exploration to sample objects (information) and feed back the results thus modifying and enriching the initial schema. A schema for Neisser defines plans for perceptual action and readiness to take in certain kinds of perceptual structure. If an evoked schema is to be effective for guiding search, it must be generated early in problem solving. How does the initial visual input from the radiograph stimulate the formation of a schema? After initial schema formation, what role does visual recognition play in evaluating targets detected during focal search? What is recognized, features, patterns, objects or what? Both perceptual and cognitive approaches have focused on features as the basic unit of cognitive processing. This leads to a bottom-up analysis by synthesis of the object to be recognized. Both approaches also talk about the importance of patterns and chunking of information which are higher-level perceptual or cognitive structures. David Marr (1982) pushed visual recognition to the top-down object-representation level, and this has been expanded by Ullman (1996). The box that one gets into in postulating models of the visual recognition process is the chicken-and-egg dilemma: whether the observer first detects a distinctive part (feature) and builds up the object percept; or, whether the object percept is globally recognized, holistically, without intervening building-block steps. This is a critical question for cognitive modeling underlying visual recognition because we build error-correcting feedback based on our theory of the information-unit building blocks. Thus, if our theoretical building blocks are features, we train by feeding back features of object to-be-recognized. And how do we confirm that the features are truly the building blocks behind visual recognition? We ask the observers to think out loud and they say they use FEATURES to recognize the object. This circular logic is prevalent in the theoretical accounts of both perceptual and cognitive approaches used to study visual recognition that are reviewed below, and the answers they generate. Different experimental methodologies have been used to try get at the answers to these questions, but visual recognition still remains a puzzle.

Flash experiments. One answer to the visual-recognition puzzle comes from so-called flash studies in which radiographic images are presented briefly (e.g., 200 ms, the typical duration of an eye fixation) using a tachistoscope (Kundel and

Nodine, 1975; Gale, Vernon, Miller *et al.*, 1990). Several studies have asked how much can be seen in a single glance by tachistiscoptically presenting radiographs to radiologists and asking for diagnosis. In 1975, Kundel and Nodine identified a key skill that characterizes radiology expertise. They found that in 200 ms experienced radiologists could accurately recognize 70 percent of the abnormalities detected under free search of a chest radiograph. Many of the abnormalities recognized in 200 ms were large, high-contrast targets (e.g., mass, pneumonia and enlarged hearts) which significantly altered the appearance of normal anatomic structures in the chest x-ray image. Small or low-contrast targets (e.g., lung nodule, histoplasmosis) were not detected in 200 ms. This led to the interpretation that a global response (akin to Gregory's "object hypothesis," 1970) involving input from the entire retina provides an overall (schematic) impression of the radiograph that initiates focal search to test image perturbations leading to a diagnostic decision (Kundel and Nodine, 1983). The initial grasp of the visual scene is compared against schemata in which stored knowledge representations and deviations from expectations of a normal chest pattern are spatially encoded and flagged, all within the average duration of a single eye fixation. Kundel and Nodine (1983) showed that differences between radiologists' and laypersons' schemas of radiographic images are reflected in their drawings of what they saw. The drawings by laypeople, who did not recognize what they were looking at, consistently depicted background features. The drawings by radiologists, who did recognize what they were looking at, depicted image objects (see Figure 19.3). Interestingly, when looking at a hidden figure (puzzle-picture of the head of a cow), unfamiliar to both groups, the drawings leading up to recognition consistently focused on background features surrounding the hidden object for both groups. Only after the cow was recognized, presumably as the result of a match to an appropriate cognitive schema, did the drawings depict the hidden object (see Figure 19.4). Correlated with shifts in focus of the drawings from features to objects was a corresponding shift in focus of eye fixations from background features to object centers.

Similar findings have been found for detecting breast lesions (Mugglestone, Gale, Cowley *et al.*, 1995). For example, Mugglestone, Gale, Cowley *et al.* compared mean overall performance (Az area, that is the area under the Receiver Operating Characteristic or ROC curve), mean percent correct recall and mean percent return to screen of 9 radiologists under flash (200 ms) and unlimited viewing. They found overall that performance was poorer under flash than unlimited viewing (0.518 vs 0.700, respectively), primarily attributable to missing subtle abnormalities that failed to standout against mixed and dense breast-parenchymal backgrounds compared to lesions in fatty breast backgrounds (49% vs 31% for flash and unlimited viewing respectively). The lower overall performance for breast images compared to chest images was primarily due to the interaction of the conspicuity of the abnormality with anatomic background structures in the image. Inconspicuous, solitary findings in both breast and chest images seem to lack perceptual saliency in flash viewing. It may also be that lack of anatomic landmarks in breast images may fail to provide a distinctive anatomic schemata to facilitate pattern recognition compared to chest images which are rich in anatomic structures. Reflections

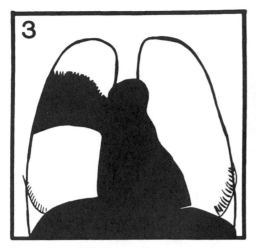 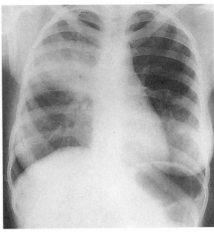

Figure 19.3: A silhouette drawing of a chest x-ray image containing a right-upper-lobe pneumonia (left), and the actual chest x-ray image containing the abnormality (right). The silhouette drawing was made by an experienced radiologist to illustrate the major finding on the chest x-ray film which was used in a flash study of image perception (Kundel and Nodine, 1975). The drawing depicts the abnormality in schematic fashion which may reflect how an experienced radiologist's cognitive schema encodes the chest-x-ray image when viewed in a 200 ms. flash presentation. The actual chest x-ray image was used in the experiment. In flash viewing, 30 percent of the observers gave an accurate diagnosis. In free viewing, diagnostic accuracy increased to 50 percent.

of these schemata are clearly illustrated in the drawings of chest-disease patterns shown in silhouette form in Kundel and Nodine (1975).

This would mean that the initial global impression for a breast image would key on conspicious features rather than anatomic landmarks, and that the global impression would be less effective in guiding focal search of the breast image. It is doubtful that the global impression can detect microcalcifications, and this was confirmed by Mugglestone, Gale, Cowley *et al.* (1995). Maybe this is why we observe that mammographers typically make two passes over a case that they are reading, the first to gather an overall impression and check for masses, and a second slow deliberate scan with a magnifying glass to catch microcalcifications.

Decision-time experiment. A second answer to the visual-recognition puzzle comes from a decision-time study of expertise in mammography which shows that experts are significantly faster and more accurate in detecting breast lesions than less-expert observers (Nodine, Kundel, Mello-Thoms, *et al.*, 1999). The initial detection, localization and classification of true lesions by experts occurred within 15 sec on average. This is much longer than flash viewing but in this case decision time included search time scanning both craniocaudal (CC) and mediolateral oblique (MLO) breast images for lesions, and detection plus localization time using a mouse-controlled cursor. The speed and accuracy of expert performance suggests to us a rapid global image impression that cues efficient focal search and supe-

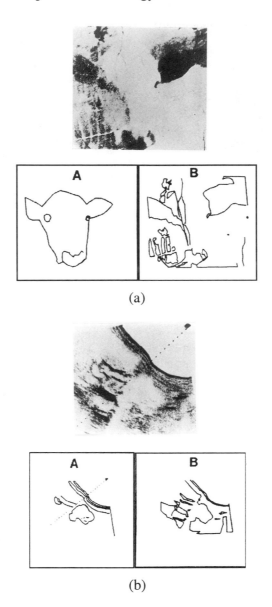

Figure 19.4: A puzzle-picture of the head of a cow (top, Figure 19.4(a)), and a longitudinal ultrasound image of the abdomen showing a dilated bile duct and the head of the pancreas (top, Figure 19.4(b)). These images were shown to 6 observers, 3 radiologists and 3 laypeople. The outline drawings under the pictures show what observers saw after 20 sec viewing. Observer A in Figure 19.4(a) (lower left) reported that he saw a "cow's head." Observer B in Figure 19.4(a) (lower right) reported that he saw an abstract picture of a "fish." The outline drawings below the picture in Figure 19.4(b) show what the observers saw after seeing the ultrasound image. Observer A in Figure 19.4(b) (lower left) was a radiologists, and reported seeing a "dilated common duct" from a pancreatic mass. Observer B in Figure 19.4(b) (lower right) was a layperson, and reported seeing an "aerial photograph." The drawings suggest that visual concepts of what observers thought they saw are driving image perception.

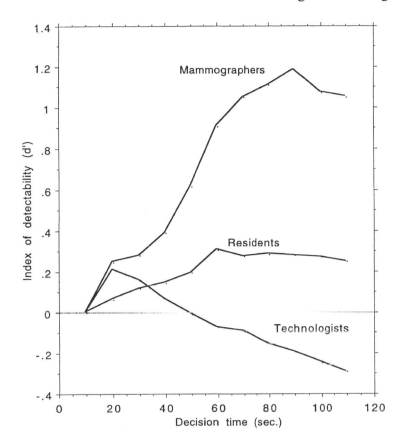

Figure 19.5: Speed-accuracy relationship as indicated by d', the index of detectability, as a function of decision time for mammographers, residents and technologists performing a combination mammography screening-diagnostic task (Nodine, Kundel, Mello-Thoms *et al.*, 1999). Overall performance as measured by d' which is the normal deviate, $z(TP)$, of true positive fraction $- z(FP)$, of the false positive fraction, increased for mammographers and to a lesser extent for residents. Overall performance decreased below chance ($d' = 0$) for technologists, meaning that false positives outnumbered true positives. Differences in performance were hypothesized as primarily due to lack of perceptual learning, which limited object recognition skills, causing competition between true malignant lesions, benign lesions, and normal image perturbations.

rior visual recognition of lesions. Initial impression, search and evaluation were more drawn out in observers with less expertise, and breakdowns in performance resulted in fewer true positives and more false positives. Figure 19.5 shows the speed-accuracy relationship related to mammography expertise.

Eye-position experiments. A third answer to the visual-recognition puzzle comes from eye-position studies of expertise in mammography (Figure 19.6) which also show that experts are faster and more accurate at detecting breast lesions (Nodine, Kundel, Lauver *et al.*, 1996; Krupinski, 1996). Using time to hit (TTH, search time to fixate a lesion) as the dependent variable, these studies show that experts

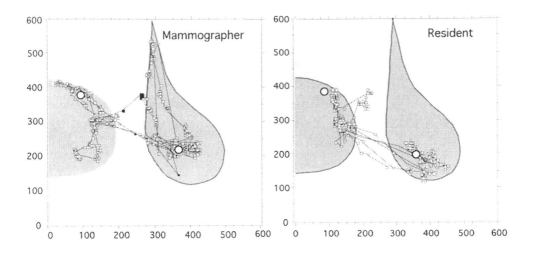

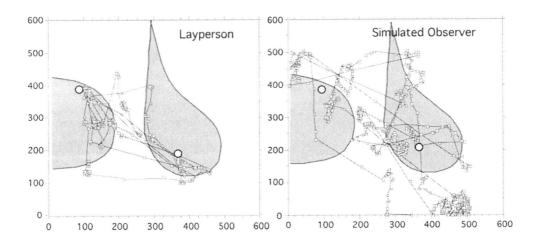

Figure 19.6: Scanning patterns of a mammographer (upper left), resident (upper right), layperson (lower left), and the simulated observer (lower right) to a digital mammographic image containing craniocaudal (CC) and mediolateral oblique (MLO) projections. The duration of the scan was limited to 16 sec in this comparison. The center of the mass in the CC view (left), and MLO view (right) are indicated by circles. The mammographer hits the mass in both views within 2 sec. The resident fixates the mass in the CC view in 1 sec, but takes almost 16 sec to fixate the mass in the MLO view. The layperson comes close to fixating the mass in both views. The simulated observer performs a random walk for 16 sec ultimately fixating the mass in the MLO view, but missing the mass in the CC view. The simulated observer scanpath uses saccade length and gaze duration data from human scanpaths. This results in fixations clustering in several regions of the display, but these clusters are independent of image content, since fixation x, y locations were randomly generated. Further details can be found in Nodine, Kundel, Lauver *et al.* (1996).

(experienced mammographers) find lesions faster than observers with less experience and training. Nodine, Kundel, Lauver *et al.* found that mammographers searching a two-view mammographic display containing CC and MLO images first fixated a mass that was reported correctly with an average TTH = 2.69 sec, whereas radiology residents required an average TTH = 4.74 sec to detect a correctly reported mass. Support for the view that the search strategy of experts was not random comes from a comparison of their TTH data with that of simulated observers that searched the breast image randomly.

Interestingly, the simulated observers took an average TTH = 4.67 sec which meant random fixations first hit an area containing a true mass after about the same search time as radiology residents. However, human observers failed to fixate only 2 percent of areas containing true masses whereas simulated observers failed to fixate 44 percent of areas containing true masses. These comparison data provide strong evidence that speed and accuracy of expert performance is tied to the rapid generation of a diagnostically-useful initial schematic representation that is effective in guiding search. We speculate that what experts recognize at first glance are unexpected oddities generated from a global characterization of the image that are flagged as regions to-be-searched by focal scanning. Thus, the goal of the initial global problem representation in radiology is not to find a target per se (because there are too many possibilities), but rather to find something odd about the image on which to focus the search strategy. Expertise comes into play in characterizing what in the image is odd. To recognize this the observer must first know what is not odd, or what is "normal." Evidence that the visual recognition of experts is tuned to differentiate odd or uncharacteristic features signalling pathology from clinically normal features comes from Myles-Worsley, Johnston, Simons *et al.* (1988). These odd features that occur in x-ray images have been called "perturbations" implying that their presence in the image disturbs the observer's image representation (schema). They found that as radiologists develop expertise in recognizing clinically-relevant abnormalities, they tend to selectively ignore normal feature variants, suggesting that detection of perturbations becomes more refined. Both perceptual and cognitive approaches agree that one of the most important signs of expertise is speed and accuracy of recognizing globally whether an image is normal or abnormal. This preceeds detailed search and analysis which leads to a specific diagnosis, and even this phase is faster in experts.

Probability-analysis experiments. A final answer to the visual-recognition puzzle comes from probability analysis of error paths in breast lesion detection (Mello-Thoms, Nodine, Kundel, 1999). What this analysis shows is that the initial decision made when examining a pair of breast images (CC and MLO views) significantly influences any subsequent analysis on that image. Namely, when the first decision is a true positive then the probability that the observer will find the same lesion on the other view is very high, with experts being significantly better than residents or technologists. Furthermore, on average, in this senario, the observer will make significantly fewer mistakes (false positives or false negatives) than if the first decision is incorrect (false positive). Moreover, when the first decision is incorrect, then the probability that the observer will find the true lesion, when one is present, is very small. Thus, beginning with error seems to promote other errors, dragging performance down. Interestingly enough, when the first decision is a false positive, in an image pair that has a true malignant lesion visible, on average the observers will make significantly fewer errors than when the first decision is a false positive in a normal image pair. In fact this difference can be quite staggering depending on the level of expertise. Experts will make about 8 times more errors when the first decision is a false positive on a normal image than when it is a false positive on an image with a malignant lesion present, whereas residents will make about 5 times more errors and technologists will make only about 2 times more errors. Maybe this is because of the confidence that experts have in their decisions, or because the image perturbation that led the expert to make the initial false positive decision on a normal image repeats itself in other areas of the image, thus misleading the expert into making other incorrect decisions. With residents and technologists this occurs to a smaller degree, probably because these two groups generate more errors on a regular basis, that is, they are more consistently fooled by image disturbances. In other words, the presence of a true lesion, even when the true lesion is not reported by the observer, seems to work as a perceptual bias for the number of false positives made.

Both the perceptual approach and the cognitive approach stress the importance of a rapid initial mental representation of the problem. Whether this is referred to as a schema or cognitive structure makes no difference because both perceptual and cognitive approaches are referring to representations of the same process. The perceptual approach uses visual-feature mappings, and the cognitive approach uses logical rule-based mappings to represent problems and generate solutions. The flash studies show that experienced radiologists have clear and unambiguous definitions of "normal," from which fast accurate recognition of deviations are globally detected.

19.5.3 Decision making

Evidence for differences in decision making as a function of level of expertise comes from two sources. First, from eye-position studies of observers who make perceptual errors in radiology, and second from our study of the speed-accuracy relationship in developing mammography expertise (Nodine, Kundel, Mello-Thoms et al., 1999).

Eye-position studies have identified three kinds of error in lung nodule detection: search errors, detection errors, and interpretation errors. Two-thirds of errors are divided between detection and interpretation, not search (Kundel, Nodine, Carmody, 1978). Visual dwell data show that missed targets (breast or chest lesions) receive as much if not more visual attention as do recognized, truly-positive targets (Krupinski, Nodine, Kundel 1998). This means that observers look at the missed target long enough to report it, but decide not to report it. Thus, over 60 percent of missed targets seem to be cognitively processed, as evidenced by both fixation clustering and prolonged visual dwelling on the missed target, yet observers fail to find sufficient evidence to report the object they evaluated as a target candidate. Analysis of eye fixations and visual dwell provides an information-theoretic account of the cause of errors of omission, false negatives, in radiology. Unfortunately it is difficult to disentangle whether the cause of the omission error was faulty recognition or decision making. Errors of commission, false positives, are also associated with prolonged dwell times that are equivalent to those found for true positives.

To shed light on this we looked at overall performance (area under AFROC) as a function of the time course of viewing mammographs by observers representing different levels of mammography expertise (Nodine, Kundel, Mello-Thoms *et al.*, 1999). We measured decision time, which is equivalent to what experimental psychologists refer to as "reaction time" (Posner, 1986), and related it to decision outcome using a combination mammography screening/diagnostic task. We have already reported above that experts were faster and more accurate performers, and that this is attributed to a well-developed prototypic normal breast schema that facilited the recognition of abnormal deviants correctly evaluated as malignant lesions. Perhaps the most interesting finding coming from this experiment is not the speed-accuracy relationship of experts, but rather that of the least expert in mammography interpretation, the mammography technologists, who had neither training nor experience reading mammograms. One technologist stands out in particular because she took the task literally and called every visible blob on every case. Her decision criterion for deciding that a malignant breast lesion was present was: Do I see a blob? She called 193 malignant lesions on 150 breast images of which 50 (26%) were correct. Her strategy appeared not to be driven by a schematic representation that maps anatomic knowledge with pathological knowledge. Rather, her strategy was driven by a simple blob-detection algorithm. In comparison, an expert (mammographer) called 97 malignant lesions of which 52 (54%) were correct. Thus, the mark of expertise is not how many correct lesions are recognized, but rather the balance between reporting true lesions and minimizing reporting false lesions. This calls on highly-tuned perceptual discrimination and differentiation which is learned through massive amounts of image-reading experience supplemented by feedback.

19.6 Connectionism—another approach to information processing

The perceptual approach and the cognitive approach to information processing deal with the reasoning process leading to decision making in very different ways. In particular the cognitive approach attempts to create a set of rules that will guide perception, evaluation and decision making. A shortcoming of this method is that different experts in the same field may have very different reasoning processes, as shown in Lesgold, Feltovitch, Glaser *et al.* (1988), Raufaste, Eyrolle, Marine (1998). This imposes tremendous difficulties to modeling the decision process, because input from each expert has to be carefully weighted and placed in the reasoning steps of a model that a computer can execute.

The cognitive approach can be seen in the first generation of AI systems, based upon predicate logic, which implied that all of the conclusions had to be drawn from a set of logical statements that basically corresponded to a game-playing scheme. Even the attribute-based representation systems, which allowed for broader mappings than the predicate logic did, used some sort of rule at each step to arrive at any conclusion. This was particularly true regarding decision trees. In predicate logic and attribute-based representations, sets of rules are designed based upon experts' verbal explanations of their analyses of medical images. This approach, however, impaired the use of artificial intelligence in problems for which no such set of rules could be consistently derived. Nonetheless, this does not imply that systems with this kind of representation are doomed to failure. There are obvious applications in which such a set of rules can be derived, and the problem is thus successfully solved.

An interesting point that can be made regarding these knowledge representations is, are human internal representations like these? That is, do humans use some logic- or attribute-based approach to solve their problems? Furthermore, these approaches seem to indicate that a serial structure is necessary, because each new conclusion can only be drawn based upon the answer to the previous question. This serial approach to brain function has been contested (Barrow, 1996). It has been shown that this approach maps the brain to a universal turing machine, which leads to restrictions regarding the speed of information processing, the robustness of the system and its lack of flexibility to deal with complex decision making tasks such as medical image interpretation (Dawson, 1998). Moreover, if indeed perception and cognition are based on a set of rules, shouldn't experts have a similarly structured set of rules? But that is not what one sees in practice, which may indicate that, although certain processes may be dealt with by the brain in this way, not necessarily all processes are analyzable in this fashion. Thus another type of knowledge representation must be considered.

The perceptual approach deals with the creation of an internal map that is based upon features that were visually extracted from the scene. This approach does not need to infer what this internal map looks like, for it only looks at the sequence of steps in and out of the internal map. It seems rational to ask an intelligent system to do this, namely, to build its own internal representation based upon a set of percepts extracted from the problem and then use these features to process the information by running through the internal map and producing a decision.

Thus, a third approach to information processing is created. Namely, it is based on the processing capabilities of the human brain, with its parallel weighted connections, that receives input and produces output, although the "how" is not entirely clear. This approach is called connectionism, and it is used by a fast growing branch of AI called artificial neural networks (or ANNs). In this chapter only one type of ANN will be considered, namely, the multi-layer perceptron (MLP), which is a multi-layer feedforward network (Haykin, 1994).

One of the major drawbacks with using the connectionist approach is that it is not clear which elements from the input patterns have a more significant contribution to the classification process. This is often called the credit-assignment problem, because the "thinking" process of the network is done at an internal (and unobservable) level, in the hidden neurons, and no insights can be gained into what actually helped the network achieve the final result. Furthermore, even if the network derives a probabilistic distribution for the data, it cannot tell the user which distribution it is, which does not help the human understanding of the problem, although some methods have been recently developed to extract knowledge embedded in ANNs (Tickle, Andrews, Galea et al., 1998).

Interestingly enough, this seems to be the way that the brain of a human expert works. For example, one may ask a distinguished radiologist how he or she arrived at a particular diagnosis, but often times they will not be able to list all of the steps that they took, or which factors weighted more heavily than others to generate a conclusion. Obviously if the problem is simple (for example, if a large malignant lesion covers a portion of the breast) then one has no doubts about what generated the particular diagnosis, but in these cases the ANNs also perform quite well, because the weight of the evidence in one dimension (in this case, size) is so overwhelming (Found and Muller, 1996). These are often not the cases in which one is interested. The secret for good performance, particularly in tasks like cancer detection, lies in the subtle lesions, in the early findings that may prevent a starting cancer from taking over.

Nonetheless, acquiring expertise in radiology requires massive amounts of practice, which is a problem for the novice radiologist or for a radiology trainee. As previously discussed, performance improves as a function of deliberate practice, that is, of self-motivated practice, as long as feedback is available to correct errors. Most of the time it is not possible to use a human expert to provide this feedback to inexperienced radiologists. In this sense the use of intelligent systems to aid these practitioners seem quite logical. The intelligent system can work as an educated second opinion, or by providing feedback to the observer about specific regions in the image.

In this section we will briefly discuss intelligent systems and artificial neural networks, as well as examine expertise in the context of ANNs. We will also discuss how to compare the performance of human experts with that of their artificially intelligent counterparts.

19.6.1 What is an intelligent system?

We will consider that an intelligent system is one that has agents (that is, elements) that allow it to successfully interact with its environment (Russell, 1996). Note that the definition as stated uses a measure of performance to determine if the system's actions in the environment lead to success or failure. It also assumes that knowledge about the environment is available to the system in a format that the system can not only use but that covers the universe of the domain of the problem. In other words, this knowledge is sufficient to allow the system to respond to its environment in an appropriate way (Partridge, 1996).

The interaction between an intelligent system and its environment as described above corresponds in psychology to a cognitive process (Fox, 1996), which is ap-

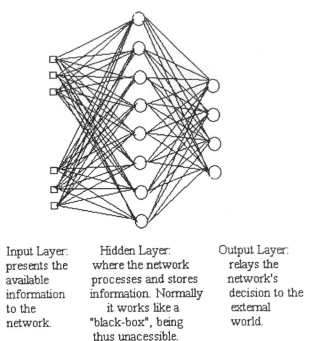

Input Layer:
presents the
available
information
to the
network.

Hidden Layer:
where the network
processes and stores
information. Normally
it works like a
"black-box", being
thus unacessible.

Output Layer:
relays the
network's
decision to the
external
world.

Figure 19.7:   A generic representation of a multilayered perceptron. This network architecture is divided into 3 parts: the input layer, which receives information provided by the environment; the hidden layer (s), which processes that information; and the output, layer which transmits the network's decision to the environment.

propriate, considering that learning is one of the hallmarks of intelligence (Russell, 1996). In other words, if a machine can learn, then, in principle, it can become intelligent. In this context intelligence refers to the ability of freeing itself from its creator, namely, from making up its own hypotheses and assumptions about the environment, even if these contradict the original hypotheses that the system was taught (Russell, 1996). In the domain of radiology expertise, this means that the system should be able to find its own unique interpretation for a given image instead of trying to match it to the ones that were used to teach the system.

Only one type of ANN will be considered here, the multi-layer perceptron (MLP). This is a very powerful network architecture that has been proven successful in a variety of contexts (Haykin, 1994). A generic representation of the MLP can be seen in Figure 19.7. As shown, this network architecture is divided into 3 parts, namely, the input layer, which receives the information provided by the environment, the hidden layer(s), which processes this information, and the output layer, which relays the network's decision to the environment.

Multi-layer perceptrons can learn in two different ways. In supervised learning the system is presented with a set of examples and the truth table, that is, a list that maps each example to its correct category. Although this method has some obvious advantages—namely, feedback is immediate, because the system instantly knows if it succeeded or if it failed—it nonetheless poses a problem in situations where no such truth table exists, that is, when there is no check on reality. In these cases unsupervised learning may be the best option. This learning technique allows the system to create its own map between "truth" and the examples presented to it. Thus, even though this is a more flexible type of learning, it has the drawback that many different classes may be created to represent objects belonging to the same category if the features that characterize these objects are not very similar. For example, many different classes could be created to represent masses in the breast, because these can be stellate, more or less dense, etc. Note that in this case, learning occurs by agreement, as opposed to by matching with a truth table as in the supervised learning case.

The process of presenting an ANN with a set of examples and letting it form its own representational map is called training. When previously unseen examples are presented to the network, its performance is judged by measuring how much and how well it learned. This process is called testing. If its responses are appropriate we deem that it learned to solve that particular problem. In this sense the learning process can be seen as a mapping between the examples domain, which offers discrete sampling about the (possibly) continuous multidimensional nature of the problem, and hypotheses formation, which allows the system to decide which action to take in the presence of a certain input. Note that in practice if the network performance during testing is below acceptance standards, it will have to be retrained. This process is equivalent to finding out that at the end of residency the performance of the residents is significantly below that of their mentors, and then attempting to improve their performance by exposing them to more cases.

Artificial neural networks have been successfully used in many areas of radiology, such as to predict breast cancer invasion (Lo, Baker, Kornguth et al., 1997), to find calcifications in mammograms (Nishikawa, Jiang, Giger et al., 1994), to detect signs of lung cancers in chest radiographs (Lo, Lin, Freeman et al., 1998), and to differentiate benign from malignant lesions in mammograms (Zheng, Greenleaf, Gisvold, 1997).

Despite this success, it is important to consider that in most of the applications of ANNs to medical image reading, the selection of the features that will guide network diagnosis is done in one of two ways. Either image features and patient data are used to represent the problem to the network, or image parameters are extracted by some preprocessing step. Unfortunately, each of these representations has drawbacks. In the first case a human specialist has to search the image looking for the appropriate parameters (examples of such features could be the presence of calcification clusters, breast density, etc.), which may not be viable if the system is to be used to aid novice radiologists or to train residents, because neither of these groups may be completely capable of deriving such predictive features from the image. Furthermore, if one needs a specialist to derive the predictive image features, then one may as well use that specialist to read the image itself, and thus skip the ANN altogether.

In the second case, exhaustive search of the image is done in order to derive the features for the ANN. As shown elsewhere (Kundel, 1987) experts do not search like this, but rather, use their prior knowledge (acquired by experience) to guide their search in a heuristic fashion, thus avoiding spending time looking in regions of the image where lesions are unlikely. One can argue that this procedure prevents total coverage of the image, and thus should increase the rate of false negatives, resulting from the presence of lesions in parts of the image where the expert failed to look. But this does not seem to be the case (Kundel, 1987). Experience seems to allow the experts to mentally generate a probabilistic map of the likelihood of lesions in different parts of the image. In taking information from this probabilistic map, the expert is in fact optimizing search using as constrains total time spent reading the image and the value of finding true lesions against the cost of missing a true lesion. Studies have shown (Nodine, Kundel, Mello-Thoms *et al.*, 1999) that experts are very fast and accurate in finding pairs of lesions given two mammographic views of the same breast, whereas residents and radiology technologists lag far behind. Furthermore, because of their lack of formal training, radiology technologists do not seem to build such probabilistic maps, but rather use what we called a "shot-gun strategy." They exhaustively examine the image and call everything that looks blob-like. As a consequence, the same criterion for lesion detection is used everywhere in the image, despite the local changes in anatomy (and thus in contrast appearance attributable to x-ray transmission), and the different likelihoods that a lesion will develop in different regions of the breast (Haagensen, 1986). This generates many incorrect decisions.

One of the biggest problems with artificial intelligence (AI) is its inability to deal with the incorporation of prior knowledge in the formation of new hypotheses. Note that this hinders the search process, because the machine cannot build the probabilistic map that experts do. This forces the search to be performed using a "shot-gun" strategy, which generates many false positives, and the results may resemble the exhaustive "blob-detector" radiology technologists described above, which is not acceptable for a system that aims to help radiologists.

19.6.2 Expertise in the context of artificial neural networks

Learning is an important part of improving performance in a decision making task such as mammography. Nodine, Kundel, Mello-Thoms *et al.* showed that human performance in reading mammograms improves as a function of individual talent and the number of mammogram cases read. Furthermore, we showed that experts have seen the largest number of cases, and also that their performance is significantly better than that of either novices or laypersons. In other words, we showed that human performance improves as a function of practice.

It is very difficult to use this measure to characterize expertise in artificial neural networks, primarily because in the vast majority of ANNs learning only occurs during the design part (a.k.a. training). This implies that, once the system has learned the input-output mapping with the examples provided to it, up to a desirable error level, it does not learn anymore. It is important to mention that this limitation is no fault of the theory of ANNs, but rather it is related to most of the algorithms currently available to train them. It is not impossible to develop a learning algorithm that permits the network to learn continuously, and in fact such algorithms do exist (e.g., the adaptive resonance algorithm). The problem is that in order to allow the network to continuously learn one has to allow for the network structure to be flexible, that is, one has to permit the network architecture to change as new classes are learned. In mathematics this is called the "stability-plasticity dilemma," because a compromise exists between how much the network architecture can change and how these changes may affect the network's stability. This problem affects all of the existing algorithms to train ANNs, and it does not have a closed-form solution. Thus, the price that one pays for keeping the network learning is the risk of either making it so big that it takes a very large amount of time to generate an outcome, or having it become unstable. As a consequence of this, the most widely used algorithms do not allow the network to learn anything new, once it has been trained.

This impacts the network's performance in two different ways. Namely, the level of error generated when the network was tested in the laboratory or elsewhere represents the best level of error that the network is ever able to achieve, primarily because the testing samples were drawn from the same population that the network was trained on and under the same conditions (i.e., film quality, image acquisition setup, acquisition technique, digitization, etc.). Second, if the conditions are changed—for example, if an intelligent system is being used for cancer detection and the incidence of cancer in the population it addresses changes for some reason—then the majority of ANNs cannot adapt on their own to the new conditions, unless they are retrained taking into account the new situation. This is undesirable, considering that finding the appropriate set of parameters for an ANN may take anywhere from a few hours to a few months or even years.

One important point to consider at this step is that there is a minority of artificial systems that can respond to perceived changes in the environment on their own. An example of this would be the adaptive resonance theory neural network, which is an unsupervised learning network capable of creating new nodes to represent the new classes it encounters at any point in time, during or after training. Although this is a great advantage as far as adaptation goes, it is important to remember that it too suffers from the drawbacks of the unsupervised learning systems, namely, it may create many unnecessary classes in response to the variations in the input patterns.

A consequence of the fact that the ANNs can only learn during training is that it possesses a static knowledge, whereas the human experts possess a dynamic knowledge. All that the network knows today it will know tomorrow, but no more, although the human experts will continue to acquire knowledge. This greatly impacts the nature of expertise that the ANN possesses, namely, it is a different kind of expert than the humans, because its expertise is unchanging.

At this point, an important question remains: how does one measure the performance of an ANN? And, how does one contrast it with the performance of the human experts?

A methodology to measure the performance of an AI system versus the performance of human observers was proposed in Haynes (1997). In this case the AI system would perform a task (reading a set of mammograms, for example) and humans with different experience levels would also perform the same task. A panel of expert judges would then rank performance, placing on the top of the list the better performances (more true lesions found, less mistakes, etc.) and on the bottom, the worse. The worst performance gets assigned a low score, and the best a high score. Observers with the same level of experience have their scores averaged, so that only one score represents each level of experience. A "skill function" is then plotted, which draws observer's experience versus the scores they received. Note that in this case the AI system is considered to be another observer. Confidence bands are also derived. Thus, to estimate the level of performance of the AI system versus the human experts, one can look at the plot and compare the AI's performance with that of the human observers that are closer to it. In this way one can make assessments such as "the ANN performed at a level of an observer with x years (or number of cases read, or whichever other measure) of experience."

One problem with such argument is that observers with the same level of experience may perform very differently, according to observer's talent, as shown in Nodine, Kundel, Mello-Thoms *et al.*, 1999. Thus, by averaging them together one is in fact misrepresenting performance at that level of experience. If, on the other hand, one uses only one observer with a given level of experience, then one is certainly risking representing that level with either the best or the worst performance, which certainly is not an acceptable measure.

Which criterion can be used then to measure the performance of an ANN? Well, certainly if one uses the same data set to test different ANNs, the one that has a smaller error is to be said to be the best. However, could one then go out and use this same data set to test human observers, and then compare these results with the ones from the ANN? The immediate answer is no, because human performance varies greatly with the level of expertise, which involves both talent and training. Thus, by saying that the ANN performed "better" than the human observers, one is in fact saying that it performed better against those particular observers which had a given level of talent and training. There are no guarantees, however, that as the number of cases seen by the observers increases, their performance would stay at the same level, and thus such a comparison is limited to that particular instant in time. On the other hand, if the human observers performed better than the ANN, nothing could be said, especially if the human observers had seen a larger number of cases than the ANN was trained with. One could say that the human observers in this case were trained with a larger (and possibly broader) data set. If the humans and the ANN had seen a similar number of cases, then one would have to be careful with the conclusions drawn, because one would have to show that this number is enough to generate human expertise (or to account for a decent training set for the machine).

What can be said, then, about expertise of an artificial neural network? One important point to consider initially is that, if all that constitutes expertise is something that can be computed, then there necessarily exists a set of rules that lead to it, because every mathematical identity can be rewritten as expressions from first-order logic (Bringsjord, 1997). Thus, if expertise is at all computable then ANNs or any other artificially intelligent system can conceptually be capable of realizing the same type of expertise as humans, and probably of achieving as good or even better performance then human experts, because of their massive computational capabilities. If on the other hand, as we propose, expertise has a component that is not computable, such as the spontaneous generation of new concepts, then artificial systems cannot simulate that component, and their expertise will be different, in kind, to that of the human expert.

Another important part of human expertise is creativity. Namely, the ability to respond appropriately to the unknown, to derive a meaningful set of actions by contrasting the novelty with what is known, is one of the hallmarks of the human experts. In this way, creativity is another characteristic that separates the human expert from the novices. In this context all three different types of creativity (Boden, 1998) are to be considered, namely, the exploratory type, which involves the generation of new ideas by the exploration of the knowledge domain; the combinatorial type, which generates new ideas by creating new associations for old ideas; and the transformational type, which involves transforming what is known to generate a concept never before conceived. By possessing one (or more) of these types of creativity a human expert can not only further the knowledge in his/her domain of expertise but also derive a meaningful strategy once he/she is faced with an unknown (or never before seen) aspect of the problem, and then learn from it (Palmer, 1997).

Intelligent systems have a great deal of difficulty dealing with the concept of creativity. As pointed out elsewhere (Boden, 1996; 1998) only the exploratory type of creativity has been dealt with in AI systems, with a small degree of success. The other two types rely heavily in the human associative memory, and most of its processes are, as of yet, not completely understood and thus cannot be replicated in a network. As a consequence of this, the intelligent systems that currently exist cannot generate a new concept on their own, and when facing the unknown may not react appropriately, because of their incapacity to adapt to the new situation.

Thus, as a summary, we can say that we believe that intelligent systems should be more and more used to do things that people do poorly, because their capabilities for massive amounts of computations is very helpful in some situations. On the other hand, in tasks were people do well, the role of the expert system may be more restricted, such as that of a tutor or a peer whose second opinion should be taken into account, but that probably should not be left alone to run the show.

19.7 Conclusions

In this chapter we described the nature of expertise, particularly referring to expertise in radiology. We showed, for example, that mammography expertise, as measured by overall performance (area under the AFROC curve) is highly dependent on the logarithm of the number of cases read. Our recent study of expertise in mammography (Nodine, Kundel, Mello-Thoms et al., 1999) also showed that residents in training develop similar decision-making strategies, as measured by their use of decision confidence ratings, as expert mammographers. From a practical standpoint this suggests that resident training in mammography is effective in providing a general framework for learning radiology reading skills. But residents were inferior to experts in recognizing true breast lesions. We hypothesize that this weakness is primarily attributable to the lack of fine-tuned visual-recognition skills which are dependent on perceptual learning. Supporting the tuning of visual recognition argument, Sowden, Davies, Roling (1998) have recently shown that massed practice detecting calcifications in positive-contrast mammograms (bright target on dark background) positively transfers to a new task in which the calcifications are displayed in negative-contrast mammograms (dark target on bright background). This suggests that perceptual learning improves perceptual sensitivity in the detection of high-contrast targets. Massed practice was defined as a detection trial followed immediately by feedback about the correctness of observer's response. This improvement in perceptual sensitivity occurred even though the amount of massed practice was limited to 720 trials followed by a transfer test. The key to improvement seems to be the feedback. The development of expertise in chess playing, which draws on similar mental representations and optimization strategies to those for radiology expertise, also supports the importance of massed practice as the primarily change agent.

When we looked at the question of what is learned when reading medical images, we showed that acquired knowledge is translated into a variety of cognitive skills and strategies. As expertise is acquired, search strategies become less exhaustive and more probabilistically driven by enriched anatomic-pathologic schemas. Visual recognition of potential targets becomes more accurate because of an expansive image-reading repertoire that defines decision thresholds for normalcy. This acts to fine-tune discrimination and generalization thus facilitating perceptual differentiation of abnormalities.

We have proposed that expert systems possess a different kind of expertise than human experts, for they are only able to generate one of the two components of human expertise, namely, the computable part, called training. This by no means hinders their utility, but care should be taken when comparing the performance of an expert system to that of a human expert.

Most radiology expertise skills and strategies find representations in the three models of information processing discussed, the perceptual approach, the cognitive approach and the connectionist approach. Although each of these approaches deals with different representations of the same underlying system, they ultimately rely on the same basic learning pinciple about how the acquisition and processing of information occurs. The essential role of experience in learning is to enrich structured knowledge in order to facilitate radiographic interpretation

Finally, all the theorizing about how radiology expertise is acquired boils down to a very simple answer: Practice, which as we have defined it in this paper means case-reading experience, enriched by feedback in the form of knowledge of results, makes the structured knowledge perfect! This is not a very deep theory of learning, but it seems to capture the essence of how expertise in radiology is acquired.

Acknowledgment

The writing of this chapter was supported, in part, by Grant DAMD17-97-1-7103 between the USAMRMC and the first author.

References

Anderson JR. *Cognitive Psychology and Its Implications*, 4th Edition. New York: WH Freeman, 1995:304.

Barrow H. "Connectionism and Neural Networks." In Boden MA (Ed.) *Artificial Intelligence*. San Diego, CA: Academic Press, 1996:135–156.

Bass JC, Chiles C. "Visual Skill: Correlation with Detection of Solitary Pulmonary Nodules." Investigative Radiology 1990;25:994–998.

Boden MA. "Creativity." In Boden MA (Ed.) *Artificial Intelligence*. San Diego: Academic Press, 1996:267–292.

Boden MA. "Creativity and Artificial Intelligence." Artificial Intelligence 1998;103:347–356.

Bringsjord S. "An Argument for the Uncomputability of Infinitary Mathematical Expertise." In Feltovich P, Ford KM, Hoffman RR (Eds.) *Expertise in Context*. Cambridge, MA: AAAI Press/The MIT Press, 1997:475–497.

Charness N, Krampe R, Mayr U. "The Role of Practice and Coaching in Entrepreneurial Skill Domains: an International Comparison of Life-Span Chess Skill Acquisition." In Ericsson KA (Ed.) *The Road to Excellence*. Mahwah, NJ: Lawrence Erlbaum Associates, 1996:51–80.

Charness N. "Expertise in Chess: the Balance Between Knowledge and Search." In Ericsson KA, Smith J (Eds.) *Toward a General Theory of Expertise*. Cambridge: Cambridge University Press, 1991:39–63.

Chase WG, Simon HA. "Perception in Chess." Cognitive Psychology 1973;4:55–81.

Chi MTH, Glaser R, Farr MJ. *The Nature of Expertise*. Hillsdale, NJ: Lawrence Erlbaum, 1988.

Dawson MRW, *Understanding Cognitive Science*. Malden, MA: Blackwell Publishers Inc., 1998.

de Groot A. *Thought and Choice in Chess*. The Hague: Mouton, 1965.

Ericsson KA, Charness N. "Expert Performance." American Psychologist 1994;49:725–747.

Found A, Muller HJ. "Searching for Unknown Feature Targets on More than One Dimension: Investigating a 'Dimension-Weighting Account'." Perception and Psychophysics 1996;58:88–101.

Fox J. "Expert Systems and Theories of Knowledge." In Boden MA (Ed.) *Artificial Intelligence*. San Diego, CA: Academic Press, 1996:157–181.

Gale AG, Vernon J, Millar K, Worthington BS. "Reporting in a Flash." British Journal of Radiology 1990;63:S71.

Gobet F, Simon, HA. Templates in Chess Memory: A Mechanism for Recalling Several Boards. Cognitive Psychology 1996;31:1–40.

Gregory RL. *The Intelligent Eye*. New York: McGraw-Hill, 1970.

Groner R, Groner M, Bischof WF. *Methods of Heuristics*. Hillsdale, NJ: LEA, 1983.

Haagensen CD. *Diseases of the Breast*, 2nd Edition-Revised reprint. Philadelphia: Saunders, 1986:380–382.

Hayes CC. "A Study of Solution Quality in Human Expert and Knowledge-Based System Reasoning." In Feltovich P, Ford KM, Hoffman RR (Eds.) *Expertise in Context*. Cambridge, MA: AAAI Press/The MIT Press, 1997:339–362.

Haykin S. "Neural Networks: A Comprehensive Foundation." Englewood Cliffs, NJ: Macmillan College Publishing Company, Inc., 1994.

Krupinski EA, Nodine CF, Kundel HL. "Enhancing Recognition of Lesions in Radiographic Images Using Perceptual Feedback." Optical Engineering 1998;37:813–818.

Krupinski EA. "Visual Scanning Patterns of Radiologists Searching Mammograms." Acad Radiol 1996;3:137–144.

Kundel HL, Nodine CF, Krupinski EA. "Computer-Displayed Eye Position as a Visual Aid to Pulmonary Nodule Interpretation." Invest Radiol 1990;25:890–896.

Kundel HL, Nodine CF, Thickman D, Toto L. "Searching for Lung Nodules: A Comparison of Human Performance with Random and Systematic Scanning Models." Invest Radiol 1987;22:417–422.

Kundel HL, Nodine CF. "A Visual Concept Shapes Image Perception." Radiology 1983;146:363–368.

Kundel HL, Nodine CF, Carmody DP. "Visual Scanning, Pattern Recognition and Decision Making in Pulmonary Nodule Detection." Investigative Radiology 1978;13:175–181.

Kundel HL, Nodine CF. "Interpreting Chess Radiographs without Visual Search." Radiology 1975;116:527–532.

Kundel HL, La Follette P. "Visual Search Patterns and Experience with Radiological Images." Radiology 1972;103:523–528.

Kundel HL, Wright DJ. "The Influence of Prior Knowledge on Visual Search Strategies During Viewing of Chest Radiographs." Radiology 1969;93:315–320.

Lesgold AM, Rubinson H, Feltovich P, Glaser R, Klopfer D, Wang Y. "Expertise in a Complex Skill: Diagnosing X-ray Pictures." In Chi MTH, Glaser R, Farr MJ (Eds.) *The Nature of Expertise*. Hillsdale, NJ: Lawrence Erlbaum, 1988:311–142.

Lesgold AM. "Acquiring Expertise." In Anderson JR, Kosslyn SM (Eds.) *Tutorials in Learning and Memory*. San Francisco: WH Freeman, 1984:31–60.

Lesgold AM, Feltovitch PJ, Glaser R, Wang Y. "The Acquisition of Perceptual Diagnostic Skill in Radiology." LRDC Technical Report PDS-1, University of Pittsburgh, 1 September, 1981.

Lo JY, Baker JA, Kornguth PJ, Iglehart JD, Floyd Jr CE. "Predicting Breast Cancer Invasion with Artificial Neural Networks on the Basis of Mammographic Features." Radiology 1997:203:159–163.

Lo SCB, Lin JSJ, Freeman MT, Mun SK. "Application of Artificial Neural Networks to Medical Image Pattern Recognition: Detection of Clustered Microcalcifications on Mammograms and Lung Cancer on Chest Radiographs." Journal of VLSI Signal Processing 1998;18:1–12.

Marr D. *Vision: A Computational Investigation into the Human Representation and Processing of Visual Information.* San Francisco: WH Freeman, 1982.

Mello-Thoms C, Nodine CF, Kundel HL. "The Effects of the First Response in Mammogram Reading: The Noise in the Head." Paper presented at Far West Imaging Society Meeting, Calgary, May, 1999.

Miller GA. "The Magic Number Seven, Plus or Minus two: Some Limits on Our Capacity for Processing Information." Psychological Review 1956;63:81–97.

Mugglestone MD, Gale AG, Cowley HC, Wilson ARM. "Diagnostic Performance on Briefly Presented Mammographic Images." In Kundel HL (Ed.) *Image Perception. Proceedings of SPIE.* 1995;2436:106–116.

Myles-Worsley M, Johnston WA, Simons MA. "The Influence of Expertise on X-Ray Processing." J Experimental Psychology: Memory and Cognition 1988;14:553–557.

Newell A, Rosenbloom PS. "Mechanisms of Skill Acquisition and the Law of Practice." In Anderson JR (Ed.) *Cognitive Skills and Their Acquisition.* Hillsdale, NJ: Lawrence Erlbaum, 1981:1–55.

Newell A. "You Can't Play 20 Questions with Nature and Win: Projective Comments on the Papers of this Symposium." In Chase WG (Ed.) *Visual Information Processing.* New York: Academic Press, 1973:283–308.

Newell A, Simon HA. *Human Problem Solving.* Englewood Cliffs, NJ: Prentice-Hall, 1972.

Neisser U. *Cognition and Reality.* San Francisco: WH Freeman, 1976:21.

Nishikawa RM, Jiang Y, Giger ML, Schmidt RA, Vyborny CJ, Zhang W, Papaioannou J, Bick U, Nagel R, Doi K. "Performance of Automated CAD Schemes for the Detection and Classification of Clustered Microcalcifications." In Gale AG, Astley SM, Dance DR, Cairns AY (Eds.) *Digital Mammography.* Amsterdam: Elsevier Science B.V., 1994.

Nodine CF, Kundel HL, Mello-Thoms C, Weinstein S, et al. "How Experience and Training Influence Mammography Expertise." Academic Radiology 1999 (submitted).

Nodine CF, Krupinski EA. "Perceptual Skill, Radiology Expertise, and Visual Test Performance with NINA and WALDO." Acad Radiol 1998;5:603–612.

Nodine CF, Kundel HL. "Using Eye Movements to Study Visual Search and to Improve Tumor Detection." Radiographics 1987;7:1241–1250.

Nodine CF, Kundel HL, Lauver SC, Toto LC. "Nature of Expertise in Searching Mammograms for Breast Masses." Acad Radiol 1996;3:1000–1006.

Palmer DC. "Selectionist Constraints on Neural Networks." In Donahoe J, Dorsel VP (Eds.) *Neural-Network Models of Cognition.* Amsterdam: Elsevier Science B. V., 1997:263–282.

Patel VL, Groen GJ. "The General and Specific Nature of Medical Expertise: A Critical Look." In Ericsson KA, Smith J (Eds.) *Toward a General Theory of Expertise*. Cambridge: Cambridge University Press, 1991:93–125.

Parasuraman R. "Effects of Practice on Detection of Abnormalities in Chest X-Rays." Proceedings Human Factors Society 1986;309–311.

Partridge D. "Representation of Knowledge." In Boden MA (Ed.) *Artificial Intelligence*. San Diego, CA: Academic Press, 1996:55–87.

Posner MI. *Chronometric Explorations of Mind*. New York: Oxford, 1986.

Proctor RW, Dutta A. *Skill Acquisition and Human Performance*. Thousand Oaks, CA: Sage, 1995:248.

Raufaste E, Eyrolle H. "Expertise et Diagnostic Radiologique: I. Avancees Theoriques." J Radiol 1998;79:227–234.

Raufaste E, Eyrolle H. "Expertise et Diagnostic Radiologique: II. Etude Empirique." J Radiol 1998;79:235–240.

Raufaste E, Eyrolle H, Marine C. "Pertinence Generation in Radiological Diagnosis: Spreading Activation and the Nature of Expertise." Cognitive Science 1998;22:517–546.

Russell S. "Machine Learning." In Boden MA (Ed.) *Artificial Intelligence*. San Diego, CA: Academic Press, 1996:89–133.

Selfridge OG. "Pandemonium: A Paradigm for Learning." In *The Mechanisation of Thought Processes*. London: HM Stationery Office, 1959.

Smoker WRK, Berbaum KS, Luebke NH, Jacoby CG. "Spatial Perception Testing in Diagnostic Radiology." AJR 1984;143:1105–1109.

Sowden P, Davies I, Roling P. "Perceptual Learning of the Detection of Features in X-Ray Images: A Functional Role for Improvements in Adults' Visual Sensitivity?" J Experimental Psychology: Human Perception and Performance 1999 (in press).

Sternberg RJ. "Costs of expertise." In Ericsson KA (Ed.) *The Road to Excellence*. Mahwah, NJ: Lawrence Erlbaum Associates, 1996:347–354.

Tickle AB, Andrews R, Golia M, Diederick J. "The Truth Will Come to Light: Directions and Challenges in Extracting the Knowledge Embedded Within Trained Artificial Neural Networks." IEEE Transactions on Neural Networks 1998;9:1057–1068.

Ullman S. *High-Level Vision: Object Recognition and Visual Cognition*. Cambridge, MA: MIT Press, 1996:161.

Wood BP. "Visual Expertise." Radiology 1999;211:1–3.

Zheng Y, Greenleaf JF, Gisvold JJ. "Reduction of Breast Biopsies with a Modified Self-Organizing Map." IEEE Transactions on Neural Networks 1997;8:1386–1396.

CHAPTER 20
Practical Applications of Perceptual Research

Elizabeth A. Krupinski
University of Arizona Health Sciences Center

CONTENTS

20.1 Introduction

A lot of the work into perceptual and observer performance issues in radiologic imaging (and medical imaging in general) began as a result of a series of studies [1, 2] done after WWII. These studies were designed to determine which of four roentgenographic and photofluorographic techniques was better for mass screening of chest images for tuberculosis. What seemed to be a rather easy and practical question to answer in a fairly straightforward investigation turned out to yield results that created more questions than answers. Inter-observer and intra-observer variabilities were so high that it could not be determined which imaging method yielded better diagnostic accuracy. Prior to this study, it was generally presumed that radiologists did not differ that much from each other in their diagnoses, and that if the same image was shown to the same radiologist at two points in time the diagnosis would not differ substantially. These studies suggested otherwise—radiologists were not as consistent as previously thought. One follow-up study [3] even tried to get radiologists to simply describe characteristics of radiographic shadows. Again there was wide inter-observer variation and moderately high intra-observer variation even on the seemingly straightforward description of lesion characteristics. This suggested that differences/errors in performance might lie in perceptual and cognitive factors rather than in technical factors such as bad technique or poor processing. Even today studies are being conducted that look at reader variability and ways to reduce it [4].

Since these early studies, much research has been done to elucidate the perceptual and cognitive processes involved in the reading of radiographic and other medical images. The previous chapters in this book described a variety of ways that image perception and observer performance have been investigated. Over the years, we have learned a lot about what types of errors are made [5, 6], under what circumstances they are more likely to be made [7–10], what the human visual system is actually capable of perceiving in an image [11, 12], and how to predict performance [13–15] with a variety of human visual system models. The goal of this chapter is to describe some practical applications of perceptual research in medical imaging. The intent is to provide some examples where perceptual research can or has made an impact in the clinical environment and to illustrate the general framework for extending perceptual research to practical applications. The intent is not to provide an exact methodology for doing the research or making the transition from the lab to clinic, because there really is no single correct method or formula to do this.

20.2 Bridging the gap between research and clinical practice

The American Heritage Dictionary [16] defines practical as "capable of being used or put into effect; designed to serve a purpose: useful, efficient." In the context of medical image-perception, the first part of the definition suggests that the results of image-perception research should somehow be implemented in the clinical environment and into the real-world task of interpreting clinical images. The second part of the definition implies that the application of the results of perceptual research should somehow improve performance or make the interpretation task easier and/or more efficient. To some extent, this treatment of practical applications in perception research follows the technology impact model (TIM) [17]. TIM measures the success of investigations in terms of the results of a technology evaluation study being able to invoke some sort of change in the mindset or practice of those responsible for medical decisions regarding patient care. This may not always be as easy as it sounds, although sometimes the application of empirical results to practical situations is quite straightforward.

There are two very broad approaches to measuring and understanding perceptual processing of medical images. The first approach uses subjective techniques. Underlying these subjective techniques are two basic assumptions. The first is that if a radiologist rates one rendition of an image as better than another rendition, it is somehow more pleasing or easier to look at. The second assumption is that if it is more pleasing or easier to look at, then it will be easier to render a correct diagnostic decision. These assumptions are generally not explicitly stated, but there have been many studies conducted with the hope that images rated as subjectively better than others will translate in the clinic into better performance. For example, the effect of image compression is a topic of great concern today because of the need to store and transfer very large digital images for picture archiving and communications systems (PACS) and teleradiology applications. A typical CR (computed radiography) image requires about 5 Mb of data, so high compression rates without loss of diagnostic information are desirable.

It is very difficult to separate image aesthetics from image quality, especially from the observer's point of view, because they may not be independent factors. For example, some radiologists prefer a blue-based film to a clear-based film to a sienna-based film. In terms of image quality (e.g., noise, spatial resolution, signal-to-noise ratio, etc.) there are no significant differences between clear, sienna, and blue-based film. The preference for one versus the other is aesthetic and is usually related to what type of film was used when the radiologist was in training. The dye added to the film does reduce eye-strain, but there have been no studies indicating that the color of the film impacts image-quality measures. It really comes down to preference or aesthetics. However, if one does not like an image from an aesthetic point of view, it can be very difficult to subjectively judge it as having good image quality if these two factors are dependently linked in the observer's mind.

An example of a typical study done to look at the effects of image compression using a subjective evaluation technique was recently done by Uchida *et al.* [18]. Radiologists looked at a series of CR hand images pairing the original uncompressed image with a compressed (20 : 1) version. They had to rate the images in terms of the depiction of bone cortex, trabeculae, soft tissue, and lesion margins, using a five-level scale that scored the original or compressed version as better. Each feature was rated separately. The diagnosis was known so diagnostic performance was not measured. Overall, there were no significant differences in the subjective ratings for original versus compressed images, although poorer image quality was noted for most structures. The authors conclude that high data compression may be clinically acceptable for CR hand images. The important caveat is that with this type of subjective evaluation, diagnostic accuracy was never actually measured so nothing can be said about whether compression will influence lesion-detection rates. It does, however, tell us something about the perception of image quality as a function of compression and is therefore important in that respect.

The second broad approach uses more objective techniques to study perception and performance. These types of studies measure diagnostic performance directly, for example using the receiver operating characteristic (ROC) paradigm or other indices of detectability. The ROC paradigm itself makes some basic assumptions about perception (i.e., the visual system's ability to discriminate signal from noise). Perception can also be measured more directly, for example using eye-position recording techniques and determining if or for how long a radiologist fixates a lesion and then correlating that perceptual information with the cognitive decision that is rendered.

An example of a study looking at image compression effects using an objective approach was done by Good *et al.* [19] using JPEG (Joint Photographic Experts Group) compressed chest images (ranging from 15 : 1 to 61 : 1). In addition to providing subjective assessments of image quality, the radiologists in the study had to determine if each of five possible abnormalities was present in the images. The results were analyzed using ROC techniques. The images were perceived to decline in image quality with increasing compression (not significantly), but there were no significant differences in diagnostic performance as a function of compression level. The radiologists rated their comfort levels lower with increasing compression, but their viewing times did not change over compression levels. Thus, although both this and the previously described study looked at the effects of compression using clinical images and radiologist observers, this one actually looked at diagnostic performance. Studies such as this, that combine subjective and objective evaluation measures, may strengthen the argument for practical clinical application of compression techniques and may make the transition from lab to clinic easier.

Both the subjective and objective techniques are quite valid ways of assessing perceptual and cognitive processes associated with reading medical images, although there is some evidence [20–22] that they may not always yield comparable results. Additionally, as noted above, subjective studies may be useful as an initial step to show that images are acceptable from a quality point of view to radiologists, but without performance data it is hard to judge the practical application of the results to the clinical environment. There is also the problem of whether they are actually independent measures. There are certainly aspects of each one that come into play when either one or the other is being measured and it is nearly impossible to completely separate them. However, studies can be conducted that emphasize one versus the other even though subjective parameters may almost always influence at least the confidence one has in a diagnostic decision. In either case, there are always the same generalization questions that arise with any study, whether there is a waiting application or not. Were there enough cases, was there enough variety of cases, were there enough observers, were there enough observers with different levels of expertise, what happens when all the extraneous variables that were controlled for in the experimental situation are now uncontrolled and, so on? These questions can really only be answered once the idea is put into actual clinical practice, but the results of empirical studies give us good reason to believe that the transition from experiment to clinic will be successful. The rest of this chapter describes a few very promising and important areas where perceptual research has the potential or already has bridged the gap between research and clinical practice with the goal of improving diagnostic decision making or improving the general diagnostic environment.

20.3 Image display and workstation design

The practice of radiology is increasingly changing from a film and light box-based to a computer and cathode ray tube (CRT) monitor-based display medium. PACS and teleradiolgy applications are becoming more and more common in radiology departments, so light boxes are being phased out and monitors are being phased in. This transition may seem straightforward and easy to some, but it is actually a rather involved [23–25] and sensitive process. In many radiology departments, most images are still read from film. Even inherently digital modalities (MRI, CT, US, Nuc Med) are printed to film. However, as monitor resolution and brightness have improved, the push for the "totally filmless" radiology department has increased. In general, it seems that most images can be read from a monitor without any loss in diagnostic accuracy [26–30]. The rest of this chapter will focus on a few image-display issues as examples of practical applications of perceptual research.

20.3.1 Choosing the "right" monitor for clinical use

There are a number of excellent articles in the literature that review various characteristics of soft-copy display in the context of human visual perception and minimal viewing standards [25, 31, 32]. Basically there are any number of physical parameters that can be measured when assessing a display for soft-copy presentation of images. Some of the more important ones [33] are: spatial resolution; contrast resolution; luminance; modulation transfer; display transfer function; veiling glare; noise (spatial and temporal); display size; image motion and flicker; and display uniformity. In many cases the physical measurements can be compared to or evaluated against well-known models of visual perception [34, 35]. In other cases, well-controlled performance studies can be conducted with human observers using phantom images as stimuli [36], and basic psychophysical relationships between display and performance can be assessed. Finally, observer performance studies that measure diagnostic accuracy in some fashion can be done with clinical images [26–30], and it is this type of study that really helps bridge the gap between research and clinical application.

As noted previously, there have been a number of studies that suggest that, for most types of images, displaying radiographic images on CRT monitors may be equivalent to displaying them on film in terms of diagnostic performance. Diagnostic accuracy may not, however, be the only benchmark by which we can measure the appropriateness of using monitors for reading x-ray images. The following study [26, 37] illustrates this point. Three bone radiologists and three orthopedic surgeons read 27 bone-trauma cases, once from film and once from a monitor. The radiologists had to search each image for fractures, dislocation or subluxation, ligamentous injury, and soft-tissue swelling or effusion. The presence/absence of each feature was rated separately for each case. Eighteen cases had soft-tissue swelling and of these 12 had an associated single fracture. Four cases showed dislocation or subluxation, 10 had evidence of ligamentous injury, and 8 had joint effusions. Nine cases had no trauma indicators. There were potentially 312 true-positive decisions and 498 true-negative decisions when the 5 trauma indicators and 6 readers were combined for the 27 cases. The 52 existing trauma indicators noted above were multuplied by 6 readers to yield 312 true positives. The nine normal cases multiplied by the 5 lesion categories by 6 readers results in 270 true negatives. For the 18 cases with swelling, there were 6 without fracture, 14 without dislocation or subluxation, 8 without ligamentous injury, and 10 without effusions. When these 38 trauma indicators are multiplied by 6 readers, the result is an additional 228 potential true negatives. Again, the readers had to indicate the presence/absence of each feature for each case. Eye position was recorded to determine if there were any aspects of visual search that might differ for film versus monitor viewing. A previous study [38] that compared monitor versus film viewing of chest radiographs found that total viewing time was about twice as long with the monitor than with film. So this study looked at total viewing time as well as various aspects of visual search while the radiologists viewed the images. Diagnostic performance did not differ statistically for film versus monitor viewing (film = 86% true positives (TP), 13% false-positives (FP); CRT = 80% TPs, 21% FPs), although performance was slightly better overall with film. Image quality was rated slightly better for film than CRT images in terms of overall quality, contrast, and sharpness, but the differences were not significant.

What did differ significantly between film and monitor viewing was total viewing time and other parameters of visual search. Average viewing time for film was 46.45 s, but was 91.15 s for monitor viewing. Again, total viewing time for the monitor was about twice as long as for film. The eye-position records provided some insight into why this difference occurred. Part of the increase in viewing time was directly related to the fact that dwell times associated with true-negative decisions were significantly longer for monitor than film viewing (see Table 20.1). This difference may not seem important if you just compare the median dwell times alone. However, on an average image there are maybe one or two true-positive, false-negative, and/or false-positive decisions with associated fixation clusters, and about 15 to 29 true-negative fixation clusters. The prolonging of individual true-negative fixation clusters has much more impact on total dwell time than lesion-associated fixations because the dwells are accumulated over many more fixation clusters.

Table 20.1: Median dwell times (ms) for decisions made viewing film versus monitor display of bone radiographs

	Film	n	Monitor	n
True Positive	1206	349	1286	328
False Negative	1204	59	938	79
False Positive	896	72	895	94
True Negative*	358	2052	532	1856

$^*X^2 = 10.67, df = 1, p = 0.001$

Time to first fixate the lesion after the image first appeared (4.67 s into search for monitor versus 2.35 s for film) also differed ($t = 4.84, df = 107, p = 0.0001$) for the two display conditions. It took longer for the radiologists to have even a single fixation fall on the lesion (whether it was detected or not) on the monitor than on film. This occurred even though the actual detection report rates were comparable for the film and monitor. One final factor contributing to extended viewing time was that 95% of fixation clusters generated during film reading were in diagnostic image areas, but only 78% of clusters in monitor reading were in diagnostic areas. On the monitor, 20% of the clusters were on the menu, increasing the overall viewing time and drawing attention away from the diagnostic areas. Figure 20.1 shows the relative portion of total viewing time spent on various image areas for film vs monitor viewing. Overall, this study demonstrated that even though diagnostic accuracy did not differ for film versus monitor viewing, there were differences in perceptual processing as revealed by differences in the various eye-position parameters. Clearly, there may be other aspects of performance that are important to consider when making the transition from film to monitor viewing than just diagnostic accuracy. Prolonged viewing times could impact significantly on workflow, could increase fatigue and could decrease overall reading efficiency. If these differences in total viewing time and other visual search parameters do not decrease as radiologists gain more experience with viewing images from monitors, some of these more basic perceptual factors may have to be considered in more depth.

The results of this study show that although diagnostic accuracy may not differ significantly for film versus monitor viewing, there are other important factors that are affected. Most current computer displays include a menu to navigate through cases. The presence of this menu can affect the way the radiologist searches an image and how much time and attention is devoted to searching diagnostic areas. When designing an interface, it is important to keep this fact in mind—the menu should not distract the reader from the diagnostic task. Perhaps other alternatives should be investigated using other modalities than vision. For example, one could use voice control or a foot pedal instead of a mouse or trackball to navigate through cases and implement image processing functions. there has not been much investi-

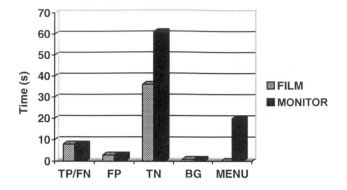

Figure 20.1: Average viewing time (s) per image broken down by image areas: TP/FN = on the lesion reported (TP) or not (FN), FP = false-positive, TN = true-negative, BG = background.

gation into these options in radiology, although these types of interfaces have been developed in other areas (e.g., interfaces for the handicapped).

Another important area where perceptual studies are being done in monitor evaluation is in terms of luminance. For example, in mammography a luminance of 3000 cd/m^2 is recommended for light boxes [39]. The maximum luminance available today for monitors is about 200 ft L. Luminance is certainly an important factor because it impacts on dynamic range, although at some point contrast itself may be the more important factor in influencing detection performance. Objects can generally be distinguished from their background when the difference in luminance is large enough. If the difference is not large enough, objects are difficult to see. However, it is not really the absolute difference in luminance, but rather the relative difference in luminance. The relative difference is expressed by the ratio of the two luminance levels (contrast ratio), or by the difference divided by the sum of the luminances (contrast). Thus, it is difficult to tell whether differences in performance as a function of display luminance are attributable to the changes in luminance alone or to the inherently related effects on contrast. In either case, there is probably a minimally acceptable luminance level for monitor viewing of radiographic images.

There have been a number of studies showing the importance of luminance with film displays [40, 41], so there is good reason to believe luminance is just as important with monitor displays. In general, studies have found that monitor luminance does not affect diagnostic performance to any significant degree. For example, Song *et al.* [42] looked at the detection of pulmonary nodules on a 100-ft L versus a 65-ft L monitor. Eight radiologists viewed 80 chest images using both monitors. ROC Az was slightly higher with the 100-ft L monitor (0.8734) than with the 65-ft L monitor (0.8597), but the difference was not statistically significant. The differences in performance for film versus monitor reading were greater for the observers who had less experience reading from soft-copy displays. Hemminger *et al.* [43] also looked at the effects of monitor luminance and detection performance

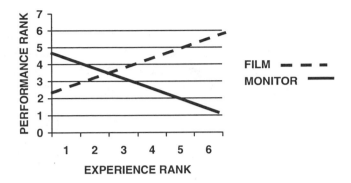

Figure 20.2: Years of experience as a board-certified radiologist and ROC Az performance using film vs monitor for viewing CR chest images.

for the detection of masses in mammograms. Simulated masses were embedded in random quadrants of cropped 512×512 portions of mammograms. Contrast of the masses with respect to background was set at 4 different levels. Luminance was changed by placing neutral density filters on the monitors, and the resulting luminances ranged from 10 ft L to 600 ft L. Twenty observers viewed 20 combinations of the 5 density filters and 4 contrast levels, for a total of 400 observations per observer. As in the previous study, there were no significant differences in performance between any of the luminance levels tested. It is possible that in both experiments statistical power was low due to not having enough cases, although the Hemminger *et al.* study had 400 observations per reader. In any study, it is very difficult to accumulate the very high number of cases needed to reveal statistical significance when the differences are small in the first place.

Krupinski *et al.* [44] have also noted a fairly high correlation between years of experience using soft-copy displays in general with performance viewing medical image from monitors. In both a radiology and a pathology study that compared traditional viewing (film for radiology and light microscope for pathology) versus monitor viewing of images, it was found that readers who had more experience with computers, video games, and other recreational uses of computers and monitors performed better with the soft-copy medical displays than those who had little or no recreational experience with computers and monitors. Those with less computer experience also tended to have been board-certified for longer and so were more experienced with the traditional modes of viewing, so they had better performance with film and light microscope viewing (see Figure 20.2).

ROC Az in the radiology studied ranged from 0.732 to 0.878 for film and 0.785 to 0.918 for monitor. ROC Az in the pathology study ranged from 0.977 to 0.996 with light microscopy and 0.981 to 0.996 for video. All readers had 20/20 vision or 20/20 corrected. In the radiology study two of the readers with less experience wore glasses and two with more experience wore glasses. In the pathology study, one reader with less experience wore glasses and two with more experience wore glasses. The results of the Song *et al.* [42] study illustrate a point that was brought up before. Experience can play a very important role in the successful transition from film to monitor viewing of medical images. The degree to which perceptual learning or adaptation plays a role has not been determined at this point, but there are indications that actual perceptual parameters are affected by changes in display parameters such as luminance and thus are subject to change through learning and experience.

Another experiment [45] was done to look specifically at whether changes in luminance actually do affect perceptual parameters in any way. For this study, 50 pairs of mammograms were displayed on two high-resolution monitors: one with a maximum luminance of 140 ftL and the other 80 ftL. Observer performance was measured using AFROC (alternative free response ROC) techniques and eye position was recorded in both display conditions. The average A_1 (area under the curve) value for 80 ftL was 0.9594, and 0.9695 for 140 ftL ($t = 1.685$, $df = 5$, $p = 0.1528$). There was no statistically significant difference in observer performance, just as the previous two studies found. Viewing times were 52.71 s versus 48.99 s ($t = 1.99$, $df = 299$, $p = 0.047$) respectively for 80 ftL versus 140 ftL. Although the difference was relatively small it was statistically significant, to some extent mirroring the difference seen in film versus monitor viewing in which the brighter film-based display had shorter viewing times than the dimmer monitor-based display. The eye-position data revealed that the average number of clusters generated during search was significantly greater for the 80-ftL monitor, but only on normal (lesion-free) images. Decision dwell times did not differ significantly for true-positive, false-negative, or false-positive decisions, although all dwell times were longer for the 80-ftL than for the 140-ftL monitor. It was interesting to note, however, that median dwell times for the TN decisions were significantly longer for the lower than the higher luminance display ($X^2 = 4.08$, $df = 1$, $p < 0.05$). These results suggest that changes in display luminance may affect the radiologists' ability to determine that normal features are indeed normal more than it affects the ability to detect a perturbation in the image and decide that it indeed represents a lesion.

The results of this study demonstrate again that although observer performance was not significantly affected by changes in the display for the part, perceptual performance was affected as reflected in the eye-position recording data. The impact of these differences in perceptual performance in the clinical environment might be significant if they result in greater fatigue, changes in workflow-or even displeasure using displays that result in longer viewing times. Another possible explanation for improved detection performance with higher luminance displays has to do with the effects of luminance on pupil size. Under low-luminance conditions, the pupil dilates so that more light photons can stimulate the photoreceptors. Under high luminance conditions, the pupil constricts to avoid over-excitation and slower recovery times of the photoreceptors. There is evidence [46] that detection of low- to moderate-contrast targets is better with smaller pupil sizes. In radiology, many lesion targets have relatively low contrast so they should be more detectable when display luminance is higher and pupil diameter is smaller. The effect of pupil size on the detection of high-contrast objects is weaker. There have not been any studies reported in the radiology literature that have looked at pupil changes as a function of display luminance. One study [47] did look at pupil diameter as a function of diagnostic decision and found that false-negative decisions were associated with increased pupil diameter, while true and false-positive decisions were associated with decreased diameter. I have looked at the eye-position data from the study [45] described above comparing the 80- and 140-ft L monitors, but have found no systematic relationships between pupil size and decision or as a function of display luminance. Pupil size changes as the radiologists scanned the mammographic image going from fatty (bright) to dense (dark) areas. The ranges of pupil diameters did not differ significantly for the two displays. Subtler differences may be more apparent upon closer examination of the data or by comparing data from individual images at specific locations on the two displays.

20.3.2 Display fidelity: why can't images look the same on different monitors?

PACS and teleradiology systems allow radiologists to send images within and between hospitals, using different monitors for viewing at every send-and-review station. Even if identical models of monitors are used at every display station, a given image can look very different from one monitor presentation to the next unless some sort of consistent quality-control measures or presentation standards are used to calibrate the displays. One display function standard that has been recommended for radiology is based on the concept of perceptual linearization. The idea of perceptual linearization was first introduced by Pizer [48, 49], such that equal steps in the gray values presented on a CRT monitor evoke equal steps in brightness sensation on the part of the human observer. Over the years, this idea has gained support and has even been implemented into the DICOM standard [50], representing a very significant perceptually based idea that has successfully bridged the gap between research and practical application in the clinical environment.

The basic idea for perceptual linearization comes from the fact that displaying images on a monitor involves two nonlinear mappings. The first mapping involves taking the recorded image data (the actual numeric values from a digital image) and transforming them into the luminance values on the screen of a CRT monitor. This mapping between the computer's command levels (ADU or analog to digital units) and the luminance represents the monitor's display function or characteristic curve. Figure 20.3 shows some examples of display functions for three different monitors calibrated using the SMPTE (Society for Motion Picture and Television Engineers) pattern. It should be obvious that different monitors have very different display functions, even when calibrated in the same manner. The second mapping involves the transformation of the display luminance to the response of the human visual system in terms of the sensation of brightness. If the combination of these two mappings is not optimal, the perceived dynamic range of the display device will not be optimal. In radiology, dynamic range or the optimal transfer of gray-scale information is crucial to the diagnostic process because the amount of

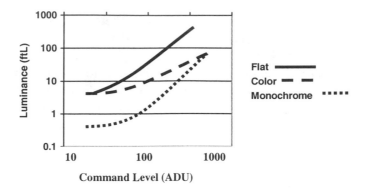

Figure 20.3: Display functions of various monitor display systems: a monochrome flat panel (2560 × 2048), a color CRT (1600 × 1200) and a monochrome CRT (1600 × 1200).

x-ray absorption by tissue is represented in the digital image by gray-scale (luminance) differences. If the absorption differences are not adequately represented on the monitor, the visual system will not be able to perceive the relevant brightness information that distinguishes lesion tissue from background tissue and lesions will be missed. The change in luminance required for a target lesion to be detected from its surround luminance as a function of the surround luminance is referred to as the luminance contrast sensitivity function (CSF).

There has been extensive work into how to perceptually linearize displays [48, 49, 51–53], which display functions are best [54, 55], does it actually improve performance (often measured in terms of the number of perceived just noticeable differences or JNDs) [55, 56]. The majority of studies have used purely psychophysical paradigms with simple geometric or grating-pattern stimuli, and have generally shown that perceptual linearization does in fact increase the number of perceived JNDs for a given display system. Many of these studies have shown examples of radiographic images on perceptually linearized versus non-linearized displays to illustrate how the linearized displays show images that look better subjectively [49, 52, 53]. Very few studies have been done, however, that have looked at the effects of perceptual linearization on performance using real radiographic images.

There are a few exceptions. Belaid *et al.* [56] had observers look at a series of complex achromatic scenes including two medical images (angiogram of the kidney and an MRI mammogram). Beside each image was a gray-scale chart. The observer's task was to determine the average gray value for specified scene locations, by matching its brightness to one of the discrete gray-scale steps shown on the gray-scale chart. The gray levels for the image backgrounds were set at high and low gray levels. Images were presented in both a perceptually linearized and in a nonlinearized version. The difference in matching performance did not differ significantly for linearized versus nonlinearized displays. Background gray level (high versus low) did have an effect on performance. Brightness matchings tended to be underestimated for the low-level displays, and tended to be overestimated with the high-level displays, especially at the lower original image values. This interactive effect of surround luminance on perceived target brightness is known as simultaneous brightness induction [58]. In other words, local background information affects brightness judgments significantly, so global linearization methods may not be as effective as hoped with visually complex scenes with numerous and diverse luminance variations (as in a radiographic image). Thus, the authors suggest that instead of using a single look-up table to try and insure perceptual linearization of all images, other rules such as using the average luminance of each individual scene must be considered for selecting the best surround luminance.

Another study [59] not only looked at whether lesion detection performance was better using a perceptually linearized display, but it also looked at whether a perceptually linearized display affected visual search parameters. Six radiologists viewed a series of 50 mammograms (18 with a single subtle mass, 18 with a single subtle microcalcification cluster, 14 lesion-free). The images were displayed once a monitor that was perceptually linearized using the Barten curve [52, 53], and once on the same monitor that was calibrated using the SMPTE pattern so that the display function was not perceptually linearized. The Barten curve is based on human contrast sensitivity and perceptual linearization principles, and it is derived from psychophysical just noticeable difference (JND) studies. Basically, the Barten curve standard refers to contrast sensitivity for a standard target consisting of a 2 deg × 2 deg square filled with horizontal or vertical bars with sinusoidal modulation of 4 cycles per degree (the peak contrast sensitivity of the human visual system). The square is placed on a uniform background whose luminance is equal to the average luminance of the target. Contrast sensitivity is defined by the threshold modulation at which the human observer can just detect the target (JND). The display function holds for the luminance rage from 0.05 to 4000 cd/m^2 and explicitly includes the luminance generated by ambient light reflected by the display. The exact details for generating the standard display curve can be found in Ref. [54]. Eye position was recorded as the radiologists searched the images for subtle microcalcification clusters and masses. Alternative free response receiver operating characteristic (AFROC) analysis indicated, as expected, that detection performance was significantly higher ($t = 5.42$, $df = 5$, $p = 0.003$) with the perceptually linearized display ($A_1 = 0.972$ on average) that with the non-linearized display ($A_1 = 0.951$ on average).

The eye-position data showed that (1) total viewing times were longer with the nonlinearized display, (2) median dwell times for all types of decisions (true and false, positive, and negative) were longer with the nonlinearized display, and (3) more fixation clusters were generated per image with the non-linearized display than with the perceptually linearized display. There were no differences for mass versus microcalcification cluster for any parameter analyzed, but the lesion free images had significantly more clusters generated per image than those that contained lesions. Again, it seems as if the radiologists had a more difficult time deciding that the lesion-free images were indeed lesion free than deciding that images contained a lesion. In other words, visual search with the perceptually linearized display was much more efficient and yielded better diagnostic accuracy than the nonlinearized display. These results confirm what previous studies found in terms of perceptual linearization improving observer performance, and it also showed that perceptual linearization can affect basic perceptual processing activities as well.

As noted previously, the advantages of standardizing image-display systems using perceptual linearization have been so well recognized from the experimental data that it is now part of the DICOM standard, and it will be used in the clinical environment for presentation of radiographic images on digital displays. There is still some question as noted previously, as to whether a single-display standard for all scenes is possible given the strong dependence of the luminance-brightness relationship on the surround luminance (the brightness-induction effect). As monitor displays are used more and more in the clinical environment, we will increasingly see the effects of perceptual linearization using many different types of images in various viewing environments.

20.3.3 Image processing and computer-aided diagnosis (CAD)

One of the main advantages of acquiring radiologic images digitally and displaying them on CRT monitors, is that image processing tools and computer-aided detection (CAD) schemes can be readily implemented. Thus, there has been a proliferation of image processing [60, 61] and CAD [62–64] tools developed in the past 20 years. With the advent of digital acquisition technologies in chest imaging (i.e., computed radiography (CR)) and the recent progress in digital mammography, clinical implementation of these tools seems likely. These tools are sometimes used in the clinic now (e.g., in CT, MRI, US), but for the most part these tools are used only in experimental situations for plain film images. Part of the problem with implementing image-analysis tools in the clinical environment is that only a few, limited studies have been conducted to demonstrate reliably their utility in improving observer performance. For the most part, results from the use of CAD and image processing in the clinical environment have been equivocal [65–69].

The need for automated image-analysis tools arises because radiologic images are generally quite complex. The detection and recognition of lesions in these images can be difficult because: (1) x-ray images are two-dimensional representations in which three-dimensional solid structures are made transparent, requiring an understanding of projective geometry to determine the true depth and location of imaged structures; and (2) lesions, especially nodules or masses, are typically embedded in a background of anatomic noise. The difficulty of the task of finding a lesion in a radiographic image is especially evident when one considers general screening. If the radiologist has no clinical history and is looking for any possible abnormality, then theoretically the entire image must be searched in order to make a complete and accurate diagnosis. Even when clinical information is available, the radiologist must read the entire image carefully for the possible presence of other abnormalities in the image. This is not to say that the radiologist must exhaustively search and fixate every part of the image (see Chapter 8), because much information is collected during the initial global view of the image and through general scanning of the image with the useful visual field. Knowledge about where lesions are likely to occur (and not occur) also make exhaustive scanning of the image unnecessary.

For general screening studies, error rates (misses) have been estimated to range from 15 to 30% with 2 to 15% false-positive rates [70–75]. Many of these missed lesions are, in retrospect, visible on the radiograph and thus are one of the major causes for malpractice suits in radiology [76–80]. Missed lesions can also result in delayed treatment and possibly increase the severity of the patient's illness. These are just a few of the many reasons why ways have been investigated to aid the human observer in detecting and classifying lesions in radiographic images.

In some cases image-processing algorithms can be designed for selective use by the radiologist, or they can be designed for automatic implementation based on some pre-analysis of the image. In either case, the occasions under which the radiologist chooses to use the tools and whether use of these tools improves diagnostic accuracy should be evaluated. To investigate this issue, many studies [81, 82] use a protocol in which an unprocessed and processed version of the same image are put side-by-side. The radiologist is asked which one they prefer. If they choose the processed image, the conclusion is generally that the processed image is better than the unprocessed. The unspoken assumption is that this translates directly into better performance, which unfortunately may not always be the case.

Studies that actually look at performance as a function of the use of image processing tell us much more about whether the images actually improve diagnostic accuracy or whether they are just perceptually pleasing for one reason or another. Pisano et al. [83, 84] have recently conducted two studies that looked at the effects of an image processing algorithm (called intensity windowing, IW) that uses intensity windowing to improve image quality. The intensity windowing technique determines a new pixel intensity by a linear transformation that maps a selected band of pixel values onto the available gray-level range of a particular display system. Their studies used 256×256 portions of real mammograms and simulated masses or calcifications. Observers saw the images in both the processed and unprocessed versions using a number of intensity settings. For both masses and calcifications there was a statistically significant improvement in detection when intensity windowing was used.

Another study [69] looked at how often radiologists used given image-processing options in addition to the question of whether image processing use improved performance. Six radiologists viewed 168 chest images with either nodules, bronchiectasis, interstitial disease, or no lesions. Images first appeared used a linear film-like display function, and the radiologists had to provide a diagnosis. After that there were 5 image processing functions available: video reverse, lung window, mediastinum window, high-pass filter, and low-pass filter. The radiologists could use any of the functions (or not) and then had to report a second decision (see Table 20.2 below for average use of the various processing functions). Diagnostic accuracy (ROC Az) did not differ significantly for decisions made with and without image processing. Overall, 93% of diagnostic decisions were not changed with image processing. Two percent of decisions changed from TP to FN, 2%

Table 20.2: Average number of times image processing functions were used per case on different types of disease categories across all radiologists

Function	Normal	Nodule	Interstitial	Bronchiectasis
Low-pass	0.05	0.05	0.06	0.01
Mediastinum	0.41	0.44	0.41	0.41
Video-reverse	0.49	0.53	0.50	0.56
High-pass	0.56	0.54	0.52	0.56
Lung	0.95	0.93	1.03	1.10
Linear	1.27	1.28	1.34	1.27

from FN to TP, 1% from FP to TN and 2% from TN to FP. The beneficial decision changes were completely balanced by the negative decision changes!

A related question was whether certain image-processing functions were used more with certain disease categories than others. This is of interest to automated image processing because it might be possible to pre-select an image processing function if the clinical history or diagnostic question prompts a given disease. If it does, processing may be applied automatically to improve lesion detectability. It is also interesting from a perceptual point of view as certain processing methods may improve lesion detectability more than others and only under certain circumstances. The study found nothing suggesting that certain disease categories are better visualized using a given processing function (see Table 20.2). In fact, there only seemed to be an effect that radiologists preferred certain functions for all images. This in itself might be useful for automated processing in the practical environment, because a radiologist could log onto a workstation and the computer would know to present all images using the preferred functions.

Contrasting the above studies, it is clear that some image processing applications do affect observer performance and others do not. Neither of these studies measured any perceptual parameters directly, but improved lesion detection (or lack of it) does suggest that perception of certain features was indeed improved by the application of image-processing algorithms. It may be difficult and time consuming to conduct observer performance studies for every new image-processing algorithm that is developed. However, the studies described above demonstrate clearly that unless the algorithms are put to the test using real clinical images in an observer performance study, it is impossible to tell if they will impact on performance.

20.3.4 All the bells and whistles? Practical aspects of user interface

Related to the issue of which image-processing functions are used and when, is the general issue of workstation design. As Langer and Wang [85] and Gay *et al.* [86] demonstrated in a recent review of ten digital image review workstations, there are quite a few aspects that need to be considered when choosing the "right" workstation. Some of them do not impact on perception or performance directly (e.g., archive size), but others do—often in ways that are not obvious at first. For example, one factor they considered was how many monitors a workstation had and obviously different manufacturers allow for different numbers of monitors. Does the number of monitors impact on perceptual performance in any way? Langer and Wang did not address this issue, but Beard *et al.* [87] did. Their study actually looked at film viewing to determine what the monitor viewing requirements might be. Radiologists viewed a series of mammograms in which each case had the left and right, craniocaudal and mediolateral, views for the current and a comparison study. All images were hung on the viewbox at the same time as they generally are in the clinical situation. Eye position was recorded as the radiologists searched the images calcifications and masses. Through their analysis of the radiologists' search patterns and the use of a magnifying glass (to estimate when and how often zoom and roam functions would be used in soft-copy display), they were able to develop a prototypical search strategy that mammographers use during mammographic search. They determined that using four monitors would probably be best from an ergonomic and perceptual point of view. For instance, the mammographers went back and forth between the various images on average between 1 and 6 times depending on the image pair (e.g., old and new craniocaudal right breast average = 6, range = 0–24). A workstation with four monitors could accommodate this volume of comparison scans much more efficiently than a single monitor that used either lower-resolution images with zoom/roam functions, or some sort of image-viewing procedure where the radiologist has to sequence through the images without being able to view them all at once.

There are certainly many other aspects of workstation design and use that can be evaluated to consider impact on performance and perception. As already noted, many studies have found significant differences in viewing times for film versus monitor display [29, 37]. Viewing times are longer when there are more functions to choose from and when there are complicated ways to access and use the menu items [38]. Compared to film reading, where the radiologist generally just needs to sit in front of an alternator and read the films as they scroll by (sometimes accessing nearby film folders), monitor reading imposes new tasks on the radiologist. Now the radiologist must truly interact with the display system. A mouse, trackball, or other interface device is generally used, creating a whole new task to be done while reading (some systems are now using voice commands, but that is also different from what they are used to). This new task represents a new attentional distraction for the radiologist. The presence of the menu on the screen also represents a new attentional distractor. All of these factors can lead to confusion if not designed properly with the radiologist in mind. Above all, the radiologist's task is to diagnose images, not to have to manipulate them in numerous ways before they can reach that diagnostic decision. If it takes too long and is too complicated to get the images displayed properly, the radiologist is unlikely to go through the trouble. The gains in diagnostic accuracy must outweigh any difficulties it takes to use workstations and any image-analysis tools on that workstation. The radiologist must be able to devote the necessary cognitive and attentional resources to the diagnostic task, without having to allocate needed resources to confusing or complicated tasks that will be distracting. Confusion and distraction can easily lead to increased viewing times, poorer workflow rates, and decreased diagnostic performance. Well-designed interfaces and easy-to-use image-analysis tools will decrease confusion and distraction, potentially increasing system use and maybe even improving diagnostic performance. The key is to keep the radiologist's mind and visual system in mind when designing image-analysis tools and image displays.

20.4 Prompting/cueing to improve diagnostic performance

A number of ways have been tried over the years to improve observer-detection performance. Automated image analysis and CAD schemes differ from past attempts in that a computer is used to analyze the radiographic image and provide detection and/or classification information to the radiologist to incorporate into the final diagnostic decision. The advantage of using computers is that they are consistent. An algorithm is developed which uses the same criteria for every case, and detection results are consistent as long as the algorithm or its thresholds are not changed. Other attempts to improve performance rely more heavily on the human observer. The human observer, however, is much more variable than the computer. Depending on any number of factors (even time of day!), radiologists will change their decision criteria and the way they search images [9], which can contribute to errors being made.

Much of the work in automated image analysis has been done in mammography [88–92], although chest imaging has also been an important area for successful use of CAD and image analysis [93, 94]. Most of work in mammography has focused on detection of microcalcification clusters. Part of the reason is that microcalcifications are generally high-contrast punctate objects that have very different properties than the surrounding breast tissue. In contrast, masses tend to be embedded in the surrounding breast tissue and have properties quite similar to the surrounding tissue. Stellate lesions are especially difficult to detect because of their irregular borders and very thin "tendrils" that emanate from the body of the lesion into the surrounding tissue. Computer detection rates for microcalcifications tend to be higher than for masses, but there is much work being done to improve detection rates and decrease false-positive rates in both of these areas [95, 96].

A number of people are also using computer analysis techniques to characterize other characteristics of mammograms. For example, there are attempts being made to characterize parenchymal patterns [97, 98], because different breast patterns are associated with differing levels of risk for developing breast cancer. Some breast-tissue classification systems have been developed for use by radiologists [99], but their use is not universal. The detection of changes in the appearance of the breast, or in the appearance of potential lesions that are being watched over time for changes in appearance, is also of great interest to those developing computer analysis techniques. The human visual system is very good at detecting change, but subtle differences in size or shape can be difficult to detect, especially since subtle changes require that attention be focused on the locus of change [100]. Lapses in attention or distractions, which often occur in reading rooms, can result in subtle lesion changes being missed. A computer does not suffer from lapses in attention or distractions, so changes in lesion shape or size might be more reliably detected using CAD schemes designed for this purpose [101].

In chest radiography, the issues for lesion detection and classification are similar to those in mammography. Radiologists look for changes over time in some cases, and in other cases they are searching for specific lesions. As in mammography, however, lesions such as nodules are embedded in the complex background of the lungs and are often quite difficult to detect. Other disease patterns such as interstitial lung abnormalities can also be quite difficult to detect and classify. CAD has had some success in detecting and characterizing lung lesions and disease entities [102–105], but the success rate is not as high as in mammography. One of the major differences between research in CAD for mammography versus chest imaging, is that research in chest imaging uses different types [106–108] of images (e.g., digitized film, CR, CT, MRI), while CAD for mammography uses almost exclusively mammography images (although there are some exceptions, see [48] for example).

20.4.1 Clinical use of CAD

The clinical success of any automated system depends on a number of issues. The information provided by the computer must be reliable. True positive rates need to be high and false positive rates low. Too many false positives will result in radiologists not trusting and becoming frustrated with the system. Too few true positives will have the same result. Ideally, one would like the automated system to confirm what has been detected by the human observer and to point out the very subtle lesions that are missed—without pointing out too many irrelevant locations.

For the most part, automated image analysis systems have been evaluated in terms of the true-positive and false-positive rates, independent of the utilization of the information by the radiologist who is making the final diagnostic decision. It is only recently that studies are being conducted that actually include the radiologist in the evaluation [109–113]. The results of these studies are generally positive. For example, a recently study by Jiang *et al.* [114] compared diagnostic performance of radiologists with and without CAD. The radiologists read 104 mammography cases for microcalcification clusters. The average ROC Az went from 0.61 without CAD to 0.75 with CAD. The difference in performance was statistically significant. They also kept track of biopsy recommendations. With CAD the radiologists recommended an average of 6.4 additional biopsies for malignant cases and 6.0 fewer for benign cases ($p = 0.003$). This study is a good example of a very practical application of research that, although its origins are in image processing and analysis, has a very strong perceptual component. CAD points out suspicious areas to the radiologist that they may or may have already looked at, but did not report on anything. The presence of the CAD prompt obviously helps alter the perception of the radiologist who now sees something in the image and recognizes it as a lesion, where previously they had not seen or recognized anything (eye-position data would of course tell us if the radiologist had actually fixated the lesion prior to CAD).

It is worth noting, however, that not all studies have found computer aids to be helpful. Mugglestone [115] compared reading mammograms with and without lesion prompts, and found that the addition of computer-generated prompts did not improve the number of lesions detected. There was a slightly lower false negative rate with prompts, but this was accompanied by an associated rise in the false positives. The authors conclude that prompting has an interfering effect since it has little influence on the true-positive rate and actually may increase the false-positive rate.

For the majority of automated image-analysis tools, the radiographic images need to be in digital form. With digitally acquired images, the raw data are easily accessed, analyzed, and manipulated. Analog (plain-film) data must be digitized, generally resulting in some degree of information loss. In either case, once the data is in digital format it can be displayed on a CRT monitor for viewing. The results of automated image-analysis schemes can also be easily displayed on the monitor. Intermediate steps (e.g., printing back to film) are required if the diagnostic images cannot be viewed satisfactorily on a monitor, which may result in loss of information or extra steps to visualize the computer data with respect to the original images.

The mammographers at our institution have noted a potential problem with computer-provided prompts when they use the R2 ImageChecker system for mammography. Because they have so much confidence in the ability of the computer to correctly identify the microcalcification clusters, they tend to find themselves "skimming" the mammograms instead of conducting a thorough microcalcification search. To see if this is really the case, a recent study by Krupinski [116] recorded the eye position of radiologists as they scanned mammograms using CAD. Cases with masses and/or microcalcification clusters were digitized and analyzed by ImageChecker. Half of the readers were experienced mammographers and half were fourth year residents. Observers were instructed to search the original film images, provide an initial diagnosis, then access and view the CAD information whenever they wanted to and provide a revised diagnosis.

On average, the mammographers accessed the CAD images after 104 s of search, and the residents accessed it after 86 s. The mammographers then spent 49 s on average searching the CAD and original images, and the residents spent 63 s. Figure 20.4 shows the average viewing time for each decision before and after CAD viewing for the mammographers and residents. It can be seen that the mammographers and residents had different viewing patterns before and after CAD. Changes in decisions also varied. For the mammographers, 50% of the original false negatives were correctly reported as lesions after CAD. For the residents 33% were correctly reported after CAD.

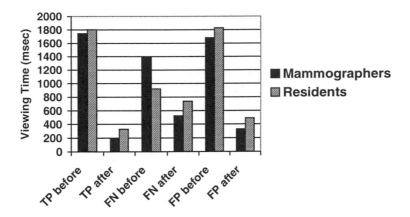

Figure 20.4: Average viewing times (msec) for true-positive (TP), false-negative (FN), and false-positive (FP) decisions by mammographers and residents before and after CAD.

These results suggest a number of interesting conclusions and implications for use of automated image-analysis schemes that cue the radiologist to particular image locations. The first is that there may be a significant difference in how the computer-provided information is used, depending on the experience of the observer. For the most part, CAD will probably be more useful for the general radiologist than for the expert mammographer. The results of this study suggest, however, that the radiologists with less mammographic experience seemed to rely more heavily on the CAD information than did the mammographers—and that this reliance on CAD affected their visual search behaviors. The residents tended to access the CAD images sooner than the mammographers and spent less time dwelling on false-negative locations before CAD. After CAD, the residents' dwells on the false-negative areas was longer than that of the mammographers, but their false negative to true positive conversion rate was lower (33% versus 50%) than the mammographers. It would seem that a thorough search of the image before CAD is presented is extremely beneficial with respect to CAD having its desired effect. Perceptually speaking, it seems as if the more a suspicious region is fixated and visually processed before CAD is presented, the easier it is to recognize that suspicious region as actually positive after CAD reinforces the suspicion by prompting it as a lesion.

The finding that lesions detected before CAD is presented receive extended dwell, but receive very little dwell once CAD is presented, is also interesting. This result confirms the idea that computer prompting is a good way to confirm the radiologists' suspicion if the level of suspicion was high enough to report the lesion in the initial search. The very short dwells on these lesions after the computer-analysis information is presented suggest that the radiologists are basically giving a quick double-checking glance to these already detected areas just to make sure the computer location and their originally detected location are one in the same. The interesting thing is that the false positives showed this same trend-extended dwell on the suspected location prior to CAD and relatively short dwell duration after CAD. With the false positives, however, the dwells after CAD were short, but slightly longer than for the true positives. With respect to performance, the mammographers changed 50% of their false positives to true negatives after CAD was presented, and the residents changed 25% of their decisions.

These results suggest a benefit of CAD that is rarely talked about—the influence of CAD on the radiologists' false positives. Because CAD and the radiologist report the same false positives areas only about one-third of the time [117], it is not surprising that the radiologists would spend more time looking at an area that they called positive but that the computer did not. This is especially true if the radiologist believes that CAD's performance is high and expects it to be right most of the time without a lot of false positives. Mammographers might believe that CAD's performance is high because of its advertised sensitivity/specificity rates when the system was purchased and by means of experience using the system and seeing how good of a "second reader" it actually is in practice. By double checking areas that the radiologist called positive, but CAD did not, the experienced mammographer seems better able to modify the initial incorrect decision than the less-experienced resident. The effect is not complete, however, because even the experienced mammographers changed only 50% of their false-positive reports to true negatives. If general radiologists are found to perform more like residents than expert mammographers, they too may have trouble changing their false-positive calls even if CAD does not confirm their suspicions.

20.4.2 Satisfaction of search and CAD: a possible pitfall?

Satisfaction of search (SOS) is a phenomenon first reported by Tuddenham [5] and subsequently studied by others [118–121], in which the radiologist fails to report multiple lesions on a radiograph after one lesion has already been detected. Although SOS has not yet been studied specifically with respect to CAD, two studies [115, 116] do suggest that SOS might occur with these tools. Mugglestone [115] found that radiologists tended to concentrate on prompted areas of mammograms and ignore unprompted areas. Unprompted lesions tended to be fixated minimally and were often missed. Krupinski [116] also found this to be true. Before CAD was presented, radiologists had a median true-negative dwell time of about 700 ms. After CAD was presented, true-negative dwell times fell to about 150 ms and the number of fixation clusters outside areas indicted by CAD was minimal. Radiologists often went back to check areas that they had called positive that CAD did not, but they did not spend much time on other areas outside the CAD-indicated regions of interest.

The findings from both of these studies suggest that an SOS effect may be occurring with automated analysis and detection schemes. The presence of the computer prompts tends to draw the radiologists' attention to the prompted areas and tends to inhibit them from searching unprompted areas. Because the computer does not have a 100% detection rate, there are lesions that will be unprompted by the computer and undetected by radiologists in an initial search of the image.

In fact, Krupinski and Nishikawa [115] found that about 5% of microcalcification clusters go undetected by both CAD and radiologists when both search the same mammogram. Therefore, radiologists need to recognize that the computer is not a perfect second reader and that they still should give an image a good second search even after the computer-generated feedback has been presented. This is especially true if, as mammographers at our institution noted, it is found that it is all too easy to give an image a cursory initial search then access the computer information for the prompts.

20.5 Color applications in radiology

A final area where the transition from film to monitor display has and will continue to yield questions for perception researchers in medical imaging is the application of color to the display of radiographic images. Traditionally, the standard for displaying radiographic images has been gray scale. Today the most color present in a radiographic film is dye (generally blue) in the film base added to reduce eyestrain for the interpreting radiologist [122]. However, with the advent of digital image acquisition and display systems there has arisen the possibility of adding color to images or even creating purely color-scale radiographic images. The latter idea is certainly only speculation at this point in time, but adding color to gray-scale radiographs is already being done in some modalities. There are a number of reasons why color images are attractive for displaying images. Levkowitz and Herman [123] suggest that while gray scale has a dynamic range of about 60 to 90 JNDs, color probably has a dynamic range of at least 500 JNDs. On the other hand, the visual system has lower spatial resolution in the color channels than in the luminance channels, so increasing dynamic range by going to color may actually be confounded by color-luminance dependencies [124, 125]. Thus, color radiography may have a lot of potential in some circumstances, but we obviously need to do a lot of clinically relevant studies to determine its ultimate success in terms of practical applications.

Perhaps the most successful application of color has been in Doppler ultrasound [126, 127]. Without going into the physics and technology of it all, Doppler ultrasound records and tracks flow information (e.g., blood flow through the vessels). Color Doppler ultrasound superimposes a color image of the flow information over the real-time gray-scale image, giving the radiologist a view of both the anatomy and functional blood flow. The same sort of technique is also beginning to be used in some MRI, CT, and nuclear medicine imaging procedures [128, 129]. Image registration, 3D imaging rendering, and areas such as virtual endoscopy [130] where color cameras can actually be used to acquire images are additional areas where color applications are appearing in radiology. Many of the studies dealing with color in radiography are generally from the engineering or image processing approach—can it be done. There are few observer performance or perception studies that look at the effects of color in radiographic image display.

One interesting study by Rehm *et al.* [131] did look at the effects of color on performance, in the context of merging/registering brain images from MRI and

PET. The technique that was used to merge the MRI and PET brain images (interleaving of alternate pixels with independent color scales) successfully registered the images. It also produced an unusual perceptual effect in which low-contrast signals (typically in the MRI image) were camouflaged, resulting in a decrease in signal-detection performance. The effect was explained by perceptual merging—if the contrast difference between adjacent pixels is not high enough, the pixels are perceptually merged into a larger "megapixel." The stimuli used in the study were uniform backgrounds, and when the target images were merged with the uniform backgrounds, the merged signal-to-background luminance was reduced. If the signal-to-background luminance ratio was near the Weber threshold (the threshold at which a simple disk of luminance can be detected against a uniform background luminance) before the interleaving merge of the images, the interleaved luminance ratio may actually fall below the threshold if conditions are right for perceptual merging. The low-contrast target that was visible prior to merging is rendered invisible. The phenomenon was observed in a psychophysical study with geometric signals and backgrounds, so the practical effect of the phenomenon with clinical images is unclear.

A number of pseudocolor scales have been tested [132–134] in a variety of other more traditional medical imaging applications with relatively little success or even enthusiasm for expanding to the clinical setting. Li and Burgess [135] conducted a rather comprehensive study looking at gray scale and 12 color scales (heated object, rainbow, and 10 variations of spiral trajectories in the CIELAB uniform color space) using signals added to white noise displays. Performance was best with the gray scale, followed closely by the color heated object scale. Performance with the other color scales was 25–30% lower than with the gray scale. The results were not very encouraging in terms of promoting studies using color mapping for actual clinical images. Should color displays prove to be useful for clinical imaging, it is important to keep in mind that shifting to color displays will require investigation into a whole new set of rules for quality control and calibration of color monitors [136] to maintain fidelity between monitors and over time.

20.6 Conclusions

As noted in the introduction, the goal of this chapter was to provide some examples of the kind of perceptually based research that has or will have practical impact on clinical reading of medical images. In some cases the practical applications have already been realized (e.g., color in MRI, PET, and ultrasound images), and in some cases we are on the verge of realizing how practical and useful some research will be (e.g., CAD). This chapter has concentrated on using examples that have to do with the ongoing transition from film to monitor based viewing of softcopy medical images in the clinical environment. This is the way of the future, so it will be extremely important to understand how technology impacts on the human observer and how the human observer adapts to new ways of viewing image data.

It is important to realize in this transition that one of the most important advantages of the digital display is that the radiologist now has a dynamic image that can be manipulated in a variety of ways that were not possible with analog (film) images. There is always the potential for new sources of error, but there is also the potential for great strides to be made in terms of creating displays that will improve the appearance of images perceptually so that they lead to better diagnostic performance. In either case, perceptual research and its practical application to the clinical environment will always have a place in medical imaging.

Here are some final thoughts on how to help bridge the gap between laboratory research and practical application of findings. The potential for automated image-analysis as an aid to the radiologist is immense. Someday we may be using automated image-analysis programs on every image that goes through a radiology department. Volume is very high in many places and a lot of cases are normal. In combination with a clinical history or presenting symptomolgy, judicious use of automated processing for the detection of specific lesions or disease features will be useful and feasible. Ideally, one might want to see a "package" system developed automatically analyzes an image for many types of lesions. If the detection algorithms could work in parallel with sufficient speed, they could work directly on the digital data from any digital modality. If the images are then viewed directly on a CRT monitor, the computer prompts could be accessed quite easily and superimposed over the image.

Most of the potential problems with using the computer to analyze images and provide information to the radiologist that were noted above can be avoided with judicious use. As long as radiologists recognize the limitations of automated analysis schemes as well as their own limitations, the use of these schemes will serve quite nicely as a reliable second reader. Radiologists need to integrate the computer output into their normal reading procedure, without changing their normal search and detection behaviors to any great extent. Careful and thorough search of images and lesions will be necessary no matter how accurate automated schemes get. In the final analysis it is the radiologist who is responsible for collecting, analyzing, and weighing all the available data and coming up with a diagnostic decision and suggesting a course of treatment.

In terms of workstation design, all of the above comments hold true. Additionally there are certain others features that become even more important when looking at the design of an entire workstation. As already noted, the amount of information on the display at one time is very important. Although there are alternatives (e.g., voice control), most current computer interfaces rely on the menu. If menus are going to continue to be the primary means of interacting with the computer, efforts need to be made to keep it as simple as possible. We have shown in a number of studies that most radiologists tend to use only a very few select image processing tools, even when there are a lot of choices available. A good interface will provide only a few basic (e.g., window, level, video-reverse) image processing tools. Others can be available, but possibly only by accessing a special menu. It is also possible to automate things. Radiologists can log on to a workstation and it will know that radiologist's preferred image appearance and hanging strategy. If we are going to adopt other types of interfaces such as voice control, these too need to be evaluated to determine how effectively they can be used by the radiologist and whether they impact on performance in any way (positively or negatively).

In every situation where image analysis is being automated or the image is being processed in some way to help the radiologist in terms of improved diagnostic accuracy, two things are important. The first is to make it simple. The more work the radiologist has to do to get the image to look like they wants it too, the less attention they are paying to diagnosing that image. The second point is to involve radiologists in as much of the development of automated image-analysis schemes and workstation design aspects as possible. This includes interviewing radiologists *and* observing them in the actual clinical setting. In the final analysis, it is the radiologist that either will or will not use whatever computer-aided tool the engineer comes up with. If it's too slow or is not useful diagnostically, it will not be used.

References

[1] Birkelo CC, Chamberlain WE, Phelps PS, Schools PE, Zachs D, Yerushalmy J. "Tuberculosis Case Finding: Comparison of Effectiveness of Various Roentgenographic and Photofluorographic Methods." JAMA 133:359–366, 1947.

[2] Garland LH. "On the Scientific Evaluation of Diagnostic Procedures." Radiology 52:309–328, 1949.

[3] Newell RR, Chamberlain WE, Rigler L. "Descriptive Classification of Pulmonary Shadows. Revelation of Unreliability in Roentgenographic Diagnosis of Tuberculosis." Am Rev Tuberc 69:566–584, 1954.

[4] Beam CA, Sullivan DC, Layde PM. "Effect of Human Variability on Independent Double Reading in Screening Mammography." Acad Radiol 3:891–897, 1996.

[5] Tuddenham WJ, "Visual Search, Image Organization, and Reader Error in Roentgen Diagnosis." Radiology 78:694–704, 1962.

[6] Kundel HL, Nodine CF, Carmody D. "Visual Scanning, Pattern Recognition and Decision-Making in Pulmonary Nodule Detection." Invest Radiol 13:175–181, 1978.

[7] Christensen EE, Murry RC, Holland K *et al.*, "The Effect of Search Time on Perception." Radiology 138:361–365, 1981.

[8] Brogdon BG, Kelsey CA, Moseley RD. "Factors Affecting Perception of Pulmonary Lesions." Radiol Clinics of N America 21:633–654, 1983.

[9] Gale AG, Marray D, Miller K, Worthington BS. "Circadian Variation in Radiology." In Gale AG, Johnson F (Eds.) *Theoretical and Applied Aspects of Eye Movement Research*. North-Holland: Elsevier Science, 1984, pp. 313–321.

[10] Berbaum KS, Franken EA, Dorfman DD, Rooholamini SA, Kathol MH, Barloon TJ, Behlke FM, Sato Y, Lu CH, El-Khoury GY, Flickenger FW,

Montgomery WJ. "Satisfaction of Search in Diagnostic Radiology." Invest Radiol 25:133–140, 1990.

[11] Burgess AE. "Prewhitening revisited," Proc SPIE 3340, 1998, pp. 55–64.

[12] Meyers KJ, Barrett HH, Borgstrom MC, Patton DD, Seeley GW. "Effect of Noise Correlation on Detectability of Disk Signals in Medical Imaging." JOSA A2:1752–1759, 1985.

[13] Abbey CK, Barrett HH, Eckstein MP. "Practical Issues and Methodology in Assessment of Image Quality Using Model Observers." Proc SPIE 3032, 1997, pp. 182–194.

[14] Jackson WB, Beebee P, Jared DA, Biegelsen DK, Larimer JO, Lubin J, Gille JL. "X-Ray Image System Design Using a Human Visual Model." Proc SPIE 2708, 1996, pp. 29–40.

[15] Eckstein MP, Abbey CK, Whiting JS. "Human Vs Model Observers in Anatomic Background." Proc SPIE 3340, 1998, pp. 16–26.

[16] Davies P. *The American Heritage Dictionary of the English Language*. New York: Dell Publishing, 1980, p. 554.

[17] Goin JE, Hermann GA. "The Clinical Efficacy of Diagnostic Imaging Evaluation Studies: Problems, Paradigms, and Prescriptions." Invest Radiol 26:507–511, 1991.

[18] Uchida K, Watanabe H, Aoki T, Nakamura K, Nakata H. "Clinical Evaluation of Irreversible Data Compression for Computed Radiography of the Hand." J Dig Imaging 11:121–125, 1998.

[19] Good WF, Maitz G, King J, Gennari R, Gur D. "Observer Performance of JPEG-Compressed High-Resolution Chest Images." Proc SPIE 3663, 1999, pp. 8–13.

[20] Rockette HE, Johns CM, Weissman JL, Holbert JM, Sumkin JH, King JL, Gur D. "Relationship of Subjective Ratings of Image Quality and Observer Performance." Proc SPIE 3036, 1997, pp. 152–159.

[21] Qu G, Huda W, Belden CJ. "Comparison of Trained and Untrained Observers Using Subjective and Objective Measures of Imaging Performance." Acad Radiol 3:31–35, 1996.

[22] Gur D, Rubin DA, Kart BH, Peterson AM, Fuhrman CR, Rockette HE, King JL. "Forced Choice and Ordinal Discrete Rating Assessment of Image Quality: A Comparison." J Dig Imaging 10:103–107, 1997.

[23] Roehrig H. "Image Quality Assurance for CRT Display Systems." J Digital Imaging 12:1–2, 1999.

[24] Blume H, Bergstrom S, Goble J. "Image Pre-Hanging and Processing Strategies for Efficient Work-Flow Management with Diagnostic Radiology Workstations." J Digital Imaging 11:66, 1998.

[25] Mertelmeier T. "Why and How is Soft Copy Reading Possible in Clinical Practice?" J Digital Imaging 12:3–11, 1999.

[26] Lund PJ, Krupinski EA, Pereles S, Mockbee B. "Comparison of Conventional and Computed Radiography: Assessment of Image Quality and Reader Performance in Skeletal Extremity Trauma." Acad Radiol 4:570–576, 1997.

[27] Elam EA, Rehm K, Hillman BJ, Maloney K, Fajardo LL, McNeill K. "Efficacy of Digital Radiography for the Detection of Pneumothorax: Comparison with Conventional Chest Radiography." AJR 158:509–514, 1992.

[28] Scott WW, Bluemke DA, Mysko WK *et al.* "Interpretation of Emergency Department Radiographs by Radiologists and Emergency Medicine Physicians: Teleradiology Workstation Versus Radiograph Readings." Radiol 197:223–229, 1995.

[29] Krupinski EA. "Differences in Viewing Time for Mammograms Displayed on Film Versus a CRT Monitor." In Karssemeijer N, Thijssen M, Hendriks J, van Erning L (Eds.) *Digital Mammography '98*. Boston: Kluwer Academic Publishers, 1998, pp. 337–343.

[30] Marx C, Fleck M, Bohm T, Gebner C, Hochmuth A, Kaiser WA. "Comparison of Conventional and Secondarily Digitized Mammograms by ROC Analysis to Evaluate a Computer System for Digital Routine Mammography." In Karssemeijer N, Thijssen M, Hendriks J, van Erning L (Eds.) *Digital Mammography '98*. Boston: Kluwer Academic Publishers, 1998, pp. 495–496.

[31] Wang J, Langer S. "A Brief Review of Human Perception Factors in Digital Displays for Picture Archiving and Communications Systems." J Dig Imaging 10:158–168, 1997.

[32] Muka E, Blume H, Daly S. "Display of Medical Images on CRT Soft-Copy Displaya: A Tutorial." Proc SPIE 2431, 1995, pp. 341–359.

[33] Roehrig H, Blume H, Ji TL *et al.* "Performance Tests and Quality Control of Cathode Ray Tube Displays." J Dig Imaging 3:134–145, 1990.

[34] Johnson JP, Lubin J, Krupinski EA, Peterson HA, Roehrig H, Baysinger A. "Visual Discrimination Model for Digital Mammography." Proc SPIE 3663, 1999, pp. 253–263.

[35] Jackson WB, Said MR, Jared DA, Larimer JO, Lubin J, Gille JL. "X-Ray Image System Designusing a Human Visual Model." Proc SPIE 303, 1997, pp. 64–73.

[36] Davies AG, Cowen AR, Bruijns TJ. "Psychophysical Evaluation of the Image Quality of a Dynamic Flat-Panel Digital X-Ray Detector Using the Threshold Contrast Detail Detectability (TCDD) Technique." Proc SPIE 3663, 1999, pp. 170–179.

[37] Krupinski EA, Lund PJ. "Differences in Time to Interpretation for Evaluation of Bone Radiographs with Monitor and Film Viewing." Acad Radiol 4:177–182, 1997.

[38] Krupinski EA, Maloney K, Bessen SC, Capp MP, Graham K, Hunt R, Lund P, Ovitt T, Standen JR. "Receiver Operating Characteristic Evaluation of Computer Display of Adult Portable Chest Radiographs." Invest Radiol 29:141–146, 1994.

[39] American College of Radiology. FDA's Final Rule for Mammography Quality Standards Effective April 28. ACR Bulletin 55:7–30, 1999.

[40] Waynant RW, Chakrabarti K, Kaczmerak R, Suleiman O, Rowberg A. "Improved Sensitivity and Specificity of Mammograms by Producing Uniform Luminance from Viewboxes." J Dig Imaging 11:189–191, 1998.

[41] Maldjian PD, Miller JA, Maldjian JA, Baker SR. "An Automated Film Masking and Illuminating System Versus Conventional Radiographic Viewing Equipment: a Comparison of Observer Performance." Acad Radiol 3:827–833, 1996.

[42] Song K, Lee JS, Kim HY, Lim T. "Effect of Monitor Luminance on the Detection of Solitary Pulmonary Nodule: ROC Analysis." Proc SPIE 3663, 1999, pp. 212–216.

[43] Hemminger BM, Dillon A, Johnston RE. "Evaluation of the Effect of Display Luminance on the Feature Detection Rates of Masses in Mammograms." Proc SPIE 3036, 1997, pp. 96–106.

[44] Krupinski EA, Weinstein RS, Rozek LS. "Experience-Related Differences in Diagnosis from Medical Images Displayed on Monitors." Telemedicine J 2:101–108, 1996.

[45] Krupinski EA, Roehrig H, Furukawa T. "Influence of Film and Monitor Display Luminance on Observer Performance and Visual Search." Acad Radiol 6:411–418, 1999.

[46] Berman SM. "Energy Efficiency Consequences of Scotopic Sensitivity." J of the Illuminating Engineering Society 4:3–14, 1992.

[47] White KP, Hutson TL, Hutchinson TE. "Modeling Human Eye Behavior During Mammographic Scanning: Preliminary Results." IEEE Transactions on Systems, Man and Cybernetics 27:494–505, 1997.

[48] Pizer SM, Chan FH. "Evaluation of the Number of Discernible Levels Produced by a Display." In DiPaola R, Kahn E (Eds.) Information Processing in Medical Imaging. Paris, France: Editions INSERM, 1980, pp. 561–580.

[49] Pizer SM, "Intensity Mappings to Linearize Display Devices." Computer Graphics and Image Processing 17:262–268, 1981.

[50] ACR/NEMA: Digital Imaging and Communications in Medicine (DICOM), Supplement 28: Grayscale Standard Display Function, Letter Ballot Text, Jan 25, 1998.

[51] Blume H, Daly S, Muka E. "Presentation of Medical Images on CRT Displays: a Renewed Proposal for a Display Function Standard." Proc SPIE 1897, 1993, pp. 215–231.

[52] Barten PGJ. "Physical Model for Contrast Sensitivity of the Human Eye." Proc SPIE 1666, 1992, pp. 57–72.

[53] Barten PGJ. Contrast Sensitivity of the Human Eye and its Effects on Image Quality. Uitgeverij HV Press, 1999.

[54] Blume H. "The ACR/NEMA Proposal for a Grey-Scale Display Function Standard." Proc SPIE 2707, 1996, pp. 344–360.

[55] Belaid N, Martens JB. "Grey Scale, the "Crispening" Effect, and Perceptual Linearization." Signal Processing 70:231–245, 1998.

[56] Belaid N, VanOverveld I, Martens JB. "Display Fidelity: Link Between Psychophysics and Contrast Discrimination Models." Spatial Vision 11:205–223, 1997.

[57] Hemminger BM, Johnston RE, Rolland JP, Muller KE. "Introduction to Perceptual Linearization of Video Display Systems for Medical Image Presentation." J Dig Imaging 8:21–34, 1995.

[58] Heinemann EG. "Simultaneous Brightness Induction." In Jameson D, Hurvich LM (Eds.) *Handbook of Sensory Physiology VII*. Berlin: Springer, 1972, pp. 146–169.

[59] Krupinski EA, Roehrig H, "Influence of Monitor Luminance and Tone Scale on Observers' Search and Dwell Patterns." Proc SPIE 3663, 1999, pp. 151–156.

[60] Bolle SR, Sund T, Stromer J. "Receiver Operating Characteristic Study of Image Preprocessing for Teleradiology and Digital Workstations." J Dig Imag 10:152–157, 1997.

[61] Oda N, Nakata H, Watanabe H, Terada K. "Evaluation of Automatic-Mode Image Processing Method in Chest Computed Radiography." Acad Radiol 4:558–564, 1997.

[62] Vittitoe NF, Baker JA, Floyd CE. "Fractal Texture Analysis in Computer-Aided Diagnosis of Solitary Pulmonary Nodules." Acad Radiol 4:96–101, 1997.

[63] Kocur CM, Rogers SK, Myers LR, Burns T. "Using Neural Networks to Select Wavelet Features for Breast Cancer Diagnosis." IEEE Engin in Med and Biol (May/June):95–102, 1996.

[64] Giger ML, Nishikawa RM, Kupinski M *et al.* "Computerized Detection of Breast Lesions in Digitized Mammograms and Results with a Clinically-Implemented Intelligent Workstation." In Lemke HU, Vannier MW, Inamura K (Eds.) *CAR '97*. New York: Elsevier Science, 1997, pp. 325–330.

[65] Mugglestone MD, Lomax R, Gale AG, Wilson ARM. "The Effect of Prompting Mammographic Abnormalities on the Human Observer." In Doi K, Giger ML, Nishikawa RM, Schmidt RA (Eds.) *Digital Mammography '96*. New York: Elsevier Science, 1996, pp. 87–96.

[66] Krupinski EA. "An Eye-Movement Study on the Use of CAD Information During Mammographic Search." In *7th Far West Image Perception Conference*, Tucson, AZ, 1997.

[67] Hendriks JH, Holland R, Rijken H *et al.* "A Pilot Study on Computer Aided Diagnosis-Assisted Reading Compared to Double Reading in Screening for Breast Cancer." Radiol 205(P):216, 1997.

[68] Jiang Y, Nishikawa RM, Schmidt RA, Metz CE, Doi K. "Improving Breast Cancer Diagnosis with Computer-Aided Diagnosis (CAD): an Observer Study." Radiol 205(P):274–275, 1997.

[69] Krupinski EA, Evanoff M, Ovitt T, Standen JR, Chu TX, Johnson J. "The Influence of Image Processing on Chest Radiograph Interpretation and Decision Changes." Acad Radiol 5:79–85, 1998.

[70] Heelan RT, Flehinger BJ, Melamed MR. "Non-Small Cell Cancer: Results of the New York Screening Program." Radiology 151:289–293, 1984.

[71] Kundel HL. "Perception Errors in Chest Radiology." Seminars in Respiratory Medicine 10:203–210, 1989.

[72] Muhm JR, Miller WE, Fontan RS, Sanderson DR, Uhlenhopp MA. "Lung Cancer Detection During a Screening Program Using Four-Month Chest Radiographs." Radiology 148:609–615, 1983.

[73] Bassett LW, Manjikian V, Gold RH. "Mammography and Breast Cancer Screening." Surg Clinics of North America 70:775–800, 1990.

[74] Bassett LW, Gold RH. *Breast Cancer Detection: Mammography and Other Methods in Breast Imaging.* New York: Grune & Stratton, 1987.

[75] Bird RE, Wallace TW, Yankaskas BC. "Analysis of Cancers Missed at Screening Mammography." Radiology 184:613–617, 1992.

[76] Berlin L. "Malpractice and Radiologists." *AJR* 135:587–591, 1980.

[77] Berlin L. "Does the "Missed" Radiographic Diagnosis Constitute Malpractice?" Radiology 123:523–527, 1977.

[78] James AE. *Medical/Legal Issues for Radiologists.* Chicago, IL: Precept Press, 1987.

[79] Kern KA. "Causes of Breast Cancer Malpractice Litigation: A 20-Year Civil Court Review." Arch Surg 127:542–546, 1992.

[80] Kravitz RL, Rolph JE, McGuigan K. "Malpractice Claims Data as a Quality Improvement Tool: I. Epidemiology of Error in Four Specialties." JAMA 266:2087–2092, 1991.

[81] Britton CA, Gabriele OF, Chang TS et al. "Subjective Quality Assessment of Computed Radiography Hand Images." J Dig Imaging 9:21–24, 1996.

[82] Kundel HL, Nodine CF, Brikman I et al. "Preliminary Observations on a History-Based Image Display Optimizer for Chest Images." Proc SPIE 1232, 1990, pp. 46–48.

[83] Pisano ED, Chandramouli J, Hemminger BM, Glueck D et al. "The Effect of Intensity Windowing on the Detection of Simulated Masses Embedded in Dense Portions of Digitized Mammograms in a Laboratory Setting." J Dig Imaging 10:174–182, 1997.

[84] Pisano ED, Chandramouli J, Hemminger BM et al. "Does Intensity Windowing Improve the Detection of Simulated Calcifications in Dense Mammograms?" J Dig Imaging 10:79–84, 1997.

[85] Langer S, Wang J. "An Evaluation of Ten Digital Image Review Workstations." J Dig Imaging 10:65–78, 1997.

[86] Gay SB, Sobel AH, Young LQ, Dwyer SJ. "Processes Involved in Reading Imaging Studies: Workflow Analysis and Implications for Workstation Development." J Dig Imaging 10:40–45, 1997.

[87] Beard DV, Bream P, Pisano ED, Conroy P, Johnston RE et al. "A Pilot Study of Eye Movement During Mammography Interpretation: Eyetracker Results and Workstation Design Implications." J Dig Imaging 10:14–20, 1997.

[88] Matsubara T, Fujita H, Hara T *et al.* "New Algorithm for Mass Detection in Digital Mammograms." In Lemke HU, Vannier MW, Inamura K, Farman AG (Eds.) *Computer Assisted Radiology and Surgery '98.* New York: Elsevier, 1998, pp. 219–223.

[89] Vilarrasa A, Gimenez V, Manrique D, Rios J. "A New Algorithm for Computerized Detection of Microcalcifications in Digital Mammograms." In Lemke HU, Vannier MW, Inamura K, Farman AG (Eds.) *Computer Assisted Radiology and Surgery '98.* New York: Elsevier, 1998, pp. 224–229.

[90] Jiang Y, Nishikawa RM, Schmidt RA, Metz CE, Giger ML, Doi K. "Benefits of Computer-Aided Diagnosis in Mammographic Diagnosis of Malignant and Benign Clustered Microcalcifications." In Karssemeijer N, Thijssen M, Hendriks J, van Erning L (Eds.) *Digital Mammography '98.* Boston: Kluwer Academic Press, 1998, pp. 215–220.

[91] Zwiggelaar R, Astley SM, Taylor CJ. "Detecting the Central Mass of a Spiculated Lesion Using Scale-Orientation Signatures." In Karssemeijer N, Thijssen M, Hendriks J, van Erning L (Eds.) *Digital Mammography '98.* Boston: Kluwer Academic Press, 1998, pp. 63–70.

[92] Bottema MJ, Slavotinek JP. "Detection of Subtle Microcalcifications in Digital Mammograms." In Karssemeijer N, Thijssen M, Hendriks J, van Erning L (Eds.) *Digital Mammography '98.* Boston: Kluwer Academic Press, 1998, pp. 209–214.

[93] Jiang H, Masuto N, Iisaku S, Matsumoto M *et al.* "A GUI System for Computer-Aided Diagnosis of Lung Cancer Screening by Using CT." In Lemke HU, Vannier MW, Inamura K, Farman AG (Eds.) *Computer Assisted Radiology and Surgery '98.* New York: Elsevier, 1998, pp. 236–241.

[94] Armato SG, Giger ML, MacMahon H. "Computerized Analysis of Abnormal Asymmetry in Digital Chest Radiographs: Evaluation of Potential Utility." J Dig Imaging 12:34–42, 1999.

[95] teBrake GM, Karssemeijer N. "Detection of Stellate Breast Abnormalities." In Doi K, Giger ML, Nishikawa RM, Schmidt RA (Eds.) *Digital Mammography '96.* New York: Elsevier, 1996, pp. 341–346.

[96] Byng JW, Yaffe MJ, Jong RA, Shumak RS, Lockwood GA, Tritchler DL, Boyd NF. "Analysis of Mammographic Density and Breast Cancer Risk from Digitized Mammograms." Radiographics 18:1587–1598, 1998.

[97] Huo Z, Giger ML, Olopade OI *et al.* "Computer-Aided Diagnosis: Breast Cancer Risk Assessment from Mammographic Parenchymal Patterns in Digitized Mammograms." In Doi K, Giger ML, Nishikawa RM, Schmidt RA (Eds.) *Digital Mammography '96.* New York: Elsevier, 1996, pp. 191–194.

[98] Priebe CE, Solka JL, Lorey RA *et al.* "The Application of Fractal Analysis to Mammographic Tissue Classification." Cancer Letters 77:183–189, 1994.

[99] Wolfe JN. "Breast Patterns as an Index of Risk for Developing Breast Cancer." AJR 126:1130–1139, 1976.

[100] Rensink RA, O'Regan JK, Clark JJ. "To See or Not to See: The Need for Attention to Perceive Changes in Scenes." Psychological Science 8:368–373, 1997.

[101] Sanjay-Gopal S, Chan H, Sahiner B *et al.* "Evaluation of Interval Change in Mammographic Features for Computerized Classification of Malignant and Benign Masses." Radiol 205(P):216, 1997.

[102] Mao F, Qian W, Clarke LP. "Fractional Dimension Filtering for Multiscale Lung Nodule Detection." Proc SPIE 3034, 1997, pp. 449–456.

[103] Xu XW, MacMahon H, Giger ML, Doi K. "Adaptive Feature Analysis of False Positives for Computerized Detection of Lung Nodules in Digital Chest Images." Proc SPIE 3034, 1997, pp. 48–436.

[104] Ishida T, Ashizawa K, Katsuragawa S, MacMahon H, Doi K. "Computerized Analysis of Interstitial Lung Diseases on Chest Radiographs Based on Lung Texture, Geometric-Pattern Features and Artificial Neural Networks." Radiol 205(P):395, 1997.

[105] Kido S, Ikezoe J, Tamura S *et al.* "A Computerized Analysis System in Chest Radiography: Evaluation of Interstitial Lung Abnormalities." J Dig Imaging 10:57–64, 1997.

[106] Zhao B, Reeves AP, Yankelevitz DF, Henschke CI. "Three-Dimensional Multi-Criteria Iterative Segmentation of Helical CT Images of Pulmonary Nodules." Radiol 205(P):168, 1997.

[107] Toshioka S, Kanazawa K, Niki N *et al.* "Computer-Aided Diagnosis System for Lung Cancer Based on Helical CT Images." Proc SPIE 3034, 1997, pp. 975–984.

[108] Behrens U, Teubner J, Evertsz CJG *et al.* "Computer Assisted Dynamic Evaluation of Contrast-Enhanced Breast-MRI." In Lemke HU, Vannier MW, Inamura K (Eds.) *Computer Assisted Radiology '96.* New York: Elsevier, 1996, pp. 362–367.

[109] Hendriks JH, Holland R, Rijken H *et al.* "A Pilot Study on Computer Aided Diagnosis-Assisted Reading Compared to Double Reading in Screening for Breast Cancer." Radiol 205(P):216, 1997.

[110] Jiang Y, Nishikawa RM, Schmidt RA, Metz CE, Doi K. "Improving Breast Cancer Diagnosis with Computer-Aided Diagnosis (CAD): An Observer Study." Radiol 205(P):274, 1997.

[111] Chan H, Sahiner B, Helvie MA *et al.* "Effects of Computer-Aided Diagnosis (CAD) on Radiologists' Classification of Malignant and Benign Masses on Mammograms: An ROC Study." Radiol 205(P):275, 1997.

[112] Strickland RN, Baig LJ, Dallas WJ, Krupinski EA. "Wavelet-Based Image Enhancement as an Instrument for Viewing CAD Data." In Doi K, Giger ML, Nishikawa RM, Schmidt RA (Eds.) *Digital Mammography '96.* New York: Elsevier, 1996, pp. 441–446.

[113] Kallergi M, Clarke LP, Qian W *et al.* "Interpretation of Calcifications in Screen/Film, Digitized, and Wavelet-Enhanced Monitor-Displayed Mammograms: a Receiver Operating Characteristic Study." Acad Radiol 3:285–293, 1996.

[114] Jiang Y, Nishikawa RM, Schmidt RA, Metz CE, Giger ML, Doi K. "Improving Breast Cancer Diagnosis with Computer-Aided Diagnosis." Acad Radiol 6:22–33, 1999.

[115] Mugglestone MD, Lomax R, Gale AG, Wilson ARM. "The Effect of Prompting Mammographic Abnormalities on the Human Observer." In Doi K, Giger ML, Nishikawa RM, Schmidt RA (Eds.) *Digital Mammography '96*. New York: Elsevier, 1996, pp. 87–92.

[116] Krupinski EA. "An Eye-Movement Study on the Use of CAD Information during Mammographic Search." Paper presented at the *7th Far West Image Perception Conference*, Tucson, AZ, 1997.

[117] Krupinski EA, Nishikawa RM. "Comparison of Eye Position Versus Computer Identified Microcalcification Clusters on Mammograms." Med Phys 24:17–23, 1997.

[118] Berbaum KS, Franken EA, Dorfman DD *et al.* "Satisfaction of Search in Diagnostic Radiology." Invest Radiol 25:133–140, 1990.

[119] Berbaum KS, Franken EA, Dorfman DD *et al.* "Cause of Satisfaction of Search Effects in Contrast Studies of the Abdomen." Acad Radiol 3:815–826, 1996.

[120] Samuel S, Kundel HL, Nodine CF, Toto LC. "Mechanism of Satisfaction of Search: Eye Position Recordings in the Reading of Chest Radiographs." Radiol 194:895–902, 1995.

[121] Berbaum KS, Franken EA, Dorfman DD, Miller EM, Caldwell RT, Kuehn DM, Berbaum ML. "Role of Faulty Search in the Satisfaction of Search Effect in Chest Radiography." Acad Radiol 5:9–19, 1998.

[122] Curry TS, Dowdey JE, Murry RC. "*Christensen's Physics of Diagnostic Radiology.*" Philadelphia: Lea & Febiger, 1990, p. 138.

[123] Levkowitz H, Herman GT. "Color Scales for Image Data." IEEE Comp Graphics and Applic 12:72–80, 1992.

[124] Granger EM, Heurtley JC. "Visual Chromaticity Modulation Transfer Function." JOSA 63:1173–1174, 1973.

[125] Mullen KT. "The Contrast Sensitivity of Human Colour Vision to Red-Green and Blue-Yellow Chromatic Gratings." J of Physiology 359:381–400, 1985.

[126] Alcazar JL, Laparte C. "In Vivo Validation of the Time Domain Velocity Measurement Technique of Blood Flow in Human Fetuses." Ultrasound in Med and Biol 24:9–13, 1998.

[127] Meilstrup JW. "Clinical Perspectives of Diagnostic Ultrasound." Proc SPIE 3664, 1999, pp. 2–6.

[128] Aoki S, Osawa S, Yoshioka N, Yamashita H, Kumagai H, Araki T. "Velocity-Coded Color MR Angiography." Am J Neuroradiology 19:691–693, 1998.

[129] Hawighorst H, Engenhart R, Knopp MV, Brix G, Grandy M *et al.* "Intracranial Meningeomas: Time and Dose-Dependent Effects of Irradiation on Tumor Microcirculation Monitored by Dynamic MR Imaging." MRI 15:423–432, 1997.

[130] Kim CY. "Reevaluation of JPEG Image Compression to Digitalized Gastrointestinal Endoscopic Color Images: a Pilot Study." Proc SPIE 3658, 1999, pp. 420–426.

[131] Rehm K, Strother SC, Anderson JR, Schaper KA, Rottenberg DA. "Display of Merged Multimodality Brain Images Using Interleaved Pixels with Independent Color Scales." J Nuc Med 35:1815–1821, 1994.

[132] Milan J, Taylor KJW. "The Application of the Temperature Scale to Ultrasound Imaging." J Clin Ultrasound 3:171–173, 1975.

[133] Chan FH, Pizer SM. "An Ultrasound Display System Using a Natural Scale." J Clin Ultrasound 4:345–348, 1976.

[134] Houston AS. "A Comparison of Four Standard Scinitigraphic TV Displays." J Nuc Med 21:512–517, 1980.

[135] Li H, Burgess AE. "Evaluation of Signal Detection Performance with Pseudocolor Display and Lumpy Backgrounds." Proc SPIE 3036, 1997, pp. 143–149.

[136] Shepherd AJ. "Calibrating Screens for Continuous Color Displays." Spatial Vision 11:57–74, 1997.

Index